USMLE STEP 1
SECRETS IN COLOR

USMLE STEP 1
SECRETS IN COLOR

FIFTH EDITION

TED O'CONNELL, MD
Chief, Department of Family and Community Medicine, Kaiser Permanente
Vallejo, Vallejo, California; Founding Program Director, Family Medicine
Residency Program, Kaiser Permanente Napa-Solano, Napa, California;
Associate Clinical Professor, Department of Community and Family
Medicine, University of California–San Francisco School of Medicine,
San Francisco, California

RYAN A. PEDIGO, MD, MHPE
Associate Residency Program Director, Department of Emergency Medicine,
Harbor-UCLA Medical Center, Torrance, California;
Assistant Professor of Emergency Medicine,
David Geffen School of Medicine at UCLA, Los Angeles, California

Senior Editors

KATIE P. CARSKY, MD, MS
MATTHEW J. CHRISTENSEN, MD
JOHN A. DAMIANOS, MD
HUBERT HUANG, MD

ELSEVIER

Elsevier
1600 John F. Kennedy Blvd.
Ste 1600
Philadelphia, PA 19103-2899

USMLE STEP 1 SECRETS IN COLOR, FIFTH EDITION

ISBN: 978-0-323-81060-9

Notice

Previous editions copyrighted 2004, 2008, 2013, 2017

Content Strategist: James T. Merritt
Senior Content Development Specialist: Malvika Shah
Publishing Services Manager: Shereen Jameel
Senior Project Manager: Prem Kumar Kaliamoorthi
Design Direction: Bridget Hoette

Printed in India

Last digit is the print number: 9 8 7 6 5 4 3 2 1

To my parents, Fran and Ted, for modeling hard work, commitment, and social justice, and for teaching me the value of a great education. And to Nichole, Ryan, Sean, and Claire. I love you.
TED O'CONNELL

To my beautiful wife, Tiffany, for her unconditional love and support to both me and Lucy.
RYAN A. PEDIGO

REVIEW BOARD

ACKNOWLEDGMENTS

We wish to acknowledge the contributors to the 4th edition of USMLE *Step 1 Secrets in Color*.

AUTHORS

Thomas A. Brown, MD

Sonali J. Bracken, MD, PhD

CONTRIBUTORS

Matthew N. Anderson, MD

Melissa Argraves, MD

Yetunde Asiedu, MD

Giana C. Bistany, MD, MS

Martina S. Burn, MD

Samantha Chirunomula, MD

Sarah E. Conway, MD

Sarah Cryer, MD

Robert D'Angelo, MD

Apeksha Dave, MD

Stephanie Davis, MD

Christopher Del Prete, MD

Joravar Dhaliwal, MD

Andrew J. Duarte, MD

Ryan P. Duggan, MD

Thomas J.S. Durant, MPT, MD

Cory Dwyer, MD

Brian P. Epling, MD

Patrick A. Field, MD

Rebecca Flugrad, MD

Eric Han, MD

Alex M. Hennessey, MD

Matthew Howe, MD

Liza Karamessinis, MD

Shirin Karimi, MD

Adam J.S. Kaye, MD

Andrew Kelsey, MD

Kaitlyn Ryan LaMarche, MD

Hien Le, MD

Aaron Lee, MD

Deirdre Lewis, MD

Maritza Montanez, MD

Henry L. Nguyen, MD

Lena M. O'Keefe, MD, MS

Meaghen Roy-O'Reilly, MD

Nicole J. Rubin, MD

Joseph M. Ryan, MD

Neda Shahriari, MD

Kelsey Sokol, MD

Eunice Song, MD

Bryan Stenson, MD

Margaret Stevenson, MD

Long Tu, MD

Hollis A. Viray, MD

Gillian Weston, MD

David S. Wong, MD

Kyle T. Wright, MD, PhD

REGARDING ERRATA

A list of errata for this book can be found at www.tedxoconnell.com and at www.BookRevision.com.

We also welcome you to visit the website to submit errors, updates, or suggestions for this book. Thank you for helping to ensure the accuracy and high quality of *USMLE Step 1 Secrets in Color*.

Ted O'Connell, MD
Ryan A. Pedigo, MD, MHPE

PREFACE

Preparing for the United States Medical Licensing Examination (USMLE) Step 1 can be an intimidating and nerve-wracking experience. We are here to help you master the material that will be tested on this exam. Truly understanding the information and concepts, rather than memorizing facts, will reduce your anxiety on test day and will provide a solid foundation for the rest of your medical career.

HOW EARLY SHOULD YOU BEGIN STUDYING FOR THE USMLE?

Students frequently ask this question, but unfortunately there is no simple way to answer it. Students commonly allocate anywhere from 2 to 6 months to study for the USMLE Step 1, but some take more time and a rare few may need less. The point is that each student should begin preparations at a time that makes sense for them. When planning your study schedule, consider how busy you estimate you will be in the months leading up to your exam (do not neglect your coursework!), how many hours per day you are willing to dedicate to productive study time, and how well you think you retain information in the short term versus the long term. Most medical students will have figured out which study styles work best for them long before they even begin to think about boards. Do not change your study habits dramatically for the USMLE if you have found methods that work well for you.

HOW WILL THIS BOOK HELP YOU PREPARE FOR STEP 1?

As you may have already figured out, there are many review books available to help you prepare for this exam. Although the content in these books may overlap quite a bit, the way that material is presented can vary dramatically from resource to resource. The trick to selecting good review products is to use those that mesh well with your learning style and the actual format of the USMLE. The more books you have in front of you, the greater the potential for confusion and the less productive you will feel. In other words, an overabundance of resources eventually will become an impediment to your studying. The most efficient test takers are the students who consolidate their study materials as time goes by. Start with a fresh copy of the newest edition of *First Aid for the USMLE Step 1*. This will be your primary resource for the USMLE Step 1. Our book is designed to supplement the information that you learn in First Aid and help you place it into clinical context through a mix of basic-concept and case-based questions. The detailed explanations we provide to our questions will offer you insight into the way that the USMLE will expect you to think through questions on test day. In addition, our book will provide you with dozens of valuable study tips (including tips from third- and fourth-year medical students and residents who have earned competitive scores on the USMLE Step 1) to facilitate your studying.

We begin each chapter with an insider's guide that will provide you with our best study strategies for that particular subject. In addition, each chapter includes a number of Step 1 Secrets that will point out the highest-yield topics to focus on for boards. It is our mission to offer you the type of valuable information that will help you master this information and perform well on test day.

NOW THAT YOU HAVE SELECTED YOUR RESOURCES, HOW SHOULD YOU GO ABOUT STUDYING FOR THE EXAM?

- Set up a study schedule as *early* as possible. Determine when you will begin studying, how much time you will dedicate to test preparation each week or month, and when you would like to cover specific subject areas in your review process. Keep in mind that you will need the last few weeks before the exam to review all of the content that you have studied.
- Make a *flexible* study schedule, especially early in your preparations. Give yourself some free time every day to enjoy other activities and relax your mind. This will increase the productivity of your study time.
- Purchase a copy of *First Aid for the USMLE Step 1* as soon as possible, and casually review it when studying for your medical school exams, especially during your second year. There is no need to place your emphasis on studying for your board exam before you are ready, but familiarizing yourself with First Aid in advance will make you feel much more comfortable when beginning your USMLE studying.
- Annotate your copy of First Aid with notes from *USMLE Step 1 Secrets* and other high-yield resources. All of your notes will therefore be in one place in the weeks leading up to your exam date, and you will have a much easier time getting through all of the material during your final review phase.
- Begin using question bank software months before your exam date. Most students use UWorld, though other question banks such as the Kaplan USMLE Step 1 Qbank are also utilized. We recommend doing both random questions and

timed blocks so you get used to the pacing of the exam. Focusing too much on questions early on will not be effective until you start to develop a strong knowledge base. As you get closer to the exam, the majority of your time should be spent doing blocks from the question banks, not only to apply the knowledge that you've learned but also to build your mental endurance.

- In the month before you take the USMLE Step 1, try to do two to three blocks per day on the question bank you are using. No matter which mode you use, you will benefit from reading all of the answer explanations at the end so you understand why the correct answer is correct and why the incorrect answers are wrong. Consider marking questions with great learning points or excellent diagrams so that you can easily find them again. Keep in mind that you can download question bank apps for your smartphone.
- The night before your exam, try to put your books away and get a good night's rest. Half of the battle will be keeping your focus through an intense, 8-hour exam day. If you feel the need to study the day before or morning of your exam as a "warmup" or to relieve some anxiety, we recommend going through the high-yield review sections at the end of First Aid or a few of your own notes. You may also consider answering a couple of practice questions, but be wary of looking at the answers at this time in case you get them wrong. Avoid cramming any information (new or old) right before your exam to prevent an anxiety attack.

WHEN WILL I GET MY RESULT?

Naturally, this is one of the most frequently asked questions among eager examinees who have completed the USMLE Step 1. Results are typically made available on the NBME website 3 to 4 weeks after your exam date (lag time is determined by the number of students who have taken the test during your window). When your result is available, you will receive an email notification from the organization that registered you for your examination.

TEN THINGS STUDENTS WISH THEY HAD KNOWN BEFORE TAKING THE USMLE STEP 1

1. Questions on the USMLE Step 1 are often slightly longer than those found in most question bank programs. Most students finish in time, but keeping on pace will be very important to your success on this exam.
2. Before the start of your exam, you will be given a small whiteboard on which to scribble formulas and perform calculations during your test. You may take a *few minutes* before you actually begin your test to jot down some notes. Determine what you will write on your whiteboard during the final week of your review so as not to waste time during your test.
3. Anatomy throws many students for a loop on Step 1 because they are often unsure how to prepare for this subject. Be sure to read our "Insider's Guide to Clinical Anatomy for the USMLE Step 1" in Chapter 26 of this book.
4. You should expect to have a small percentage of questions on topics that you have never seen or studied. You may also get four to five questions on the same topic. If you do not know the answer, take your best guess and move on. Do not let yourself become flustered or frustrated, otherwise you may miss some easy questions.
5. You are allowed 45 minutes of break time during your exam, but you can gain extra break time by skipping the tutorial (15 minutes; you can watch a similar tutorial on the NBME website before your exam date) or finishing a block before the allotted time expires. Most students find an hour of break time to be adequate, but you should spend some time before your exam planning out how you will allot your time. Do not forget that you are expected to include lunch in your break time.
6. Bring snacks. You will be facing a long day. We suggest that you eat a small lunch and a few snacks in between blocks rather than one big lunch (some students will otherwise become lethargic during the afternoon). Be wary of selecting high-sugar snacks (the last thing you need while taking the USMLE is a sugar crash!).
7. Although it is no secret that you should dress in comfortable clothing while sitting for your exam, students often do not know that they should wear as little jewelry and clothing with as few pockets as possible. To prevent the use of prohibited items, most testing centers will scan you with a metal wand and ask you to turn out your pockets each time you re-enter the examination room following a break. This is not only a frustrating process but is also a waste of your break time. You will get through this inspection much more quickly with less jewelry and fewer pockets. Also remember to bring your ID and locker key with you every time you leave the test center.
8. All NBME exams are different! Do not be fooled by students who tell you that their questions were identical to those in the USMLE World, Kaplan Qbank, USMLE Consult, or USMLERx. There is no guarantee that your experience will be the same as theirs. The more questions you do, the better prepared you will be. We recommend that you reserve at least 1000 practice questions to answer in conditions that closely simulate the exam (full blocks, random assortment, and timed mode).
9. When scheduling your exam date, keep in mind that having more time to study will not necessarily improve your performance. Every individual has a peak performance window, and trying to study past this window *may* hurt your score. For those of you who have more flexibility than your friends when planning your exam date, be careful about delaying boards for too long. It is possible that you will find it increasingly more difficult to concentrate on studying once your friends have moved past this stage. It is also not advisable to delay your exam too long after you have completed the second year of medical school because you may spend more time relearning the basics.

10. You should arrive at your testing center 30 minutes before your start time. If you speed through the registration process, you may be allowed to begin your examination early. This may be a good option for some students, particularly those who would otherwise spend the time building anxiety. Another good option for anxiety relief is to sign up for a practice examination at your testing site a few weeks before your actual exam date. To do this, you must request a permit from the NBME website.

ONE FINAL NOTE

Although it will be a challenging task, studying for the USMLE Step 1 will also be a rewarding experience that will prepare you for a successful transition into your clinical years. Students often say that they feel incredibly accomplished (and intelligent!) after sitting for this examination. Before you know it, the USMLE Step 1 will be behind you, and you will be well on your way to a wonderful career in medicine.

Wishing you the best on this exam and in your career,

Ted O'Connell, MD
Ryan A. Pedigo, MD, MHPE

A NOTE FROM THE AUTHORS

On the USMLE examinations, and throughout medical education, associations are often made between disease processes and certain racial and ethnic groups or even socioeconomic status. These associations become linked with individual groups and can perpetuate stereotypes, misinformation, and racism. In essence, physicians in training are taught to link key words, phrases, and ideas for the purposes of making associations on examinations and in clinical contexts.

Associations made with certain terms or disease processes, without qualifications or explanation, can cause those of us in health care to believe that being of part of a particular group causes an individual to have a predilection for health problems and disease process. The reasons a disease process is more prevalent in certain racial, ethnic, and socioeconomic groups may be due in large part to long-standing social inequities, health disparities, structural racism, oppression, adverse childhood experiences, politics, environment, and likely many other factors. It is vitally important to remember that an increased prevalence should not be assumed to be intrinsically linked to being part of any particular group.

Because *USMLE Step 1 Secrets in Color* is designed to help prepare you for success on the USMLE Step 1 exam, some of these key words and linkages remain in this book out of necessity, because the linkages are so prevalent on standardized exams. However, we have tried to remove these whenever possible. Despite this, we encourage you to consider the broader social issues outlined above and work within the health care system to call out and try to eliminate inappropriate associations between disease processes and individual groups of people. We owe it to our patients and to society to do this and to be better going forward.

Ted O'Connell, MD
Ryan A. Pedigo, MD, MHPE

TABLE OF CONTENTS

CARDIOLOGY

BASIC CONCEPTS—HEMODYNAMICS

1. **What are the mathematical determinants of the arterial blood pressure?**
   The mean arterial pressure (MAP) is determined by the amount of blood the heart pumps into the arterial system in a given time (e.g., cardiac output [CO]) and the resistance the arteries exert (e.g., total peripheral resistance [TPR]). Mathematically, this is expressed as MAP = CO × TPR. Consequently, all drugs that lower blood pressure (BP) work by affecting either CO, TPR, or both.
   Note: The primary determinant of systolic blood pressure (SBP) is CO, whereas the primary determinant of diastolic blood pressure (DBP) is TPR. Because approximately one-third of the cardiac cycle is spent in systole and two-thirds in diastole, the MAP can also be calculated as MAP = 1/3 SBP + 2/3 DBP.

2. **What are the primary determinants of CO?**
   CO is the amount of blood pumped by the ventricles per unit time. It is determined by the volume of blood ejected during each ventricular contraction (stroke volume [SV]) and how frequently the ventricular contractions occur (heart rate [HR]), expressed as CO = HR × SV. The HR can be affected by a variety of factors but is principally under the control of the autonomic nervous system. Medications that inhibit the activity of β_1-adrenergic receptors (i.e., beta-blockers) can reduce CO by decreasing HR and SV.
   Note: In addition to their negative inotropic effect, the more cardioselective (nondihydropyridine) calcium channel blockers (CCBs; verapamil, diltiazem) can also reduce HR by slowing impulse transmission through the atrioventricular (AV) node. They achieve part of their antihypertensive effect through this mechanism.

3. **What are the three main factors that affect SV?**
   The three primary determinants of SV are preload, contractility, and afterload.

4. **What is preload, and how does it affect SV?**
   Preload is the degree of tension (load) on the ventricular muscle when it begins to contract. The primary determinant of preload is end-diastolic volume, which represents the volume of blood in the ventricle at the very end of diastole, right before systole begins. End-diastolic volume can be estimated by measuring atrial pressure, as the amount of pressure measured in each atrium is directly correlated to the volume of fluid contained within the associated ventricle.
   The most widely accepted theory explaining the relationship of preload and SV is the Frank-Starling mechanism, which demonstrates that increased preload results in increased SV. One proposed mechanism is that increased end-diastolic volumes result in stretching of ventricular muscle fibers, increasing overlap of actin and myosin within sarcomeres, which allows for a stronger ventricular contraction and thus a larger SV. This mechanism allows the heart to maintain its ejection fraction (EF) in the face of increased preload. It is important to note that the Frank-Starling law only holds true in a physiologic range of end-diastolic volumes. Eventually, increasing end-diastolic volumes will result in a decrease in SV. This occurs in congestive heart failure (CHF), which is graphically represented in Fig. 1.1.
   A general rule to understand about cardiac hemodynamics is that preload is primarily affected by venous return, whereas afterload is primarily affected by the arterial system. Preload increases with increased blood volume, venoconstriction (often secondary to sympathetic activation), passive leg raising, and decreased intrathoracic pressure (i.e., during inspiration). Preload decreases with venodilators (e.g., nitrates), decreased blood volume (e.g., diuresis, hemorrhage), Valsalva maneuver (i.e., expiration against a closed glottis), and compression of venous supply (e.g., later stages of pregnancy).
   Note: Certain maneuvers, such as exercise or quickly standing from a seated position, will alter preload and/or afterload, which will affect SV, CO, and ultimately MAP (Fig. 1.2).

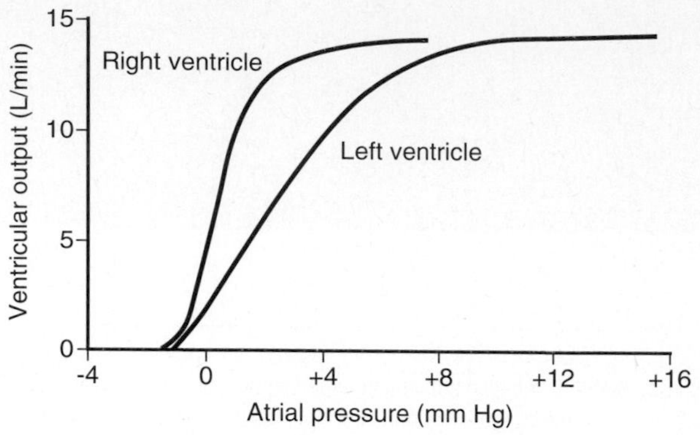

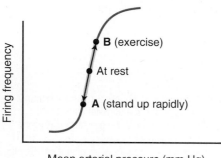

Figure 1.1. Ventricular output as a function of end-diastolic volume (reflected by atrial pressure). *(From Guyton AC, Hall JE.* Textbook of Medical Physiology. *11th ed. Philadelphia: WB Saunders; 2006:112.)*

Figure 1.2. Control of blood pressure by the baroreceptor reflex. *(From Brown TA.* Rapid Review Physiology. *Philadelphia: Mosby; 2007:144.)*

Note: Another theory to explain the Frank-Starling relationship proposes that cardiac troponin becomes increasingly sensitive to cytosolic calcium at greater sarcomere lengths, thereby resulting in increased calcium binding and increased force of muscle contraction.

5. **What is contractility, and how does it affect SV?**
Contractility is a measure of how forcefully the ventricle contracts at a given preload. Naturally, a more forceful contraction will eject a greater fraction of blood from the ventricle, thereby increasing SV. Contractility is principally influenced by the activities of the sympathetic nervous system (e.g., β_1-adrenergic receptors) and parasympathetic nervous system (e.g., muscarinic [M_2] cholinergic receptors) on ventricular myocytes. By antagonizing the sympathetic input to the myocardium, beta-blockers exert part of their antihypertensive effect by reducing contractility, which reduces SV, CO, and oxygen demand. Contractility also increases as the intracellular concentration of calcium (Ca^{2+}) increases, which is indirectly achieved by digoxin and by decreased concentrations of extracellular sodium (Na^+). This mechanism will be explained in further detail in the discussion regarding digoxin. In addition to beta-blockade, contractility is decreased by systolic dysfunction, hypoxia, calcium channel blockade, and acidosis.

6. **What is afterload, and how does it affect SV?**
Afterload is the ventricular wall stress that occurs during systolic ejection. Afterload is commonly simplified to the resistance that the ventricles need to overcome to eject blood from the heart (i.e., aortic pressure). The aortic pressure is undoubtedly a major factor in determining afterload, but the ventricular wall thickness and chamber radius also contribute. The law of Laplace states that wall stress, or tension (σ), is proportional to pressure (P) and radius (r) and inversely proportional to wall thickness (h).

$$\sigma \propto \frac{P - r}{h} \qquad [1.1]$$

Afterload is most commonly described in terms of the left ventricle, but the same principles can be applied to the right ventricle when discussing pulmonary hypertension (Table 1.1).

7. **What are the primary determinants of peripheral resistance?**
The resistance across a blood vessel (Eq. 1.2) is determined by blood viscosity (η), vessel length (l), and vessel radius (r).

$$R = 8\eta l/\pi r^4 \qquad [1.2]$$

Table 1.1. Hemodynamic Changes Associated With Common Cardiac Pathologies

CONDITION	EFFECT ON P, r, OR h	EFFECT ON AFTERLOAD (σ)
Hypertension (systemic HTN, vasoconstrictors)	↑ P	↑ Afterload
Hypotension (↓ blood volume, vasodilators)	↓ P	↓ Afterload
LVH (diastolic heart failure)	↓ r, ↑ h	↓ Afterload However, a common cause of LVH is HTN
Dilated cardiomyopathy (systolic heart failure)	↑ r, ↓ h	↑ Afterload
Aortic stenosis	↑ P, because of additional transvalvular pressure gradient	↑ Afterload
Pulmonary HTN	↑ P in the right ventricle	↑ Afterload on the right ventricle

σ, Tension; ↓, decreased; ↑, increased; *h*, wall thickness; *HTN*, hypertension; *LVH*, left ventricular hypertrophy; *P*, pressure; *r*, radius.

The total resistance across a network of vessels can be related to the concept of circuits:

In series: $R_{total} = R_1 + R_2 + R_3 \ldots$
In parallel: $1/R_{total} = 1/R_1 + 1/R_2 + 1/R_3 \ldots$

The vasculature of the body is a complex network of blood vessels in series and in parallel. For the purposes of your USMLE Step 1 exam, if asked, calculating the total resistance within a network will be simplified to only a few vessels.

The TPR is the sum of all individual resistances. The TPR is principally mediated by arteriolar diameter, which is modified by arteriolar vasoconstriction and vasodilation. As seen in Eq. 1.2, resistance to blood flow through a vessel is inversely proportional to the fourth power of the radius. Consequently, small changes in arteriolar diameter (and thus radius) will have profound effects on blood flow.

The sympathetic nervous system promotes arteriolar vasoconstriction by stimulating α_1-adrenergic receptors. This increases Ca^{2+} influx (via calcium channels) into arteriolar smooth muscle and stimulates smooth muscle contraction. Therefore α_1-adrenergic receptors and arteriolar Ca^{2+} channels are targets for antihypertensive drugs.

In all organs except for the lungs, arteriolar vasodilation is promoted by tissue hypoxia and by the accumulation of metabolic waste (e.g., adenosine) that is produced when oxygen demand increases (e.g., during exercise). This vasodilation allows supply to meet demand.

Note: In general, there is no direct parasympathetic innervation of the vasculature. However, vasodilation of arterioles can be caused by the administration of exogenous cholinomimetics. These drugs act on muscarinic receptors (M3 receptors) present on endothelial cells, which stimulate release of nitric oxide (NO) when activated. NO diffuses to the adjacent smooth muscle, resulting in vasodilation and decreased peripheral resistance.

8. **What is the mechanism by which the sympathetic nervous system responds to a reduction in BP?**
The baroreceptor reflex is a feedback mechanism that allows the autonomic nervous system to rapidly respond to changes in BP. The purpose is to maintain BP during sudden changes in pressure (e.g., when quickly standing up from a seated position). Baroreceptors are stretch receptors located in arteries that adjust the frequency of their signal proportional to the stretch of the vessel. The two main locations of the baroreceptors are at the carotid sinus and the aortic arch, which send signals to the solitary nucleus of the medulla oblongata via the glossopharyngeal (cranial nerve [CN] IX) and vagus (CN X) nerves, respectively (Fig. 1.3). Increased signals to the solitary nucleus inhibit sympathetic outflow and excite parasympathetic outflow. The carotid sinus baroreceptors are more sensitive and therefore have a stronger effect on changes in BP. The aortic arch baroreceptors are less sensitive and only respond to *increases* in BP. The two reflex-loop scenarios can be simplified with the following flow charts:

↓ BP → ↓ stretch of carotid sinus baroreceptor → ↓ firing of afferent nerve → ↓ parasympathetic efferent firing and ↑ sympathetic efferent firing → ↑ BP via ↑ contractility, ↑ HR, and ↑ vasoconstriction.

↑ BP → ↑ stretch of carotid sinus and aortic arch baroreceptor → ↑ firing of afferent nerve → ↑ parasympathetic efferent firing and ↓ sympathetic efferent firing → ↓ BP via ↓ contractility, ↓ HR, and ↓ vasoconstriction.

Note: The aortic arch and carotid sinuses also have chemoreceptors, which should not be confused with the baroreceptors. Chemoreceptors work to maintain P_{O_2}, P_{CO_2}, and pH.

9. **How do the α_1-receptor antagonists work?**
The α_1-receptor antagonists are a collection of medications named with the suffix *-zosin* (e.g., prazosin, terazosin, doxazosin). These medications prevent peripheral vasoconstriction by antagonizing the α_1-receptors that are normally stimulated by the sympathetic nervous system. α_1-Receptors are located on vascular smooth muscle cells and coupled to G_q proteins. Antagonists cause decreased release of inositol triphosphate (IP_3) and subsequently prevent the release of Ca^{2+} from intracellular stores, resulting in smooth muscle relaxation and arteriolar vasodilation.

α_1-Receptors are also responsible for contraction of the pupillary dilator muscle and intestinal/bladder sphincters. Thus α_1-receptor antagonism can also lead to miosis and increased bowel or bladder movement.

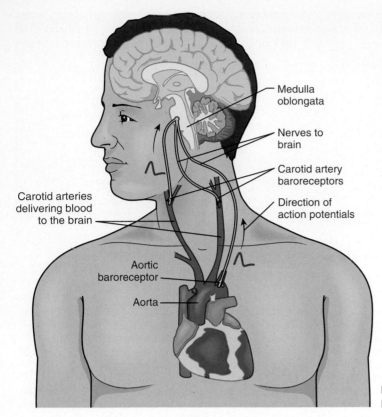

Figure 1.3. Diagram of the baroreceptor reflex pathway.

10. How do the α_1-receptor antagonists cause orthostatic hypotension?

Upon standing from a supine or sitting position, blood will pool in the venous system of the lower extremities unless a competent sympathetic nervous system can appropriately compensate. This compensation is ordinarily stimulated by the baroreceptor reflex, which promotes peripheral venoconstriction and increased HR as described previously. However, α_1-receptor antagonists will block this reflexive vasoconstriction, leading to the transient hypotension and lightheadedness (from cerebral hypoperfusion) that is associated with orthostatic hypotension as the result of decreased venous return and reduced MAP. Reflex tachycardia will still occur despite α_1-receptor antagonism because reflex tachycardia is mediated by beta-receptors.

   Note: Reflex tachycardia occurs in an attempt to maintain CO. Recall that CO = HR $\times$ SV. Thus when SV is reduced due to decreased venous return (i.e., decreased preload), HR must increase to compensate and maintain CO.

11. What hemodynamic changes occur during exercise?

Exercise requires more oxygen to be delivered to skeletal muscle to meet its increased metabolic demand. This delivery is accomplished mainly by an increase in CO secondary to increases in both SV and HR. Contraction of the lower limb muscles pushes blood toward the right atrium and increases venous return. MAP is only modestly increased during exercise despite the large increase in CO because systemic vascular resistance (SVR) significantly decreases as a result of widespread vasodilation in skeletal muscle. Local cellular metabolites (e.g., adenosine, hydrogen [H^+] ion, CO_2) are largely responsible for this vasodilation.

12. Describe how CO and venous return will change under the four clinical scenarios listed below. Which clinical scenarios would shift the CO and venous return curves to the points labeled 1, 2, 3, and 4 in Fig. 1.4?

   1. **Exercise:** Lower limb muscles push blood toward the right atrium and increase venous return. Sympathetic activity increases CO by increasing HR, SV, and contractility.
   2. **AV fistula:** Increased venous return from an AV fistula will shift the venous return curve to the right. CO will slightly increase as a result of the increased preload (Frank-Starling mechanism); it is important to understand that this increase is therefore *not* due to a change in contractility or inotropy. If these AV anastomoses were much larger, the operating point of the heart would be shifted to (1) because it would cause a large decrease in SVR and stimulate the activity of the sympathetic nervous system, increasing inotropy; these large anastomoses are sometimes referred to as *AV shunts*.
   3. **Compensated heart failure:** Patients with this condition have elevated right atrial pressures as the result of an increased volume status caused by renin-angiotensin-aldosterone system (RAAS) activity. Cardiac function is decreased (decreased

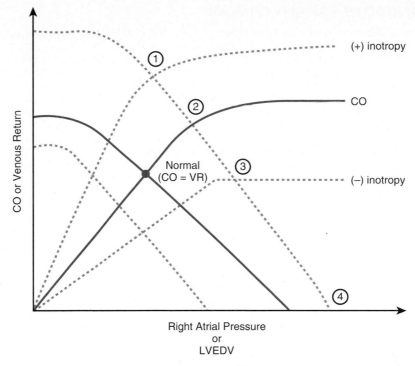

Figure 1.4. Cardiac output (CO) and venous return curves. *LVEDV,* Left ventricular end-diastolic volume; *VR,* venous return.

inotropy) as a result of the underlying heart failure, but they can maintain a near-normal CO at rest with the increased volume (Frank-Starling mechanism).

4. **Ventricular fibrillation:** Ventricular fibrillation causes equalization of all pressures. Right atrial pressure increases to become equal to the mean systolic filling pressure. CO in ventricular fibrillation falls to zero.

BASIC CONCEPTS—EXCITATION-CONTRACTION COUPLING

1. What is the source of cytosolic Ca^{2+} during ventricular systole?

   During the plateau phase (phase 2) of the ventricular myocyte action potential, voltage-gated Ca^{2+} channels allow Ca^{2+} influx from the extracellular fluid into the cytosol, stimulating further Ca^{2+} release from the sarcoplasmic reticulum. This phenomenon is referred to as *calcium-induced Ca^{2+} release.* In fact, the majority of the cytosolic Ca^{2+} comes from the sarcoplasmic reticulum, not the extracellular fluid. This mechanism of Ca^{2+} release is in contrast to release from skeletal muscle, where depolarization of the cell membrane triggers sarcoplasmic Ca^{2+} release without entry of extracellular Ca^{2+} into the cytosol.

2. What is the function of Ca^{2+} in cardiac muscle contraction?

   Cytosolic Ca^{2+} binds to troponin C, inducing a conformational change that moves tropomyosin away from the myosin-binding sites that are present on the actin filament, which allows for the sliding mechanism of contraction to occur. The force of contraction is proportional to the intracellular Ca^{2+} level. Note that unlike skeletal muscle, cardiac muscle is dependent on extracellular Ca^{2+} influx for contraction to occur.

   The cardioselective nondihydropyridine CCBs (e.g., verapamil, diltiazem) reduce contractility by antagonizing extracellular Ca^{2+} entry and inhibiting the subsequent calcium-induced Ca^{2+} release that occurs in heart muscle. This action is another mechanism by which CCBs work to lower BP.

   Note: The nondihydropyridine CCBs also decrease HR by suppressing AV node conduction.

3. What is the mechanism by which β-adrenergic stimulation increases cardiac contractility?

   Norepinephrine (NE) acts on β-adrenergic receptors to activate adenylyl cyclase, which stimulates a signaling cascade that ultimately results in the production of cAMP. This promotes cAMP-dependent phosphorylation of a number of proteins via protein kinase A (PKA). Phosphorylation of L-type Ca^{2+} channels results in increased Ca^{2+} entry into the myocyte. In addition, β-adrenergic stimulation results in phosphorylation and inhibition of a protein called *phospholamban*, which normally inhibits the sarco/endoplasmic reticulum calcium adenosine triphosphatase, or ATPase (SERCA). Inhibiting phospholamban increases Ca^{2+} reuptake by the sarcoplasmic reticulum, which allows for myocyte relaxation and enables the heart to beat faster. Such rapid ventricular relaxation at elevated HRs is important to ensure adequate ventricular filling during the shorter diastolic periods. Overall, the goal of sympathetic stimulation is to increase CO by increasing both HR and SV.

BASIC CONCEPTS—ARRHYTHMIAS

1. **What is the relationship between the various phases of the ventricular myocyte action potential and the various ion fluxes across the cell membrane?**

    The phases of the ventricular myocyte action potential and the ion fluxes associated with each phase are outlined in Fig. 1.5. In phase 0, the sharp rise in membrane voltage is due to sodium (Na^+) influx. Phase 1 involves a brief repolarization that is due to the transient outward flow of potassium (K^+) that follows Na^+ channel inactivation. In phase 2, the action potential plateaus because of a balance between Ca^{2+} influx and K^+ efflux. During phase 3, there is rapid repolarization because of unopposed K^+ efflux. Phase 4 is the resting potential, which is maintained predominantly through the opening of K^+ channels. Intracellular concentrations of K^+ are maintained at high levels in cardiac myocytes because of the action of membrane-bound Na^+-K^+-ATPase. The opening of K^+ channels during phase 4 leads to passive K^+ efflux (i.e., down its concentration gradient). Because the cell is permeable only to K^+ at this time, negatively charged counterions are unable to follow these K^+ ions as they diffuse outward, causing the cell to become increasingly negative in charge. Therefore the effluxed K^+ ions are attracted back toward the interior of the cell to maintain resting potential. Because phase 4 is dominated by K^+ permeability, it therefore has a value close to the K^+ reversal potential (-85 mV).

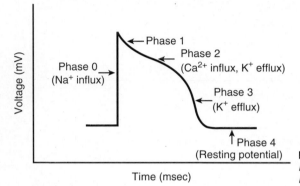

Figure 1.5. Phases of the ventricular myocyte action potential. *(From Brown TA, Brown D. USMLE Step 1 Secrets. Philadelphia: Hanley & Belfus; 2004:77.)*

Note: The antiarrhythmic agents all work by affecting one or more components of the ventricular myocyte action potential. Class I antiarrhythmics block Na^+ channels and therefore antagonize phase 0. Class III antiarrhythmics work by blocking K^+ channels, which prolongs phase 3 depolarization. Some class IA and all class III antiarrhythmics increase action potential duration as well as the QT interval. Toxicity of these agents can lead to *torsades de pointes*, an arrhythmia associated with long QT syndrome, hypokalemia, and hypomagnesemia.

2. **What is the relationship between the various phases of the nodal cell action potential and the various ion fluxes across the cell membrane?**

    The phases of the nodal cell action potential and the ion fluxes associated with each phase are outlined in Fig. 1.6. Nodal cells possess a unique sodium (Na^+) channel, the I_f channel, which allows them to spontaneously discharge without stimulation. The I_f channel is open during the resting phase (phase 4), allowing for Na^+ influx that causes a gradual rise in membrane potential. Eventually, the membrane potential reaches a threshold that triggers the influx of Ca^{2+} through voltage-gated Ca^{2+} channels (this upstroke is termed *phase 0*). Nodal cells do not contain a plateau phase; thus, the phase 2 seen in the ventricular myocyte action potential is absent from the nodal cell action potential. Phase 3, or the downstroke, represents the inactivation of Ca^{2+} channels and the opening of K^+ channels, allowing for K^+ efflux and repolarization of the membrane.

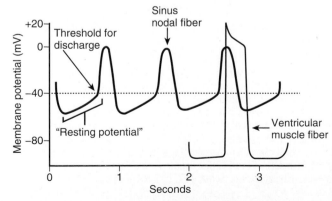

Figure 1.6. Rhythmic discharge of a sinus nodal fiber. The sinus nodal action potential is also compared with that of a ventricular muscle fiber. *(From Guyton AC, Hall JE. Textbook of Medical Physiology. 11th ed. Philadelphia: WB Saunders; 2006:117.)*

Note: The nondihydropyridine CCBs (i.e., verapamil, diltiazem) reduce HR by antagonizing these slow Ca^{2+} channels on the sinoatrial (SA) node. These drugs are considered class IV antiarrhythmics.

3. **Through what mechanism does sympathetic stimulation increase heart rate?**
The release of NE from sympathetic neurons causes activation of β_1-adrenergic receptors in nodal tissue. These receptors stimulate production of cAMP, resulting in an increase in I_f and a positive chronotropic effect on the heart. In essence, sympathetic stimulation increases the cellular influx of Na^+ ions and decreases the efflux of K^+ ions, thus increasing the slope of the resting potential in the nodal cells. When the slope of phase 4 is increased, the threshold for the upstroke is reached faster, resulting in a faster HR. Beta-blockers reduce HR by antagonizing this effect.
Note: Beta-blockers are considered class II antiarrhythmics.

4. **What are the classes of antiarrhythmic medications, and how do their mechanisms of action and potential side effects vary?**
Antiarrhythmic medications are organized by class in Table 1.2 alongside the mechanisms of action and most commonly tested side effects of each class.

Table 1.2. Antiarrhythmic Medications

CLASS	MECHANISM OF ACTION	PROTOTYPE AGENT(S)	COMMONLY TESTED SIDE EFFECTS
IA	Inhibits Na^+ and K^+ channels, prolongs QRS complex and QT interval, prolongs ERP	Quinidine, procainamide	Lupus-like syndrome (procainamide); cinchonism (quinidine); torsades de pointes
IB	Inhibits Na^+ channels, shortens repolarization, ↓ QT interval	Lidocaine	
IC	Inhibits Na^+ channels, prolongs QRS complex	Flecainide, propafenone	Contraindicated in patients with ischemic or structural heart disease
II	Beta-blockers; ↑ PR interval, ↓ automaticity (↓ slope of phase 4 depolarization in nodal cells)	Propranolol, metoprolol, atenolol, esmolol, carvedilol, bisoprolol	May mask hypoglycemic episodes; may precipitate α-adrenergic crises in patients with pheochromocytoma or cocaine toxicity; dyslipidemia (metoprolol)
III	Inhibits K^+ channels	Amiodarone, sotalol, ibutilide	Pulmonary fibrosis, corneal deposits, gray man syndrome, hepatotoxicity, or thyroid dysfunction (amiodarone); torsades de pointes (sotalol, ibutilide)
IV	Inhibits Ca^{2+} channels, ↑ PR interval, ↓ automaticity	Nondihydropyridine CCBs (verapamil, diltiazem)	Flushing, constipation

There is considerable overlap regarding the mechanisms of action of these antiarrhythmics. For the sake of simplicity, only the *primary* mechanism of action is considered in this classification.
↓, Decreased; ↑, increased; *CCBs,* calcium channel blockers; *ERP,* effective refractory period.

CASE 1.1

A 60-year-old Caucasian man presents to his physician for his third visit in 2 months with a blood pressure of approximately 155/95 mm Hg on each occasion. Physical examination is unremarkable. After discussing various lifestyle modifications, a 3-month trial of diet and exercise fails to reduce his blood pressure.

1. **What are the two types of hypertension and which does this patient most likely have?**
The two types of hypertension are essential (also called *primary* or *idiopathic*) and secondary. Essential hypertension is thought to account for approximately 80% to 90% of cases of hypertension. When approaching a patient with hypertension, it is important to consider the underlying medical conditions that may cause secondary hypertension. Potential causes of secondary hypertension that you should keep in mind include renal artery stenosis; primary hyperaldosteronism; Cushing syndrome; pheochromocytoma; coarctation of the aorta; chronic renal disease; excessive alcohol use; pregnancy; increased intracranial pressure; and various medications such as monoamine oxidase (MAO) inhibitors, oral decongestants, nonsteroidal anti-inflammatory drugs (NSAIDs), and oral contraceptives. If causes of secondary hypertension are ruled out, then essential hypertension is diagnosed by exclusion.

2. **How is hypertension defined, and what are the potential complications?**

Hypertension was redefined in the updated American College of Cardiology/American Heart Association (ACC/AHA) guidelines published in 2017. There are now four blood pressure categories for adults, based on SBP and DBP. These updated guidelines are presented in Table 1.3.

Table 1.3. 2017 ACC/AHA Hypertension Guidelines

CATEGORY	BLOOD PRESSURE RANGES	GOAL BLOOD PRESSURE
Normal	SBP: <120 mm Hg **and** DBP: <80 mm Hg	Maintain current blood pressure
Elevated	SBP: 120–129 mm Hg **and** DBP: <80 mm Hg	Maintain current blood pressure
Hypertension stage 1	SBP: 130–139 mm Hg **or** DBP: 80–89 mm Hg	SBP: <130 mm Hg **and** DBP: <80 mm Hg
Hypertension stage 2	SBP: ≥140 mm Hg **or** DBP: ≥90 mm Hg	SBP: <130 mm Hg **and** DBP: <80 mm Hg

ACC/AHA, American College of Cardiology/American Heart Association; *DBP*, diastolic blood pressure; *SBP*, systolic blood pressure.

Note: Patients with SBP and DBP in two separate categories are considered to be in the higher of the two categories.

Evidence suggests that the risk for complications in hypertensive disease is a continuum, increasing as BP rises. It is also largely influenced by comorbid conditions. Major complications of hypertension include accelerated atherosclerosis, premature cardiovascular disease, diastolic (and to a lesser extent, systolic) heart failure, stroke, intracerebral hemorrhage, chronic kidney disease, end-stage renal disease, retinopathy, and acute hypertensive crisis.

Note: A blood pressure *below* 130/80 mm Hg is the target BP for all hypertensive adults, including those with comorbid conditions, according to the 2017 ACC/AHA guidelines. This includes patients with comorbidities such as existing atherosclerotic or cardiovascular disease, diabetes mellitus, chronic kidney disease, heart failure, and peripheral artery disease.

3. **How is hypertension managed?**

The details of hypertension management, like most clinical management discussions, are more applicable to the USMLE Step 2 CK exam than USMLE Step 1. Therefore this topic is thoroughly discussed in the USMLE Step 2 Secrets textbook and only needs a brief introduction here in the event you encounter one of the few management-related questions that are still included on the USMLE Step 1 exam. Nonpharmacologic interventions (e.g., lifestyle modifications) are considered first-line therapy for all categories of hypertension. The updated ACC/AHA guidelines separate pharmacologic options into *primary* and *secondary* agents. The 2017 ACC/AHA recommendations for lifestyle changes, primary pharmacotherapy, and secondary pharmacotherapy are listed in Table 1.4.

Note: Beta-blockers should not be used as monotherapy for primary hypertension. Beta-blockers may decrease BP, but recent studies have shown that they do not adequately prevent stroke compared with other pharmacologic options.

STEP 1 SECRET

While not related to this patient case, it is very high yield for the USMLE Step 1 to know which antihypertensive medications are safe to use during pregnancy. These medications are labetalol, hydralazine, nifedipine, and methyldopa. Remember these antihypertensives with the mnemonic **lower hypertension in new mothers with labetalol, hydralazine, nifedipine, and methyldopa.**

CASE 1.2

A 48-year-old man is newly diagnosed with both type 2 diabetes mellitus (DM) and hypertension. To help control his blood sugar, he is started on metformin.

Table 1.4. 2017 ACC/AHA Recommendations for Hypertension Management

INTERVENTION	DESCRIPTION
Lifestyle modifications	Reduced dietary sodium intake Reduced alcohol intake (men <2 drinks/day; women <1 drink/day) DASH diet Regular exercise (90–150 minutes/week)
Primary pharmacotherapy	Thiazide diuretic ACE inhibitor or ARB CCB: both DHP and non-DHP
Secondary pharmacotherapy	Loop diuretic Potassium-sparing diuretic Aldosterone antagonist diuretic Direct renin inhibitor β-Receptor blocker α-Receptor blocker Direct arterial vasodilator

ACC/AHA, American College of Cardiology/American Heart Association; *ACE,* angiotensin-converting enzyme; *ARB,* angiotensin receptor blocker; *CCB,* calcium channel blocker; *DASH,* dietary approaches to stop hypertension; *DHP,* dihydropyridine.

1. How would the fact that this patient also has type 2 DM influence treatment for his hypertension?
   DM is a comorbid condition whose pathophysiology must be considered when choosing a first-line medication. Angiotensin-converting enzyme (ACE) inhibitors or angiotensin receptor blockers (ARBs) are the preferred first-line antihypertensive medications in patients with DM because ACE inhibitors and ARBs have been shown to reduce the progression of proteinuria (and the subsequent nephropathy) in this patient population.
   Diabetes is a major cardiovascular risk factor. Tight blood pressure control is critical in patients with diabetes to reduce the mortality risk from macrovascular disease (e.g., myocardial infarction, stroke). Tight blood pressure control also reduces the risk of microvascular complications such as retinopathy, nephropathy, and neuropathy.

2. What are the mechanisms by which ACE inhibitors and ARBs lower blood pressure?
   ACE inhibitors prevent the conversion of angiotensin I to angiotensin II. Angiotensin II directly contributes to peripheral vasoconstriction, stimulation of thirst, renal sodium reabsorption in the proximal tubule, and aldosterone production (Fig. 1.7), all of which are antagonized by ACE inhibitors. ARBs act as an angiotensin II receptor antagonist. Another

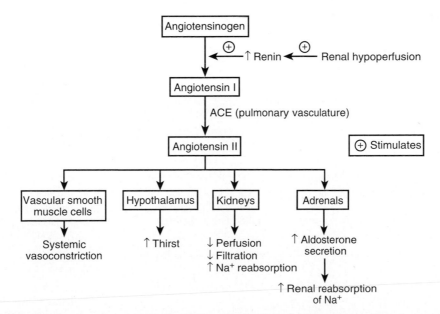

Figure 1.7. Enzymatic cascade and physiologic effects of the renin-angiotensin-aldosterone system. ↓, Decreased; ↑, increased; *ACE,* angiotensin-converting enzyme. *(From Brown TA.* Rapid Review Physiology. *Philadelphia: Mosby; 2007:148.)*

proposed mechanism that may explain why ACE inhibitors and ARBs successfully treat hypertension in patients with diabetes is by preventing the efferent arteriolar constriction that angiotensin II is known to cause. Preventing efferent arteriolar constriction in this way reduces glomerular filtration pressure and lowers glomerular filtration rate (GFR), which lessens glomerular damage and is a key aspect of renal-protective hypertension management strategies.

3. Why might the use of beta-blockers be relatively contraindicated in this patient?
Beta-blockers are not recommended for use in patients with diabetes because they could mask important signs of hypoglycemia (e.g., tremor and palpitations) that indicate impending hypoglycemic crisis, which are mediated through the sympathetic nervous system. Beta-blockers also antagonize epinephrine-stimulated hepatic gluconeogenesis and glycogenolysis, which may further exacerbate a hypoglycemic state. This is especially a concern with patients with diabetes who are prescribed second-generation sulfonylureas, dipeptidyl peptidase (DPP-4) inhibitors, or insulin, as these medications are also known to precipitate hypoglycemic episodes.

Note: Although beta-blockers could mask many of the symptoms associated with hypoglycemia, they will not prevent the diaphoresis commonly seen in severe hypoglycemia, because sweat glands are innervated by sympathetic cholinergic nerves rather than sympathetic adrenergic nerves.

4. What effect might a thiazide diuretic have on this patient's glycemic control?
Diuretics commonly worsen *hyper*glycemia in patients with diabetes. Although the mechanism remains uncertain, this increase in serum glucose is likely related to a combination of hypokalemia and intravascular volume depletion that occurs with initiation of diuretic therapy. Hypokalemia can contribute to impaired glucose tolerance because potassium is a necessary cotransporter for glucose uptake, meaning a hypokalemic state reduces insulin secretion, stimulates insulin resistance, and impairs cellular glucose uptake.

The intravascular volume depletion resulting from diuresis reduces CO, which stimulates epinephrine production by the sympathetic nervous system, which promotes insulin resistance and reduces glucose uptake by the liver and skeletal muscle.

While this is seldom seen clinically, for the purpose of your USMLE Step 1 exam, you should also note that thiazide diuretics should be used cautiously in patients with diabetes because they may theoretically increase the risk of hyperlipidemia and hyperuricemia.

CASE 1.2 CONTINUED:

The patient is started on lisinopril, which he initially tolerates well. After about a month he develops a dry cough and wonders if it is somehow related to his new medication.

5. What is the mechanism by which ACE inhibitors, such as lisinopril, can cause a cough?
ACE not only converts angiotensin I into angiotensin II but is also crucial in the degradation pathway of bradykinin in the blood. Accumulation of bradykinin as the result of ACE inhibitor use is believed to be the primary cause of this cough. It is thought that the accumulated bradykinin stimulates nociceptors in the airways through an unknown mechanism, thereby initiating the cough reflex. This undesirable side effect can be avoided by using an ARB such as losartan.

6. Cover all but the left-most column of Table 1.5, and for each antihypertensive drug listed, name the drug class, mechanism of action, and most commonly tested side effects of each.

Table 1.5. Antihypertensive Drugs

DRUG	DRUG CLASS	PRIMARY MECHANISM OF ACTION	PRIMARY SIDE EFFECTS
Hydralazine	Direct arterial vasodilator	↑ cGMP leading to smooth muscle relaxation and afterload reduction	Lupus-like syndrome Reflex tachycardia
Lisinopril Accupril Benazepril	ACE inhibitor	↓ ATII production ↓ Peripheral resistance ↓ Aldosterone secretion	Dry cough Hyperkalemia Angioedema (↑ bradykinin) Acute kidney injury (↓ GFR)
Losartan Valsartan	ARB	Inhibit ATII action in tissues	
Methyldopa Clonidine	α_2-Receptor agonist	↓ CNS sympathetic outflow	Sedation, depression Rebound hypertension (following abrupt withdrawal of clonidine)

Table 1.5. Antihypertensive Drugs—cont'd

DRUG	DRUG CLASS	PRIMARY MECHANISM OF ACTION	PRIMARY SIDE EFFECTS
Acebutolol Atenolol Betaxolol Bisoprolol Esmolol Metoprolol Nebivolol	Selective β_1-receptor blocker	Negative chronotropic and inotropic effects (reduced CO)	Bradycardia/heart block Sexual dysfunction Bronchospasm (at high doses) Depression (at high doses)
Nadolol Pindolol Propranolol Timolol	Nonselective β-blocker	Negative chronotropic and inotropic effects (reduced CO)	Bronchospasm Bradycardia/heart block CHF Exercise intolerance
Prazosin Terazosin Doxazosin	α_1-Receptor antagonist	↓ Peripheral resistance	Postural hypotension
Labetalol Carvedilol	Combined α- and β-receptor blocker	Combined effect of α_1-blockers and β-blockers	
Diltiazem Verapamil	Non-DHP CCB	↓ CO ↓ Peripheral resistance (diltiazem)	Bradycardia/heart block
Amlodipine Nifedipine	DHP CCB	↓ Peripheral resistance (more specific for vascular smooth muscle than cardiac muscle)	Reflex tachycardia
Hydrochlorothiazide Chlorthalidone	Thiazide diuretic	Inhibits sodium and water reabsorption in distal convoluted tubule	Hypokalemia Hyperuricemia Hyperglycemia Hyperlipidemia Hypercalcemia
Furosemide Bumetanide	Loop diuretic	Inhibits Na^+-Cl—-2 K^+ pump in thick ascending limb of loop of Henle	Hypokalemia Hyperuricemia Hyperglycemia Hypocalcemia Ototoxicity
Spironolactone Eplerenone	Aldosterone receptor antagonist diuretic	Antagonizes action of aldosterone	Hyperkalemia Gynecomastia (spironolactone)

↓, Decreased; ↑, increased; *ACE*, angiotensin-converting enzyme; *ARB*, angiotensin receptor blocker; *ATII*, angiotensin II; *CCB*, calcium channel blocker; *cGMP*, cyclic guanosine monophosphate; *CHF*, congestive heart failure; *CNS*, central nervous system; *CO*, cardiac output; *DHP*, dihydropyridine; *GFR*, glomerular filtration rate.

SUMMARY BOX: ANTIHYPERTENSIVE PHARMACOTHERAPY IN TYPE 2 DIABETES MELLITUS

- Angiotensin-converting enzyme (ACE) inhibitors are first-line therapy for hypertension in patients with type 2 diabetes mellitus because of their nephroprotective actions. The primary side effect of ACE inhibitors is a dry cough, which is likely the result of bradykinin accumulation.
- Beta-blockers are relatively contraindicated for treating hypertension in patients with diabetes because of the concern that they may mask the symptoms of a hypoglycemic crisis.
- Thiazide diuretics should be used cautiously in patients with diabetes because of their potential risk of inducing hyperlipidemia and hyperuricemia in this patient population.

CASE 1.3

A 65-year-old man with an unremarkable past medical history is evaluated for a 6-month history of chest pain with exertion. His pain resolves immediately with rest and/or sublingual nitroglycerin. The pain is a substernal pressure sensation that remains localized and does not radiate to the arms, shoulder, or jaw. Physical exam is unrevealing.

1. **What is the most likely diagnosis?**
   The most likely diagnosis in this patient is angina pectoris. Angina pectoris is chest pain caused by impaired blood flow to the myocardium, usually because of stenosis of the coronary arteries by atheromatous plaques. The resulting transient myocardial ischemia promotes anaerobic respiration and the release of waste products (e.g., lactic acid) that cause cardiac pain.
      Note: Recall that visceral cardiac pain is sensed by sympathetic fibers that travel parallel to the coronary vessels and enter the spinal cord between C8 and T4. Be alert for "silent" cardiac ischemia in patients with autonomic neuropathy (e.g., patients with diabetes) or patients who have received a heart transplant (in which the autonomic fibers have been severed).

CASE 1.3 CONTINUED:

The patient states that his episodes of chest pressure generally last around 5 minutes but never longer than 15 minutes. They often occur when he uses the push mower to mow the lawn on the steep part of the yard or when he rides his bicycle up a hill but not when he is walking, sitting, or sleeping. He thinks the severity and pattern of chest pain have stayed pretty much the same since he first noticed it 6 months ago.

2. **Does this patient have stable or unstable angina? How are these two diagnoses different, and which is more serious?**
   This patient has stable angina. In stable angina, a constant and predictable level of physical exertion elicits the reported chest pain (or anginal equivalent such as dyspnea). Stable angina usually lasts between 2 and 5 minutes, and occasionally over 10 minutes, but rarely over 15 minutes or less than 1 minute. It is always promptly relieved by rest. In contrast, unstable angina is characterized by chest pain that is unrelieved by rest or that occurs after only mild exertion and can last longer than 15 minutes. Unstable angina is more serious because it indicates a disruption within the atheromatous plaque(s) in the coronary arteries that is causing ischemia. It may also involve the formation of a nonocclusive thrombus. When unstable angina develops, the patient should be emergently evaluated to rule out an impending myocardial infarction (MI).

3. **How can angina occur in the absence of coronary atherosclerosis?**
   Vasospastic angina (also called Prinzmetal or *variant* angina) is transmural cardiac ischemia as the result of sporadic vasospasm of the coronary arteries. It should be suspected in a patient who has anginal symptoms at rest. Vasospastic angina is thought to be chemically mediated by an increased production of thromboxane A_2 (TXA_2) by platelets or an increased production of endothelin-1 in damaged endothelial cells. Severe anemia could also theoretically produce angina because of reduced delivery of oxygen to the heart and increased demand on the heart to pump more blood as a result of the reduced oxygen-carrying capacity of the blood. On rare occasions, patients with pheochromocytoma without coronary artery disease can experience severe coronary vasospasm resulting in cardiac ischemia and, at times, even MI. Last, ventricular hypertrophy may cause subendocardial ischemia and angina because the increase in myocardial perfusion is usually not as great proportionally as the degree of myocardial hypertrophy.
      Note: Cocaine use can also produce angina secondary to coronary vasoconstriction. This is mediated by α-adrenergic activation, increased endothelin (a vasoconstrictor), and decreased production of NO (a vasodilator).

4. **What are the principal physiologic determinants of myocardial oxygen supply?**
   Myocardial oxygen supply is dependent on coronary artery perfusion and arterial oxygen-carrying capacity.
   - Coronary artery perfusion is primarily dependent on the amount of time spent in diastole, diastolic perfusion pressure, thickness of the myocardium, and the vascular resistance of the coronary arteries.
   - Arterial oxygen-carrying capacity is largely dependent on the hemoglobin concentration and the efficiency of gas exchange in the lungs.
      Although severe anemia or hypoxemia can substantially decrease myocardial oxygen supply, supply is more often limited as a result of inadequate myocardial perfusion. This can result from tachycardia (faster heart rates mean decreased time spent in diastole, which is the period when nearly all coronary blood flow occurs), inadequate diastolic perfusion pressure (resulting from hypotension), dehydration, valvular abnormalities (e.g., regurgitation), or an increased left ventricular end-diastolic pressure (LVEDP), which occurs in concentric and eccentric hypertrophy.

5. **What are the principal physiologic determinants of myocardial oxygen demand?**
   Any factor that affects the hemodynamics of the cardiovascular system can affect myocardial oxygen demand. Thus oxygen demand is increased as HR, contractility, afterload, and sympathetic activity increase. To compensate for elevated oxygen demand, the heart increases coronary blood flow, which in turn increases oxygen delivery. Recall that oxygen extraction from the coronary arteries is very efficient (assumed to be 100%), so the only way to increase oxygen delivery to the heart is to alter coronary blood flow.

6. **Which factors contribute to a myocardial oxygen demand that exceeds supply in this patient?**
   Demand is increased by the sympathetic-mediated increase in HR as well as the increased contractility in response to exertion. At the same time, supply is decreased because an elevated HR means reduced diastolic filling time, giving sclerotic coronary arteries less time to deliver oxygenated blood to the myocardium. Normally, coronary arteries can sufficiently dilate to maintain adequate myocardial blood flow. In patients with angina pectoris, coronary artery narrowing from atherosclerosis prevents adequate myocardial perfusion, causing transient ischemia and the clinical symptoms described by this patient.

7. Why is nitroglycerin effective in eliminating anginal pain?

Nitroglycerin is converted within endothelial cells to NO, which is also referred to as *endothelium-derived relaxation factor* (EDRF) because of its vasodilatory effects. Perhaps the most important reason nitroglycerin effectively eliminates anginal pain is its ability to reduce myocardial oxygen demand through venous dilation (decreasing preload) and arteriolar dilation (reducing afterload). For the USMLE Step 1 exam, however, it is important to understand that the effect of nitroglycerin is much greater on reducing *preload* than afterload because it dilates veins more than arteries. In any case, decreasing preload and afterload reduces cardiac contractility and myocardial wall tension, which additionally allows greater myocardial perfusion during diastole. Nitroglycerin and other organic nitrates also exert effects directly on the coronary vasculature, including vasodilation of the coronary arteries and relief of coronary artery spasm. The precise mechanisms by which nitrates reduce symptoms of anginal pain therefore will depend on which pathologic mechanism is responsible for the angina in a given patient (e.g., atherosclerotic occlusion vs. vasospasm).

   Note: High doses of nitrates can produce *reflex tachycardia*, which occurs as a spontaneous sympathetic response in the setting of hypotension, and this can further exacerbate anginal pain by increasing myocardial oxygen demand. Because nitrates relax both vascular and nonvascular smooth muscle, they can relieve the pain of both angina and esophageal spasm, making it difficult to distinguish between these two conditions based solely on their response to nitrates. The compensatory tachycardia that develops because of nitroglycerin-mediated vasodilation can be prevented with beta-blockers.

8. What are the mechanisms by which beta-blockers decrease myocardial oxygen demand and therefore may treat the symptoms of angina?

Beta-blockers exert negative chronotropic and inotropic effects on the heart. Perfusion of the myocardium increases with the longer time spent in diastole, secondary to a beta-blocker's negative chronotropic effect. An additional benefit of a beta-blocker is its antagonism of the β_1-adrenergic receptors that normally stimulate renin release in the RAAS pathway. This inhibition of renin release will decrease systemic vascular resistance and therefore decrease afterload. The heart's oxygen demand will decrease with the lowered resistance it has to overcome.

CASE 1.3 CONTINUED:

An exercise stress test is performed to investigate the possibility of coronary artery disease and to assess the patient's level of cardiopulmonary function. While he is on the treadmill, the electrocardiogram (ECG) reveals ST-segment depression, which is determined to be evidence of early cardiac ischemia. This occurs when his HR and BP have both increased ~50% above baseline.

9. How could a similar evaluation be made in a patient who cannot tolerate an exercise stress test (e.g., orthopedic condition, diabetic foot ulcer, chronic lung disease)?

Pharmacologic agents can be used to simulate the stress of exercise. Dobutamine (a synthetic catecholamine) has positive inotropic and chronotropic effects on the heart. Its administration is physiologically similar to physical exertion because both will cause an increase in myocardial oxygen demand. Adenosine (a potent coronary vasodilator with a short half-life) is more commonly used with positron emission tomography (PET) scanning. Together these create an accurate image of coronary perfusion.

SUMMARY BOX: ANGINA PECTORIS

- The three main forms of angina are stable, unstable, and variant (Prinzmetal). Distinguishing between these patterns has important implications for prognosis and treatment.
- An imbalance between myocardial oxygen supply and demand underlies the pathophysiology of angina pectoris.
- Nitroglycerin's primary mechanism of action is the dilation of peripheral veins, which reduces preload and therefore lowers myocardial oxygen demand. It also has direct effects on the coronary arteries, which makes nitroglycerin a useful agent when managing any of the three forms of angina.

CASE 1.4

A 52-year-old man presents to the emergency department for evaluation of a crushing substernal pressure sensation for the past hour. He is obese and diaphoretic. The pain radiates to his left arm and jaw. He is concerned because he usually gets chest pain only after exercising, which is typically relieved by rest. However, this pain has not resolved despite numerous attempts to relax. Additionally, he feels nauseated, which is new compared to past episodes.

1. What is the most likely diagnosis in this patient and why?

Based on his presentation, acute coronary syndrome is at the top of the differential list, which includes unstable angina, non-ST elevation myocardial infarction (NSTEMI), and ST elevation myocardial infarction (STEMI). Although this episode could represent unstable angina, it is absolutely critical to evaluate for MI in all patients with this presentation. The typical presentation of MI involves crushing substernal pain for longer than 30 minutes that is not relieved by rest or nitroglycerin. This diagnosis should be considered immediately because a timely intervention is essential to the patient's outcome. Acute MI is a leading cause of death in adults in the United States and has a high incidence rate in men between the ages of 40 and 65 years.

2. What are some common risk factors for coronary artery disease?
    Common risk factors for coronary artery disease (CAD) include older age (men >45, women >55), hypertension, dyslipidemia (e.g., high low-density lipoprotein [LDL], low high-density lipoprotein [HDL]), smoking, DM, and a first-degree family member (e.g., parent or sibling) with history of premature heart disease (CAD in men <55 years old, women <65 years old). Other less robust but still generally accepted risk factors include obesity, sedentary lifestyle, high-fat diet, and persistently high stress levels.

CASE 1.4 CONTINUED:

An ECG reveals ST-segment elevation in two consecutive leads. A chest x-ray study does not show mediastinal widening or other abnormalities. The patient is given morphine, oxygen, nitroglycerin, metoprolol, and aspirin. The consulting cardiologist decides that the patient is a suitable candidate for emergent angioplasty, and he is taken to the cardiac catheterization laboratory.

3. What kind of MI is this patient experiencing?
    He is experiencing an STEMI. The pathophysiology classically involves complete occlusion of a coronary artery resulting in transmural tissue infarction, meaning the full thickness of the wall has been deprived of oxygen. Studies have shown that emergent angioplasty will improve mortality in patients with STEMI if performed in a timely fashion. Unlike the classic patient with STEMI, subendocardial MIs only affect a portion of the ventricular wall thickness and typically lack ST-segment elevation, and are thus referred to as *non-STEMI* (NSTEMI). NSTEMIs are caused by an incomplete occlusion or a transient total occlusion of a coronary artery. Patients with NSTEMIs also have elevations in cardiac enzymes as the result of myocardial damage, and these patients may also benefit from cardiac catheterization, although not on the same emergent basis as a STEMI.

4. In addition to analysis of the ECG, what serum tests should be ordered to confirm or rule out an acute MI?
    When a patient presents to the emergency department with a suspected MI, an ECG is the first step for diagnosis. Serum levels of cardiac enzymes, which leak out of damaged or ischemic myocardial tissue, are also helpful to diagnose a suspected acute MI. These cardiac enzymes may be more sensitive indicators of MI but may not elevate to diagnostic levels until several hours after the onset of chest pain. These enzymes include troponin I, creatine kinase MB fraction (CK-MB), and myoglobin, with each having unique specificities and different times for peak elevation (Fig. 1.8). Myoglobin rises soon after the onset of cardiac pain. Although it is a very early marker, it is nonspecific for MI. Troponin I begins to rise after approximately 4 hours and is the most specific for acute MI; it also remains elevated for the longest period of time (7–10 days). CK-MB has good specificity and begins to rise with troponin. It does not remain elevated nearly as long as troponin does, which is clinically useful in diagnosing a *recurrent* MI.

    Because these enzymes remain elevated for some time, they may be more useful than an ECG, which provides only a snapshot of the heart's electrical activity at a particular moment in time, in a patient who presents a few days after experiencing MI-like symptoms.

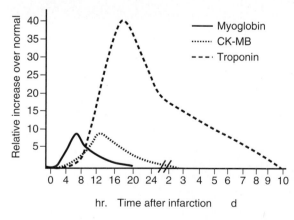

Figure 1.8. Timeline of cardiac marker production following myocardial infarction. *CK-MB,* Creatine kinase MB fraction; *d,* days; *hr,* hours. *(From Henry JB. Clinical Diagnosis and Management by Laboratory Methods. 20th ed. Philadelphia: WB Saunders; 2001:297.)*

CASE 1.4 CONTINUED:

The patient's angiogram shows a 95% narrowing of the left anterior descending (LAD) coronary artery. Angioplasty is performed, and a drug-eluting stent is successfully placed, restoring patency to the vessel. After 3 days in the hospital, the patient is discharged with prescriptions for lisinopril, lovastatin, clopidogrel, and metoprolol in addition to daily aspirin and as-needed nitroglycerin he was already taking.

5. **What other treatment option is available besides angioplasty to restore coronary blood flow? What are the major contraindications to its use?**
Thrombolytic therapy with tissue plasminogen activator (tPA) or streptokinase is also possible but must be performed within a certain time frame to be effective. It is not used unless coronary catheterization is unavailable and the patient presents within the necessary time frame. Thrombolytic therapy is contraindicated in patients at high risk for hemorrhage (e.g., recent major surgery, bleeding disorder, anticoagulant use, severe hypertension, recent hemorrhagic cerebrovascular accident [CVA]).

    Note: Bleeding caused by thrombolytic therapy can be treated with *aminocaproic acid*, which inhibits the activation of plasminogen.

STEP 1 SECRET

Knowing the antidotes for common drug overdoses will be useful for the USMLE Step 1.

6. **What is the physiologic rationale for giving beta-blockers to patients with a history of MI?**
As discussed previously, beta-blockers lower myocardial oxygen demand, making the heart less susceptible to infarction. Additionally, because infarction creates an area of fibrosis that can produce an arrhythmia, beta-blockers are also useful for their antiarrhythmic properties. However, if the infarction involves the tissues of the conduction pathway and results in heart block, beta-blocker use may be contraindicated. Overall, beta-blockers have been shown to reduce mortality when given after an MI.

7. **How might an MI lead to the following short- and long-term sequelae?**
   A. **Pulmonary edema** can result from two problems: (1) The weakened left ventricle (LV) might no longer be able to effectively pump blood into the aorta, resulting in a reduced ejection fraction (EF). This is termed *systolic dysfunction.* (2) The LV could still pump effectively but might become stiff (noncompliant) as a result of the infarct (and ongoing ischemia), thus necessitating increased ventricular filling pressures to achieve an adequate end-diastolic volume. This is termed *diastolic dysfunction.* Regardless of the precise cause (LV pump failure or noncompliance), the increased left ventricular filling pressures cause a backpressure of blood in the left atrium and pulmonary circulation. Ultimately, the resulting elevated hydrostatic pressures in the pulmonary capillaries lead to transudation of fluid into the pulmonary interstitium and alveolar space.

       Initially, this interstitial fluid is completely removed by the pulmonary lymphatics. However, when the pulmonary capillary hydrostatic pressure increases too much (typically >30 mm Hg), the ability of the lymphatics to remove excess fluid is overcome, and interstitial fluid and intra-alveolar fluid accumulate, resulting in pulmonary edema. Pulmonary edema reduces oxygen diffusion across the pulmonary membrane, causing hypoxemia. This further exacerbates the failing heart. This is one reason why oxygen therapy may be beneficial after a severe MI.
   B. **Arrhythmias.** Leakage of electrolytes from the necrotic myocardial cells results in electrolyte imbalances that can precipitate arrhythmias. These arrhythmias are most common *within a few days after the MI.*
   C. **Murmur.** If the MI causes rupture of the ventricular septum or a papillary muscle, then the new-onset murmur of a ventricular septal defect (VSD) or valvular regurgitation would be auscultated (both of which are holosystolic murmurs).
   D. **Ventricular rupture.** The inflammatory reaction in the infarcted site weakens the myocardial wall. Ventricular rupture typically occurs *3 to 7 days after* the infarct and can result in hemopericardium (i.e., blood in the pericardial sac).
   E. **Pericarditis.** The inflammatory reaction to necrotic myocardium can also cause pericarditis (usually *within the first week after the MI*). Suspect this if the patient has a pericardial friction rub.
   F. **Dressler syndrome,** an autoimmune process that occurs secondary to leakage of intracellular proteins from necrotic myocardial cells, is a type of pericarditis that develops *1 to 10 weeks after an MI.* Consider this diagnosis whenever you see a patient who presents with pleuritic chest pain, fever, and symptoms of pericardial effusion several weeks after MI.

STEP 1 SECRET

Pay attention to the duration of symptoms after the suspected myocardial infarction (MI) because this will guide your evaluation of complications. Vignettes may include a patient who has had an MI and can ask for the complication with its correlated histology.

8. **What is sudden cardiac death, and why are patients with a history of MI predisposed to it?**
Sudden cardiac death is defined as death *within 1 hour* of onset of symptoms (usually as the result of a lethal arrhythmia such as ventricular fibrillation). This is most commonly associated with nonocclusive clots, which typically cause subendocardial infarcts. Subendocardial infarcts are often referred to as *non–Q wave MIs* or *NSTEMIs.*

SUMMARY BOX: CORONARY ARTERY DISEASE

- Major modifiable coronary risk factors include hypertension, smoking, and dyslipidemia, and major nonmodifiable risk factors include age, male gender under age 65, and family history of premature heart disease.
- Cardiac muscle enzymes such as creatine kinase MB fraction (CK-MB) and cardiac-specific troponins are sensitive indicators of myocardial infarction (MI) if measured at least 4 hours after the onset of symptoms.
- Patients who are post-MI are at increased risk for another MI as well as a number of other complications, including pulmonary edema, ischemic myocardial rupture, pericarditis, new-onset murmurs, arrhythmias, and sudden cardiac death.

CASE 1.5

A 72-year-old woman with a long history of poorly controlled hypertension and diabetes presents with a 1-month history of worsening fatigue and dyspnea. Initially, she experienced difficulty breathing only with exertion, but recently it occurs even at rest. She admits to supporting herself with two pillows at night to help with breathing (two-pillow orthopnea).

1. **What disorder is at the top of your differential diagnosis list?**
   These symptoms describe a classic presentation of heart failure, but before jumping straight to that diagnosis, be sure to consider alternative causes such as myocardial ischemia, lung disease, anemia, and atrial fibrillation. Diagnosis of heart failure is largely based on a careful history, physical examination, and tests that assess cardiac function.

CASE 1.5 CONTINUED:

On physical examination, she has distended neck veins, bibasilar pulmonary crackles, and bilateral lower extremity edema. Her apical impulse is displaced laterally beyond the midclavicular line, and an S_3 gallop is appreciated on auscultation. On chest x-ray, the cardiac silhouette appears slightly enlarged, and an echocardiogram reveals an EF of 38% with no valvular abnormalities. Serum levels of brain natriuretic peptide (BNP) are substantially elevated.

2. **In pathophysiologic terms, what is heart failure?**
   Heart failure results from either (1) pathologically depressed CO or (2) normal CO that can only be maintained at elevated ventricular filling pressures, which pathologically increases venous hydrostatic pressures. It therefore follows that there are two major categories of symptoms seen in heart failure: those resulting from depressed CO (i.e., systolic heart failure) and those resulting from fluid accumulation caused by increased filling pressures (i.e., diastolic heart failure). Heart failure is also categorized according to the side of the heart that has failed to function. Left-sided heart failure results in a decrease in the inotropic ability of the heart to pump the necessary amount of blood to the rest of the body. It can be compensated for by the RAAS, which will increase intravascular volume, venous return, and contractility to maintain CO. When these compensatory mechanisms can no longer meet the body's metabolic demands, it is termed *decompensated heart failure.* Symptoms such as fatigue, lethargy, and weakness are due to inadequate CO and worsen with exertion.

   Whether the heart failure is compensated or decompensated, ventricular pressures become elevated, which may cause pulmonary edema and lead to dyspnea (as experienced by this patient). If left-sided heart failure is not treated, the pulmonary pressures will remain elevated and can cause the right side of the heart to fail; this is called *biventricular failure.* This leads to a similar backup of blood in the venous circulation, resulting in jugular venous distention, hepatomegaly, and pitting edema.

   Heart failure that manifests with these symptoms is called *congestive heart failure* (CHF). Notice that this patient has signs of both left- and right-sided heart failure.

   Note: The most common cause of right-sided heart failure is left-sided heart failure. Other, less common causes of right-sided heart failure include pulmonary hypertension, tricuspid regurgitation, pulmonary stenosis, and septal defects.

3. **What are the differences between systolic and diastolic heart failure? Which does this patient most likely have?**
   Heart failure can be broadly classified as systolic (pump) failure or diastolic (filling) failure. Systolic heart failure is characterized by insufficient contractility of the ventricles, with an EF below 40%. For this reason, systolic heart failure is also known as *heart failure with reduced ejection fraction,* often abbreviated HFrEF. Diastolic heart failure is characterized by poor ventricular compliance (decreased *lusitropy*), resulting in insufficient filling of ventricles during diastole. Hence, diastolic failure is also known as *heart failure with preserved ejection fraction,* often abbreviated HFpEF. It is estimated that approximately two-thirds of patients with heart failure have systolic failure and one-third have diastolic failure. However, because most patients with systolic dysfunction have components of diastolic dysfunction as well, this classification scheme is characterized by substantial overlap.

   This patient's reduced EF and S_3 heart sound make systolic heart failure the most likely diagnosis.

   Note: The EF is defined as SV divided by end-diastolic volume (SV/EDV) and is normally 55% to 75%. This is typically determined by echocardiogram.

4. What is the etiology of heart failure?

Systolic heart failure is associated with myocardial damage or ischemia as well as volume-overloaded states such as valvular regurgitation and kidney disease. Diastolic heart failure is usually associated with pressure overload (e.g., hypertension) and myocardial ischemia, but it may also be caused by infiltrative diseases (e.g., amyloidosis, hemochromatosis, sarcoidosis).

5. The body's response to heart failure is initially helpful but becomes maladaptive with time. For each of the following physiologic responses observed in heart failure, describe both the adaptive and pathologic results.

1. Increased sympathetic activity

Adaptive: Increased sympathetic activity results in tachycardia and increased contractility of the heart, both of which increase CO. Interestingly, patients in heart failure secrete three to four times more NE per day than normal healthy individuals. Recall that the determinants of CO are given by the equation

$$CO = HR \times SV \qquad [1.3]$$

Additionally, in the setting of reduced CO (e.g., systolic heart failure), vasoconstriction caused by elevated sympathetic activity helps maintain sufficient arterial pressure to provide adequate perfusion to critical organs. Remember, the determinants of arterial pressure are CO and TPR:

$$MAP = CO \times TPR \qquad [1.4]$$

Pathologic: The sympathoadrenal activation seen in the context of a failing heart results in a reduced amount of time spent in diastole. This decreases the time available for coronary perfusion (supply) in a setting where the load on the heart (demand) is already being increased by sympathetic activity. Over time, the increased load results in cardiac remodeling and worsening cardiac function, which is exacerbated by a decreased blood supply. Additionally, the sympathetically mediated chronic vasoconstriction in skeletal muscles that occurs during heart failure and the decreasing CO are largely responsible for the muscle fatigue observed in these patients.

2. Fluid retention

Adaptive: The kidneys sense reduced CO through decreases in renal perfusion and GFR. They respond by activating the RAAS to retain fluid and expand plasma volume. This elevation in intravascular volume increases venous return to the heart and subsequently increases preload. This response has a positive inotropic effect on the heart via the Frank-Starling relationship and will increase CO.

Pathologic: The increased preload from fluid retention places an increased workload on the heart. This can precipitate symptoms of angina secondary to insufficient coronary perfusion. Excessive preload stretches the myocardium to a point of suboptimal overlap of actin and myosin filaments in the sarcomeres, counterintuitively reducing contractility. Finally, fluid retention can also cause complications associated with excessive volume expansion (e.g., pulmonary edema).

Note: Because nitrates and diuretics both decrease preload (as well as afterload to some degree), they help alleviate the symptoms of CHF associated with excessive volume expansion.

3. Myocardial hypertrophy

Adaptive: The value of this process depends on the type of overload that occurs in heart failure. In a pressure-overloaded heart (from hypertension or aortic stenosis), there is *concentric* hypertrophy (circular thickening of the myocardium) that strengthens ventricular contractions in the setting of a significant afterload. In pressure-overloaded ventricles, the increased systolic wall stress causes addition of sarcomeres in parallel, which reduces the stress on each individual sarcomere according to the law of Laplace (wall stress = pressure × radius/thickness). In a volume-overloaded heart, the increase in diastolic wall stress from increased end-diastolic volume causes poor alignment of sarcomere fibrils (past the adaptive point of the Frank-Starling relationship), so sarcomeres are added in series to expand the chamber volume and optimize fiber alignment. This is described as *eccentric* hypertrophy.

Pathologic: Oxygen demand of the hypertrophied heart is increased, which may exacerbate an existing ischemic condition. In fact, the vascular supply to the heart often does not increase proportionately to the muscular hypertrophy. Additionally, the thickened myocardium requires a larger distance for oxygen to diffuse, which is already exacerbated by the elevated ventricular diastolic pressures of heart failure. This reduces the gradient for oxygen diffusion from the coronary arteries through the myocardium. Hypertrophy also reduces ventricular compliance, which can cause or worsen diastolic dysfunction. The sympathetic nervous system and angiotensin II are involved in mediating the ventricular remodeling found in hypertrophy and in ventricular dilation.

Note: If an adequate CO is restored by these compensatory mechanisms, the heart failure is said to be *compensated.* If these physiologic reflexes alone cannot restore adequate CO, the heart failure is said to be *decompensated.*

6. Given the pathophysiologic adaptations described in the previous question, why might beta-blockers be beneficial in heart failure?

Beta-blockers have many effects that additively decrease the overall cardiac workload and improve function of an ailing heart:

1. Inhibit sympathetic activity
   a. Decrease preload by preventing sympathetic-mediated venoconstriction

    b. Decrease contractility and HR
    c. Decrease afterload
  2. Decrease renin secretion
    a. Decrease fluid retention and afterload
  3. Decrease cardiac remodeling

7. **How is digoxin believed to increase cardiac contractility in patients with heart failure?**
Similar to skeletal muscle fibers, cardiac muscle fibers contract when the intracellular Ca^{2+} levels rise. Digoxin increases the intracellular Ca^{2+} through an indirect mechanism involving ion exchanges. By directly inhibiting the Na^+/K^+ pump, digoxin increases intracellular Na^+. Because the extracellular/intracellular Na^+ gradient drives the Na^+/Ca^{2+} exchanger, in the presence of high intracellular Na^+ less Ca^{2+} is pumped out of the cell, increasing intracellular Ca^{2+} and therefore increasing contractility.

    Note: In contrast to drugs such as ACE inhibitors and beta-blockers, which have been shown to reduce mortality, digoxin has been shown to improve cardiac performance and quality of life without an improvement in mortality risk. It is not a first-line agent in the treatment of heart failure.

STEP 1 SECRET

Digoxin is a high-yield drug for the USMLE Step 1. In addition to its mechanism of action, it is important to know the commonly tested side effects of digoxin. These include cholinergic effects (e.g., diarrhea, vomiting, increased PR interval), arrhythmias, and blurry yellow vision. Digoxin toxicity is treated by stopping the medication and administering potassium (K^+), magnesium (Mg^{2+}), and antidigoxin antigen-binding (Fab) fragments. Lidocaine is given for digoxin-induced arrhythmias.

8. **In Table 1.6, cover the right-hand column and give the mechanism of action for each of the listed drugs used to manage CHF.**

Table 1.6 Drugs Used for Congestive Heart Failure

DRUG	DRUG CLASS	MECHANISM OF ACTION
Digoxin	Cardiac glycoside	↑ inotropic effect, ↓ chronotropic effect (due to vagus nerve [CN X] stimulation), ↑ EF
Bisoprolol Carvedilol Metoprolol (extended release)	Selective β_1-receptor blocker	↓ chronotropic effect, ↓ inotropic effect, ↓ myocardial demand
Benazepril Captopril Cilazapril Enalapril Enalaprilat Fosinopril Lisinopril Moexipril Perindopril Quinapril Ramipril Trandolapril	ACE inhibitor	↓ aldosterone, ↓ plasma volume, ↓ actions of ATII
Candesartan Eprosartan Irbesartan Losartan Olmesartan Telmisartan Valsartan	ARB	Inhibits actions of ATII

↓, Decreased; ↑, increased; *ACE*, angiotensin-converting enzyme; *ARB*, angiotensin receptor blocker; *ATII*, angiotensin II; *EF*, ejection fraction; *CN*, cranial nerve.

9. What is "high-output" heart failure?

High-output heart failure refers to the *inability* of the heart to *maintain an elevated cardiac output* in pathologic situations that demand it, such as in hyperthyroidism, AV malformations, Paget disease (of bone), anemia, and sepsis.

Note: In the case of AV malformations, the dramatic drop in TPR when going from a high-pressure arteriole to a low-pressure venule demands an increase in CO to maintain MAP. This elevated CO causes an increased workload on the heart which, when maintained for a long time, can cause progressive cardiac dysfunction.

SUMMARY BOX: HEART FAILURE

- Heart failure is a complex clinical syndrome that represents a final common pathway for a variety of pathologic processes that impair cardiac function.
- Heart failure is classified by two general types: systolic (pump) and diastolic (filling) dysfunction, with considerable clinical overlap between the two.
- The initially adaptive physiologic responses (e.g., increased sympathetic activity, fluid retention, myocardial hypertrophy) become maladaptive when prolonged, leading to progressive deterioration of cardiac function.
- When thinking about heart failure, categorize the findings according to whether they suggest left-sided versus right-sided heart failure, preserved versus reduced ejection fraction (EF), and compensated versus decompensated cardiac output (CO).

CASE 1.6

A 50-year-old man presents complaining of chest pain that has occurred with gradually diminishing levels of physical exertion, as well as two recent episodes of syncope while golfing. Cardiovascular examination reveals a blood pressure of 120/90 mm Hg, a loud crescendo-decrescendo systolic murmur best appreciated at the upper right sternal border (with radiation to both carotid arteries), and a weak and delayed carotid upstroke. An ECG reveals left ventricular hypertrophy, and an echocardiogram reveals a bicuspid aortic valve with reduced valvular orifice (<1 cm^2).

1. What is the most likely diagnosis?

This patient likely has aortic stenosis, a common valvular disorder in which excessive narrowing of the aortic valve increases afterload. If left untreated, aortic stenosis may result in angina, exertional syncope, dyspnea (from heart failure), and increased cardiovascular mortality. Symptoms are often, but not always, seen when the area of the aortic orifice is less than 1 cm^2 (normal area is 3 cm^2).

2. What likely predisposed this patient to developing aortic stenosis?

Stenosis generally occurs only in elderly patients secondary to calcification, which is referred to as *senile calcific aortic stenosis*. However, congenitally bicuspid or even unicuspid valves (as opposed to the normal tricuspid aortic valve) calcify and narrow at an earlier age, usually in the late 40s or in the 50s, as happened with this patient.

3. What causes heart murmurs, and why does this patient have one?

Heart murmurs are caused by turbulent blood flow, which occurs at elevated flow velocities. In this case, the stenotic aortic valve forces the heart to contract more forcefully, which generates a significant pressure gradient between the left ventricle and the aorta, creating high-flow velocities across the aortic valve with every heartbeat. When a patient with aortic stenosis performs a maneuver that decreases preload (e.g., Valsalva maneuver) or increases afterload (hand grip exercise) the associated murmur will decrease in intensity. This is due to the decrease in velocity/flow across the valve. Rapid squatting will increase venous return to the heart, thereby increasing preload and intensifying the murmur. The intensity of the murmur does not necessarily indicate the severity of the disease.

Note: Carotid bruits are due to the same mechanism as murmurs, with the stenotic lumen causing increased flow velocities and resulting in turbulent blood flow that can be auscultated near each carotid bifurcation.

4. What compensatory left ventricular changes occur as a result of aortic stenosis?

Cardiomyocytes respond to pressure and volume overload stressors differently. In response to volume overload (e.g., aortic regurgitation), sarcomeres within myocytes are added in series, which has the effect of increasing ventricular lumen volume—an adaptive response termed *eccentric hypertrophy*. In contrast, aortic stenosis is characterized by a pathologically elevated afterload and thus leads to pathophysiologic changes that resemble those observed with systemic hypertension. The myocardium responds to an increased afterload by adding sarcomeres in parallel, resulting in a hypertrophied myocardium that is better able to eject blood against increased resistance. This adaptive response is termed *concentric hypertrophy*. One of the drawbacks of hypertrophy is that the thickened myocardium is typically less compliant, requiring increased filling pressures and predisposing to dyspnea and pulmonary edema.

5. **Why does this patient have a weak, delayed carotid upstroke with a narrowed pulse pressure on physical examination? Think about how the left ventricular pressure-volume loop changes in aortic stenosis.**

   In aortic stenosis, a significant proportion of cardiac work is devoted to generating sufficient force to overcome the valvular resistance. Consequently, a smaller proportion of cardiac work is used to eject blood, resulting in decreased SV and reduced pulse pressure. This is also affected by the amount of time available for ejection, because more of the time that should be spent in systole is instead consumed by isovolumetric contraction. Additionally, ventricular hypertrophy can impair diastolic filling, which reduces preload. Recall that elevated preload normally compensates for decreased SV via the Frank-Starling mechanism.

   A pressure-volume loop comparing changes in LV pressure and volume throughout the cardiac cycle in a normal heart and one with aortic stenosis is shown in Fig. 1.9. Note that in aortic stenosis, higher pressures must be generated during isovolumetric contraction (phase 2) to overcome the increased afterload. This leaves correspondingly less energy and time available for the ejection phase (phase 3), and therefore the SV in aortic stenosis (uncompensated) is reduced. This reduced SV explains the weak and delayed carotid upstroke (*pulsus parvus et tardus*) and the decreased pulse pressure evident on physical examination.

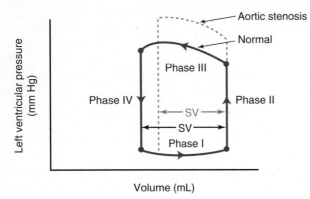

Figure 1.9. Pressure-volume changes in aortic stenosis. *SV,* Stroke volume. *(From Brown TA.* Rapid Review Physiology. *Philadelphia: Mosby; 2007:128.)*

STEP 1 SECRET

You should practice interpreting diagrams depicting pressure-volume loops in relation to the events in the cardiac cycle, as you are likely to see at least one on your USMLE Step 1 exam.

---

6. **As a result of aortic stenosis, do ventricular myocytes spend more time in isotonic or isometric (isovolumetric) contraction?**

   Myocytes spend more time in isometric (isovolumetric) contraction to overcome the increased afterload caused by the stenotic aortic valve. Because the time available for electrical and mechanical ventricular systole is finite, this results in a shortened isotonic ejection phase.

7. **Explain the cause of this patient's presenting complaints. What is most likely causing his episodes of syncope? What is most likely causing his chest pain?**

   Patients with stenotic aortic valves have left ventricular outflow obstruction that limits their ability to augment CO. This particularly occurs in the setting of exercise or other exertional activity, when the increased metabolic demand necessitates increased CO. Because the CO cannot be adequately increased, there will be relative cerebral hypoperfusion and symptoms of syncope. His chest pain likely is due to the accumulation of metabolic waste products (e.g., lactic acid) that are generated during the anaerobic respiration that cardiomyocytes experience when stressed by this increased workload.

8. **What are some causes of increased myocardial oxygen *demand* in aortic stenosis?**

   The physiologic consequences of aortic stenosis are outlined in Fig. 1.10. The increased left ventricular mass requires more oxygen for normal contractile function. In addition, the increased left ventricular pressure that develops to overcome the outflow obstruction increases the workload on the LV. This raises the myocardial volume of oxygen (MV_{O_2}) demand.

9. **What are some causes of decreased myocardial oxygen *supply* in aortic stenosis?**

   As HR increases to compensate for a depressed CO, less time is spent in diastole, which is when the majority of coronary perfusion occurs. Additionally, owing to decreased compliance, the left ventricular diastolic pressure typically increases in the setting of aortic stenosis, which further reduces coronary perfusion. Finally, aortic pressure is reduced because of the decreased SV, which decreases coronary blood flow because the coronary arteries originate from the aorta.

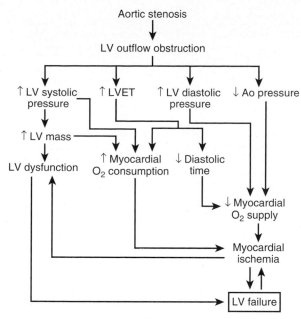

Figure 1.10. Causes of increased myocardial oxygen demand and decreased myocardial oxygen supply in the setting of aortic stenosis. *Ao,* Aortic; *LV,* left ventricular; *LVET,* left ventricular ejection time. *(From Boudoulas H, Gravanis MB.* Cardiovascular Disorders: Pathogenesis and Pathophysiology. *St. Louis: Mosby; 1993:64.)*

10. **Why is atrial fibrillation a particularly dangerous complication in aortic stenosis, aside from the risk of embolic stroke?**

    Aortic stenosis often results in elevated left atrial pressures and subsequent dilation of the left atrium. Dilation of the left atrium compresses the conducting fibers, thereby predisposing patients to atrial fibrillation.

    Under normal physiologic circumstances, the "atrial kick" (the additional ventricular filling that occurs as a result of atrial contraction) does not provide a significant percentage of the CO. However, in situations in which the ventricular filling is impaired (e.g., aortic stenosis), this extra filling by the atrial kick is essential to sustain an adequate CO. Because this patient's CO is already compromised, atrial fibrillation would impair the ability of the atria to provide that atrial kick, further reducing CO and potentially precipitating severe heart failure.

11. **Describe the murmur of aortic stenosis.**

    Aortic stenosis is characterized by a systolic crescendo-decrescendo ejection murmur best appreciated at the upper right sternal border. It may radiate to the carotid arteries.

    As previously stated, the murmur of aortic stenosis is enhanced by maneuvers that increase preload (e.g., squatting, passive leg raising). As a general rule of thumb, left-sided murmurs increase on exhalation, and right-sided murmurs increase on inspiration.

    If aortic stenosis results in the formation of a noncompliant ventricle, an S_4 heart sound may be heard. Atrial fibrillation will prevent the S_4 heart sound from developing.

STEP 1 SECRET

Murmur characteristics are a favorite topic for the USMLE Step 1. Be sure that you can distinguish murmurs according to location, characteristic symptoms, and maneuvers used to alter their sounds. Remember to practice listening to audio files of the most common murmurs. These murmurs include those accompanying aortic stenosis, pulmonary stenosis, aortic regurgitation, mitral regurgitation, tricuspid regurgitation, mitral valve prolapse, hypertrophic cardiomyopathy, ventricular septal defect, and patent ductus arteriosus.

SUMMARY BOX: AORTIC STENOSIS

- Aortic stenosis most commonly presents as a crescendo-decrescendo systolic murmur heard loudest at the upper right sternal border and radiating to both carotid arteries. A delayed carotid upstroke and narrowed pulse pressure (*pulsus parvus et tardus*) are associated findings.
- Decreased cardiac output (in decompensated states) and increased myocardial oxygen demand are important consequences of aortic stenosis. It follows that the natural history of this condition leads to angina, syncope, heart failure, and premature death if not identified and managed appropriately.

CASE 1.7

A 56-year-old moderately obese, postmenopausal woman with type 2 diabetes mellitus (DM) is evaluated during her annual examination. Physical examination is significant for abdominal obesity and a curvilinear patch of darkly pigmented skin around her neck. Blood tests reveal elevated LDL cholesterol, low HDL cholesterol, markedly elevated triglycerides, and a fasting plasma glucose level of 145 mg/dL.

1. This patient's constellation of symptoms is consistent with what syndrome, and what is its significance?

   These symptoms are consistent with metabolic syndrome (also called *insulin resistance syndrome* or *syndrome X*). This syndrome is increasingly prevalent in the United States and is significant because patients with metabolic syndrome are at increased risk of premature death from cardiac disease. As defined by the 2001 National Cholesterol Education Program (ATP III) and updated in 2005 by the American Heart Association/National Heart, Lung, and Blood Institute (AHA/NHLBI), metabolic syndrome is diagnosed by the presence of at least three of the following five features:

   • Central obesity (waist circumference >35 inches in women, >40 inches in men)
   • Triglyceride levels ≥150 mg/dL
   • HDL cholesterol <50 mg/dL in women, <40 mg/dL in men
   • Fasting blood glucose ≥100 mg/dL
   • Blood pressure ≥130/85 mm Hg

       It is clear that patients who fulfill criteria for metabolic syndrome are at significant risk for increased morbidity and mortality associated with cardiovascular disease and DM. Hence the diagnosis of metabolic syndrome can help identify patients who should be treated with stringent cardiovascular risk factor modification strategies. Management of metabolic syndrome consists of controlling each of the component factors individually: weight loss, improving lipid profiles, decreasing blood glucose, and decreasing blood pressure.

2. Part of this woman's presentation is dyslipidemia, a disorder of lipoprotein metabolism. What is the structure of a lipoprotein, where are lipoproteins synthesized, and what are the major types of lipoproteins?

   Lipoproteins are macromolecular structures composed of an inner core of cholesterol esters and triglycerides (TGs; the latter may also be referred to as *triacylglycerols*) and an outer core of apolipoproteins (APOs), phospholipids, and unesterified free cholesterol. The major types of lipoproteins include chylomicrons, very low-density lipoproteins (VLDLs), intermediate-density lipoproteins (IDLs), LDL, and HDL. Chylomicrons are synthesized within intestinal enterocytes, whereas VLDL is synthesized within the liver. IDL and LDL are both generated via VLDL catabolism throughout the systemic circulatory system. HDL is synthesized by the liver and intestine.

3. What are the functions of the various forms of lipoproteins? How are they removed from the circulation?

   Chylomicrons deliver dietary TGs to adipose tissue, skeletal muscle, and cardiac muscle; cholesterol-rich chylomicron remnants are then taken up by the liver.

   VLDL delivers liver-synthesized TGs to adipose tissue, skeletal muscle, and cardiac muscle; it is removed by intravascular conversion to IDL and ultimately LDL.

   LDL delivers cholesterol to cells throughout the body; it is removed by internalization via LDL receptor (principally in the liver).

   Note: Defects or premature internalization of the LDL receptor cause *familial hypercholesterolemia*.

   HDL facilitates the return of excess cholesterol from cells to the liver for biliary excretion; it is removed via hepatic uptake.

CASE 1.7 CONTINUED:

The patient implements new lifestyle modifications upon physician recommendation, focusing on a low-fat, low-cholesterol diet and walking for 45 minutes 5 days per week. After 3 months, her follow-up visit reveals that her weight and lipid profile are largely unchanged. As a result, she is prescribed simvastatin. Before she takes her first dose, her liver enzymes are checked.

4. What is the mechanism of action of simvastatin and other statin medications?

   Statins inhibit 3-hydroxy-3-methylglutaryl (HMG) CoA reductase, which is the enzyme responsible for catalyzing the rate-limiting step in cholesterol synthesis. Not only do these drugs reduce cholesterol synthesis, they also upregulate the expression of LDL receptors on the surface of hepatocytes, which promotes increased cholesterol uptake and further lowers serum cholesterol levels. Statins are the most potent pharmacologic agents for lowering LDL cholesterol. They also cause a modest reduction of TGs but have only a small effect on increasing high-density lipoprotein cholesterol (HDL-C). Statins are increasingly being investigated for their role in decreasing inflammation in blood vessels, further preventing vascular disease.

5. Adding which other class of cholesterol-lowering drugs to this patient's regimen should only be done with great caution?

Because statins and fibrates can independently cause muscle damage (myositis) and liver damage (hepatotoxicity), these risks are increased when the two classes are prescribed and taken together. Hepatotoxicity is evaluated by periodically monitoring the hepatic enzymes alanine transaminase (ALT) and aspartate transaminase (AST). Routine monitoring of transaminases is not necessary if a statin is being used alone. If myopathy or rhabdomyolysis is suspected, creatine phosphokinase (CPK) levels can be evaluated.

6. What is the cause and clinical significance of this woman's hypertriglyceridemia?

TGs come from two sources: those consumed in the diet (dietary) and those synthesized by the liver (nondietary). Dietary TGs are broken down in the gut and then reformed in intestinal enterocytes, where they are packaged in chylomicrons. Chylomicrons enter the lymphatics and eventually drain into the venous circulation via the thoracic duct. Nondietary TGs are primarily synthesized in the liver and enter the bloodstream packaged in VLDLs.

   TGs are an independent risk factor for coronary vascular disease. One theoretic mechanism for this finding may be attributed to the transfer of TGs to HDL by cholesterol ester transfer protein (CETP). TG-rich HDL is rapidly catabolized by lipoprotein lipase, which results in a decrease in HDL levels whenever TGs are elevated.

7. What enzymatic mechanism clears TGs from the circulation?

Lipoprotein lipase is an enzyme present on the luminal surface of capillary endothelial cells in adipose tissue, skeletal muscle, and cardiac muscle that catalyzes the release of fatty acids from the TGs that are contained within chylomicrons and VLDL. The released fatty acids then diffuse out of the circulatory system and into the surrounding cells.

   Note: Insulin stimulates the synthesis of lipoprotein lipase. If insulin production is impaired, as in type 1 diabetes, then TGs accumulate in the circulation and hasten the development of atherosclerosis.

8. What is the clinical significance of elevated LDL levels?

Elevated levels of serum LDL have been associated with a number of pathophysiologic conditions including atherosclerosis; chylomicronemia; obesity; Alzheimer dementia; xanthomas; and dyslipidemia associated with diabetes, insulin resistance, and infection.

   Note: Become familiar with the key physical exam findings associated with hyperlipidemia: xanthomas, tendinous xanthoma, and corneal arcus. These are often mentioned in USMLE Step 1 vignettes that test your knowledge about hyperlipidemia.

9. What is the clinical significance of this patient's low levels of HDL-C)?

Low serum HDL-C is another risk factor for coronary heart disease. HDL-C is involved in reverse cholesterol transport, in which excess cholesterol is transported from peripheral tissues and atheromatous plaques to the liver for conversion into bile salts or unaltered excretion in the bile. Recall that biliary excretion is the only major mechanism for cholesterol removal from the body. Additionally, there is growing evidence to support a role for HDL-C in preventing LDL oxidation. This could be an important finding because oxidized LDL is the atherogenic form (i.e., macrophages do not phagocytose normal LDL, only oxidized LDL. These macrophages then transform into the lipid-laden foam cells that accumulate to become an atherosclerotic plaque.).

   Note: Unlike normal LDL, oxidized LDL can be taken up by scavenger receptors, thus promoting pathologic cholesterol accumulation and atherosclerosis.

   Plasma HDL levels can increase with exercise, moderate alcohol consumption, and pharmacologic agents such as niacin (most notably), as well as fibrates and statins to a lesser degree.

   Note: A ratio of total cholesterol to HDL cholesterol can be used to predict coronary vascular disease (CVD) risk. An optimal ratio is ≤3.5. A person with total cholesterol of 180 mg/dL but an HDL of only 30 mg/dL would have a ratio of 6, which would place that person at higher risk for developing CVD than an individual with the same total cholesterol level but higher HDL level.

10. What is the mechanism of action of the lipid-lowering fibrates/fibric acid derivatives (e.g., gemfibrozil, fenofibrate)?

These agents are PPAR-alpha (peroxisome proliferator-activated receptor-α) agonists that lead to increased synthesis of lipoprotein lipase, causing a significant reduction in TG level. They also increase the expression of enzymes involved in fatty acid oxidation, which results in a decrease in the availability of TGs for VLDL synthesis. Last, they increase levels of APO A-I and APO A-II, both of which promote increased HDL levels. Fibrates have little effect on LDL directly.

   Note: Commonly tested side effects of fibrates include hepatotoxicity, cholesterol gallstones, and myositis.

11. How does niacin influence the lipid profile? What are the concerns about using niacin?

Niacin (nicotinic acid) is a water-soluble B vitamin that can lower lipoprotein(a) levels by 25% and so can be used for patients with lipoprotein(a) excess. There is no evidence, though, that a reduction in lipoprotein(a) with niacin reduces clinical events. Large randomized trials have raised serious concerns about the safety and efficacy of niacin in combination with statin therapy, and by extension about niacin monotherapy. Niacin can increase glucose levels, can induce hyperuricemia, can produce hypotension in patients treated with vasodilators, can increase plasma homocysteine levels, and may increase the risk of infection.

   Note: A major side effect of niacin is facial and upper body flushing (niacin rush), which is suspected to be due to increased prostaglandin synthesis. Taking aspirin or another type of NSAID before the niacin to reduce the synthesis of these vasodilatory prostaglandins can minimize this flushing. Do not confuse this reaction with the flushing observed with vancomycin, which causes red person syndrome and can be prevented with antihistamine use before administration.

12. **How do the bile-sequestering resins (e.g., cholestyramine, colestipol, colesevelam) lower LDL cholesterol levels?**
    The bile-sequestering resins bind bile acids in the intestine and prevent their reuptake in the distal ileum. This stimulates increased hepatic synthesis of bile acids. Because bile acids are formed from cholesterol, increasing their synthesis will increase cholesterol catabolism, upregulate LDL receptor expression on hepatocytes, and decrease serum cholesterol levels.
    Note: These drugs impair the bile-mediated emulsification, digestion, and absorption of fats, fat-soluble vitamins (vitamins A, D, E, and K), and certain drugs. Consequently, adverse effects of bile-sequestering resins commonly include bloating, flatulence, abdominal pain, steatorrhea, deficiencies of fat-soluble vitamins, and inadequate oral bioavailability of some drugs including warfarin, thiazides, and select statins. Decreased bile acid reabsorption also promotes the formation of cholesterol gallstones, which is enhanced by coadministration with fibrates.

OTHER RELATED QUESTION

13. **What is the cause of the disorder of lipid metabolism known as *abetalipoproteinemia*?**
    Abetalipoproteinemia is an autosomal recessive genetic disorder characterized by the absence of lipoprotein APO B, resulting in a deficiency of lipoproteins APO B-48 and APO B-100. This is clinically significant because APO B-48 is critical to chylomicron synthesis, and APO B-100 is critical for the secretion of VLDL and LDL into the systemic circulation. Chylomicrons, VLDL, and LDL will therefore be absent in patients with abetalipoproteinemia. Because chylomicrons cannot be produced and secreted without APO B-48, intestinal biopsy will reveal large, lipid-vacuolated enterocytes. Symptoms include steatorrhea, weight loss, potential anemia, and malabsorption of fat-soluble vitamins. Retinitis pigmentosa may develop as a result of vitamin A deficiency. Vitamin E deficiency can specifically present with neurologic symptoms as the result of spinocerebellar and corticospinal degeneration.

SUMMARY BOX: METABOLIC SYNDROME AND DYSLIPIDEMIAS

- Metabolic syndrome is characterized by abdominal obesity, dyslipidemia, insulin resistance, and hypertension. It is an indicator for increased cardiovascular risk.
- Management of metabolic syndrome consists of treating each of its components with lifestyle modifications and pharmacologic agents to control weight, improve lipid profiles, heighten insulin sensitivity, and lower blood pressure.
- Cholesterol-lowering medications include statins (most potent for lowering low-density lipoprotein cholesterol [LDL-C]), fibrates, bile-sequestering bile acid resins, and, very rarely, niacin.

CHAPTER 2

PULMONOLOGY

Insider's Guide to Pulmonology for the USMLE Step 1
Pulmonology is a favorite subject for the USMLE Step 1 because it provides a lot of opportunity to integrate across disciplines. Therefore you should expect to find pulmonology questions on related subjects such as microbiology, cardiology, and clinical anatomy. We especially recommend spending some time with an anatomy atlas to refamiliarize yourself with chest x-ray films. However, this does not mean that USMLE test makers will forget to include questions regarding pulmonary physiology and pathology. In fact, many pulmonology questions on Step 1 will require you to apply conceptual knowledge of pathophysiology. In other words, avoid memorizing a ton of detailed information for this subject. Instead, focus on reasoning through the pathophysiology of various conditions as they relate to the lung (e.g., *why* compliance increases with emphysema, *why* altitude changes alter pH, *why* certain diseases alter the alveolar-arterial oxygen gradient [AaDo$_2$]?). You will notice that the key point is to constantly ask yourself "why?" when studying for this subject!

BASIC CONCEPTS—MECHANICS OF BREATHING

1. What are the driving forces for the following types of airflows?
    A. Inspiratory airflow?
        A negative intrapleural pressure (i.e., the pressure outside the lungs but still within the chest) is created by the opposing tendencies of the chest wall to expand and the lung to collapse. This negative intrapleural pressure is transmitted to the alveoli such that there is a pressure gradient between alveolar air spaces and the external environment, resulting in airflow into the lung.
        Muscles involved in normal inspiration include the diaphragm and external intercostals. In the setting of forced inspiration, accessory muscles such as the scalene and sternocleidomastoid muscles are employed.

    B. Expiratory airflow?
        An increase in intrapleural pressure (i.e., becomes less negative) is created by passive relaxation of the diaphragm and elastic recoil of the lungs and chest wall.
        In the case of forced expiration, contraction of the abdominal muscles (rectus abdominis, internal and external obliques, transversus abdominis) can also increase the intrapleural pressure. The internal intercostals are also involved in forced expiration by pulling the ribs down.

2. What are the forces of resistance for the following types of airflows?
    A. Inspiratory airflow?
        Airway resistance, compliance resistance, and tissue resistance are the forces of resistance for inspiration (Fig. 2.1); the sum of these forces determines the total work of breathing (pressure x volume).

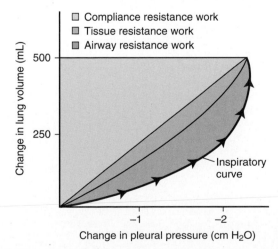

Figure 2.1. Relative contributions of the three types of resistance to the total work of breathing. *(From Brown TA.* Rapid Review Physiology. *2nd ed. Philadelphia: Mosby; 2012.)*

Airway resistance is generated by the friction between rapidly moving gas molecules and the walls of the airways. It is typically a small component of the work of breathing. Airway resistance is greater in the large airways because they are *arranged in series,* whereas the small airways are *arranged in parallel.*
The total resistance (R_T) of a specific number (n) of resistors in series is equal to the sum of their individual resistances such that:

$$R_T = R_1 + R_2 + R_3 + \cdots + R_n \qquad [2.1]$$

By contrast, the total resistance (R_T) of a specific number (n) of resistors in parallel is calculated as:

$$1/R_T = 1/R_1 + 1/R_2 + 1/R_3 + \cdots + 1/R_n \qquad [2.2]$$

Compliance resistance is generated as the lungs inflate and overcome their intrinsic elastic recoil (i.e., a measurement of the elastic resistance of the system). The work to overcome this resistance (compliance work) normally accounts for the largest proportion of the work of breathing. Note that compliance work is reduced in obstructive lung disease (less elastic recoil to overcome) and increased in restrictive lung disease (increased stiffness and limited expansion).
Tissue resistance is generated as the pleural surfaces slide over each other during respiration. This resistance is normally minimal because of the presence of pleural fluid. Note that tissue resistance can increase markedly in conditions in which the pleural surfaces become adherent to each other, as may occur with an empyema.
B. Expiratory airflow?
Reduction in airway diameter associated with increased intrathoracic pressures affects resistance during expiration. Expiration is typically a passive process because this resistance is small and is easily overcome by the energy provided by elastic recoil of the lung and chest wall. However, in certain conditions in which airway diameter is pathologically reduced (e.g., asthma) or the forces of elastic recoil of the lung are reduced (e.g., emphysema), expiration may become an active process requiring use of accessory muscles.

3. What does pulmonary compliance measure?
Compliance is a measure of lung distensibility. Compliant lungs are easy to distend. Compliance is inversely proportional to wall stiffness. The higher the compliance, the easier it is to fill the lungs. Compliance (C) can be measured as the change in volume (ΔV) required for a fractional change in pressure (ΔP):

$$C = \Delta V / \Delta P \qquad [2.3]$$

The properties of compliance and elastance (tendency of the lung to recoil inward; see question 5) are inversely proportional to one another. In conditions in which elastance decreases (e.g., emphysema), compliance will automatically increase. Compliance can be decreased by pulmonary fibrosis, pneumonia, and pulmonary edema, among other causes.

4. With respect to the compliance curve of the lungs, how might breathing at an elevated functional residual capacity in chronic obstructive pulmonary disease result in less "efficient" breathing? What is hysteresis on the compliance curve?
Fig. 2.2 shows a compliance curve of the lungs. Note that the lungs are most compliant in the midportion of the inspiratory curve (steepest slope, greatest change in volume per unit change in pressure). Breathing at an elevated functional residual capacity (FRC), as patients with chronic obstructive pulmonary disease (COPD) are prone to do for a variety of reasons, is less efficient and requires more work. Hysteresis describes the difference between compliance of the lung during inspiration and expiration. The lung volume at any given pressure during inspiration is always less than the lung volume at the same pressure during expiration. The difference in compliance (change in volume over change in pressure) is due to the additional energy required to overcome resistance during inspiration.

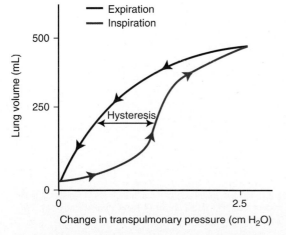

Figure 2.2. Compliance curve of the lungs: lung volume plotted against changes in transpulmonary pressure (the difference between pleural and alveolar pressure). *(From Brown TA: Rapid Review Physiology. 2nd ed. Philadelphia: Mosby; 2012.)*

5. **What does pulmonary elastance measure? How is pulmonary elastance altered in restrictive and obstructive lung diseases and why?**
    Elasticity is the property of matter that makes it resist deformation. As elasticity increases, increasingly greater pressure changes will be required to distend the lungs. Pulmonary elastance (E) can be calculated as the change in pressure (ΔP) divided by the change in volume (ΔV):

    $$E = \Delta P/\Delta V \tag{2.4}$$

    In restrictive lung diseases such as silicosis and asbestosis, which are characterized by parenchymal fibrosis, pulmonary elastance increases. In COPD, which is characterized by parenchymal destruction, elastance decreases.

6. **How does surfactant affect alveolar surface tension?**
    Water molecules lining the surface of alveoli are attracted to each other and are repelled by the hydrophobic air molecules. The attractive force between water molecules generates surface tension, which in turn produces a *collapsing pressure* that promotes alveolar collapse. Surfactant is composed of phospholipids (mainly lecithin and sphingomyelin) that reduce the collapsing pressure by minimizing the interaction between alveolar water molecules (Fig. 2.3).

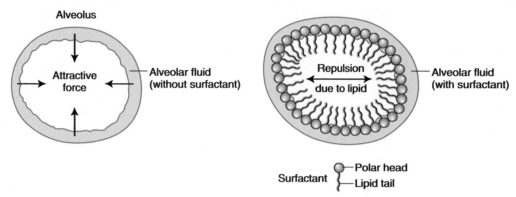

Figure 2.3. Role of surfactant in reducing alveolar surface tension. Note the orientation of the hydrophilic "head" in the alveolar fluid and the hydrophobic "tail" in the alveolar air. *(From Brown TA. Rapid Review Physiology. 2nd ed. Philadelphia: Mosby; 2012.)*

7. **Why are smaller alveoli more prone to collapse, and how is this relevant to neonatal respiratory distress syndrome?**
    Laplace's law states that the collapsing pressure (P) is directly proportional to surface tension (T) and inversely proportional to the alveolar radius (R), such that smaller alveoli will experience a larger collapsing pressure:

    $$P = 2T/R \tag{2.5}$$

    The combination of small alveoli and inadequate surfactant production in premature infants contributes to respiratory failure in neonatal respiratory distress syndrome (NRDS).
    Fetal amniotic fluid can be measured for lecithin and sphingomyelin content, the ratio of which can serve as an indicator of fetal lung maturity. A ratio of less than 1.5 is a strong predictor of NRDS. Maternal steroids can be given if the fetus is between 24 and 34 weeks of gestation in order to increase fetal lung maturity before delivery if they are at risk of preterm delivery within 7 days.

8. **What is minute ventilation?**
    Minute ventilation is the total volume of air that enters and exits the lung each minute. The normal (resting) minute ventilation is a function of tidal volume and respiratory rate:

    $$\text{Minute ventilation} = \text{Respiratory rate} \times \text{Tidal volume} \tag{2.6}$$

    Example:

    $$= 12 \text{ breaths/min} \times 500 \text{ mL/breath}$$
    $$= 6 \text{ L/min}$$

9. **What is dead space? What is the difference between anatomic dead space and physiologic dead space?**
    Dead space refers to lung volume that is ventilated but not perfused by deoxygenated blood, such that there is no potential for gas exchange in this space. The anatomic dead space is lung volume that receives ventilation but in which there are no pulmonary capillaries available for gas exchange. This anatomic dead space includes the nasal cavity, pharynx, larynx, trachea, bronchi, and conducting bronchioles, often referred to as the *conducting airways*. Anatomic

dead space is involved with warming, humidifying, and filtering air without participating in gas exchange. The physiologic dead space includes both the anatomic dead space and the alveoli that are ventilated but not perfused (alveolar dead space), so no gas exchange occurs in them either.

The majority of physiologic dead space can be attributed to the apex of the lung because of poor perfusion at the apex compared with the base. Exercise decreases physiologic dead space by improving perfusion to the entire lung.

10. Why is the alveolar minute ventilation a much better representation of *functional* ventilation?
Alveolar minute ventilation is the volume of air that enters and exits the alveoli per minute. To calculate this rate, the physiologic dead space has to be taken into account and subtracted from the tidal volume. The typical anatomic dead space is about 150 mL, and alveolar dead space is minimal in healthy people.

$$\text{Alveolar ventilation} = \text{Respiratory frequency} \times (\text{Tidal volume} - \text{Anatomic dead space}) \qquad [2.7]$$
$$= 12 \text{ breaths/min} \times (500 \text{ mL/breath} - 150 \text{mL})$$
$$= 4.2 \text{ L/min}$$

The alveolar ventilation is a much better representation of *functional* ventilation because the alveoli are where gas exchange occurs.

STEP 1 SECRET

You are expected to know basic formulas such as those listed in the preceding questions. They will not be provided to you on the USMLE. A computerized calculator will be available for your use.

BASIC CONCEPTS — VENTILATION-PERFUSION MATCHING

1. What does the ventilation/perfusion ratio measure, and what is its approximate value? What is an ideal value for this ratio?
The ventilation/perfusion ratio ($\dot{V}/\dot{Q}$) measures how well pulmonary ventilation and pulmonary perfusion are matched, indicating how efficiently oxygenation of blood is occurring in the pulmonary capillaries. Normally, the lungs receive most of the cardiac output (≈ 5 L/min), and the prototypical 70-kg man has an alveolar ventilation rate of roughly 4 L/min (as shown in question 10). A ventilation rate of 4 L/min and a pulmonary perfusion rate of 5 L/min yield a $\dot{V}/\dot{Q}$ ratio of 0.8, which implies suboptimal matching of pulmonary ventilation and perfusion. A $\dot{V}/\dot{Q}$ ratio of 1 is ideal and represents optimal matching of pulmonary ventilation and perfusion.

The $\dot{V}/\dot{Q}$ ratio can be applied to the lungs as a whole, or to separate areas of the lungs, and is a measure of the efficiency of ventilation in those separate areas as well. Regional differences in ventilation and perfusion exist across various zones of the lungs because of the force of gravity. In an upright subject, both blood flow and ventilation are decreased at the apex of the lung and increased at the base of the lung. However, the decrease in perfusion is greater than the decrease in ventilation at the apex of the lung, leading to an increased $\dot{V}/\dot{Q}$ ratio. Likewise, the $\dot{V}/\dot{Q}$ ratio at the base is decreased because the increase in perfusion is greater than the increase in ventilation. This difference leads to an apical $\dot{V}/\dot{Q}$ ratio of roughly 3, while the basal $\dot{V}/\dot{Q}$ ratio is closer to 0.6.

During exercise, the greater increase in alveolar ventilation and lesser increase in cardiac output lead to a more uniform $\dot{V}/\dot{Q}$ ratio from apex to base that more closely approximates the ideal $\dot{V}/\dot{Q}$ ratio of 1.0.

2. What conditions cause an increase in the $\dot{V}/\dot{Q}$ ratio?
The $\dot{V}/\dot{Q}$ ratio increases whenever pulmonary ventilation is proportionately greater than pulmonary perfusion. As just discussed, exercise is a normal situation in which ventilation increases proportionally more than perfusion, and in this case it optimizes the $\dot{V}/\dot{Q}$ ratio. A pathologic condition that increases the $\dot{V}/\dot{Q}$ ratio is a pulmonary embolus. In this condition, patients are often tachypneic (respiring rapidly), which increases ventilation. The clot in the lungs also reduces pulmonary perfusion, so both of these processes increase the $\dot{V}/\dot{Q}$ ratio. In fact, the $\dot{V}/\dot{Q}$ ratio in the blocked segment would theoretically approach infinity because blood flow to that region is completely blocked ($\dot{Q} = 0$). The pathologic consequence of an increased $\dot{V}/\dot{Q}$ ratio is that ventilation is "wasted" in lung areas that are not adequately perfused.

3. What causes a decrease in the ventilation/perfusion ratio?
Generally, any lung disease in which the process of ventilation itself is compromised will decrease the amount of oxygen that the pulmonary blood flow receives, predisposing the patient to hypoxemia. This is deleterious because less oxygen diffuses into the blood that flows through the lungs. Additionally, less carbon dioxide can be "blown off," predisposing to hypercapnia. An example is asthma, in which the bronchoconstriction that occurs impairs ventilation and reduces the $\dot{V}/\dot{Q}$ ratio.

Patients with decreased $\dot{V}/\dot{Q}$ ratio will respond to oxygen administration. However, a $\dot{V}/\dot{Q}$ ratio of 0 generally implies an obstructed mainstem bronchus that will not respond to oxygen.

4. What effect does COPD usually have on the ventilation/perfusion ratio?
Airway obstruction in COPD can reduce ventilation relative to perfusion, decreasing the $\dot{V}/\dot{Q}$ ratio. However, pulmonary capillary loss in COPD can increase ventilation relative to perfusion, causing an increased $\dot{V}/\dot{Q}$ ratio. In fact, if these two

processes are occurring in the same patient, this patient can have a normal $\dot{V}/\dot{Q}$ ratio despite severe ventilation/perfusion mismatches in different parts of the lung!

5. **What is the difference between an anatomic shunt and a physiologic shunt?**
   Most anatomic shunts occur within the heart when deoxygenated blood from the right side of the heart crosses the septum and mixes with oxygenated blood from the left side of the heart. This mixture results in varying degrees of hypoxemia that cannot be improved with the administration of 100% O_2.

   In a physiologic shunt, deoxygenated blood bypasses the gas-exchanging unit. Atelectasis can occur in many lung diseases, including pneumonia. In atelectasis, ventilatory obstruction to the gas-exchanging unit leads to a subsequent loss of volume and a $\dot{V}/\dot{Q}$ ratio of 0.

BASIC CONCEPTS — GAS EXCHANGE

1. **What influences the diffusion of gases from the alveoli into the pulmonary capillaries and vice versa?**
   Gas diffusion across a membrane (the pulmonary membrane in this case) is described by Fick's law of diffusion:

$$V_{gas} = \frac{A \times D (P_1 - P_2)}{T} \qquad [2.8]$$

where V_{gas} is the volume of gas that traverses the membrane per unit time, A is the surface area of the membrane, D is the diffusivity coefficient of the particular gas in the particular membrane, $P_1 - P_2$ is the partial pressure difference of the specific gas across the membrane, and T is the thickness of the membrane.

   It is important to recognize that all pulmonary diseases that create respiratory dysfunction affect one or more of the parameters in the diffusion equation. For example, in asthma, the impaired ventilation reduces the pressure gradient for oxygen across the membrane. In emphysema, ventilation is impaired (reducing the pressure gradient), and the surface area of the pulmonary membrane is reduced from loss of alveoli.

   Note: The *diffusing capacity* of the pulmonary membrane is defined as the volume of gas (typically measured using carbon monoxide) that can diffuse across the pulmonary membrane per mm Hg pressure difference across the membrane. It can be seen from Fick's law that the diffusing capacity is dependent on the surface area, gas diffusivity, and membrane thickness.

2. **What is the alveolar-arterial oxygen gradient, and what is the clinical significance of its magnitude?**
   The alveolar-arterial oxygen gradient ($P_{AO_2} - P_{aO_2}$, sometimes designated AaD_{O_2}) is a measure of the difference in oxygen tension, or partial pressure, between the alveoli and arterial blood. In a healthy person, a typical alveolar oxygen tension (P_{AO_2}) might be roughly 110 mm Hg, whereas the arterial oxygen tension (P_{aO_2}) might be roughly 100 mm Hg. In such a healthy person, this slight 10 mm Hg difference in the partial pressure of oxygen between these two "compartments" reflects the highly efficient diffusion of oxygen across the pulmonary membrane. AaD_{O_2} increases by 3 mm Hg with every decade of life past the age of 30 but should never exceed 25 mm Hg. A high alveolar-arterial oxygen gradient implies the presence of pulmonary disease that is causing impaired diffusion of alveolar oxygen across the pulmonary membrane, resulting in hypoxemia. In contrast, AaD_{O_2} can appear normal in a patient who is hypoventilating.

3. **How is the AaD_{O_2} calculated?**

$$AaD_{O_2} = \text{Alveolar oxygen partial pressure} - \text{Arterial oxygen partial pressure}$$

where

$$P_{AO_2} = F_{iO_2}(P_B - P_{H_2O}) - (P_{aCO_2})/R \qquad [2.9]$$

where P_{AO_2} = alveolar partial pressure of oxygen; F_{iO_2} = the fraction of inspired oxygen (usually 0.21); P_B is barometric pressure (usually 760 mm Hg); P_{H_2O} is water vapor pressure (usually 47 mm Hg); P_{aCO_2} = alveolar pressure of carbon dioxide, which equals the arterial pressure of carbon dioxide because of rapid diffusion across the alveolar membrane; and R = the respiratory quotient (usually 0.8; the ratio of carbon dioxide to oxygen consumption).

4. **What are the primary determinants of respiratory drive?**
   Respirations do not occur without input from the nervous system, which comes from the medullary respiratory center (or from conscious drive). The respiratory center responds to input from central and peripheral chemoreceptors. Chemoreceptors in the carotid bodies and at the aortic arch bifurcation can detect changes in $PaCO_2$, PaO_2, and $[H^+]$. Hypoxia, hypercapnia, and acidemia stimulate these peripheral chemoreceptors, which then transmit to and stimulate the respiratory center to increase the rate and depth of respirations. Central chemoreceptors are stimulated by hypercapnia by way of CO_2 diffusing across the blood-brain barrier and dissolving to form carbonic acid, thereby lowering the pH of the central nervous system (CNS). Central chemoreceptors do not respond directly to hypoxia.

Note: The predominant mechanism of respiratory suppression of barbiturates, benzodiazepines, opioids, and general anesthetics is to make the medullary respiratory center less responsive to increases in Pa_{CO_2}.

5. **How does increasing or decreasing the arterial P_{CO_2} (Pa_{CO_2}) affect pH?**
   When CO_2 dissolves in water, the following reaction occurs:

$$CO_2 + H_2O \xleftrightarrow{\text{CA}} HCO_3^- + H^+ \qquad [2.10]$$

where CA is carbonic anhydrase.
   If additional CO_2 is added, the reaction shifts to the right, creating more hydrogen ions, which decrease the pH of the solution. Conversely, removal of CO_2 pushes the reaction to the left, resulting in removal of H^+ from solution, with an overall increase in pH. It is this reaction that the lungs exploit to compensate for alterations in arterial pH.
   By increasing or decreasing ventilation, and thereby affecting the arterial P_{CO_2} levels, the pH can be raised or lowered.

6. **What is respiratory acidosis? Respiratory alkalosis?**
   In respiratory acidosis, the lungs are not ventilating well, and the CO_2 that builds up shifts Eq. 2.10 to the right, lowering the pH to an abnormal level. Examples of causes of respiratory acidosis include airway obstruction or hypoventilation secondary to opioid toxicity. In respiratory alkalosis, the lungs are blowing off too much CO_2, shifting the same equation to the left and raising the pH to an abnormal level. Respiratory alkalosis can be caused by hyperventilation, for example, secondary to salicylate toxicity (early) or high altitude. In both cases, the respiratory rate and depth are pathologically mismatched to the physiologic demands/needs.
   The kidneys attempt to compensate for respiratory acidosis by retaining bicarbonate or, for respiratory alkalosis, by increasing bicarbonate excretion, exploiting the other side of this chemical reaction. Unlike the process of respiratory compensation, renal compensation is slow and can take several days to be complete.

STEP 1 SECRET

Recognizing various acid-base disorders not only is a USMLE favorite but also will be a very useful skill during your clinical years!

---

7. **What are the forced expiratory volume and the FEV_1/FVC ratio?**
   The forced expiratory volume (FEV_1) is the maximum amount of air that can be expired *in 1 second* following a full inspiration. The forced vital capacity (FVC) is the total amount of air that can be forcibly expired following a full inspiration. The FEV_1/FVC ratio is therefore the percent volume of air that can be expired in 1 second relative to the maximum expiration.

8. **What is the principal difference between "restrictive" and "obstructive" lung disease with respect to the FEV_1/FVC ratio?**
   In restrictive lung disease (e.g., pulmonary fibrosis), decreased pulmonary compliance limits *inspiratory* volumes. Although expiration is not impaired, the limited inspiratory volumes result in smaller FEV_1 and FVC volumes. Furthermore, the increased pulmonary elastic recoil results in a smaller decrease in FEV_1 than in FVC, resulting in a normal or modestly increased FEV_1/FVC ratio.
   In obstructive lung disease, *expiratory* airflow is impaired secondary to airway narrowing and from decreased pulmonary elastic recoil in emphysematous COPD. FEV_1 is decreased proportionally more than FVC, resulting in a reduced FEV_1/FVC ratio.
   Table 2.1 lists some examples of obstructive and restrictive lung diseases.

Table 2.1. Obstructive and Restrictive Lung Diseases

OBSTRUCTIVE LUNG DISEASES	RESTRICTIVE LUNG DISEASES
Chronic bronchitis	Neuromuscular diseases (poliomyelitis, myasthenia gravis, Duchenne
Emphysema	muscular dystrophy, Guillain-Barré syndrome)
Asthma	ARDS
Bronchiectasis	Neonatal respiratory distress syndrome
Cystic fibrosis	Sarcoidosis
	Idiopathic pulmonary fibrosis
	Goodpasture syndrome
	Wegener granulomatosis
	Drug toxicity
	Pleural diseases

ARDS, Acute respiratory distress syndrome.

STEP 1 SECRET

You may be asked to interpret spirometry readings and flow volume diagrams on the USMLE. It is important to know how to determine the FEV$_1$/FVC ratio from one of these diagrams to identify the category of pulmonary disease a patient may have. You should be able to tell this from the shape of the diseased curve compared with a normal curve.

CASE 2.1

A 23-year-old woman is evaluated for a chronic cough and episodes of dyspnea and chest tightness. The cough is worse at night and often wakes her from deep sleep. She denies ever smoking but does report seasonal allergies and worsened respiratory symptoms when pollen levels are high.

1. **What disorder do you suspect?**
   Chronic cough in a young adult, particularly a cough that worsens at night and is associated with dyspnea and chest tightness, is classic for asthma. However, gastroesophageal reflux disease and myocardial ischemia (though the latter is unlikely) need to be considered as well.

CASE 2.1 CONTINUED:

While the patient is asymptomatic, a physical examination is entirely unremarkable. Pulmonary function testing is initially normal, but in response to a methacholine challenge, she experiences moderate respiratory distress, and her FEV$_1$/FVC ratio drops to 55%. After treatment with an albuterol inhaler, her symptoms resolve and her FEV$_1$/FVC ratio normalizes.

2. **What is the diagnosis? How is this condition classified?**
   The diagnosis is asthma, which can be classified as extrinsic (allergic, type I) or intrinsic (nonallergic, type II) asthma. Extrinsic asthma commonly begins in children who have a family history of allergies and asthma, whereas intrinsic asthma usually begins in adult life and can be associated with chronic bronchitis, exercise, or cold air. The distinction between intrinsic and extrinsic, although useful from a pathophysiologic perspective, is of limited value clinically because most patients present with a spectrum of overlapping characteristics, including elevated immunoglobulin E (IgE) levels in those with nonallergic asthma.

3. **What is the pathophysiologic process causing symptoms in this woman?**
   This patient likely has extrinsic (i.e., allergic) asthma because she reports seasonal allergies. Allergic asthma is initiated by a type I hypersensitivity reaction. Antigens from the environment enter the lungs and bind IgE antibodies on mast cells and basophils. This stimulates cross-linking of membrane-bound IgE antibodies, resulting in cellular degranulation and release of cytokines. Histamine (via G$_q$-linked H$_1$ receptors) and other proinflammatory mediators cause *reversible* bronchoconstriction and airway obstruction, leading to respiratory symptoms. Her symptom of chest tightness is likely related to this diffuse bronchoconstriction.

4. **About 5% of patients with asthma are sensitive to aspirin, and some may even develop fatal bronchospasm from ingesting aspirin. What is currently believed to be the biochemical basis of this?**
   Aspirin inhibits cyclooxygenase (COX) and therefore prevents the synthesis of prostaglandins, while shunting substrates into the leukotriene pathway in some inflammatory cells. Pulmonary leukotrienes are potent bronchoconstrictors and therefore may exacerbate bronchospasm in asthmatics (and even nonasthmatics).
   Note: Patients with asthma who also have rhinitis and nasal polyps are particularly sensitive to this effect of aspirin and may need to avoid aspirin altogether. Many of these patients have a similar reaction to ibuprofen and naproxen (NSAIDs). They should be instructed to take acetaminophen for analgesia.

5. **What is exercise-induced asthma?**
   Patients who have exercise-induced asthma become short of breath during aerobic exercise. Unlike other forms of asthma, exercise-induced asthma is not associated with airway hyperresponsiveness or with airway remodeling. The exact mechanism of the condition is unknown, but it is likely related to the heating and humidifying of large volumes of air during exercise. Patients may find some relief with bronchodilator use before the onset of exercise.

6. **What is the explanation for the decreased FEV$_1$/FVC ratio in this woman?**
   This ratio is reduced in asthma because bronchoconstriction increases airway resistance and impairs the *rate* of expiratory airflow. Mediators include leukotrienes, interleukins (e.g., interleukin-4, -13 [IL-4, IL-13]) histamine, and eosinophils. The epithelium becomes fragile, and there is thickening of the basement membrane. Glucocorticoids inhibit this inflammation.

7. **Why does methacholine cause her FEV$_1$/FVC ratio to decrease?**
   The common denominator in the different types of asthma is *hyperreactivity of the tracheobronchial tree*, especially to inflammatory mediators. Methacholine is a direct cholinergic agonist that can cause bronchoconstriction via muscarinic

receptor–mediated effects. Patients with asthma will respond to lower doses of methacholine than the general population. Often, a bronchodilator such as albuterol is administered before a repeat methacholine challenge. The degree of reversibility of decreased FEV_1/FVC ratio can be useful in distinguishing asthma from other causes of obstructive lung disease, such as COPD.

8. **What is residual lung volume, and how is it affected in an asthma attack?**
Residual lung volume is the volume of air left in the lung after a maximal expiration. The elevated resistance to expiratory airflow that develops during bronchoconstriction does not allow normal expiration of the usual percentage of alveolar gas at typical intrathoracic pressures, resulting in an increased residual volume. This increase in residual volume is typical of obstructive airway diseases. Note that the increase in residual volume in emphysema is caused by *air trapping* in the smaller airways and not hypertrophy or bronchoconstriction as in asthma.

9. **Why is wheezing generally heard most during expiration in asthma?**
During expiration, the increase in intrathoracic pressure further decreases the diameter of airways that are already narrowed from bronchoconstriction, making it more difficult for air to flow, creating a turbulent and noisy airflow. Note that in acute asthmatic attacks, both inspiratory and expiratory wheezes are caused by bronchospasm.
    The pathophysiology of wheezing is different in COPD, in which bronchospasm rarely occurs. Rather, extensive parenchymal destruction promotes airway collapse during expiration because of the higher intrathoracic pressures, resulting in more of an expiratory wheeze.

10. **With respect to the pathophysiology of asthma, what are the two mechanistic targets of pharmacologic intervention?**
Because bronchoconstriction and pulmonary inflammation play such an important etiologic role in asthma, pharmacotherapy in asthma is primarily aimed at stimulating bronchodilation (or preventing bronchoconstriction) and at inhibiting the pulmonary inflammatory process. We discuss the specific drugs employed for these purposes later.

11. **Quick review: Cover the two columns on the right side of Table 2.2, and identify the class of drug and mechanism of action for the listed antiasthmatic drugs.**

Table 2.2. Medications Used for Treatment of Asthma

AGENT(S)	DRUG CLASS	MECHANISM OF ACTION
Albuterol	β_2-Agonist (short-acting)	Bronchodilation by β_2 stimulation of adenylyl cyclase, which triggers cAMP formation. This leads to PKA opening Ca^{2+} channels, causing hyperpolarization and bronchodilation
Salmeterol	β_2-Agonist (long-acting)	Bronchodilation through same mechanism as albuterol, increased duration (12+ hours) due to lipid solubility
Cromolyn sodium	Mast cell stabilizer	Prevents release of histamine and other proinflammatory substances
Ipratropium	Anticholinergic (short-acting antimuscarinic)	Quaternary analog of atropine. Inhibits bronchoconstriction
Montelukast	Leukotriene receptor antagonist	Inhibits activity of proinflammatory leukotrienes
Zileuton	5-Lipoxygenase inhibitor	Inhibits synthesis of leukotrienes from arachidonic acid
Beclomethasone, fluticasone	Glucocorticoid	Antiinflammation via inhibition of a variety of proinflammatory agents

cAMP, Cyclic adenosine monophosphate; *PKA,* protein kinase A.

12. **Why are albuterol and salmeterol preferable to isoproterenol in treating asthma?**
Although all three of these drugs are beta-agonists, only albuterol and salmeterol are selective β_2-agonists, the adrenergic receptor type present in the lungs that mediates bronchodilation. Isoproterenol has both β_2- and β_1-agonist activity and can therefore stimulate cardiac β_1-receptors, resulting in tachycardia and palpitations.
    Note: Beta-blockers should generally be avoided in patients with asthma because they can precipitate or exacerbate bronchospasm. If use of a beta-blocker is warranted, selective β_1-receptor blockers (e.g., atenolol, esmolol, extended release metoprolol, nebivolol) should be administered because they have less effect on respiratory function.

13. This patient was prescribed a combination inhaler that contains a β_2-agonist and a corticosteroid. A month or so later she noticed a white cheesy exudate on her soft palate and pharynx. What probably happened?

The patient likely developed oropharyngeal candidiasis (the causative agent is *Candida albicans*). This infection is due to glucocorticoid-mediated suppression of the local immunologic response. For this reason, it is suggested that patients rinse their mouths after using inhaled corticosteroids.

14. Why is cromolyn sodium useful in the prevention but not the treatment of asthmatic attacks?

Cromolyn sodium inhibits mast cell degranulation and the release of histamines and prostaglandins that occurs in an allergic-response asthmatic attack. However, once the mast cells have degranulated (i.e., following an acute asthma attack), this agent has no significant effect on the activity of the inflammatory mediators that are released. Essentially, it is too late to use cromolyn sodium once symptoms have developed.

15. What histologic changes would be expected in the bronchial smooth muscle and mucosa if a biopsy were performed in this patient?

1. *Smooth muscle hyperplasia/hypertrophy* secondary to recurrent bronchoconstriction
2. *Mucosal edema* (with a relative *eosinophilia*) secondary to a chronic subacute inflammatory process
3. *Curschmann spirals* (whorls of desquamated epithelium found in the mucus of patients with asthma)
4. *Charcot-Leyden crystals* (degranulated eosinophil membranes found in the mucus of patients with asthma)
5. *Goblet cell hyperplasia* to facilitate mucus secretion during exacerbations

16. What is theophylline, and what are some of the drawbacks of its use?

Theophylline is a methylxanthine derivative (meaning it has a structure similar to caffeine and purine bases) that can be used in the treatment of asthma. Its effectiveness is due to its bronchodilatory and antiinflammatory actions, although the precise mechanisms by which it mediates these actions are beyond the scope of this book. Because theophylline is such an inexpensive drug, it remains the drug of choice in the treatment of asthma in many nonindustrialized countries and is still occasionally used in the United States for the treatment of asthma that has been refractory to beta-agonists, steroids, and other newer agents. Unfortunately, theophylline has a narrow therapeutic index and can precipitate seizures, cardiac arrhythmias, and even death. Plasma theophylline levels must be monitored regularly, and toxicity is treated with beta-blockers.

SUMMARY BOX: ASTHMA PRESENTATION

- Wheezing, cough (that is often worse late at night or early in the morning), chest tightness, and dyspnea
- Symptoms are often triggered or worsened by exercise, cold air, or inhaled noxious particles.
- History of prolonged upper respiratory tract infections
- Diagnosis
  - Disproportionate decrease in the FEV_1/FVC ratio in response to methacholine
- Pathology
  - Smooth muscle hypertrophy secondary to recurrent bronchoconstriction and mucosal edema (with a relative eosinophilia) secondary to a chronic subacute inflammatory process
  - Curschmann spirals and Charcot-Leyden crystals are found in the mucus of patients with asthma.
- Treatment
  - Glucocorticoids (inhaled and oral)
  - β_2-Agonists (short-acting and long-acting)
  - Mast cell stabilizers
  - Anticholinergics
  - Leukotriene receptor antagonists
  - 5-Lipoxygenase inhibitors
  - Theophylline

CASE 2.2

A 36-year-old man who works on a farm is evaluated for a several-month history of worsening dyspnea with exertion. He is diagnosed with asthma and given an albuterol inhaler to be used when symptomatic. The patient has now returned to your office upset that his inhaler "doesn't do a darned thing!"

---

1. What are some potential causes of this man's symptoms?

He may be using the inhaler incorrectly. He may also have COPD, hypersensitivity pneumonitis, congestive heart failure (CHF), coronary artery disease, pulmonary hypertension, an infectious process, malignancy, or anemia. More information is clearly needed.

CASE 2.2 CONTINUED:

At the next visit he continues to inform you: "Doc, I don't understand it. I just bought this farm a month ago, and every time I go out there, I get short of breath after only a few hours. I've never had trouble breathing like this before. When I'm at the farm I can hardly work outside."

2. **What is the most likely diagnosis at this time?**
   Acute attacks of dyspnea with a clear exposure history and lack of response to albuterol are suggestive of hypersensitivity pneumonitis (also known as *extrinsic allergic alveolitis*).

3. **What is the pathophysiology of this disorder, and why does not albuterol help?**
   Hypersensitivity pneumonitis is an acute immune-mediated inflammatory disease of the lung; it results from an allergic reaction to a wide variety of allergens and causes acute shortness of breath. It is characterized by diffuse inflammation of the interstitium, terminal bronchioles, and alveoli. It subsumes a wide variety of diseases with the same underlying etiology and pathogenesis but can be due to exposure to different allergens (e.g., farmer's lung, pigeon handler's lung, humidifier lung). Unlike in asthma, only the terminal bronchioles are affected (which lack the smooth muscle of larger bronchioles), explaining why albuterol may not be helpful. Note that the "allergic" reaction is *not* IgE-mediated.

4. **How is hypersensitivity pneumonitis treated?**
   The most crucial aspect of treatment is avoidance of exposure to allergens. If there is continuous exposure to the offending allergen and continual alveolar inflammation (alveolitis), the chronic inflammation can ultimately result in irreversible pulmonary fibrosis.

SUMMARY BOX: HYPERSENSITIVITY PNEUMONITIS

- Presentation
  - Wheezing and dyspnea. Symptoms are often triggered or worsened by a variety of antigens including occupational exposures (as noted in the text).
- Epidemiology
  - Often called "farmer's" or "bird breeder's" lung because it has been noted in these populations.
- Diagnosis
  - History of exposure to a provoking allergen such as inhaled organic dust
  - Imaging: Diffuse infiltrates seen on chest x-ray film with appropriate symptoms and, if disease course is progressive, restrictive patterns on pulmonary function tests (PFTs) from eventual fibrosis
- Pathology
  - Biopsy may show poorly formed, noncaseating granulomas or mononuclear cell infiltrates.
- Complications:
  - Untreated hypersensitivity pneumonitis can progress to irreversible pulmonary fibrosis.
- Treatment
  - Most often reversible if diagnosed early and offending agent removed

CASE 2.3

A 37-year-old man with a known history of allergic asthma is evaluated in the emergency department for respiratory distress and low-grade fever. His albuterol inhaler has not alleviated his symptoms in recent days. A chest x-ray shows diffuse pulmonary infiltrates, and laboratory workup reveals a marked eosinophilia and elevated IgE levels.

1. **What is the suspected diagnosis?**
   Allergic bronchopulmonary aspergillosis (ABPA) is suspected. The presentation of fever, eosinophilia, and pulmonary infiltrates is classic for ABPA, a condition caused by a hypersensitivity response to the fungus *Aspergillus fumigatus*. ABPA predominantly occurs in patients with asthma.
   Note: Several other fungi can also cause identical clinical and laboratory findings but do so less commonly than *Aspergillus*.

2. **What other tests can be done to more confidently establish this diagnosis?**
   Skin sensitivity tests to the fungus *Aspergillus fumigatus*, as well as *Aspergillus*-specific serum IgE tests, may be performed.

3. **What is the cause of the pulmonary infiltrate?**
   There is marked infiltration of the pulmonary parenchyma with eosinophils in this disease, which is why this disease is known as one of the "eosinophilic pneumonias."
   Note: The eosinophilic pneumonias encompass a spectrum of diseases of different causes, all of which have in common eosinophilic infiltration of the lung and, often, peripheral blood eosinophilia, as in this patient. ABPA and other eosinophilic pneumonias are treated with corticosteroids.

SUMMARY BOX: ALLERGIC BRONCHOPULMONARY ASPERGILLOSIS

- Presentation
  - Allergic bronchopulmonary aspergillosis (ABPA) typically occurs in patients with asthma and manifests with dyspnea, fever, eosinophilia, and infiltrates on chest x-ray.
- Treatment
  - Corticosteroids are the mainstay of treatment.

CASE 2.4

A 70-year-old previously healthy man is evaluated for a 3-day history of fever, cough, and fatigue. The cough produces "rusty"-colored sputum. Lab results show a white blood cell (WBC) count of 18,000 cells/μL (normal = 4500–10,000 cells/μL), and the chest x-ray is shown in Fig. 2.4.

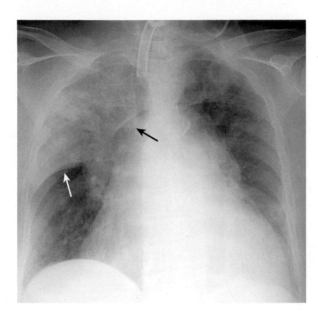

Figure 2.4. Chest x-ray for patient in Case 2.4. White arrow points at the inferior margin of the upper lobe, which is sharply demarcated. Black arrow points to the aortic border, which is silhouetted by the fluid density of the pneumonia. *(From Herring W. Learning Radiology: Recognizing the Basics. 4th ed. Philadelphia: Elsevier; 2020: 70-76, Fig. 9.3.)*

1. What is the most likely diagnosis?
   Lobar (typical) pneumonia from *Streptococcus pneumoniae* is the likely diagnosis. The patient's fever, increased WBC count, and chest x-ray appearance are all suggestive of lobar (typical) pneumonia. The x-ray indicates a right upper lobe pneumonia. The inferior margin of the upper lobe is sharply demarcated as a result of the fissures that divide the lobes (*white arrow*). The border of the aorta is silhouetted by the fluid density of the pneumonia (*black arrow*).

   On the USMLE, whenever you get a description of "rusty"-colored sputum, you should reflexively think of streptococcal pneumonia. *S. pneumoniae* is a gram-positive organism often associated with lobar pneumonia in this age group. Another cause of lobar pneumonia is *Klebsiella pneumoniae*, which will likely present with red currant jelly sputum in a patient with alcohol use disorder or diabetes. These patients are at increased risk for pneumonia caused by *K. pneumoniae* because of their weakened immune system. It is extremely high yield to remember the classic description of these two types of sputum.

2. How would your differential diagnosis change if the patient presented with a 2-week history of low-grade fever, cough, and diffuse patchy infiltrates seen on chest x-ray?
   This presentation is more typical of atypical (interstitial) or walking pneumonia. It typically follows a more indolent course than for lobar pneumonia and is often seen in adolescents and adults. Often, chest x-ray appearance is much worse than might be expected from the patient's symptoms. Bacterial causes of atypical pneumonia include *Mycoplasma pneumoniae*, *Chlamydia pneumoniae*, and *Legionella pneumophila*. Viral causes include respiratory syncytial virus (RSV) and adenovirus.

3. What are some common causes of pneumonia in different age groups?
   See Table 2.3.

CASE 2.5

A 75-year-old woman with a long history of cigarette smoking is evaluated for gradually worsening shortness of breath with exertion over many years.

Table 2.3. Common Causes of Pneumonia

NEONATES (<4 WEEKS)	CHILDREN (4 WEEKS–18 YEARS)	ADULTS (18–40 YEARS)	ADULTS (40–65 YEARS)	ELDERLY
Group B streptococci *Escherichia coli* *Listeria monocytogenes*	Viruses (respiratory syncytial virus, influenza, parainfluenza) *Mycoplasma* *Chlamydia pneumoniae* *Streptococcus pneumoniae*	*Mycoplasma* *C. pneumoniae* *S. pneumoniae*	*S. pneumoniae* *Haemophilus influenzae* Anaerobes Viruses *Mycoplasma*	*S. pneumoniae* Influenza virus Anaerobes *H. influenzae* Gram-negative rods

1. **What is the differential diagnosis?**
   Given her smoking history, this sounds like COPD or lung cancer. However, always consider cardiovascular causes of shortness of breath including coronary artery disease, CHF, and anemia.

CASE 2.5 CONTINUED:

Physical examination reveals a cachectic elderly woman who is unable to speak in complete sentences because of respiratory distress. A prolonged expiratory phase is noted. Lung fields are hyperresonant on percussion. A chest x-ray is shown in Fig. 2.5. Pulmonary function tests (PFTs) reveal an FEV_1/FVC ratio of 45%. An electrocardiogram (ECG) indicates right ventricular hypertrophy. Blood tests reveal an elevated hemoglobin and hematocrit.

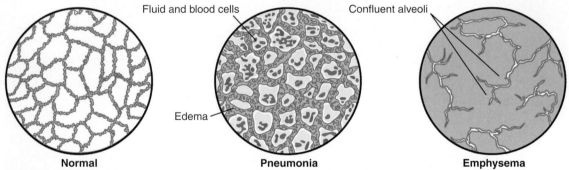

Fluid and blood cells Confluent alveoli

Edema

Normal **Pneumonia** **Emphysema**

Figure 2.5. Pulmonary changes in emphysema. *(From Hall JE. Guyton and Hall Textbook of Medical Physiology. 13th ed. Philadelphia: Elsevier; 2016: 549-557, Fig 43-5.)*

2. **What is the diagnosis?**
   All of the preceding findings are suggestive of COPD, an obstructive lung disease associated with exposure to cigarette smoke. Expiration is normally a passive process, but because of parenchymal destruction in COPD, the lungs lose their elastic recoil, and expiration becomes inefficient and prolonged, resulting in air-trapping and pursed-lip breathing. Pursed-lip breathing serves to maintain the pressure within the lungs such that the airways remain open rather than collapsing and contributing to air trapping (more on this later). The reduced FEV_1/FVC ratio also suggests an obstructive process and argues against the other diagnostic possibilities. Finally, even the elevated hemoglobin would be an expected physiologic compensation for the hypoxemia associated with emphysema.

3. **What is the pathophysiologic explanation for the decreased FEV_1/FVC ratio in this woman?**
   The widespread destruction of alveolar septa and alveolar elastin in emphysema causes decreased elastic recoil of the alveoli, which is one of the major forces for expiratory airflow. This compromised expiratory airflow in COPD decreases both FEV_1 and FVC, with a particularly greater effect on FEV_1. Therefore the ratio of FEV_1 to FVC is decreased. Decreased FEV_1 to FVC ratio is the hallmark of an obstructive lung disease. When approaching a question on the boards, always look at the FEV_1/FVC ratio. If it's less than 70%, then you have a diagnosis of an obstructive process, and you can narrow down your answer choices.

4. **Why is the patient so thin?**
   Because of premature airway collapse and air trapping, the patient must breathe above her FRC. Deviations in breathing pattern above FRC (with obstructive) or below FRC (with restrictive) lung disease are inefficient and require significant muscular effort and use of accessory muscles, resulting in increased caloric expenditure.

5. **What is the most likely cause of emphysema in this woman?**
Chronic cigarette smoking is the most common cause of emphysema. Smoking damages the respiratory airways, resulting in the release of proteases by activated alveolar macrophages and neutrophils. These proteases degrade alveolar elastin and collagen, resulting in alveolar destruction and loss of elastic recoil during expiration.
   Note: Cigarette smoke is also thought to directly inhibit alveolar elastin synthesis and to inhibit the activity of α_1-antitrypsin, a protease inhibitor synthesized and secreted by the liver.

6. **Would a biopsy of this woman's lung reveal enlarged or reduced respiratory airways?**
Airways would appear enlarged. The destruction of alveolar elastin that occurs in emphysema results in permanent abnormal enlargement of the airspaces distal to the terminal bronchiole (see Fig. 2.5). This is accompanied by destruction of their alveolar walls without obvious fibrosis. This process causes the hyperlucency or darkness on chest x-ray film (Fig. 2.6) because there is both more air in the lungs and less lung tissue.

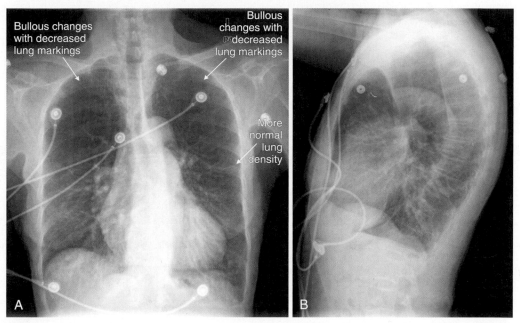

Figure 2.6. Bullae in chronic obstructive pulmonary disease (COPD). A, Posterior-anterior (PA) chest x-ray. B, Lateral chest x-ray. *(From Broder J.* Diagnostic Imaging for the Emergency Physician. *Philadelphia: Saunders; 2011, Fig. 5-46.)*

7. **How do centriacinar and panacinar emphysema differ in terms of morphology and etiology?**
Centriacinar emphysema is much more common than panacinar emphysema and is typically acquired secondary to a long history of cigarette smoking. In centriacinar emphysema, respiratory bronchioles are abnormally enlarged, whereas the distal alveoli are spared. Centriacinar emphysema preferentially affects the upper lobes in the early stages, while panacinar emphysema involves all lung fields, particularly the lung bases. Panacinar emphysema is associated with α_1-antitrypsin deficiency and involves abnormal enlargement of the distal alveoli, alveolar ducts, and respiratory bronchioles. This disease should be suspected in any adult with symptoms of emphysema but minimal exposure to cigarettes. Also remember that α_1-antitrypsin deficiency can cause histologic and pathologic changes to the liver.

8. **Why may administration of large volumes of concentrated O_2 to this woman cause hypercapnia?**
Patients with COPD often have higher CO_2 and lower oxygen saturations at baseline because of the increased dead space, which impairs gas exchange, resulting in hypercapnia and hypoxemia. These patients therefore become used to a certain level of hypercapnia and hypoxemia. Increasing oxygen can reduce ventilatory drive, resulting in hypercapnia. In addition, studies suggest that oxygen administration may lead to changes in $\dot{V}/\dot{Q}$ matching, with oxygen administration and the Haldane effect (oxygen displaces CO_2 from hemoglobin) responsible for oxygen-induced hypercapnia.

9. **How does emphysema cause the right ventricular hypertrophy seen on this patient's ECG?**
First, recall that the pulmonary vessels respond to hypoxia by constricting and diverting blood flow from poorly ventilated to well-ventilated regions of the lung. When small areas of the lung are damaged or filled with fluid, this is an appropriate adaptive response. However, in COPD, the widespread hypoxia results in diffuse vasoconstriction. The diffuse vasoconstriction and the destruction of septal capillaries cause pathologically elevated pulmonary arterial pressures. Just as systemic hypertension often leads to left ventricular hypertrophy, pulmonary hypertension can lead to right ventricular hypertrophy.

10. **Why is an individual with α_1-antitrypsin deficiency at increased risk for developing emphysema?**
    α_1-Antitrypsin is a protein secreted by the liver that inhibits the activity of various proteolytic enzymes in the serum. Some of these enzymes, such as neutrophil elastase, degrade alveolar elastin. Widespread alveolar elastin degradation in the lungs then produces early-onset emphysema throughout the entire acinus (panacinar emphysema). Generally, this disease should be suspected in a nonsmoker who develops emphysema at an early age.
    Note: α_1-Antitrypsin deficiency is not a true deficiency state; rather than being secreted by the liver, α_1-antitrypsin accumulates in periodic acid-Schiff (PAS)-positive granules in the hepatocytes. This can eventually lead to hepatocellular carcinoma. Consider this diagnosis whenever you see a patient with symptoms of emphysema who also demonstrates symptoms of liver failure.

11. **Why do patients with COPD breathe through pursed lips?**
    Normally, the equal pressure point (EPP), the point at which intrapleural pressure and alveolar pressure are equal, falls in the cartilaginous airways close to the mouth, preventing bronchial collapse (cartilage resists collapse). In patients with emphysema, alveolar pressure falls as a result of decreased elastic recoil pressure. The pressure in the alveolus (P_A) is defined by the relationship

$$P_A = P_{el} + P_l \qquad [2.11]$$

where P_{el} = elastic recoil pressure and P_l is the pressure across the lung. Decreased alveolar pressure shifts the EPP into small, noncartilaginous airways that are prone to collapse on expiration. Breathing through pursed lips elevates alveolar pressure and pushes the EPP back toward the mouth to prevent expiratory airway collapse and air trapping.

12. **What pharmacologic agents are used to treat COPD?**
    See Table 2.4.

SUMMARY BOX: CHRONIC OBSTRUCTIVE PULMONARY DISEASE

- Presentation
  - Progressive insidious dyspnea
  - Note that emphysema and chronic bronchitis fall on a continuum for patients with chronic obstructive pulmonary disease (COPD), so there may be overlapping symptoms, and most often patients have characteristics of both diseases.
  - On physical examination, these patients will have hyperresonance of the chest, wheezes, decreased breath sounds bilaterally, prolonged expiratory phase, and pursed-lip breathing.
  - Pulse oximetry on room air at rest or with minimal exertion may be decreased.
- Epidemiology
  - Most commonly seen in heavy smokers (centriacinar) with the exception of those who have α_1-antitrypsin deficiency (panacinar)
- Diagnosis
  - Chest x-ray may show hyperinflation and hyperlucency of the lungs, increased anteroposterior diameter ("barrel chest"), and flattening of the diaphragm.
  - FEV_1/FVC ratio $<70\%$, with minimal improvement following the administration of bronchodilators
  - Patients are often hypoxemic, and this results in a modest polycythemia.
- Pathology
  - Destruction of lung parenchyma results from pathologic activation of proteases.
  - The destruction of alveolar elastin results in permanent abnormal enlargement of the air spaces distal to the terminal bronchiole.
  - This is accompanied by destruction of their alveolar walls but without obvious fibrosis.
- Complications
  - Right ventricular hypertrophy with pulmonary hypertension, hypoxemia necessitating supplemental oxygen, and (rarely) spontaneous pneumothorax from rupture of a surface bleb
- Treatment
  - Inhaled bronchodilators (beta-agonists and muscarinic antagonists) given alone, in combination, or with addition of inhaled glucocorticoids. The long-acting bronchodilators are used for regular treatment, and short-acting bronchodilators are used for symptom relief as needed.
  - Supplemental oxygen is the only treatment shown to improve survival.
- Prognosis
  - Progressive disease that will not resolve
  - The rate of decline in pulmonary function can be greatly reduced with smoking cessation.

CASE 2.6

A 55-year-old man who has not had regular medical care presents to the walk-in clinic with concerns of a chest cold, noting daily morning productive cough for the past 2 years. He has smoked one pack of cigarettes daily since the age of 20.

Table 2.4. Medications Used for Treatment of Chronic Obstructive Pulmonary Disease

MEDICATION CLASS	EXAMPLES	MECHANISM OF ACTION	CLINICAL USE
Short-acting beta-agonist	Albuterol Levalbuterol	Bronchodilation by β_2 stimulation of adenylyl cyclase, which triggers cAMP formation. This leads to PKA opening Ca^{2+} channels, causing hyperpolarization and bronchodilation	Relief of acute symptoms
Short-acting muscarinic antagonist	Ipratropium	Bronchodilation through same mechanism as albuterol, increased duration due to lipid solubility	Relief of acute symptoms
Long-acting beta-agonist	Salmeterol Formoterol Arformoterol Indacaterol Vilanterol Olodaterol	Bronchial smooth muscle relaxation by selective action on β-2 receptors	Long-term symptom and exacerbation control
Long-acting muscarinic antagonist	Tiotropium Aclidinium Umeclidinium Glycopyrrolate Revefenacin	Bronchodilation through inhibition of acetylcholine at muscarinic receptors in bronchial smooth muscle	Long-term symptom and exacerbation control
Glucocorticoids	Budesonide Fluticasone Mometasone	Reducing inflammation via inhibition of a variety of proinflammatory agents	Long-term symptom and exacerbation control

cAMP, Cyclic adenosine monophosphate; *PKA,* protein kinase A.

1. **What is the likely diagnosis?**
   Chronic bronchitis is the likely diagnosis. Chronic bronchitis can be diagnosed in patients with a productive cough for at least 3 months in 2 consecutive years and evidence of obstruction. Acute exacerbations are often precipitated by bacterial or viral upper respiratory infection. A history of smoking is typical.

2. **Why may cigarette smoking predispose to chronic lung infections?**
   The toxins in cigarette smoke paralyze the mucociliary tract, resulting in impaired mucous clearance from the airways. Furthermore, pseudostratified, ciliated cells are replaced with goblet cells. This "preneoplastic" condition is true squamous metaplasia, creating an environment susceptible to infection.

CASE 2.6 CONTINUED:

The patient notes that the cough produces whitish phlegm and that about 3 weeks ago he developed a runny nose, sore throat, and fever. He has also noted chest tightness and worsening shortness of breath. His physical examination is notable for wheezing, bibasilar crackles on inspiration, and cyanotic appearance.

3. **What is the pathogenesis of chronic bronchitis?**
   Chronic bronchitis is caused by chronic irritation of the airways by inhaled substances (e.g., cigarette smoke) and repeated infections of the airways. Histopathologically, there is hypertrophy of submucosal glands and goblet cells, resulting in mucous hypersecretion in both large and small airways, which reduces their diameters and makes expiration more difficult. Mucous hypersecretion is reflected by an elevated Reid index (normal is less than 40%; generally >50% in chronic bronchitis), which is defined as gland depth/total thickness of the bronchial wall between the epithelium and underlying cartilage. It objectively measures smooth muscle hypertrophy.

4. **What is the basis of the reduced FEV_1/FVC ratio in chronic bronchitis?**
   Hypertrophy of mucus-secreting glands and mucous hypersecretion leads to reduction of airway diameter. These changes are the principal causes of expiratory airflow limitation, with minimal effect on elastic recoil of the alveoli. This leads to a decreased FEV_1 with smaller changes in FVC, thus resulting in a reduced FEV_1/FVC ratio.
      The bronchial wall biopsy specimen from a normal patient (Fig. 2.7A) shows normal pseudostratified columnar epithelium with scattered goblet cells overlying smooth muscle and a submucosal gland. The bronchial wall biopsy specimen from a patient with chronic bronchitis (Fig. 2.7B) shows infiltration of the submucosa by inflammatory cells (*In*) overlying hypertrophied smooth muscle (*M*) with hypertrophy of the mucous glands (*G*). Surface epithelial hyperplasia (and even metaplasia) are also common findings.

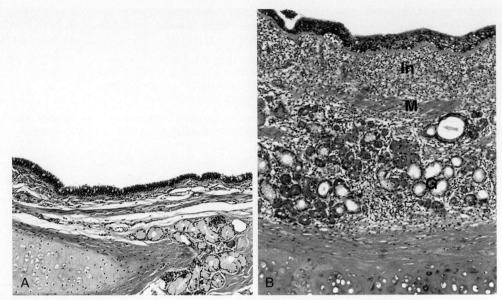

Figure 2.7. A, Bronchial wall from normal patient. B, Bronchial wall from a patient with chronic bronchitis. *(From O'Dowd G, Bell S, Wright S. Wheater's Pathology: A Text, Atlas, and Review of Histopathology, 6th ed. Philadelphia: Elsevier; 2020: 133–149.e8, Fig. 12.9.)*

5. **What is an acute exacerbation of COPD? What classes of medications should be avoided or prescribed with great caution in these situations?**
   An acute exacerbation of COPD entails the acute onset of significantly greater dyspnea and alterations in blood gases such as worsening hypoxemia or hypercapnia. These exacerbations are usually due to respiratory infections such as acute bronchitis or pneumonia. Drugs that suppress respiration, such as opioid analgesics, benzodiazepines, and barbiturates, should be avoided in these patients. Beta-blockers, which inhibit catecholamine-mediated bronchodilation, also should be avoided.

6. **What acid-base abnormality is commonly found in patients with COPD, and what is its origin?**
   Respiratory acidosis secondary to hypercapnia stemming from alveolar hypoventilation is commonly found. As a compensatory response, the kidneys excrete additional hydrogen ions and reabsorb bicarbonate to increase the pH. Always remember that a compensatory response will never completely return a pH to normal or "overcompensate."

7. **How might mechanical ventilation lead to respiratory alkalosis?**
   If tidal volumes and respiratory rate are set too high, this may "float" the patient to the other end of the spectrum, causing him to blow off too much CO_2 and go into respiratory alkalosis. The kidneys will attempt to compensate for this by excreting more bicarbonate to lower the pH back to normal.
   Note: Respiratory acidosis or alkalosis can develop rapidly, over minutes to hours. However, renal compensation occurs more slowly and can take several days for complete compensation. Again, remember that there is never complete compensation.

SUMMARY BOX: CHRONIC BRONCHITIS

- Presentation
  - Productive cough, cyanosis, crackles, and wheezing
- Diagnosis
  - Productive cough for 3 months in at least 2 consecutive years
  - Pulmonary function tests (PFTs) yield an FEV_1/FVC ratio <70%, with only slight improvement following the administration of bronchodilators.
  - Patients are often hypoxemic and hypercapnic.
- Pathology
  - Hypertrophy of submucosal glands and goblet cells, resulting in mucous hypersecretion in both large and small airways, which reduces airway diameter and obstructs expiratory airflow
  - The Reid index (gland depth/total thickness of bronchial wall) objectively measures smooth muscle hypertrophy.
- Complications
  - May ultimately lead to right ventricular hypertrophy and right-sided heart failure secondary to pulmonary hypertension

---

SUMMARY BOX: CHRONIC BRONCHITIS—cont'd

- Treatment
  - Bronchodilators and corticosteroids are mainstays of treatment.
  - Antibiotics may be necessary for acute exacerbations of chronic bronchitis, which are often triggered by an infection.
  - Drugs that suppress respiration, such as opioid analgesics, benzodiazepines, and barbiturates, should be used very cautiously in these patients.
- Prognosis
  - As with emphysema, this is a progressive disease that does not resolve. Again, the rate of decline is reduced with smoking cessation.

CASE 2.7

A 50-year-old man who works in a shipyard and has a 40-pack-year history of tobacco smoking is evaluated for a several-year history of gradually worsening dyspnea. He denies orthopnea, paroxysmal nocturnal dyspnea, and edema.

1. **What is the likely diagnosis?**
   This patient likely has either pulmonary fibrosis from asbestos exposure (asbestosis), COPD, or malignancy related to cigarette exposure. We need more information.

CASE 2.7 CONTINUED:

PFTs show an FVC <50% of predicted for his age, height, and gender and an FEV_1/FVC ratio of 85%. His chest x-ray and computed tomography (CT) scan are shown in Fig. 2.8.

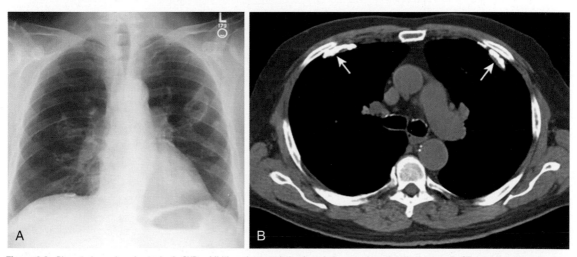

Figure 2.8. Pleural plaque in asbestosis. A, CXR exhibiting characteristic pleural plaques along the diaphragm. B, CT revealing pleural plaques as dense calcifications along the pleural surface. *(From Torigian DA, Lau CT, Miller WT. Radiology Secrets Plus. 4th ed. Philadelphia: Elsevier; 2017: 181-188, Fig. 21-5.)*

2. **What is the diagnosis?**
   Remember that FEV_1/FVC >80% is diagnostic of restrictive lung disease. Given his exposure history and this pattern on PFTs, he presumably has asbestosis.

3. **What are the pneumoconioses?**
   The pneumoconioses are a group of lung diseases caused by the inhalation of various types of dust particles in different occupational settings. The dust particles set off an inflammatory alveolitis, which, if the exposure continues, may lead to pulmonary fibrosis. Steroids may offer some relief in the early inflammatory stage but are of no benefit in the later fibrotic stage. The two most important pneumoconioses to be familiar with for the USMLE are asbestosis and silicosis.
   Asbestos was commonly used as an insulator because of its fire-resistant properties. The classic patient worked with insulation in a shipyard or in the construction industry. Asbestosis is an interstitial lung disease that results in pulmonary fibrosis. Asbestos exposure also predisposes to certain malignancies (see next question). Be able to

recognize the pleural plaques (see Fig. 2.8), which appear as irregular linear or curvilinear calcifications on chest x-ray (A) and as curvilinear dense calcifications along the pleural surface on CT scan (B). Also be able to identify "ferruginous bodies" (also known as asbestos bodies once the presence of asbestos is confirmed) that are commonly seen on the boards and are diagnostic for asbestos exposure (Fig. 2.9).

The other pneumoconiosis to know is silicosis, which is seen in patients who have been occupationally exposed to fine airborne silica, as is often seen in jobs that require stone cutting or sandblasting. Reflexively think of silicosis in any patient who has "eggshell" calcifications of the hilar lymph nodes.

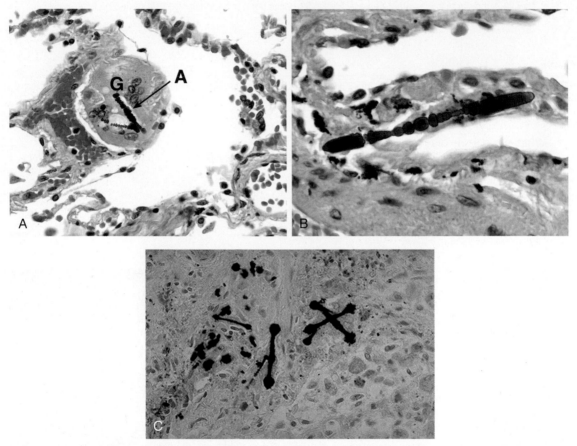

Figure 2.9. A, High-power view of alveolar space containing giant cell (G) with typical asbestos bodies (A). B, Beaded hemosiderin proteinaceous coat over asbestos fiber with beaded appearance and fine central core at higher magnification. C, Prussian blue iron stain of ferruginous bodies (also known as asbestos bodies). *(From O'Dowd G, Bell S, Wright S. Wheater's Pathology: A Text, Atlas, and Review of Histopathology. 6th ed. Philadelphia: Elsevier; 2020: 133-149.e8, Fig. 12.15 and Klatt EC. Robbins and Cotran Atlas of Pathology. 3rd ed. Philadelphia: Elsevier; 2015: 107-158.e8, Fig. 5-40.)*

4. **What is the most likely malignancy in a smoker who has been exposed to asbestos?**
   The most common malignancy in patients who have been exposed to asbestos Is bronchogenic carcinoma, especially in patients who have also smoked. In contrast, mesothelioma is a rare cancer of the pleural lining of the lungs that is not independently associated with smoking.

5. **What are some other common causes of pulmonary fibrosis?**
   A great variety of factors may cause pulmonary fibrosis, including silicosis, granulomatous diseases of the lung (e.g., sarcoidosis), connective tissue diseases (e.g., lupus, rheumatoid arthritis), and certain medications (e.g., amiodarone, bleomycin, methotrexate). It is also commonly idiopathic.

6. **What is the pathophysiologic explanation for the reduction in FVC in this man?**
   Fibrosis of the alveolar walls and septa make the alveoli less compliant. The alveoli therefore do not expand as well, resulting in a reduced inspiratory volume. This inability to take a deep breath translates into reduced expiratory volume and reduced FEV_1 and FVC values. However, unlike obstructive disorders, the effect on FVC is much greater than the effect on FEV_1, and thus the FEV_1/FVC ratio is normal or even increased (>80%; normal is 70%–75%).

7. What lung biopsy finding may be present in this patient that is unique to asbestosis?

Ferruginous bodies (or asbestos bodies), which are fibers of asbestos lined by hemosiderin deposits, may be seen. These yellow-to-brown, rod-shaped bodies stain positively with Prussian blue. You should be able to recognize an asbestos body in a histopathology image.

SUMMARY BOX: ASBESTOSIS

- Symptoms
  - Exertional dyspnea; with advanced disease, dyspnea at rest, dry cough, chest pain, and recurrent respiratory tract infections
- Diagnosis
  - Look for history of exposure, chronically worsening dyspnea, and classic changes on chest x-ray (e.g., pleural plaques).
- Pathology
  - Ferruginous bodies (or asbestos bodies), which are fibers of asbestos lined by hemosiderin deposits. These yellow-to-brown, rod-shaped bodies stain positively with Prussian blue.

CASE 2.8

A 45-year-old woman reports chronic fatigue and shortness of breath with exertion. Her history is significant for rather heavy menstrual bleeding (menorrhagia). She has never smoked. She shows no signs of cyanosis, and the only notable finding on physical examination is conjunctival pallor. Laboratory tests show hemoglobin (Hb) of 7.5 g/mL (normal range is 12–15 g/dL). Blood work reveals low plasma iron, ferritin, and increased total iron-binding capacity.

1. What is the likely cause of this woman's dyspnea?

Severe iron deficiency anemia, probably secondary to heavy menstrual flows, is the likely cause of the dyspnea. As patients get older, always consider gastrointestinal (GI) bleeding as another source of iron deficiency anemia. If a 70-year-old man presented with a similar picture of anemia, this would be colon cancer until proven otherwise.

2. What is the difference between the Pao_2 and the arterial oxygen content?

The Pao_2 is the partial pressure of oxygen *dissolved* in arterial plasma, also referred to as *oxygen tension.* The partial pressure of arterial oxygen is principally mediated by adequate ventilation and gas exchange. Remember that plasma is the acellular component of blood and does not include the red blood cells (RBCs).

The arterial oxygen content, on the other hand, is a measure of the total quantity of oxygen in a given volume of blood. You should remember that very little oxygen is carried in the plasma. Instead, the majority is carried in the hemoglobin-rich RBCs. The hemoglobin does not affect the partial pressure of oxygen in arterial blood but does mediate the amount of oxygen that is carried in blood at a given partial pressure of oxygen. Because each gram of Hb can bind approximately 1.34 mL of O_2 at normal Pao_2, the average person with an Hb of 15 g/dL has an arterial O_2 content of approximately 20 mL O_2/100 mL (i.e., 15 g Hb/dL $\times$ 1.34 mL O_2/g Hb = 20.1 mL O_2/dL, or 20.1 mL O_2/100 mL). Anemia is defined as having an Hb of less than 14 mg/dL for males and 12 mg/dL for females. In anemia, a reduction in Hb will clearly reduce the arterial oxygen content (Table 2.5).

Table 2.5. Pulmonary and Respiratory Terminology	
Pao_2 (mm Hg)	Partial pressure of alveolar oxygen
Pao_2 (mm Hg)	Partial pressure of dissolved oxygen in arterial blood
Arterial oxygen content (mg/dL)	Total quantity of oxygen bound to hemoglobin in volume of arterial blood
SaO_2 (% saturation)	Percentage of oxygen-binding sites on hemoglobin with oxygen bound (in decimal format)

You should know the formula for total oxygen content:

$$O_2 \text{ content} = [Hb] \times 1.34 \text{ mL } O_2/\text{g Hb} \times SaO_2 + 0.003 \text{ mL}/O_2/100 \text{ mL blood/mm Hg} \times 100 \text{ mg Hg} \qquad [2.12]$$

As you can see, Pao_2 directly contributes very little to total oxygen content. However, adequate Pao_2 is required to saturate Hb in the lungs.

CASE 2.8 CONTINUED:

Arterial O_2 saturation by pulse oximetry on room air is 99%.

3. **What does arterial oxygen saturation measure?**
Arterial oxygen saturation is a measure of the percentage of oxygen-binding sites on Hb that have oxygen bound to them. As mentioned previously, it is determined by the Pa_{O_2}, with higher Pa_{O_2} values associated with greater oxygen saturation. It is critical that you remember that a patient with anemia will have normal oxygen saturation but decreased oxygen content.
   Note: many factors other than the Pa_{O_2} can influence the affinity of Hb for oxygen. See Fig. 2.10 for examples of factors that can contribute to "leftward shift" and "rightward shift" of the oxygen dissociation curve.

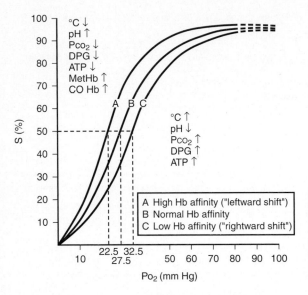

Figure 2.10. Curve B is from a normal adult at 38°C, pH 7.40, and Pco_2 35.0 mm Hg. Curves A and C illustrate the effect on the affinity for oxygen (P_{50}) of variations in temperature (°C), pH, Pco_2, 2,3-diphosphoglycerate (DPG), adenosine triphosphate (ATP), methemoglobin (MetHb), and carboxyhemoglobin (CO Hb). Curve A is of the newborn. *(From Duc G. Assessment of hypoxia in the newborn: suggestions for a practical approach. Pediatrics. 1971;48(3):469-481.)*

4. **Why does not this woman's anemia make her cyanotic?**
Cyanosis is caused by the presence of at least 5 g/dL of arterial *deoxy*hemoglobin, which occurs at a low Pa_{O_2}. In a person with only anemia, there will be normal oxygen saturation and minimal deoxyhemoglobin. Our patient's O_2 saturation is 99%, indicating good respiratory function. Theoretically, an anemic patient must reach an even lower oxygen saturation to present as clinically cyanotic. For a patient with a normal Hb of 15 g/dL to reach 5 g/dL of deoxyhemoglobin, they would have to be at an O_2 saturation of 66%, which is very low. For an anemic patient with an Hb of 10 g/dL, they would have to have an O_2 saturation of 50%. If you can understand these calculations, you should be able to understand both anemia and cyanosis.
   Methemoglobinemia is another potential cause of cyanosis. In conditions such as pyruvate kinase deficiency or glucose-6-phosphate dehydrogenase (G6PD) deficiency or following exposure to oxidizing drugs such as benzocaine or dapsone, the mechanisms that defend against oxidative stress within the RBCs are overwhelmed, and the ferrous ion (Fe^{2+}) of the heme moiety of Hb is oxidized to the ferric state (Fe^{3+}). This converts Hb to methemoglobin, which is unable to bind oxygen and is therefore dark brown. For any patient with "chocolate-colored blood," think about methemoglobinemia.

5. **How is the anemia contributing to this woman's dyspnea?**
The peripheral chemoreceptors cannot "sense" the low arterial oxygen content; they can only sense the Pa_{O_2}, which is normal because ventilation is unimpaired. However, the low oxygen content promotes anaerobic respiration, which lowers arterial pH and increases respiratory drive, causing dyspnea and reducing Pco_2.

RELATED QUESTIONS

6. **What are typical values for arterial and venous Po_2, and what do they represent with respect to the hemoglobin dissociation curve?**
At a normal arterial Po_2 of 100 mm Hg, hemoglobin is fully saturated. This corresponds to the "loading" portion of the hemoglobin dissociation curve, which occurs in the pulmonary capillaries (Fig. 2.11). In the peripheral capillaries, O_2 diffuses rapidly from the blood to the tissues, such that the Po_2 in venous blood drops to approximately 40 mm Hg, corresponding to Hb that is only approximately 75% saturated (i.e., bound to three molecules of O_2).

STEP 1 SECRET

Know how to interpret oxygen dissociation curves and what factors shift the curve to the left or to the right. This is a commonly tested principle on the USMLE.

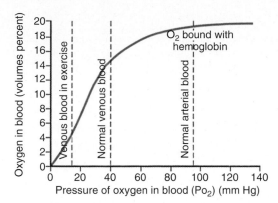

Figure 2.11. Oxyhemoglobin dissociation-curve.

7. Would exposure to carbon monoxide be expected to affect the Pa_{O_2}? Explain.

No. Carbon monoxide exhibits its effect by binding to Hb and preventing oxygen from dissociating from Hb (leftward shift) but will not affect the amount of oxygen dissolved in plasma. Therefore exposure to carbon monoxide should not alter Pa_{O_2}, although the O_2 *saturation* will decrease. Because CO causes a left shift of the oxygen dissociation curve, patients have increased venous O_2 saturation. Think strongly about CO poisoning for any patient with cherry red lips and nail beds.

8. Differentiate between external and internal respiration. Which is affected by anemia?

Gas exchange between the alveoli and blood in the pulmonary capillaries is referred to as *external respiration,* whereas the exchange of gases between capillary blood and the interstitial fluid is referred to as *internal respiration. Cellular respiration* refers to the exchange of gases between the cells and the interstitial fluid. External respiration may be compromised by low atmospheric oxygen (e.g., high altitude) or poor alveolar ventilation (e.g., pneumonia). Internal and cellular respiration, by contrast, will be affected by anemia because less oxygen will be transferred from the capillary blood to the interstitium and cells. Another cause of defective cellular respiration is cyanide toxicity, which poisons the electron transport chain. Despite having "cyan" in its name, cyanosis, like carbon monoxide poisoning, can lead to a cherry red patient secondary to increased venous O_2. Be on the lookout for cyanide toxicity in a firefighter or patient with smoke inhalation injury.

STEP 1 SECRET

In a patient with smoke inhalation injury, be on the lookout for the three poisonings we've talked about: carbon monoxide poisoning, cyanide toxicity, and methemoglobinemia.

SUMMARY BOX: ANEMIA

- Presentation
  - Classic features include tachycardia, fatigue, dyspnea on exertion, and conjunctival pallor on physical examination without signs of cyanosis.
- Epidemiology
  - Can be seen in any patient prone to blood loss (women with menorrhagia), anyone prone to hemolysis (mechanical heart valves), or patients with familial hemoglobinopathies
- Diagnosis
  - Hemoglobin less than 14 mg/dL for males and 12 mg/dL for females
- Pathophysiology: Pa_{O_2} is the partial pressure of oxygen dissolved in arterial blood; it is also known as the oxygen tension. The PA_{O_2} is the alveolar oxygen tension.
  - The arterial oxygen content measures the total amount of oxygen in blood and is primarily determined by the concentration of hemoglobin (Hb).
  - The arterial oxygen saturation reflects the extent of Hb saturation with oxygen. It is determined by the Pa_{O_2}, with a higher Pa_{O_2} causing greater oxygen saturation, although many other factors (e.g., temperature, 2,3-diphosphoglycerate [DPG]) can influence the affinity of Hb for O_2.
  - Cyanosis is caused by the presence of at least 5 g/dL of deoxyhemoglobin. Severely anemic patients are not typically cyanotic if their Pa_{O_2} is normal.
  - Methemoglobinemia results from conditions associated with impaired ability of red blood cells (RBCs) to defend against oxidative stressors, such as pyruvate kinase and glucose-6-phosphate dehydrogenase (G6PD) deficiency or exposure to oxidizing agents such as benzocaine. Be on the lookout for the description of "chocolate-colored blood."
  - Carbon monoxide binds Hb avidly and prevents oxygen from dissociating from Hb. It therefore does not typically cause cyanosis or alter the Pa_{O_2}. Consider CO poisoning in any patient who has cherry red lips and nail beds.

CASE 2.9

A 35-year-old male victim of multiple blunt trauma is in shock because of splenic rupture. The patient undergoes surgery and is transferred to the intensive care unit (ICU). The next day, he becomes acutely short of breath. A chest x-ray shows diffuse bilateral pulmonary infiltrates, and arterial blood gas analysis reveals severe hypoxemia. A pulmonary artery catheter threaded through his superior vena cava (SVC), right atrium, and right ventricle and into his pulmonary artery shows a normal pulmonary capillary wedge pressure.

1. What is the anticipated diagnosis?
   He most likely has acute respiratory distress syndrome (ARDS). ARDS is the final common pathway reaction to various serious injuries to the lung. ARDS is diagnosed by the presence of acute-onset respiratory failure, bilateral diffuse pulmonary infiltrates, severe hypoxemia, and the coexistence of a disease known to cause it.

2. What are the etiology and pathogenesis of this disease?
   ARDS occurs secondary to a wide variety of causes, including sepsis, shock, severe pancreatitis, gastric aspiration, pneumonia, trauma, and near drowning. The common link in all these conditions is widespread pulmonary capillary endothelial damage. This leads to inflammation and fluid extravasation into the alveoli and interstitium, resulting in significant alveolar and interstitial edema and, consequently, severe hypoxemia.

3. What is the histology of this condition?
   Alveoli in ARDS are pink and thickened, an appearance called *hyaline membranes*. Hyaline membranes are proteinaceous alveolar exudates that line the periphery of alveoli (Fig. 2.12, *arrows*). Be able to recognize this pathognomonic image of ARDS. In the setting of ARDS, many alveoli are collapsed, while others are distended.

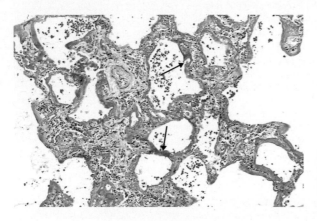

Figure 2.12. Diffuse alveolar damage of acute respiratory distress syndrome (ARDS); arrows indicate hyaline membranes. *(From Kumar V. Robbins and Cotran Pathologic Basis of Disease. 9th ed. Philadelphia: Elsevier Saunders; 2015: 669-726, Fig. 15-4.)*

4. How is this condition managed?
   ARDS is managed with supportive therapy with a ventilator to maintain oxygenation and treatment of the underlying disease that is causing it. Unfortunately, this condition can be very challenging to treat, in part because delivering a high Fio_2 (fraction of inspired oxygen) via a ventilator can produce damaging free radicals that further exacerbate the condition.

5. What is the diffusion equation, and which parameter is influenced most by the high concentration of inspired oxygen?
   Recall that the diffusion Eq. (2.8) relates an increase in diffusion rates (V_{gas}) to increases in the partial pressure gradient ($P_1 - P_2$) of a gas across the membrane, increased solubility of the gas (D), or an increased surface area (A) available for diffusion. It also relates increase in diffusion rate (V_{gas}) to decreases in membrane thickness (T), and vice versa. The high Fio_2 increases the partial pressure gradient of oxygen across the pulmonary membrane, which attenuates the reduction in diffusion that occurs because of the increased membrane thickness (from edema).

6. Both CHF and ARDS can cause significant pulmonary edema. How does the cause of pulmonary edema differ in these two settings?
   In CHF, increased hydrostatic pressure from fluid backing up in the pulmonary system causes pulmonary edema. Note that in this situation, the pulmonary capillary wedge pressure would be elevated from the fluid backup (typically as a result of a stiff left ventricle). In contrast, in ARDS, increased capillary permeability is the basis for the edema, so pulmonary capillary wedge pressure should be normal.

7. Why is it necessary to be particularly cautious in giving fluids to this patient?
   Excessive fluids can push someone into CHF. The resulting increase in pulmonary edema can seriously compromise already inadequate respiratory function (increased edema makes the diffusion barrier even thicker).

RELATED QUESTION

8. Using the diffusion equation, explain why each of the conditions in Table 2.6 is associated with hypoxemia.

Table 2.6. Conditions Causing Hypoxemia

CONDITION	EXPLANATION FOR HYPOXEMIA
Neuromuscular respiratory insufficiency	Decreased ventilation reduces change in pressure (ΔP)
Pulmonary edema	Increased thickness (T) of pulmonary membrane/diffusion barrier
Emphysema	Reduced surface area (A) of pulmonary membrane from alveolar degradation Reduced pressure gradient (ΔP) from impaired ventilation
Pneumonia	Decreased oxygen diffusion due to pulmonary edema (i.e., T increases in diffusion equation) and reduced "available" surface area (A) of pulmonary membrane
Asthma	Reduced pressure (ΔP) secondary to ventilatory insufficiency
Neonatal respiratory distress syndrome	Reduced surfactant increases surface tension in alveoli, causing alveoli to collapse, impairing ventilation (ΔP) and reducing surface area (A) of pulmonary membrane
Acute respiratory distress syndrome (i.e., diffuse alveolar damage)	Presence of diffuse pulmonary infiltrates increases thickness (T) of pulmonary membrane

SUMMARY BOX: ACUTE RESPIRATORY DISTRESS SYNDROME

- Presentation
  - A patient with acute respiratory distress syndrome (ARDS) will have progressive hypoxemia despite oxygen therapy.
- Epidemiology
  - Suspect ARDS in patients who are in the intensive care unit (ICU), especially those who have sepsis, pancreatitis, or shock.
- Diagnosis
  - Bilateral lung opacification on CXR of unclear etiology following lung insult
  - Hypoxemia is almost always present
- Treatment
  - Mechanical ventilation in the ICU
  - Supportive care (e.g., mechanical ventilation) and treatment of the underlying condition

CASE 2.10

A 75-year-old woman with a 90-pack-year history of cigarette smoking reports a 6-month history of hemoptysis, shortness of breath, fatigue, and an unintentional 30-lb weight loss. Chest x-ray reveals increased anteroposterior (AP) diameter and flattening of the diaphragm and also reveals a large mass in her right upper lobe. Biopsy establishes that the mass is malignant. Laboratory tests show plasma sodium of 125 mEq/L (normal range is 135–145 mEq/L) and urine osmolarity of 450 mOsm.

1, What type of lung cancer does this woman likely have?
   Small cell carcinoma of the lung is most likely. Various paraneoplastic syndromes can occur in the setting of lung cancer. The syndrome of inappropriate secretion of antidiuretic hormone (SIADH) is most commonly observed in small cell lung carcinoma. Hypercalcemia is more characteristic of squamous cell carcinoma. This woman's hyperosmolar urine in a setting of hyponatremia is consistent with SIADH, which makes small cell carcinoma more probable.

STEP 1 SECRET

The USMLE frequently presents paraneoplastic syndromes, especially those related to lung cancers! Be sure that you can recognize symptoms of paraneoplastic syndromes caused by various malignancies.

2. **If a patient with small cell carcinoma develops bilateral ptosis (droopy eyelids), as well as neuro-muscular weakness, what paraneoplastic syndrome should be suspected?**
Lambert-Eaton syndrome occurs quite frequently in small cell carcinoma. It results from antibodies that attack the voltage-gated calcium channels on the terminal bouton of presynaptic motor neurons. Remember that myasthenia gravis and Lambert-Eaton affect different sites of the motor neuron. The best way to remember this is that L comes before M. Lambert-Eaton is presynaptic, and myasthenia gravis is postsynaptic.

3. **If a lung tumor is growing at the apex of the lung and compressing the cervical sympathetic chain on that side, what manifestations might one see?**
The cervical sympathetic chain supplies the superior tarsal muscle (which elevates the eyelid), the dilator pupillae, and the sweat glands of the face. Therefore cutting off this nerve supply results in ipsilateral ptosis, miosis, and anhydrosis (i.e., Horner syndrome). Note the distinction from Lambert-Eaton syndrome, in which the ptosis is bilateral.
   Note: Tumors in the apex of the lung are known as *Pancoast tumors.* They are most commonly seen with squamous cell carcinoma of the lung. Another commonly seen complication of lung tumors is SVC syndrome (often associated with small cell carcinoma), in which the SVC is compressed by the growing tumor. This impairs venous drainage from the head and upper limbs, resulting in swelling and purple discoloration of the arms and face.

4. **What are the two principal classifications of lung cancer, and how does this affect treatment?**
Small cell lung cancer (SCLC) and non–small cell lung cancer (NSCLC) are the two principal classifications. The therapeutic and prognostic considerations do not differ for subtypes of non–small cell cancers, and all are generally treated with surgery. Small cell carcinomas can almost never be surgically resected but respond transiently to radiation therapy. (See Case 10.4 in Chapter 10, Oncology, for more information.)

5. **How can squamous cell carcinoma cause hypercalcemia without any bony metastases?**
This type of lung cancer is known to release parathyroid hormone–related peptide (PTHrP), which stimulates bone resorption in much the same fashion as parathyroid hormone (PTH) does.

DIFFERENTIAL DIAGNOSIS

6. **If a patient with small cell carcinoma has hypertension, hypernatremia, hypokalemia, abdominal striae, and a "buffalo hump," what should be suspected?**
Cushing syndrome should be suspected due to ectopic adrenocorticotropic hormone (ACTH) production, another common paraneoplastic syndrome in small cell carcinoma.

SUMMARY BOX: SMALL CELL CANCER OF THE LUNG

- Presentation
  - Dyspnea; rapid, unexplained weight loss; and any symptoms caused by a paraneoplastic syndrome
- Diagnosis
  - Chest x-ray study, computed tomography (CT) scan, and biopsy. Various paraneoplastic syndromes such as syndrome of inappropriate secretion of antidiuretic hormone (SIADH) are associated with small cell carcinoma.
- Pathology
  - Cells are generally small, have little cytoplasm, and are round or oval, often resembling lymphocytes. Small cell cancer of the lung is also called *oat cell cancer* because of its appearance.
- Treatment
  - Small cell cancers often metastasize quickly and are therefore not amenable to resection. They are, however, responsive to radiation.

CASE 2.11

A 38-year-old woman presents for evaluation of a several-week history of nonproductive cough and shortness of breath with exertion. She also reports generalized fatigue, night sweats, and unintentional weight loss. Physical examination reveals erythematous cutaneous nodules on the lower extremities and mild hepatosplenomegaly. A chest x-ray shows bilateral hilar lymphadenopathy. Blood work reveals hypercalcemia.

1. **What must be included in the differential diagnosis?**
Both lymphoma and sarcoidosis must be included in the differential diagnosis.

CASE 2.11 CONTINUED:

These findings prompt the physician to request a mediastinal lymph node biopsy, which reveals noncaseating granulomas.

2. Now what is the most likely diagnosis?

Sarcoidosis, a systemic granulomatous disease of unknown cause, is the most likely diagnosis. Common features in exam question stems are hilar lymphadenopathy, hypercalcemia, and noncaseating granulomas. Sarcoidosis is three to four times more common in African Americans than in Caucasians.

STEP 1 SECRET

Sarcoidosis is a commonly tested topic for Step 1. Be able to recognize the symptoms of sarcoidosis, hilar lymphadenopathy on x-ray, and the appearance of granulomas on an image.

3. How can sarcoidosis cause cor pulmonale (right ventricular failure)?<

As an inflammatory pulmonary disease, sarcoidosis can cause widespread pulmonary fibrosis with obliteration of the pulmonary vascular bed, resulting in significant pulmonary hypertension. The pulmonary vasoconstriction that occurs in hypoxemia from pulmonary fibrosis may also contribute to this process.

4. How is pulmonary hypertension defined?

Normal pulmonary artery pressure is between 10 and 14 mm Hg. In pulmonary hypertension, the pulmonary artery pressure increases to greater than 25 mm Hg at rest or 35 mm Hg during exercise. This increase in the pulmonary artery pressure can cause atherosclerosis, medial hypertrophy, and intimal fibrosis of the pulmonary arteries.

5. What is the difference between primary and secondary pulmonary hypertension?

Primary pulmonary hypertension is due to an inactivating mutation in the *BMPR2* gene. The *BMPR2* gene normally acts to inhibit vascular smooth muscle proliferation. Primary pulmonary hypertension is often observed in young women.

Secondary pulmonary hypertension, on the other hand, is a consequence of chronic lung disease that is distinct from pulmonary hypertension itself. Examples include the destruction of lung parenchyma seen in COPD, the increase in pulmonary resistance seen in mitral stenosis, the decrease in cross-sectional area of the pulmonary vasculature bed seen with recurrent thromboemboli or hypoxic vasoconstriction, and the inflammation and medial hypertrophy seen with certain autoimmune diseases (e.g., sarcoidosis).

6. How can sarcoidosis cause a restrictive cardiomyopathy?

Granulomatous infiltration of the myocardium can cause fibrosis and reduced ventricular compliance. This is fairly similar to the pathogenesis of restrictive cardiomyopathy that develops from infiltration in amyloidosis and hemochromatosis.

Note: Because elevated levels of angiotensin-converting enzyme (ACE) are frequently associated with sarcoidosis, the diagnostic workup often includes a measurement of serum ACE. The hypercalcemia that develops in sarcoidosis is due to increased production of 1,25-dihydroxyvitamin D_3 by the macrophages in granulomas. Sarcoidosis is also associated with Bell palsy.

SUMMARY BOX: SARCOIDOSIS

- Symptoms
  - May be generalized or focused depending upon the organ(s) involved. With lung involvement, dyspnea on exertion and wheezing may be present. Skin changes including erythema nodosum, plaques, maculopapular eruptions, and subcutaneous nodules appear commonly. Anterior uveitis and polyarthritis also may be present.
- Diagnosis
  - Based on clinical (see symptoms), radiologic (bilateral hilar lymphadenopathy), and histologic findings (noncaseating granulomas)
- Pathology
  - Noncaseating granulomas that can involve almost any organ system
- Treatment
  - Glucocorticoids are the first-line treatment followed by chemotherapeutic agents based upon the organ system and extent of involvement.

CASE 2.12

A 27-year-old man who is stabbed in the chest in a bar fight is taken to the emergency department by ambulance. He is conscious with rapid breathing (tachypnea), hypotension, and pleuritic chest pain. There is tracheal deviation to the left, jugular venous distention, right-sided hyperresonance to percussion, and decreased breath sounds over the right lung. A chest x-ray shows decreased vascular markings on the right side. A needle thoracostomy is performed immediately to decompress the lung, and then a chest tube is inserted to stabilize breathing.

1. **What is the diagnosis?**

   A pneumothorax is the diagnosis. More specifically, because this patient has tracheal deviation to the opposite side of the affected lung, he likely has a tension pneumothorax. Note that spontaneous pneumothorax normally causes tracheal deviation to the same side of the collapsed lung to fill the pleural space now unused by the lung. Tension pneumothorax is typically caused by penetrating injuries to the chest wall that cause defects in either parietal or visceral pleura, allowing air into the pleural cavity during inspiration. In a tension pneumothorax, the defect serves as a one-way valve, allowing air to enter but not exit. Increased intrathoracic pressure causes mediastinal shifting and compression of the SVC and inferior vena cava. Compression of these vessels causes reduced venous return. Reduced venous return results in cardiac and pulmonary symptoms, explaining the signs of tracheal deviation, jugular venous distention, and hypotension.

2. **Why should the chest tube be inserted immediately superior to the lower rib in the intercostal space in which it is inserted?**

   This position is necessary to avoid the neurovascular bundle (from top to bottom: vein, artery, nerve) that runs on the inferior aspect of each rib.

3. **What is the pressure inside the pleural cavity (intrapleural space) normally?**

   The pleural pressure is normally negative, which helps maintain the lungs in expanded form. When either the visceral or parietal pleura is punctured, the influx of air under atmospheric pressure abolishes the vacuum and results in a positive intrapleural pressure, which collapses the lung.

4. **How does hypoxia-induced vasoconstriction help compensate, to some extent, for the respiratory dysfunction caused by pneumothorax?**

   The blood that would ordinarily go to the collapsed (hypoxic) lung gets shunted to the opposite lung. This shunting reduces local $\dot{V}/\dot{Q}$ mismatch and subsequent hypoxemia.

5. **Is this patient more likely to be experiencing respiratory acidosis or respiratory alkalosis? Explain.**

   Decreased effective ventilation secondary to a collapsed lung will cause hypercapnia and respiratory acidosis.

   Note: A pneumothorax can cause a *mixed* respiratory and metabolic acidosis because of both impaired ventilation, which increases plasma CO_2 levels, and increased anaerobic metabolism in the tissues from reduced oxygen delivery, which increases plasma levels of acids such as lactic acid.

6. **What effect will a pneumothorax have on the serum ionized calcium level?**

   A pneumothorax will increase the serum ionized calcium level because acidosis causes displacement of calcium from binding sites on albumin (via increased competition with hydrogen ions for these binding sites). In contrast, alkalosis leads to the ionized form of albumin, which can bind free calcium and reduce serum ionized calcium concentrations. Hypoalbuminemia also results in low levels of serum ionized calcium secondary to increased affinity of albumin for calcium.

SUMMARY BOX: PNEUMOTHORAX

- Symptoms
  - Sudden onset of severe dyspnea with sharp pain in one's side
- Diagnosis
  - The trachea and mediastinum will shift away from the side of the pneumothorax. Physical signs include a distended unilateral chest, hyperresonance, and absence of breath sounds.
- Pathology
  - Commonly associated with emphysema, asthma, connective tissue disorders such as Marfan syndrome, and trauma, so the pathologic features vary according to the cause
- Treatment
  - Insert chest tube, stabilize breathing, and treat underlying cause.

CHAPTER 3

NEPHROLOGY

Insider's Guide to Nephrology for the USMLE Step 1
Nephrology can be a tricky subject for many medical students because mastering renal physiology requires comfort with and even manipulation of several formulas. Luckily, the scope of nephrology-related questions on the USMLE tends to be somewhat limited. Focus heavily on the subjects listed in First Aid and then use the cases in this chapter to test your understanding of the material. Be sure to understand detailed principles regarding nephron function and activation of the renin-angiotensin-aldosterone system. Concerning renal pathology, commonly tested subjects include renal failure, nephritic versus nephrotic syndromes, urinary tract infections (UTIs), and nephrolithiasis.

BASIC CONCEPTS

1. What are the major functions of the kidney?

   The kidney's major functions are regulation of body fluid volume, osmolality, electrolyte balance, acid-base balance, and hormone synthesis. It accomplishes these functions by recycling the body's extracellular fluid many times per day and removing/excreting unneeded and/or toxic substances and reclaiming needed substances. For example, the vast majority of filtered water, sodium, and bicarbonate are normally reclaimed by the body. However, in certain situations, the kidneys can substantially alter the handling of these substances. The kidneys also play an important endocrine function, synthesizing vitamin D and the hormone renin.

2. Describe the gross anatomic features of the kidney in Fig. 3.1.

   The kidneys are paired organs that lie in the retroperitoneal space. The kidney is surrounded by a fibrous capsule covering an *outer cortex* and an *inner medulla*. The cortex and medulla primarily consist of *nephrons*, the functional units of the kidneys, of which there are approximately 1 million per kidney. The medulla divides into structures known as *renal pyramids*, the apices of which terminate in papillae. The papillae are located at the cusp of the inner medulla and drain into pouches called *minor and major calyces*, which eventually lead to the *renal pelvis* (the upper portion of the ureter).

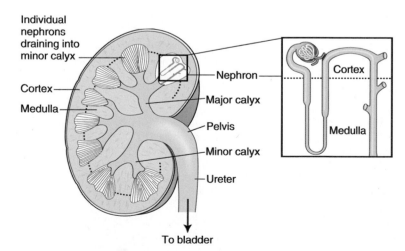

Figure 3.1. Structure of the kidney. The *inset* shows the location of the nephron. *(From Brown TA. Rapid Review Physiology. 2nd ed. Philadelphia: Mosby; 2012, Fig. 6-1.)*

3. Describe the vascular supply of the nephron in Fig. 3.2.

   To continuously recycle the plasma and, by extension, the entire extracellular fluid compartment, the kidneys receive approximately 20% to 25% of the cardiac output despite making up less than 2% of body weight. The blood supply to the kidneys comes from the renal arteries, which stem from the abdominal aorta. The renal arteries branch into

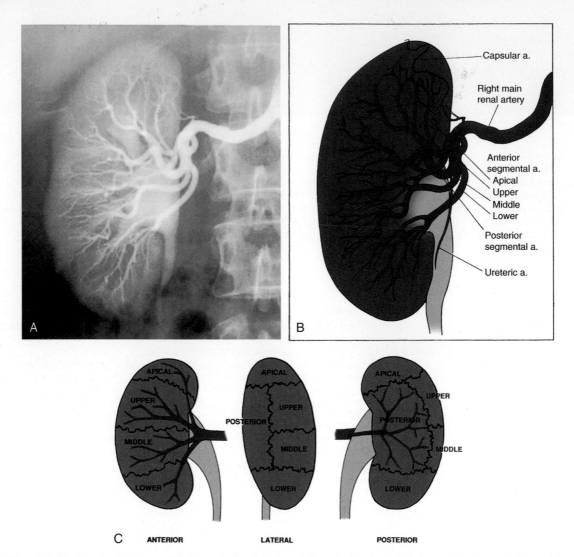

Figure 3.2. Blood supply of the kidney. A–B, Segmental branches of the right renal artery demonstrated by renal angiogram. C, Segmental circulation diagram of right kidney. D, Intrarenal arterial anatomy. *(From Partin AW. Campbell-Walsh Urology. 12th ed. Philadelphia: Elsevier; 2021:1865-1876.e1, Fig. 84-16, eFig. 84-17.)*

segmental arteries, which further divide into interlobar arteries (not to be mistaken with interlobular arteries). These give rise to the arcuate arteries, which lie between the renal cortex and medulla and arc around the outside of the renal pyramids. Arcuate arteries give off cortical radial arteries, which are also known as interlobular arteries. Cortical radial arteries end in capillary networks, but they also give off lateral branches that become afferent arterioles. Afferent arterioles lead into the glomerular capillaries, efferent arterioles, peritubular capillaries (surround proximal and distal tubules in the cortex), and vasa recta (descend to the loop of Henle in the medulla).

Clinical Pearl

The vasa recta perfuse the renal papillae at a very slow rate to maintain the countercurrent mechanism, the process of generating an osmotic gradient in order to absorb water from the tubular fluid to concentrate urine. Also, oxygen content in the papillae tends to be lower than in other parts of the kidney. This combination of relative hypoxemia and slow blood flow predisposes the papillae to thrombosis and ischemic papillary necrosis, characterized clinically by flank pain and gross hematuria. Myriad conditions can cause renal papillary necrosis, including **P**yelonephritis, **O**bstructive nephropathy, **S**ickle cell crisis, **T**uberculosis, **C**hronic liver disease, **A**nalgesics, **R**enal transplant rejection, **D**iabetes, and **S**ystemic vasculitis; think POSTCARDS.

4. **What are the filtration forces at the level of the glomerulus that determine the glomerular filtration rate?**

   Filtration forces at the glomerulus include the hydrostatic pressure in the glomerular capillaries and the Bowman space, as well as oncotic pressure in the glomerular capillary and the Bowman capsule. The glomerular filtration rate (GFR) represents the summation of all nephrons' filtration rates within both kidneys, indicating how well the kidneys are functioning. The formula for GFR is shown in Eq. 3.1 (Fig. 3.3).

   $$GFR = K_f ([P_G] - [\Pi_G + P_B])$$ [3.1]

   where
   K_f = filtration coefficient, a constant
   P_G = hydrostatic pressure in the glomerular capillaries
   P_B = hydrostatic pressure in the Bowman space
   Π_G = oncotic pressure in the glomerular capillaries
   Π_B = oncotic pressure in the Bowman space (omitted because proteins are not filtered; normally, this is zero)
   Individual forces can be affected in pathologic states. For example, minimal change disease can increase the oncotic pressure in the Bowman space (Π_B) by increasing the protein content within the space. Obstructive nephropathy can decrease the Bowman hydrostatic pressure (P_B). Hypertension can increase the glomerular hydrostatic pressure (P_G), and hypoalbuminemia can decrease the glomerular oncotic pressure (Π_G).

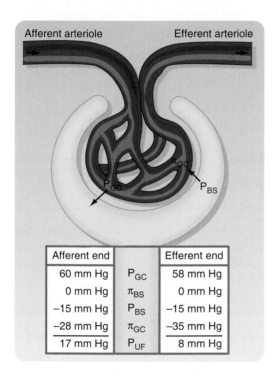

Afferent end		Efferent end
60 mm Hg	P_{GC}	58 mm Hg
0 mm Hg	π_{BS}	0 mm Hg
−15 mm Hg	P_{BS}	−15 mm Hg
−28 mm Hg	π_{GC}	−35 mm Hg
17 mm Hg	P_{UF}	8 mm Hg

Figure 3.3. Filtration forces at the glomerulus. π_{BS}, Oncotic pressure in the Bowman space; π_{GC}, oncotic pressure in the glomerular capillaries; P_{BS}, hydrostatic pressure in the Bowman space; P_{GC}, hydrostatic pressure in glomerular capillary; P_{UF}, net ultrafiltration pressure. *(From Koeppen BM, Stanton BA. Berne and Levy Physiology. 7th ed. Philadelphia: Elsevier; 2018: 581-602, Fig. 33-17.)*

5. **How does the renal *clearance* of a substance relative to GFR provide information about the renal handling (i.e., secretion, reabsorption) of that substance?**

   After filtration at the glomerulus, as substances travel down the nephron, their tubular concentration may vary due to *net* secretion or reabsorption. The clearance value for a given substance provides useful information about the renal handling of that substance (Fig. 3.4). Substances are generally handled in three ways.

   A substance such as inulin, which is filtered completely at the glomerulus but neither reabsorbed nor secreted (much like creatinine), will have a renal clearance that approximates GFR. By contrast, urea is significantly reabsorbed along the nephron and will have a clearance less than GFR because much of the filtered urea is returned to the plasma. Substances with net secretion will have clearance rates greater than GFR because they are removed from the filtered plasma at the glomerulus and unfiltered plasma in the peritubular capillaries (Fig. 3.5).

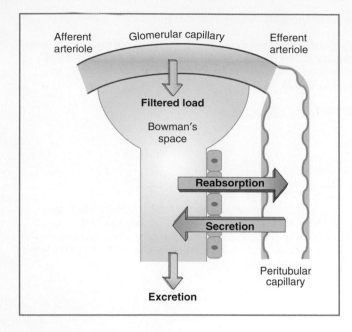

Figure 3.4. Filtration, reabsorption, and secretion along the nephron. *(Adapted from Costanzo LS.* Physiology. *6th ed. Philadelphia: Elsevier; 2018: 245-310, Fig. 6.12.)*

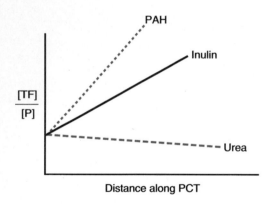

Figure 3.5. Because of the reabsorption of water, the tubular fluid concentration of inulin increases roughly threefold compared with plasma concentration along the proximal convoluted tubule (PCT). Because inulin is neither secreted nor reabsorbed, substances that become concentrated more than inulin (e.g., PAH) are secreted, and substances that become less concentrated than inulin (e.g., urea) are reabsorbed. *[P],* Plasma concentration; *PAH,* para-aminohippuric acid; *[TF],* tubular fluid concentration. *(From Brown TA.* Rapid Review Physiology. *2nd ed. Philadelphia: Mosby; 2012, Fig. 6-12.)*

6. **Why does creatinine clearance from the plasma reasonably approximate GFR?**
   Recall that creatinine is continuously formed as a breakdown product in skeletal muscle and released into the bloodstream. Similar to inulin, it is freely filtered at the glomerulus and neither reabsorbed nor secreted significantly. In actuality, creatinine is slightly secreted but is a good approximation for GFR and therefore renal function [i.e., ability to remove toxins from the blood]. The amount filtered across the glomerulus (PCr × GFR) is approximately equal to the amount that is excreted in urine (UCr × V) (see Fig. 3.6).

7. **How is renal blood flow regulated, and what are the interrelationships between renal blood flow, GFR, and filtration fraction?**
   The kidneys autoregulate renal blood flow over a wide range of systemic arterial pressure by altering the resistance in the afferent and efferent arterioles. If systemic arterial pressure and therefore renal artery pressure drops, the resulting reduction in renal plasma flow will prompt moderate constriction of the efferent arteriole. This compensatory mechanism increases glomerular hydrostatic pressure and filtration fraction to minimize any reduction in GFR (Fig. 3.7 and Table 3.1).
   Note: More details on this concept are found in Chapter 4 (Fluids and Electrolytes).

Clinical Pearl

Prostaglandins are potent vasodilators that help counter-regulate the vasoconstrictor effects induced by angiotensin II (Ang II) and the sympathetic nervous system (SNS). Because nonsteroidal antiinflammatory drugs (NSAIDs) block the production of prostaglandins, they can cause renal injury at high doses as a result of severe decreases in renal blood flow.

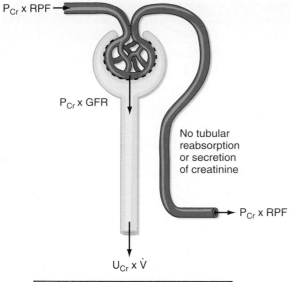

P_{Cr} x RPF

P_{Cr} x GFR

No tubular
reabsorption
or secretion
of creatinine

P_{Cr} x RPF

U_{Cr} x $\dot{V}$

| Amount filtered | = | Amount excreted |
| P_{Cr} x GFR | | U_{Cr} x $\dot{V}$ |

Figure 3.6. Renal handling of creatinine. *GFR,* Glomerular filtration rate; *P_{Cr},* plasma creatinine concentration; *RPF,* renal plasma flow; *U_{Cr},* urine creatinine concentration; *$\dot{V}$,* volume of urine produced. *(From Koeppen BM, Stanton BA. Berne and Levy Physiology. 7th ed. Philadelphia: Elsevier; 2018: 581-602, Fig. 33.13.)*

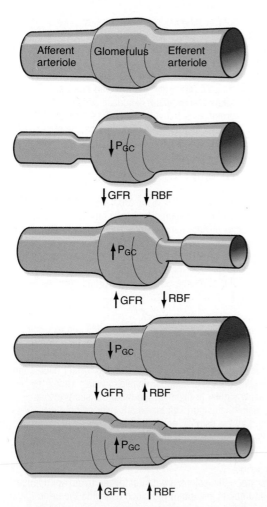

Afferent
arteriole

Glomerulus

Efferent
arteriole

↓P_{GC}

↓GFR ↓RBF

↑P_{GC}

↑GFR ↓RBF

↓P_{GC}

↓GFR ↑RBF

↑P_{GC}

↑GFR ↑RBF

Figure 3.7. Effects of afferent and efferent vasoconstriction on glomerular forces and glomerular filtration rate (GFR). *P_{GC},* Hydrostatic pressure in glomerular capillary; *RBF,* renal blood flow. *(From Koeppen BM, Stanton BA. Berne and Levy Physiology. Philadelphia: Elsevier; 1994: 581-602, Fig. 33.21.)*

Table 3.1. Regulation of RPF, GFR, and Filtration Fraction

EFFECT	RPF	GFR	FILTRATION FRACTION (GFR/RPF)
Constriction of afferent arteriole	↓	↓	No change
Constriction of efferent arteriole	↓	↑	↑

GFR, Glomerular filtration rate; *RPF,* renal plasma flow.

8. **In brief, what are the functions of the major nephron segments? What hormones act on these segments?**

The filtered load enters the tubules at the Bowman capsule. It traverses the systems in the following order: proximal tubule, thick ascending limb of the loop of Henle, distal tubule, and collecting ducts.

Proximal tubule. The proximal tubule participates in the majority of solute reabsorption via isosmotic reabsorption of solutes and water through the action of Na-glucose, Na-amino acid, Na-phosphate active cotransport, and Na-H exchange. As solutes are reabsorbed at the proximal tubule, the interstitium becomes hyperosmotic while the tubular fluid becomes dilute and hypoosmotic. Water is isosmotically reabsorbed because of the permeability of proximal tubular cells. Therefore increased sodium reabsorption at the proximal tubule leads to increased water reabsorption. Ang II regulates Na-H exchange, increasing Na^+ reabsorption and H^+ excretion. Atrial natriuretic peptide (ANP) decreases Na^+ reabsorption. Parathyroid hormone (PTH) inhibits the action of Na-phosphate cotransport.

Thick ascending loop of Henle (TALH). The TALH reabsorbs solute through the Na-K-2Cl symporter (triporter). The TALH is impermeable to water, leading to dilution of the tubular fluid, and is essential to the countercurrent exchange mechanism. Regulation of the TALH is flow-dependent (increased flow leads to increased solute reabsorption).

Distal tubule. The initial segment of the distal tubule is water-impermeable and reabsorbs NaCl via Na-Cl cotransport to further dilute tubular fluid. PTH works at the distal tubule to promote calcium absorption. The late distal tubule contains principal cells and intercalated cells (see subsequent discussion). Regulation of the distal tubule is flow-dependent (increased flow leads to increased solute reabsorption).

Collecting duct. The collecting duct is composed of two cell types: principal cells and intercalated cells. Principal cells reabsorb sodium through epithelial sodium channels (ENaC), secrete potassium, and are involved in water reabsorption. Aldosterone stimulates the opening of ENaC, leading to sodium reabsorption. Increased sodium reabsorption through ENaC causes a negative luminal potential, which promotes (positively charged) potassium secretion. Antidiuretic hormone (ADH) leads to water reabsorption at the collecting duct through the insertion of aquaporins in the basolateral membrane of principal cells. Intercalated cells secrete either H^+ (α-intercalated cells) or bicarbonate (β-intercalated cells) and play a critical role in acid-base balance (see Chapter 5, Acid-Base Balance).

9. **What is the countercurrent exchange mechanism, and how does it allow for the creation of dilute or concentrated urine?**

The *countercurrent exchange mechanism* refers to the spatial relationship of the TALH, distal tubule, and collecting duct and their blood supply, the *vasa recta.* One must remember that water moves between cells based on osmotic forces to understand the creation of dilute and concentrated urine. A hyperosmolar environment will draw water out of the tubules and therefore concentrate the urine. The body adjusts water reabsorption and, by extension, urine concentration by regulating how much water is allowed to leave the tubules by altering their permeability. As urine passes through the tubules, solutes and water are reabsorbed as described in question 1. Recall that the TALH is impermeable to water; therefore, only solute (NaCl) is reabsorbed, leaving dilute urine in the tubules. As the solute is reabsorbed, this creates a hyperosmotic interstitium in the medulla (Fig. 3.8).

10. **What is the role of ADH in the production of concentrated or dilute urine?**

In the deep medulla, the interstitial osmolality reaches 1200 mOsm/L, while in the cortex, the osmolality approximates 300 mOsm/L (same as plasma). In the deep medulla, where maximum solute reabsorption has occurred, the urine's osmolality is around 1200 mOsm/L; however, when it reaches the water-permeable cortex, it is normally equilibrated with plasma. Further solute reabsorption can occur in the distal tubule after an excess water load and further dilutes the urine to 30 to 60 mOsm/L. Under normal circumstances, the collecting duct is also impermeable to water. Therefore without modification, the kidney will produce urine with an osmolality similar to plasma (300 mOsm/L; see previous discussion). However, with the release of ADH (see previous discussion), aquaporin channels are inserted onto the luminal membrane of collecting duct cells, and water is reabsorbed by the osmotic action of the previously mentioned hyperosmolar medullary interstitium. Therefore the maximum urine osmolality is around 1200 to 1400 mOsm/L (Figs. 3.9 and 3.10).

11. **Differentiate between nephritic and nephrotic syndrome.**

Nephritis indicates inflammation of the nephron. Thus glomerular nephritic lesions are characterized by an abundance of leukocytes. Inflammation leads to injury of glomerular walls, promoting escape of red blood cells into the urine

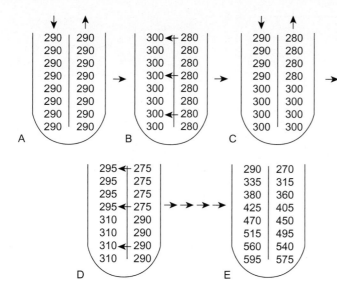

Figure 3.8. Countercurrent exchange system. A, In a countercurrent system with a hairpin bend (e.g., the loop of Henle), the fluid begins isosmolar throughout both the descending and ascending limbs. B, Active transport of solutes from the ascending lumen through the interstitium to the descending lumen creates a single effect transverse gradient across the interstitium between the limbs (20 mOsm/kg H_2O). C, Fluid continues to flow down the descending limb and up the ascending limb. D, Active transport from the ascending limb continues. The transverse gradient is reestablished (20 mOsm/kg H_2O). E, The cycle of panel C and panel D is repeated over and over. The bottom of the loop progressively increases in osmolality so that the vertical gradient (Panel E: bottom of loop 575–595 vs. top of loop 270–290) far exceeds the transverse gradient (still 20 mOsm/kg H_2O). For the countercurrent mechanism to work efficiently, two requirements must be met: the fluid must be moving slowly, and the two vertical "limbs" of the "U" must be contiguous. *(From Sands JM, Layton HE. Seldin and Giebisch's The Kidney. 5th ed. London: Elsevier; 2013: 1463-1510, Fig. 43.7.)*

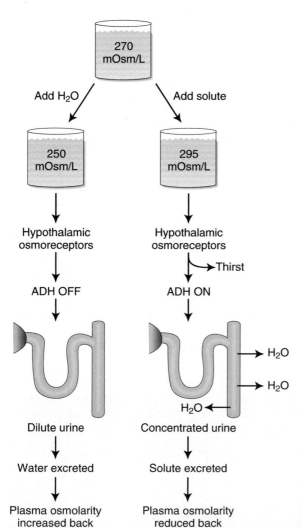

Figure 3.9. Renal response to water and solute loads. The addition of water decreases plasma osmolality, which triggers the hypothalamic osmoreceptors to turn off the production of antidiuretic hormone (ADH), which results in the excretion of the excess water as dilute urine. The addition of solute increases plasma osmolality. This triggers ADH release, which stimulates thirst and the reabsorption of water in the collecting duct by insertion of aquaporins. *(From Brown TA. Rapid Review Physiology. 2nd ed. Philadelphia: Mosby; 2012, Fig. 6-29.)*

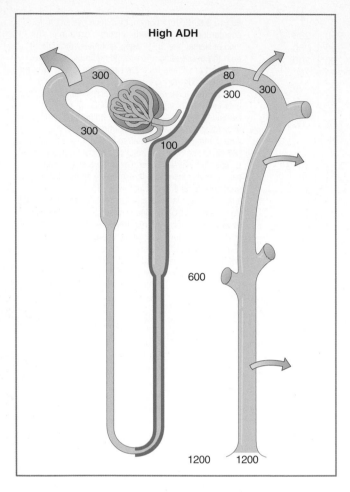

High ADH

300

300

300

80
300 300

100

600

1200   1200

Figure 3.10. Production of concentrated urine with the presence of ADH. *ADH,* Antidiuretic hormone. *(From Costanzo L. Physiology. 6th ed. Philadelphia: Elsevier; 2018: 245-310, Fig. 6.42.)*

(in the form of casts). Damage to the nephron also leads to decreased urine output and proteinuria (up to 3 g/day). However, proteinuria is much more severe in nephrotic syndrome (see later). Nephritic syndrome is also associated with hypertension as a result of excess fluid retention. The hallmark of nephrotic syndrome is "nephrotic range proteinuria," or more than 3 g of protein spilled into the urine within 24 hours. Because of protein loss in the urine, nephrotic patients have signs of hypoalbuminemia (low blood protein). Applying the principle of Starling forces (see Chapter 4), a decrease in intravascular oncotic pressure (due to the low albumin) will promote water loss from the vasculature, leading to edema. Morning periorbital edema is a huge clue to a nephrotic process. Because the intravascular oncotic pressure decreases, the liver compensates by increasing lipoproteins production, leading to hyperlipidemia.

The signs and symptoms of nephritic versus nephrotic syndrome are summarized in Table 3.2.

Table 3.2. Signs and Symptoms of Nephritic and Nephrotic Syndrome

NEPHRITIC SYNDROME	NEPHROTIC SYNDROME
Hematuria	Proteinuria (>3 g in 24 hr)
Hypertension	Edema
Low level proteinuria	Hyperlipidemia
Decreased urine output	Lipiduria
	Hypoalbuminemia

STEP 1 SECRET

It is important to be able to distinguish between nephritic and nephrotic syndromes based on a question stem. Understanding the differences between nephritis and nephrosis will allow quick elimination of wrong answer choices come test day.

CASE 3.1

A 78-year-old man is evaluated for a several-day history of lower abdominal pain. He admits to urinary difficulties over the last few years, including difficulty initiating his urinary stream, weak stream, waking several times at night to urinate (nocturia), and postvoid dribbling. He notes that he has not urinated in the past 2 days. He denies taking any tricyclic antidepressants, antipsychotics, antihistamines, or sympathomimetic agents. On physical examination, his bladder is palpably enlarged, and a digital rectal examination reveals an enlarged prostate. Microscopic urine examination shows no hematuria or crystalluria. Plasma creatinine is significantly elevated. Abdominal ultrasound reveals a markedly distended bladder and enlargement of the renal pelvises.

1. What is the probable cause of this patient's problems?

   This patient has acute urinary retention, most likely secondary to occlusion of the bladder neck by benign prostatic hyperplasia (BPH). The elevated plasma creatinine concentration strongly suggests acute kidney injury (AKI).

2. What are the three etiologic classifications of AKI?

   AKI is classified as prerenal, renal (intrinsic), or postrenal (obstructive). This man's AKI clearly has an obstructive etiology. In this case, acute bladder distention caused by long-standing BPH caused urine to back up to the kidneys, resulting in bilateral hydronephrosis (dilated renal pelvises) and AKI. Fig. 3.11 shows severe hydronephrosis from long-standing obstruction, with marked dilatation of the renal pelvis and calyces and loss of cortical parenchyma.

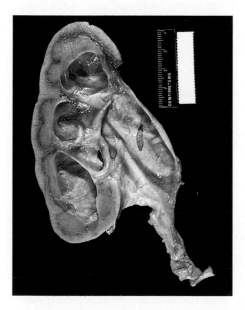

Figure 3.11. Hydronephrosis of the kidney, with marked dilation of the pelvis and calyces and thinning of the renal parenchyma. *(From Kumar V, Abbas AK, Aster JC. Robbins and Cotran Pathologic Basis of Disease. 9th ed. Philadelphia: Elsevier Saunders; 2015: 897-957, Fig. 20-48.)*

3. Why was reviewing the medication list so important in this patient?

   Multiple classes of drugs can cause urinary retention secondary to cholinergic blockade, which inhibits contraction of the detrusor muscle. Tricyclic antidepressants (e.g., amitriptyline, imipramine), phenothiazine antipsychotics (including low-potency "typical" antipsychotics such as chlorpromazine and thioridazine), and first-generation antihistamines (e.g., diphenhydramine) are all older "dirty" agents that act on a multitude of receptor types, including muscarinic acetylcholine receptors. Anticholinergic actions such as dry mouth, constipation, and urinary retention are possible side effects of these medications. Recall that the detrusor muscle of the bladder is stimulated to contract by parasympathetic (cholinergic) innervation. The anticholinergic agent atropine has a similar effect. The anticholinergic effects of the widely used agents oxybutynin and tolterodine are used therapeutically to control urge incontinence. Sympathomimetics (e.g., oral decongestants such as pseudoephedrine), on the other hand, can cause urinary retention by increasing α-adrenergic tone of the internal urethral sphincter. Opiates (i.e., narcotics) have many anticholinergic-like side effects (in addition to constipation, pupillary constriction, etc.) and can cause acute urinary retention when given in high doses.

SUMMARY BOX: OBSTRUCTIVE ACUTE KIDNEY INJURY

- Epidemiology: Common in older men with benign prostatic hyperplasia (BPH)
- Presentation: Sudden-onset suprapubic or abdominal pain with inability to urinate
- Pathophysiology: Typically from detrusor blockage from BPH but can be due to neurogenic bladder, medication side effects, or even (rarely) bilateral obstructing nephrolithiasis
- Diagnosis: Suggestive history, enlarged bladder on exam, hydronephrosis on ultrasound or computed tomography (CT), and prompt emptying of the bladder upon catheterization
- Treatment: Depends on the cause; alpha-blockers such as tamsulosin are commonly used to relax the detrusor neck and prostate, and in rare cases, transurethral resection of the prostate (TURP) or other surgical intervention is needed

---

CASE 3.2

A 68-year-old man unexpectedly collapses and is rushed to the hospital via ambulance and is found to have ruptured an abdominal aortic aneurysm. During surgery, the abdominal aorta is clamped at a level superior to the renal arteries for a little over an hour. The next morning he is found to have a severe acute decline in his renal function, with a blood urea nitrogen (BUN) of 75 mg/dL and creatinine of 3.2 mg/dL. His calculated glomerular filtration rate (GFR) is depressed to ≈10 mL/min (normal >100 mL/min), his urine output is diminished to ≈200 mL in 24 hours (despite being normotensive), and urine microscopy reveals "muddy brown" granular casts.

---

1. What is the probable diagnosis?
   Acute tubular necrosis (ATN) secondary to prolonged ischemia during the operation is the probable diagnosis.

2. What is the pathophysiology of ATN?
   In ATN, tubular epithelial cells are damaged by ischemia or nephrotoxins and slough off from the tubular basement membrane. The sloughed tubular epithelial cells block the lumen of the renal tubules, forming epithelial "muddy brown" casts and impeding urine flow. Additionally, the denuded areas of basement membrane allow back-leakage of the filtered fluid. Although this back-leakage does not change the amount of fluid filtered across the glomerular membrane, it does change the amount of waste products that are excreted, changing the *calculated* GFR. Both the obstruction to flow and back-leakage contribute to reduced urine output in ATN.

Clinical Pearl

Nephrotoxic agents causing acute tubular necrosis (ATN) include the chemotherapeutic agent cisplatin, aminoglycoside antibiotics, acyclovir, protease inhibitors, the antifungal amphotericin B, intravenous radiographic contrast media, heavy metals (Fanconi syndrome), uric acid from tumor lysis syndrome, and the heme pigments myoglobin and hemoglobin.

---

3. What are the three phases of ATN?
   In the *initiation phase*, the injurious agent or condition is present, but the deterioration of renal function has not yet begun or is just beginning. In the *maintenance phase*, GFR is reduced and oliguria persists. During this time, uremic complications are likely to manifest. Finally, in the *recovery phase*, renal tubular epithelial cells proliferate, repopulate the denuded areas, and urine output normalizes.

4. How can the fractional excretion of sodium help differentiate prerenal azotemia from ischemic ATN?
   In prerenal azotemia, inadequate renal perfusion reduces GFR, but the reduced perfusion is not so severe as to cause cellular damage. The kidneys respond to hypoperfusion by retaining Na^+, causing a reduction in the fractional excretion of Na^+ to below 1%. The fractional excretion of sodium ($FENa^+$) is simply the percent of the filtered load of sodium that is excreted. It can be calculated as shown in Eq. 3.2:

$$FENa^+ = C_{Na}/GFR = (U_{Na} \times V/P_{Na}) / (U_{Cr} \times V/P_{Cr}) = (U_{Na} \times P_{Cr}) / (P_{Na}/U_{Cr})$$ [3.2]

   where
   C_X = clearance of substance X; volume of plasma from which substance X is cleared per unit time
   U_X = excretion rate of substance X
   V = urine volume
   P_X = plasma concentration of substance X
   Cr = creatinine

If the hypoperfusion is severe enough, prerenal azotemia will result in ischemic damage to the tubular epithelium that is characteristic of ATN. In ATN, many of the tubular cells are no longer functional, and the kidney is unable to retain Na^+ in the setting of decreased GFR. As a result, the $FENa^+$ in ATN is typically greater than 2%. In addition to the $FENa^+$, the BUN/Cr ratio can sometimes be useful in distinguishing between prerenal azotemia and ATN. Urea is primarily reabsorbed in the proximal tubule. In the setting of low extracellular volume (ECV), the increased Na^+ reabsorption in the proximal tubule (as stimulated by Ang II, the SNS, and intrinsic glomerular processes) will pull additional urea out of the filtrate through bulk flow. Thus BUN can be used as a marker for proximal Na^+ reabsorption. Creatinine, in contrast, is less affected by Na^+ reabsorption (recall that creatinine is a useful marker for GFR because it is not significantly reabsorbed). In prerenal azotemia, one expects a BUN/Cr ratio elevated to greater than 20. In ATN, in which the reabsorption of Na^+ and urea is impaired, this ratio is often less than 10.

Clinical Pearl

Although the blood urea nitrogen/creatinine (BUN/Cr) ratio is more readily available (because it requires only standard blood tests instead of both urine and blood), it is significantly less accurate than the fractional excretion of sodium ($FENa^+$) and can change independent of renal function. A classic example is a gastrointestinal (GI) bleed in which large amounts of hemoglobin are broken down in the GI tract into urea and reabsorbed into the circulation, elevating the BUN level and the BUN/Cr ratio in a manner that is independent of renal function.

---

5. **How might rhabdomyolysis cause ATN?**

Rhabdomyolysis is acute extensive destruction of skeletal muscle cells; it can occur with trauma (especially prolonged crush injuries), drugs (e.g., statins), extreme physical exertion, and a host of other scenarios. With muscle injury, large amounts of the O_2 storage protein myoglobin are released into the circulation and, upon arrival to the kidneys, leads to renal failure via multiple mechanisms. First, myoglobin is directly toxic to renal tubular epithelial cells. Second, myoglobin can precipitate severe Ang II-induced vasoconstriction, resulting in an ischemic component to the ATN. Third, myoglobin can precipitate in the renal tubules and cause obstruction.

Clinical Pearl

In order to prevent renal injury in the setting of rhabdomyolysis, aggressive fluid hydration is initiated with intravenous (IV) normal saline. Contrast-induced acute tubular necrosis (ATN) is similar to myoglobin-induced ATN in that it involves both direct toxic and vasoconstrictive/ischemic components. Of interest, the $FENa^+$ in contrast-induced nephropathy is often less than 1%, suggesting that the primary pathogenesis may occur via vasoconstriction. Contrast-induced ATN may be prevented or minimized with precontrast hydration, though studies are limited.

SUMMARY BOX: ACUTE TUBULAR NECROSIS

- Epidemiology
  - Common in elderly patients with compromised renal function in the setting of hypotension, sepsis
  - Rhabdomyolysis and chemical damage can also damage the tubules
  - Most common cause of intrinsic renal failure
- Presentation: Acute kidney injury with diminished urine output and "muddy brown" granular casts on microscopy
- Pathophysiology
  - Ischemic insult resulting from low flow states
  - Direct toxicity most commonly from nephrotoxic drugs such as amphotericin and cisplatin
- Diagnosis
  - Muddy brown casts in the urinary sediment
  - Fractional excretion of sodium ($FENa^+$) greater than 2%

CASE 3.3

A 53-year-old Caucasian woman develops mediastinitis following coronary bypass surgery. She becomes septic with multiple organ failure and requires intensive care unit (ICU) admission, intubation, pressor support, and hemodialysis. Her sternal wound appears infected and is surgically debrided. Cultures grow methicillin-sensitive *Staphylococcus aureus*. After 1 week, she is discharged home on long-term intravenous nafcillin. Ten days after discharge, she returns to the emergency department complaining of several days of fever, nausea, malaise, and rash. On physical examination, she is febrile to 38.7°C (101.7°F), and she has a full-body, intensely erythematous maculopapular rash. Initial laboratory findings are notable for an elevated creatinine of 3.9 mg/dL. She has a modest leukocytosis with a differential of 62% neutrophils, 22% lymphocytes, 12% eosinophils, and 4% monocytes.

1. **What is the most likely cause of her AKI?**

Acute interstitial nephritis (AIN) caused by nafcillin is the most likely cause. AIN is commonly an allergic reaction to a drug such as antibiotics, particularly β-lactams (especially penicillins and cephalosporins) and sulfonamides; NSAIDs; and proton pump inhibitors (PPIs) such as omeprazole and pantoprazole. AIN is less commonly caused by infections and is rarely a manifestation of an autoimmune disease (e.g., sarcoidosis).

In a setting of AKI, the triad of fever, rash, and peripheral eosinophilia following initiation of a new medication is highly suggestive of AIN, but all three of these nonrenal manifestations are present in only a minority of patients. Urine microscopy may show white blood cells (WBCs), WBC casts, and red blood cells (RBCs). Urine eosinophils are highly suggestive but may not be present in all cases. When the diagnosis of AIN is unclear, biopsy can be performed, but often empiric therapy with corticosteroids is attempted first.

STEP 1 SECRET

*Remembering the most common conditions that cause eosinophilia can be helpful. These conditions include helminthic infections, asthma and allergic disorders, drug-induced AIN, and certain forms of malignancy (e.g., Hodgkin lymphoma). Remember, if you see eosinophils on your exam, do not WAIL: think **W**orms, **A**llergy, **I**nterstitial **N**ephritis, and **L**ymphoma.*

2. **What are the major types of NSAID-induced renal toxicity?**

NSAIDs can cause a bewildering array of renal side effects.

The most common renal toxicity of NSAIDs is hemodynamically mediated (ischemic) AKI. In the normal kidney, vasodilatory prostaglandins, such as PGI_2 (prostacyclin) and PGE_2, are produced to help maintain adequate renal perfusion through vasodilatory action at the afferent arteriole. The enzyme cyclooxygenase (COX) is required for prostaglandin production. The inhibition of COX-1 or COX-2 by NSAIDs can decrease prostaglandin production, which results in vasoconstriction of the renal arterioles, renal hypoperfusion, and a dramatic decrease in GFR. Risk factors for NSAID-induced kidney injury include age greater than 65 years, baseline renal dysfunction, and intravascular volume depletion (e.g., diuretic use and cirrhosis). This is partly because such patients with renal dysfunction or volume depletion depend more heavily than normal on prostaglandin production to maintain adequate renal perfusion. Interstitial nephritis, as described in the previous question, is a less common cause of NSAID-induced renal toxicity. Interestingly, NSAID-induced AIN often lacks the peripheral eosinophilia present in other types of AIN. In addition to interstitial nephritis, NSAIDs can rarely cause nephrotic syndrome. This typically manifests as minimal change disease in an adult taking NSAIDs, but other types of glomerular processes (e.g., membranous nephropathy) are possible as well.

STEP 1 SECRET

Patients with advanced age, renal dysfunction, or low effective circulating volume (e.g., congestive heart failure) are at the highest risk for NSAID-induced acute kidney injury.

SUMMARY BOX: ACUTE INTERSTITIAL NEPHRITIS AND NSAIDS

- Presentation: Fever, rash, and peripheral eosinophilia in a setting of acute kidney injury (AKI) after the introduction of a new drug
  - Urine eosinophils clinch the diagnosis
- Causes: Numerous, but think NSAIDs, certain antibiotics, and proton pump inhibitors (PPIs)
- Treatment: Removal of the offending drug usually suffices

CASE 3.4

A 65-year-old woman with a long history of poorly controlled hypertension is evaluated for a persistently elevated plasma creatinine for 6 months. Additional laboratory findings include hyperkalemia, hyperphosphatemia, metabolic acidosis, and borderline low calcium level. Hemoglobin A_{1c} and fasting glucose values are both normal. Urine microscopy does not reveal any hematuria or casts.

1. **What is most likely causing this patient's BUN and creatinine elevation?**

She has chronic kidney disease (CKD) resulting from a long history of poorly controlled hypertension. Hypertension is the second-most common cause of CKD. Renal failure from hypertension is particularly common in African American patients. The pathologic changes associated with long-standing hypertension are termed *hypertensive nephrosclerosis* (also known as *benign nephrosclerosis* or *hyaline arteriolar nephrosclerosis*). As shown in Fig. 3.12, hyaline arteriosclerosis is associated with hyaline deposition, marked thickening of the walls, and a narrowed lumen.

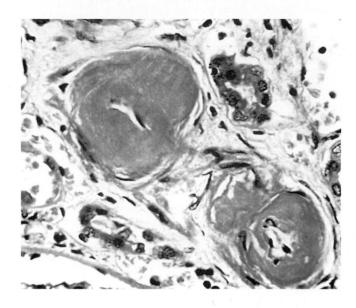

Figure 3.12. Hyaline arteriolosclerosis. High-power view of two arterioles with hyaline deposition, marked thickening of the walls, and a narrowed lumen. *(Courtesy Dr. M.A. Venkatachalam, Department of Pathology, University of Texas Health Sciences Center, San Antonio, TX. From Kumar V, Abbas AK, Aster JC. Robbins Basic Pathology. 10th ed. Philadelphia: Elsevier; 2018: 549-581, Fig. 14.18.)*

2. What is the importance of normal fasting glucose and hemoglobin A_{1c} levels when determining the differential diagnosis?
This finding essentially rules out a component of diabetic nephropathy, the most common cause of CKD.

3. What is the difficulty in establishing that this patient's CKD was definitively due to hypertension, even if no other specific disease processes can be identified on renal biopsy?
The difficulty stems from the fact that hypertension is both a potential cause and a potential result of renal disease. Furthermore, renal biopsy findings can be nonspecific if renal insufficiency is chronic and may fail to distinguish between other precipitating insults. For example, her CKD may have been due to an episode of glomerulonephritis that permanently damaged the kidneys, resulting in her hypertension. Nevertheless, hypertension, regardless of its cause, contributes to progressive loss of renal function.

4. How could this woman's CKD explain the following findings?
Metabolic acidosis. The kidneys normally excrete a large quantity of nonvolatile acids, including both inorganic acids (e.g., ammonium and hydrogen ions) and organic acids (e.g., sulfate and phosphate). Thus metabolic acidosis occurs in CKD as these acids accumulate in the body.

   Hyperkalemia. Normally, aldosterone drives the secretion of potassium (in exchange for sodium) in the distal tubule. CKD predisposes to hyperkalemia, both because there are fewer nephrons capable of engaging in potassium secretion and because as GFR decreases, less potassium is filtered.

   Anemia. Would you expect a microcytic, normocytic, or macrocytic anemia? Renal erythropoietin synthesis is compromised in severe CKD, resulting in anemia. We would expect normocytic anemia because a lack of erythropoietin reduces the rate of erythropoiesis.

5. How does this woman's CKD explain her borderline hypocalcemia?
Generally, renal dysfunction leads to the accumulation of electrolytes that are normally excreted by the kidneys, resulting in hyperkalemia, hyperphosphatemia, and acidosis typical of advanced CKD. Calcium differs in that its serum levels may be *decreased* in advanced CKD as a result of several processes. First, the kidney is the site of 1,25-dihydroxyvitamin D (i.e., calcitriol) synthesis from 25-hydroxyvitamin D, via the activity of renal α_1-hydroxylase in the proximal tubule. Because 1,25-dihydroxyvitamin D is the active form that stimulates intestinal calcium absorption, loss of renal parenchyma reduces synthesis of this compound and reduces intestinal calcium absorption. Second, as GFR declines, renal phosphate excretion declines and leads to hyperphosphatemia. This elevated serum phosphate can complex with serum calcium and reduce free ionized calcium levels. In addition, the increased phosphate, through negative feedback, also inhibits the synthesis of 1,25-dihydroxyvitamin D. Recall that 1,25-dihydroxyvitamin D increases serum levels of *both* Ca^{2+} and phosphate by promoting the intestinal absorption of both substances. On the other hand, PTH increases serum calcium levels while promoting phosphate excretion at the level of the kidney. However, in clinical practice, hypocalcemia with CKD may not occur because of the rapid compensatory increase in serum PTH levels mediated by the parathyroid glands.

Note: There are two forms of vitamin D: plant-derived vitamin D_2 (ergocalciferol) is acquired in our diets; vitamin D_3 is made endogenously in our skin in a reaction that is catalyzed by ultraviolet rays (i.e., sunlight). To become biologically active, both vitamin D_2 and D_3 must be hydroxylated twice. The first hydroxylation is unregulated and occurs in the liver to produce the 25-hydroxyvitamin D diol form. The second step, which is impaired in advanced CKD, is highly regulated and produces the 1,25-dihydroxyvitamin D triol form (hence the name calci*triol*).

STEP 1 SECRET

Hypocalcemia in advanced chronic kidney disease (CKD) is due to (1) decreased synthesis of the active form of vitamin D (1,25-dihydroxyvitamin D) in the proximal tubule, (2) complexed free calcium by elevated phosphate levels, and (3) inhibition of active vitamin D synthesis by the elevated phosphate. Advanced CKD results in secondary hyperparathyroidism. Elevated parathyroid hormone (PTH), in turn, can cause abnormal bone formation (osteitis fibrosa cystica), whereas deficiency of activated vitamin D can (in adults) lead to osteomalacia. The full spectrum of bony changes resulting from high PTH, low Ca^{2+}, and chronic acidosis is called renal osteodystrophy.

6. **Would PTH levels be increased or decreased in this patient?**
   PTH levels are increased in advanced CKD because PTH is released in response to hypocalcemia (or hyperphosphatemia). This increase in PTH is reactive in nature (i.e., an appropriate response to the hypocalcemia and hyperphosphatemia of advanced CKD) and is termed *secondary hyperparathyroidism*. Patients in early CKD often have a high PTH level with relatively normal serum calcium. However, in advanced CKD, as both 1,25-hydroxyvitamin D levels decrease and phosphate levels increase to a greater extent, the progressively elevated PTH levels are unable to compensate, and severe hypocalcemia develops.

Clinical Pearl

Primary hyperparathyroidism, in which an abnormality of the parathyroid gland (typically glandular hyperplasia or an adenoma) results in increased PTH levels, causes *hypercalcemia* rather than hypocalcemia.

---

7. **How does PTH normally act to regulate serum Ca^{2+}? How are PTH levels normally regulated?**
   PTH acts to increase serum Ca^{2+} while maintaining serum phosphate levels by stimulating bone reabsorption to release Ca^{2+} and phosphate into circulation. It also promotes the synthesis of vitamin D by stimulating the activity of α_1-hydroxylase in the proximal tubule. Active 1,25-dihydroxyvitamin D then increases intestinal absorption of Ca^{2+} and phosphate and, at high levels, promotes bone resorption, again acting to increase serum levels of both Ca^{2+} and phosphate. Finally, PTH stimulates Ca^{2+} reabsorption at the level of the kidney while strongly promoting *phosphate excretion*.
   Thus PTH acts directly and indirectly in bone, the GI tract, and the kidneys to increase plasma Ca^{2+}. However, because the phosphate released from bone and absorbed from the GI tract is excreted in the kidneys, the combination of PTH and vitamin D activation tends to have no net effect on serum phosphate.
   Generally, PTH release is stimulated by low Ca^{2+} levels and is inhibited by the active 1,25-dihydroxy form of vitamin D via negative feedback (Fig. 3.13).

8. **What are the potential pathologic manifestations of hyperparathyroidism that develops in advanced CKD?**
   The *chronically* high PTH levels in advanced CKD stimulate bone resorption, which can result in osteoporosis, as well as abnormal cysts in areas of demineralized bone (*osteitis fibrosa cystica*). So, a relatively normal PTH level is an important therapeutic goal in the chronic management of advanced CKD in order to prevent bone disease. Additionally, the high PTH levels may accelerate vascular calcification, including the coronary arteries, through disordered calcium and phosphate homeostasis. The myocardium, valves, and conduction system are also subject to accelerated calcification. These patients may be at an increased risk of cardiovascular events and even death. Agents such as active vitamin D analogs that have negative feedback on PTH release, as well as newer agents that suppress PTH release by mimicking the action of calcium on the parathyroid gland (e.g., cinacalcet), can be used to maintain normal PTH levels.

STEP 1 SECRET

Parathyroid hormone (PTH) and vitamin D are routinely tested topics on the USMLE. It is important to understand the difference between primary and secondary hyperparathyroidism and to know which conditions elevate PTH and vitamin D levels.

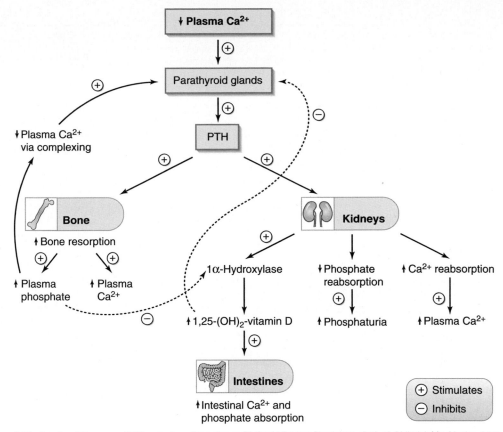

Figure 3.13. Parathyroid hormone (PTH) overview. *(From Brown TA.* Rapid Review Physiology. *2nd ed. Philadelphia: Mosby; 2012: 128.)*

9. **Why is this patient also predisposed to osteomalacia?**
   Osteomalacia is a disease of adults resulting from activated vitamin D deficiency, causing *impaired mineralization* of newly deposited osteoid matrix in bone, resulting in malleable bones (malacia). If this vitamin D deficiency and impaired mineralization occur before closure of the epiphyseal plates in prepubertal children, it is referred to as *rickets*.
   Renal osteodystrophy includes the spectrum of bony changes that result from advanced CKD and includes osteitis fibrosa cystica caused by secondary hyperparathyroidism, osteomalacia from impaired vitamin D synthesis and decreased mineralization, and bone loss from the need to buffer the metabolic acidosis in advanced CKD.

10. **Does this woman have azotemia or uremia?**
    This patient has azotemia. *Azotemia* refers to increased BUN and creatinine in an asymptomatic person. If this patient were symptomatic, she have uremia. Uremia is a *clinical syndrome* consisting of a constellation of symptoms or complications attributable to renal failure. Possible manifestations include nausea, pruritus, malaise, seizures, confusion (uremic encephalopathy), bleeding (from uremia-induced platelet dysfunction), pericarditis, and fluid overload.

11. **If this patient were uremic, and a friction rub was detected on physical examination, what might you suspect?**
    Uremic pericarditis, characterized by a fibrinous exudate within the pericardial space, might be suspected. The suspicion of pericarditis is supported by the presence of a friction rub on examination and chest pain that is relieved by sitting forward (as leaning forward elevates the heart from the diaphragmatic portion of the pericardium).

SUMMARY BOX: ADVANCED CHRONIC KIDNEY DISEASE

- Presentation: Normocytic anemia, hyperkalemia, metabolic acidosis, hypocalcemia, hyperphosphatemia, secondary hyperparathyroidism
- Causes: Numerous causes, but hypertension and diabetes are the most common
- Uremia: *Clinical syndrome* of specific symptoms or complications attributable to renal failure such as nausea, pruritus, malaise, seizures, confusion, bleeding, pericarditis, and fluid overload

CASE 3.5

A 32-year-old woman with a history of hypertension presents for evaluation of right-sided flank pain. She denies urinary symptoms such as dysuria, urgency, and frequency. Physical examination is unremarkable. Labs reveal an elevated creatinine level. A urinalysis shows the presence of red blood cells (RBCs) and protein. Renal ultrasound shows enlarged kidneys with numerous cysts. The patient then recalls that her mother had some kind of kidney disease.

1. What is the diagnosis?

   Autosomal dominant (adult) polycystic kidney disease (ADPKD) is the diagnosis. ADPKD is due to mutation in *PKD1* or *PKD2* (less common, milder symptoms, later onset). Note the diffuse, bilateral distribution of cysts in ADPKD shown in Fig. 3.14. Be familiar with this high-yield image for Step 1.

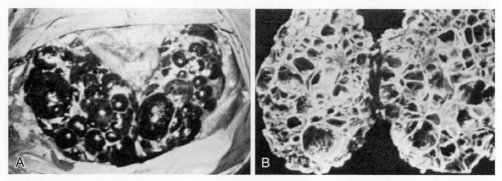

Figure 3.14. A. Autosomal dominant polycystic kidney disease (ADPKD) gross pathology revealing cystic structures visible from the outside of the specimen bilaterally. **B.** Parenchyma replaced by numerous cortical and medullary cysts. *(Courtesy F.E. Cuppage, Kansas City, KS; From Torres VE, Harris PC.* Brenner and Rector's The Kidney. *11th ed. Philadelphia: Elsevier; 2020: 1490-1534.e13, Fig. 45.5.)*

2. What is the primary complication of this disease?

   End-stage renal disease (ESRD) is the primary complication. Renal transplant is curative.

3. Why must urinary tract infections be treated aggressively in patients with this disease?

   Patients with ADPKD are treated aggressively to prevent pyelonephritis, which can be remarkably difficult to treat in these patients as the cysts are filled with mostly stagnant urine, which is an excellent breeding ground for bacteria. These cysts are difficult for antibiotics to penetrate; therefore, early and aggressive intervention is essential for good outcomes.

4. If this patient suddenly develops a severe headache, what vascular abnormality must be suspected?

   Intracranial (berry) aneurysms are associated with ADPKD. Rupture of a berry aneurysm classically results in acute onset of a severe "worst-of-my-life" headache, a subarachnoid hemorrhage. Presumably, the mutations in the polycystin gene that causes tissue to separate in the kidneys and form cysts also predispose vascular connective tissue to separate and form aneurysms. While the prevalence of berry aneurysms in patients with ADPKD is typically 5%, it is even higher in patients with a first-degree relative with known history of ruptured intracranial aneurysm. ADPKD is also associated with polycystic liver disease, mitral valve prolapse, and colonic diverticula for similar reasons.

STEP 1 SECRET

The relationship between berry aneurysm formation and autosomal dominant (adult) polycystic kidney disease (ADPKD) is a commonly tested Step 1 principle.

5. Other than the pattern of inheritance, how does ADPKD differ from autosomal recessive polycystic kidney disease?

   Autosomal recessive (*infantile*) polycystic kidney disease (ARPKD) typically presents in infancy, although there are less severe childhood and adolescent forms. It is always associated with liver abnormalities, including hepatic cysts and congenital hepatic fibrosis. In many patients, congenital fibrosis leads to portal hypertension and liver dysfunction. Patients can develop renal failure in utero, leading to Potter syndrome (failure of kidney development and subsequent lack of amniotic fluid production). Hepatic cysts (and less commonly, cysts in other organs, e.g., the pancreas and lungs) do occur in ADPKD, but they are *not* associated with liver fibrosis or organ dysfunction.

Note: Patients with ADPKD have large kidneys, while patients with ARPKD have small kidneys.

6. What is tuberous sclerosis, and how can it be differentiated from ADPKD?

Tuberous sclerosis is a genetic disease that is also inherited in an autosomal dominant manner. In this disease, multiple cysts (and tumors) form in the kidneys. The disorder is additionally characterized by a variety of central nervous system (CNS) abnormalities, including intellectual disability and seizures (resulting from cerebral "tuber" formation), as well as a variety of characteristic dermatologic lesions such as ash-leaf macules, adenoma sebaceum (i.e., angiofibromas), shagreen patches (connective tissue nevi), and subungual and periungual fibromas. Tuberous sclerosis is associated with a variety of findings including astrocytomas, renal angiomyolipomas, pulmonary lymphangioleiomyomatosis (LAM), retinal hamartomas, and cardiac rhabdomyomas.

7. What is von Hippel-Lindau syndrome, and how can it be differentiated from ADPKD?

Like ADPKD, ARPKD, and tuberous sclerosis, von Hippel-Lindau (VHL) syndrome is characterized by multiple cysts in both kidneys. It is an autosomal dominant disorder characterized by a tendency to form multiple types of neoplasms and hamartomas. It is caused by a mutation in the VHL gene, which normally functions in tumor suppression. In addition to cysts of the kidneys and other organs, affected patients develop hemangioblastomas of the CNS (Lindau tumors) and the retina, pheochromocytomas, and pancreatic tumors. The renal cysts are often complicated by the development of renal cell carcinoma, frequently bilateral.

STEP 1 SECRET

In addition to type I and II neurofibromatosis, tuberous sclerosis and VHL syndrome are high-yield topics for Step 1. Be able to identify the various tumors associated with these conditions.

---

8. What is medullary cystic disease, and how can it be differentiated from ADPKD?

In medullary cystic disease, the cysts are confined to the medulla; the cysts are not present throughout the kidney as in ADPKD. This rare cystic disease is also characterized by severe renal dysfunction. On ultrasound, the kidneys appear small, and the majority of patients develop kidney stones.

9. Quick review: Cover the right four columns in Table 3.3. What are the characteristic features of each of the cystic kidney diseases?

Table 3.3. Cystic Kidney Diseases

DISEASE	SITE OF CYSTS IN KIDNEY	MODE OF INHERITANCE	AGE AT ONSET	KEY ASSOCIATED FEATURES
ADPKD	Throughout	AD	Adulthood	Intracranial berry aneurysm and asymptomatic hepatic cysts
ARPKD	Throughout	AR	Infancy	Hepatic cysts and congenital hepatic fibrosis with possible portal hypertension and liver dysfunction
Tuberous sclerosis	Throughout	AD	Childhood	Mental retardation, seizure disorder, renal angiomyolipomas, cardiac rhabdomyomas, dermatologic lesions
Von Hippel-Lindau disease	Cortex (mostly)	AD	Teens to young adulthood	CNS and retinal hemangioblastomas, bilateral renal cell carcinoma
Medullary cystic disease	Medulla	AD	Childhood	Some develop gout as a result of increased uric acid

AD, Autosomal dominant; *ADPKD,* autosomal dominant polycystic kidney disease; *AR,* autosomal recessive; *ARPKD,* autosomal recessive polycystic kidney disease; *CNS,* central nervous system.

10. **Why is medullary sponge kidney not included in Table 3.3?**
    True cysts do not form in medullary sponge kidney. Rather, segments of the collecting tubules become abnormally dilated in the medulla at the tips of the renal papillae. The primary complication of these dilations is a predisposition to nephrolithiasis and pyelonephritis as a result of urinary stasis. Isolated hematuria or urinary tract infections (UTIs) can also occur. This disorder is seen primarily in adults and, compared with medullary cystic disease, is relatively common.

11. **What is the most common cause of renal cysts?**
    Most renal cysts are *incidental* nonneoplastic simple cysts that are not associated with a particular disease. Such simple cysts are more common with increasing age, occurring in up to 33% of people older than 50 years, and require no further workup.
    Cysts are particularly common in patients on hemodialysis, increasing in incidence, size, and number with duration of dialysis. Dialysis-associated cysts are also generally asymptomatic but can be complicated by hematuria.

SUMMARY BOX: CYSTIC KIDNEY DISEASE

- Autosomal dominant (adult) polycystic kidney disease (ADPKD) is the most common cystic renal disease.
  - Characterized by colicky abdominal or flank pain; hematuria; early-onset hypertension; and, ultimately, end-stage renal disease
  - Associated with increased risk of pyelonephritis, intracranial (berry) aneurysms, and asymptomatic hepatic cysts
- Autosomal recessive (infantile) polycystic kidney disease (ARPKD): Less common; associated with cysts in the liver, pancreas, and lungs, as well as liver dysfunction because of congenital hepatic fibrosis
- Other cystic kidney diseases: tuberous sclerosis, von Hippel-Lindau (VHL) syndrome, medullary cystic disease

---

CASE 3.6

A 5-year-old boy is brought to the clinic by his parents, who are concerned because he has been lethargic recently and appears "swollen" to them. Physical examination is significant for whole body edema (anasarca). Labs reveal hyperlipidemia and hypoalbuminemia. Urinalysis reveals the presence of proteins and lipids in the urine but no red blood cells (RBCs). Urine microscopy reveals the structure shown in Fig. 3.15.

---

1. **What is the likely diagnosis in this child and why?**
   Nephrotic syndrome, characterized by massive proteinuria (>3 g/24 hours), hypoalbuminemia resulting in severe edema (sometimes described as morning facial puffiness or scrotal edema by USMLE exam writers), and hyperlipidemia are likely diagnoses. Because of lipiduria and subsequent cholesterol precipitation, urine microscopy may show the presence of fatty casts and oval fat bodies with attached lipid droplets, which exhibit a Maltese cross pattern under polarized light (see Fig. 3.15). The massive proteinuria can make urine appear foamy or frothy. Although slight hematuria is sometimes seen in nephrotic syndrome, it is typically transient and much less severe than that associated with nephritic syndrome.
   The cause of hyperlipidemia is unclear but may relate to increased protein synthesis by the liver in response to the loss of serum proteins. In fact, elevated lipoprotein synthesis is often responsible for the onset of hyperlipidemia. Because of the preferential loss of antithrombin III in the urine, nephrotic syndrome is associated with an increased risk of clotting (particularly venous thromboembolism). In general, however, thrombotic complications of nephrotic syndrome are rare in children and tend to occur in adults with other risk factors for clotting.

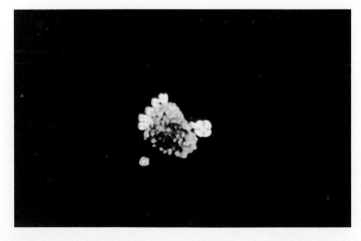

Figure 3.15. Urine microscopy for patient in Case 3.6, exhibiting oval fat bodies with attached lipid droplets. *(From McPherson RA.* Henry's Clinical Diagnosis and Management by Laboratory Methods. *23rd ed. St. Louis: Elsevier; 2017: 442-480.e3, Figure 28-14.)*

2. **What is the likely cause of nephrotic syndrome in this patient?**
   Minimal change disease (MCD; also known as *nil disease* or *lipoid nephrosis*) is the most common cause of nephrotic syndrome in children and commonly occurs following infections (especially respiratory infections).

3. **Assuming MCD as the underlying pathologic condition, what would you expect gross histologic examination to reveal if a renal biopsy were performed?**
   The kidney would be *normal* or nearly normal on light microscopy, hence the term *minimal change disease*. The pathologic diagnosis is generally made using electron microscopy, which demonstrates diffuse flattening ("effacement") of the podocyte foot processes, resulting in loss of the selective permeability of the glomerulus and leading to proteinuria (Fig. 3.16).

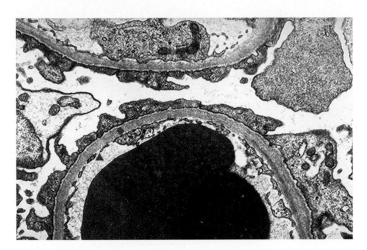

Figure 3.16. Fusion of the podocytes on electron microscopy. Normal-thickness basement membrane (*diamond*) and normal fenestrated endothelium (*arrowhead*) are present around a capillary loop with two RBCs (*star*). The epithelium that overlies the basement membrane exhibits fusion of the podocytes (*cross*, +), which should be separated by slit pores. This finding occurs in all glomerular diseases that present with the nephrotic syndrome. RBCs, Red blood cells. *(From Klatt EC.* Robbins and Cotran Atlas of Pathology. *3rd ed. Philadelphia: Elsevier; 2021: 261-298.e4, Fig. 10-42.)*

Note: Focal segmental glomerular sclerosis (FSGS), another important cause of nephrotic syndrome, would also show diffuse effacement of the podocyte foot processes on electron microscopy. However, light microscopy would reveal areas of sclerosis in some, but not all, glomeruli (i.e., focal sclerosis). FSGS is unlikely in a young child, but it is the most common cause of primary nephrotic syndrome in adults of African descent. It is also associated with human immunodeficiency virus (HIV) infection, obesity, and heroin use (Table 3.4).

Table 3.4. Summary of Primary Renal Diseases That Manifest as Idiopathic Nephrotic Syndrome

| | MINIMAL CHANGE NEPHROTIC SYNDROME | FOCAL SEGMENTAL SCLEROSIS | MEMBRANOUS NEPHROPATHY | *Membranoproliferative Glomerulonephritis* | |
				CLASSICAL (FORMERLY TYPE I)	DENSE DEPOSIT DISEASE (FORMERLY TYPE II)
Incidence*					
Children	80%	10%	< 5%	7%	2%
Adults	5%–10%	20%	25%–30%	12%	2%
Clinical Manifestations					
Age (years)	2–6, some adults	2–10, some adults	40–50	5–30	5–25
Nephrotic syndrome	100%	70% at presentation	80%	60%–70%	60%–70%
Asymptomatic proteinuria	0	30%	20%	30%–40%	30%–40%
Hematuria	30% (micro)	50% (micro)	60%	50%–80%	50%–80%

Continued

Table 3.4. Summary of Primary Renal Diseases That Manifest as Idiopathic Nephrotic Syndrome—cont'd

	MINIMAL CHANGE NEPHROTIC SYNDROME	FOCAL SEGMENTAL SCLEROSIS	MEMBRANOUS NEPHROPATHY	*Membranoproliferative Glomerulonephritis*	
				CLASSICAL (FORMERLY TYPE I)	DENSE DEPOSIT DISEASE (FORMERLY TYPE II)
Hypertension	30%	30%–50% (20% early)	Variable, not infrequent	35%	35%
Time to progression to renal failure	Does not progress	10 years	25% in 10 years	10–20 years	5–15 years
Laboratory findings	Manifestations of nephrotic syndrome	Manifestations of nephrotic syndrome	Renal vein thrombosis, cancer, SLE, hepatitis B	None	Partial lipodystrophy
	↑ BUN in 15%–30%	↑ BUN in 20%–40%	Manifestations of nephrotic syndrome	Low C1, C4, C3–C9	Normal C1, C4; low C3–C9
Light microscopy	Normal	Focal sclerotic lesions	Thickened GBM, spikes	Thickened GBM ("tram-tracking"), endocapillary proliferation	Lobulation
Immunofluorescence	Negative	IgM, C3 in lesions	Fine granular IgG, C3	Granular IgG, C3	C3 only (linear or granular)
Electron microscopy	Foot process fusion	Foot process fusion	Subepithelial dense deposits	Mesangial and subendothelial deposits	Dense deposits
Response to steroids	90% (>50% relapse)	40%–60% complete or partial remission	May slow progression	Variable	Variable

aApproximate incidence as a cause of idiopathic nephrotic syndrome. About 15%–30% of cases of adult nephrotic syndrome are due to various diseases that usually manifest with acute glomerulonephritis.

↑, Elevated; *BUN,* blood urea nitrogen; *C,* complement; *GBM,* glomerular basement membrane; *Ig,* immunoglobulin; *SLE,* systemic lupus erythematosus.

Modified from Goldman L. *Goldman-Cecil Medicine,* 26th ed. Philadelphia: Elsevier; 2020, 753–763.e2.

4. **Why might this boy be susceptible to infections with this illness?**
   Because of heavy proteinuria, immunoglobulins are lost in the urine (in addition to albumin), leading to hypogammaglobulinemia.

5. **How should this boy be managed? Should a renal biopsy be performed?**
   Nephrotic syndrome caused by MCD typically responds *extremely* well to glucocorticoids such as prednisone. Because MCD causes a majority (roughly 80%) of nephrotic syndrome cases in children, renal biopsy is generally *not* needed. However, if there is not adequate response to steroids, renal biopsy should be considered to rule out other causes. Of note, FSGS characteristically responds *poorly* to steroids. Thus FSGS should be suspected in any patient (particularly any older patient) with presumed MCD who does not respond rapidly to steroids.

6. **What are the other major causes of nephrotic syndrome?**
   There are five major causes of nephrotic syndrome. Three are primary renal diseases; two are systemic diseases capable of producing nephrotic syndrome. Although they all cause nephrotic syndrome, some have nephritic characteristics. In other words, there is a spectrum between nephrotic and nephritic syndromes.

   The primary renal diseases are MCD (the most common cause of nephrotic syndrome in children), FSGS (the most common cause in adults of African ancestry), and membranous nephropathy (the most common cause of nephrotic syndrome in Caucasian adults).

FSGS, of the three, is the most nephritic; in other words, it is most likely to be associated with some degree of hypertension, hematuria, or kidney injury (see Case 3.7 for more on nephritic syndrome). MCD, in contrast, is completely nephrotic.

Membranous nephropathy is usually idiopathic but can be associated with hepatitis B and C infection, autoimmune disease (particularly lupus), malignancy (particularly carcinomas and Hodgkin lymphoma), or drugs (e.g., NSAIDs, captopril, and gold salts) because of their immunogenicity. Light microscopy reveals basement membrane thickening, and electron microscopy shows characteristic dense deposits on the epithelial side of the basement membrane (so-called "spike and dome" appearance; Fig. 3.17).

The systemic diseases are diabetes and amyloidosis. Although diabetes is a major cause of nephrotic syndrome (because diabetes is so common), nephrotic syndrome is rather uncommon among patients with diabetes. Amyloidosis is the least common of the five.

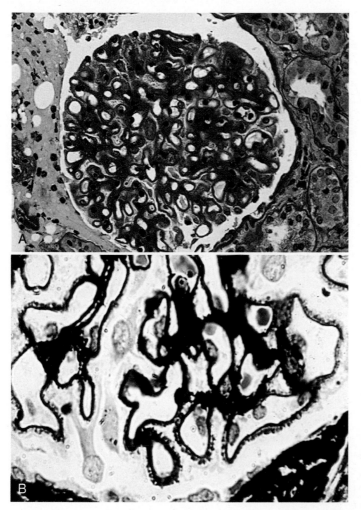

Figure 3.17. Membranous nephropathy. A, Light micrograph of membranous nephropathy demonstrating thickening of the glomerular capillary wall but no hypercellularity. B, Silver stain of idiopathic membranous nephropathy showing spike formation along the outer aspect of the glomerular basement membrane corresponding to projections of the basement membrane between the epimembranous deposits. *(From Goldman L.* Goldman-Cecil Medicine. *26th ed. Philadelphia: Elsevier; 2020: 753-763.e2, Fig. 113-4.)*

STEP 1 SECRET

Glomerulonephritic syndromes are a favorite topic for the test makers. In addition to differentiating between nephritic and nephrotic syndromes based on clinical and laboratory information and knowing which syndromes are associated with which diseases (e.g., association of hepatitis B and C with membranous nephropathy), you should be able to identify each type of glomerulonephritis by light microscopy, electron microscopy, and immunofluorescence (if applicable).

SOME DIFFERENTIAL DIAGNOSIS CONCEPTS

7. What condition might you suspect in a 6-year-old girl who presents with abdominal pain, joint pain, hematuria (or melena) and proteinuria, and palpable purpura on her buttocks and lower extremities?
Henoch-Schönlein purpura (HSP) is a small-vessel vasculitis of children that commonly follows an upper respiratory tract infection. Presumably, the mucosal immune stimulation caused by the upper respiratory tract infection stimulates the production of immunoglobulin A (IgA). This disease is characterized by IgA deposition in small vessels of the GI tract, glomeruli, joints, and skin. In addition to hematuria and proteinuria, renal involvement can progress to hypertension and, uncommonly, AKI.

Clinical Pearl

Palpable purpura always suggests a *vasculitic* process because inflammation of the small vessels of the skin allows red blood cells (RBCs) to extravasate (i.e., leak) into the dermis and form the palpable lesion. In Henoch-Schönlein purpura (HSP), the rash tends to be present on the buttocks and lower extremities in a "waist-down" distribution and can be accidentally mistaken for child abuse or trauma.

SUMMARY BOX: GLOMERULAR DISEASE

- Nephrotic syndrome
  - Characterized by massive proteinuria (>3 g/24 hours), hypoalbuminemia, edema (often anasarca), hyperlipidemia, lipiduria, and (in adults) increased risk of venous thromboembolism (loss of antithrombin III)
  - Most common subtype in children is minimal change disease (MCD), which responds to steroids
  - Most common subtype in Caucasian adults is membranous nephropathy; it is associated with hepatitis B, lupus, and various carcinomas
- Nephritic syndrome
  - Characterized by modest proteinuria (<3 g/24 hours), hematuria, renal insufficiency, hypertension, and urinary dysmorphic red blood cells (RBCs) and/or RBC casts on urine microscopy

---

CASE 3.7

A 42-year-old man is evaluated for a pre-employment physical. He had a bad sore throat recently but currently feels well. Blood pressure is 152/90 mm Hg. Physical examination is unrevealing. Labs show an elevated BUN and creatinine. Urinalysis reveals hematuria and moderate proteinuria. Antistreptolysin O (ASO) and anti-DNase B titers are markedly elevated. Labs from a previous visit 3 months ago revealed normal BUN and creatinine levels.

---

1. What is the most likely diagnosis?
The most likely diagnosis is acute nephritic syndrome (acute glomerulonephritis) characterized by a relatively sudden onset of *mild to moderate proteinuria* (i.e., <3 g/24 hours), *hematuria, renal insufficiency* (elevated creatinine), and *hypertension.*
Urine microscopy will also often show dysmorphic RBCs and RBC casts (Fig. 3.18).

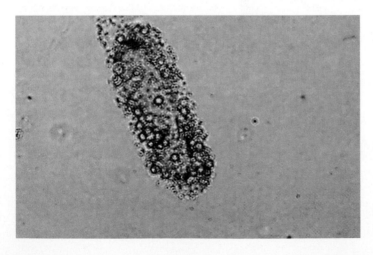

Figure 3.18. Erythrocyte cast (×200). (*From McPherson RA. Henry's Clinical Diagnosis and Management by Laboratory Methods. 23rd ed. St. Louis: Elsevier; 2017: 442-480.e3, Figure 28-17.*)

2. **What segment of the nephron is involved in acute glomerulonephritis? How does this compare with nephrotic syndrome?**

The glomerulus is involved. The presence of dysmorphic RBCs (which are deformed by passage through the damaged glomeruli) or RBC casts (which form within the renal tubules) indicates that hematuria is of a *glomerular* origin.

The glomerulus is also the primary site of injury in nephrotic syndrome, but in general, different sides of the glomeruli are damaged. In nephrotic syndrome, podocyte foot processes and glomerular basement membrane (GBM) are most damaged (exemplified by foot process effacement seen in MCD or FSGS), whereas the endothelium and basement membrane are typically more involved in glomerulonephritis. It is the endothelial damage that allows for the leakage of RBCs through the glomerulus that is typical of glomerulonephritis.

Again, nephrotic and nephritic syndromes are two ends on the spectrum of glomerular disease. Certain diseases are very characteristically nephrotic (i.e., MCD), others are very nephritic (i.e., rapidly progressive or crescentic glomerulonephritis), and most others fall somewhere in between.

3. **What was the likely cause of this man's sore throat, and what is its relationship to the renal dysfunction?**

Streptococcal pharyngitis caused by group A β-hemolytic streptococcus (i.e., *Streptococcus pyogenes*). The patient now has a poststreptococcal glomerulonephritis (PSGN). This condition is caused by antibody-antigen complex deposition in the glomerulus, resulting in inflammatory destruction of the glomerulus (primarily mediated via complement activation). For the USMLE, look for subepithelial hump-like deposits along the capillary basement membranes, as depicted by the *straight arrow* in Fig. 3.19.

In some patients, in whom the history of a prior infection may be difficult to elicit, antibody evidence of recent streptococcal infection can help make the diagnosis. The two most common antibodies tested for are those directed against the streptococcal antigens streptolysin O (diagnostic but not prognostic) and DNase B. The immune complex formation also results in the consumption of complement, which is reflected in a decrease in serum complement levels.

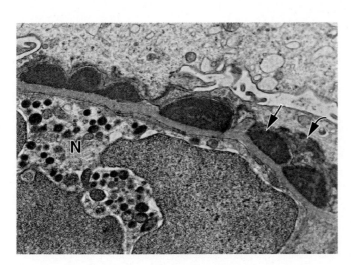

Figure 3.19. Electron micrograph of a portion of a glomerular capillary from a patient with acute poststreptococcal glomerulonephritis (PSGN) showing subepithelial dense deposits (*straight arrow*), condensation of cytoskeleton in adjacent epithelial cytoplasm (*small curved arrow*), and a neutrophil (*N*) marginated against the basement membrane with no intervening endothelial cytoplasm (magnification ×5000). *(From Alan SL, et al. Brenner and Rector's The Kidney. 11th ed. Philadelphia: Elsevier; 2020: 1007-1091.e32, Fig. 31.25.)*

4. **Would it alter the diagnosis of his renal disorder if the patient had recently had cellulitis rather than pharyngitis?**

This is not likely. Streptococcal infections of the skin and soft tissue can also cause a PSGN. Note that this contrasts with acute rheumatic fever, which exclusively follows streptococcal pharyngitis.

5. **What is the treatment for PSGN?**

Supportive care is the treatment for PSGN. Hypertension must be controlled with medications and salt restriction. In general, steroids or immunosuppressive agents (used in many other glomerular diseases) are *not* used. Prognosis is generally much better in children than in adults.

Note: In contrast with rheumatic fever, the incidence of PSGN is *not* decreased by antibiotic administration.

6. **How would the diagnosis change if a renal biopsy revealed "glomerular crescents"?**

Glomerular crescents are the hallmark of crescentic or rapidly progressive glomerulonephritis (RPGN), which, as the name suggests, is a form of rapidly evolving glomerular disease that frequently responds poorly to treatment and progresses to renal failure. Crescents are formed by clusters of rapidly proliferating parietal epithelial cells, fibrin, and infiltrating leukocytes (Figs. 3.20 and 3.21).

The major types of RPGN are distinguished using immunofluorescence. Pauci-immune glomerulonephritis is the most common cause of RPGN. Its name derives from the fact that on renal biopsy, immune complexes are *not* seen on

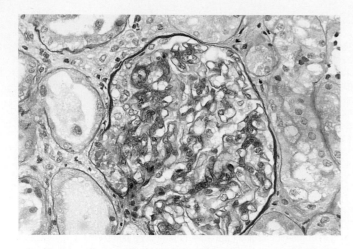

Figure 3.20. Normal glomerulus. *(From Damjanov I. Pathology for the Health-Related Professions. 5th ed. St. Louis: Elsevier; 2017: 317, Fig. 31-5.)*

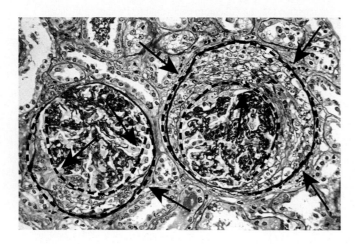

Figure 3.21. Crescentic glomerulonephritis (periodic acid–Schiff [PAS] stain). *Arrows* point to a proliferation of parietal epithelial cells and leukocytes (shown as a dotted line) in the Bowman capsule, occupying approximately 50% of the entire urinary space. The cells encase and compress the glomerular tuft. *(Courtesy Dr. MA Venkatachalam, University of Texas Health Sciences Center, San Antonio, TX; From Kumar V. Robbins and Cotran Pathologic Basis of Disease. 9th ed. Philadelphia: Elsevier Saunders; 2015: 897-957, Fig. 20-10.)*

immunofluorescence. Pauci-immune glomerulonephritis is commonly associated with vasculitic conditions such as granulomatosis with polyangiitis and the similar disorder microscopic polyangiitis. These conditions are associated with positive antineutrophil cytoplasmic antibodies (ANCA); granulomatosis with polyangiitis is usually c-ANCA positive (diffuse *cy*toplasmic staining pattern), whereas microscopic polyangiitis tends to be p-ANCA positive (*p*erinuclear cytoplasmic pattern). Granulomatosis with polyangiitis usually presents with a triad of glomerulonephritis and involvement of both the upper and lower respiratory tracts. The respiratory disease is usually in the form of oral ulcers or purulent or bloody nasal discharge along with pulmonary nodules, infiltrates, or cavities.

Goodpasture syndrome is another form of RPGN caused by antibodies directed against the GBM. These anti-GBM antibodies form immune complexes that can be seen on immunofluorescence as *linear* deposits of IgG and C3. These anti-GBM antibodies can also react with the alveolar basement membrane of the lungs to cause pulmonary hemorrhage (and subsequent hemoptysis) in addition to glomerulonephritis.

RPGN can also represent the end stage of many other forms of immune complex–mediated glomerulonephritis. In such a case, immunofluorescence typically reveals "lumpy-bumpy" granular (i.e., nonlinear) deposition along the glomeruli.

STEP 1 SECRET

Granulomatosis with polyangiitis presents with upper respiratory symptoms (nares and lungs), but Goodpasture syndrome (lungs only) does not. Goodpasture syndrome involves linear deposits along the glomerular basement membrane (GBM), but granulomatosis with polyangiitis does not. You will be given at least one of these two pieces of information on your USMLE examination if the question requires you to distinguish between the two diagnoses.

7. **What is the most common cause of glomerulonephritis worldwide?**

   IgA nephropathy (i.e., Berger disease) is overall the most common primary glomerular disease (nephritic or nephrotic). This disorder is similar to HSP but without any extrarenal manifestations. Renal biopsy typically shows immune complex deposition (primarily composed of IgA) within the mesangium (the same mesangioproliferative picture seen on biopsy in HSP).

   Affected patients often present with chronic asymptomatic microscopic hematuria and trace proteinuria, with exacerbations characterized by *gross hematuria* occurring after viral infections or GI illness. IgA nephropathy is a disorder that can present with features of both nephrotic and nephritic syndromes.

STEP 1 SECRET

Although similar in presentation to poststreptococcal glomerulonephritis (PSGN), IgA nephropathy can be distinguished based on history. PSGN occurs weeks after an upper respiratory infection, whereas IgA nephropathy occurs within days. This is a favorite concept for the USMLE!

8. **What syndrome do you suspect in a 13-year-old boy with microscopic hematuria and hearing loss?**

   Alport syndrome (i.e., hereditary nephritis) would be suspected. Although less common, Alport syndrome is clinically similar to IgA nephropathy in that it presents with asymptomatic microscopic hematuria. It is caused by mutations in type IV collagen normally found in the GBM and elsewhere, and it is inherited in an X-linked manner (can be either dominant or recessive). Alport syndrome is associated with abnormal hearing and vision (i.e., sensorineural hearing loss and lens abnormalities). Diagnosis can be made with skin biopsy because of the presence of type collagen IV in the skin. If performed, renal biopsy typically shows fragmentation of the basement membrane in a "basket weave" pattern with no specific pattern of immunofluorescence seen on light microscopy.

   As an aside, there are only a few medications that can cause both ototoxicity and nephrotoxicity. These drugs include loop diuretics (e.g., furosemide), vancomycin, cisplatin, and aminoglycosides.

9. **Quick review: Cover the right column in Table 3.5 and attempt to diagnose the cause of the glomerulonephritis based on the laboratory findings and history provided in the left column.**

Table 3.5. Differential Diagnosis for Glomerulonephritis

FINDINGS ON LABORATORY TESTS AND HISTORY	LIKELY CAUSE OF GLOMERULONEPHRITIS
Anti-GBM antibodies, hematuria, and hemoptysis	Goodpasture syndrome (i.e., anti-GBM disease)
c-ANCA–positive with a history of bloody nasal discharge and hemoptysis	Granulomatosis with polyangiitis
Defect in type IV collagen with congenital hearing and ocular impairment	Alport syndrome
Massive proteinuria and edema in an adult with hepatitis B	Membranous nephropathy
Hematuria, episodic abdominal pain, joint pain, and a lower extremity purpuric rash	Henoch-Schönlein purpura

c-ANCA, Cytoplasmic antineutrophil cytoplasmic antibodies; *GBM,* glomerular basement membrane.

SUMMARY BOX: POSTSTREPTOCOCCAL GLOMERULONEPHRITIS

- Acute nephritic syndrome occurring 1 to 2 weeks after streptococcal sore throat or skin/soft tissue infection
- Diagnosis: Antistreptolysin O (ASO) or anti-DNase B titers to document recent infection
- Therapy: Not commonly needed; typically resolves without specific therapy
- Do not confuse with IgA nephropathy!

CASE 3.8

A 45-year-old man is evaluated for a several-hour history of severe left-sided flank pain that radiates into his groin. He reports some mild nausea but denies vomiting or diarrhea. On physical examination, he is writhing in pain, but an abdominal exam is otherwise unrevealing. Urine microscopy reveals gross hematuria without red blood cell (RBC) casts, dysmorphic RBCs, or WBC casts. Labs reveal mild hypercalcemia.

1. **What is the most likely diagnosis?**
   Nephrolithiasis is the most likely diagnosis. The severe flank pain (i.e., renal colic) and urologic (i.e., nonglomerular) hematuria are suggestive of nephrolithiasis, which can be confirmed by noncontrast CT. Hypercalcemia is one of many risk factors for nephrolithiasis.

2. **What are the most common causes of nephrolithiasis?**
   Dehydration, hypercalciuria, and primary hyperparathyroidism. Other causes include *Proteus* infection (struvite stones; Fig. 3.22), hyperuricosuria (uric acid stones; Fig. 3.23), and impaired absorption of basic amino acids (cystine stones; Fig. 3.24)

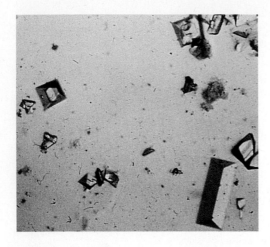

Figure 3.22. Coffin lid crystals of magnesium ammonium phosphate (struvite). *(From Feehally J, et al. Comprehensive Clinical Nephrology. 6th ed. Philadelphia: Elsevier; 2019: 689-703.e1, Fig. 57.3 D.)*

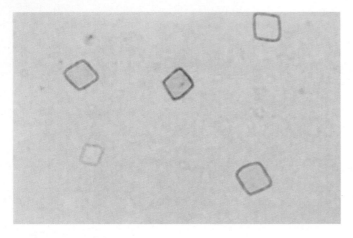

Figure 3.23. Uric acid crystals (×160). *(From McPherson RA. Henry's Clinical Diagnosis and Management by Laboratory Methods. 23rd ed. St. Louis: Elsevier; 2017: 442-480.e3, Fig. 28-28.)*

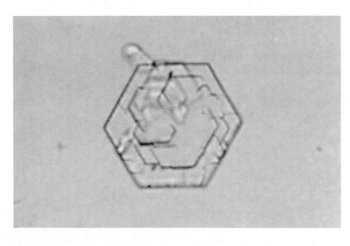

Figure 3.24. Hexagonal cystine crystals, which indicate cystinuria (×200). *(From McPherson RA. Henry's Clinical Diagnosis and Management by Laboratory Methods. 23rd ed. St. Louis: Elsevier; 2017: 442-480. e3, Fig. 28-38.)*

The majority of kidney stones are calcium stones (calcium oxalate or calcium phosphate), followed by struvite stones (magnesium ammonium phosphate), then uric acid stones and cystine stones.

3. **How can nephrolithiasis cause renal failure?**
Complete obstruction of a ureter or ureteric pelvis increases the hydrostatic pressure in the ureters, and ultimately the renal tubules. Increased hydrostatic pressure diminishes net filtration pressure at the glomerulus, causing an acute decline in the GFR. However, if the other kidney is intact and healthy, it can compensate for the decreased GFR in the obstructed kidney.
　　Recall that obstruction of urine flow out of a kidney causes hydronephrosis, in which the renal pelvis and calyces dilate significantly (pelvicaliectasis). Hydronephrosis is usually detected on renal ultrasound or CT scan.

4. **What are the two most common causes of hypercalcemia?**
Primary hyperparathyroidism is the predominant cause in the community, whereas malignancy-induced hypercalcemia predominates in hospitalized patients. These two conditions account for over 90% of hypercalcemia cases.
　　Recall that primary hyperparathyroidism is usually caused by a parathyroid adenoma (majority of cases), hyperplasia (10% of cases), or carcinoma (rarely). Hypercalcemia is the most common metabolic derangement that complicates malignancy, occurring in 10% to 20% of patients with cancer. Breast cancer and multiple myeloma can produce hypercalcemia by metastasizing to bone and causing lytic destruction; others, such as squamous cell cancer of the lung (and other organs) and renal cell carcinoma, secrete an ectopic hormone known as *parathyroid hormone–related peptide* (PTHrP). A popular mnemonic for the complications of hyperparathyroidism is "stones, bones, moans, groans, and psychiatric overtones," referring to the increased risk for renal calculi, peptic ulcers (presumably from increased gastric acid secretion), pathologic fractures, vague bone pains, muscle aches or weakness, malaise, fatigue, and psychosis. Hypercalcemia can cause polydipsia and polyuria (from osmotic diuresis), constipation, and hypertension (from increased smooth muscle tone).

Clinical Pearl

A mnemonic for causes of hypercalcemia is **CHIMPANZEES**: excess **C**alcium ingestion, **H**yperparathyroidism or **H**yperthyroidism, **I**atrogenic (i.e., drug-induced, as from thiazide administration) or **I**mmobilization, **M**yeloma, **P**aget disease of bone, **A**ddison disease, **N**eoplasm, **Z**ollinger-Ellison syndrome (typically in association with multiple endocrine neoplasia type I syndrome), **E**xcess vitamin D, **E**xcess vitamin A, **S**arcoid and other granulomatous diseases. Many of these conditions, although potential causes of hypercalcemia, are more commonly associated with normal serum calcium.

---

5. **Why is hypercalcemia secondary to hyperparathyroidism less likely to cause renal calculi formation than other causes of hypercalcemia?**
Generally, the risk of calcium oxalate stone formation in the urine is proportional to the *urine* calcium concentration. Although primary hyperparathyroidism increases urine calcium concentration, it does so to a lesser extent because PTH promotes hypercalcemia by stimulating renal tubular calcium reabsorption.

6. **Why does UTI with bacteria such as *Proteus mirabilis* predispose patients to struvite stone formation?**
Struvite stones precipitate at *higher* urinary pH. *Proteus* species express the enzyme urease, which cleaves urea to form ammonia and carbon dioxide. The ammonia released increases the urinary pH and forms the ammonium that can precipitate as part of the struvite stones. Struvite stones, like calcium oxalate stones, are radiopaque.
　　Note: Struvite stones are often large, at times occupying all the renal calyces to form characteristic "staghorn" calculi.

7. **How does urinary pH influence the precipitation of uric acid stones?**
As a weak acid, uric acid is *less* soluble in its (neutral, protonated) uric acid form than in the (unprotonated, negatively charged) urate form. Decreasing urinary pH increases the concentration of the less soluble uric acid form, thereby facilitating crystallization (particularly at a pH of 5–5.5).
　　The diuretic acetazolamide can help dissolve uric acid stones, as inhibition of carbonic anhydrase prevents bicarbonate reabsorption and increases urinary pH.
　　Uric acid stones are associated with hyperuricemia and hyperuricosuria. Thus in addition to increased fluid intake (as used with all stone types) and urine alkalinization, allopurinol can help prevent the recurrence of uric acid stones by decreasing uric acid synthesis (via inhibition of the enzyme xanthine oxidase).

8. **What is cystinuria, and how does it lead to cystine stones?**
Cystinuria is a genetic disease in which there is a defect in the transporter responsible for the absorption of the *basic* amino acids cystine, ornithine, lysine, and arginine. Because cystine is not as soluble as these other amino acids, it precipitates selectively in this disease.
　　Cystinuria is distinct from the disease homocystinuria. In the latter case, a genetic defect in homocysteine catabolism causes extreme elevations in plasma and urine homocysteine concentrations.
　　Cystine and uric acid stones are both "organic stones," which are typically radiolucent and cannot be visualized using x-rays but can be seen with CT scan. This contrasts with most calcium-containing stones, which are radiopaque and can be visualized using x-rays.

9. How does Crohn disease lead to an increased risk of kidney stones?

Crohn disease frequently involves the terminal ileum, which is the primary site of bile salt reabsorption. Because bile salts and fat normally extensively bind calcium, increased levels of bile salt in the intestinal lumen resulting from malabsorption decreases the levels of free calcium in the gut. Less free calcium is available to bind oxalate, which, in turn, is left unbound and absorbed in the gut. As a result, patients with Crohn disease tend to hyperabsorb oxalate. This excess oxalate is excreted in the urine, and the high urinary oxalate concentration predisposes to calcium oxalate stone formation.

SUMMARY BOX: NEPHROLITHIASIS

- Presents with "renal colic" and urologic (i.e., nonglomerular) hematuria; can cause obstruction and, if bilateral, renal failure
- Pathology: Stones are composed of (in order of decreasing incidence) calcium, struvite, uric acid, and cysteine.
- Diagnosis: Computed tomography
- Mechanisms of hypercalcemia include:
  - Direct lysis of bone (as in myeloma or breast cancer)
  - Ectopic production of parathyroid hormone (PTH)-related peptide (as in squamous cell lung cancer)
  - Excess production of activated vitamin D by macrophages (by lymphomas or granulomatous diseases)
  - Less common causes include calcium ingestion, milk-alkali syndrome, thiazide diuretics, Paget disease, hypervitaminosis D or A, and endocrine disorders (Addison disease or hyperthyroidism)
- Struvite stones consist of magnesium ammonium phosphate and precipitate at a high urinary pH. As a result, they often complicate infections caused by urease-producing (i.e., urea-cleaving and ammonia-releasing) organisms like *Proteus*. "Staghorn" calculi are usually composed of struvite.
- Uric acid stones precipitate at *lower* urine pH, and as a result, the carbonic anhydrase inhibitor acetazolamide can be used to dissolve them.
- Cystinuria is a defect in tubular basic amino acid reabsorption that results in recurrent cystine stones.
- Crohn disease leads to bile acid malabsorption, which predisposes to both gallstones and kidney (calcium oxalate) stones.

CASE 3.9

A 38-year-old woman complains of sudden-onset urinary symptoms, including burning with urination, frequent urination, urgency, and a feeling of incomplete bladder emptying, as well as nausea, vomiting, and right-sided back pain. On physical examination she has a fever of 39.2°C (102.5°F) and right-sided costovertebral angle tenderness. Urinalysis reveals numerous WBCs, bacteria, and white blood cell (WBC) casts. She is admitted to the hospital and prescribed ciprofloxacin. She is also told to drink plenty of fluids.

---

1. What is the most likely diagnosis?

Acute pyelonephritis is the most likely diagnosis. Although WBC casts can be seen with other causes of renal parenchymal inflammation (e.g., AIN), WBC casts in the setting of dysuria and flank pain are pathognomonic for acute pyelonephritis.

2. What is the most common source of infection in pyelonephritis?

In most cases, infections are the result of ascending infection from the bladder and urinary tract. A minority of infections are from hematogenous dissemination. The most common infectious agents are fecal flora that has colonized the vaginal introitus, predominantly *Escherichia coli*. In sexually active young women, infection with *Staphylococcus saprophyticus* (coagulase-negative staphylococcus) is the second most common. Among cases of hematogenous seeding of the renal parenchyma, coagulase-positive *S. aureus* is the most common pathogen.

3. Why are pregnant women with asymptomatic bacteriuria treated more aggressively than non-pregnant women with the same condition?

Although asymptomatic bacteriuria rarely causes problems in nonpregnant women (typically not treated in nonpregnant women), pregnant women with this condition are more susceptible to pyelonephritis. Aside from the dangers of developing bacteremia and sepsis, pyelonephritis also increases the risk of premature delivery.

4. Why are pregnant women with bacteriuria more susceptible to pyelonephritis?

Pregnancy results in relaxation of the basal tone of the ureteral smooth muscle because of increased levels of progesterone. This ureteral dilation or physiologic hydronephrosis increases urine pooling and, in turn, the risk of ascending infection.

5. How does AIN differ from acute pyelonephritis?

AIN, like pyelonephritis, is characterized by inflammation of the renal interstitium. However, rather than infection, it is caused by an allergic reaction, most commonly a drug hypersensitivity. Although infectious agents (less commonly than drugs) can also precipitate AIN, the infectious process itself is minimally involved in the pathogenesis, whereas the immunologic hypersensitivity to the infectious agent is paramount. AIN can also be a manifestation of autoimmune disorders such as sarcoid (albeit rarely).

See Case 3.3, question 1, for a review of AIN as a cause of intrinsic AKI.

6. Why are UTIs in men younger than 50 often evaluated aggressively?
These infections are usually due to urologic abnormalities because younger men are ordinarily resistant to UTIs (with the exception of sexually transmitted diseases). Women are predisposed to UTIs because of the shorter length of the female urethra and the proximity of the vagina and perineum to the urethral meatus.

Note: In men older than 50, BPH causes greater urinary retention and stasis of bladder urine, which facilitates bacterial overgrowth.

SUMMARY BOX: ACUTE PYELONEPHRITIS

- Signs and symptoms: Urinary tract infection (UTI) symptoms, fever, and nausea and vomiting
- Pathology: Usually results from ascending urinary infection caused by fecal flora, most commonly *Escherichia coli*. In young women, *Staphylococcus saprophyticus* is second only to *E. coli*. Hematogenous infection of the kidneys is most commonly caused by *Staphylococcus aureus*.
  - Pregnancy predisposes to ascending urinary infection; thus, asymptomatic bacteriuria in pregnancy is treated to prevent pyelonephritis and the subsequent risk of sepsis and preterm delivery.
  - Men older than 50 years are predisposed to UTI from benign prostatic hyperplasia (BPH)-related urinary retention and stasis. Likewise, adult men under 50 with a UTI should be evaluated for sexually transmitted infections (STIs) or urinary anomalies.
- Diagnosis: Costovertebral angle tenderness on examination and WBC, bacteria, and WBC casts in the urine (highly suggestive)

CHAPTER 4

FLUID AND ELECTROLYTES

Insider's Guide to Fluid and Electrolytes for the USMLE Step 1

Many of the important concepts that were introduced in Chapter 3 (Nephrology) are further explored in Chapters 4 (Fluid and Electrolytes) and 5 (Acid-Base Balance). Concepts relating to fluid and electrolytes make up a large portion of the renal physiology and pharmacology material tested on the USMLE Step 1. You will soon see that this is *not* a section that requires memorizing lots of small details. Instead, it demands a thorough understanding of the mechanisms of action of various hormones and drugs involved in regulating fluid and electrolyte balance. Know which segments of the nephron are affected by these individual hormones and drugs. If applicable, it is a good idea to categorize how each hormone or drug affects glomerular filtration rate (GFR), renal plasma flow (RPF), filtration fraction (FF), and so on. For those of you who do not have a strong background in renal physiology, you may need to read through the discussion in this chapter a few times to fully grasp all of the material.

BASIC CONCEPTS—RENAL FILTRATION AND TRANSPORT PROCESSES

1. What forces govern the glomerular filtration rate at the level of the glomerulus?

   The forces that govern the glomerular filtration rate (GFR) at the level of the glomerulus are the same forces that direct fluid movement in the systemic capillaries. Forces that drive fluid across the glomerular membrane include the hydrostatic pressure in the glomerular capillaries and the oncotic pressure in the Bowman space (Fig. 4.1). Because there is usually very little protein in the Bowman space, the contribution from the filtrate's oncotic pressure is typically negligible. Forces that oppose fluid movement across the glomerular membrane are the hydrostatic pressure in the Bowman space and the plasma oncotic pressure.

   Glomerular hydrostatic pressure and, in turn, GFR will change based on the behavior of the afferent and efferent arterioles. The afferent arteriole delivers blood to the glomerulus, while the efferent arteriole returns filtered blood from the glomerulus back to systemic circulation. To keep this straight in your mind, remember the alliteration *afferent*

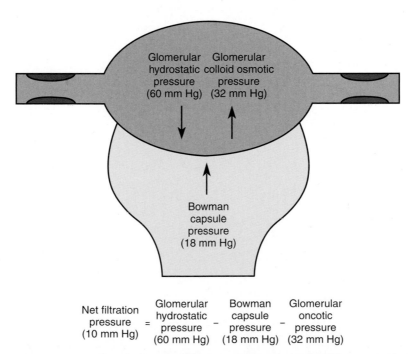

Figure 4.1. Summary of forces that drive filtration through the glomerular capillaries. The values shown are estimates for healthy adult humans. *(From Guyton AC, Hall JE. Textbook of Medical Physiology. 11th ed. Philadelphia: WB Saunders; 2007.)*

arrives, efferent exits. Because the glomerulus is located between the afferent and efferent arterioles, changes in the caliber of the arterioles tend to have opposite effects on the glomerulus. Either dilation of the afferent arteriole or constriction of the efferent arteriole will increase glomerular pressure and filtration. Conversely, constriction of the afferent arteriole or dilation of the efferent arteriole will decrease glomerular pressure and GFR.

2. **Describe the relationship between glomerular filtration rate and renal blood flow.**
   Renal blood flow (RBF) can be calculated as shown in Eq. 4.1:

$$\text{Renal blood flow (RBF)} = \frac{\text{Renal artery pressure} - \text{Renal venous pressure}}{\text{Renal vascular resistance}} \qquad [4.1]$$

The major resistance vessels within the kidney are the afferent and efferent arterioles, and an isolated constriction of either will increase renal vascular resistance and subsequently decrease RBF. Unlike RBF, GFR will either increase or decrease depending on the relative degree of contraction and dilation of each arteriolar vessel:

Increasing afferent resistance: ↓ GFR, ↓ RBF
Decreasing afferent resistance: ↑ GFR, ↑ RBF
Increasing efferent resistance: ↑ GFR, ↓ RBF
Decreasing efferent resistance: ↓ GFR, ↑ RBF

Factors that regulate the afferent and efferent arterioles are discussed later.
   Note: Most circulating vasoconstricting and vasodilating agents act on the afferent arteriole. An important exception, however, is angiotensin II, which acts preferentially to vasoconstrict the *efferent* arteriole. Thus angiotensin II works to preserve GFR in a setting of decreased renal perfusion. Angiotensin-converting enzyme (ACE) inhibitors decrease GFR by inhibiting the formation of angiotensin II and therefore blunting its effect on the efferent arteriole.
   In addition to the oncotic and hydrostatic pressures, the surface area and integrity of the glomerular membranes are also important determinants of GFR. Mathematically, these factors are represented through a filtration constant. These factors are most relevant in disease states in which the glomeruli are damaged. The formula for calculating GFR is given in Chapter 3 (Nephrology).

STEP 1 SECRET

To help you recall the function of angiotensin II on the glomerular arteriole system, just remember the acronym **ACE***:* **a***ngiotensin II* **c***onstricts the* **e***fferent arteriole.*

3. **How do angiotensin-converting enzyme inhibitors and angiotensin receptor blockers affect glomerular filtration rate?**
   ACE inhibitors and angiotensin receptor blockers (ARBs) tend to acutely decrease GFR. Blocking the action of angiotensin II prevents vasoconstriction of the efferent arteriole, which decreases intraglomerular pressure and, in turn, decreases filtration.
   Although ACE inhibitors and ARBs usually cause a decrease in GFR (manifesting as an increase in plasma creatinine) in the short term, they have an important beneficial effect on preserving renal function in individuals with diabetes mellitus and other chronic kidney diseases. This benefit likely results from the fact that a decrease in glomerular pressure may, over the long term, decrease the wear on the glomeruli despite acutely reducing GFR. Because of this long-term benefit, a certain degree of creatinine elevation is tolerated when starting an ACE inhibitor or ARB.

4. **How do prostaglandins and nonsteroidal antiinflammatory drugs influence RBF?**
   While prostaglandins do not exert significant effects on RBF under normal physiologic conditions, they play an important role under conditions of hypovolemia and stress and in the elderly by limiting afferent/efferent arteriole vasoconstriction. Because they have a more prominent effect on the afferent arteriole, prostaglandins cause net afferent dilation, which results in an increase in RBF. Both acute and chronic nonsteroidal antiinflammatory drugs (NSAID) use inhibits prostaglandin synthesis, which prevents this compensatory afferent vasodilation and therefore reduces RBF under conditions of high angiotensin II and sympathetic stimulation. This can potentially result in renal ischemia and acute kidney injury (AKI). Signs of AKI include weight gain (as the result of fluid retention) and elevated laboratory values of serum creatinine, blood urea nitrogen (BUN), and potassium levels.

5. **What is meant by the term** *filtration fraction,* **and how will an isolated increase of the glomerular capillary oncotic pressure affect the FF?**
   The FF is the percent of plasma passing through the glomerular capillaries that is actually filtered by the glomerulus. Think of it as, quite literally, the *fraction* of plasma that gets *filtered*. It can be calculated as shown in Eq. 4.2:

$$\text{Filtration fraction (FF)} = \frac{\text{Glomerular filtration rate}}{\text{Renal plasma flow}} \qquad [4.2]$$

In a typical healthy adult, FF is about 20%. Because the glomerular capillary oncotic pressure opposes filtration, increasing it will decrease the net filtration pressure and decrease the FF.

6. **What are the three layers of the glomerular "filter," and how do they contribute to the renal filtration of blood at the glomerulus?**

The three components of the glomerular filter include the *endothelial cells* of the glomerular capillaries, the underlying *basement membrane*, and the *glomerular epithelial cells* (also called *podocytes*). These components each contribute to renal filtration in distinct ways.

The endothelium of the glomerular capillaries is *fenestrated*, meaning porous. Along with the relatively high hydrostatic pressure present in the glomerular capillaries, the fenestration of these capillaries allows for the filtration of large volumes of plasma across the capillary bed.

The underlying basement membrane is a collection of type IV collagen and heparin sulfate. It is negatively charged, which helps prevent the filtration and subsequent urinary loss of large plasma proteins, which are also negatively charged. Importantly, these negatively charged proteins include albumin, which is why hypoalbuminemia can occur in various types of glomerular diseases (e.g., nephrotic syndromes).

The glomerular epithelial cells (podocytes) serve as the final layer of the glomerular filter. These specialized cells have cytoplasmic extensions called *foot processes,* with intervening slit-pores, that together envelop the glomerular capillaries and form a final barrier for filterable molecules to traverse before entering the capsular space of the glomerulus.

Note: The glomerulus also contains macrophage-like mesangial cells and mesangial matrix interspersed between these layers (Fig. 4.2). The function of the mesangium is not very well understood, though it may serve both a structural role and a housekeeping role. Regardless, the mesangium can be an important site of glomerular disease.

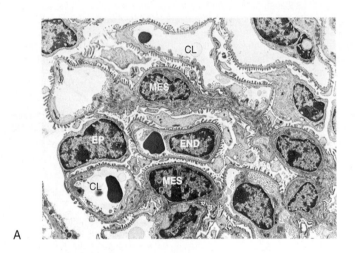

A

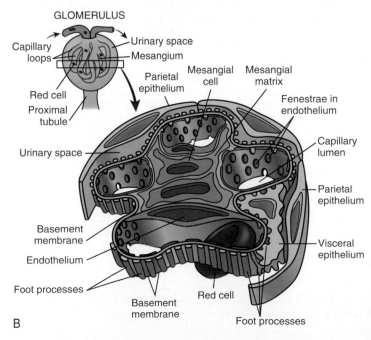

B

Figure 4.2. A, Low-power electron micrograph of the renal glomerulus. CL, Capillary lumen; END, endothelium; EP, visceral epithelial cells with foot processes; MES, mesangium. B, Schematic representation of a glomerular lobe. *(Courtesy Dr. Vicki Kelley, Brigham and Women's Hospital, Boston, MA.)*

7. **What is the significance of the creatinine clearance, and how is it measured?**

Because creatinine is neither reabsorbed nor secreted to a clinically significant degree, the creatinine clearance can be used to approximate GFR and is therefore an important indicator of renal function.

The clearance of any substance is defined as the volume (V) of plasma that is cleared of that substance per unit of time. For example, a creatinine clearance rate of 125 mL/min implies that, every minute, creatinine is being completely removed and excreted (by the kidneys) from 125 mL of plasma. As shown in Eq. 4.3, the clearance (C) of a substance can be calculated by dividing the urinary excretion rate of that substance by the substance's plasma concentration. The urinary excretion rate of a substance can be determined from its concentration in urine and the urine flow rate.

$$C = \frac{\text{Urinary flow rate (mL/min)} \times \text{Urinary creatinine concentration (Ucr)}}{\text{Plasma creatinine concentration (Pcr)}} \qquad [4.3]$$

$$= \frac{V \times Ucr}{Pcr}$$

You can easily derive this formula by recalling that all creatinine that appears in the urine is a result of the removal of creatinine from plasma:

$$\text{Rate of creatinine removal from plasma} = \text{Rate of creatinine excretion in urine}$$

$$Pcr \times C = V \times Ucr$$

$$C = \frac{V \times Ucr}{Pcr} \qquad [4.4]$$

Clinically, a single plasma creatinine level is used frequently, along with a patient's weight, age, and gender (and, in some equations, race [though this is hotly debated and being eliminated], and serum albumin as a measure of nutrition status), to estimate creatinine clearance and GFR. These additional factors are included to estimate the rate of creatinine production, which depends on muscle mass (because creatinine is a by-product of the muscle energy storage molecule creatine). Note that these equations work well only when the patient's renal function is at a steady state. They become less accurate when renal function is rapidly changing, as in AKI.

SUMMARY BOX: GENERAL CONCEPTS IN RENAL FILTRATION AND TRANSPORT PROCESSES

- Renal blood flow (RBF) and hydrostatic pressure within the glomerular capillaries are regulated by vasoconstriction and vasodilation of the afferent and efferent arterioles.
- Most circulating vasoactive substances act to constrict or dilate the afferent arteriole. Angiotensin II is unique in that it acts primarily to constrict the *efferent* arteriole.
- Nonsteroidal antiinflammatory drugs (NSAIDs) can decrease renal plasma flow (RPF) and potentially cause renal ischemia by impairing prostaglandin synthesis, thereby preventing dilation of the afferent arteriole.
- Angiotensin-converting enzyme (ACE) inhibitors and angiotensin receptor blockers (ARBs) may acutely decrease glomerular filtration rate (GFR), but their effect on lowering glomerular pressure helps preserve renal function over the long term in patients with diabetes mellitus and chronic kidney disease.
- Components of the glomerular filter include (1) the capillary endothelial cells, (2) the negatively charged basement membrane, and (3) the epithelial cells (podocytes) and the intervening mesangium.
- Creatinine clearance is an important indicator of GFR because creatinine is neither secreted nor reabsorbed by the kidney to a clinically significant degree.
  - Estimates of creatinine clearance are *inaccurate* in the setting of a rapidly changing GFR (i.e., acute kidney injury).

BASIC CONCEPTS—RENAL CONTROL OF EXTRACELLULAR FLUID BALANCE

1. **What are the extracellular fluid compartments of the body, and how do their relative sizes compare to the intracellular fluid compartment?**

The extracellular fluid (ECF) consists of the interstitial fluid and plasma.

Overall, total body water in a healthy young man is roughly 60% of body weight (whereas in a woman it is about 50%). For an "average" 70-kg man, total body water is therefore approximately 42 L (recall that 1 L of water weighs 1 kg). About two-thirds of the total body water is found intracellularly; the other one-third makes up the ECF volume. Thus a 70-kg man has about 14 L of ECF: $(70 \times 0.6) \times \frac{1}{3}$. Plasma volume accounts for about one-third to one-fourth of the ECF (approximately 4 L in a 70-kg individual), whereas the remaining 10 L is interstitial fluid.

2. **How do the kidneys regulate extracellular fluid volume?**

The kidneys regulate ECF *volume* by adjusting the rate of excretion of *sodium* (Na^+). In contrast, the kidneys regulate body fluid *osmolarity* and *sodium concentration* by altering the excretion of *free water* (i.e., water without sodium). This is one of the most important concepts in renal physiology: In the normal state, *volume* is regulated through *sodium balance,* whereas *osmolarity* and *sodium concentration* are regulated through *water balance.*

To be more precise, it is the effective circulating volume (ECV) that is regulated by the body, not the ECF volume. This is because the body has no way to directly follow ECF volume levels. Instead, various pressure and volume detectors located throughout the circulatory system (e.g., in the atria, the aortic arch, the carotid sinus, and the afferent arterioles of the kidney) monitor the ECV and, through various mechanisms, stimulate or inhibit Na^+ excretion accordingly. ECV is *not* a measurable volume; it represents the volume of arterial blood that is effectively perfusing tissue. ECV is generally proportional to ECF, but notable exceptions occur during congestive heart failure (CHF), cirrhosis, and nephrotic syndrome.

The renin-angiotensin-aldosterone system (RAAS) is possibly the most important of these regulatory mechanisms.

3. **What is the normal role of the renin-angiotensin-aldosterone system?**
The role of the RAAS is to ensure adequate organ perfusion. It accomplishes this through a series of signaling pathways that ultimately act to maintain an appropriate plasma volume and blood pressure.

RAAS is activated in response to decreased ECV. Specifically, reduced renal blood flow is sensed by a group of specialized smooth muscle cells located in the wall of the afferent arterioles (part of the juxtaglomerular apparatus). This sensing mechanism functions so that a decrease in afferent arteriolar perfusion will stimulate renin production and secretion.

Once released into systemic circulation, renin enzymatically cleaves the serum precursor protein angiotensinogen into angiotensin I, which, in turn, is cleaved in the lungs and elsewhere by the endothelial ACE into the physiologically active peptide angiotensin II. Angiotensin II is a potent vasoconstrictor that acts to directly increase blood pressure; in fact, it is the most potent physiologic vasoconstrictor known. Angiotensin II also has a direct effect to promote Na^+ reabsorption in the proximal tubule. A third action of angiotensin II is stimulation of aldosterone release from the adrenal cortex. Aldosterone stimulates the reabsorption of Na^+ (coupled to the secretion of K^+ or H^+) in the distal tubule of the nephron. This retained Na^+ (or, more specifically, the fluid volume that accompanies it) helps restore ECV.

4. **What is the role of the sympathetic nervous system in maintaining effective circulating volume?**
In addition to helping maintain blood pressure via systemic vasoconstriction, the sympathetic nervous system stimulates Na^+ retention in response to low ECV through several mechanisms. First, sympathetically mediated vasoconstriction of the afferent arteriole causes decreased GFR, which promotes Na^+ retention through RAAS activation. This is regulated by the macula densa (a collection of specialized cells that line the distal tubule), which senses a decreased delivery in Na^+ load secondary to decreased blood pressure and stimulates renin release. The sympathetic fibers to the afferent arteriole also directly stimulate renin release through activation of β_1-adrenergic receptors. Finally, the sympathetic nervous system (like angiotensin II) promotes Na^+ reabsorption in the proximal tubule.

5. **How does antidiuretic hormone regulate extracellular fluid volume?**
Under normal conditions, antidiuretic hormone (ADH) does *not* work to regulate ECF volume. Instead, ADH normally functions to regulate the reabsorption of free water in the collecting duct in response to changes in body fluid *osmolarity*. This occurs via interactions with vasopressin 2 (V2) receptors in the basolateral membrane of the collecting duct, leading to insertion of aquaporins (water channels) in the apical membrane, rendering it permeable to water.

However, when ECV is severely compromised (decreased by 5%–10% of normal), secretion of ADH by the posterior pituitary is stimulated. Thus with significant hypovolemia, the function of ADH changes to help preserve fluid volume rather than correct a deranged osmolarity.

This ability of ADH to sacrifice osmolarity to help maintain ECV is an exception to the preceding rule, which asserts that water balance is regulated to maintain osmolarity while Na^+ balance is regulated to maintain fluid volume. When volume is low enough, the body abandons this usual division of labor and retains both Na^+ *and* water, regardless of osmolarity. This change is illustrated by disease states such as CHF, nephrotic syndrome, and cirrhosis. Because these three diseases are characterized by decreased ECV, hyponatremia commonly occurs in each condition as a result of chronically elevated ADH levels, because the body prioritizes the restoration of fluid volume over osmolarity in these critical circumstances.

CASE 4.1

A 78-year-old man is evaluated for refractory hypertension. His current antihypertensive regimen includes a thiazide diuretic, an ACE inhibitor, a beta-blocker, and an α_1-receptor antagonist. Physical examination is significant for a blood pressure of 184/105 mm Hg and auscultation of an abdominal bruit.

1. **What disease does this patient most likely have, and what is its underlying cause?**
This elderly patient likely has renovascular hypertension secondary to renal artery stenosis (RAS), which is most commonly the result of atherosclerosis of the renal arteries. Fibromuscular dysplasia of the renal arteries, a less common disease that primarily affects middle-aged women, also produces renovascular hypertension by occluding the lumen of the renal arteries.

CASE 4.1 CONTINUED:

A renal angiogram reveals a 95% occlusion of the left renal artery, confirming a diagnosis of renal artery stenosis (RAS). Renal angioplasty is performed to relieve the occlusion, and the patient's blood pressure subsequently normalizes.

2. **How does the renin-angiotensin-aldosterone system contribute to renovascular hypertension?**
If one kidney is significantly hypoperfused because of renal artery narrowing, it will release abnormally high levels of renin into the systemic circulation. This will increase systemic angiotensin II and aldosterone levels, which will cause

widespread vasoconstriction and significant Na^+ and water retention as discussed previously. Both of these actions result in increased blood pressure. In essence, renovascular hypertension is the result of the kidneys "misunderstanding" and acting as if the local hypoperfusion they are experiencing is a reflection of whole body hypoperfusion, leading to inappropriate fluid retention and chronically elevated blood pressure.

3. **How do the kidneys regulate effective circulating volume and blood pressure independently of the renin-angiotensin-aldosterone system?**

   Along with renin, angiotensin II, aldosterone, ADH, and the sympathetic nervous system as described previously, additional mechanisms for regulating ECV and blood pressure exist.

   At higher arterial pressures, the kidneys are better perfused, which directly results in increased GFR. Increased GFR alone increases the volume of urine that is produced, thereby reducing the ECF volume and blood pressure. This phenomenon is referred to by some as a *pressure natriuresis.* At lower arterial pressures, the reduced renal perfusion reduces GFR and increases tubular reabsorption of Na^+ and water (glomerulotubular balance), helping to expand ECF volume and restore the blood pressure.

   Atrial natriuretic peptide (ANP) is yet another hormonal signal that helps regulate ECV and blood pressure. High ECV mechanically expands the cardiac atria, stimulating the release of ANP and thereby promoting natriuresis (i.e., Na^+ excretion) by the kidneys in an effort to decrease ECV. In the setting of low ECV, ANP release is inhibited.

4. **If angiotensin II promotes vasoconstriction, why does the angiotensin II released during hypovolemic states not reduce glomerular filtration rate?**

   The preferential action of angiotensin II on the *efferent* (rather than the afferent) arteriole elegantly allows it to maintain GFR despite causing widespread vasoconstriction and reduced renal perfusion. Although vasoconstriction of the efferent arteriole reduces renal blood flow, it also increases the hydrostatic pressure of the glomerulus, which increases the net filtration pressure and maintains the GFR.

STEP 1 SECRET

If it has not become apparent yet, it is critical to know that angiotensin II maintains glomerular filtration rate (GFR) by preferentially constricting the efferent arteriole. Note that angiotensin II will also increase filtration fraction (FF) because of the increased GFR and reduced renal plasma flow (RPF) (Eq. 4.2).

5. **Why should angiotensin-converting enzyme inhibitors or angiotensin receptor blockers be avoided in patients with bilateral renal artery stenosis?**

   The normal role of angiotensin II in maintaining GFR in the face of hypovolemia is even more pronounced in the setting of bilateral RAS.

   Kidneys with bilateral RAS are dependent on angiotensin II–mediated constriction of the efferent arteriole to maintain glomerular filtration pressure and GFR. This tonic angiotensin-mediated constriction of the efferent arteriole is driven by high plasma levels of angiotensin II. Administering an ACE inhibitor (or an ARB) in this setting will cause the efferent arteriolar vasoconstriction to abruptly cease, causing GFR in both kidneys to drop precipitously and possibly induce AKI.

SUMMARY BOX: RENAL CONTROL OF EXTRACELLULAR FLUID BALANCE

- Extracellular fluid (ECF) volume, or, more precisely, *effective circulating volume* (ECV), is regulated by adjusting the rate of *sodium* (Na^+) excretion.
- *Osmolarity* is regulated by adjusting the rate of *free water* excretion.
- The body will always attempt to maintain Na^+ balance before water balance.
- ECV and blood pressure are regulated by the renin-angiotensin-aldosterone system (RAAS), the sympathetic nervous system, atrial natriuretic peptide (ANP), and intrinsic renal mechanisms.
- When ECV is decreased by 5% to 10% of baseline, antidiuretic hormone (ADH) release is stimulated, helping maintain volume while potentially sacrificing osmolarity.
- Renal artery stenosis (RAS) leads to hypertension via chronic RAAS activation.
  - RAS is most commonly caused by atherosclerosis. In younger women, renal hypertension may be caused by fibromuscular dysplasia.
  - Angiotensin-converting enzyme (ACE) inhibitors and angiotensin receptor blockers (ARBs) should be avoided in patients with bilateral RAS because of these patients' dependence on high levels of circulating angiotensin II to preserve glomerular filtration rate (GFR).

RENAL CONTROL OF EXTRACELLULAR FLUID OSMOLARITY

CASE 4.2

A 48-year-old man with a history of cholelithiasis but without any current abdominal pain or nausea is admitted to the hospital for an elective cholecystectomy. Presurgical workup reveals a serum sodium concentration of 125 mEq/L (normal 135–145 mEq/L). He complains of occasional fatigue, anorexia, and mild confusion. Physical examination is unremarkable. Urinalysis reveals an elevated urine osmolarity.

1. **What is the most likely diagnosis, and what is its cause?**

   Syndrome of inappropriate antidiuretic hormone secretion (SIADH) is the most likely diagnosis. Unexplained hyponatremia in a setting of increased urine osmolarity strongly suggests SIADH.

   In SIADH, excessive release of ADH from the posterior pituitary causes unnecessary free water retention in the collecting duct of the nephron. This additional water dilutes the plasma, resulting in decreased osmolarity and hyponatremia and *inappropriately* concentrates the urine (as opposed to the *appropriate* concentration of urine as a compensatory response to hypovolemia).

CASE 4.2 CONTINUED:

Further questioning reveals a 40-pack-per-year history of cigarette smoking. He denies any recent vomiting or diarrhea, has a normal albumin level, and shows no signs of heart failure. He denies taking diuretics or other medications. A chest x-ray film reveals a 3-cm spiculated pulmonary nodule near the hilum of the right lung.

2. **What additional disease states are associated with SIADH?**

   SIADH is associated with many diseases and disorders. For the USMLE Step 1, ectopic secretion of ADH by small cell carcinoma of the lung is the classic cause. In addition to this paraneoplastic syndrome, SIADH can be seen in a variety of nonmalignant diseases of the lung, including tuberculosis, pneumonia, pneumothorax, chronic obstructive pulmonary disease (COPD), and asthma.

   SIADH can also occur from lesions or tumors of the pituitary or hypothalamus, as well as in the setting of other intracranial pathologies such as head trauma, stroke, intracranial bleeds, and infection. It has also been associated with pain, nausea, and the postoperative state.

   Importantly, SIADH may also occur as a medication side effect, particularly with the antineoplastic agent cyclophosphamide or psychotropic medications such as antiepileptics, antipsychotics, and antidepressants (including selective serotonin reuptake inhibitors [SSRIs]).

3. **What is the function of antidiuretic hormone?**

   ADH (previously known as *vasopressin)* has two primary functions that correspond to its two names: the maintenance of plasma osmolarity and the maintenance of plasma volume and blood pressure.

   As discussed previously, to maintain plasma osmolarity, ADH is secreted in response to increased plasma osmolarity and stimulates the insertion of water channels (aquaporins) into the luminal membranes of the collecting ducts to facilitate free water resorption. This is the *antidiuretic* function of the hormone.

   Recall that ADH also helps maintain plasma volume and blood pressure in the setting of dramatically decreased ECV. In addition to increasing water reabsorption to expand ECV, it also works to directly maintain blood pressure through arterial vasoconstriction, hence the older term *vasopressin.*

4. **Why is the antidiuretic hormone release in SIADH considered "inappropriate"?**

   The excess ADH release seen in SIADH is considered "inappropriate" because its release is not occurring in response to its appropriate physiologic stimuli, which are increased osmolarity and hypovolemia. Rather, the ADH secretion occurs in an unregulated, autonomous fashion, independent of osmolarity or volume status, and is thus considered to be "inappropriate."

   In general, patients with SIADH are either euvolemic or only mildly hypervolemic. This counterintuitive phenomenon occurs because despite the elevated ADH levels, the body's other mechanisms for regulating volume status are preserved. In particular, the increased ADH-stimulated water reabsorption is countered by decreased activity of the RAAS and sympathetic nervous system and increased levels of brain natriuretic peptide (BNP), such that ECV and ECF volumes are maintained near normal.

   Euvolemia in spite of elevated ADH levels is important for two reasons. First, it reinforces the notion that *volume* is regulated through *sodium balance,* whereas *osmolarity* and *sodium concentration* are regulated through *water balance*. Second, it helps distinguish SIADH from other causes of hyponatremia that are generally associated with pronounced hypovolemia or hypervolemia (more specifically, a reduced ECV [e.g., profuse diarrhea, CHF, nephrotic syndrome]).

5. **What is the result of inadequate antidiuretic hormone release?**

   An inadequate level of ADH is the characteristic feature of central diabetes insipidus (DI), in which the posterior pituitary does not secrete sufficient ADH. DI is marked by excessive renal loss of free water, resulting in dilute urine, increased plasma osmolarity, and *hypernatremia.*

   DI can be generally divided into two major categories: central DI or nephrogenic DI. The inadequate ADH release of central DI is seen with head trauma, surgery, or other intracranial processes such as infection, tumor, or stroke. Central DI is treated with a synthetic analog of ADH called *desmopressin* (or DDAVP). This drug binds specifically to V2 receptors on the collecting duct that mediate the renal effects of ADH.

   Nephrogenic DI results from the inability of the kidneys to respond to ADH and can be caused by drug toxicity (e.g., lithium), hypercalcemia, an intrinsic mutation of the renal ADH receptor, and various other conditions. Nephrogenic DI, by definition, will *not* respond to DDAVP. The underlying cause of nephrogenic DI must be corrected, although salt restriction and thiazide diuretics (to block renal diluting ability) may be helpful.

STEP 1 SECRET

Distinguishing central diabetes insipidus (DI) from nephrogenic DI is high yield for the USMLE Step 1 and can be determined based on the body's response to the synthetic ADH analog desmopressin (DDAVP). Remember that nephrogenic DI will respond poorly to DDAVP, because the problem lies within the kidney itself. The body already has plenty of circulating ADH, and adding synthetic ADH in the form of DDAVP will not change anything. On the other hand, central DI will show a full response to DDAVP, because the fundamental problem is inadequate production (or release) of ADH. Address this deficiency by administering DDAVP and you have fixed the problem.

6. **How does hyponatremia cause the central nervous system symptoms described by this patient (e.g., fatigue, anorexia, and confusion)?**
   Na^+ concentration is the primary determinant of plasma and interstitial fluid osmolarity. Hyponatremia induces an osmotic shift of fluid into cells, including into neurons, in an attempt to restore osmotic homeostasis. This can result in cerebral edema and precipitate a wide variety of neurologic effects. If hyponatremia is severe, coma and convulsions may occur.

7. **Why must the hyponatremia be corrected slowly in this patient?**
   Overly rapid correction of hyponatremia (e.g., increasing serum Na^+ concentration by more than 12 mEq in a 24-hour period) is thought to place patients at risk for the development of osmotic demyelination syndrome (ODS), a disorder that can result in flaccid quadriplegia, dysphagia, facial weakness, coma, and, in some cases, death. A rare but classic manifestation of pons destruction in ODS is "locked-in syndrome," in which a conscious patient demonstrates paralysis of all muscles except those involved in eye opening and vertical gaze. The pathophysiology of ODS is believed to involve the overly rapid osmotic shift of fluid back out of brain cells in response to a rapid increase in plasma osmolarity, resulting in the death of myelin-producing oligodendrocytes and loss of myelin in the pons and other regions of the brain. In fact, magnetic resonance imaging (MRI) studies have shown that multiple areas of the brain are damaged with the overly rapid correction of hyponatremia, leading to symptoms including cognitive and psychiatric dysfunction. This disorder is classically seen in patients with significant alcohol use disorder who are suspected to be predisposed to this condition as a result of chronic malnutrition.
   Overly rapid correction of *hypernatremia* also leads to serious central nervous system (CNS) pathology, but in the form of *cerebral edema* rather than ODS. Again, it is prudent to avoid correcting serum Na^+ concentration faster than 0.5 mEq/L per hour.

8. **Why was it important to ask about vomiting, diarrhea, or diuretic use?**
   These are all causes of Na^+ wasting that can result in hyponatremia. Note that in these cases there are significant fluid losses also, resulting in *hypovolemic* hyponatremia. In contrast, SIADH is associated with a euvolemic or mildly hypervolemic hyponatremia (see previous question 4).
   Other causes of hypovolemic hyponatremia include salt wasting from mineralocorticoid deficiency (i.e., adrenal insufficiency) and "third-spacing" events (e.g., severe burns, pancreatitis, or bowel obstruction).
   Note: In this setting, the ADH release is *appropriate*, as it is stimulated by hypovolemia and decreased ECV.

9. **Why was it important to measure the serum albumin level and look for evidence of heart failure?**
   Hypoalbuminemia (from liver disease or nephrotic syndrome) and heart failure can each cause fluid retention and hyponatremia, resulting in *hypervolemic* hyponatremia.
   In this setting, ADH release is appropriate because, despite total body hypervolemia, these conditions are characterized by decreased ECV.

10. **How would levels of plasma antidiuretic hormone, plasma osmolarity, and urine osmolarity help distinguish between SIADH, diabetes insipidus, and psychogenic polydipsia?**
    These features are compared in Table 4.1.

SUMMARY BOX: RENAL CONTROL OF EXTRACELLULAR FLUID OSMOLARITY

- Antidiuretic hormone (ADH, vasopressin) has two primary effects: (1) increased aquaporin expression to stimulate free water reabsorption in the collecting duct (its *antidiuretic* function) and (2) systemic vasoconstriction (its *vasopressor* function).
- Under normal conditions, ADH is released in response to increased osmolarity. ADH release is also stimulated by a significant decrease (i.e., a drop of 5%–10% or more) in effective circulating volume (ECV). Release of ADH that is not caused by either of these stimuli is considered "inappropriate."
- The classic cause of hyponatremia secondary to syndrome of inappropriate antidiuretic hormone secretion (SIADH) is ectopic ADH secretion by a small cell carcinoma of the lung. Other causes include pituitary or hypothalamic lesions, various other lung and central nervous system (CNS) diseases, drug side effects, pain, nausea, and the postoperative state.
- Hyponatremia and high ADH levels can occur in congestive heart failure (CHF), cirrhosis, or nephrotic syndrome. Other causes of hyponatremia include Na^+ wasting via the gastrointestinal tract (e.g., vomiting or diarrhea) or kidneys (e.g., from diuretic use). In these diseases, ADH release is considered appropriate because of the reduced ECV.
- Inadequate ADH activity causes diabetes insipidus (DI), resulting in free water wasting and hypernatremia. DI is either *central* (inadequate ADH release) or *nephrogenic* (inability of the kidney to respond to adequate ADH release).

Table 4.1. Distinguishing Features of SIADH, DI, and Psychogenic Polydipsia

SYNDROME	PLASMA ADH	PLASMA OSMOLARITY	URINE OSMOLARITY	PATHOPHYSIOLOGIC EXPLANATION	CLASSIC USMLE STEP 1 ASSOCIATION
SIADH	High	Low	Inappropriately high	ADH causes excess water reabsorption by the kidneys, creating an inappropriately concentrated urine in the setting of low plasma osmolarity	Small cell carcinoma of the lung; cyclophosphamide use
Central DI	Low	High	Low	Lack of hypothalamic ADH secretion causes wasting of free water in excess of sodium, resulting in hyperosmolar plasma	Head trauma (disruption of the pituitary stalk); pituitary tumor
Nephrogenic DI	High	High	Low	Inability of the kidneys to respond to ADH results in wasting of free water and hyperosmolar plasma	Lithium toxicity; ADH receptor mutation
Psychogenic polydipsia	Low	Low	Maximally dilute (about 50 mOsm)	Enormous free water intake overwhelms ability of normal kidneys to excrete free water despite creating a maximally dilute urine	Schizophrenia or other psychiatric disease

ADH, Antidiuretic hormone; *DI*, diabetes insipidus; *SIADH*, syndrome of inappropriate antidiuretic hormone (secretion).

PHARMACOLOGY OF DIURETICS

1. How do diuretics work to lower extracellular fluid volume?

All diuretics act by inhibiting the reabsorption of Na^+ at various defined points along the nephron, thereby increasing the rate of Na^+ excretion and lowering the ECF volume. In other words, all diuretics are natriuretics.

The effect of any particular diuretic is ultimately limited, however, as the decrease in ECF volume means reduced Na^+ delivery to the nephron, such that the initially increased rate of Na^+ excretion eventually returns to baseline (i.e., equal to the rate of Na^+ intake). A new steady state is achieved at a lower ECF volume; continued administration of the diuretic is required to maintain this new equilibrium.

2. What percentage of the filtered sodium is reabsorbed at each point along the nephron under normal physiologic conditions (i.e., in the absence of diuretics)?

The majority of Na^+ resorption occurs in the proximal tubule, and each subsequent segment reabsorbs progressively less. The currently accepted percentages of Na^+ resorption that occurs along the nephron are listed in Table 4.2. Notice that roughly 99% of filtered Na^+ is normally reabsorbed. In general, the proximal tubule and ascending loop of Henle are relatively permeable and reabsorb large amounts of Na^+ (and the water that accompanies it) via relatively low-energy-requiring mechanisms, whereas the subsequent segments tend to be less permeable and require higher-energy mechanisms to actively "extract" increasingly smaller amounts of Na^+ against progressively higher concentration gradients.

These percentages are important in that the potency of each type of diuretic depends not only on the amount of Na^+ reabsorption that can be potentially inhibited in each region of the nephron but also on the resorptive capacity of the nephron segments *distal* to the site of diuretic action. These distal segments tend to compensate for the inhibition of proximal Na^+ reabsorption by increasing their own resorptive activity. For example, although one might predict that inhibition of proximal tubular Na^+ reabsorption (e.g., by carbonic anhydrase inhibitors) would result in the greatest diuresis, it tends to produce only a small diuresis because the downstream nephron segments respond to the increased Na^+ delivery with their own increased reabsorption.

Diuretics that act in the distal tubule and cortical collecting duct (i.e., the K^+-sparing diuretics) are also weak diuretics because they can influence, at most, only 10% to 15% of the filtered Na^+ load. Loop diuretics are therefore the most potent diuretics, in part because a large amount of Na^+ is reabsorbed in the loop of Henle *and* in part because the distal tubule and collecting duct downstream are limited in their ability to compensate. Note, however, that the primary reason why loop diuretics are the most potent diuretics is that they impair the generation of the medullary interstitial osmotic gradient that typically drives the concentration of urine (see question 3, next).

Table 4.2. Sodium (Na$^+$) Reabsorption Along the Nephron

SEGMENT	PERCENTAGE
Proximal tubule	60
Loop of Henle	25
Distal tubule	10
Collecting duct	4

3. In which region of the nephron does each of the following major diuretic types act (carbonic anhydrase inhibitors, osmotic diuretics, loop diuretics, thiazide diuretics, and K$^+$-sparing diuretics)? What are their mechanisms of action and major uses?

The details of renal Na$^+$ transport and the mechanisms of each diuretic type are best remembered when learned in progressive order starting with the most proximal region of the nephron and advancing distally, in the same order that an Na$^+$ molecule may encounter each region as it is excreted.

Carbonic anhydrase inhibitors (CAIs), such as acetazolamide, effectively act to inhibit NaHCO$_3$ (sodium bicarbonate) reabsorption in the proximal tubule through a complex mechanism that is further outlined in Chapter 5 (Acid-Base Balance). CAIs are not commonly used as diuretics in part because, as mentioned earlier, they have a weak diuretic effect as a result of their proximal site of action. Furthermore, because CAI administration may induce a metabolic acidosis that ultimately decreases the amount of filtered bicarbonate that is reabsorbed, its small diuretic effect is rapidly lost. In addition to the treatment or prevention of altitude sickness, CAIs are also used to treat open-angle glaucoma, as carbonic anhydrase is involved in the synthesis of aqueous humor of the eye, and the inhibition of carbonic anhydrase would therefore reduce intraocular pressure.

Osmotic diuretics also act primarily in the proximal tubule. Osmotic diuretics are substances that are freely filtered at the glomerulus but are poorly reabsorbed along the nephron. They inhibit Na$^+$ and water reabsorption by increasing the osmolarity of the tubular fluid, thereby pulling water into the urinary system and counteracting the concentration gradient that typically drives the reabsorption of water and Na$^+$ from the proximal tubule. The most commonly used osmotic diuretic is mannitol, which can be used in the acute treatment of cerebral edema, elevated intracranial pressure, or elevated intraocular pressure (as in acute closed-angle glaucoma). Certain endogenous substances (e.g., glucose, urea, and calcium) can act as osmotic diuretics when present at very high serum levels (i.e., glucose in diabetes or urea in chronic kidney disease).

Loop diuretics, such as furosemide, block the Na$^+$/K$^+$/2Cl$^-$ cotransporter present on the luminal surface of the thick ascending limb of the loop of Henle. Loop diuretics are the most potent diuretics currently available, not only because of their site of action, but because the inhibition of Na$^+$ transport in the loop of Henle abolishes the countercurrent mechanism used to generate the concentrated medullary interstitium that drives the maximal concentration of urine. In addition to impairing concentrating ability, they also block the nephron's diluting ability because they act to block the reabsorption of Na$^+$ in the water-impermeable thick ascending limb. Loop diuretics are first-line agents in the treatment of fluid overload caused by cardiac, hepatic, or renal disease (e.g., CHF, cirrhosis, or nephrotic syndrome). They are particularly useful in the treatment of acute cardiogenic pulmonary edema because loop diuretics also have rapid venodilator effects that effectively decrease cardiac preload.

Thiazide diuretics, such as hydrochlorothiazide, act to block the Na$^+$/Cl$^-$ cotransporter on the luminal surface of the early distal tubule (i.e., the cortical diluting segment). Again, because they inhibit Na$^+$ reabsorption at a water-impermeable segment of the nephron, thiazides impair the nephron's diluting ability; unlike loop diuretics, however, they do not affect the ability of urine to concentrate. They are relatively potent diuretics. Their major use is in the treatment of hypertension; in fact, they are considered first-line agents for this use because they are very inexpensive and were shown in the largest antihypertensive trial to date (ALLHAT Study) to effectively reduce cardiovascular mortality relative to calcium-channel blockers, ACE inhibitors, and alpha-blockers.

There are two subtypes of K$^+$-sparing diuretics. They both inhibit the activity of a specific type of Na$^+$ channel (the amiloride-sensitive channel) on the luminal surface of the principal cells of the late distal tubule and cortical collecting duct (Fig. 4.3). The expression of these surface channels is normally increased by the activity of aldosterone. Amiloride and triamterene act by directly blocking these Na$^+$ channels (through an aldosterone-independent action), whereas spironolactone and eplerenone act by blocking the mineralocorticoid receptor upon which aldosterone normally acts (through an aldosterone-dependent action). Because Na$^+$ reabsorption in the distal tubular cells is linked to K$^+$ excretion (via the basolateral Na$^+$/K$^+$-ATPase), this particular mechanism of inhibited Na$^+$ reabsorption results in retention of K$^+$ as well. K$^+$-sparing diuretics are the weakest diuretics; as such, they are typically used as adjuncts to other diuretics in the treatment of fluid overload and hypertension. They are particularly useful in preventing the hypokalemia that may be caused by other diuretics. The two aldosterone antagonists (spironolactone and eplerenone) also have an important role in the treatment of CHF, for which they have been documented to have a mortality risk benefit (as do beta-blockers and ACE inhibitors). The aldosterone antagonists are also particularly useful in the treatment of fluid overload related to cirrhosis, which, like CHF, is characterized by low ECV and high aldosterone levels. They can also be used in the specific treatment of other causes of hyperaldosteronism.

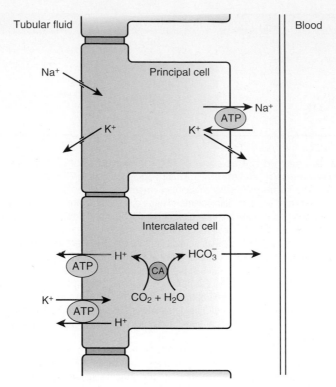

Figure 4.3. Transport pathways in principal cells and H^+-secreting intercalated cells of the distal tubule and collecting duct. ATP, Adenosine triphosphate; CA, carbonic anhydrase. *(From Koeppen BM, Stanton BA. Renal Physiology. 4th ed. Philadelphia: Mosby; 2007.)*

4. How does each major diuretic type affect the concentrations of serum electrolytes?

All diuretics increase K^+ excretion except, as their name implies, the K^+-sparing diuretics. Hypokalemia is particularly common with the stronger loop and thiazide diuretics. There are multiple mechanisms for diuretic-induced hypokalemia. First, proximally acting diuretics increase the flow rate of fluid past the principal cells of the late distal tubule, which lowers the K^+ concentration of the tubular fluid and thereby promotes K^+ excretion. Similarly, proximally acting diuretics increase distal delivery of Na^+, which also promotes K^+ excretion by increasing the rate of exchange of Na^+ for K^+ (Fig. 4.4). Diuretics also indirectly promote hypokalemia by decreasing ECV, which leads to increased aldosterone levels and aldosterone-stimulated K^+ excretion in an attempt to retain Na^+. CAIs also promote hypokalemia via induction of a metabolic acidosis. In the late distal tubule, K^+ and H^+ are secreted in exchange for reabsorbed Na^+ such that increased distal delivery of H^+ results in decreased H^+ excretion and a concomitant increase in K^+ excretion. See Chapter 5, Acid-Base Balance, for more on the interaction between K^+ levels and acid-base balance.

Hyponatremia can occur as a side effect of either loop or thiazide diuretics. Both of these diuretic types impair the nephron's diluting ability (i.e., the nephron's ability to separate water and Na^+). Diuretic-induced hyponatremia occurs particularly with thiazides in elderly patients, whose kidneys tend to have a decreased diluting ability at baseline.

The effects of diuretics on calcium (Ca^{2+}) and magnesium (Mg^{2+}) balance are relatively complicated and involve, among other mechanisms, changes in the luminal voltage gradients. However, the most clinically relevant effects are the dramatic *increase* in Ca^{2+} *excretion* (i.e., *decrease* in Ca^{2+} *serum concentration*) caused by loop diuretics and the unique ability of thiazides to *decrease* Ca^{2+} excretion (i.e., *increase* Ca^{2+} *serum concentration*). Loop diuretics are frequently used with intravenous fluids in the treatment of severe or symptomatic hypercalcemia (e.g., hypercalcemia of malignancy). Thiazides have unique effects on Ca^{2+} balance because the distal tubule is the only segment of the nephron in which Ca^{2+} reabsorption does *not* occur in parallel with Na^+ reabsorption. Thiazides inhibit Na^+ reabsorption by blocking the Na^+/Cl^- cotransporter on the apical membrane of the distal tubule. The subsequent decreased epithelial Na^+ concentration increases the activity of the Na^+/Ca^{2+} antiporter on the basolateral membrane. This moves Ca^{2+} into the interstitium as it pulls Na^+ into the epithelial cell and creates the gradient for more Ca^{2+} to be absorbed from the lumen. Because thiazides tend to cause hypercalcemia by decreasing urinary Ca^{2+} concentration, they can be used to prevent calcium kidney stone formation. Recall that elevated serum Ca^{2+} predisposes to calcium stone formation only by promoting elevated *urinary* Ca^{2+}. In contrast with the differing effects on Ca^{2+}, loop and thiazide diuretics can *both* cause clinically relevant hypomagnesemia.

Finally, each of the major diuretic types has a predictable effect on acid-base balance. CAIs, by inhibiting bicarbonate reabsorption, tend to promote metabolic acidosis. The stronger thiazide and loop diuretics, by producing decreased ECV, tend to promote a contraction alkalosis. Contraction alkalosis refers to the increase in bicarbonate reabsorption

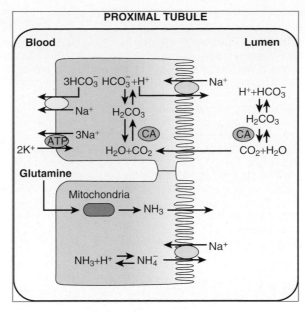

PROXIMAL TUBULE

Figure 4.4. Proximal tubule. *(From Goldman L, Ausiello D. Cecil Textbook of Medicine. 22nd ed. Philadelphia: WB Saunders; 2004.)*

that occurs with fluid loss and subsequent Na^+ reabsorption. K^+-sparing diuretics tend to favor a generally mild acidosis by promoting H^+ retention in a manner similar to their ability to promote K^+ retention (i.e., inhibition of Na^+ reabsorption in the late distal tubule prevents the secretion of K^+ and H^+ that would normally occur in exchange for Na^+). See Chapter 5, Acid-Base Balance, for more on the effects of diuretics on acid-base balance.

5. What are the other relatively common or important side effects of diuretics?
One of the most common side effects of diuretics is a direct extension of their therapeutic effect: overdiuresis and hypovolemia. Prerenal azotemia from overdiuresis is by far the most common type of diuretic-induced nephrotoxicity.

Multiple commonly used diuretics can cause hypersensitivity reactions associated with the sulfonamide residues they contain. These diuretics include acetazolamide, thiazides, and most loop diuretics (including furosemide). Similarly, loop diuretics and thiazides can cause allergic interstitial nephritis, albeit rather uncommonly. Ethacrynic acid is unique among the loop diuretics in that it does not contain a sulfonamide residue and hence would have no allergic cross-reactivity with other loop diuretics or sulfonamides.

The potent loop diuretics have the most potential for volume depletion and electrolyte abnormalities. Loop diuretics also tend to promote hyperuricemia, which, along with diuretic-induced hypovolemia, can aggravate or trigger gout. Loop diuretics can also cause ototoxicity, but usually only with large, rapidly administered intravenous doses. Ototoxicity is rare in the doses commonly used in clinical practice today.

Thiazides are similar to loop diuretics in their potential to exacerbate hyperuricemia and gout. Thiazides can also somewhat exacerbate hyperlipidemia or hyperglycemia, though generally not to a clinically relevant degree.

Spironolactone is a relatively nonspecific inhibitor of corticosteroid receptors, with significant antiandrogen effects in addition to its antimineralocorticoid effects. These antiandrogenic effects can manifest as gynecomastia and erectile dysfunction in men and hirsutism or breast tenderness in women. These nonspecific effects can be clinically useful in the treatment of acne vulgaris and hirsutism (i.e., spironolactone may both cause and treat hirsutism). In contrast, eplerenone selectively blocks only the mineralocorticoid receptors and therefore does not have these antiandrogen effects.

STEP 1 SECRET

The mechanisms of action, clinical uses, and notable side effects of diuretics are extremely important to understand when studying for the USMLE Step 1. This importance is probably no secret to you at this point. The detailed discussion in this chapter speaks for itself!

SUMMARY BOX: PHARMACOLOGY OF DIURETICS

- All diuretics lower extracellular fluid (ECF) volume by inhibiting the tubular reabsorption of sodium (Na^+).
- The potency of each diuretic depends both upon the capacity for Na^+ reabsorption at that particular nephron segment and upon the resorptive capacity of the downstream segments that may compensate for the diuretic's action.
- Carbonic anhydrase inhibitors (e.g., acetazolamide) and osmotic diuretics (e.g., mannitol) act primarily in the proximal tubule.
- Loop diuretics (e.g., furosemide) are the most potent diuretics and act by blocking Na^+ reabsorption in the thick ascending limb of the Loop of Henle, which impairs the nephron's ability to concentrate urine. They are first-line agents in the treatment of fluid overload as a result of cardiac, hepatic, or renal disease.
- Thiazide diuretics (e.g., hydrochlorothiazide) block Na^+ reabsorption in the early distal tubule and are first-line agents in the treatment of hypertension.
- K^+-sparing diuretics either directly block Na^+ reabsorption in the late distal tubule or cortical collecting duct (amiloride, triamterene) or do so indirectly by blocking the activity of aldosterone on mineralocorticoid receptors (spironolactone, eplerenone).
- All diuretics except the K^+-sparing diuretics amiloride, triamterene, spironolactone, and eplerenone tend to increase K^+ excretion and may cause hypokalemia.
- Loop diuretics can dramatically increase calcium excretion, whereas thiazides increase calcium reabsorption.

ACID-BASE BALANCE

BASIC CONCEPTS

1. **Why is the extracellular concentration of hydrogen ions so tightly regulated?**

   Hydrogen (H^+) ions are extremely reactive and, if present in significant amounts, will denature and inactivate the proteins that are essential to other physiologic functions. The H^+ ion concentration within the body's fluid compartments must therefore be held within a very narrow range and at a very low concentration to prevent this from occurring. Such tight control is accomplished by the presence of extracellular and intracellular buffers, removal of volatile acids by the lungs, and excretion of nonvolatile acids by the kidneys. Plasma concentrations of other cations and anions, by contrast, are present at much higher levels.

2. **How does the body prevent or react to derangements in acid-base balance?**

   Maintaining appropriate acid-base balance is the job of the bicarbonate/carbon dioxide (HCO_3^-/CO_2) buffer system. This system relies on three functional components to prevent or react to derangements in acid-base balance: the extracellular fluid (ECF), the lungs, and the kidneys. The ECF buffers immediately, the lungs buffer within minutes, and the kidneys buffer within days. Each of these is described in more detail in the following questions.

   It is important to understand that these buffering systems are generally responding to an acid load. This is because the dietary metabolism of proteins produces a small acid load (approximately 50–100 mEq) in the form of nonvolatile acids such as sulfate (SO_4^{2-}) and phosphate (PO_4^{3-}). These nonvolatile acids are excreted in the urine in the form of ammonium (NH_4^+) and titratable acids.

3. **What is the role of the HCO_3^-/CO_2 buffer system in maintaining acid-base balance?**

   This system is the first line of defense in maintaining acid-base balance. When the body detects an acid-base imbalance, carbonic acid (H_2CO_3) rapidly dissociates into either carbon dioxide (CO_2) or bicarbonate (HCO_3^-), as shown in Eq. 5.1.

   $$H_2O + CO_2 \rightleftarrows H_2CO_3 \rightleftarrows H + HCO_3^- \tag{5.1}$$

   Buffering systems work most efficiently near the pKa of the buffer. The pKa is defined as the pH at which half the acid is dissociated; in other words, the pH at which $[CO_2] = [HCO_3^-]$ for the above reaction. The HCO_3^-/CO_2 buffer system is an effective buffering system because the end products of the reaction (CO_2 and HCO_3^-) can be rapidly excreted by the lungs and kidneys, respectively. This is discussed in more detail later in this chapter.

4. **What is the role of the lungs in maintaining acid-base balance?**

   The lungs act quickly as the second line of defense in maintaining acid-base balance. The lungs contribute to acid-base balance by manipulating the concentration of CO_2. Acid-base derangements resulting from elevated or depressed CO_2 levels are said to be *respiratory* in nature (e.g., respiratory acidosis or respiratory alkalosis, respectively). In acid-base disorders resulting from abnormal HCO_3^- concentrations (e.g., metabolic acidosis or metabolic alkalosis), the lungs can attempt to compensate by expelling or retaining CO_2. These changes in CO_2 will be reported as a change in the partial pressure of CO_2 (P_{CO_2}); P_{CO_2} will decrease as CO_2 is expelled and increase as CO_2 is retained. Note that the ability of the lungs to fully compensate for a metabolic alkalosis is limited, as the excessive retention of CO_2 (hypercapnia) would have serious adverse effects. Table 5.1 outlines how to calculate the expected compensatory response of the lungs in the context of metabolic acid-base disturbances.

5. **What is the role of the kidneys in maintaining acid-base balance?**

   The kidneys are the third and last line of defense in maintaining acid-base balance. Acid-base derangements resulting from elevated or depressed HCO_3^- levels are said to be *metabolic* in nature (e.g., metabolic alkalosis or metabolic

Table 5.1. Respiratory Compensation for Metabolic Acid-Base Disturbances

CONDITION	PRIMARY CHANGE	EXPECTED COMPENSATION
Metabolic acidosis	Decreased HCO_3^-	Decreased $Pco_2 = 1.2 \times \Delta HCO_3^-$
Metabolic alkalosis	Increased HCO_3^-	Increased $Pco_2 = 0.7 \times \Delta HCO_3^-$

acidosis, respectively). Because the lungs can only secrete volatile acids in the form of CO_2, it remains up to the kidneys to secrete the nonvolatile acids. As previously mentioned, these are produced in small amounts (relative to CO_2 production) by the daily metabolism of dietary proteins. These nonvolatile acids are excreted in the urine in the form of NH_4^+ and titratable acids.

In acid-base disorders resulting from abnormal CO_2 concentrations (e.g., respiratory acidosis or respiratory alkalosis), the kidneys can attempt to compensate by expelling or retaining HCO_3^-. The acute and chronic compensation mechanisms used by the kidneys under these circumstances are outlined in Table 5.2. Unlike the lungs, renal compensation takes at least 3 days to complete.

Table 5.2. Renal Compensation for Respiratory Acid-Base Disturbances

CONDITION	PRIMARY CHANGE	EXPECTED COMPENSATION
Acute respiratory acidosis	Increased Pco_2	Increased $HCO_3^- = 0.2 \times \Delta Pco_2$
Chronic respiratory acidosis	Increased Pco_2	Increased $HCO_3^- = 0.35 \times \Delta Pco_2$
Acute respiratory alkalosis	Decreased Pco_2	Decreased $HCO_3^- = 0.2 \times \Delta Pco_2$
Chronic respiratory alkalosis	Decreased Pco_2	Decreased $HCO_3^- = 0.5 \times \Delta Pco_2$

6. With the understanding that a typical buffering system works best at a pH near its pKa, why is the HCO_3^-/CO_2 buffering system so effective despite its pKa of 6.1 being so far from the plasma pH of 7.4?

As discussed in question 3, this buffer system is effective because the lungs and kidneys are able to quickly and efficiently excrete CO_2 and HCO_3^-, respectively. This can be demonstrated through Eq. 5.1, which can be shifted to the left when the lungs excrete CO_2 or to the right through protein buffering of H^+ ions, renal excretion of H^+, and renal excretion of HCO_3^-.

7. Discuss the relationship between plasma HCO_3^-, Pco_2, and pH.

Understanding this relationship is the key to getting acid-base questions correct on the USMLE Step 1 and all future board exams. For the purposes of your exam, think of plasma HCO_3^- as the representation of "base" in the body and the Pco_2 as the representation of "acid" in the body; the reality is much more complicated in clinical practice, but this simplification will hold true as you encounter acid-base exam questions and serves as a foundation for you to begin your analysis of each acid-base question. The reported pH serves as the indication of how lopsided the current acid-base imbalance may be. HCO_3^- and Pco_2 have a direct relationship, meaning as one increases (to a pathologic degree), the other will also increase (in an attempt to compensate). The same is true as either value decreases. Because pH is proportional to total body base concentration and inversely proportional to total body acid, the pH will increase (i.e., become more alkalotic) as HCO_3^- increases or Pco_2 decreases and will decrease (i.e., become more acidotic) as HCO_3^- decreases or Pco_2 increases.

Armed with this knowledge and the understanding that physiologic pH is approximately 7.40, you are ready to begin interpreting lab values and identifying primary acid-base disturbances. First look at the pH to determine whether an acidosis or alkalosis is present, then look to the given values of HCO_3^- and Pco_2 to determine which is the likely culprit. Fig. 5.1 outlines this in greater detail.

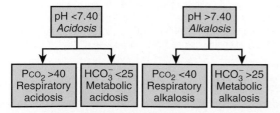

Figure 5.1. Determining the primary acid-base abnormality. HCO_3^-, Serum concentration of bicarbonate; Pco_2, partial pressure of carbon dioxide. (From Piccini JP, Nilsson KR. The Osler Medical Handbook. 2nd ed. Baltimore: Johns Hopkins University; 2006.)

A change in HCO_3^- of 10 mEq/L up or down causes pH to increase or decrease by 0.15 units, respectively. A change in P_{CO_2} of 10 mm Hg up or down causes pH to decrease or increase by 0.08 units acutely and by 0.03 units if the alteration is chronic.

8. **Why is net renal acid excretion necessary to maintain acid-base homeostasis?**
   Metabolism of carbohydrates and fats yields primarily carbon dioxide, which is easily excreted by the lungs. In contrast, metabolism of the dietary proteins found in meat and other protein-rich foods generates a large quantity of nonvolatile acids (e.g., lactate, sulfate, phosphate) that cannot be excreted by the lungs. These nonvolatile acids must be excreted somehow to prevent the development of a metabolic acidosis, and net renal acid excretion is how this is accomplished.

9. **What mechanisms do the kidneys use to prevent acidosis in the face of this acid load?**
   In general, the kidneys act to prevent acidosis through the net excretion of acid and reabsorption of base. This is accomplished through four major mechanisms: the kidneys (1) efficiently reabsorb *filtered* HCO_3^- in the proximal tubule (through a mechanism that is coupled with H^+ ion secretion into the tubular fluid), (2) synthesize HCO_3^- to be retained and the acid NH_4^+ to be secreted, (3) secrete titratable buffers such as ammonia and phosphate (which bind H^+ ions and increase the acid excretory capacity of the urine without causing a precipitous drop in urinary pH), and (4) actively pump acid (in the form of H^+ ions) into the tubular fluid at the distal tubule.

10. **How are bicarbonate (HCO_3^-) and ammonium (NH_4^+) generated de novo by the kidney?**
    The deamination of glutamine in the proximal tubule generates two NH_4^+ molecules and two HCO_3^- molecules. These NH_4^+ molecules function as an acid and are secreted into the tubular lumen, while the HCO_3^- molecules function as a base and are reabsorbed into the systemic circulation.

    Glutamine deamination is stimulated when the cells of the proximal tubule sense an acidotic state (e.g., elevated levels of H^+ ions or CO_2). Thus this mechanism appropriately increases the de novo synthesis of HCO_3^- (to be retained) and NH_4^+ (to be secreted) in response to acidotic conditions.

11. **How do the kidneys reabsorb filtered bicarbonate (HCO_3^-)?**
    The full cycle is outlined in Fig. 5.2. H^+ ions are secreted into the lumen of the proximal tubule (primarily via countertransport with Na^+), where they react with HCO_3^- in the filtrate to form carbonic acid (H_2CO_3). This carbonic acid rapidly dissociates into carbon dioxide (CO_2) and water (H_2O) through the action of carbonic anhydrase. Both CO_2 and H_2O can readily and passively diffuse back into the cell, where the reverse reaction takes place intracellularly; CO_2 reacts with H_2O and carbonic anhydrase to regenerate carbonic acid, which then dissociates into HCO_3^- and an H^+ ion. The HCO_3^- is then resorbed into the interstitial space and ultimately returned to the venous circulation, while the H^+ ion is secreted back into the tubular lumen by countertransport with Na^+ to begin the cycle again.

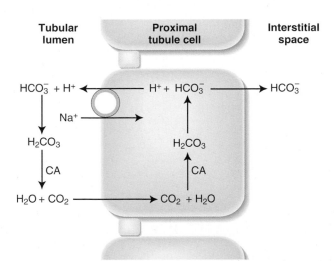

Figure 5.2. Mechanism of bicarbonate resorption. *CA,* Carbonic anhydrase; *CO₂,* carbon dioxide; *H⁺,* hydrogen ion; *HCO₃⁻,* bicarbonate; *H₂CO₃,* carbonic acid; *H₂O,* water; *Na⁺,* sodium ion. *(From Brown TA. Rapid Review Physiology. 2nd ed. Philadelphia: Elsevier; 2011.)*

Clinical Pearl
Acetazolamide is an inhibitor of carbonic anhydrase, the enzyme that catalyzes the rapid dissociation of carbonic acid in the tubular fluid into CO_2 and H_2O and facilitates an essential step in the reabsorption of HCO_3^-. Therefore the net effect of inhibiting carbonic anhydrase is increased urinary excretion of HCO_3^-, as HCO_3^- cannot be resorbed without functional carbonic anhydrase. Because this negatively charged HCO_3^- is excreted with an accompanying Na^+ molecule via the Na^+/HCO_3^- cotransporter, acetazolamide is also a diuretic (albeit a weak one). Carbonic anhydrase functions in the proximal tubule because it is anchored to the luminal surface of the plasma membrane of proximal tubular epithelial cells.

This pharmacotherapeutic mechanism of action essentially mimics the pathophysiology seen in proximal (type II) renal tubular acidosis (RTA), in which HCO_3^- reabsorption by the tubular epithelium is impaired. The result of decreased HCO_3^- reabsorption is a mild metabolic acidosis. This ability of acetazolamide to create a mild metabolic acidosis can be used therapeutically in the treatment or prevention of the respiratory alkalosis that may develop at elevated altitudes (i.e., acute mountain sickness). It is also useful to treat conditions such as cystinuria (acetazolamide alkalinizes urine to prevent cystine stone formation) and glaucoma (acetazolamide decreases aqueous humor secretion to reduce intraocular pressure).

12. **What is an anion gap, and how is it calculated?**
The anion gap (AG) is the difference between the plasma concentration of one specific cation (Na^+) and the sum of the plasma concentrations of two specific anions (HCO_3^- and Cl^-) (Eq. 5.2). Other plasma cations and anions that are commonly provided on a list of laboratory values include potassium (K^+), calcium (Ca^{2+}), magnesium (Mg^{2+}), sulfate (SO_4^{2-}), phosphate (PO_4^{3-}), organic anions (e.g., lactate), and plasma proteins such as albumin, but do not let these additional numbers confuse you; not one of these additional ions is relevant when calculating an AG.

$$AG = [Na^+] - [(HCO_3^- + Cl^-)] \qquad [5.2]$$

Inserting typical values for Na^+ (140 mEq/L), HCO_3^- (24 mEq/L), and Cl^- (108 mEq/L) yields the following:

$$AG = [Na^+] - [(HCO_3^- + Cl^-)]$$
$$= 140 - (24 + 108)$$
$$= 8$$

At first glance, you may be tempted to think that this positive value for the AG suggests that the plasma contains more cations than anions. However, because of the need to maintain electroneutrality, we know intuitively this is not the case. What explains this positive AG is the presence of negative charges on plasma proteins (primarily albumin), which are unmeasured in standard laboratory analyses and not included in the AG calculation despite the fact that they are present and active in the patient's plasma. This concept bears repeating. The plasma concentration of albumin is the primary reason for the positive AG calculation. If the plasma concentration of albumin were to drop significantly, fewer unmeasured negative anions would be present and the AG would need to be adjusted downward accordingly.

It so happens that under typical conditions the unmeasured cations (K^+, Ca^{2+}, Mg^{2+}) balance out the unmeasured anions (PO_4^{3-}, SO_4^{2-}, lactate), with the exception of the negative charges on albumin.

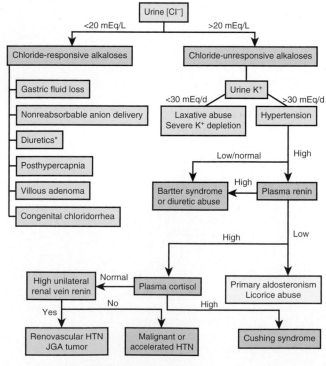

Figure 5.3. Diagnostic algorithm for metabolic alkalosis. The algorithm is based on the urine chloride concentration. *HTN*, Hypertension; *JGA*, juxtaglomerular apparatus. *(From Brenner BM. Brenner and Rector's The Kidney. 7th ed. Philadelphia: WB Saunders; 2004.)*

* After diuretic therapy

To further clarify the concept of the AG, let us revisit the concept of electroneutrality as it pertains to the AG. Electroneutrality dictates that the concentrations of all plasma cations and anions, both measured and unmeasured, need to be equal; that is, that the sum of all ionic charges must ultimately be zero (i.e., *electrically neutral*). With respect to calculation of the AG, the following should therefore be true:

Measured cations + unmeasured cations = measured anions + unmeasured anions

Rearranged to:

Measured cations − measured anions = unmeasured anions − unmeasured cations

Simplified to:

AG = unmeasured anions − unmeasured cations

Now you should hopefully understand why the AG can be represented with the equations AG = [Na$^+$] − [(HCO$_3^-$ + Cl$^-$)] or AG = unmeasured anions − unmeasured cations. They represent the same thing!

STEP 1 SECRET

While the acceptable anion gap (AG) range may slightly vary between institutions, for the purposes of your USMLE Step 1 exam, **consider any AG that is calculated to be greater than 16 mEq/L to be an elevated anion gap.** *Almost all clinically significant increases in AG are caused by an increased production of unmeasured anions such as lactate. While in theory a decrease in unmeasured cations can increase the AG, in practice this is seldom seen, as Ca^{2+}, Mg^{2+}, and K$^+$ are present in such small concentrations that even in the setting of hypocalcemia or hypokalemia, the AG will not be increased to a significant degree.*

CASE 5.1

A patient has the following laboratory results: Na$^+$, 140 mEq/L; K$^+$, 4.2 mEq/L; HCO$_3^-$, 12 mEq/L; Cl$^-$, 100 mEq/L; glucose, 86 mg/dL.

1. Calculate the AG for this patient. What specific information does this patient's AG tell you?
   Remember, no matter how many laboratory values you are given, only three ion concentrations are used to calculate the AG: Na$^+$, HCO$_3^-$, and Cl$^-$. This patient's AG is calculated as follows:

$$AG = [Na^+] - [(HCO_3^- + Cl^-)]$$
$$= 140 - (12 + 100)$$
$$= 28$$

   Remember that as far as the USMLE is concerned, a normal AG range is from approximately 8 to 16 mEq/L. Given this patient's low HCO$_3^-$ of 12 (normal is ~24 mEq/L) and elevated AG of 28 mEq/L, even without measuring the pH we know this patient is experiencing a high anion gap metabolic acidosis (HAGMA), which means excess unmeasured anions are being created. Using this as a starting point, you will be able to infer the specific cause of this patient's condition based on the additional clinical information provided to you in the vignette (e.g., presence of renal failure, ingestion of acid), as discussed later in this case.

2. Why does the production of unmeasured anions result in HAGMA?
   The production and accumulation of an unmeasured organic acid or anion causes an elevated AG because the plasma concentrations of Cl$^-$ and/or HCO$_3^-$ are reduced proportionally to how much unmeasured anion is created.

3. How do you know if there is an additional metabolic acid-base disturbance present in addition to the HAGMA you have already identified?
   The delta-delta can be used to determine if there is an additional metabolic acid-base disturbance present. For every 1 mEq of anion contributing to the changing AG, the concentration of HCO$_3^-$ should fall by 1 mEq from its normal value of approximately 24 mEq/L. Therefore the change in AG (e.g., the expected AG minus the reported AG, or ~12 mEq/L minus the calculated AG) should equal the change in HCO$_3^-$ (e.g., expected HCO$_3^-$ minus reported HCO$_3^-$, or 24 mEq/L minus 12 mEq/L, in this case) if the HAGMA is the only metabolic disturbance present. However, if a discrepancy exists, more than one metabolic disturbance is present. This is the concept of the delta-delta, which simply represents the comparison of the change in AG (ΔAG) to the change in bicarbonate (ΔHCO$_3^-$). The delta-delta should be interpreted as follows (Fig. 5.3):
   - If ΔAG = ΔHCO$_3^-$, then the HAGMA you already identified is the only metabolic acid-base disorder present.
   - If ΔAG < ΔHCO$_3^-$, then there is a hyperchloremic metabolic acidosis present *in addition to* the identified HAGMA (because the *change* in bicarbonate is *greater* than expected).
   - If ΔAG > ΔHCO$_3^-$, then there is a metabolic alkalosis present *in addition to* the HAGMA (because the *change* in bicarbonate is *smaller* than expected).

4. **What are the typical causes of HAGMA?**

While there are dozens of HAGMA-inducing disorders you may experience on your clinical rotations, the causes of HAGMA that are high yield for the USMLE can be remembered using the mnemonic **MUDPILES**:

Methanol

Uremia

Diabetic ketoacidosis (DKA)

Polyethylene glycol

Isoniazid or **I**ron toxicity

Lactic acidosis

Ethanol or **E**thylene glycol

Salicylates

As mentioned previously, the accumulation of an unmeasured organic acid or anion will result in an elevated anion gap by proportionally reducing the plasma concentrations of Cl^- and/or HCO_3^-. Methanol and ethylene glycol are metabolized to formic acid (which may cause visual disturbances) and oxalic acid (which may cause kidney dysfunction), respectively. The AG seen in renal failure results from the accumulation of phosphates, sulfates, and other organic anions, which reduce Cl^- and/or HCO_3^- concentration. Salicylates include aspirin and other derivatives of salicylic acid; look for a vignette that describes a patient with chronic joint pain who takes aspirin daily. The antituberculosis drug isoniazid is also a derivative of an organic acid (isonicotinic acid) that may induce HAGMA in addition to the vitamin B_6 deficiency with which it is classically associated.

It is important to remember that there are many causes of lactic acidosis. Sepsis, seizures (with increased muscle contraction or impaired breathing), medications (e.g., metformin), ischemia of limbs or organs (especially small bowel ischemia), cyanide or carbon monoxide poisoning, and circulatory or respiratory failure can all cause lactic acidosis and therefore lead to HAGMA.

In addition, recall that ketosis can result from starvation and chronic alcohol abuse in addition to the classic diabetic ketoacidosis, albeit much less commonly and usually with a much less severe acidosis. In chronic alcohol abuse, this is most often seen a few days after heavy binge drinking in the setting of poor food intake. There are numerous mechanisms involved, including depletion of nicotinamide adenine dinucleotide (NAD^+) by hepatic oxidation of alcohol, reduced nutrient intake, and dehydration (which decreases urinary ketone excretion).

STEP 1 SECRET

The **MUDPILES** *mnemonic is a must-know for Step 1. Among these common causes of metabolic acidosis, diabetic ketoacidosis and lactic acidosis are USMLE favorites.*

5. **Why does a non-AG metabolic acidosis create an acidotic state without generating an elevated AG?**

Rather than producing unmeasured anions as in HAGMA, a non-AG (normal gap) metabolic acidosis is caused by processes that reduce plasma HCO_3^- concentration but proportionally increase plasma Cl^- concentration. This is why a non-AG metabolic acidosis is also referred to as *hyperchloremic acidosis*.

For example, consider the ingestion of a strong acid such as hydrochloric acid (HCl). The HCl immediately releases its H^+ ion, which is buffered by HCO_3^- of the HCO_3^-/CO_2 buffer system, resulting in an mEq-for-mEq replacement of HCO_3^- with Cl^-. Renal or intestinal losses of HCO_3^-, as with diarrhea or type 2 RTA, can also cause a non-AG metabolic acidosis. In diarrhea, the decreased transit time of the bicarbonate-rich fluid prevents much of the HCO_3^- from being reabsorbed in exchange for Cl^-, thereby causing a hyperchloremic (non-AG) metabolic acidosis. Additionally, the volume depletion caused by diarrhea stimulates the renin-angiotensin-aldosterone system (RAAS), resulting in Na^+ retention and increased retention of Cl^- in exchange for HCO_3^-. In type 2 RTA, impaired HCO_3^- reabsorption by the proximal tubular cells results in urinary HCO_3^- wasting and subsequent hyperchloremic (non-AG) metabolic acidosis. Renal and nonrenal causes of hyperchloremic (non-AG) metabolic acidosis can often be distinguished from one another based on whether the urine anion gap is positive or negative, as discussed below.

Clinical Pearl

The urine anion gap (UAG) (Eq. 5.3) can be used to distinguish renal from intestinal causes of hyperchloremic metabolic acidosis. In the setting of metabolic acidosis, the appropriate response of the kidney is to ramp up ammonia production to generate new HCO_3^- and excrete excess acid as NH_4^+ (ammonium). This NH_4^+ is generally paired with chloride (Cl^-) to maintain electroneutrality in the urine. Therefore the concentration of Cl^- in the urine can be used to approximate the concentration of NH_4^+ in the urine and indicate if the kidneys are appropriately excreting acid. If the UAG is negative, it indicates that NH_4^+ (an unmeasured cation) is being appropriately excreted into the urine. If the UAG is positive, it indicates that the kidneys are unable to excrete excess acid, suggesting that renal tubular acidosis (RTA) is present.

$$UAG = \left[NA^+ \right]_u + \left[K^+ \right]_u - \left[Cl^- \right]_u$$ [5.3]

STEP 1 SECRET

You are expected to know the major causes of high anion gap (AG) and non-AG metabolic acidosis previously discussed for the USMLE Step 1.

6. How do you diagnose an acid-base disorder?

We suggest that you follow the diagnostic algorithm outlined in Fig. 5.4 when faced with any acid-base questions on the USMLE Step 1 exam.

CASE 5.2

An older woman has had diarrhea for 2 days. She is tachypneic on physical examination.

1. Based only on this limited information, what acid-base disturbance might you suspect in this patient?

Diarrhea results in the loss of bicarbonate-rich intestinal fluids, so we should suspect that a metabolic acidosis may be present. As discussed in Case 5.1, because of compromised distal intestinal exchange of HCO_3^- for Cl^-, the rapid excretion of diarrheal fluid would be expected to cause a hyperchloremic metabolic acidosis. Because the pathogenesis does not involve production of unmeasured anions, this would cause a non-AG metabolic acidosis. In response to the volume depletion caused by the diarrhea, stimulation of the RAAS would promote Na^+ retention in an attempt to restore intravascular volume. This Na^+ resorption is powered by a Na^+/H^+ ATPase pump such that Na^+ retention increases renal loss of HCO_3^- with concomitant exchange for Cl^-, further contributing to a hyperchloremic metabolic acidosis.

Now to explain this patient's tachypnea. If our suspicions of an underlying metabolic acidosis are correct, this patient's tachypnea represents the "blowing off" of excess CO_2 by the lungs in an attempt to compensate for the metabolic acidosis.

CASE 5.2 CONTINUED:

The patient's laboratory values are as follows:

pH: 7.20
P_{CO_2}: 19 mm Hg
$[HCO_3^-]$: 7 mEq/L
$[Cl^-]$: 120 mEq/L
$[Na^+]$: 140 mEq/L
Albumin: 4 g/dL

2. What is the primary acid-base disorder?

Following the diagnostic pathway outlined in Fig. 5.4, the laboratory results reveal a non-AG metabolic acidosis, which is consistent with our suspicions based on the patient's 2-day history of diarrhea.

Remember, your first step when faced with any acid-base question should be to look at the pH to identify your patient's current status; here, you realize that it is abnormally low, meaning our patient has an acidemia. Next, determine whether the acidemia is the result of respiratory or metabolic causes by checking the reported HCO_3^- and P_{CO_2} levels. In this case, HCO_3^- and P_{CO_2} are both low. HCO_3^- is a base, and therefore decreased levels of HCO_3^- will result in a metabolic acidosis. CO_2, on the other hand, is an acid. Low levels of CO_2 will decrease acid levels and should result in a respiratory alkalosis if it were the primary disorder. However, because the patient's pH is not in the alkalotic range, we know this low CO_2 is not the primary acid-base disturbance, but in fact is the body's attempt to compensate for the true primary disorder. Therefore this patient has a metabolic acidosis with respiratory compensation. In this situation, the body tries to correct for the decreased pH of metabolic acidosis through hyperventilation and loss of CO_2. In contrast with metabolic compensation by the kidneys, respiratory compensation occurs immediately.

Because this patient has a metabolic acidosis, we must assess the AG. In this patient, the AG $= 140 - (120 + 7) =$ 13 mEq/L (normal range $= 8-16$ mEq/L), confirming that this a non-AG metabolic acidosis. Note that this is consistent with our suspicions based on the patient's history of diarrhea.

3. Why does diarrhea cause a metabolic acidosis?

Diarrhea results in the loss of bicarbonate-rich fluid. Intestinal fluid is fairly rich in HCO_3^-, but normally much of this is reabsorbed via a Cl^-/HCO_3^- exchange process in the colon. Diarrhea shortens intestinal transit time, limiting the opportunity for colonic Cl^-/HCO_3^- exchange, and thereby increases the concentration of HCO_3^- in the stool. This loss of HCO_3^- is thus electrically balanced by an increase in serum Cl^- concentration. This hyperchloremic state leaves the AG unchanged.

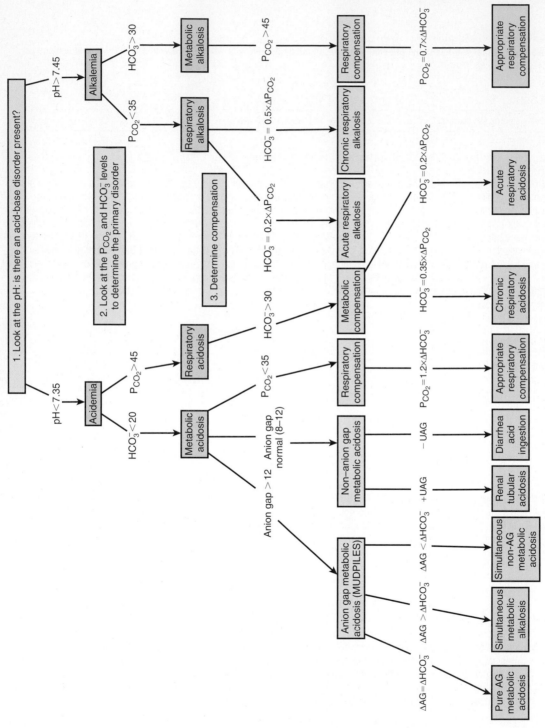

Figure 5.4. Diagnostic algorithm for acid-base disorders. *AG*, Anion gap; *UAG*, urine anion gap.

4. If this patient were found to have a positive urine anion gap, what diagnosis would be suspected?

RTA should be the suspected diagnosis in patients with a positive urine anion gap (UAG) (Eq. 5.3). See Table 5.3 for descriptions of the three types of RTA.

Table 5.3. Classification of Renal Tubular Acidosis (RTA)

TYPE OF RTA	PATHOPHYSIOLOGY	URINE pH	DEGREE OF ACIDOSIS	SERUM K^+	BICARBONATE EXCRETION (AFTER BICARBONATE LOAD)
Type I (distal RTA)	Inability to secrete H^+ in distal tubule	>5.3	Severe (serum HCO_3^- often <10 mEq/L)	Decreased	<3%
Type II (proximal RTA)	Deficit of carbonic anhydrase and HCO_3^- reabsorption in proximal tubule, can begin to reabsorb bicarbonate after pH decreases below a threshold level. May lead to impaired proximal tubular reabsorption of other nutrients (e.g., glucose, phosphate, amino acids)	<5.3	Modest (serum HCO_3^- 12–16 mEq/L)	Decreased	>15%
Type IV (hyperkalemic RTA)	Hypoaldosteronism or aldosterone resistance	<5.3	Mild (serum HCO_3^- 14–20 mEq/L)	Increased	<3%

5. Is there appropriate respiratory compensation or is a mixed disorder present in this patient?

The body attempts to compensate for metabolic acidosis by decreasing P_{CO_2} (e.g., excreting volatile acid) through hyperventilation. Such respiratory compensation is virtually immediate. Using the equation in Table 5.1, the expected change in $P_{CO_2} = 1.2 \times (24 - HCO_3^-) = 1.2 \times (24 - 7) = 20.4$. The actual change in this case is $(40 - 19) = 21$, reflecting appropriate compensation.

In looking at Table 5.1, it is apparent that the lungs can more readily excrete CO_2 than retain it in response to metabolic acid-base disturbances. This ability to rapidly excrete CO_2 is important because excessive CO_2 retention can lead to severe hypercapnia, mental status changes, coma, and death.

Note: While compensation during any acid-base disturbance may occur, it will never fully resolve the primary disturbance.

6. What would it mean if appropriate respiratory compensation were not present, and this patient's P_{CO_2} was instead 30 mm Hg?

With all other laboratory values remaining the same, if this patient had a P_{CO_2} of 30 mm Hg, a mixed disorder would be present—that is, more than one primary acid-base disorder occurring at the same time. A P_{CO_2} of 30 mm Hg in this case would represent inappropriate retention of CO_2, indicating a concomitant respiratory acidosis in addition to the metabolic acidosis you already identified.

SUMMARY BOX: METABOLIC ACIDOSIS AS THE RESULT OF DIARRHEA

- Results in non–anion gap metabolic acidosis
- Compensation: Lungs blow off CO_2
- Change in $P_{CO_2} = 1.2 \times$ change in HCO_3^- (see Table 5.1)
- Urine anion gap (UAG) (Eq. 5.3) expected to be negative

SUMMARY BOX: METABOLIC ACIDOSIS

1. Metabolic acidosis is defined as pH < 7.35 with $HCO_3^- < 22$ mEq/L
2. Look at the Pco_2 to determine if the degree of respiratory compensation is appropriate or if a mixed disorder is present. The expected change in $Pco_2 = 1.2 \times (24 - HCO_3^-)$.
3. Determine the anion gap (AG):

$$AG = [NA^+] - [(Cl^- + HCO_3^-)] = \text{unmeasured anions} - \text{unmeasured cations}$$

4. If a non-AG metabolic acidosis is confirmed, search for etiological clues in the history (e.g., diarrhea) and determine the urine anion gap (UAG):

$$UAG = (U_{Na} + U_K) - U_{Cl} = \text{unmeasured anions} - \text{unmeasured cations}$$

CASE 5.3

You are called to consult on a postsurgical patient in the intensive care unit (ICU) who has developed sudden-onset dyspnea and hypoxemia. Breath sounds are clear. Pulse is elevated at 130 beats/min.

1. **Based only on this limited information, what acid-base disturbance might you suspect in this patient?**
   Recent surgery, immobility, sudden-onset hypoxemia, respiratory distress, tachycardia, and clear lung sounds, which argue against congestive heart failure (CHF) and pneumonia, all point toward pulmonary embolism (PE). A PE classically causes hyperventilation, which would blow off CO_2 and result in a respiratory alkalosis. The compensatory renal response, which would take multiple days to occur, would be to increase HCO_3^- excretion.

CASE 5.3 CONTINUED:

The following laboratory values are reported for this patient:
   pH: 7.50
   Pco_2: 20 mm Hg
   $[HCO_3^-]$: 20 mEq/L

2. **What is the primary acid-base disorder?**
   Following the diagnostic pathway outlined in Fig. 5.4, the elevated pH with decreased Pco_2 indicates that the primary disorder is a respiratory alkalosis.

3. **What is the differential diagnosis in this patient?**
   Intensive care unit (ICU) patients are at increased risk for PE because they are immobile and more often have serious diseases such as CHF (stasis), recent surgery (injury to endothelium), or cancer (hypercoagulable state). Therefore a PE is the most likely cause of this patient's condition. The sudden change of vital signs further supports this diagnosis.
      As discussed, hypoxia from a PE leads to hyperventilation and subsequent respiratory alkalosis. However, hypoxia and hyperventilation can occur in virtually any form of lung disease, including pneumonia, pulmonary edema (as caused by CHF or acute respiratory distress syndrome [ARDS]), or restrictive lung disease. Pain, anxiety, and various central nervous system (CNS) disorders are common causes of respiratory alkalosis in the ICU that occur in the absence of hypoxia. Patients with asthma are interesting because although they can develop hypoxia, these patients very dramatically hyperventilate during asthma attacks, such that a degree of respiratory alkalosis develops that is often out of proportion to the hypoxia.
      It is important to note that if hyperventilation persists, respiratory muscle fatigue can arise, leading to CO_2 accumulation and respiratory acidosis (a process referred to as *hypercapnic respiratory failure*). Recognize that in order to transition from respiratory alkalosis (pH > 7.45) to respiratory acidosis (pH < 7.35), the patient's measured pH will transiently fall within the normal range (pH 7.35–7.45). **Do not let this fool you!** If the pH of a patient with respiratory alkalosis appears to resolve on its own, your patient is not spontaneously recovering; they are experiencing respiratory muscle fatigue and will continue to decompensate if you do not intervene.

STEP 1 SECRET

The USMLE loves to ask questions about pulmonary embolism (PE) because it is such a critical diagnosis. Remember that patients with a PE are tachypneic; this hyperventilation leads to excess removal of CO_2 from the bloodstream and predisposes to a respiratory alkalosis.

4. **Is there appropriate compensation or is this a mixed disorder?**
Because the full effect of renal compensation for respiratory disturbances is not immediate, for acid-base disturbances with a respiratory cause one must first determine if the disturbance is acute or chronic. In this patient, the respiratory alkalosis is acute. The appropriate compensation for any respiratory alkalosis is to decrease serum HCO_3^- through increased renal excretion. Using the equation in Table 5.2, the appropriate acute change in $HCO_3^- = 0.2 \times \Delta P_{CO_2} = 0.2 \times (40 - 20) = 0.2 \times 20 = 4$. The actual change in this case can be calculated by subtracting the reported plasma HCO_3^- concentration from 24 (the expected value for HCO_3^-), which is $24 - 20 = 4$; therefore, there is appropriate acute metabolic compensation.

STEP 1 SECRET

It is not likely that the USMLE will ask you to calculate the degree of renal or pulmonary compensation for an acute or chronic acid-base disorder using the formulas listed in Tables 5.1 and 5.2. However, these are important formulas to know for your clinical years, particularly because they can help you spot mixed disorders.

5. **Does the degree of compensation allow you to draw any conclusions as to the duration of the condition?**
Yes. Even if the history of an acute process was not available in this patient, we could conclude from the reported laboratory values that this respiratory alkalosis is acute. If this were a more chronic presentation, as occurs at high altitude or in pregnant women (because of the progesterone-induced increase in tidal volume), the kidneys would have responded by excreting more HCO_3^-. The decrease in HCO_3^- would have been $0.5 \times \Delta P_{CO_2} = 10$. Because it would take a couple of days for the kidneys to fully adjust to this patient's respiratory alkalosis, we know that the onset of this patient's condition occurred acutely.

If you are attempting to remember the preceding numbers, it is useful to realize that the kidneys more easily and more rapidly excrete HCO_3^- than retain HCO_3^- when responding to respiratory acid-base disturbances. Thus renal compensation for a respiratory alkalosis is both more complete and more rapid than the compensation for a respiratory acidosis (see Table 5.2 and Fig. 5.5).

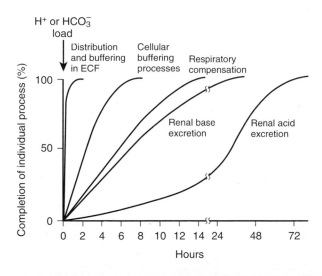

Figure 5.5. Time course of acid-base compensatory mechanisms. In response to a metabolic acid or alkaline load, individual approaches to completion of distribution and extracellular buffering mechanisms, cellular buffering events, and respiratory and renal regulatory processes are presented as a function of time. *ECF,* Extracellular fluid. *(From Brenner BM.* Brenner and Rector's The Kidney. *7th ed. Philadelphia: WB Saunders; 2004.)*

SUMMARY BOX: RESPIRATORY ALKALOSIS

- Etiology: Hyperventilation (e.g., pain, anxiety, CNS disease), hypoxemia (e.g., lung disease), or both (e.g., acute asthma attack)
- Maximal renal compensation requires a few days.
- It is easier for the kidneys to excrete HCO_3^- than to retain it when a respiratory acid-base disturbance exists, resulting in greater compensation for respiratory alkalosis than for respiratory acidosis.

CASE 5.4

A 41-year-old woman is evaluated for a preemployment physical and is found to have a significantly elevated blood pressure.

1. **Given her hypertension, if this patient were to have a concurrent acid-base disturbance, which acid-base disturbance would be most likely?**
   If this patient has an acid-base disturbance, it will likely be related to her hypertension, as the boards love questions about secondary causes of hypertension. Conditions associated with excess mineralocorticoids and glucocorticoids can cause secondary hypertension through plasma volume expansion. These conditions expand plasma volume in part by promoting renal resorption of filtered Na^+, which promotes H^+ ion secretion and therefore HCO_3^- synthesis. Thus we might expect a metabolic alkalosis to be present in a patient with secondary hypertension.

   The expected respiratory compensation for a metabolic alkalosis would be hypoventilation in an attempt to retain CO_2. However, because appropriate ventilation is required for oxygen exchange across the pulmonary membrane, respiratory compensation via hypoventilation would be limited.

CASE 5.4 CONTINUED:

Laboratory results are as follows:
   pH: 7.55
   HCO_3^-: 35 mEq/L
   P_{CO_2}: 19 mm Hg

2. **What is the primary acid-base disorder?**
   Following the diagnostic pathway outlined in Fig. 5.4, you should note that the pH is in the alkalotic range with elevated HCO_3^- and reduced P_{CO_2}, all of which are consistent with a metabolic alkalosis. Whether respiratory compensation is appropriate remains to be seen.

3. **What is the differential diagnosis in this patient?**
   The very broad differential diagnosis for this patient should include loss of gastric secretions (i.e., vomiting), diuretics, volume depletion, hypokalemia, mineralocorticoid excess, Cushing syndrome, excessive licorice consumption, rare diseases of intrinsic renal dysfunction (e.g., Bartter, Gitelman, and Liddle syndromes), and 11β-hydroxysteroid dehydrogenase (11β-HSD) deficiency (Fig. 5.6). Patients who are in the ICU and who have a chronic respiratory acidosis corrected too quickly can also develop a similar picture because their kidneys, which have become used to excreting a large acid load to compensate, will take several days to readjust.

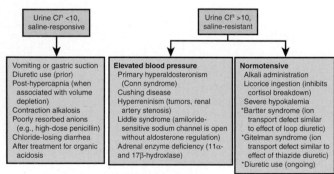

Figure 5.6. Differential diagnosis of metabolic alkalosis. *(From Piccini JP, Nilsson KR. The Osler Medical Handbook. 2nd ed. Baltimore: Johns Hopkins University; 2006.)*

4. **What is the pathophysiology of each of the conditions in the differential diagnosis?**
   - Volume depletion (*contraction alkalosis*)
     - Na^+ and HCO_3^- reabsorption are directly linked in the proximal tubule by the Na^+/HCO_3^- cotransporter. Volume depletion induces Na^+ resorption in an attempt to restore fluid volume and thereby leads to increased HCO_3^- reabsorption as well.
     - Volume depletion stimulates the RAAS. The resulting increase in aldosterone promotes Na^+ reabsorption in exchange for K^+ and H^+ in the distal tubule.
   - Hypokalemia
     - K^+ and H^+ compete for secretion in the distal tubule; hypokalemia stimulates K^+ retention, resulting in increased H^+ secretion.

- Hypokalemia also causes a transcellular shift of K^+ out of cells in an attempt to replete the low serum K^+ concentration, which is electrically balanced (in part) by a shift of H^+ intracellularly, directly lowering serum H^+ concentration.
    - The intracellular shift of H^+ also results in intracellular acidification, which stimulates increased ammonia production at the proximal tubule, ultimately resulting in increased excretion of H^+ in the form of NH_4^+.
- Loss of gastric secretions
    - Loss of gastric H^+ will directly cause an increase in HCO_3^- and an increase in pH.
    - Loss of gastric Cl^- will prevent HCO_3^- secretion in the distal tubule and collecting duct, as fewer Cl^- ions will be available for Cl^-/HCO_3^- exchange by intercalated cells.
    - Loss of gastric secretions may cause volume depletion.
- Diuretics (loop diuretics and thiazides only): Remember that acetazolamide and, to a lesser extent, K^+-sparing diuretics tend to cause an acidosis.
    - Volume depletion
    - Hypokalemia
- Mineralocorticoid excess: The action of aldosterone in the distal tubule results in increased H^+ (and K^+) secretion in exchange for Na^+ as aldosterone attempts to restore intravascular volume.
- Cushing disease: An excess of corticosteroids will activate the mineralocorticoid receptor.
- 11β-HSD deficiency: Defect of the enzyme that normally breaks down cortisol into cortisone within aldosterone-responsive cells causes cortisol to build up and activate the mineralocorticoid receptor.
- Licorice: "Real" licorice (black licorice, not Twizzlers red candy) contains a substance that inhibits 11β-HSD.

5. Is there appropriate compensation, or is there a mixed disorder?
There is not appropriate compensation. Per Table 5.1, the expected respiratory compensation for a metabolic alkalosis would be an increase in P_{CO_2} of $0.7 \times \Delta HCO_3^- = 0.7 \times 10 = 7$ mm Hg, meaning the P_{CO_2} should be approximately 47 mm Hg to be considered appropriate compensation in this patient. P_{CO_2} in this case is lower than expected in the setting of a metabolic alkalosis; therefore, a mixed disorder is present.

CASE 5.4 CONTINUED:

When the patient is further questioned at her follow-up appointment, she also admits to having polyuria, polydipsia, muscle weakness, and headaches. She has the following laboratory values:

$[K^+]$: 3.1 mEq/L
$[Na^+]$: 149 mEq/L
Aldosterone-renin ratio (ARR): >20

6. Based on this new information, what is the most likely diagnosis?
The presentation and laboratory values are classic for primary hyperaldosteronism (Conn syndrome). Conn syndrome should be suspected in any patient with hypertension and concurrent hypernatremia and hypokalemia.

This patient's hypokalemia and hypernatremia and, to a lesser extent, her signs and symptoms can be seen in all syndromes of high aldosterone activity, including secondary hyperaldosteronism (e.g., renin-secreting tumor, CHF, renovascular disease) and nonaldosterone mineralocorticoid excess (e.g., Cushing syndrome, 11β-HSD deficiency, licorice ingestion, exogenous mineralocorticoids). However, only in primary hyperaldosteronism is the ARR as markedly elevated as it is here (>20). In secondary hyperaldosteronism, both renin and aldosterone are increased, while in nonaldosterone mineralocorticoid excess they are both decreased. In either case, unlike in primary hyperaldosteronism, the ARR remains relatively unchanged.

SUMMARY BOX: METABOLIC ALKALOSIS

- If associated with hypertension, consider the following:
    - Primary hyperaldosteronism (Conn syndrome); look for hypokalemia and hypernatremia
    - Secondary hyperaldosteronism
        1. Renin-secreting tumor
        2. CHF
        3. Renovascular disease (e.g., renal artery stenosis)
- Nonaldosterone mineralocorticoid excess
    1. Cushing syndrome
    2. 11β-hydroxysteroid dehydrogenase (11β-HSD) deficiency
    3. Licorice ingestion
    4. Exogenous mineralocorticoids

- Other considerations
  - Loss of gastric secretions (e.g., vomiting or nasogastric suctioning): Causes metabolic alkalosis through three separate but additive mechanisms: direct loss of H^+, loss of Cl^-, and volume depletion
  - Diuretics
  - Volume depletion
- Respiratory compensation
  - Expected increase of $P_{CO_2} = 0.7 \times \Delta HCO_3^-$
  - Compensation is limited as the result of hypoventilation-induced hypercapnia

CASE 5.5

An 18-year-old man presents with 2 days of fatigue, abdominal pain, and vomiting. Physical examination reveals a thin young man in modest respiratory distress with a sweet odor to his breath and a heart rate of 130 beats/min.

1. **Based only on this limited information, what acid-base disorder might you suspect in this patient?**
   A vague complaint like this can be challenging in the clinical setting. In a thin and young patient with this presentation, type 1 diabetes mellitus should be near the top of the differential diagnosis. The sweet-smelling breath likely indicates the production of ketones (e.g., acetone) by the liver with removal by the lungs. The tachycardia is likely a reflexive response to the volume depletion that resulted from the hyperosmolar diuresis caused by this patient's suspected hyperglycemia. Then again, this young man may have unintentionally or intentionally ingested toxic amounts of ethylene glycol, aspirin, or another noxious substance. Clearly, review of the laboratory results is in order.

CASE 5.5 CONTINUED:

This patient's laboratory results are as follows:
   pH: 7.15
   $[Na^+]$: 140 mEq/L
   $[Cl^-]$: 90 mEq/L
   $[HCO_3^-]$: 20 mEq/L
   P_{CO_2}: 36 mm Hg
   $[K^+]$: 5.2 mEq/L
   Blood urea nitrogen (BUN): 52 mg/dL

2. **What is the primary acid-base disorder in this patient?**
   The low pH is in the acidotic range, and low HCO_3^- with near-normal P_{CO_2} is consistent with a metabolic acidosis. However, we would expect respiratory compensation to cause a substantial reduction in P_{CO_2} (recall from Table 5.1 that the expected compensation of $P_{CO_2} = 1.2 \times \Delta HCO_3^-$) such that with appropriate respiratory compensation we would expect a P_{CO_2} of approximately 35.

3. **What is the next step in diagnosis of this disorder?**
   Calculate the AG! It is critical to distinguish between high AG and non-AG metabolic acidosis because the differentials for each are dramatically different.
   Remember AG = $[Na^+] - [(Cl^- + HCO_3^-)]$. In this patient, AG = $140 - (90 + 20) = 30$ mEq/L.

STEP 1 SECRET

You will be expected (but not necessarily instructed) to calculate AG on the USMLE Step 1 if the diagnosis involves metabolic acidosis. Be on the lookout for this type of question!

4. **How can there be such a large AG with such an *extremely* low pH when the disturbance in HCO_3^- is so minimal?**
   This effect is caused by a superimposed metabolic alkalosis. Remember the delta-delta concept from Case 5.1: for every 1 mEq of anion contributing to the changing AG, HCO_3^- should fall by 1 mEq from its normal value. Therefore the change in AG should equal the change in HCO_3^- concentration if the HAGMA is the only metabolic disturbance present.

However, if a discrepancy in the delta-delta exists, more than one metabolic acid-base disturbance is present. The delta-delta should be interpreted as follows:

- If $\Delta AG = \Delta HCO_3^-$, the HAGMA is the sole metabolic acid-base disorder.
- If $\Delta AG < \Delta HCO_3^-$, there is a hyperchloremic metabolic acidosis in addition to the HAGMA already identified (because the *change* in HCO_3^- is *greater* than expected).
- If $\Delta AG > \Delta HCO_3^-$, there is a metabolic alkalosis in addition to the HAGMA already identified (because the *change* in HCO_3^- is *smaller* than expected).
- In this case, the $\Delta AG = 30 - 12 = 18$ mEq/L. The ΔHCO_3^- is $24 - 20 = 4$ mEq/L. Thus $\Delta AG > \Delta HCO_3^-$, indicating a "hidden" metabolic alkalosis.

5. **If respiratory compensation is incomplete, are the lungs therefore part of the problem (i.e., is there a superimposed respiratory acidosis)?**
   To answer this question we need to review the delta. This looks like a primary metabolic acidosis (pH < 7.4 and bicarbonate < 25).

6. **Is there appropriate compensation, or is this a mixed disorder?**
   The reported P_{CO_2} (36 mm Hg) is decreased by 4 from the expected value of 40 mm Hg, which is consistent with appropriate respiratory compensation per Table 5.1 ($1.2 \times \Delta HCO_3^- = 1.2 \times 4 = 4.8$).

CASE 5.5 CONTINUED:

Additional questioning reveals that this patient has a history of polyuria and polydipsia.

7. **What is the most likely diagnosis?**
   DKA in patient with undiagnosed type 1 diabetes is the most likely diagnosis. DKA is a favorite of the USMLE, so you need to understand it well. This condition occurs mainly in patients with type 1 diabetes mellitus, although it can occasionally occur in very ill patients with type 2 diabetes. It is not uncommon for children or adolescents to present in DKA without previously being diagnosed with type 1 diabetes mellitus. In fact, about 20% of patients presenting with DKA have no known previous history of diabetes. The clinical manifestations consist of polyuria and polydipsia (the result of hyperglycemia-induced osmotic diuresis); gastrointestinal (GI) symptoms such as nausea, vomiting, abdominal pain, and ileus (because of the effects of hyperglycemia and electrolyte disturbances on the GI tract); Kussmaul respirations (deep and rapid breathing pattern, attempting to compensate for the metabolic acidosis); sweet or fruity odor on the breath (acetone, a volatile ketone body, being expired by the lungs); signs of volume depletion such as tachycardia and hypotension (the result of diuresis and vomiting); and changes in mental status (from acidosis and electrolyte disturbances).

   The laboratory findings in a typical case include high AG metabolic acidosis (from the ketoacids, e.g., β-hydroxybutyrate [β-HB]), pseudohyponatremia (because of hyperglycemia), increased BUN (because of volume depletion), increased serum glucose, elevated serum and urine ketones (measured as serum β-HB or on urine dip), and leukocytosis (which may reflect an infection that triggered the episode).

   Total body potassium is usually reduced (as a result of the osmotic diuresis and volume depletion). However, serum K^+ levels are usually normal or even elevated at presentation as a result of the transcellular shift of K^+ out of cells (caused by both the lack of insulin and the acidosis).

   In this case, the superimposed metabolic alkalosis is due to vomiting and volume contraction. Remember that vomiting rids the body of gastric acid, thus increasing pH. Metabolic alkalosis can be especially dangerous because the body's compensatory response involves CO_2 retention by hypoventilation, which may lead to hypoxemia (recall that increased P_{CO_2} results in an obligatory decrease in partial pressure of oxygen [P_{O_2}]).

   Although DKA often occurs when a patient with type 1 diabetes fails to take insulin, it is also quite often precipitated by a triggering event. Infections such as pneumonia, urinary tract infection (UTI), and skin or soft tissue infection are particularly common. Other serious illnesses such as myocardial infarction (MI) or pancreatitis can serve as triggers as well.

   The hyperglycemia seen in DKA is due to increased gluconeogenesis and increased glycogenolysis by the liver in the setting of decreased consumption of glucose by the peripheral tissues, all a result of insufficient insulin relative to glucagon and the other counterregulatory hormones. The ketosis also arises from the inability of the peripheral tissues to utilize glucose. The lack of available glucose stimulates the release of free fatty acids by peripheral adipose tissues into the bloodstream. The fatty acids are then converted in the liver to the ketones β-HB and acetoacetate so that they can be used for energy by vital organs such as the CNS and heart, which normally depend on glucose for energy.

8. **What is the correct treatment for a patient in DKA?**
   Patients in DKA are treated with insulin, aggressive intravenous hydration, potassium repletion (if the reported serum K^+ is normal or low), and management of the precipitating event (when applicable).

CASE 5.6

A 38-year-old homeless man with chronic alcohol abuse comes into the emergency department with nausea, vomiting, and blurry vision. He denies any recent ingestion of alcohol, saying that he "ran out of booze." His blood alcohol level is undetectable. His laboratory values are as follows:

> pH: 7.29
> [Na$^+$]: 135 mEq/L
> [Cl$^-$]: 100 mEq/L
> [HCO$_3$$^-$]: 14 mEq/L
> Glucose: 90 mg/dL

1. What is the most likely diagnosis?

   This man likely has methanol intoxication. His AG is 21 mEq/L, recalling that AG = [Na$^+$] − [(Cl$^-$ + HCO$_3$$^-$)] = 135 − (100 + 14) = 135 − 114 = 21. Visual impairment in the setting of a high AG metabolic acidosis is highly suggestive of methanol poisoning (see **MUDPILES** mnemonic). Methanol is found in windshield wiper fluid and is therefore an easily accessible alcohol. It is also found in shellac and varnish. Methanol, like ethanol, is metabolized by the enzyme alcohol dehydrogenase. The formic acid that results is a mitochondrial toxin that acts by inhibiting cytochrome oxidase of oxidative phosphorylation. The retina, optic nerve, and basal ganglia are especially vulnerable. In the first 6 hours following ingestion, the signs and symptoms of methanol intoxication resemble those of ethanol intoxication. After this period, visual disturbances and depressed consciousness become prominent. Physical examination might reveal papilledema. Blurry vision in the setting of elevated AG metabolic acidosis are the buzzwords to recognize for methanol ingestion on the USMLE.

CASE 5.6 CONTINUED:

This homeless man returns to the emergency department 6 weeks later with apparent inebriation and signs of pulmonary edema and cardiovascular collapse. He again denies alcohol consumption. In addition, he is found to have calcium oxalate stones on urine microscopy, and his urine fluoresces when observed under a Wood lamp.

2. Now what is the most likely diagnosis?

   Now this man likely has ethylene glycol intoxication. Ethylene glycol can be found in antifreeze and deicing solutions. Antifreeze in the United States commonly has an additive that produces the Wood lamp fluorescence. Alcohol dehydrogenase is again the metabolizing enzyme, producing oxalic acid. Oxalic acid can combine with calcium to produce crystals in the urine seen on microscopic examination. If extensive crystal precipitation occurs within the kidneys, acute kidney injury can result. In severe cases, renal failure occurs, along with depressed consciousness, coma, and cardiopulmonary collapse.

3. What is the treatment for this patient?

   Fomepizole inhibits alcohol dehydrogenase and is therefore very effective to reverse both methanol and ethylene glycol toxicity because it can prevent the buildup of the toxic metabolites (formic and oxalic acids, respectively). Intravenous ethanol also works in theory, as high ethanol levels would competitively inhibit the metabolism of methanol or ethylene glycol by alcohol dehydrogenase and prevent the production of these toxic metabolites. In severe cases of methanol or ethylene glycol ingestion such as those resulting in severe acidemia with end-organ damage (e.g., visual disturbances, acute kidney injury), hemodialysis is indicated because it directly removes methanol, ethylene glycol, and their acid metabolites from the circulation.

STEP 1 SECRET

*As mentioned throughout this book, drug side effects and toxicities are extremely high yield for the USMLE Step 1. Knowing antidotes to common drug overdoses (e.g., fomepizole for methanol, ethanol, and ethylene glycol poisoning) is an easy way to earn points on the USMLE. Remember, **fome**pizole is for overdoses of **m**ethanol and **e**thylene glycol.*

CASE 5.7

A patient with a history of depression is brought into the emergency department with nausea, vomiting, and tinnitus. Her laboratory values are as follows:

> [Na$^+$]: 140 mEq/L
> [K$^+$]: 3.5 mEq/L
> [Cl$^-$]: 104 mEq/L

[HCO$_3^-$]: 16 mEq/L
Glucose: 100 mg/dL
pH: 7.50
P$_{CO_2}$: 20 mm Hg
P$_{O_2}$: 125 mm Hg

1. **What is the most likely diagnosis?**
   This patient has a mixed disorder consisting of a respiratory alkalosis and a high AG metabolic acidosis.
   The pH is in the alkalotic range, and the low P$_{CO_2}$ in the setting of the increased pH suggests a respiratory alkalosis. The AG in this case is 20 mEq/L; recall that AG = [Na$^+$] − [(Cl$^-$ + HCO$_3^-$)] = 140 − (104 + 16) = 20. Remember that an elevated AG, even in the setting of a normal or elevated pH, *always* reflects a metabolic acidosis. For that reason, it is often worthwhile to calculate the AG in acid-base problems regardless of the given pH.
   The prototypical mixed acid-base disorder that appears on the USMLE is salicylate toxicity (e.g., aspirin overdose). In this case, the patient's history of depression suggests a risk of suicidal ideation, while the tinnitus in particular is a major clue for salicylate poisoning. On the USMLE, you should always consider aspirin toxicity in a patient with the combination of an AG metabolic acidosis and respiratory alkalosis (**Note:** Initial aspirin overdose directly activates the respiratory center in the medulla, resulting in hyperventilation and a respiratory alkalosis).
   Although aspirin is itself an acid, most of the AG produced in aspirin toxicity occurs from the lactic acid buildup that results from aspirin's ability to interfere with cellular metabolism when ingested at toxic levels.
   Side effects of aspirin can be recalled using the mnemonic **ASPIRIN**: **A**sthma, **S**alicylism, **P**eptic ulcers, **I**ntestinal bleeding, **R**eye syndrome, **I**diosyncratic reactions, and **N**oise (tinnitus).

SUMMARY BOX: HAGMA

- Causes: **MUDPILES: M**ethanol, **U**remia, **D**iabetic ketoacidosis, **P**olyethylene glycol, **I**soniazid and **I**ron supplements, **L**actic acidosis, **E**thylene glycol, and **S**alicylate toxicity
- If ΔAG = ΔHCO$_3^-$, then the HAGMA is the sole metabolic acid-base disorder.
- If ΔAG < ΔHCO$_3^-$, then there is a non-AG metabolic acidosis present in addition to the HAGMA already identified (because the *change* in HCO$_3^-$ is *greater* than expected).
- If ΔAG > ΔHCO$_3^-$, then there is a metabolic alkalosis present in addition to the HAGMA already identified (because the *change* in HCO$_3^-$ is *smaller* than expected).
- HAGMA + blurry vision: Think methanol ingestion
- HAGMA + urine with oxalate crystals and/or Wood lamp fluorescence: Think ethylene glycol ingestion.
- HAGMA + respiratory alkalosis ± tinnitus: Think aspirin toxicity.
- Remember the common causes of lactic acidosis: Sepsis, circulatory or respiratory failure, limb or organ ischemia (especially small bowel), cyanide or carbon monoxide toxicity, and hepatic failure are all USMLE favorites.

CASE 5.8

The emergency department admits a patient with congestive heart failure presenting in severe respiratory distress. His laboratory values are as follows:
   pH: 7.0
   P$_{CO_2}$: 60 mm Hg
   [HCO$_3^-$]: 28 mEq/L

1. **What is the primary acid-base disorder?**
   Following the diagnostic pathway outlined in Fig. 5.4, you should recognize that the pH is in the acidotic range with markedly elevated P$_{CO_2}$, indicating a respiratory acidosis.

2. **What is the differential diagnosis in this patient?**
   The differential diagnosis of CO$_2$ retention is very broad, and includes not only lung disease but also central hypoventilation from any cause (e.g., sedatives, CNS trauma, pickwickian syndrome), neuromuscular disorders (e.g., myasthenia gravis, Guillain-Barré syndrome, amyotrophic lateral sclerosis [ALS], muscular dystrophy, poliomyelitis), upper airway obstruction (e.g., acute airway obstruction, laryngospasm, obstructive sleep apnea), CHF, and thoracic cage abnormalities (e.g., pneumothorax, flail chest, scoliosis).
   Note: Lung disease generally impairs gas exchange through dead space (lung that is ventilated but not perfused) or shunting (lung that is perfused but not ventilated) or, most commonly, a combination of both (i.e., ventilation-perfusion mismatch). Disorders with prominent dead space ventilation (e.g., emphysema) tend to cause prominent and early CO$_2$ retention. Disorders with prominent intrapulmonary shunting (e.g., asthma, pulmonary edema, pneumonia, atelectasis, or pulmonary embolism) tend to cause prominent hypoxia but can result in hypercapnia later as well.

3. What is the most likely diagnosis in this patient?

From the limited amount of information we are given, acute pulmonary edema as the result of CHF is the most likely explanation. An intrapulmonary shunt is created when alveoli are filled with fluid, such as in pneumonia, pulmonary edema (from ARDS or CHF), or atelectasis. Intrapulmonary shunts generally lead to hypoxemia, which often in turn stimulates hyperventilation and a *decreased* (or normal) Pco_2. However, when the shunt fraction is very large or when the increased hyperventilation and increased work of breathing lead to muscle fatigue, respiratory acidosis is the result.

4. Is there appropriate compensation, or is this a mixed disorder?

The increase in HCO_3^- is $28 - 24 = 4$ mEq/L. An acute respiratory acidosis would be expected to raise bicarbonate by $0.2 \times \Delta Pco_2 = 0.2 \times 20 = 4$ mEq/L (see Table 5.2). Therefore there is appropriate compensation. Recall that maximal compensation by the kidney in the setting of a respiratory acidosis takes about 3 days.

CASE 5.8 CONTINUED:

The patient is intubated and admitted to the intensive care unit. He steadily improves over the next couple of days and then suddenly develops a respiratory acidosis again.

5. How can you determine if this exacerbation is due to central hypoventilation from sedation or due to a ventilation-perfusion (V/Q) mismatch, such as worsening of his pulmonary edema or development of a ventilator-associated pneumonia?

Often the history will reveal an obvious cause of a respiratory acidosis. However, it can get very tricky when there are multiple possible causes that fit with the patient's history. To determine if the patient's hypercapnia is a result of sedation or of lung pathology, you can check the patient's alveolar-arterial O_2 gradient (A-a gradient). A normal or unchanged A-a gradient indicates that the lungs are exchanging gases normally and that the impairment is from a separate process, such as central hypoventilation as the result of excessive sedation or neuromuscular disease. Lung disease resulting in $\dot{V}/\dot{Q}$ mismatch will reveal an increased A-a gradient.

SUMMARY BOX: RESPIRATORY ACIDOSIS

- Differential diagnosis = lung disease (usually via ventilation/perfusion mismatch), central hypoventilation, neuromuscular disorders, upper airway obstruction, and thoracic cage abnormalities.
- Maximal compensation (e.g., HCO_3^- retention) by the kidney takes about 3 days.
- Dead space ventilation (e.g., in emphysema) results in hypercarbia early.
- Disorders involving intrapulmonary shunts (e.g., asthma, pulmonary edema, pneumonia, atelectasis, or pulmonary embolism [PE]) only result in hypercarbia when a large shunt or respiratory muscle fatigue develops.
- Increased alveolar-arterial (A-a) gradient suggests a $\dot{V}/\dot{Q}$ abnormality and a lung defect.
- Normal/unchanged A-a gradient suggests an underlying central hypoventilation or neuromuscular disorder.

GASTROENTEROLOGY

BASIC CONCEPTS

1. The three major fuel sources used by the body are carbohydrates, fats, and proteins. Where does digestion of these macromolecules primarily occur?
   See Table 6.1.

Table 6.1. Digestion of Major Fuel Sources

MACROMOLECULE	STRUCTURAL FORM DURING INTAKE	SITE OF BREAKDOWN	STRUCTURAL FORM ABSORBED
Carbohydrates	Simple and complex carbohydrates	Begins in the mouth but primarily occurs in the small intestine	Monosaccharides
Fats	Triglycerides	Mostly in the small intestine (less than 10% occurs in the mouth and stomach)	Free fatty acids
Proteins	Polypeptides	Begins in the stomach but primarily occurs in the small intestine	Amino acids and small peptides

2. What are the anatomic layers of the gut wall (Fig. 6.1)?
   From the lumen moving outward, the layers of the gastrointestinal (GI) tract are as follows: (1) mucosa, comprising the mucosal epithelium, lamina propria, and muscularis mucosae; (2) submucosa, which contains the submucosal (Meissner) nerve plexus; (3) muscularis propria, comprising an inner circular smooth muscle layer, myenteric (Auerbach) nerve plexus, and outer longitudinal smooth muscle layer; and (4) serosa (intraperitoneal organs) or adventitia (retroperitoneal organs), which is the fibrous outer covering.
   Note: The taeniae coli are band-like muscles composing the outer longitudinal smooth muscle layer of the large intestine, except in the appendix and the rectum.

3. Digestion of food begins in the mouth. What are the constituents of saliva?
   Saliva contains α-amylase, which begins the process of carbohydrate digestion, and lingual lipase, which initiates lipid digestion. It also contains mucins that lubricate food. In addition, saliva contains many molecules that are important for preventing bacteria from entering the digestive tract, including immunoglobulins, potassium bicarbonate, and lysozyme. Saliva is produced by the acinar cells of the parotid, submandibular, and sublingual glands and is initially produced as an isotonic solution. As the secretions move along the salivary duct, they are modified by the columnar epithelial cells that line the duct; Na^+ and Cl^- are reabsorbed into the body, while K^+ and HCO_3^- are secreted into the saliva. Because duct cells are impermeable to water, the final result is that saliva is hypotonic to plasma. When saliva secretion is stimulated, myoepithelial cells contract and eject saliva into the mouth.

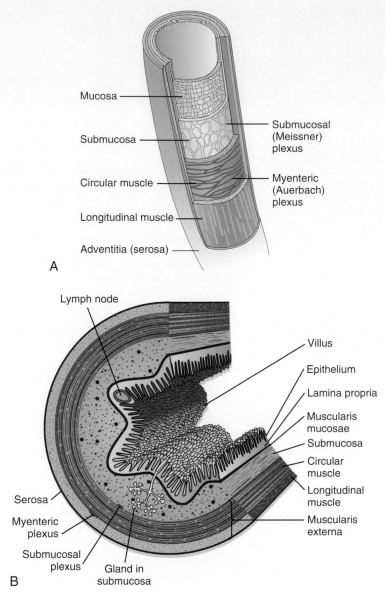

Figure 6.1. A–B, Two different views of the layers of the gut wall. *(A from Brown TA. Rapid Review Physiology. Philadelphia: Mosby; 2007. B from Koeppen BM, Stanton BA.* Berne and Levy Physiology. *6th ed. Updated ed. Philadelphia: Mosby; 2010, Fig. 26-2.)*

4. From the mouth, food passes through the esophagus and to the stomach. How is this passage of food regulated?

   The process of deglutition (swallowing) is complex. After the neurologic and mechanical initiation of deglutition, which propels macerated food from the mouth and posterior oropharynx into the esophagus, the passage of food is regulated via coordinated actions of the upper esophageal sphincter (UES) and lower esophageal sphincter (LES). Relaxation of the UES allows food to enter the esophagus from the pharynx, where it makes its way through the esophagus via a series of coordinated movements referred to as *peristalsis*. Peristalsis is orchestrated by the myenteric plexus of the enteric nervous system and propels the bolus of food toward the LES, which is constricted between meals to prevent reflux of acidic gastric contents into the esophagus. In response to swallowing and subsequent distention of the esophagus, the LES relaxes, allowing the bolus of food to pass into the stomach.

5. What is the primary function of the stomach?

   Although the stomach functions primarily as a reservoir for food waiting to be digested in the small intestine, it also prepares the food for digestion by converting it into an acidic substance known as *chyme*. Table 6.2 summarizes the functions of the major cell types involved in gastric secretions.

Table 6.2. Major Cell Types in the Stomach

CELL TYPE	PRODUCT	FUNCTION	STIMULI	INHIBITORS
G cell	Gastrin	Stimulates activity of parietal cells	Presence of food in the stomach	Low pH
Parietal cell	Hydrochloric acid (HCl) Intrinsic factor	Converts pepsinogen into pepsin (active form), denatures proteins, kills bacteria, binds vitamin B_{12} to prevent its degradation in the small intestine	Gastrin, histamine, parasympathetic stimulation	Antihistamines, anti-cholinergic drugs Proton pump inhibitors inhibit secretion of HCl into the gastric lumen
Mucous cell	Mucus and bicarbonate	Protects the gastric lining from the surrounding acidic environment	Prostaglandins	NSAIDs
Chief cell	Pepsinogen (inactive form)	Converts large polypeptides into smaller peptides and amino acids	Intake of food	—

NSAIDs, Nonsteroidal antiinflammatory drugs.

6. **How are pancreatic enzymes stored and activated?**

Pancreatic enzymes are made and stored in the pancreatic acinar cells in the form of inactive zymogens. When they are stimulated to be released, they are released into the duodenum through the sphincter of Oddi at the ampulla of Vater.

In the small intestine, pancreatic enzymes are activated. First, brush border enzyme enterokinase activates trypsinogen into trypsin. Then trypsin activates other pancreatic enzymes.

Pancreatic secretion is isotonic to plasma because it has the same Na^+ and K^+ concentrations as plasma. However, it has much higher HCO_3^- concentration and lower Cl^- concentration than plasma. The HCO_3^- is important because it enables pancreatic enzymes to increase the pH of contents in the small intestine, protecting the small intestine from damage that would otherwise be caused by the acidic chyme.

7. **What are the functions of the GI hormones?**

See Table 6.3.

Table 6.3. Functions of GI Hormones

HORMONE	FUNCTION	SITE OF SECRETION	STIMULUS FOR RELEASE
Cholecystokinin (CCK)	Stimulates the contraction of the gallbladder and relaxation of the sphincter of Oddi so bile can be secreted into intestine Stimulates pancreatic enzyme secretion Inhibits gastric emptying (allowing more time for digestion)	I cells of duodenum and jejunum	Fatty acids and monoglycerides in the duodenum and jejunum
Secretin	Stimulates pancreatic enzyme and HCO_3^- secretion	S cells of duodenum	Acidification of duodenal contents
Glucose-dependent insulinotropic peptide (GIP)	Stimulates insulin release (This is why oral glucose is more effective than intravenous glucose in causing insulin release.)	K cells of duodenum and jejunum	Fatty acids, amino acids, and, importantly, *orally administered* glucose

GI, Gastrointestinal.

8. **What are bile salts, and what is their function?**

Bile salts are amphipathic molecules that are formed from the degradation of cholesterol in the liver. They solubilize fats in meals by forming micelles, which have a hydrophilic head that is dissolved in the aqueous solution and a hydrophobic tail that is on the inside of the micelle along with the fat (Fig. 6.2). The micelle has two functions to aid in fat digestion: (1) It creates a bigger surface area on which pancreatic lipase can work (emulsification), and (2) it facilitates the delivery of fatty acids to the intestinal enterocytes for absorption. As a point of interest, bile is the primary method the body has for eliminating cholesterol.

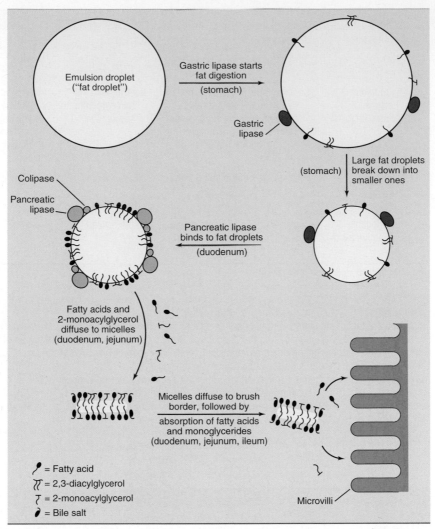

Figure 6.2. Sequence of events in fat digestion. A small amount of fat is hydrolyzed by gastric lipase in the stomach, but pancreatic lipase is the major enzyme of fat digestion. Bile salts containing micelles are required for efficient absorption of fatty acids, monoglycerides, and other dietary lipids. *(From Meisenberg G, Simmons WH. Principles of Medical Biochemistry. 3rd ed. Philadelphia: Saunders; 2012.)*

9. **What is enterohepatic circulation, and why is it important in the digestion of fats?**
   Enterohepatic circulation refers to the circulation of bile salts, drugs, and other substances excreted from the liver, taken up by enterocytes of the small intestine, and returned to the liver. Because bile salts are necessary for digestion of fats, impairment of the enterohepatic circulation will compromise fat digestion, leading to the sequelae of fat malabsorption. In Crohn disease, for example, inflammation of the terminal ileum prevents the reabsorption of bile salts to the liver. If the liver is not able to synthesize enough new bile salts to meet demand, patients will have impaired fat digestion and fatty stools (steatorrhea).

10. **What defines the foregut, midgut, and hindgut anatomically (Fig. 6.3)? Which main arteries provide the blood supply to each segment? Which nerves supply these regions?**
    The foregut comprises the upper GI tract beginning at the esophagus down to a site in the second part of the duodenum just distal to the ampulla of Vater (where the common bile duct empties into the intestinal lumen). Its main vascular supply comes from the celiac artery. The midgut extends from the second part of the duodenum down to the splenic flexure of the colon and is served by the superior mesenteric artery. The hindgut extends from the splenic flexure of the colon to the anus and is supplied by the inferior mesenteric artery. The foregut and midgut are innervated by the vagus nerve, and the hindgut is innervated by the pelvic nerve.
    Note: The pancreas and liver are embryologic outgrowths of the foregut and share the vascular supply of the foregut (i.e., celiac artery). Although the spleen is not an embryologic derivative of the foregut (it is of mesodermal origin), it too is supplied by the celiac artery.

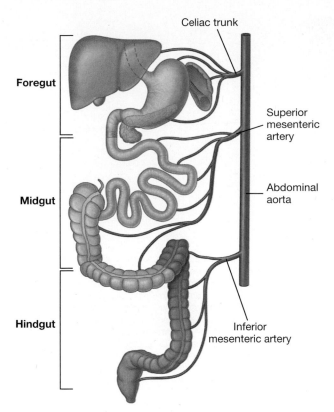

Celiac trunk

Foregut

Superior
mesenteric
artery

Abdominal
aorta

Midgut

Hindgut

Inferior
mesenteric artery

Figure 6.3. Divisions of the gastrointestinal tract into the foregut, midgut, and hindgut, summarizing the primary arterial supply to each segment. *(From Drake RL, Vogl AW, Mitchell AWM.* Gray's Basic Anatomy. *Philadelphia: Churchill Livingstone; 2013.)*

Embryology Pearl

The pancreas and liver are embryologic outgrowths of the foregut and share the vascular supply of the foregut (i.e., celiac artery). Although the spleen is not an embryologic derivative of the foregut (it arises in the mesentery of the stomach, so it is of mesodermal origin), it too is supplied by the celiac artery.

CASE 6.1

A 45-year-old obese man presents with a 2-year history of chest discomfort following heavy meals. He describes the discomfort as a substernal burning sensation that radiates to his neck. The discomfort worsens when he is lying down in bed at night. He mentions that he also has a chronic cough and hoarse voice in the morning.

---

1. What is the differential diagnosis?
   The differential diagnosis includes gastroesophageal reflux disease (GERD), esophageal spasm, achalasia, and angina associated with coronary artery disease. Note that myocardial ischemia/infarction should be part of the differential diagnosis in any case in which there is chest discomfort/pain, especially considering that this patient is a middle-aged, obese male, all of which are risk factors for heart disease. GERD characteristically presents with pyrosis (heartburn), which can mimic myocardial ischemia, and waterbrash, the regurgitation of sour material into the mouth. The symptoms of GERD are typically exacerbated by eating large meals, bending over, or being recumbent in bed. In addition to heartburn, patients with GERD can also present with chronic cough from gastric acid irritation of the tracheobronchial tree and a hoarse voice in the morning from the gastric acid irritation of the vocal cords at night.

CASE 6.1 CONTINUED:

Physical examination is significant for obesity. There is no chest wall tenderness. Cardiac examination is unremarkable except for auscultating bowel sounds in the patient's chest. A cardiac stress test is negative for inducible ischemia. A barium swallow is as shown in Fig. 6.4.

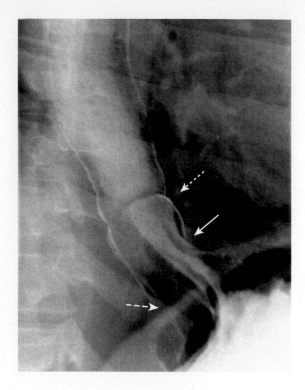

Figure 6.4. Sliding hiatal hernia. A bulbous collection of contrast representing the herniated stomach is evident above the diaphragm. Gastric folds are present in the hernia, identifying it as part of the stomach (*solid white arrow*). Notice the esophagus does not narrow as it normally does when passing through the esophageal hiatus (*dashed white arrow*). Just above the hernia is a thin, web-like filling defect characteristic of a Schatzki ring (*dotted white arrow*). The Schatzki ring marks the level of the esophagogastric junction. *(From Herring W.* Learning Radiology: Recognizing the Basics. *2nd ed. Philadelphia: Saunders; 2012.)*

2. Based on the findings in Fig. 6.4, what is the patient's likely diagnosis?

   A sliding hiatal hernia is the likely diagnosis. In a sliding hiatal hernia, the gastroesophageal junction herniates upward through the esophageal hiatus in the diaphragm. The additional lower esophageal sphincteric pressure that is normally provided by the diaphragm is then lost, allowing reflux of gastric contents to occur more easily. This contrasts with a paraesophageal hiatal hernia, in which a portion of the gastric fundus rolls into and herniates through the diaphragm but the gastroesophageal junction remains in place. Although paraesophageal hiatal hernias usually do not cause reflux because they do not affect LES tone, they are more serious because they can become incarcerated (strangulated) and ischemic.

3. Discuss the pathophysiology of GERD.

   GERD is caused by the reflux of acidic or bilious gastric contents into the esophagus, which irritates the esophageal mucosa and causes pain. Many factors can predispose to reflux. One of the most important factors is abnormal transient relaxation of the LES unrelated to swallowing. A continually relaxed (atonic) LES will also allow reflux. Increased intra-abdominal pressure (due to obesity, pregnancy, Valsalva maneuver, etc.), increased gastric volume (due to eating a large meal or gastroparesis), and decreasing distance of gastric contents from the gastroesophageal junction (occurring when lying down or with hiatal hernia) may exacerbate reflux of gastric contents into the esophagus.

CASE 6.1 CONTINUED:

The patient is started on a 1-week therapeutic trial of omeprazole, which provides substantial relief. He is therefore started on a long-term course of omeprazole.

4. Cover the far-left column of Table 6.4 and attempt to name the medications used in the treatment of GERD based on the class of medication, the mechanism of action, and the primary side effects listed in the table.

5. Why may the omeprazole this patient was given increase his risk for hypergastrinemia?

   Proton pump inhibitors (PPIs) such as omeprazole inhibit gastric hydrochloric acid (HCl) secretion by irreversibly inhibiting the hydrogen potassium adenosine triphosphate (H^+/K^+-ATPase) pump on gastric parietal cells. This raises gastric pH, which disinhibits gastric secretion by the G cells, resulting in hypergastrinemia.

Table 6.4. Medication Used for Treatment of Gastroesophageal Reflux Disease

MEDICATION	CLASS	MECHANISM OF ACTION	PRIMARY SIDE EFFECT
Cimetidine Ranitidine Nizatidine Famotidine	Histamine H_2 receptor antagonists	Inhibits histamine-stimulated release of hydrochloric acid by blocking H_2 receptors on parietal cells	Cimetidine inhibits hepatic cytochrome P-450 enzymes and causes gynecomastia
Metoclopramide	D_2 receptor antagonist Antiemetic Prokinetic	Prokinetic drug (increases gastric emptying and LES tone); contraindicated in patients with small bowel obstruction	Parkinsonian symptoms, seizures
Omeprazole Lansoprazole Rabeprazole	Proton pump inhibitors	Irreversibly inhibits the parietal cell H^+/K^+-ATPase pump, thus decreasing acid secretion into the gastric lumen	Hypergastrinemia, increased risk of pneumonia and infection with *Clostridioides difficile*. Decreased serum Mg^{2+}

H^+/K^+-ATPase, Hydrogen-potassium adenosine triphosphate; *LES,* lower esophageal sphincter.

CASE 6.1 CONTINUED:

Unfortunately, the patient is lost to follow-up, but he shows up at his physician's office 3 years later reporting 6 months of progressively worsening dysphagia to solids and unintentional weight loss. He says he tried to be diligent about taking his omeprazole for the first month but soon stopped taking his pills and learned to tolerate the discomfort.

6. **Which complications of GERD could be responsible for the patient's difficulty swallowing?**
   Esophageal stricture results from fibrosing and scarring of the esophageal mucosa from chronic irritation and inflammation by gastric acid. This scarring narrows the lumen, which prevents a food bolus from passing through, causing food to get stuck. Another complication of GERD is Barrett esophagus, which refers to metaplasia of the esophageal epithelium (from a stratified squamous epithelium to the nonciliated columnar, goblet cell–containing epithelium that is normally found lower in the GI tract; Fig. 6.5). Barrett esophagus can progress to esophageal adenocarcinoma (EAC) of the lower one-third of the esophagus; this usually presents with progressive dysphagia and weight loss.

Clinical Pearl

Barrett esophagus is the most important risk factor for the development of adenocarcinoma of the esophagus; in fact, patients with Barrett esophagus have a 30-fold increase in their risk compared with the general population. However, despite this increase in risk over the general population, a small percentage (~1%) of patients with Barrett esophagus develop esophageal adenocarcinoma.

---

7. **Differentiate between the two types of esophageal cancers, adenocarcinoma and squamous cell carcinoma, in terms of risk factors and location.**
   Adenocarcinoma typically occurs in the lower one-third of the esophagus. Barrett esophagus and chronic irritation of esophageal epithelium from untreated GERD are risk factors for this type of cancer.
   Squamous cell carcinoma usually occurs in the upper two-thirds of the esophagus. Smoking and alcohol, especially together (synergistic effect), increase the risk for this type of cancer.
   Esophageal cancers cause progressive dysphagia to solids and liquids; they tend to cause symptoms in the later stages of development and thus have a poor prognosis (with 5-year survival of ~20%).

8. **Why would a patient with Sjögren syndrome be more susceptible to esophageal pathology in GERD?**
   Sjögren syndrome is an immune-mediated disease characterized by lymphocytic infiltration of the lacrimal and salivary glands, causing dry eyes (keratoconjunctivitis sicca) and dry mouth (xerostomia) as a result of deficient secretions. Because saliva is rich in bicarbonate, it functions to neutralize acid in the esophagus. The absence of this protective function predisposes patients with this condition to esophageal damage with even minimal gastroesophageal reflux. Sjögren syndrome is also associated with esophageal dysmotility.

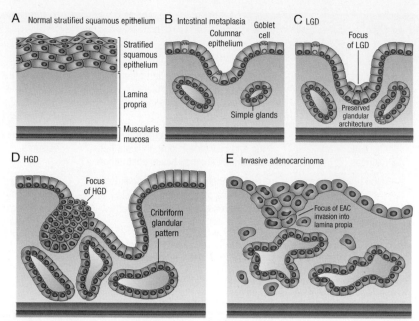

Figure 6.5. Stages involved in progression of Barrett esophagus to esophageal adenocarcinoma (EAC). A, Normal stratified squamous epithelium of the esophagus. B, Intestinal metaplasia in which the stratified squamous epithelium is replaced by columnar lined epithelium containing goblet cells. C, Low-grade dysplasia (LGD) characterized by enlargement and/or elongation of the nuclei, mild nuclear hyperchromasia, nuclear stratification, pleomorphism, increased mitoses, and lack of surface maturation. Glandular architecture is simple and there is maintenance of polarity. D, High-grade dysplasia (HGD) in which there is a marked increase in the nuclear cytoplasmic ratio, nuclear stratification, pleomorphism, abnormal mitoses, and lack of surface maturation. Development of glandular crowding, cribriform glands, and loss of nuclear polarity occurs. E, EAC, whereby abnormal cells invade the basement membrane into the lamina propria and beyond. *(Reprinted by permission from Anaparthy R, Sharma P. Progression of Barrett oesophagus: role of endoscopic and histological predictors.* Nat Rev Gastroenterol Hepatol. *2014;11:526.)*

STEP 1 SECRET

Gastroesophageal reflux disease (GERD) and its complications are a Step 1 favorite. Chest pain following meals and nocturnal cough should clue you into this diagnosis.

SUMMARY BOX: GASTROESOPHAGEAL REFLUX DISEASE

- Symptoms: Substernal chest pain (heartburn) that is worse after large meals or when lying down, chronic cough, hoarse voice, sour taste in mouth
- Risk factors: More common in obese or pregnant individuals because of increased intra-abdominal pressure
- Pathophysiology: Inappropriate relaxation of the lower esophageal sphincter (LES) or elevated intra-abdominal pressure results in regurgitation of acidic gastric contents into the esophagus, leading to esophageal irritation.
- Gastroesophageal reflux disease (GERD) is a common consequence of sliding hiatal hernias secondary to decreased LES tone.
- Diagnosis: History, barium swallow, and lack of evidence to support cardiac ischemia
- If a sliding hiatal hernia is present, bowel sounds may be auscultated in the chest.
- Treatment: Largely pharmacologic (proton pump inhibitors [PPIs]), H_2 receptor antagonists), lifestyle modifications (propping self up at night, avoiding large meal close to sleep, avoiding triggers such as alcohol, caffeine, spicy food), surgery for refractory GERD
- Complications: Esophageal stricture, esophageal ulceration, Barrett esophagus, and adenocarcinoma

CASE 6.2

A 50-year-old woman presents to her physician with a report of recent dysphagia to solids and liquids for over 2 years.

1. In pathophysiologic terms, how do you approach dysphagia?
   Dysphagia can be approached broadly in terms of oropharyngeal or esophageal etiology.

Oropharyngeal dysphagia is caused by difficulty initiating a swallow reflex from either neurologic or muscular problems. Typical causes include stroke, amyotrophic lateral sclerosis (ALS; Lou Gehrig disease), and myasthenia gravis. Patients usually have coughing or choking with dysphagia of oropharyngeal etiology and may have a history of aspiration pneumonia. Esophageal dysphagia is caused by food getting stuck in the esophagus after being swallowed. This is due to either mechanical obstruction or esophageal dysmotility. History can often distinguish between an obstructive etiology and a motility disorder. Patients with an obstructive etiology (e.g., esophageal adenocarcinoma) will have progressive dysphagia, which begins with an inability to swallow solid foods and progresses to an inability to swallow both solids and liquids. Patients with a dysmotility disorder (e.g., achalasia, scleroderma-like esophagus, diffuse esophageal spasm) will have trouble swallowing solids and liquids from the onset of disease.

CASE 6.2 CONTINUED:

Given this patient's long-standing dysphagia to solids and liquids, a motility disorder is suspected. Further history reveals occasional chest pain with eating, nocturnal cough, and an unintentional 15-lb weight loss in the past 2 months despite a preserved appetite. She was recently admitted to the hospital for treatment of pneumonia. Esophageal manometry shows increased LES pressure with incomplete LES relaxation and a complete absence of peristalsis in the lower esophagus. A barium swallow is shown in Fig. 6.6.

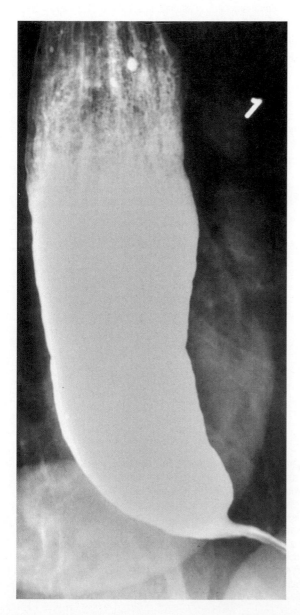

Figure 6.6. Barium swallow of patient in Case 6.2. *(From Cummings CW, Flint PW, Haughey BH, et al. Otolaryngology: Head and Neck Surgery. 4th ed. Philadelphia: Mosby; 2005.)*

2. What is the likely diagnosis in this woman? Describe the pathophysiology of this disease.
Achalasia is the likely diagnosis. The initial dysphagia to solids and liquids, barium swallow showing the classic "bird's beak" appearance, and esophageal manometry findings of aperistalsis and increased LES pressure are classic for achalasia. The LES is normally tonically constricted, generating enough intraluminal pressure to prevent the reflux of gastric contents into the esophagus. During the esophageal phase of swallowing, the LES relaxes in response to a food bolus descending through the esophagus, a phenomenon referred to as *receptive relaxation*. In achalasia, there is destruction of the submucosal myenteric plexus, which mediates receptive relaxation and also mediates esophageal peristalsis (hence the aperistalsis). Although the exact mechanism of increased LES tone in patients with achalasia is not known, research suggests that these patients have loss of nitric oxide–secreting neurons, a key factor in LES relaxation. Proposed mechanisms include immune-mediated, viral, and genetic. The failure of the LES to relax together with the failure of the distal esophagus to undergo peristalsis allows food to accumulate and dilate the lower esophagus, creating the bird's beak appearance on barium swallow (see Fig. 6.6).

3. For what type of cancer are patients with achalasia at increased risk?
Patients with achalasia are at increased risk for esophageal squamous cell carcinoma.

4. Chagas disease is also known to be a cause of achalasia (pseudoachalasia or secondary achalasia). What is the pathologic mechanism, and what organism is the primary culprit?
Chagas disease (American trypanosomiasis) can cause destruction of the myenteric plexus in the esophagus by the protozoal parasite *Trypanosoma cruzi* (particularly common in South America). In addition to achalasia, Chagas disease can cause megacolon by destroying the myenteric plexus of the colon.

5. What was the likely cause of this woman's previous episode of pneumonia?
The pneumonia was likely caused by aspiration of esophageal contents, especially while sleeping, because of the presence of undigested material in the esophagus.

6. In addition to pneumatic dilatation of the lower esophageal sphincter and surgical or endoscopic myotomy, injection of botulinum toxin into the lower esophageal sphincter is a treatment option for this woman. What is this drug's mechanism of action in this context?
Much of the tonic constriction of the LES is due to vagal cholinergic innervation. Because botulinum toxin exerts its effects by inhibiting the release of acetylcholine from nerve endings, it reduces this input to LES tone.

SUMMARY BOX: ACHALASIA

- Symptoms: Dysphagia (to solids and liquids), chest pain associated with eating, nocturnal cough, unintentional weight loss despite preserved appetite
- Risk factors: Acquired causes include infection with *Trypanosoma cruzi* (Chagas disease).
- Pathophysiology: Motility disorder caused by destruction of the myenteric plexus
- Diagnosis: Barium swallow, which shows a "bird's beak" appearance. Esophageal manometry will show distal aperistalsis and increased lower esophageal sphincter (LES) tone.
- Treatment: Pneumatic dilation, esophagomyotomy, and injection of botulinum toxin into the LES
- Complications: Pneumonia secondary to aspiration, esophageal squamous cell carcinoma

---

CASE 6.3

A 33-year-old man is evaluated for a 2-month history of burning epigastric pain that develops an hour or so after meals. The pain is particularly bothersome at night and often awakens him from sleep. The patient denies any alterations in bowel habits.

---

1. What is the differential diagnosis?
The differential diagnosis for postprandial epigastric pain includes biliary colic, GERD, functional dyspepsia, and peptic ulcer disease (PUD). Biliary colic is severe, acute-onset right upper quadrant pain caused by gallstones and is usually precipitated by fatty meals. It has a higher frequency in women but is still common in men. GERD may cause epigastric or substernal discomfort that worsens with large meals or when lying flat. Functional dyspepsia can produce epigastric pain and bloating that is worsened by stress or food and is unrelated to bowel habits, but it cannot be due to another etiology such as PUD or gastritis. PUD encompasses both gastric and duodenal ulcers. Duodenal ulcers, which are more common, typically cause the most pain 1 to 3 hours after a meal, when the acidic chyme enters the small bowel. Pain may also occur at night because of circadian rhythm–induced acid secretion. Food or antacids can relieve the epigastric pain. Gastric ulcers have a more variable presentation, but epigastric pain is typically precipitated by food, and therefore patients may experience weight loss because of food avoidance.
Based on the patient's history, a duodenal ulcer is the most likely diagnosis.

CASE 6.3 CONTINUED:

After a brief history and physical examination, the physician prescribes an antacid and schedules a follow-up visit in 2 weeks to see if this treatment provides relief.

2. If you were this man's physician, what would you have done differently in the treatment of this patient?

The patient with epigastric pain warrants a thorough history and physical examination, looking for any red-flag symptoms, such as GI bleeding, anemia, dysphagia, persistent vomiting, or unintentional weight loss, because these problems could point toward more serious pathologic processes such as malignancy. The two usual culprits for PUD are nonsteroidal antiinflammatory drugs (NSAIDs) and the bacterium *Helicobacter pylori*. A more thorough history could have discovered if the patient were taking NSAIDs, which you would have recommended that he stop taking. Testing for *H. pylori* would also be advised to guide treatment and prevent recurrence.

In the absence of red-flag symptoms in a young adult with suspected PUD, visualization of the ulcer by upper endoscopy or barium swallow is not necessary, and the patient can be empirically treated with a PPI (e.g., omeprazole).

3. How are NSAIDs thought to predispose to the formation of ulcers? What alternatives exist to lessen GI side effects?

Because of their action on cyclooxygenase-1 (COX-1), a side effect of NSAIDs is that they inhibit the production of prostaglandins in the gastric mucosa. These prostaglandins normally function to protect the gastric mucosa from the acidic environment by increasing mucus and bicarbonate secretion and by stimulating local vasodilation, which maintains mucosal perfusion and prevents ischemic injury. As a result, patients on NSAIDs are prone to GI irritation, bleeding, and ulceration.

Two options exist to circumvent this problem: (1) NSAIDs can be taken with misoprostol, PPIs, or H$_2$ receptor antagonists (rarely done), or (2) selective COX-2 inhibitors can be used instead of NSAIDs when the goal is to reduce inflammation. Recall that the constitutively expressed COX-1 is present in multiple tissues while the inducible form, COX-2, is present *primarily* in inflammatory cells. Unfortunately, COX-2 inhibitors can be prothrombotic and exacerbate hypertension, increasing the risk of stroke and myocardial infarction. This major side effect led to rofecoxib being pulled from the US market in 2004.

CASE 6.3 CONTINUED:

The patient misses his 2-week appointment and returns 7 months later looking pale and tired. The antacids initially provided some relief, but now the pain is back and is worse than before. In addition, the patient has noticed he has dark, tarry stools and feels tired all the time.

4. Based on the appearance of the stool, is this more likely an upper GI bleed or a lower GI bleed?

It is more likely an upper GI bleed (UGIB), likely caused by a bleeding duodenal ulcer. UGIB is anatomically distinguished from a lower GI bleed (LGIB) in that it occurs proximal to the ligament of Treitz, which marks the division between the duodenum and jejunum. UGIB presents with either hematemesis or melena. Melena occurs because the hemoglobin has time to be broken down by bacteria in the gut to give dark, tarry stools. LGIB presents with hematochezia (bright red rectal bleeding) because bacteria do not have the time to break down hemoglobin. However, brisk UGIBs such as bleeding esophageal varices can present with hematochezia because blood stimulates GI motility and decreases transit time.

STEP 1 SECRET

Gastrointestinal bleeds are a common cause of anemia, as is evidenced by this patient's symptoms of paleness and fatigue (see Chapter 12, Anemias). Be on the lookout for this popularly used vignette on Step 1.

5. What are the major complications of PUD?

Hemorrhage is the most common complication of PUD and can present as hematemesis or melena. Potential sources of hemorrhage include a posterior penetrating duodenal ulcer (gastroduodenal artery) or penetrating gastric ulcer on the lesser curvature (left gastric artery). Perforation into the abdominal cavity usually presents as sudden onset of pain with peritonitis; irritation of the diaphragm may have referred pain to the shoulder via the phrenic nerve. A chest x-ray or kidney, ureter, and bladder (KUB) x-ray will usually demonstrate free air under the diaphragm. Gastric outlet obstruction can rarely result from chronic ulcers and typically presents with persistent vomiting and weight loss.

While duodenal ulcers are generally benign, gastric ulcers should be biopsied during upper endoscopy to rule out gastric adenocarcinoma (intestinal type). Benign ulcers are small with a sharp punched-out appearance, while malignant ulcers tend to appear large with heaped up margins. Chronic gastritis, *H. pylori*, and dietary nitrosamines (found in smoked foods) predispose to development of the intestinal type of gastric adenocarcinoma. Intestinal-type gastric adenocarcinoma is associated with metastases to the left supraclavicular node (Virchow node) and the periumbilical region (Sister Mary Joseph nodule).

Note 1: Gastric adenocarcinoma can be intestinal type (discussed previously) or diffuse type. Diffuse type is characterized by signet ring cells and desmoplasia, which results in thickening of stomach walls (linitis plastica). It metastasizes to Virchow node and bilateral ovaries (Krukenberg tumor).

Note 2: Pancreatic adenocarcinoma also metastasizes to Virchow (signal, sentinel) node, located in the left supraclavicular fossa.

CASE 6.3 CONTINUED:

Laboratory evaluation reveals a hemoglobin level of 10 g/dL. An upper endoscopy reveals a well-demarcated, clean-based ulcer in the proximal duodenum, as shown in Fig. 6.7.

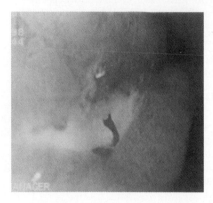

Figure 6.7. Gastric ulcer *(white base)* with bleeding vessel. *(From Goldman L, Ausiello D. Cecil Textbook of Medicine. 22nd ed. Philadelphia: WB Saunders: 2004.)*

6. What are the potential etiologies of duodenal and gastric ulcers?
   Duodenal ulcers (more likely than gastric ulcers) are due to *H. pylori* 90% of the time. They can also be due to Zollinger-Ellison syndrome (ZES), which is a non-β islet cell tumor of the pancreas that secretes gastrin.

   Gastric ulcers are due to *H. pylori* 80% of the time. They can also be due to NSAID use.

   The differential diagnosis for ulcers is malignancy. While duodenal ulcers are almost never malignant, gastric ulcers can be caused by adenocarcinoma.

7. How can the urea breath test be used to determine the etiology of this patient's ulcer?
   H. pylori is a bacterium that causes duodenal and stomach ulcers. It produces the enzyme urease, which breaks down urea to liberate carbon dioxide and ammonia. The ammonia allows *H. pylori* to alkalinize its local environment; this is important for survival of the organism in the acidic stomach. *H. pylori* can be detected by having a patient ingest [13]C- or ^{14}C-labeled urea; if the patient has *H. pylori*, their breath will contain radiolabeled CO_2 from the breakdown of ingested urea. *H. pylori* infection can also be detected by serum antibodies to this organism, but this test does not discriminate between current and previous infection unless immunoglobulin M (IgM) is specifically requested. It is also possible to look for *H. pylori* antigen in the stool.

8. During endoscopy, if multiple duodenal ulcers had been found in our patient, what disease should be suspected and what test should be performed?
   Whenever there are multiple peptic ulcers, they are refractory to aggressive therapy, or the ulcers are located in abnormal positions such as the jejunum, ZES should be suspected. The increased gastrin secretion by these tumors causes excessive secretion of acid. A markedly elevated gastrin level, usually with levels greater than 1000 pg/mL (fasting levels <150 pg/mL), is indicative of ZES. The secretin test will also show a paradoxical increase in gastrin.

Clinical Pearl

Recall that patients on proton pump inhibitors (PPIs) may also have substantially elevated gastrin levels, so it may be difficult to immediately differentiate between a patient on a PPI and one with Zollinger-Ellison syndrome (ZES). For this reason, when testing for gastrin levels, the patient should be off PPIs for at least 1 week before a blood draw.

CASE 6.3 CONTINUED:

The patient's urea breath test is positive, and he is therefore prescribed "triple therapy."

9. Why was our patient prescribed triple therapy?

The patient has an *H. pylori* infection that needs to be eradicated to reduce the rate of recurrence of peptic ulcer and the risk of developing gastric adenocarcinoma. Triple therapy typically includes two antibiotics (often clarithromycin and amoxicillin) and a PPI. Because of increasing global resistance to clarithromycin, patients living in high-resistance areas may be treated with "quadruple therapy," which features bismuth, metronidazole, tetracycline, and a PPI.

CASE 6.3 CONTINUED:

At his 4-week follow-up, the patient denies any abdominal symptoms but does comment that he has noticed fatty enlargement of his breasts. He reports that in addition to the medications prescribed, he has been taking over-the-counter cimetidine.

10. What is the most likely cause of his gynecomastia?

One of the distinctive side effects of cimetidine (H_2 receptor antagonist) is gynecomastia, along with prolactin release, impotence, and decreased libido in men. Another noteworthy fact about cimetidine is that it inhibits one of the hepatic cytochrome P-450 enzymes, which makes it particularly dangerous when given with warfarin because warfarin is metabolized through this pathway. Thus patients on cimetidine and warfarin may have elevated prothrombin times (PTs).

STEP 1 SECRET

Know which drugs upregulate and downregulate the hepatic cytochrome P-450 enzymes. These drugs have been known to show up on many USMLE forms (Table 6.5).

Table 6.5. Cytochrome P-450 Inhibitors and Inducers

INHIBITORS	INDUCERS
Cimetidine	Barbiturates
Macrolides	Quinidine
Azole antifungals	Rifampin
Isoniazid	Phenytoin
Sulfonamides	Griseofulvin
Grapefruit juice	Carbamazepine
Protease inhibitors	St. John's wort
Ciprofloxacin	Chronic alcohol use

11. What alternative pharmacologic treatment strategies exist for patients with peptic ulcer disease?
   1. PPIs, such as omeprazole, lansoprazole, and pantoprazole
   2. Other H_2 receptor antagonists, such as ranitidine, famotidine, and nizatidine (these are less effective than PPIs)
   3. Anticholinergics, such as atropine (inhibits HCl secretion)
   4. Mucosal protective agents, such as misoprostol (PGE1 analog) and bismuth/sucralfate (binds to base of ulcer to provide physical protection)
   5. Antacids, such as calcium carbonate, magnesium hydroxide, and aluminum hydroxide

---

Pharmacology Pearl

Magnesium causes diarrhea, whereas aluminum causes constipation, so these two compounds are often mixed together in antacid formulations to balance these effects.

SUMMARY BOX: PEPTIC ULCER DISEASE

- Peptic ulcer disease (PUD) classically presents with pain after eating (gastric ulcers) or pain relieved by meals (duodenal ulcers).
- Diagnosis is made based on symptoms, history of nonsteroidal anti-inflammatory drug (NSAID) use, upper endoscopy, and barium swallow. Use the urea breath test, IgM serum antibody, or stool antigen test to diagnose current *Helicobacter pylori* infection.

SUMMARY BOX: PEPTIC ULCER DISEASE—cont'd

- PUD is mainly caused by *H. pylori* and NSAIDs. Gastric ulcers may also be due to malignancy, so they should be biopsied. Think Zollinger-Ellison syndrome with markedly elevated gastrin levels, multiple ulcers, ulcers refractory to therapy, or ulcers in unusual locations (ileum and jejunum).
- Hemorrhage and perforation are major complications of PUD. Melena indicates a upper gastrointestinal bleed (UGIB). Hematochezia indicates a lower GI bleed (LGIB) or a brisk UGIB.
- Treatment of PUD involves treating the underlying cause. If *H. pylori* is the cause, give the patient triple therapy of a proton pump inhibitor (PPI) and two antibiotics. If the patient is on NSAIDs, stop them and give the patient a PPI (generally preferred), misoprostol, or a H_2 receptor antagonists to reduce GI side effects. For antiinflammatory effects, selective cyclooxygenase-2 (COX-2) inhibitors reduce GI side effects but have cardiovascular risks.
- The H_2 receptor antagonist cimetidine inhibits P-450 (contraindicated with warfarin) and causes gynecomastia.

CASE 6.4

A 42-year-old obese woman presents with a history of epigastric pain that has worsened in the past week and is exacerbated by food. She has lost 20 lb over the past 2 months and has felt a little feverish in the past week. She has also been bothered by nausea and vomiting.

1. What is the differential diagnosis for postprandial epigastric pain?

   The differential diagnosis for postprandial epigastric pain in the presence of nausea and vomiting includes gallstone disease, GERD, PUD, pancreatitis, acute gastritis, and functional dyspepsia. Gallstone disease, including biliary colic and acute cholecystitis, is the leading diagnosis because the patient has several risk factors: obesity, middle age, female sex, and recent weight loss (which may have been lost due to fasting, which is another risk factor), which predispose her to gallstone formation. Also, pain associated with biliary colic is exacerbated by eating (classically associated with fatty foods). GERD, PUD (particularly gastric ulcers), and acute gastritis are also all typically exacerbated by food. Functional dyspepsia (especially postprandial pain syndrome) can cause pain, nausea, and vomiting after meals but would not be associated with fever or weight loss.

CASE 6.4 CONTINUED:

Upon further questioning, the patient clarifies that she is not eating because of the pain food causes rather than because of a lack of appetite. She also admits to drinking six alcoholic drinks per day and taking ibuprofen regularly for lower back pain.

2. How does this information alter the differential diagnosis?

   Now, gastric ulcers, acute gastritis, and acute pancreatitis are the most likely diagnoses. Gastric ulcers are related to NSAID use and are associated with weight loss, but alcohol does not usually play a significant role in their pathogenesis. NSAIDs and alcohol are major risk factors for acute gastritis, and the pain from food usually leads to anorexia and weight loss. Acute pancreatitis as a result of alcohol use or gallstones is another concern.

CASE 6.4 CONTINUED:

Physical examination reveals mild epigastric tenderness. Serum lipase is within normal limits. A urease breath test is negative. Endoscopy is positive for punctate erosions in the antrum (Fig. 6.8), and a tissue biopsy reveals diffuse inflammation of the gastric mucosa with no evidence of malignancy.

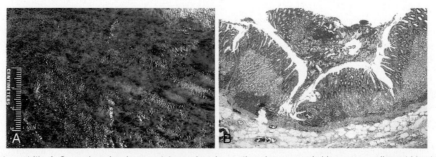

Figure 6.8. Acute gastritis. A, Gross view showing punctate erosions in an otherwise unremarkable mucosa; adherent blood is dark because of exposure to gastric acid. B, Low-power microscopic view of focal mucosal disruption with hemorrhage; the adjacent mucosa is normal. *(From Kumar V, Abbas AK, Fausto N. Robbins and Cotran Pathologic Basis of Disease. 7th ed. Philadelphia: WB Saunders; 2005.)*

3. Based on these findings, the diagnosis of acute gastritis is confirmed. What are the two primary classifications of this disease?

Acute gastritis can be divided into infectious and noninfectious gastritis. Noninfectious gastritis (as in this case) is caused by exposure to toxins and drugs (e.g., ethanol, NSAIDs) and severe physiologic stress (e.g., burns, head trauma, surgery). Infectious gastritis is typically caused by *H. pylori*.

CASE 6.4 CONTINUED:

You counsel the patient about cutting back on alcohol and stopping NSAIDs, which the patient does, and her symptoms resolve within weeks. Years later, the patient brings her 68-year-old mother to you because she thinks you are "the greatest doctor in the world" after solving her "belly" problem. The patient's mother has been experiencing fatigue, memory difficulties, and numbness and tingling in her feet for the past 6 months.

4. What is the differential diagnosis for the mother's symptoms?

The differential diagnosis is broad but includes depression, dementia, vitamin B_{12} (cobalamin) deficiency, diabetic peripheral neuropathy, and alcoholic peripheral neuropathy. Depression could explain the memory difficulties, especially in the elderly (pseudodementia), and the fatigue. Dementia is consistent with memory difficulties. Vitamin B_{12} deficiency can cause memory difficulties and paresthesias, as this patient describes, and the anemia associated with vitamin B_{12} deficiency can explain the fatigue. Diabetic and alcoholic peripheral neuropathies can cause paresthesias in the extremities.

CASE 6.4 CONTINUED:

Physical examination is significant for epigastric tenderness and impaired vibratory sense and proprioception in the lower extremities. Her hemoglobin is 9.5 g/dL, and mean corpuscular volume (MCV) is 105 fL. A peripheral blood smear is shown in Fig. 6.9.

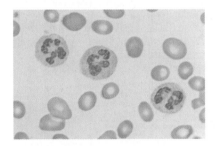

Figure 6.9. Peripheral blood smear for patient in Case 6.4. *(From Hoffman R, Benz EJ Jr, Shattil SJ, et al.* Hematology: Basic Principles and Practice. *4th ed. Philadelphia: Churchill Livingstone; 2005.)*

5. What most likely explains the macrocytic anemia in the peripheral blood smear shown in Fig. 6.9?

Vitamin B_{12} deficiency is the likely explanation. This woman has a macrocytic (MCV >100 fL), megaloblastic (peripheral smear showing hypersegmented neutrophils with >5 lobes) anemia. This could be caused by either vitamin B_{12} or folate deficiency. Given this woman's neurologic symptoms, vitamin B_{12} deficiency is most likely. Vitamin B_{12} is required for DNA synthesis in rapidly proliferating erythrocyte progenitor cells.

STEP 1 SECRET

Fig. 6.9 is a high-yield image for Step 1. Immediately associate hypersegmented neutrophils with folate and vitamin B_{12} deficiency. If neurologic findings are mentioned in the clinical vignette, vitamin B_{12} deficiency is likely.

CASE 6.4 CONTINUED:

A serum vitamin B_{12} (cobalamin) level is 120 pg/mL (normal ≥300 pg/mL).

6. What are the various causes of vitamin B_{12} deficiency?

Vitamin B_{12} deficiency is caused by either (1) a nutritional deficiency or (2) a malabsorption syndrome.

1. Dietary sources of vitamin B_{12} include red meat, fortified cereals, and dairy products. Nutritional deficiency can be seen in elderly patients with "tea and toast" diets and in patients with chronic alcohol abuse (secondary to nutritional deficiency).

2. Absorption of vitamin B_{12} depends on several proteins. In the saliva, vitamin B_{12} binds with R-binder and is transported to the duodenum; in the duodenum, pancreatic enzymes separate B_{12} from R-binder so that vitamin B_{12} can bind to intrinsic factor (IF; made by parietal cells of the stomach). Vitamin B_{12} bound to IF is absorbed in the terminal ileum. Malabsorption syndromes that cause vitamin B_{12} deficiency include pernicious anemia, celiac disease, bacterial overgrowth, infection with the tapeworm *Diphyllobothrium latum*, Crohn disease, and pancreatic insufficiency. Pernicious

anemia (type A chronic gastritis) is caused by immune-mediated destruction of parietal cells in the fundus and body of the stomach, which decreases the amount of IF (and HCL acid) produced. Through various mechanisms, celiac disease, bacterial overgrowth, and Crohn disease affect absorption at the terminal ileum. Pancreatic insufficiency results in a deficiency in pancreatic enzymes that normally separate vitamin B_{12} from R factor, which is important for allowing IF to bind vitamin B_{12}.

Note: Reserves of vitamin B_{12} are long-lasting (2–7 years) even with severe malabsorption.

7. **What test can help with diagnosing the cause of vitamin B_{12} deficiency?**
The Schilling test can help determine the cause of malabsorption in patients with vitamin B_{12} deficiency. The first stage of the Schilling test is to saturate all the blood and tissue vitamin B_{12} binding sites with an intramuscular injection of vitamin B_{12}. Radiolabeled vitamin B_{12} is then given orally. In the absence of vitamin B_{12} malabsorption, the vitamin B_{12}/IF complex would normally be absorbed in the terminal ileum and excreted in the urine because all tissue and blood vitamin B_{12} binding sites are saturated. If the level of urine radioactivity is low (suggesting that malabsorption is indeed present), then the second stage of the test is repeated with oral vitamin B_{12} plus IF, which specifically determines whether the patient has pernicious anemia (recall that because the parietal cells produce IF, supplementation with IF should increase vitamin B_{12} absorption in patients with pernicious anemia). If the urine radioactivity is still low after the second stage, then a third stage uses oral vitamin B_{12} plus either antibiotics or pancreatic enzymes to test for bacterial overgrowth or pancreatic insufficiency, respectively.

Note: Even though the Schilling test is now rarely used, you are still expected to understand the principles behind it for the USMLE.

CASE 6.4 CONTINUED:

The patient's Schilling test shows normal vitamin B_{12} absorption with the addition of IF, and the diagnosis of pernicious anemia is therefore made.

8. **What are the two primary classifications of chronic gastritis?**
Chronic gastritis is also subdivided into two types: type A (immune-mediated) and type B (infectious). Type A chronic gastritis is caused by immune-mediated destruction of parietal cells in the fundus and body of the stomach. Type B chronic gastritis is associated with *H. pylori* colonization of the gastric antrum. Type B chronic gastritis is more common than type A, accounting for approximately 80% of the cases of chronic gastritis. Type A causes pernicious anemia (as described previously) and achlorhydria (HCl deficiency), which can result in G cell hyperplasia from elevated gastrin levels and predispose to enteric infections, especially *Salmonella*. Both types of chronic gastritis are risk factors for the development of gastric adenocarcinoma.

SUMMARY BOX: ACUTE/CHRONIC GASTRITIS

- Patients with acute gastritis typically present with pain and a history of nonsteroidal antiinflammatory (NSAID) use, alcohol use, or recent burns (Curling ulcer). Chronic gastritis may or may not cause pain; if type A (immune mediated), patients have symptoms of anemia and B_{12} deficiency, and if type B (infectious *Helicobacter pylori*), patients will have increased risk of ulcers. Diagnosis is based on obtaining a detailed past medical history, upper endoscopy, and barium swallow and checking for autoantibodies against parietal cells (chronic type A) and checking for *H. pylori* (chronic type B).
- In acute gastritis, there is disruption of the mucosal barrier, leading to inflammation and pain.
- In chronic type A gastritis, destruction of parietal cells leads to decreased production of intrinsic factor (pernicious anemia) and hydrochloric acid (achlorhydria). Patients may develop vitamin B_{12} deficiency, which would present with neurologic symptoms and megaloblastic anemia with polysegmented neutrophils.
- The Schilling test can help distinguish among the various malabsorption syndromes causing vitamin B_{12} deficiency.

CASE 6.5

A 38-year-old man with a history of alcohol use disorder presents to the emergency department with sudden-onset, severe epigastric pain that radiates to his back. He also reports nausea and vomiting.

1. **What is the differential diagnosis for abdominal pain radiating to the back?**
The differential diagnosis includes acute pancreatitis, ruptured abdominal aortic aneurysm, perforated duodenal ulcer, biliary colic, and renal colic. In a middle-aged man with heavy alcohol use, acute pancreatitis is more likely.

CASE 6.5 CONTINUED:

Physical examination is significant for fever 38.3°C (101°F), tachycardia, blood pressure (BP) of 98/60 mm Hg, epigastric tenderness, and absent bowel sounds. Laboratory tests reveal elevated serum lipase, hypocalcemia, and a leukocytosis.

2. **What is the diagnosis? What are the causes of this disease?**

Acute pancreatitis characteristically presents with epigastric pain radiating to the back, elevated lipase and amylase, and leukocytosis. Although uncommon, acute pancreatitis may also be associated with hypocalcemia; this is because as the pancreas undergoes liquefactive necrosis, the surrounding fat undergoes fat necrosis, which involves fatty acid saponification of calcium salts. This process essentially chelates calcium, resulting in hypocalcemia.

Acute pancreatitis is caused by alcohol abuse and gallstones. Other, less common but well-established causes of acute pancreatitis include severe hypertriglyceridemia (typically >2000 mg/dL), marked hypercalcemia, abdominal trauma (that compresses the pancreas), medications, iatrogenic causes (e.g., following endoscopic retrograde cholangiopancreatography [ERCP]), and annular pancreas (developmental malformation in which the pancreas forms a ring around the proximal part of the duodenum). You may actually be expected to know that a scorpion bite is yet another cause of pancreatitis!

Patients with acute pancreatitis will almost always have elevated serum amylase and lipase (lipase is more specific).

3. **What is a potential complication of acute pancreatitis?**

Acute pancreatitis can lead to the formation of a fibrous pseudocyst that surrounds the pancreas; if this cyst ruptures, patients can experience hemorrhage, disseminated intravascular coagulation (DIC), acute respiratory distress syndrome (ARDS), and multiorgan failure.

4. **How can gallstones cause pancreatitis?**

Gallstones can pass into the lower common bile duct and obstruct the egress of bile into the intestine. The bile can then back up into the pancreatic duct, irritating and inflaming the pancreatic tissue. The pancreatic duct also cannot empty, so pancreatic secretions may build up and contribute to the inflammatory process.

Note: Patients with cystic fibrosis often develop chronic pancreatitis because thick pancreatic secretions can block the pancreatic duct.

CASE 6.5 CONTINUED:

The patient spends 4 days in the hospital and is discharged home feeling well. However, he continues to drink alcohol, and several years later, he is evaluated for a 2-month history of abdominal pain, diarrhea, and weight loss. An abdominal x-ray study is shown in Fig. 6.10.

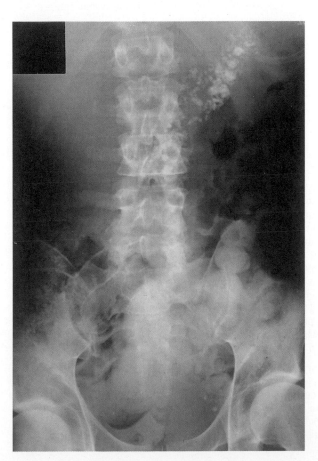

Figure 6.10. Calcification in pancreas. *(From Noble J.* Textbook of Primary Care Medicine. *3rd ed. St. Louis: Mosby; 2001.)*

5. **What is the likely diagnosis in this case, and what is the most common cause of this disease?**
The combination of chronic alcohol use, abdominal pain, diarrhea, weight loss, and pancreatic calcifications on an abdominal x-ray film is classic for chronic pancreatitis. Alcohol is the most common cause of chronic pancreatitis (gallstones are *not* a major cause, unlike for acute pancreatitis).
   Note: Patients with chronic pancreatitis will not always have elevated serum amylase and lipase because of a burned out pancreas; these are much more reliable for acute pancreatitis.
   Please note that an abdominal x-ray would never reasonably be ordered to evaluate suspected chronic pancreatitis. Its inclusion here is purely for teaching purposes.

6. **What are the primary complications of chronic pancreatitis?**
The sequelae of chronic pancreatitis include fat malabsorption, fat-soluble vitamin deficiency (vitamins A, D, E, and K), persistent diarrhea, and insulin-dependent diabetes mellitus. A lack of pancreatic lipase that helps fat digestion in the small intestine results in fat malabsorption and fat-soluble vitamin (A, D, E, and K) deficiency. These and other poorly absorbed nutrients are then available to be catabolized/fermented by the bacterial flora in the large intestine. The final products of this catabolism are typically osmotically active and draw water into the lumen of the intestine, leading to an osmotic diarrhea. Diabetes mellitus results from chronic inflammation, eventually destroying the β cells of the islets of Langerhans.

SUMMARY BOX: ACUTE/CHRONIC PANCREATITIS

- Acute pancreatitis classically presents as epigastric pain radiating to the back.
- Major causes of acute pancreatitis are gallstones, alcohol, trauma, hypercalcemia, hypertriglyceridemia, and scorpion stings. Mumps, immune-mediated diseases, and certain drugs can also increase the risk for acute pancreatitis.
- In acute pancreatitis, laboratory results will show elevated amylase and lipase (lipase has higher specificity) and leukocytosis.
- Pathophysiology involves backup of bile and pancreatic enzymes, leading to irritation and autodigestion of the pancreas. Complications of acute pancreatitis can be the formation of a pseudocyst that ruptures, leading to hemorrhage, disseminated intravascular coagulation (DIC), acute respiratory distress syndrome (ARDS), and multiorgan failure.
- Chronic pancreatitis is chronic inflammation of the pancreas, most commonly caused by alcohol abuse and also seen with cystic fibrosis. Diagnosis is more difficult to make because patients often do not have elevated serum amylase and lipase.
- Chronic pancreatitis can lead to persistent diarrhea; diabetes mellitus; fat malabsorption; steatorrhea; and vitamin A, D, E, and K deficiencies.

CASE 6.6

A 2-week-old boy is brought to the emergency department with nonbilious projectile vomiting that began earlier in the day. The prenatal course, birth, and postnatal course were unremarkable.

---

1. **What is the differential diagnosis for projectile vomiting in a newborn?**
The differential diagnosis includes infantile hypertrophic pyloric stenosis, tracheoesophageal fistula, esophageal atresia, duodenal atresia, annular pancreas, and gastroenteritis. The most likely diagnosis in this case is infantile hypertrophic pyloric stenosis, which usually presents with nonbilious projectile vomiting around 2 to 4 weeks of life. Tracheoesophageal fistula is an abnormal communication between the trachea and esophagus that usually presents with coughing and cyanosis during the first feeding. The fistula typically occurs at the midlevel of the esophagus, which is where the lungs bud off from the foregut during embryologic development. Esophageal atresia is another embryologic esophageal disorder in which the esophagus ends in a blind pouch, resulting in food accumulation and reflux into the airway, also causing coughing and cyanosis during the first feedings. Duodenal atresia typically presents with vomiting within the first day of life, and the vomitus tends to be bilious if the atresia occurs below where the common bile duct enters the second part of the duodenum. Finally, annular pancreas is caused by the ventral and dorsal pancreatic buds being abnormally fused around the second part of the duodenum, which can result in duodenal obstruction and projectile vomiting within the first few days of life.

2. **What acid-base and electrolyte disorder can be caused by prolonged vomiting in this baby, and how does it develop?**
Hypochloremic hypokalemic metabolic alkalosis can develop. Because gastric parietal cells secrete hydrochloric acid into the lumen of the stomach, prolonged vomiting can deplete the body of both hydrogen and chloride ions. The alkalosis that develops is caused by the loss of hydrochloric acid and the simultaneous retention of the bicarbonate that is generated when the parietal cells make hydrochloric acid.

CASE 6.6 CONTINUED:

Physical examination reveals a firm, palpable olive-like mass in the epigastric region, and ultrasound reveals a thickened and elongated pylorus muscle (Fig. 6.11).

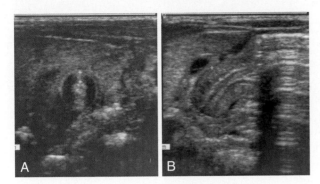

Figure 6.11. A, Transverse sonogram demonstrating a pyloric muscle wall thickness of greater than 4 mm *(distance between crosses)*. B, Horizontal image demonstrating a pyloric channel length greater than 14 mm *(wall thickness outlined between crosses)*. *(From Kliegman RM, Behrman RE, Jenson HB, et al. Nelson Textbook of Pediatrics. 18th ed. Philadelphia: WB Saunders; 2007.)*

3. What is the most likely diagnosis?
   Hypertrophic pyloric stenosis is the most likely diagnosis because of findings on physical examination and ultrasound.

STEP 1 SECRET

"Palpable olive-like mass" in the epigastric region is a popular buzzword for pyloric stenosis (although rarely appreciated in clinical practice). The mass is the result of muscular hypertrophy of the pyloric sphincter.

CASE 6.6 CONTINUED:

The infant undergoes surgical pyloromyotomy. One week later, the mother returns to the physician because the infant is experiencing severe diarrhea after being breastfed.

4. What is the most likely cause of the diarrhea?
   Dumping syndrome is caused by the delivery of excessive amounts of hyperosmotic chyme from the stomach to the small intestine, which may occur with a dysfunctional pyloric sphincter. The intestine is unable to process such a large quantity of chyme, resulting in an osmotic diarrhea, which may cause diarrhea, dizziness, weakness, and tachycardia following meals.
   Note: Dumping syndrome may also occur following gastric bypass surgery. Because the meal is delivered to the small intestine more quickly than usual, the increased tonicity of the small intestine causes a large fluid shift into the gut lumen. This increases the motility of the small intestine and results in diarrhea. In severe cases, the luminal shift of fluid stimulates blood flow to the intestine, which decreases total blood volume. Hypotension and reflex tachycardia can result.

SUMMARY BOX: HYPERTROPHIC PYLORIC STENOSIS

- Infantile hypertrophic pyloric stenosis typically presents in 2- to 4-week-old infants with nonbilious projectile vomiting; stenosis is not present at birth and takes time to develop.
- Diagnosis is based on physical examination and ultrasound.
- Prolonged vomiting may result in a hypochloremic hypokalemic metabolic acidosis resulting from vomiting of gastric acid and subsequent volume contraction leading to activation of the renin-angiotensin-aldosterone system (RAAS).
- Treatment is surgical pyloromyotomy.
- Dumping syndrome can result from a dysfunctional pyloric sphincter after surgical pyloromyotomy.
- Tracheoesophageal fistula presents with coughing and cyanosis with the first feeding.
- Duodenal atresia presents in the first day of life, demonstrates a "double-bubble" sign on radiographs (Fig. 6.12) and can cause bilious vomiting. It is associated with Down syndrome.

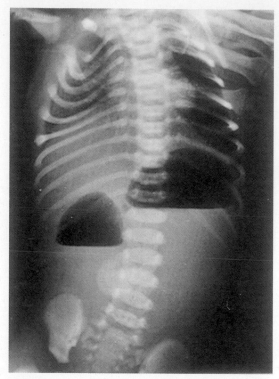

Figure 6.12. "Double bubble" in duodenal atresia. *(From McIntosh N, Helms PJ, Smyth RL, Logan S.* Forfar and Arneil's Textbook of Pediatrics. *7th ed. Philadelphia: Elsevier; 2008.)*

CASE 6.7

A 33-year-old woman reports a long-standing history of diarrhea, flatus, and abdominal pain. More recently, she has experienced unintentional weight loss despite a preserved appetite. She has never left the United States.

1. What is the differential diagnosis?
   The differential diagnosis includes inflammatory bowel disease (IBD), celiac disease, giardiasis, irritable bowel syndrome (IBS), Whipple disease, tropical sprue, disaccharidase (lactase) deficiency, and abetalipoproteinemia. From the history, IBD, giardiasis, and celiac disease are the most likely possibilities given the red flag feature of recent weight loss on a background of chronic diarrhea and abdominal pain. Weight loss does not typically occur in IBS and lactase deficiency. Whipple disease is unlikely because it typically occurs in older men and includes a migratory arthropathy. Tropical sprue is unlikely because the patient has not traveled outside of the United States. Abetalipoproteinemia is unlikely because it normally presents within the first few months of life.

CASE 6.7 CONTINUED:

Physical examination is unremarkable. Stool examination for ova and parasites is negative. A complete blood count (CBC) reveals microcytic anemia. A pathology report from a small intestinal biopsy (Fig. 6.13A) describes an intestinal mucosa significant for villous atrophy, lymphocytic infiltration of the lamina propria, and hyperplastic crypts. The woman is told she has a malabsorption syndrome and is put on a special diet devoid of wheat, barley, and rice. Six months later, a repeat biopsy shows complete resolution of mucosal damage to the small intestines (Fig. 6.13B), and she is encouraged to stay on her current diet.

2. What is the most likely diagnosis in this case?
   Celiac disease is caused by hypersensitivity to the gliadin in gluten, which is present in wheat, barley, rice, and many processed foods. Exposure to gliadin in a susceptible person causes gliadin to be presented by antigen-presenting cells on major histocompatibility complex (MHC) class II; thus, helper T cells are thought to mediate damage to the intestinal mucosa. Celiac disease is associated with the HLA-DQ2 and HLA-DQ8 alleles.

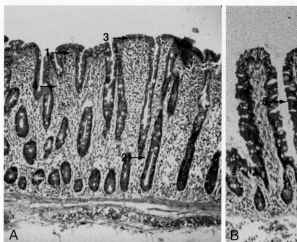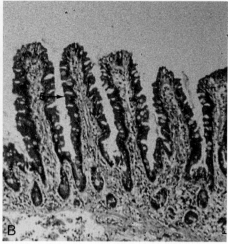

Figure 6.13. A, Duodenal biopsy specimen from patient in Case 6.7. The histologic features of severe villus atrophy *(arrow 1)*, crypt hyperplasia *(arrow 2)*, enterocyte disarray *(arrow 3)*, and intense inflammation of the lamina propria and epithelial cell layer *(arrow 4)* are evident. B, Repeat duodenal biopsy after 6 months on a strict gluten-free diet. There is marked improvement, with well-formed villi *(arrow 5)* and a return of the mucosal architecture toward normal. *(From Feldman M, Friedman LS, Brandt LJ. Sleisenger and Fordtran's Gastrointestinal and Liver Disease. 10th ed. Philadelphia: Elsevier; 2016.)*

Note: Patients with celiac disease may have small, herpes-like vesicles on the skin known as *dermatitis herpetiformis*.

3. **How is celiac disease diagnosed?**

   Screening for celiac disease is done by assessing for antibodies that are associated with the disease. The most sensitive and specific antibody is antitissue transglutaminase IgA. Of note, celiac disease is also associated with IgA deficiency, so a patient with celiac disease with IgA deficiency would have a false-negative anti-TTG antibody test; thus, anti-TTG should always be tested in conjunction with a total IgA level. Other celiac disease antibodies include antigliadin IgA and antiendomysial IgA. Definitive diagnosis requires endoscopy, which grossly features duodenal scalloping, and biopsy, which reveals blunted villi. Celiac disease (celiac sprue, nontropical sprue) is confirmed by resolution of mucosal damage following a gluten-free diet (Fig. 6.14).

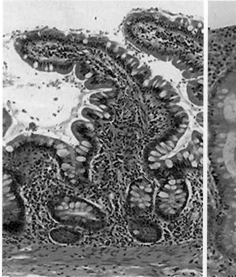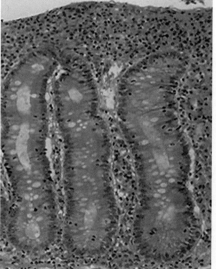

Figure 6.14. Celiac disease (sprue), microscopic. Compare normal small intestinal mucosa *(left panel)* and mucosa in celiac disease *(right panel)* with blunting and flattening of villi (in severe cases, loss of villi with flattening of the mucosa, as shown here), loss of crypts, increased mitotic activity, loss of the brush border, and infiltration with CD4 cells producing cytokines. *(From Klatt EC. Robbins and Cotran Atlas of Pathology. 3rd ed. Philadelphia: Elsevier; 2015, Fig. 7-84.)*

4. How is celiac disease associated with microcytic anemia in this patient?

Celiac disease typically affects the proximal small bowel (duodenum and jejunum) where iron and folate are absorbed. This can result in iron-deficiency (microcytic) anemia and a folate-deficiency (macrocytic) anemia. In this case, the iron malabsorption is greater than the folate, as is typically seen. Vitamin B_{12} malabsorption, which can also cause macrocytic anemia and neurologic symptoms, can occur with more severe celiac disease that affects the terminal ileum (although this is rare).

5. How do the signs, symptoms, and intestinal biopsy findings in Whipple disease differ from celiac disease?

Whipple disease is due to infection with *Tropheryma whipplei*. It typically occurs in men over the age of 40. The signs and symptoms are similar, but intestinal biopsy shows lipid vacuolation with infiltration of PAS (periodic acid–Schiff)-positive macrophages with small bacilli in Whipple disease. As mentioned previously, patients will often present with a migratory arthropathy affecting the larger joints.

6. With respect to etiology and symptomatology, how does celiac disease differ from tropical sprue?

Both these diseases have the same symptoms, but tropical sprue does not respond to a gluten-free diet. Intestinal biopsy findings are similar in both diseases, although tropical sprue affects the entire small intestine, and celiac disease mostly concentrates in the proximal small bowel. In addition, tropical sprue is most commonly found, as its name implies, in the tropics (e.g., Southeast Asia, Central and South America, Caribbean). Although an infectious organism is suspected, the precise etiology of tropical sprue remains unknown. Broad-spectrum antibiotics remain the treatment of choice for tropical sprue.

SUMMARY BOX: CELIAC DISEASE/DIARRHEA

- Celiac disease typically presents with abdominal pain, diarrhea, and flatus. Patients may also have dermatitis herpetiformis. Neurologic symptoms such as gluten ataxia may also be present.
- Screening for celiac disease includes the anti-TTG IgA antibody along with total IgA levels.
- Biopsy of the duodenum reveals flattened villi. Diagnosis is confirmed with resolution of symptoms and intestinal damage after a gluten-free diet.
- Celiac disease is caused by T-cell–mediated damage in response to gliadin in gluten; damage is predominantly in the duodenum.
- Celiac disease presents similarly to tropical sprue. However, tropical sprue is infectious in origin, it does not improve with cessation of gluten, and it tends to cause damage mostly in the jejunum and ileum.
- Celiac disease often causes an iron-deficiency anemia, although rarely it can cause folate- or vitamin B_{12}–deficient anemia (because iron is absorbed in the duodenum, while folate and vitamin B_{12} are absorbed in the jejunum and ileum).
- Whipple disease has a similar presentation to celiac disease, although it typically occurs in men older than 40, and intestinal biopsy shows characteristic intestinal mucosa infiltrated with PAS (periodic acid–Schiff)-positive macrophages.

CASE 6.8

A 32-year-old woman of Ashkenazi Jewish descent reports a long history of abdominal pain and diarrhea. On a typical day, she usually passes 15 to 20 loose stools. In the past few weeks, she has lost 15 lb and has experienced several episodes of bloody diarrhea. She denies pain with bowel movements (tenesmus) but does experience pain following meals.

1. What is the differential diagnosis?

The differential diagnosis includes IBD (Crohn disease and ulcerative colitis), infectious colitis (e.g., *Shigella*, *Campylobacter*, *Escherichia coli*, *Clostridioides difficile*), and mesenteric ischemia. Crohn disease and ulcerative colitis are both characterized by abdominal pain, frequent loose stools, bloody diarrhea, and weight loss. The diarrhea tends to be nonbloody in Crohn disease if the colon is not involved. Infectious colitis is likely if the patient has significant travel history (*Shigella*, *Campylobacter*, *E. coli*) or has taken antibiotics recently (*C. difficile*). Mesenteric ischemia is more common in adults older than 50 with atherosclerotic disease; pain is acute and usually occurs following a meal.

CASE 6.8 CONTINUED:

Physical examination is significant for mild fever as well as tenderness in the right lower quadrant (RLQ). Laboratory studies show an elevated erythrocyte sedimentation rate (ESR) as well as decreased plasma levels of vitamin B_{12}, vitamin D, and vitamin K. Colonoscopy reveals a "cobblestone" appearance of the mucosa and the presence of lesions in the terminal ileum and proximal colon. Biopsy of the terminal ileum reveals granulomas and transmural chronic inflammation.

2. What is the diagnosis?

Crohn disease is the diagnosis, which can be made based on the patient's history of bloody diarrhea and presence of classic pathologic features of the disease, such as a "cobblestone" appearance of the intestinal mucosa, absence of continuous lesions along the bowel (so-called *skip lesions*), granulomas, and transmural inflammation.

3. Compare and contrast the characteristics of Crohn disease and ulcerative colitis. Try testing yourself by covering the entries in the appropriate columns of Table 6.6 for each respective characteristic.

Table 6.6. Characteristics of Crohn Disease and Ulcerative Colitis

FEATURE	CROHN DISEASE	ULCERATIVE COLITIS
Associations	↑ Prevalence in Ashkenazi Jews (though most cases occur in non-Jews)	Patient who recently quit smoking
Location in gastrointestinal tract	Anywhere (most commonly terminal ileum), usually spares rectum, and has "skip" lesions; typically gives right lower quadrant (RLQ) pain	Begins in rectum, extends proximally upward, is limited to colon, and is continuous; typically gives left lower quadrant (LLQ) pain
Wall thickness involved	Transmural inflammation, "cobblestone" appearance of mucosa; granulomas; "string sign" on imaging because of thickening of bowel wall	Mucosal and submucosal inflammation only, friable pseudopolyps on gross appearance; crypt abscesses; "lead pipe" on imaging due to loss of haustra
Complications	Malabsorption, strictures, fistulas, abscess,↑ risk of colon cancer (if colonic involvement)	Toxic megacolon, hemorrhage, primary sclerosing cholangitis, ↑↑ risk of colon cancer
Dermatologic manifestations	Erythema nodosum and pyoderma gangrenosum	Pyoderma gangrenosum and erythema nodosum
Other nonintestinal manifestations	Migratory polyarthritis, aphthous ulcers, uveitis, perianal fistulas, ankylosing spondylitis, and calcium oxalate renal calculi (due to increased oxalate absorption)	Aphthous ulcers, uveitis, and ankylosing spondylitis

STEP 1 SECRET

Thoroughly learn the information provided in Table 6.6. The USMLE commonly asks students to differentiate between Crohn disease and ulcerative colitis.

4. In what special situation does transmural inflammation of the colon occur in ulcerative colitis?
Transmural inflammation of the colon occurs in toxic megacolon, which is a medical emergency. Surgery (usually a colectomy with ileoanal anastomosis) is required to prevent peritonitis and sepsis and restore some semblance of normal bowel activity. Toxic megacolon is associated with *C. difficile* infection, especially in ulcerative colitis.

5. What congenital disorder results in constipation and a severely dilated colon (similar to toxic megacolon)? What is the etiology of this disease?
Hirschsprung disease (congenital megacolon, aganglionic megacolon) is caused by failure of the neural crest cells that form the submucosal and myenteric plexuses to migrate to the colon (Fig. 6.15). The rectum is always involved because neural crest cells migrate caudally along the intestine. Newborns will have a failure to pass meconium and an empty rectal vault on digital exam. A rectal suction biopsy will show lack of ganglion cells (suction is used for this biopsy to ensure that the submucosal tissue is isolated). Hirschsprung disease is associated with Down syndrome. Treatment involves surgical resection of the aganglionic segment.

6. How can Crohn disease cause deficiencies of the fat-soluble vitamins?
Crohn disease commonly involves the terminal ileum, where vitamin B_{12} is absorbed and bile salts are reabsorbed. Damage to the terminal ileum decreases reabsorption of bile salts; if the liver is unable to produce enough new bile salts for proper fat absorption, the patient will have decreased absorption of fat and fat-soluble vitamins (A, D, E, and K). Surgical resection of the ileum can also cause these vitamin deficiencies.

7. Why might cholestyramine help with this patient's diarrhea?
Cholestyramine is a bile acid sequestrant that binds bile salts and makes them osmotically inactive. It was originally used to treat hypercholesterolemia (before statins) because it prevents reabsorption of bile salts. Patients with Crohn disease already have poor bile salt absorption, but cholestyramine can help with their diarrhea by preventing their bile salts from being osmotically active in the colon.
Note: Cholestyramine does decrease bile salt and thus fat and fat-soluble vitamin absorption.

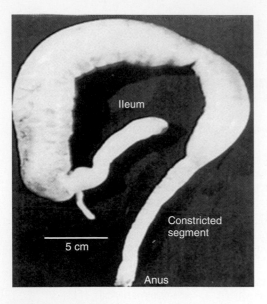

Figure 6.15. Colon from a 1-month-old infant with Hirschsprung disease. The characteristic megacolon appears proximal to a constricted terminal segment. Histologic evaluation found a normal appearing enteric nervous system in the megacolon and absence of enteric neurons in the constricted terminal segment. *(From Wood JD. Hirschsprung's disease (congenital megacolon). In: Johnson LR, ed.* Encyclopedia of Gastroenterology. *Elsevier: New York; 2004:388-391.)*

CASE 6.8 CONTINUED:

The patient is started on infliximab (an antitumor necrosis factor [TNF] α monoclonal antibody) for treatment of her active Crohn disease.

8. The patient asks about therapy with sulfasalazine, and her physician explains that this is used for ulcerative colitis but is controversial for Crohn disease. What pharmacokinetic properties of sulfasalazine make it particularly suited to treating ulcerative colitis?
   Sulfasalazine is a precursor of the active compound 5-aminosalicylic acid, a nonsteroidal antiinflammatory agent that can reduce inflammation in the bowel. However, if 5-aminosalicylic acid itself is given orally in sufficient quantities to reduce inflammation in the large bowel, significant gastric irritation will develop. Sulfasalazine avoids this problem because it is not broken down into 5-aminosalicylic acid until it reaches the distal ileum and colon. Sulfasalazine is also poorly absorbed from the GI tract, thus increasing the concentration of active drug that reaches the large bowel.

9. What extraintestinal complication of ulcerative colitis should be suspected in a patient who presents with signs of obstructive jaundice?
   Primary sclerosing cholangitis, which is caused by fibrosis of the large bile ducts, is a rare complication associated with both ulcerative colitis and Crohn disease. For the USMLE, associate primary sclerosing cholangitis with ulcerative colitis.

CASE 6.8 CONTINUED:

Several years later, the patient is seen by her physician for progressively worsening lower back pain. X-ray films of the pelvis and lumbar spine are shown in Fig. 6.16.

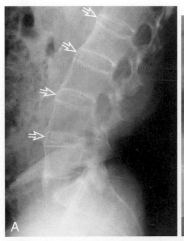
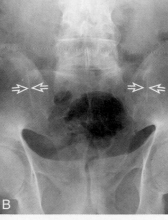

Figure 6.16. Ankylosing spondylitis. A, A lateral view of the lumbar spine demonstrates calcific bridging across the disk spaces *(arrows)*, causing the typical "bamboo spine" appearance. B, Anteroposterior view of the pelvis shows that the region of the sacroiliac joints *(arrows)* is not easily visualized owing to fusion of both sacroiliac joints. *(From Mettler FA.* Essentials of Radiology. *2nd ed. Philadelphia: WB Saunders; 2005.)*

10. **What extraintestinal complication of IBD should be suspected?**
    Ankylosing spondylitis, with the characteristic "bamboo spine" appearance and bilateral sacroiliitis, is more commonly associated with Crohn disease than with ulcerative colitis.

11. **Will a complete colectomy alleviate the extraintestinal complications of IBD?**
    No. The extraintestinal manifestations (i.e., arthritis, sclerosing cholangitis) often persist.

SUMMARY BOX: INFLAMMATORY BOWEL DISEASE

- Inflammatory bowel disease (IBD; Crohn disease and ulcerative colitis) typically presents with abdominal pain, bloody (or mucous) diarrhea, and unintentional weight loss.
- Crohn disease has a higher prevalence among Ashkenazi Jews. Ulcerative colitis might occur after a person *stops* smoking.
- IBD is diagnosed via endoscopy with biopsy and is postulated to be due to abnormal immune response to the gut microbiome.
- Crohn disease most commonly involves the terminal ileum but can affect any part of the gastrointestinal tract ("mouth to anus"); it is associated with "skip" lesions, transmural inflammation, and cobblestone appearance. Ulcerative colitis causes a continuous lesion that occurs only in the colon; it is associated with mucosal and submucosal inflammation (it is not transmural) and results in pseudopolyp formation.
- Treatment of IBD generally involves monoclonal antibodies (biologic agents).

CASE 6.9

A 13-year-old girl with a history of ovarian cysts is brought to the emergency department because of severe abdominal pain. She was awakened from sleep several hours earlier with pain that she states is now in the right lower abdomen. She also reports nausea and loss of appetite.

1. **What is the differential diagnosis?**
   The differential diagnosis includes acute appendicitis, ovarian torsion, ruptured ovarian cyst, ectopic pregnancy, pelvic inflammatory disease (PID), *Yersinia enterocolitis*, mesenteric adenitis, acute onset of IBD, Meckel diverticulitis, and right-sided diverticulitis. In this girl with a history of ovarian cysts, ruptured ovarian cysts or ovarian torsion is on the top of the differential. Acute appendicitis should also be considered in any person with right lower quadrant (RLQ) abdominal pain. Ectopic pregnancy would also warrant investigation with a pregnancy test. Right-sided diverticulitis would be unlikely in someone this young.

CASE 6.9 CONTINUED:

Physical examination is significant for a temperature of 37.9°C (100.2°F), and the patient's abdomen is tender to palpation at the McBurney point. Laboratory evaluation reveals a mild leukocytosis and a negative β-hCG (human chorionic gonadotropin). A pelvic ultrasound reveals a small ovarian cyst on the left ovary with adequate blood flow to both ovaries and no pelvic free fluid. A computed tomography (CT) scan reveals a thickened and inflamed appendix (Fig. 6.17).

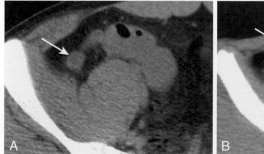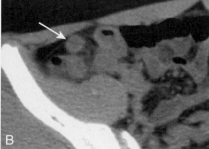

Figure 6.17. Two patients, with and without acute appendicitis. Axial noncontrast CT images in two different patients show a fluid-filled appendix of borderline size (*arrow*, A and B). Pathologic correlation shows a normal appendix in the patient seen in (A) and acute appendicitis in the patient in (B). *(From Brown MA. Imaging acute appendicitis. Semin Ultrasound CT MR. 2008;29:293-307.)*

2. **What is the diagnosis?**

Acute appendicitis is the diagnosis. Although the patient's initial presentation may be suggestive of ovarian torsion or a ruptured ovarian cyst, the physical examination findings and the CT scan confirm the diagnosis of acute appendicitis. Other physical examination findings indicative of appendicitis are positive psoas/obturator signs and positive Rovsing sign.

3. **What is the most common cause of appendicitis?**

Appendicitis is most often caused by obstruction of the lumen of the appendix, most commonly by a fecalith, but obstruction can also be due to lymphoid hyperplasia, tumors, or an intestinal stricture. Obstruction of the appendiceal lumen leads to bacterial overgrowth and acute inflammation. Polymorphonuclear cells (PMNs) are seen in the wall of the appendix.

4. **Note that Meckel diverticulitis can present similarly to appendicitis. What is its pathophysiology?**

Early in development, the midgut receives nutrients from the yolk sac via the vitelline duct. The duct should involute by around 7 weeks of development. When the duct only partially involutes, the remainder is the Meckel diverticulum.

About 50% of these diverticula are lined with heterotopic gastric or pancreatic tissue. The gastric mucosa can secrete acid, eventually creating adjacent intestinal ulcerations that can bleed and cause pain that mimics acute appendicitis. Alternatively, diverticula can lead to intussusception, incarceration, or perforation.

Note: Recall the law of the "three 2s" pertaining to Meckel diverticulum: it affects about 2% of the population, is about 2 inches long, and is located about 2 feet from the ileocecal valve.

CASE 6.9 CONTINUED:

The patient is taken to the operating room for a laparoscopic appendectomy and returns home the same day.

5. **What type of cancer of the appendix is occasionally seen as an incidental finding during an appendectomy? What substance do these tumors secrete, and what syndrome can it cause?**

Carcinoid tumors, which are neoplasms of neuroendocrine cells, can be an incidental finding during an appendectomy. They secrete large quantities of serotonin, resulting in elevated levels of the metabolite 5-hydroxyindoleacetic acid (5-HIAA), which can be easily detected. Intestinal carcinoid tumors can cause watery diarrhea but do not cause systemic symptoms until they metastasize to the liver because the liver contains monoamine oxidase (MAO) that degrades serotonin. After metastasis to the liver, patients develop carcinoid syndrome, which is a constellation of symptoms including episodic flushing, diarrhea, wheezing, and right-sided heart valve lesions (the lungs also contain MAO so patients do not develop left-sided heart problems).

Note: The appendix is the most common site of gut carcinoid tumors.

STEP 1 SECRET

Carcinoid syndrome is a favorite on boards. It usually presents after metastasis to the liver and is associated with the symptoms of wheezing, diarrhea, flushing, and right-sided heart murmurs that increase on inspiration.

6. **Although not described in the preceding case, pain from appendicitis classically begins around the umbilicus and then migrates to the RLQ. What is the neuroanatomic explanation for this pattern?**

The initial pain from appendicitis is due to activation of visceral pain receptors in the inflamed appendix and *visceral peritoneum*. The sensory nerves that carry this information synapse on spinal neurons that also receive sensory signals from the anterior abdominal wall in the periumbilical area. Because the origin of the signal cannot be discerned, the brain misinterprets the visceral pain as a poorly localized pain arising from the periumbilical area (T10 dermatome). Later, when the *parietal peritoneum* adjacent to the appendix becomes inflamed, the pain becomes sharper and is more accurately localized to the RLQ by somatic pain fibers. This exact position is referred to as the *McBurney point*, which is located two-thirds of the distance between the umbilicus and the anterior superior iliac spine. You should know this reference point for the USMLE *and* for your clinical years.

7. **What is the principal danger if appendicitis remains untreated?**

Perforation can occur, causing peritonitis (acute abdomen) and possibly abdominal abscess formation. Perforation may be detected by the presence of free air on an abdominal x-ray study or as air under the hemidiaphragm on a chest x-ray.

SUMMARY BOX: APPENDICITIS

- Appendicitis presents with periumbilical pain that later migrates to the right lower quadrant (RLQ). Patients are typically anorexic and may have nausea, vomiting, and a low-grade fever.
- Physical examination shows tenderness at the McBurney point, positive psoas/obturator signs, and positive Rovsing sign. Imaging (typically computed tomography [CT] scan) confirms diagnosis.
- Appendicitis is caused by obstruction from lymphoid hyperplasia or a fecalith that results in bacterial overgrowth and inflammation.
- Complications of appendicitis include perforation and abscess formation.
- Treatment is appendectomy.

CASE 6.10

A 50-year-old man visits the emergency department with a history of severe colicky abdominal pain, vomiting, and constipation. Past medical history is unremarkable with the exception of an appendectomy 6 years prior.

1. What is the differential diagnosis for this patient's condition?
   This presentation is classic for small bowel obstruction (SBO). General causes of bowel obstruction include surgical adhesions, hernia, tumor, volvulus, intussusception, Crohn disease, gallstone ileus, stricture, congenital malformation, and infectious enteritis.

2. What is the most likely cause of this patient's condition?
   Given this patient's past surgical history of appendectomy and otherwise unremarkable medical history, a surgical adhesion is the most likely cause of this patient's SBO. Adhesions are fibrous bands that form after injury during surgery. They connect organs and tissues that are otherwise not normally connected. Abdominal adhesions can result in small bowel obstruction if they tug on or kink the bowel and prevent the passage of bowel contents.

3. What would be expected on abdominal auscultation in this patient? How would you manage this patient?
   High-pitched, tinkling bowel sounds are generally heard in the early stages of an SBO, which eventually progress to absent bowel sounds, indicating a complete obstruction. Management involves IV fluid replacement, pain control, and decompression by placement of a nasogastric tube. Surgery may be needed if patient's SBO does not resolve within 72 hours.

STEP 1 SECRET

You may be given a multimedia question with a finding of tinkling bowel sounds on abdominal examination. Associate this with small bowel obstruction (SBO), and use the medical history to prioritize your differential diagnosis.

SUMMARY BOX: SMALL BOWEL OBSTRUCTION

- Small bowel obstruction (SBO) presents with colicky abdominal pain, abdominal distention, constipation, and vomiting.
- Surgical adhesions are the most common cause of small bowel obstruction.
- Physical examination of a patient who presents with small bowel obstruction will reveal a high-pitched tinkling sound on auscultation of the abdomen or absent bowel sounds with a complete obstruction.

HEPATOLOGY

BASIC CONCEPTS

1. Review the anatomy of the hepatic lobule and portal triad. In what manner do blood and bile flow through a lobule?

   A central hepatic vein is located at the center of each hepatic lobule. Multiple portal triads (hepatic artery, portal venule, bile duct) surround this central vein. Hepatocytes are arranged in sheets of single-cell thickness and are surrounded by blood-filled sinusoids. Blood flows from the hepatic artery and portal vein toward the central vein through the sinusoids. Bile is formed by the hepatocytes and emptied into bile canaliculi in the lateral wall of the hepatocyte. The bile flows from here toward the bile ducts (Fig. 7.1).

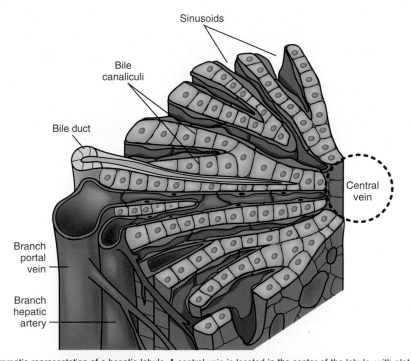

Figure 7.1. Diagrammatic representation of a hepatic lobule. A central vein is located in the center of the lobule, with plates of hepatocytes disposed radially. Branches of the portal vein and hepatic artery are located on the periphery of the lobule, and blood from both perfuses the sinusoids. Peripherally located bile ducts drain the bile canaliculi that run between the hepatocytes. *(From Bloom W, Fawcett DW. A Textbook of Histology. 10th ed. Philadelphia: WB Saunders; 1975.)*

Blood flows from the portal triad toward the central vein, and bile flows from the hepatocytes toward the portal triads. Knowing the structure of the hepatic lobule is clinically relevant. The hepatocytes located near the portal triad (zone 1) are closest to the oxygenated blood supply and are thus the first cells affected by toxins that reach the liver via the bloodstream (e.g., in the case of acetaminophen overdose). On the other hand, hepatocytes closest to the central vein (zone 3) are the farthest from the oxygenated blood supply of the lobule and are thus the first cells affected by ischemia.

2. **What is the chemical difference between conjugated and unconjugated bilirubin, and how are these substances formed?**
Bilirubin is a breakdown product of the heme moiety found in red blood cells (RBCs), bone marrow, liver, and mitochondrial cytochrome enzymes. Unconjugated bilirubin is bilirubin formed in the peripheral tissues. Given its hydrophobicity, it is poorly soluble and circulates in plasma bound to albumin. In the liver, unconjugated bilirubin is combined (conjugated) with glucuronic acid to form conjugated bilirubin, a much more soluble product.
Note: Jaundice is a yellowish discoloration of the skin, mucous membranes, and sclerae resulting from elevated levels of either conjugated or unconjugated bilirubin.

3. **Why is unconjugated bilirubin not normally excreted in the urine?**
Recall that unconjugated bilirubin is hydrophobic and circulates in the bloodstream bound to albumin. Albumin, a negatively charged protein, cannot cross a healthy glomerular basement membrane because the glycosaminoglycans that form this membrane are negatively charged and repel the albumin.

4. **What are the main causes of jaundice, and how does each affect the type of hyperbilirubinemia observed?**
See Table 7.1 for the causes of jaundice and the characteristics of each.

STEP 1 SECRET

You should be able to differentiate between the causes and presentations of conjugated and unconjugated hyperbilirubine-mias shown in Table 7.1. This is a commonly tested principle on the USMLE. For those of you who do not fully understand the details of Table 7.1, we have provided our handy approach to reasoning through the causes of jaundice.

Table 7.1 Causes of Jaundice

JAUNDICE TYPE	TYPE OF HYPERBILIRUBINEMIA	URINE (CONJUGATED BILIRUBIN)	UROBILINOGEN FORMATION	URINE AND STOOL COLOR
Hemolytic	Unconjugated (<20% conjugated bilirubin)	↑	↑	Normal
Hepatocellular	Conjugated/unconjugated (20%–50% conjugated bilirubin)	↑	↓	Normal
Obstructive	Conjugated	↑	↓	Normal urine, clay-colored feces

SECRET TO DIAGNOSING COMMON CAUSES OF JAUNDICE

In order to understand jaundice, you must first understand the pathway of bilirubin formation and excretion. RBC breakdown leads to the formation of unconjugated bilirubin, which is bound to albumin in the bloodstream. This unconjugated bilirubin (also known as *indirect bilirubin*) is water insoluble (therefore, it cannot be excreted into urine). The unconjugated bilirubin is then taken up by the liver and conjugated to glucuronic acid by the enzyme uridine diphosphate (UDP) glucuronyl transferase. This forms a water-soluble product called *conjugated bilirubin* (also known as *direct bilirubin*). Conjugated bilirubin is then excreted into the bile, which is formed in the liver. Bile itself is composed of bile salts, bilirubin, phospholipids, cholesterol, electrolytes, and water. It is stored in the gallbladder, where it is concentrated. When bile is secreted into the gut lumen, the conjugated bilirubin in the bile is deconjugated by bacterial flora into urobilinogen. Urobilinogen has three possible fates: (1) it is excreted into feces, where it gives stool its characteristic brown color; (2) it returns to the liver via the enterohepatic (portal) circulation; or (3) it is reabsorbed via the systemic circulation and excreted by the kidney, giving urine its characteristic yellowish color.

Now that you have the background on bilirubin formation and excretion, we can begin to explore the causes of jaundice. Jaundice refers to the pathologic yellowing of the skin and eyes (scleral icterus), which results from an increase in bilirubin in the blood. Jaundice may be the result of any abnormality along the aforementioned pathway. It can therefore occur as a result of (1) excessive bilirubin production, (2) decreased hepatic uptake or conjugation of unconjugated bilirubin, (3) decreased hepatocellular secretion of bilirubin into bile, and/or (4) impaired or obstructed bile flow. If this makes sense to you, it becomes formulaic to tease apart the various causes of jaundice. All you have to do is match the various causes of jaundice listed in Table 7.1 to these basic mechanisms.

Let us start with item 1 on our list: increased bilirubin production. The most notable cause of increased bilirubin production is hemolytic jaundice, which leads to an unconjugated hyperbilirubinemia. Why does this occur? Hemolysis refers to the accelerated breakdown of RBCs, which rapidly increases unconjugated bilirubin levels in the bloodstream. The liver, which must uptake and conjugate all of this bilirubin, has trouble keeping up with the rapid rate of bilirubin production. As a result, indirect bilirubin levels increase in the bloodstream. Do not confuse this with hepatocellular jaundice. The liver, in this case, is perfectly functional! It can uptake and conjugate bilirubin, but it cannot do so at the required pace. In fact, absolute amounts of conjugated bilirubin and urobilinogen increase above normal because of the increased production and conjugation of unconjugated bilirubin. The bilirubin that is conjugated is responsible for maintaining urobilinogen concentrations in urine and feces. Thus both are normally colored.

Decreased hepatic uptake and conjugation of bilirubin (items 2 and 3 in our list) are additional causes of jaundice. Consider a scenario in which the liver does not function normally, such as in viral hepatitis. This leads to hepatocellular jaundice because the "sick" liver is unable to perform its normal task of conjugating bilirubin. Some bilirubin will be conjugated (thus maintaining the normal color of urine and feces), but unconjugated bilirubin levels will also increase above normal. Note that conjugated bilirubin in the liver also leaks out into the bloodstream through the damaged hepatic tissue. It is *never* normal to see elevated bilirubin (whether unconjugated or conjugated) in the bloodstream. If this finding appears on laboratory tests, it is a red flag for disease.

The final cause of jaundice mentioned in Table 7.1 is obstructive jaundice. Obstructive jaundice occurs when conjugated bilirubin is unable to be excreted into the gut either because of impaired liver secretion of bile (see item 3) or impaired bile flow (see item 4). The most common cause of obstructive jaundice is bile duct obstruction (e.g., gallstones, pancreatic tumor). In obstructive jaundice, bile backs up into the liver, causing engorgement and rupture of intrahepatic ducts. This leads to spillage of conjugated bilirubin into sinusoidal blood and, ultimately, the systemic circulation. Thus conjugated and unconjugated bilirubin levels become elevated while urobilinogen levels decrease as a result of inadequate concentrations of conjugated bilirubin in the gut lumen. Urine color remains normal (conjugated bilirubin in the systemic circulation is water soluble and can be excreted by the kidneys), but stool becomes clay-colored because of the lack of urobilinogen excretion into feces.

Now that you have a better understanding of the causes of jaundice, revisit Table 7.1 and attempt to fill it in on your own.

1. **Which veins feed into the portal vein?**
Venous return from the foregut, midgut, and hindgut feeds into the portal vein from the gastric veins, splenic vein, and superior and inferior mesenteric veins. Consequently, portal hypertension can cause venous congestion in any and all of these vascular beds (e.g., congestive splenomegaly from splenic vein, esophageal varices from gastric veins).

2. **What are the signs and symptoms of portal hypertension?**
Portal hypertension leads to increased resistance to flow in the systemic venous system. As a result, blood cannot pass freely from the portal system to the systemic system and backs up into the portacaval anastomoses, which causes them to become engorged, dilated, or varicose. The location of these anastomoses determines the specific effects that result from portal hypertension. These symptoms and signs are listed in Table 7.2. Clinical findings of portal hypertension include ascites (secondary to increased hydrostatic pressure in the venous system), esophageal varices, hepatorenal syndrome, and splenomegaly (due to decreased drainage of venous blood from the spleen). Splenomegaly can result in anemia, thrombocytopenia, or pancytopenia as a result of cellular sequestration within the engorged spleen. Spontaneous bacterial peritonitis (note that ascitic fluid is a perfect culture medium for bacteria) is a significant and dangerous consequence of portal hypertension.

Table 7.2 Portal Hypertension: Anastomoses and Related Signs	
PORTACAVAL ANASTOMOSIS	**CLINICAL SIGN**
Left gastric vein with esophageal vein (branch of azygos vein)	Esophageal varices (leading to heavy bleeding/hematemesis)
Paraumbilical vein with epigastric vessels	Caput medusae
Superior rectal vein with middle and inferior rectal veins	Internal hemorrhoids (unlike external hemorrhoids, these are not painful because the visceral nerves that are above the dentate line sense pressure and not pain)

Note: Portal hypertension results from prehepatic, intrahepatic, and posthepatic causes. Cirrhosis is a common cause of intrahepatic portal hypertension, while portal vein thrombosis is a prehepatic cause. Right-sided heart failure and Budd-Chiari syndrome (see next question) are common precursors of posthepatic portal hypertension.

3. **How does Budd-Chiari syndrome arise, and what are its consequences?**
   Budd-Chiari syndrome occurs when the hepatic venous outflow becomes obstructed, usually because of thrombosis of the inferior vena cava. Polycythemia vera, pregnancy, and clotting disorders predispose to thrombus formation and can lead to hepatic venous outflow obstruction. The obstruction may result in portal hypertension with a classic presentation of abdominal pain, ascites, and hepatomegaly. Although this may be confused with right-sided heart failure, Budd-Chiari syndrome does *not* cause jugular venous distention because it affects only the inferior vena cava.

4. **What are the common liver biochemical tests, and what do they indicate?**
   See Table 7.3.

Table 7.3 Common Liver Biochemical Tests

ENTITY MEASURED	LAB TEST	SIGNIFICANCE OF TEST
Measure of synthetic liver function	Prothrombin time (PT)	Clotting factors are manufactured by hepatocytes. PT is not typically prolonged until severe liver damage occurs.
	Serum albumin	Albumin is manufactured by hepatocytes. Severe liver damage can result in a decrease in serum albumin.
Measure of liver damage/injury	Aspartate transaminase (AST) Alanine transaminase (ALT)	Damage to hepatocytes causes leakage of aminotransferases, causing elevation of serum AST/ALT. ALT is usually more elevated than AST in viral infections, whereas AST is usually twice as great as ALT in patients with liver damage secondary to alcohol abuse.
Measure of liver and biliary tree damage/injury	Alkaline phosphatase (ALP)	Elevated with damage to the bile duct and liver. Produced in the liver, bile duct, bone, kidney, and placenta; relatively nonspecific for liver injury.
	γ-Glutamyl transferase (GGT)	Elevated with damage to bile duct/liver; more specific marker than ALP. May also be elevated secondary to alcohol abuse (marker of mitochondrial damage).
Measure of function clearance of the liver	Bilirubin	Elevated unconjugated and conjugated bilirubin can result from hepatocyte damage because of the decreased ability of the liver to conjugate bilirubin and congestion of the canaliculi, obstructing movement of bilirubin into the gut lumen.

CASE 7.1

You are working in the emergency department when a man presents at 5 a.m. vomiting blood (hematemesis). At first glance, you can see that his mental status is impaired, his skin is jaundiced, and he has scleral icterus. Because you recognize him as the man you frequently see drinking from a brown paper bag in the park, you think you know why he is here.

1. **What is the most common cause of upper gastrointestinal bleeding?**
   Ulcers or erosions commonly cause upper gastrointestinal (GI) bleeding. These can occur in the stomach, duodenum, or esophagus (rarely) and develop when acid secretion overruns protective factors (mucous and bicarbonate secretion). Infection with *Helicobacter pylori*, use of nonsteroidal antiinflammatory drugs (NSAIDs), and cigarette smoking all disrupt the protective factors. In other cases, there is hypersecretion of gastric acid, such as that seen in Zollinger-Ellison

syndrome (gastrinoma). Other causes of upper GI bleeding include Mallory-Weiss tear, a perforated esophagus (Boerhaave syndrome), and ruptured esophageal or gastric varices.

2. **Why should a Mallory-Weiss tear be included in the differential diagnosis?**
   Mallory-Weiss tears are mucosal lacerations that extend through the gastroesophageal junction caused by excessive vomiting. Mallory-Weiss tears are another common cause of hematemesis in people with conditions causing excessive vomiting (e.g., heavy alcohol use, bulimia). However, they do not typically cause massive hematemesis, as seen with ruptured esophageal varices, and will usually heal without surgical intervention.

3. **What is scleral icterus?**
   Scleral icterus is yellow discoloration (icterus) seen in the "whites of the eye" (sclerae), an indication of increased bilirubin in the serum. The sclerae are often the first places that jaundice is observed on physical examination. Jaundice usually indicates hepatic or cholestatic pathology, but it may also indicate bleeding or hemolysis.
   Note: Vitamin A toxicity can cause yellow discoloration of the skin, but this is distinct from the scleral icterus observed with jaundice.

4. **To confirm your suspicion about severe liver disease in this patient, what physical examination findings might you expect and why?**
   1. Gynecomastia and testicular atrophy
      - Results from impaired ability of the damaged liver to metabolize estrogen, leading to hyperestrogenism
   2. Spider angiomata and palmar erythema
      - Results from impaired ability of the damaged liver to metabolize estrogen, as estrogen weakens the vascular walls
   3. Asterixis
      - Results (in part) from impaired ability of the damaged liver to metabolize ammonia into urea in the urea cycle. Excess ammonia can cause a flapping tremor when the wrist is extended (asterixis), a potential sign of hepatic encephalopathy.
   4. Enlarged liver
      - May be palpated with alcoholic hepatitis, but once cirrhosis develops, the liver will become firm and shrunken
   5. Signs of portal hypertension
      - Ascites results from increased portal pressure and subsequent engorgement of the splanchnic vasculature. Increased hydrostatic pressure within these vessels causes fluid to leak from the vasculature into the interstitium. Additionally, decreased production of albumin causes a decreased oncotic pressure within the vasculature, promoting fluid movement from the vasculature into the interstitium.
      - Hemorrhoids may result from a portacaval anastomosis between the superior rectal vein and the inferior rectal vein (see Table 7.2).
      - Caput medusae (engorged veins radiating from the umbilicus) can result from blood being diverted from the portal vein into the periumbilical veins that run along the round ligament of the liver to the anterior abdominal wall (see Table 7.2).
      - Splenomegaly results from a congested splenic vein that cannot effectively drain blood from the spleen.

CASE 7.1 CONTINUED:

On physical examination, you do indeed find spider angiomata on his face and thorax, gynecomastia, and periumbilical caput medusae. His abdomen is distended, his spleen is enlarged, he has pedal and periorbital edema, and his breath has a sweet, feculent odor.

5. **What is the pathophysiology of his ascites, pedal edema, and periorbital edema?**
   In severe liver disease, there is inadequate production of albumin, the major determinant of plasma oncotic pressure. Consequently, fluid reabsorption from the interstitium back into the capillary beds is reduced. This explains his pedal and periorbital edema. In addition to the reduced capillary oncotic pressure, the increased venous pressure in the portal system from portal hypertension causes greater intracapillary hydrostatic pressure, which opposes movement of fluid from the interstitium into the capillaries and results in ascites.

6. **What is the pathogenesis of the suspected cause of hematemesis in this patient?**
   The pathogenesis is ruptured esophageal varices (see Table 7.2). This patient has portal hypertension secondary to alcohol-induced cirrhosis. This creates portacaval anastomoses, in which the pressure in the portal venous system diverts blood from the portal system into the systemic circulation at sites where there are anastomoses. In this patient's case, blood from the gastric veins backed up into his esophageal tributaries, which became distended and eventually ruptured (Fig. 7.2).
   Note: The round ligament of the liver (ligamentum teres hepatica) is an embryologic remnant of the umbilical vein. The major morphologic characteristics of cirrhosis are extensive fibrosis with nodules of regenerating hepatocytes.

7. **How might you explain this patient's breath odor?**
   This sign of advanced liver failure may be due to the presence of aromatic toxins (e.g., ammonia) in the blood (recall the impairment in the urea cycle previously discussed). As a result of portal hypertension, there can be shunting of blood away from the liver (portosystemic shunting) toward the lungs. This creates a musty breath called *fetor hepaticus* (i.e., "breath of the dead").

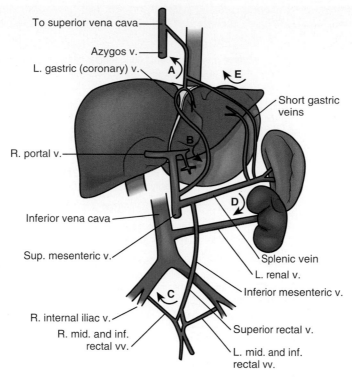

To superior vena cava

Azygos v.

L. gastric (coronary) v.

A

E

Short gastric veins

R. portal v.

B

Inferior vena cava

Sup. mesenteric v.

Splenic vein

L. renal v.

Inferior mesenteric v.

D

R. internal iliac v.

R. mid. and inf. rectal vv.

C

Superior rectal v.

L. mid. and inf. rectal vv.

Figure 7.2. Diagram of the portal circulation. The most important sites for the potential development of portosystemic collaterals are shown. A, Esophageal submucosal veins, which are supplied by the left gastric vein and drain into the superior vena cava via the azygous vein. B, Paraumbilical veins, which are supplied by the umbilical portion of the left portal vein and drain into abdominal wall veins near the umbilicus. These veins may form caput medusae at the umbilicus. C, Rectal submucosal veins, which are supplied by the inferior mesenteric vein through the superior rectal vein and drain into the internal iliac veins through the middle (*mid.*) and inferior (*inf.*) rectal veins. D, Splenorenal shunts, which are created spontaneously or surgically. E, Short gastric veins, which are supplied by the esophageal submucosal veins and drain into the splenic vein. *(From Feldman M, Friedman LS, Brandt LJ. Sleisenger & Fordtran's Gastrointestinal and Liver Disease. 8th ed. Philadelphia: WB Saunders; 2006.)*

CASE 7.1 CONTINUED:

When two large-bore intravenous (IV) lines are started to administer fluids, a fairly large hematoma develops at the IV site. Laboratory tests reveal an elevated conjugated bilirubin, unconjugated bilirubin, and prothrombin time (PT); low blood urea nitrogen (BUN); and a normal creatinine level. Serologic tests for hepatitis B and C, as well as antismooth muscle antibodies, are negative. Serum iron, transferrin, iron saturation (%), ferritin, and ceruloplasmin are all within normal limits.

8. What is the value of the following tests: hepatitis serology, iron studies, ceruloplasmin, and antimitochondrial antibodies?
   These tests all identify different causes of liver cirrhosis. Hepatitis B and C both can cause liver cirrhosis. Iron studies can test for hemochromatosis, ceruloplasmin tests for Wilson disease, and antismooth muscle antibodies test for autoimmune hepatitis, all of which can lead to liver cirrhosis.

> **Clinical Pearl**
> All of the previously identified causes of liver cirrhosis increase the risk for hepatocellular carcinoma (HCC), as do α_1-antitrypsin deficiency and aflatoxin exposure. Note that aflatoxin is a toxin produced by the fungus *Aspergillus*.

9. Assuming he is not taking any anticoagulants, what is the most likely reason this patient developed a large hematoma at the IV site?
   The liver is where most of the clotting factors are produced. Severe liver disease impairs their production and processing, producing a coagulopathy. Notice that his PT was elevated because of this.

10. List all the laboratory findings you would expect in a patient with liver failure.
    See Table 7.4 for the laboratory findings in liver failure and their underlying mechanisms.

Table 7.4 Common Findings in Patients With Liver Failure

LABORATORY VALUE	MECHANISM
Elevated or normal LFT values	Liver enzymes may be elevated during initial damage, but if cirrhosis is present or the liver shrinks over time, liver enzyme levels may appear normal in the context of decreased hepatic tissue.
Elevated PT	The liver is the site of coagulation factor production. With severe liver damage, PT becomes elevated.
Elevated serum bilirubin concentration	The liver is responsible for bilirubin uptake. Liver failure causes a spike in serum bilirubin concentration because of decreased hepatic uptake.
Hypoalbuminemia	The liver is the predominant site of albumin production. Decreased serum protein concentration may clinically manifest as ascites.
Fasting hypoglycemia	Impaired gluconeogenesis and glycogenolysis during fasting.
Elevated estrogen levels	The liver is the site of estrogen breakdown. Liver damage elevates estrogen levels, which can lead to testicular atrophy and formation of spider angiomata.
Elevated ammonia levels with decreased BUN	The liver produces the enzymes involved in the urea cycle, which converts ammonia to urea. Elevated ammonia levels can result in hepatic encephalopathy, marked by confusion, loss of consciousness, asterixis, irritability, tremor, and coma. Increased ammonia also can result in fetor hepaticus ("breath of the dead"), which is characteristic of liver disease.

BUN, Blood urea nitrogen; *LFT,* liver function test; *PT,* prothrombin time.

11. **Would you expect the ascitic fluid to be a transudate or an exudate?**
    The ascitic fluid would be a transudate. A transudate develops when fluid moves across a membrane as a result of hemodynamic forces. Because there is no alteration in the permeability of the membranes that the fluid is moving across, the fluid that accumulates has low protein content. In contrast, exudates are fluid collections that develop because of alterations in membrane/vessel permeability, so proteins and cells can move across membranes and accumulate in the extravascular fluid collections. Because ascites is caused by lowered oncotic pressure (secondary to hypoalbuminemia) and portal hypertension, both of which alter hemodynamic forces but not vessel permeability, the result is a transudate. Table 7.5 lists the differences between transudates and exudates.

Table 7.5 Transudates Versus Exudates

FLUID TYPE	MECHANISM	COMMON CAUSES	CHARACTERISTICS
Transudate	Disturbances of hydrostatic or oncotic pressures	Nephrotic syndrome Liver failure CHF	Clear fluid, protein-poor, specific gravity <1.012, fluid (LDH)/plasma (LDH) ratio <0.6, often results in pitting edema
Exudate	Increased vessel permeability; often mediated by acute-phase cytokines	Inflammation Septic shock	Cloudy fluid, protein-rich, specific gravity >1.020, fluid (LDH)/plasma (LDH) ratio >0.6

CHF, Congestive heart failure; *LDH,* lactate dehydrogenase.

STEP 1 SECRET

Transudates and exudates can both result in edema. You should know the difference between transudates and exudates and the causes of each. These comparisons are listed for you in Table 7.5.

12. **How does liver cirrhosis cause the following abnormalities?**
    1. Unconjugated (indirect) and conjugated (direct) hyperbilirubinemia
       Because there are fewer functional hepatocytes, there is a reduced ability to take up and conjugate bilirubin, which results in an unconjugated hyperbilirubinemia. Additionally, bilirubin that is conjugated may leak back into the bloodstream because of hepatocyte damage. This concept is explained in further detail later in the chapter.
    2. Reduced BUN, fetor hepaticus, and mental status changes

The liver is a major site of amino acid metabolism and is the site of the urea cycle. As discussed previously, the urea cycle metabolizes ammonia to urea. Liver damage impairs ammonia detoxification, resulting in reduced urea (BUN), as well as increased levels of ammonia. The elevated blood ammonia, which can enter the brain, can alter cerebral metabolism and neurotransmission and contribute to confusion (hepatic encephalopathy) (see Table 7.4).

Clinical Pearl

Lactulose is broken down to lactic acid in the colon, causing acidification of the microenvironment, which converts absorbable ammonium (NH_4) to unabsorbable ammonia (NH_3), which is then excreted in the feces. Hence, individuals with severe cirrhosis are often prescribed lactulose to minimize their risk for developing hepatic encephalopathy. The antibiotic rifaximin is another option, which acts by killing gut flora that produce ammonia.

---

13. **How does alcohol consumption lead to hepatitis?**

    Ethanol is metabolized in the hepatocyte using alcohol dehydrogenase (ADH). A by-product of this process is acetaldehyde. Acetaldehyde compromises the ability of the hepatocyte to protect itself from free radical damage. ADH can only metabolize a fixed amount of ethanol; thus, excess ethanol will lead to excess acetaldehyde. This acetaldehyde permits free radicals to damage the hepatocyte membrane, leading to inflammation of the liver. This kind of alcoholic hepatitis is present in approximately 1% of the US population.

14. **Why are ethanol and fomepizole used to treat methanol poisoning and ethylene glycol poisoning?**

    Methanol and ethylene glycol are metabolized through the same pathway as ethanol, and the intermediate substances that are formed in this process (formaldehyde from methanol and oxalic acid from ethylene glycol) are very toxic. Ethanol competes with both methanol and ethylene glycol for metabolism by ADH, thereby reducing the rate of formation of the toxic metabolites. Fomepizole further inhibits conversion of methanol or ethylene glycol to their toxic intermediates by directly inhibiting ADH.

15. **How is alcoholic hepatitis treated?**

    As one might guess, the patient must discontinue alcohol consumption. Because people with chronic alcohol consumption are more likely to be deficient of thiamine (vitamin B_1) and folate than the general population, individuals with alcoholic hepatitis should be treated with supplemental thiamine and folate.

SUMMARY BOX: ALCOHOLIC HEPATITIS

- Presentation: Vomiting with potential hematemesis, jaundice, scleral icterus, fetor hepaticus
- Epidemiology: Affects approximately 1% of the population
  - Risk factors: Commonly occurs in individuals with a history of alcohol abuse
- Pathophysiology: Metabolism of ethanol occurs in the liver, producing acetaldehyde. Acetaldehyde causes damage to hepatocyte membranes and compromises the liver's defense against free radicals, leading to damage of hepatocytes with resulting inflammation of the liver.
  - Diagnosis: History, physical exam, and derangements in liver function studies (prothrombin time [PT], albumin, bilirubin)
  - Complications: Esophageal varices, hepatic encephalopathy, coagulopathy, thrombocytopenia, ascites, cirrhosis
  - Treatment: Discontinue alcohol consumption, replenish folate and thiamine. Give lactulose or rifaximin for hepatic encephalopathy.

CASE 7.2

The third-year medical student that you are supervising in your primary care clinic does the initial history and examination on an 18-year-old man. Review of systems is significant for malaise and anorexia. Physical examination reveals generalized jaundice, as well as the presence of golden brown rings at the limbus of the cornea as shown (Fig. 7.3). This reminds the student of a disease for which she cannot recall the name.

1. **To what disease is the student referring?**

    The student is referring to Wilson disease (hepatolenticular degeneration), a genetic disease of copper metabolism. The golden brown corneal deposits (typically seen through slit-lamp examination of the eyes) observed with this disease are termed *Kayser-Fleischer rings* and result from copper deposition in the corneal limbus.

2. **What laboratory tests and further physical examination components would you like to do to strengthen your suspicion for this disease?**

    In addition to hepatic enzymes, you will want to order a serum ceruloplasmin, total serum copper, free copper, and urine copper. A slit-lamp examination would help confirm the suspected eye abnormality.

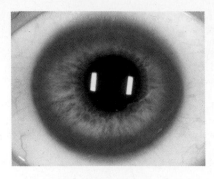

Figure 7.3. Ocular examination of patient in Case 7.2. *(From Goldman L, Ausiello D. Cecil Textbook of Medicine. 22nd ed. Philadelphia: WB Saunders; 2004.)*

CASE 7.2 CONTINUED:

Laboratory workup reveals reduced total serum copper but an increased level of free copper. Increased urinary copper excretion is also demonstrated. Slit-lamp examination confirms the presence of Kayser-Fleischer rings. Your suspicion for Wilson disease is now quite high.

3. **Describe the pathogenesis of Wilson disease.**
   In Wilson disease, there is a genetic deficiency in ceruloplasmin, which normally functions to bind plasma copper. This results in low-to-normal total plasma copper but elevated free (unbound) copper in the serum and urine. Increased free copper can deposit in the lenticular nuclei in the brain (leading to neuropsychiatric symptoms), cornea (promoting development of Kayser-Fleischer rings), liver (leading to cirrhosis and potential HCC), and other organs throughout the body.
   > **Note:** There are over 200 mutations of the *ATP7B* gene that are known to cause Wilson disease, which is inherited in an autosomal recessive manner. It usually manifests at a young age (between 6 and 20 years). Prenatal genetic screening is available within an affected family if the responsible mutation has been identified. In the United States, it is estimated that 1 in 30,000 individuals are affected by Wilson disease and 1 in 90 are carriers of mutations that cause Wilson disease.

4. **How is the diagnosis of Wilson disease definitively made?**
   A liver biopsy showing an elevated free copper concentration is required. Histologic staining for copper can also be done, but this test is not as sensitive, and a negative result does not exclude the diagnosis because copper can be deposited heterogeneously. The biopsy will also show piecemeal necrosis and lymphocytosis, which can evolve to cirrhosis.
   > **Note:** Total serum copper levels are *decreased* secondary to decreased ceruloplasmin levels. Elevated free copper levels are toxic and thus responsible for the symptoms observed in Wilson disease.

5. **If this patient remains untreated, what neurologic manifestations may develop?**
   Because of the degeneration of the lenticular nuclei (putamen and globus pallidus) in the basal ganglia, a Parkinson-like syndrome, characterized by tremors, dysarthria, bradykinesia, and spasticity, can develop. Psychiatric symptoms including changes in affect and behavior are also possible.

6. **What is the treatment for Wilson disease, and how does it work?**
   Copper chelation therapy with lifelong use of D-penicillamine or trientine hydrochloride is the treatment for Wilson disease. These drugs bind to copper and remove it from tissue. Oral administration of zinc, which competes with copper for intestinal absorption, is commonly used in combination with copper chelation therapy.

SUMMARY BOX: WILSON DISEASE

- Presentation: Malaise, jaundice
- Epidemiology: Usually manifests between 6 to 20 years of age
  - 1 in 30,000 individuals are affected
  - 1 in 90 are carriers of mutations causing Wilson disease
- Pathophysiology: Autosomal recessive mutation in the *ATP7B* gene that results in decreased ceruloplasmin, which leads to increased circulating levels of unbound copper in the serum. This copper can deposit in the lenticular nuclei (brain), cornea, joints, liver, and kidneys and cause dysfunction in each of these organ systems.
- Diagnosis: History, physical exam (presence of corneal deposits seen through slit-lamp examination), hepatic enzymes, liver biopsy revealing increased free copper levels, copper studies (decreased ceruloplasmin, decreased total serum copper, increased free copper in the serum and urine)
- Complications: Parkinson-like syndrome (tremors, dysarthria, bradykinesia, spasticity), psychiatric disturbances
- Treatment: Lifetime copper chelation therapy (D-penicillamine or trientine hydrochloride) and oral administration of zinc

CASE 7.3

A 32-year-old man develops fever, nausea, vomiting, malaise, anorexia, and abdominal pain within a few weeks of returning to the United States from vacationing in a developing country. He also mentions that his urine appears particularly dark.

1. In terms of infections, what do you include in the differential diagnosis for a patient who has recently traveled out of the country?
   You must broaden your differential diagnosis to include diseases endemic to certain areas, such as schistosomiasis in sub-Saharan Africa; infections potentially obtained from local food, such as *Vibrio cholerae* infection from drinking contaminated water in South America; diseases associated with wildlife, such as plague (*Yersinia pestis*) in countries with infected rodents; and infection from insects, such as malaria transmitted by *Anopheles* mosquitoes in tropical and subtropical countries. Sexually transmitted infections, such as human immunodeficiency virus/acquired immunodeficiency syndrome (HIV/AIDS), can be more abundant in other countries. These are just a few examples, but it is important to remember to consider such possibilities in travelers.

CASE 7.3 CONTINUED:

The patient states that he ate some shellfish that was harvested from a bay in which sewage enters. He was bitten by several mosquitoes and thinks he may have been infected with malaria. He had not received any immunizations before leaving for his vacation. On physical examination, he is jaundiced and has tender hepatomegaly. Laboratory studies reveal a peripheral smear negative for malaria, marked elevations of aspartate transaminase (AST) and alanine transaminase (ALT) (>1000), mildly elevated alkaline phosphatase (ALP), and elevated direct and indirect bilirubin. A hepatitis profile reveals positive anti-HAV IgM (hepatitis A virus immunoglobulin M), negative anti-HAV IgG (hepatitis A virus immunoglobulin G), and negative HBsAg (hepatitis B surface antigen).

2. What is the most likely diagnosis?
   Acute hepatitis A infection is the most likely diagnosis. Hepatitis A is an enterically transmitted virus that is highly endemic in parts of the developing world where sanitation is poor (i.e., Mexico, parts of Asia, Africa, South America). It is usually transmitted from an infected food handler who does not thoroughly wash their hands before handling food others will consume. Hepatitis A virus enters hepatocytes, where it replicates and leads to immune-mediated damage of the cells.

3. Why is there an elevation of both conjugated and unconjugated bilirubin?
   In viral hepatitis, the unconjugated hyperbilirubinemia is caused by a reduction in the ability of the infected hepatocytes to take up unconjugated bilirubin. The conjugated hyperbilirubinemia is caused by leakage of conjugated bilirubin from infected hepatocytes into the systemic circulation.

4. Explain how the results of the hepatitis profile facilitate the diagnosis of an acute infection rather than a chronic one.
   IgM is the first antibody isotype produced in response to a new infectious agent and remains in the circulation for about 12 weeks in hepatitis A infection. A previous infection would have been negative for anti-HAV IgM and positive for anti-HAV IgG because the IgG isotype is produced later in the infection and is the typical product of memory B cells.

5. Should the patient be concerned about developing a chronic infection or hepatic cirrhosis?
   No, because in the vast majority of cases, hepatitis A is a self-limiting infection that does not develop into a chronic infection or lead to cirrhosis. Generally, the prognosis with hepatitis A is very good, and only supportive therapy is required for full recovery. However, hepatitis B and C viruses can cause both chronic infection and cirrhosis.

6. How would you expect liver "function" test patterns to differ between parenchymal liver disease and cholestatic (biliary) disease?
   Generally, in diseases that primarily affect the liver parenchyma, both AST and ALT are elevated to a greater extent than ALP and GGT. In biliary (cholestatic) diseases, the converse is generally the case, with ALP and GGT being elevated to a greater extent than AST and ALT.

7. Now let us review some characteristic features of the different hepatitis viruses.
   See Table 7.6.

STEP 1 SECRET

Hepatitis is very commonly tested on the USMLE. You must know all the characteristics of the different hepatitis viruses. The one that confuses students most is hepatitis B because it is associated with a variety of antigens and antibodies that are either positive or negative depending on the stage of the disease. Do not worry! We discuss hepatitis B in extensive detail later in this chapter.

Table 7.6 Characteristics of Hepatitis Viruses

HEPATITIS VIRUS	TYPE OF VIRUS	TRANS-MISSION	CHRO-NICITY	CIR-RHOSIS	HEPATOCELLULAR CARCINOMA RISK	COMMENTS
A	ssRNA	Fecal-oral	No	No	No	May cause cholestasis
B	dsDNA	Parenteral	Yes	Yes	Yes	
C	ssRNA	Parenteral	Yes	Yes	Yes	Most common cause of posttransfusion hepatitis
D	ssRNA	Parenteral	Yes	Yes	Yes	Requires hepatitis B virus to replicate; can cause fulminant hepatitis
E	ssRNA	Fecal-oral	No	No	No	20% mortality rate in pregnant women

dsDNA, Double-stranded DNA; *ssRNA,* single-stranded RNA.

8. Can hepatitis A be prevented?

Yes. A live inactivated vaccine for hepatitis A is available. It is included in the vaccine recommendations of the Centers for Disease Control and Prevention (CDC) for all children over 1 year of age, as well as for children and adults traveling to certain developing nations.

Note: Infection with hepatitis A confers lifelong immunity against future HAV infections.

SUMMARY BOX: ACUTE HEPATITIS A

- Presentation: Prodrome (fatigue, anorexia, nausea and vomiting, myalgias) followed by icteric phase (dark urine, light stool, jaundice)
- Epidemiology: Transmitted via fecal-oral route; disease incidence and prevalence vary temporally and geographically (higher rates in Mexico and urban areas in Asia, Africa, and South America)
- Diagnosis: Elevated serum transaminases (in acute hepatitis, [AST] and [ALT] can exceed 1000 IU/L), presence of [HAV] antibodies ([IgM] for roughly 12 weeks after acquiring hepatitis A infection; [IgG] becomes present shortly after IgM and persists for several years), clinical symptoms (anorexia, nausea/vomiting, fever, myalgias, jaundice, dark urine)
- Pathophysiology: Hepatitis A (single-stranded RNA virus) enters the hepatocyte, where it replicates. This leads to immune-mediated destruction of virally infected hepatocytes.
- Complications: Cholestasis. Note: Hepatitis A is *not* associated with chronic hepatitis.
- Treatment: Supportive. Note: A vaccine to prevent hepatitis A is available.
- Prognosis: Excellent, generally there is no recurrence or chronic form of hepatitis A.
- Long-term immunity is acquired from an HAV infection.

CASE 7.4

A 3-day-old, full-term baby presents with jaundice that started on his face and in his eyes and spread to his body. On physical examination, there are no hematomas present. Laboratory tests show elevated indirect bilirubin, a negative direct Coombs test, normal reticulocyte count (for his age), and normal complete blood count (CBC). Enzyme assays for UDP glucuronyl transferase activity are within normal limits.

---

1. What is the most likely diagnosis?

Physiologic jaundice of the newborn is the most likely diagnosis. The unconjugated hyperbilirubinemia suggests either hemolysis or a liver that cannot adequately process the bilirubin load. The negative direct Coombs test helps exclude more serious hemolytic diseases of newborns in which the body produces autoantibodies against the newborn's native RBCs. Hemolytic diseases of newborns also cause CBC abnormalities, including anemia from extensive hemolysis and neutropenia and thrombocytopenia from suppression of myelopoiesis and platelet production in favor of erythropoiesis. Normal UDP glucuronyl transferase activity excludes congenital enzyme deficiencies.

2. Why does physiologic jaundice develop?

In the process of converting from RBCs with fetal hemoglobin to RBCs with adult hemoglobin, there is an approximately six-fold increase in the amount of unconjugated bilirubin presented to the liver. The neonatal liver often does not have the capacity to completely take up and conjugate this amount of bilirubin because of a physiologic deficiency of UDP glucuronyl transferase, resulting in a transient "physiologic" jaundice with unconjugated hyperbilirubinemia and possible kernicterus (deposition of bilirubin into the brain). The condition is fairly common, affecting 2% to 6% of newborns. Treatment involves phototherapy, which converts the unconjugated bilirubin into a water-soluble form that can be excreted in the urine.

Note: This condition is more common among breastfed babies because breast milk contains deconjugating enzymes. In this case it is referred to as *breastmilk jaundice*.

3. Why did the physician check for hematomas on physical examination?
Breakdown of RBCs in hematomas and subsequent bilirubin formation can be a cause of jaundice. Hematomas, resulting from minor birth trauma, are not uncommon in newborns.

4. Why are a normal reticulocyte count and a normal CBC important in the diagnostic workup for this neonate?
Hemolytic anemia can cause jaundice and will generally show an elevated reticulocyte count, as well as decreased hematocrit and hemoglobin levels.

5. What is the most serious complication of neonatal jaundice and how does it develop?
Kernicterus is the most serious complication of neonatal jaundice. Insoluble unconjugated bilirubin is deposited in the brain and can result when the bilirubin concentration is especially high. Kernicterus is dangerous because it can lead to irreversible brain damage.

CASE 7.4 CONTINUED:

The mother and baby return to the office when the child is 1 week old for a scheduled follow-up visit with a lactation consultant. The jaundice has resolved, but the anxious first-time mother is concerned about long-term consequences for the baby.

6. Are there long-term risks associated with physiologic jaundice of the newborn?
No. Most newborns will appear somewhat jaundiced in the first few days of life and this does not predispose them to any future disorders, hepatic or otherwise. The mother should be reassured. However, had the jaundice been severe and the bilirubin concentration greater than 20 mg/dL, there would be an increased risk for kernicterus, which can lead to long-term complications. Infants with significantly elevated bilirubin may require phototherapy or even exchange transfusion to bring bilirubin levels down.

7. Would you expect physiologic jaundice to be exacerbated or attenuated by Gilbert syndrome?
Physiologic jaundice would be exacerbated by Gilbert syndrome, which is characterized by mildly decreased UDP glucuronyl transferase activity that results in increased unconjugated bilirubin levels.

8. What is the hereditary syndrome with a more serious deficiency of UDP glucuronyl transferase than Gilbert syndrome?
Crigler-Najjar syndrome, which also causes an unconjugated hyperbilirubinemia, has a more serious deficiency of UPD glucuronyl transferase than Gilbert syndrome. Two forms of Crigler-Najjar syndrome have been described. Type 1 is caused by a genetic mutation that leads to the absence of UDP glucuronyl transferase and is characterized by high levels of unconjugated hyperbilirubinemia and kernicterus. Patients with type 1 Crigler-Najjar generally die within the first few years of life if not treated. Type 2 is a less severe form of the condition, caused by a deficiency of UDP glucuronyl transferase. Affected patients demonstrate a lower degree of hyperbilirubinemia and have a much smaller risk of kernicterus.

Note: Phenobarbital can be used to treat type 2 Crigler-Najjar syndrome because it upregulates UDP glucuronyl transferase production, thereby increasing the capacity of the liver to conjugate bilirubin.

9. What are the hereditary forms of conjugated hyperbilirubinemia, and what is the major histologic difference between them?
Dubin-Johnson and Rotor syndromes are the hereditary forms of conjugated hyperbilirubinemia. Dubin-Johnson syndrome is characterized by black, coarse pigmentation of centrilobular hepatocytes, causing the liver to appear grossly black. Dubin-Johnson syndrome is caused by a problem with excretion of conjugated bilirubin. Rotor syndrome is a milder form of the disease in which patients generally do not have a black liver. Table 7.7 outlines the differences between the hereditary forms of bilirubin metabolism and transport.

SUMMARY BOX: PHYSIOLOGIC JAUNDICE OF THE NEWBORN

- Presentation: Scleral icterus, jaundice
- Epidemiology: Rates vary depending on definition of jaundice, but the condition is common (2%–6%).
- Diagnosis: Clinical appearance, exclusion of other, more severe conditions on the differential
- Pathophysiology: Infants have erythrocytes with a decreased life span (in comparison to adult erythrocytes). Increased turnover of RBCs) leads to increased production of bilirubin. Neonates also have a physiologic deficiency of UDP glucuronyl transferase. The combination of these two factors leads to an increase in unconjugated bilirubin in the newborn.
- Complications: Kernicterus (usually when bilirubin levels exceed 20 mg/dL)
- Treatment: Phototherapy or exchange transfusion, if the bilirubin levels are extremely elevated (usually above 20 mg/dL).
- Prognosis: Excellent if treated appropriately

Table 7.7 Hereditary Disorders of Hepatic Bilirubin Metabolism and Transport

FEATURE	GILBERT SYNDROME	CRIGLER-NAJJAR TYPE I SYNDROME	CRIGLER-NAJJAR TYPE II SYNDROME	DUBIN-JOHNSON SYNDROME	ROTOR SYNDROME
Incidence	6%–12%	Very rare	Uncommon	Uncommon	Rare
Gene affected	*UGT1A1*	*UGT1A1*	*UGT1A1*	*MRP2*	Unknown
Metabolic defect	↓ Bilirubin conjugation	No bilirubin conjugation	↓↓ Bilirubin conjugation	Impaired canalicular export of conjugated bilirubin	Impaired canalicular export of conjugated bilirubin
Plasma bilirubin (mg/dL)	≤3 in absence of fasting or hemolysis, nearly all unconjugated	Usually >20 (range, 17–50), all unconjugated	Usually <20 (range, 6–45), nearly all unconjugated	Usually <7, about one-half conjugated	Usually <7, about one-half conjugated
Liver histologic appearance	Usually normal, occasional ↑ lipofuscin	Normal	Normal	Coarse pigment in centrilobular hepatocytes, leading to a grossly black liver	Normal
Other features	↓ Bilirubin concentration with phenobarbital	No response to phenobarbital	↓ Bilirubin concentration with phenobarbital	↑ Bilirubin concentration with estrogens, ↑↑ urinary coproporphyrin I/III ratio, slow BSP elimination kinetics with secondary rise	Mild ↑ urinary coproporphyrin I/III ratio, very slow BSP elimination kinetics without secondary rise
Prognosis	Normal Jaundice may be evident only with fasting and stress	Death in infancy if untreated	Usually normal	Normal	Normal
Treatment	None	Phototherapy as a bridge to liver transplantation	Phenobarbital for ↑↑ bilirubin concentration	Avoid estrogens	None available

BSP, Sulfobromophthalein; *MRP2,* multidrug resistance–associated protein-2 gene; *UGT1A1,* bilirubin UDP glucuronyl transferase gene.
From Feldman M, Friedman LS, Brandt LJ. *Sleisenger and Fordtran's Gastrointestinal and Liver Disease.* 8th ed. Philadelphia: WB Saunders; 2006.

CASE 7.5

A 45-year-old woman presents to the clinic with reports of a flu-like illness. The patient is currently employed as a nurse and has recently had to take several days off for sick leave. She states that approximately 1 month ago, she started feeling fatigued and feverish. Soon she developed an "achy" abdominal pain in the right upper quadrant (RUQ). Last week she noticed that her urine was darker than usual.

1. **What structures are located in the RUQ?**
   The liver; the gallbladder and biliary tree; the first, second, and third parts of the duodenum; the head of the pancreas and pancreatic duct; the hepatic flexure of the colon; and the right hemidiaphragm are located in the RUQ.

2. **With this initial concern of RUQ pain, what is your differential diagnosis?**
   There are several causes of acute RUQ pain—biliary disease (colic, cholecystitis, ascending cholangitis), hepatitis, acute pancreatitis, peptic ulcer disease, dyspepsia, lower lobe pneumonia, or an atypical presentation of myocardial infarction. In a 45-year-old woman, a gallstone should be high on your differential list. Her report of darkened urine suggests conjugated bilirubinuria and further supports an obstruction. It is also possible that this clinical picture could be caused by an intrahepatic process.

   > **Clinical Pearl**
   > Using anatomic cues is important for building a differential diagnosis, but abdominal pain does not always follow anatomic division. Pathology in other anatomic locations can present as right upper quadrant (RUQ) pain, such as a dissecting abdominal aortic aneurysm, a right lower lobe pneumonia, gynecologic pathology, or an atypical appendicitis, to name a few.

3. **What is cholangitis?**
   Cholangitis is an infection of the biliary tree, usually occurring as a result of a stone in the common bile duct. It requires aggressive treatment because patients can become septic quickly.

4. **What is the Charcot triad for cholangitis?**
   The Charcot triad consists of (1) fever, (2) RUQ pain, and (3) jaundice and is present in approximately 50% of patients with cholangitis. The fever is due to the response to infection, the jaundice is due to obstruction of the common bile duct (or other bile ducts), and the cause of RUQ pain is obvious. RUQ pain secondary to ascending cholangitis can radiate to the shoulder or tip of the scapula.

   > **Clinical Pearl**
   > Occasionally, patients may develop the Reynold pentad of cholangitis, which includes the Charcot triad plus altered mental status and hypotension.

CASE 7.5 CONTINUED:

On further questioning, you learn that the patient is quite concerned about being infected with human immunodeficiency virus (HIV) because of a needlestick exposure a few months earlier. On physical examination you appreciate a jaundiced, ill-appearing woman with RUQ tenderness to palpation.

5. **How does the preceding information alter the differential diagnosis?**
   Given the needlestick exposure, the concern now should be an infection such as HIV or, even more likely, viral hepatitis (B or C). One would want to check liver enzymes and serologic findings for viral hepatitis, as well as HIV at this point. These tests may also help clarify whether her pain is related to gallbladder disease and if an abdominal ultrasound is necessary.

   > **Clinical Pearl**
   > Risk of human immunodeficiency virus (HIV) transmission after percutaneous exposure to HIV-infected blood is about 0.003%. Risk of hepatitis C virus (HCV) transmission is 1.8% following percutaneous exposure to HCV-infected blood, and risk of hepatitis B virus (HBV) transmission (if the person exposed percutaneously to HBV-infected blood is not immune) ranges from 23% to 62%, depending on the hepatitis B surface antigen (HBsAg)/hepatitis B e antigen (HBeAg) status.

CASE 7.5 CONTINUED:

ALT and AST are markedly elevated, but the alkaline phosphatase and GGT are within normal limits. Hepatitis serologic assays reveal the following findings:
   HBsAg: positive
   Anti-HBs antibody: negative
   Anti-HBc-IgM: positive
   Anti-HBc-IgG: negative
   Anti-HCV: negative

6. What is the diagnosis?

The diagnosis is acute hepatitis B infection (see Secrets for Diagnosing Stages of Hepatitis B Infection below). Hepatitis B can be acute or chronic (>6 months). Acute hepatitis B often manifests weeks to months after infection with constitutional symptoms, RUQ abdominal pain, and jaundice. Because hepatitis B can be transmitted parenterally, the patient was likely infected by the needlestick.

Note: Hepatitis B has an incubation period of 30 to 180 days. Onset of illness is usually preceded by a serum sickness prodrome (e.g., fever, malaise, arthralgias/myalgias, GI distress, headaches).

7. What is the difference between acute and chronic hepatitis B infection?

As opposed to acute infection, chronic hepatitis B infection is marked by the persistence of hepatitis B surface antigen (HBsAg) in the blood for a minimum of 6 months after exposure. More specific differences between acute and chronic infection are discussed further in Secrets for Diagnosing Stages of Hepatitis B Infection.

SECRETS FOR DIAGNOSING STAGES OF HEPATITIS B INFECTION

The easiest way to think about hepatitis B is to first recall the three types of antigens associated with this infection. These are surface antigen (HBsAg), core antigen (HBcAg), and an antigen that circulates in the blood during viral replication called *hepatitis B e antigen* (HBeAg). HBcAg is not clinically useful because it is not detectable in serum, so you need not worry about that one. HBsAg is the most important of the three. It is the first antigen to appear after infection and the last antigen to disappear, and if it is present in serum, the patient *is infected* with hepatitis B virus (although you cannot tell quite yet whether this indicates an acute, chronic, or carrier state infection). HBeAg is your infectivity marker. This is especially important in pregnant women. The presence of HBeAg indicates a high infectivity rate. Approximately 90% of neonates will acquire hepatitis B infection from the mother if she is HBeAg-positive.

Let us imagine that your patient is acutely infected with HBV. Within 2 to 8 weeks after exposure, serum HBsAg will become positive (core antigen will also be positive, but remember that we cannot see this). HBeAg becomes positive soon after, and anti-HBV core antibody IgM (anti-HBc-IgM) is then produced. This antibody is clinically important for two reasons; one we will mention now and the other we will mention later. Think of anti-HBc antibody as your chronicity marker (remember "C" for chronicity). If a patient is positive for anti-HBcAg of the IgM isotype, it indicates acute/recent infection. If anti-HBc-IgG is present, the patient has chronic disease (>6 months of infection) or has recovered from disease (you will need to look at anti-HBs antibody levels to determine this). Of note, anti-HBc-IgM is a *nonprotective* antibody.

Most people with HBV will not develop chronic hepatitis because their immune system will eventually fix the problem that it caused in the first place. The immune system will start to make antibodies to HBsAg (anti-HBs) and HBeAg (anti-HBe). In this case, the antibody isotype is of minimal importance. What is important is that when this starts to happen, the patient will enter the *window period*. The best way for understanding the window period is to picture the following scenario: Let us say you have concentration of HBsAg in your serum. As the body produces anti-HBs antibodies, the HBsAg precipitates out of serum via immune complex formation. When the concentration of anti-HBs antibody equals that of HBsAg, all of the antigen precipitates out, and HBsAg becomes undetectable in serum. This also applies to HBeAg and its respective antibody.

To summarize, the window period marks the time when the patient produces surface and "e" antibodies in equal concentrations to their antigens such that neither antibody nor antigen is detectable in serum (Fig. 7.4).

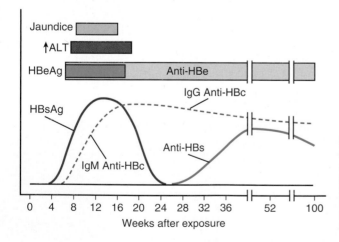

Figure 7.4. Schematic diagram of hepatitis B virus. *ALT,* Alanine transaminase; *anti-HBc,* hepatitis B core antibody; *anti-HBe,* hepatitis B e antibody; *anti-HBs,* hepatitis B surface antibody; *HBeAg,* hepatitis B e antigen; *HBsAg,* hepatitis B surface antigen; *HBs,* IgG, immunoglobulin G; *IgM,* immunoglobulin M. *(From Longo DL, Fauci AS, Kasper DL, et al.* Harrison's Principles of Internal Medicine. *18th ed. New York: McGraw-Hill; 2012.)*

How can you diagnose HBV infection during the window period? This is when anti-HBc antibody again becomes important. The *only* marker that is positive during the window period is anti-HBc antibody, and it can thus be used to test for infection during the window period.

Table 7.8 Interpretation of Hepatitis B Serologic Test Results

HBSAG	ANTI-HBC	ANTI-HBS	INTERPRETATION
−	−	−	Susceptible (never infected)
−	IgG	IgG	Immune because of natural infection
−	−	IgG	Immune because of hepatitis B immunization
+	IgM	−	Acutely infected
+	IgG	−	Chronically infected

Anti-HBc, Hepatitis B core antibody; *anti-HBs,* hepatitis B surface antibody; *HBsAg,* hepatitis B surface antigen; *IgG,* immunoglobulin G; *IgM,* immunoglobulin M; +, positive; −, negative.

Note: An individual who has been vaccinated against HBV will be positive only for anti-HBs antibody and not anti-HBc antibody because only HBsAg is used to vaccinate.

Once the window period has ended, levels of anti-HBs antibody and anti-HBe antibody rise over the levels of antigen, and these antibodies will become detectable in the serum. If a patient has detectable levels of anti-HBs antibody, *they are in the recovery phase or have been previously immunized against HBV.* How do you distinguish between a cured patient versus an immunized patient? Easy! Look for anti-HBc-IgG.

The only other thing that you need to know is what a carrier will look like. These are people who are positive for HBsAg but do not have anti-HBs antibodies, although they are otherwise asymptomatic. This tends to occur in immunocompromised patients, because these are people whose CD8+ T cells will not attack the viral antigens on hepatocytes and cause symptoms of the disease. Carriers can, however, pass the disease onto others.

We hope this makes more sense to you now and recommend rereading this section while studying Fig. 7.4 and Table 7.8 to test yourself.

1. Why are the AST and ALT values elevated in this patient?
   Viral hepatitis is an inflammatory disease of the liver. The viral particles infect hepatocytes, and in an effort to clear the infection, the host immune system destroys infected cells. Hepatocyte necrosis causes a massive leakage of hepatic enzymes. The AST and ALT are markers of hepatocyte death, *not liver function.* Thus the popularly used but technically inaccurate term *transaminitis* indicates an increased AST and ALT. In comparison, a "cholestatic" pattern suggests an obstructive process (intra- or extrahepatic) with elevated ALP and GGT.

2. What other viruses would you consider screening for in this patient?
   Screening for hepatitis D should be considered. Hepatitis D is a uniquely **d**efective virus: It requires coinfection with hepatitis B in order to replicate. A serum test for antihepatitis D Ab is indicated when HBsAg is positive.

3. What is the most common mode of transmission in HBV-endemic areas (e.g., Southeast Asia, China, and Africa)?
   Vertical transmission to neonates from HBV carrier mothers is the most common mode of transmission. Recall that mothers who are HBeAg-positive have the highest risk of perinatal transmission to their children.

   In the United States, sexual contact is the most common mode of transmission. Most neonatal infections become chronic, whereas only a small percentage of infections acquired in adulthood do. HBV is thought to be 10 times more infectious than HCV and 100 times more infectious than HIV.

4. If a patient with hepatitis B infection also presented with arthralgias, mononeuritis, fever, abdominal pain, renal disease, and hypertension, what disease might you suspect?
   Polyarteritis nodosa (PAN) is often associated with HBV. Although only a small percentage of HBV patients will develop PAN, almost one-third of patients with PAN have acute or, more commonly, chronic HBV. Membranous glomerulonephritis and membranoproliferative glomerulonephritis are also sometimes associated with HBV.

STEP 1 SECRET

If symptoms of polyarteritis nodosa (PAN) are suggested in a clinical vignette on the USMLE, the question stem will most likely mention hepatitis B association.

5. When is the HBV vaccine typically given?
   Universal vaccination of all children in the United States is recommended. The first of three doses is usually given at birth, the second at 1 to 2 months, and the third at 6 to 18 months. Children born to HBsAg-positive mothers should also be given hepatitis B immunoglobulin within 12 hours of birth to achieve passive immunity. Members of other high-risk groups, including health care workers, should also be vaccinated if they previously were not.

6. **How is viral hepatitis treated?**

   Acute hepatitis B does not always require treatment, but when it does, it is treated with antiviral therapy. Chronic hepatitis B is also treated with antiviral therapy. A number of agents are available that you do not need to know for Step 1. The hepatitis B vaccine is now routinely administered to children and high-risk individuals such as yourself (health care workers). Hepatitis C is also treated with antiviral therapy, and choice of agent is guided by viral genotype. Antiviral therapy is also available for hepatitis C. Regimen selection is guided by genotype and other patient factors; you do not need to know the specifics for USMLE Step 1. The best treatment for hepatitis D consists of the prevention of hepatitis B infection. At this time, hepatitis E is treated with supportive care.

7. **What are some other infectious causes of hepatitis?**

   Less common causes of hepatitis are given in Table 7.9.

Table 7.9 Less Common Causes of Hepatitis	
PATHOGENIC CATEGORY	**POTENTIAL ETIOLOGIC DISORDER(S)**
Amebic	*Entamoeba histolytica* abscess
Bacterial	Pyogenic hepatic abscess—may be caused by gram-positive aerobic cocci in neonates and gram-negative rods in adults
Parasitic	Leptospirosis, schistosomiasis, liver flukes (trematodes), toxoplasmosis
Viral	Cytomegalovirus (CMV), Epstein-Barr virus (EBV), herpes simplex virus (HSV), varicella-zoster virus (VZV) infections

8. **Describe the association between viral hepatitis and HCC.**

   Both chronic hepatitis B and hepatitis C infections have been strongly associated with HCC. Hepatitis C is estimated to be the causative agent behind approximately one-half of HCC cases.

SUMMARY BOX: HEPATITIS B VIRUS PRESENTATION: FEVER, JAUNDICE, AND RIGHT UPPER QUADRANT PAIN

- Epidemiology: Responsible for 5% to 10% of end-stage liver disease and up to 50% of hepatocellular carcinoma
- Diagnosis: Hepatitis B serologies, clinical presentation (signs of cirrhosis and portal hypertension as discussed previously in chronically infected patients; fever, jaundice, hepatomegaly in acutely infected patients), derangements of serum aminotransferases, liver function studies (prothrombin time [PT], bilirubin, albumin), γ-glutamyl transferase (GGT)
- Pathophysiology: Immune-mediated destruction of virally infected hepatocytes
- Complications: Cirrhosis, hepatocellular carcinoma
- Treatment: The goal of treatment is long-term suppression of the virus; antiviral therapies
- Prognosis: Variable. Good prognostic factors are undetectable hepatitis B virus (HBV) DNA load and loss of hepatitis B e antigen (HBeAg).

CASE 7.6

A 60-year-old male smoker who was infected with hepatitis B in his late 20s presents to your clinic. He had been feeling well until recently and has avoided seeing a doctor for the past 10 years.

1. **To what ailments are persons infected with hepatitis B susceptible?**

   The ones that should come immediately to mind are cirrhosis and HCC. Others include glomerulonephritis (from antibody-antigen [Ab-Ag] deposition in the glomerulus and subsequent inflammation) and PAN (from immune complex deposition in the blood vessels).

   Note: Hepatitis D virus is also parenterally and sexually transmitted, and infection can occur only with concomitant hepatitis B infection.

CASE 7.6 CONTINUED:

The patient decides to see his gastroenterologist because over the past 2 months he has noticed a dull epigastric pain that is now nearly constant, and he is feeling increasingly fatigued. He notes an unintentional 30-lb weight loss in recent months and a yellow discoloration of his skin.

2. **How does this additional information change the differential diagnosis? What specific laboratory tests might you want to order to further investigate?**
   Fatigue and unintentional weight loss should always make you consider malignancy in your differential diagnosis, especially in older patients. In a patient with a history of hepatitis B infection we need to consider HCC, which can present with jaundice, RUQ pain, ascites, and nausea. α-Fetoprotein (AFP) is a nonspecific serum marker for HCC. It may also be present with certain paraneoplastic syndromes (described subsequently in question 7).

CASE 7.6 CONTINUED:

In addition to the usual liver enzyme blood tests, a test for AFP is ordered. The AFP is markedly elevated at 1200 ng/mL (normal <10 ng/mL).

3. **What is the likely diagnosis, and how can it be confirmed?**
   HCC is the most likely diagnosis. HCC is the most common primary hepatic malignancy; it is the fifth most common cancer in men and the eighth most common in women. Histologic diagnosis is definitive, and samples can be obtained by fine-needle aspiration (FNA) or percutaneous biopsy.

4. **What other type of malignancy will produce a markedly elevated AFP?**
   Nonseminomatous germ cell tumors (think yolk sac tumor) and HCC are the only primary malignancies that will yield an AFP value greater than 500 ng/mL; liver metastases can also yield a value this high. AFP is also used in prenatal screening for Down syndrome (decreased levels) and neural tube defects (increased levels).
   Note: AFP is *not* diagnostic. It can be suggestive of the aforementioned conditions and can be used to monitor treatment for the same conditions.

5. **What are some risk factors for HCC?**
   The four major risk factors that have been identified as risk factors for HCC are chronic hepatitis B infection, chronic hepatitis C infection, cirrhosis, and dietary exposure to aflatoxin B_1. Aflatoxin B_1 is derived from *Aspergillus* species that can contaminate foodstuffs in tropical and subtropical regions of Africa and Asia. There are several minor risk factors, including cigarette smoking, oral contraceptive steroids, Wilson disease, α_1-antitrypsin deficiency, and hereditary hemochromatosis.

6. **Where are likely sites for metastatic HCC?**
   Likely sites for metastatic HCC are the lungs, regional lymph nodes, and adrenal glands. The liver is the most common site for metastases of other malignancies because of the high degree of blood supply to the liver from the portal venous system. In addition to malignancies in organs whose blood supply feeds into the portal system, lung and breast cancers often metastasize to the liver.
   You can generally differentiate primary cancer from metastatic cancer with imaging techniques by the presence of single versus multiple tumors within the organ of interest, respectively.

7. **What paraneoplastic syndromes are associated with HCC?**
   HCC is associated with the production of insulin-like factor, erythropoietin, and parathyroid hormone–related peptide (PTHrP). Clinical findings may include polycythemia and constitutive hypoglycemia. Note that the latter contrasts with liver failure secondary to noncancerous causes, which leads to fasting hypoglycemia only.

8. **In a woman who takes oral contraceptives and has a single hepatic nodule detected on ultrasound and a normal AFP, what kind of neoplasm might you suspect?**
   Hepatocellular adenomas are benign neoplasms that were very rare before oral contraceptives became widely used. Steroid use is also associated with hepatocellular adenoma risk. Hepatic angiography can be useful in making the diagnosis because many hepatocellular adenomas are avascular. Surgical resection is recommended because of the risk of rupture and, in a very small percentage of cases, transformation to HCC.

SUMMARY BOX: HEPATOCELLULAR CARCINOMA

- Presentation: Jaundice, tender hepatomegaly, ascites
- Epidemiology:
  - Most common primary hepatic malignancy
  - Fifth most common cancer in men and eighth most common in women worldwide
- Diagnosis: Hepatocellular carcinomas can be difficult to diagnose; elevated AFP is suggestive, histologic appearance of affected areas of the liver are diagnostic. Samples may be obtained with fine-needle aspiration (FNA). Imaging may be useful.
- Pathophysiology: Arises from several different pathways, including cirrhosis, environmental and carcinogenic exposures, genetic predisposition, and so forth
- Complications: Metastasis is common to the lungs, regional lymph nodes, and adrenal glands.
- Treatment: Surgical resection, liver transplantation, chemotherapy
- Prognosis: Generally pretty grim

CASE 7.7

A 19-year-old college student presents with nausea, vomiting, and abdominal pain. Initially, she is slightly confused and withdrawn, making it difficult to collect a good history, but she does tell you that she was at a fraternity party two nights ago and got "pretty drunk." She denies using any other drugs at the party. You do a pelvic examination and a rectal examination to assess for occult blood and order stat laboratory tests including a CBC, basic metabolic panel, liver enzymes, urinalysis, urine pregnancy test, and lipase. You also prepare to do an abdominal ultrasound.

1. **What are some of the common causes of acute abdominal pain with nausea and vomiting?**
   See Table 7.10.

Table 7.10 Common Causes of Acute Abdominal Pain

CAUSATIVE CONDITION	NATURE OF PAIN/ASSOCIATED FINDINGS
Acute appendicitis	Pain may be located in the periumbilical area or in the RLQ; anorexia is common.
Acute cholecystitis	Pain is located in the RUQ, and ultrasound imaging may show gallstones.
Acute gastroenteritis	Diarrhea often is a prominent component, and its characteristics, along with characterization of its onset with regard to meals, can help determine the underlying disorder.
Acute pancreatitis	Epigastric pain radiates to the back, associated with anorexia, nausea, and vomiting; plasma amylase and lipase (a more specific marker) levels may be elevated (although often not in chronic pancreatitis).
Acute salpingitis	Bilateral adnexal pain is common, with cervical motion tenderness on bimanual examination.
Biliary colic	RUQ pain is intermittent; ultrasound imaging may show gallstones.
Ectopic pregnancy	Nausea and vomiting often are absent, and a urine pregnancy test is positive; pelvic ultrasound imaging is used to rule out an intrauterine pregnancy and will sometimes reveal an adnexal mass or blood.
Intestinal obstruction	Pain often is diffuse and crampy in nature.
Perforated duodenal ulcer	Pain usually is epigastric; dark, tarry blood may be found in the stool.
Renal colic	Flank and costovertebral angle pain are severe; hematuria is common.

RLQ, Right lower quadrant; *RUQ,* right upper quadrant.

CASE 7.7 CONTINUED:

Pelvic and rectal examinations are unrevealing with stool negative for blood. Laboratory tests reveal a mild anemia and thrombocytopenia, as well as significantly elevated transaminases. The urine pregnancy test is negative, and other laboratory tests are normal. Abdominal ultrasound is unremarkable. You present these findings to the patient, telling her that it appears that her liver seems to have been damaged. Somewhere along the way, you garnered her trust and she now tells you more about the party. She saw her boyfriend kissing one of her sorority sisters, and after chugging three more beers, she went back to her dorm and took a bunch of acetaminophen before sleeping to avoid a hangover in the morning. After learning this, you order laboratory tests for total bilirubin and PT, which are elevated and prolonged, respectively.

2. **What is the most likely diagnosis and suspected etiology?**
   She has fulminant hepatic failure (FHF, or acute liver failure) resulting from acetaminophen toxicity. FHF is defined as the rapid development of hepatocellular dysfunction and mental status changes in a patient without previously known liver disease.
   Note: FHF often manifests as a coagulopathy or encephalopathy. Coagulopathy occurs because the liver is not able to adequately produce clotting factors and/or because of platelet destruction. Cerebral edema may lead to encephalopathy of varying severity. Indeed, the duration of time before encephalopathy begins is sometimes used to characterize the severity of FHF. Hypoglycemia, infections, and renal failure are other complications that can arise from FHF.

3. **What is the mechanism of hepatic damage in acetaminophen toxicity?**
   Acetaminophen is oxidized by the cytochrome P-450 system into *N*-acetyl-*p*-benzoquinone imine (NAPQI). NAPQI is toxic to liver cells but is normally detoxified in a phase II reaction by glutathione. If a toxic dose of acetaminophen is ingested, the glutathione supply is depleted, leaving NAPQI to cause liver damage.

4. What is the antidote for acetaminophen toxicity?

It is important to know that all patients who present with FHF should be considered for liver transplant because of high morbidity and mortality. In cases of acetaminophen toxicity, prompt treatment of the overdose reduces the likelihood of need for transplant. In addition to supportive treatment, acetaminophen toxicity should be treated with N-acetylcysteine, the sooner the better. Poisoning severity can be determined by plotting timed serum concentration on the Rumack-Matthew nomogram. Treatment within 8 hours of ingestion is nearly 100% hepatoprotective. Acetylcysteine substitutes for glutathione and detoxifies NAPQI. Activated charcoal should be given if the patient presents within 4 hours after ingestion. The charcoal absorbs toxins such as acetaminophen in the stomach. The effectiveness of activated charcoal drops sharply if more than 1 hour has passed from the time of toxin ingestion.

5. What is the maximum daily dosage of acetaminophen for adults?

The maximum dose for adults is 4 g/day. The maximum dose in patients with liver disease is lower (typically 2 g/day). The maximum dose for children is variable by age. Acetaminophen is an ingredient in many medications, such as cold and flu formulations. Patients may not realize this and can accidentally overdose when using multiple medications.

STEP 1 SECRET

You do not need to know brand names or medication dosages for the USMLE.

6. Why should patients with alcohol use disorder avoid acetaminophen?

Alcohol consumption increases the activity of the enzyme that metabolizes acetaminophen into NAPQI, which, as you know, is hepatotoxic. Chronic alcohol use can also deplete glutathione stores in the liver, thus reducing its protection against damage caused by reactive oxygen species.

7. What other potentially hepatotoxic drugs should you know for the USMLE?

There are far too many potentially hepatotoxic drugs to mention here, but some of the more commonly used ones include the following: amiodarone, amoxicillin, chlorpromazine, ciprofloxacin, erythromycin, fluconazole, isoniazid, methotrexate, methyldopa, statins, niacin, rifampin, salicylates, and valproic acid, as well as several antiretrovirals and anticancer drugs. It is also worth reminding you that many drugs undergo hepatic metabolism and their dosages should be adjusted in patients with liver disease. Always consider drug-induced liver injury (DILI) when faced with a patient who presents with liver failure and extremely high (>1000) hepatic enzymes.

SUMMARY BOX: ACETAMINOPHEN-INDUCED FULMINANT LIVER FAILURE

- Presentation: Nausea and vomiting, abdominal pain (not appearing until >24 hours following ingestion)
- Epidemiology: Most common cause of fulminant hepatic failure (FHF) in the United States
- Diagnosis: It is a diagnosis of exclusion. Expect to see hyperbilirubinemia, elevated transaminases, prolonged pro-thrombin time, acetaminophen level. History of acetaminophen ingestion is important. Liver biopsy may be useful.
- Pathophysiology: Depletion of glutathione supply, resulting in abundance of the toxic metabolite of acetaminophen, *N*-acetyl-*p*-benzoquinone imine (NAPQI)
- Complications: Encephalopathy, hemorrhage (due to coagulopathy), infection, acute kidney injury, metabolic imbalances (namely hypoglycemia), death
- Treatment: Activated charcoal (if identified soon after ingestion) and acetylcysteine; evaluate for liver transplant
- Prognosis: With appropriate therapy, mortality is less than 2% and hepatic failure is less than 4%.

CASE 7.8

A 41-year-old obese mother of four reports nausea, vomiting, fever, and right-sided upper abdominal pain after eating fatty meals. On physical examination, she is not jaundiced, has a temperature of 38.1°C (100.5°F), and experiences sharp pain on inspiration when pressure is applied to the lower edge of her right costal cartilage (Murphy sign). Laboratory tests show a leukocytosis with a left shift.

1. What diagnosis do you suspect?

Cholecystitis (inflammation of the gallbladder), which is usually due to obstruction of the gallbladder neck or cystic duct by a gallstone, is likely. However, other diagnoses such as ascending cholangitis should be considered.

2. What risk factors for gallstones does the patient exhibit?

This classic presentation includes the risk factors that can be remembered as the four **F**'s: **f**emale, **f**at (although not politically correct, this is a useful mnemonic because obesity is a significant risk factor), **f**ertile, **f**orties (age).

3. Why do patients with gallstones experience pain, particularly after eating a high-fat meal?

Entry of fatty acids into the duodenum stimulates the release of cholecystokinin (CCK), which causes gallbladder contraction. This creates pain by increasing biliary pressure against an obstructing stone.

CASE 7.8 CONTINUED:

Ultrasound of the RUQ reveals a distended gallbladder with pericholecystic fluid containing gallstones and also demonstrates a sonographic Murphy sign. She is admitted to the hospital and placed on antibiotics, and a surgery consult is obtained.

4. **What is a sonographic Murphy sign?**

A sonographic Murphy sign is tenderness with pressure from the ultrasound probe directly over where the gallbladder is visualized. This response can be negative in greater than 50% of cases of acute cholecystitis. In contrast, the Murphy sign on physical examination refers to a maneuver in which the physician places the hands below the costal margin at the right midclavicular line (immediately below the level of the gallbladder) after instructing the patient to exhale. The patient is asked to breathe in, and the diaphragm and abdominal contents are shifted downward as the lungs expand. The gallbladder now makes contact with the examiner's hands, which causes the patient to involuntarily stop inspiration if gallbladder disease (e.g., inflammation, gallstones) is present. This is considered a positive Murphy sign. A Murphy sign is not generally positive with cholangitis.

Note: Ultrasound is the imaging of choice to evaluate for gallstones and cholecystitis. It is quick and noninvasive and can be done at the bedside.

CASE 7.8 CONTINUED:

A laparoscopic cholecystectomy is scheduled and carried out without complication during the same hospitalization.

5. **What are the most common types of gallstones?**

Cholesterol monohydrate (80%) and calcium bilirubinate (20%) are most common. Cholesterol stones are generally light in color and radiolucent. Bilirubin stones are black and almost always radiopaque.

Clinical Pearl

Radiolucent substances are difficult to detect on x-ray film because radiant energy, such as x-rays, passes easily through them. The resulting dark spots on an x-ray blend in with the background and are difficult to discern. In contrast, radiopaque substances absorb x-rays and can be visible as light spots or *opacifications* on x-ray.

---

6. **Why does an obstructing stone in the common bile duct predispose to jaundice, whereas a stone in the cystic duct generally does not?**

A stone in the common bile duct (choledocholithiasis) can completely prevent the flow of bile to the intestines (cholestasis), causing biliary backpressure that damages the liver and results in hyperbilirubinemia and jaundice. However, a stone in the cystic duct will only prevent bile from flowing into or out of the gallbladder, leaving bile flow from the liver to the intestines unimpeded (Fig. 7.5).

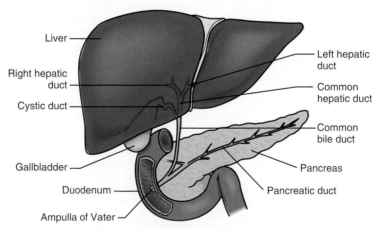

Figure 7.5. Biliary tree anatomy. *(From* Bile Duct Cancer. *American Cancer Society. 2014. Available at: http://www.cancer.org/cancer/bileductcancer/detailedguide/bile-duct-cancer-what-is-bile-duct-cancer.)*

7. **Where in the pancreas would a neoplasm causing obstructive jaundice most likely be located and why?**

It would be in the head of the pancreas. The common bile duct runs through the head of the pancreas on its way to the second part of the duodenum and can get obstructed along the way. The USMLE loves this anatomic relationship between the pancreas and the common bile duct. Note that the classic presentation of pancreatic head masses is one of "painless jaundice" in a patient with malaise and unintentional weight loss.

8. How can cholestasis cause pale stools?

Conjugated bilirubin is normally metabolized to urobilinogen (clear color) by colonic bacteria and ultimately to stercobilin (brown color) via auto-oxidation, which causes the normal stool color. Neither of these processes occurs if bile does not reach the intestines.

9. Define steatorrhea and explain why it can develop from complete obstruction of the common bile duct.

Steatorrhea, typically characterized by tarry, foul-smelling stools, refers to the presence of a significant amount of fat in stool. Bile acids first emulsify fats so that they can be digested by pancreatic lipases and then form micelles of the digested fatty acids before delivering them to the intestinal mucosa for absorption. Consequently, impaired delivery of bile to the intestines interferes with all these processes and causes steatorrhea.

10. What prevents the formation of cholesterol stones in the normal physiologic setting?

Bile salts and phospholipids solubilize cholesterol and prevent it from precipitating out of solution. In fact, for patients with small stones who are poor surgical candidates, oral bile acids are given to facilitate dissolution of the stone. Decreased bile salt and phospholipid concentrations or increased cholesterol concentrations can all lead to stone formation.

11. Why are people with Crohn disease predisposed to the development of cholesterol stones?

Crohn disease often involves the terminal ileum, where bile salts are reabsorbed. Because these salts are important in the solubilization of cholesterol, reduced reabsorption of bile salts in the terminal ileum facilitates stone formation.

12. Which cholesterol-lowering drugs bind bile acids in the intestine? Explain how these drugs lower serum cholesterol.

Cholestyramine and colestipol, which are nonabsorbable ionic resins, bind bile acids in the intestine and are eliminated in the feces, promoting the excretion of bile salts. As a result, more bile acids need to be produced de novo. Because serum cholesterol is used as a substrate for bile acids, bile acid synthesis results in reduced plasma cholesterol. Recall that the formation of bile salts is the only method available to the body to eliminate cholesterol.

13. How can infection with *Clonorchis sinensis* also lead to obstructive jaundice?

This trematode infects the hepatobiliary tree. Chronic inflammation from this infection can cause fibrotic strictures within the bile ducts that impede the egress of bile.

SUMMARY BOX: BILIARY DISEASE

- Terminology:
  - Cholelithiasis: Presence of stones in the gallbladder or cystic duct
  - Cholecystitis: Inflammation of the gallbladder
  - Choledocholithiasis: Stones in the common bile duct
  - Cholangitis: Inflammation of the biliary tree
- Presentation:
  - Cholelithiasis: Generally asymptomatic, can begin to develop biliary colic
  - Cholecystitis: Biliary colic with right upper quadrant (RUQ) pain that can become more persistent, nausea and vomiting, fever
  - Choledocholithiasis: Biliary colic with pain that can become more persistent, nausea and vomiting, fever, mild jaundice
  - Cholangitis: RUQ pain, fever, jaundice (may progress to hypotension and altered mental status)
- Epidemiology: Most gallstones are cholesterol stones. Calcium bilirubinate stones are the next most common type.
- Diagnosis:
  - Ultrasound is the initial imaging of choice for suspected biliary disease.
  - Charcot triad: Fever, RUQ pain, and jaundice; it is associated with acute cholangitis but is present in only about 50% of patients
- Pathophysiology: Formation of stones, generally either cholesterol stones or bilirubin stones, and subsequent obstruction of various parts of the biliary tree by the stones
- Complications: Biliary colic: Ingestion of fatty meals stimulates cholecystokinin (CCK) release. This stimulates gallbladder contraction against an obstructing stone, causing RUQ pain.
- Treatment: Cholecystectomy is the definitive treatment for these conditions. Patients with cholangitis may need to have their common bile duct stented and be stabilized on antibiotics before surgery.
- Prognosis: Excellent if treated in a timely manner. Cholangitis can be fatal if not treated.

CASE 7.9

A mother brings her 4-year-old child into your office and reports that he has been lethargic, sleepy, irritable, and quiet for the past few days. He has also displayed heavy vomiting that has not been relieved by fasting. You ask if the child has been feverish at all. "Not anymore," his mother answers. "He just got over the chickenpox a few days ago and had several high fevers during that time, but we gave him aspirin around the clock and the fevers eventually resolved."

1. **What is the most likely diagnosis?**
   This is a classic presentation of Reye syndrome, which is a rare but serious childhood hepatoencephalopathy. It is associated with salicylate (active ingredient in aspirin) administration in children, especially following viral infection. For this reason, aspirin use is almost never recommended for children. However, a notable exception to this guideline is giving aspirin to decrease risk of coronary artery aneurysm in children with Kawasaki disease.

2. **What is the pathophysiology of Reye syndrome?**
   Aspirin metabolites can reversibly inhibit a mitochondrial enzyme involved in β oxidation of fatty acids, leading to buildup of fatty acids and microvesicular fatty change in the liver. This may induce hepatic damage and disrupt other processes that occur in the liver such as gluconeogenesis, glycogenolysis, and the urea cycle. Clinical manifestations of these disruptions include hypoglycemia and encephalopathy or coma with increased ammonia levels in the blood.

3. **List the components of the postinfectious triad associated with Reye syndrome.**
   Encephalopathy, fatty liver degeneration, and transaminase elevation occur.

SUMMARY BOX: REYE SYNDROME

- Presentation: Vomiting, diarrhea, lethargy, irritability
- Epidemiology: Fewer than two cases per year in the United States. Note: Children should *never* receive aspirin (exception: prevention of coronary artery aneurysm with Kawasaki disease).
- Diagnosis: Diagnosis of exclusion. Must be considered in children with vomiting, altered mental status, and salicylates in blood. Clinical symptoms of Reye syndrome include lethargy, irritability, somnolence, heavy vomiting, and coma.
- Pathophysiology: Aspirin metabolites inhibit β oxidation of fatty acids in the liver, causing hepatocyte damage.
- Complications: Brain herniation, cardiac and respiratory failure, acute renal failure, death
- Treatment: Supportive.
- Prognosis: Mortality is less than 20% if treated appropriately.

ENDOCRINOLOGY

BASIC CONCEPTS

1. **What are the four major classes of chemical signaling?**
   The four major classes of chemical signaling are *endocrine*, *paracrine*, *neurocrine*, and *autocrine* (Fig. 8.1). *Endocrine* secretions (i.e., hormones) affect their target organs at a considerable distance from their site of secretion. Upon release from the cell in which they are produced, these hormones are carried through the bloodstream to other areas of the body, where they induce a response on their target tissue. *Paracrine* secretions act locally on cells and tissues directly adjacent to the cell that produced the signal and have the ability to affect multiple cells at once. Paracrine communication is particularly important in endocrine tissues such as the pancreatic islets, where constant communication between adjacent cells (e.g., α and δ cells) is critical for optimal functioning. *Neurocrine* secretions involve the secretion of peptides into the blood from specialized neurons. Hypothalamic peptides (e.g., thyrotropin-releasing hormone [TRH], gonadotropin-releasing hormones [GnRH], corticotropin-releasing hormone [CRH]) released into the pituitary portal system exemplify this type of signaling. *Autocrine* secretions are secretions from a cell that bind to receptors on that same cell to exert regulatory actions on itself.

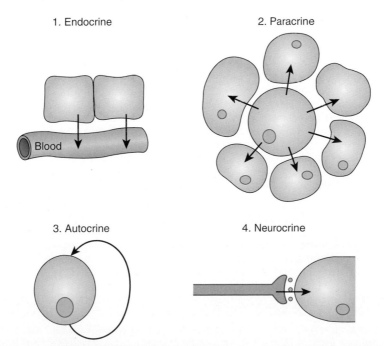

Figure 8.1. The four pathways by which chemical signals are delivered to cells. *(From Meszaros JG, Olson ER, Naugle JE, et al.* Crash Course: Endocrine and Reproductive Systems. *Philadelphia: Mosby; 2006.)*

2. **What is the cellular mechanism of action of the steroid hormones?**
   Steroid hormones are *lipophilic*, which allows them to passively diffuse across the cellular membrane and form complexes with cytosolic and/or nuclear receptors. These bound complexes activate transcriptional mechanisms that alter gene expression and protein translation (Fig. 8.2). Because steroid hormones rely on this intermediary process, it can take hours to days for their effects to manifest. Steroid hormones are created in three primary locations: the *adrenal cortex*, *gonads*, and *placenta*. Examples of steroid hormones include testosterone, estrogen, progesterone, cortisol, and aldosterone, which are all built from *cholesterol*. Although thyroid hormone is not classified as a steroid hormone, it uses the same cellular mechanism as the steroids.

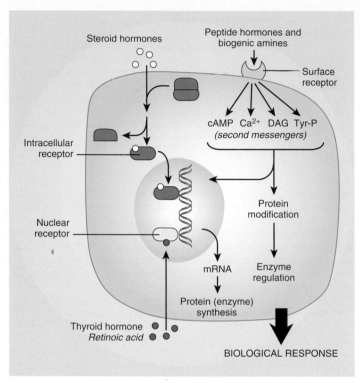

Figure 8.2. Peptide and steroid hormone mechanisms of action. Ca^{2+}, Calcium; *cAMP*, cyclic adenosine monophosphate; *DAG*, diacylglycerol; *mRNA*, messenger RNA; *Tyr-P*, phosphorylated tyrosine residue. *(From Goldman L, Ausiello D. Cecil Textbook of Medicine. 22nd ed. Philadelphia: WB Saunders; 2004.)*

3. **What is the cellular mechanism of action of the peptide hormones and catecholamines?**
   The peptide hormones and catecholamines are not lipophilic and thus *cannot* passively diffuse across the cell membrane. They bind to cell surface receptors and induce a cascade of biochemical events such as activation or inhibition of enzymes, alteration of membrane proteins, and mediation of cellular trafficking (see Fig. 8.2). Unlike the hours to days that it takes for steroid hormones to produce an effect, these processes can occur within seconds to minutes. Peptide hormones can stimulate gene expression as well. Examples of peptide hormones include insulin, parathyroid hormone (PTH), vasopressin (antidiuretic hormone or ADH), and oxytocin. Examples of catecholamines include dopamine, norepinephrine, and epinephrine. Table 8.1 shows a comparison of polypeptide and steroid hormones.

4. **What are the four primary classes of membrane-spanning receptors to which peptide hormones bind?**
   The four primary classes of membrane-spanning receptors to which peptide hormones bind are (1) tyrosine and serine kinase receptors, (2) receptor-linked kinases, (3) G protein–coupled receptors, and (4) ligand-gated ion channels (Fig. 8.3 and Table 8.2). These receptors all have unique intracellular cascades that result in cellular change.

STEP 1 SECRET

Classes of receptors used by various hormones are commonly tested on the USMLE Step 1 exam. We recommend memorizing the information listed in Table 8.2. It is important to know not only which hormones bind to which class of receptors but also the downstream signaling pathways that are ultimately activated or inhibited.

Table 8.1. Comparison of the Different Types of Hormones

	POLYPEPTIDES	STEROIDS
Size	Medium-large	Small
Ability to cross cell membrane	No	Yes
Receptor type	Cell surface	Intracellular
Solubility	Water	Fat
Action	Protein activation	Protein synthesis
Transport in the blood	Dissolved in the plasma	Bound to plasma proteins

From Meszaros JG, Olson ER, Naugle JE, et al. *Crash Course: Endocrine and Reproductive Systems.* Philadelphia: Mosby; 2006.

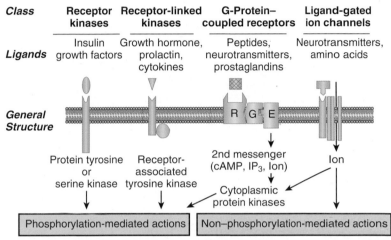

Figure 8.3. The four major classes of membrane receptors for hormones and neurotransmitters. *cAMP,* cyclic Adenosine monophosphate; *E,* effector enzyme; *G,* G protein; *IP₃,* inositol triphosphate; *R,* receptor.

Table 8.2. Classes of Receptors Used by Various Hormones

RECEPTOR CLASS	HORMONES AND RELATED SUBSTANCES
cAMP	LH, FSH, ACTH, TSH, PTH, hCG, CRH, MSH, GHRH, glucagon
cGMP	NO, ANP, BNP
IP₃	GnRH, oxytocin, TRH, angiotensin II
Steroid receptor	Estrogen, testosterone, glucocorticoids, vitamin D, aldosterone, progesterone, T_3/T_4
Tyrosine kinase	Insulin, growth factors (e.g., IGF, PDGF), GH, prolactin

ACTH, Adrenocorticotropic hormone; *ANP,* atrial natriuretic peptide; *BNP,* brain natriuretic peptide; *cAMP,* cyclic adenosine monophosphate; *cGMP,* cyclic guanosine monophosphate; *CRH,* corticotropin-releasing hormone; *FSH,* follicle-stimulating hormone; *GH,* growth hormone; *GHRH,* growth hormone–releasing hormone; *GnRH,* gonadotropin-releasing hormone; *hCG,* human chorionic gonadotropin; *IGF,* insulin-like growth factor; *IP₃,* inositol triphosphate; *LH,* luteinizing hormone; *MSH,* melanocyte-stimulating hormone; *NO,* nitric oxide; *PDGF,* platelet-derived growth factor; *PTH,* parathyroid hormone; *T₃,* triiodothyronine; *T₄,* thyroxine; *TRH,* thyrotropin-releasing hormone; *TSH,* thyroid-stimulating hormone.

5. How do tyrosine kinase receptors transmit their messages?
As depicted in Fig. 8.4, the binding of a peptide hormone to the extracellular domain of a tyrosine kinase receptor initiates a signal transduction cascade by promoting autophosphorylation of the kinase receptor and subsequent phosphorylation of downstream target proteins, thereby activating or inhibiting these proteins. Examples of tyrosine kinase receptors include the insulin receptor and several receptors involved in the development of cancer (e.g., RET, ROS).

6. How do ligand-gated ion channels work?
Activation of ligand-gated ion channels results in an influx (or efflux) of ions into (or out of) the cell. The nicotinic acetylcholine receptor on skeletal muscle is an example of such a receptor. Binding of acetylcholine to this receptor results in an influx of principally sodium ions into the cell.

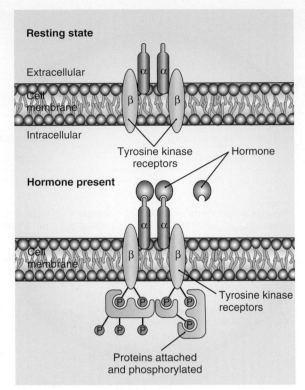

Figure 8.4. Mechanism of activation of a tyrosine kinase receptor. *(From Meszaros JG, Olson ER, Naugle JE, et al.* Crash Course: Endocrine and Reproductive Systems. *Philadelphia, Mosby; 2006.)*

7. How do G proteins transmit their signals?

The binding of a hormone (or other receptor agonist) to G protein–coupled receptors (GPCRs) induces a conformational change that causes a trimeric subunit complex (designated α-β-γ) to act. There are three types of GPCRs: G_s, G_i, and G_q. For all three classes, the G_α subunit exchanges guanosine diphosphate (GDP) for guanosine triphosphate (GTP), signaling the trimer to separate. The dissociated G_β and G_γ subunits then activate or inhibit enzymes (adenylyl cyclase, phospholipase) and ion channels (Ca^{2+} channels) according to two distinct pathways: the cyclic adenosine monophosphate (cAMP) pathway and the phosphatidylinositol (IP_3/DAG) pathway (Fig. 8.5). G-protein-linked messengers influence both the sympathetic and parasympathetic systems, along with dopamine, histamine, vasopressin, and various other agonists.

Note: Adenylyl cyclase synthesizes cAMP from adenosine triphosphate (ATP), which then activates various target proteins. As the subscript suggests, G_s receptors *stimulate* adenylyl cyclase, whereas G_i receptors *inhibit* adenylyl cyclase. G_q acts through a completely different enzyme cascade, exerting its effects through the IP_3/DAG pathway.

STEP 1 SECRET

G proteins are an incredibly high yield topic on the USMLE Step 1 exam. Study the pathways for G_s, G_i, and G_q signaling depicted in Fig. 8.5. You should know the details of these pathways, including the predominant cellular changes that occur with activation of each protein (e.g., cyclic adenosine monophosphate [cAMP] increases with G_s activation, cyclic adenosine monophosphate [cAMP] decreases with Gi activation, and intracellular [Ca^{2+}] increases with G_q activation). Connect this information to Table 8.2 to understand which specific G protein pathways are used by major hormones and receptor agonists.

---

8. Why is the total serum hormone level not an accurate reflection of hormone activity?

Many of the hormones found in the serum are inactive because they are attached to serum binding proteins. It is only the *free* hormone that is biologically active. Another important factor that affects hormone activity is the concentration of cellular hormone receptors available for binding each specific hormone and mediating its action.

9. Describe the concepts of positive and negative feedback. What is a feedback loop?

Hormone synthesis and release are governed at multiple levels. Hormone synthesis/release from an organ of interest typically involves regulation by a pituitary hormone, which itself is regulated by a hypothalamic hormone. This general pathway structure is commonly referred to as a *hypothalamic-pituitary axis (HP axis). Positive feedback* occurs when a

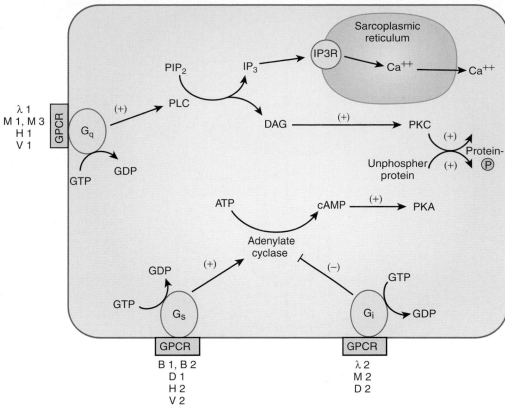

Figure 8.5. Signal transduction by G proteins. G protein–coupled receptors bind to various extracellular ligands that activate intracellular signal transduction cascades, leading to activation (G_s) or inhibition (G_i) of the cAMP signal pathway, as well as activation of the phosphatidylinositol signal pathway (G_q). Downstream effector molecule activation may stimulate release of intracellular calcium from the sarcoplasmic reticulum or promote activation of protein kinases, the latter of which influence the activity of a variety of enzymes that orchestrate cellular metabolism and function. α, Alpha GPCR; ATP, adenosine trisphosphate; β, beta GPCR; *cAMP*, cyclic adenosine monophosphate; *D*, dopamine GPCR; *DAG*, diacylglycerol; *GDP*, guanosine diphosphate; G_i, G_i protein; *GPCR*, G protein–coupled receptor; G_q, G_q protein; G_s, G_s protein; *GTP*, guanosine triphosphate; *H*, histamine GPCR; IP_3, inositol 1,4,5-trisphosphate; *IP3R*, inositol 1,4,5-trisphosphate receptor; *M*, muscarinic GPCR; *P*, phosphorylated protein; PIP_2, phosphatidylinositol 4,5 bisphosphate; *PKA*, protein kinase A; *PKC*, protein kinase C; *V*, vasopressin GPCR.

downstream product increases/accelerates the production of an upstream reactant, while *negative feedback* occurs when a downstream product reduces/inhibits the production of an upstream reactant. Although most physiologic processes utilize negative feedback in regulation, positive feedback does occur in ovulation, lactation, and with contractions during childbirth. Regulation can occur at the level of the organ, pituitary, or hypothalamus—termed *primary, secondary,* and *tertiary regulation,* respectively. The general schematic for regulation using the thyroid hormone axis as an example is shown in Fig. 8.6.

CASE 8.1

A 38-year-old woman arrives in the emergency department reporting nausea, lethargy, dizziness, diarrhea, and vomiting. One month ago, she had a complication during cesarean section delivery that left her in hemorrhagic shock. Fortunately, she was able to deliver successfully. Physical examination is unremarkable except for sparse axillary and pubic hair and depigmentation of both areolae. She also mentions that she has trouble lactating. A pituitary hormone panel shows global hypopituitarism. A magnetic resonance imaging (MRI) scan of the brain shows an empty sella turcica.

1. What is the diagnosis?
   The diagnosis is Sheehan syndrome (or postpartum pituitary gland necrosis) caused by ischemic infarction of the anterior pituitary gland. This results in a postpartum hypopituitarism that affects all of the downstream organs that rely on the hormones released by the anterior pituitary gland to properly function.

2. Why is the anterior pituitary gland more susceptible to infarction in postpartum hemorrhage than in hemorrhagic shock unrelated to pregnancy?
   During pregnancy, there is hyperplasia of the lactotrophs (prolactin-secreting cells) in the anterior pituitary gland without a proportional increase in the blood supply. As a result, decreased blood supply to the anterior pituitary gland after postpartum hemorrhage is inadequate in perfusing the hyperplastic lactotrophs, causing infarction and necrosis.

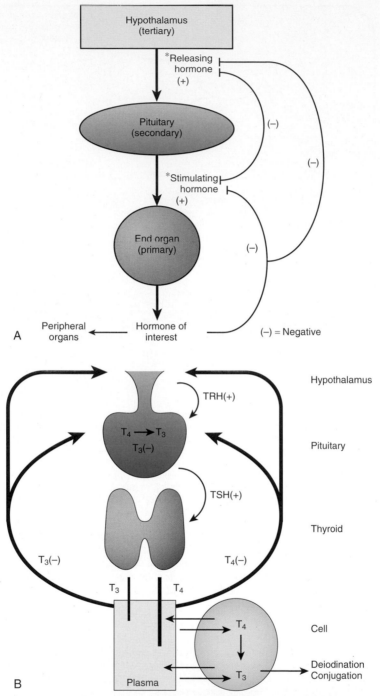

Figure 8.6. Hypothalamic-pituitary-end organ (HPO) axis and feedback loops. A, Normal hormonal physiology. Release of hormones of interest by end organs (e.g., thyroid, gonads, adrenal gland) is influenced by production of stimulatory hormones by the pituitary gland and hypothalamus. Hormones produced by the HPO axis regulate their own release by decreasing production of upstream hormones when downstream hormones are present in sufficient quantities, a concept referred to as *negative feedback*. Dysfunction of the end organ in producing hormone is referred to as a *primary problem*, while dysfunction at the level of the pituitary gland or hypothalamus is referred to as a *secondary* or *tertiary* problem, respectively. *Hormones secreted from the hypothalamus and pituitary gland are *often but not always* referred to as *releasing hormones* and *stimulating hormones*, respectively. B, Thyroid hormone release as an example of normal hormone physiology. Under normal conditions, thyrotropin-releasing hormone (TRH) is released from the hypothalamus, which causes the release of thyroid-stimulating hormone (TSH) from the anterior pituitary. TSH then causes the thyroid gland to release triiodothyronine (T_3) and thyroxine (T_4), which act on various peripheral organs. T_3 and T_4 also regulate TSH and TRH secretion through negative feedback mechanisms. In *primary* hypothyroidism (i.e., due to *thyroid* dysfunction), production of T_3 and T_4 is low, leading to lack of negative feedback on the pituitary gland, which ultimately results in elevated TSH levels as the pituitary unsuccessfully attempts to stimulate adequate T_3 and T_4 production. In *secondary* hypothyroidism (i.e., due to *pituitary* dysfunction), production of TSH is low, resulting in insufficient production (and therefore low serum levels) of T_3 and T_4. *(From Goldman L, Ausiello D.* Cecil Textbook of Medicine. *22nd ed. Philadelphia: WB Saunders; 2004.)*

3. Why is the posterior pituitary typically spared in Sheehan syndrome?

The posterior pituitary gland (neurohypophysis) is typically spared in Sheehan syndrome because it differs in embryologic origin from the anterior pituitary gland and therefore has a different blood supply. Remember, the embryologic origin of the anterior pituitary is the *Rathke pouch* (an endodermal evagination from the roof of the mouth), whereas the posterior pituitary is derived from a ventral outgrowth from the primitive hypothalamus. Table 8.3 reviews the functions of the posterior pituitary hormones.

Table 8.3. Hormones Secreted by the Posterior Pituitary

HORMONE	SYNTHESIZED BY	STIMULATED BY	INHIBITED BY	TARGET ORGAN	EFFECT
ADH	Supraoptic vasopressinergic neurons	Raised osmolarity; low blood volume	Low osmolarity	Kidney	Increases permeability of the late distal tubule and collecting duct to reabsorb water
Oxytocin	Paraventricular oxytocinergic neurons	Stretch receptors in the nipple and cervix; estrogen	Stress	Uterus and mammary glands	Smooth muscle contraction leading to birth or milk ejection

ADH, Antidiuretic hormone.
From Meszaros JG, Olson ER, Naugle JE, et al. *Crash Course: Endocrine and Reproductive Systems*. Philadelphia: Mosby; 2006.

4. Secretion of which pituitary hormones may be affected in this woman?

The hormones secreted by the anterior pituitary include **f**ollicle-stimulating hormone (FSH), **l**uteinizing hormone (LH), **a**drenocorticotropic hormone (ACTH), **t**hyroid-stimulating hormone (TSH), **p**rolactin, **e**ndorphins, and **g**rowth hormone (GH). **FLAT PEG** is a useful mnemonic to remember these hormones. **Note**: The *basophilic* hormones can be remembered easily with the mnemonic **B-FLAT**: **b**asophilic-**F**SH, **L**H, **A**CTH, **T**SH. The acidophilic hormones are therefore prolactin and GH.

Depending on the extent of the infarction, some to all of the anterior pituitary hormones may be affected (Fig. 8.7). This patient has trouble lactating, which is consistent with decreased prolactin secretion. Whenever you see a patient who is unable to lactate shortly after delivery, consider Sheehan syndrome. Her axillary and pubic hair is sparse because of decreased gonadotropin (FSH, LH) secretion causing decreased androstenedione production by *theca* cells, which ultimately decreases testosterone production. The hair follicles have 5α-reductase activity to convert testosterone to dihydrotestosterone (DHT), which is important for axillary and pubic hair growth. However, because there is less testosterone to begin with, less DHT will be made, which explains her sparse axillary hair and pubic hair. Furthermore, the patient is also weak and lethargic, which is consistent with hypocortisolism (due to decreased ACTH secretion), as well as secondary hypothyroidism (due to decreased TSH secretion).

5. Why may hypothalamic hormone secretion increase following an infarction of the anterior pituitary?

The loss of anterior pituitary hormone secretion alters the negative feedback loop that is usually in place (see Fig. 8.6). This *disinhibits* the hypothalamus, often leading to unregulated increases in hypothalamic hormone production. Table 8.4 reviews the functions of the anterior pituitary hormones.

6. Why would not hypothalamic dopamine secretion be elevated following an anterior pituitary infarction?

In contrast with the other hypothalamic hormones, dopamine primarily exerts inhibitory effects and functions to reduce the anterior pituitary secretion of prolactin. When prolactin production decreases secondary to anterior pituitary infarction, the resulting hypoprolactinemia leads to a decrease in hypothalamic dopamine production as well.

SUMMARY BOX: SHEEHAN SYNDROME

- Epidemiology: Postpartum women who experienced excessive bleeding during delivery
- Symptoms: Agalactorrhea, amenorrhea after delivery, loss of pubic and axillary hair, symptoms of secondary hypothyroidism and adrenal insufficiency (e.g., weakness, fatigue, and low blood pressure)
- Pathophysiology: Infarction of the anterior pituitary leading to necrosis and panhypopituitarism
- Diagnosis: Blood tests to measure anterior pituitary hormone levels including **f**ollicle-stimulating hormone (FSH), **l**uteinizing hormone (LH), **a**drenocorticotropic hormone (ACTH), **t**hyroid-stimulating hormone (TSH), **p**rolactin, **e**ndorphins (which share POMC origin with ACTH and MSH), and **g**rowth hormone (GH). Remember these with the acronym **FLAT PEG.**
- Treatment: Lifelong replacement therapy of estrogen, progesterone, thyroid, and adrenal hormones

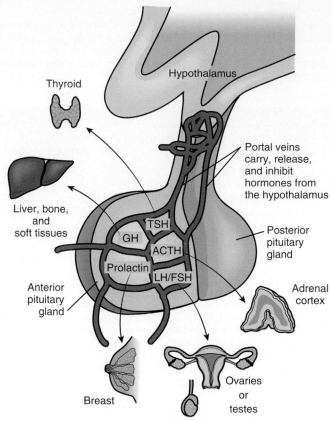

Figure 8.7. Hormones of the anterior pituitary gland and their respective target organs. *ACTH,* Adrenocorticotropic hormone; *FSH,* follicle-stimulating hormone; *GH,* growth hormone; *LH,* luteinizing hormone; *TSH,* thyroid-stimulating hormone.

Table 8.4. Hormones Synthesized and Secreted by the Anterior Pituitary

HORMONE	SYNTHESIZED BY	STIMULATED BY	INHIBITED BY	TARGET ORGAN	EFFECT
GH	Somatotrophs	GHRH	GHIH and IGF-1	Liver	Stimulates IGF-1 production and opposes insulin
TSH	Thyrotrophs	TRH	T_3	Thyroid gland	Stimulates thyroxine release
ACTH	Corticotrophs	CRH	Glucocorticoids	Adrenal cortex	Stimulates glucocorticoid and androgen release
LH + FSH	Gonadotrophs	GnRH, sex steroids	Prolactin, sex steroids	Reproductive organs	Release of sex steroids
Prolactin	Lactotrophs	PRH and TRH	Dopamine	Mammary glands and reproductive organs	Promotes growth of these organs and initiates lactation
MSH	Corticotrophs	—	—	Melanocytes in skin	Stimulates melanin synthesis

ACTH, Adrenocorticotropic hormone; *CRH,* corticotropin-releasing hormone; *FSH,* follicle-stimulating hormone; *GH,* growth hormone; *GHIH,* growth hormone–inhibiting hormone; *GHRH,* growth hormone–releasing hormone; *GnRH,* gonadotropin-releasing hormone; *IGF,* insulin-like growth factor; *LH,* luteinizing hormone; *MSH,* melanocyte-stimulating hormone; *PRH,* prolactin-releasing hormone; T_3, triiodothyronine; *TRH,* thyrotropin-releasing hormone; *TSH,* thyroid-stimulating hormone.
From Meszaros JG, Olson ER, Naugle JE, et al. *Crash Course: Endocrine and Reproductive Systems.* Philadelphia: Mosby; 2006.

CASE 8.2

A 32-year-old woman reports bumping into things often and bilateral milky nipple discharge (galactorrhea). She has not had her menses for the past 9 months and is worried about her milky nipple discharge and amenorrhea despite repeated negative home pregnancy tests. She denies any history of mental illness or treatment with neuroleptic (antipsychotic) medication. Laboratory workup confirms that she is not pregnant, but her serum prolactin level is significantly elevated. MRI scan of the brain reveals a mass in the sella turcica.

1. What is the diagnosis?

   This patient can be diagnosed with a *prolactinoma*. A prolactinoma is a pituitary adenoma caused by hyperplasia of lactotrophs; it is the most common type of hypersecreting pituitary adenoma. Table 8.5 reviews pituitary adenomas.

Table 8.5. Disorders Caused by the Deficiency or Excess of Anterior Pituitary Hormones

HORMONE	DEFICIENCY	EXCESS
GH	Dwarfism in children or adults GH deficiency syndrome	Gigantism in children, acromegaly in adults
LH and FSH	Gonadal insufficiency (decreased sex steroids)	Extremely rare but causes infertility
ACTH	Adrenocortical insufficiency (decreased cortisol and adrenal androgens)	Cushing disease (increased cortisol and adrenal androgens)
TSH	Hypothyroidism (decreased thyroid hormones)	Extremely rare but causes hyperthyroidism (increased thyroid hormones)
Prolactin	Hypoprolactinemia (failure in postpartum lactation)	Hyperprolactinemia (impotence in males, amenorrhea in females, and decreased libido)

ACTH, Adrenocorticotropic hormone; *FSH,* follicle-stimulating hormone; *GH,* growth hormone; *LH,* luteinizing hormone; *TSH,* thyroid-stimulating hormone.
From Meszaros JG, Olson ER, Naugle JE, et al. *Crash Course: Endocrine and Reproductive Systems.* Philadelphia: Mosby; 2006.

2. Why is this patient frequently bumping into things?

   Growth of the anterior pituitary causes compression of the optic chiasm, leading to *bitemporal hemianopsia*, which compromises her peripheral vision.

3. What are the normal physiologic functions of prolactin preceding, during, and following pregnancy?

   Preceding pregnancy: Prolactin levels are normal because of tonic hypothalamic inhibition by dopamine in the tuberoinfundibular pathway. During puberty, prolactin promotes the development of the mammary ducts.

   During pregnancy: Prolactin levels are high secondary to high estrogen levels (e.g., estriol secreted by the placenta), which stimulate breast maturation and lactogenesis. However, actual lactation is prevented by high estrogen and progesterone, which downregulate prolactin receptors.

   Following pregnancy: At parturition, estrogen and progesterone levels drop, disinhibiting the prolactin receptors and allowing the high level of serum prolactin to initiate lactation. The baby's suckling action is necessary to maintain the prolactin level and milk production. Prolactin will also inhibit GnRH secretion by negative feedback on the hypothalamus, leading to decreased levels of LH/FSH and ultimately leading to anovulation. Fig. 8.8 outlines the other physiologic functions of prolactin.

4. Why does this patient have galactorrhea, whereas pregnant women with similar levels of serum prolactin generally do not have this problem?

   Although prolactin stimulates milk production, the high concentrations of estrogen and progesterone that are present during pregnancy downregulate prolactin receptors, which prevents the galactorrhea that is experienced by nonpregnant patients. In contrast, this patient has hyperprolactinemia in the absence of elevated levels of estrogen and progesterone, which leads to galactorrhea.

   Note: Milk letdown occurs after childbirth because the placenta secretes large amounts of estrogen and progesterone during pregnancy. Levels of both hormones decrease once this structure is expelled after delivery. Additionally, oxytocin is secreted in response to suckling, which stimulates contraction of myoepithelial cells around the glandular tissue of the breast and ultimately leads to milk ejection.

5. Hyperprolactinemia can also occur in men. What symptoms might be expected in men?

   In men, inhibition of GnRH secretion by prolactin decreases gonadotropin (i.e., LH and FSH) production, resulting in loss of testosterone production by Leydig cells. This can cause decreased libido, erectile dysfunction, generalized malaise, and depression. Notably, galactorrhea can also rarely occur in men in response to certain stimuli, such as severe stress and prolonged starvation.

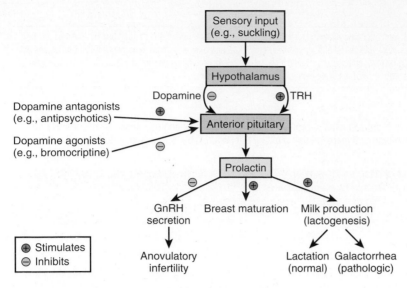

Figure 8.8. Physiologic actions of prolactin. *GnRH,* Gonadotropin-releasing hormone; *TRH,* thyrotropin-releasing hormone. *(From Brown TA. Rapid Review Physiology. Philadelphia: Mosby; 2007.)*

6. How does elevated prolactin prevent pregnancy (i.e., what is the mechanism of infertility and amenorrhea in this patient)?
   Prolactin inhibits the hypothalamic release of GnRH, which decreases FSH and LH secretion from the anterior pituitary. The consequent reduction of FSH and LH eliminates the ovulatory cycle, resulting in infertility and amenorrhea.

7. Why is it clinically relevant to ask this patient about a history of schizophrenia and the use of antipsychotic medications?
   Several antipsychotics (particularly typical antipsychotics such as haloperidol and chlorpromazine) can cause hyperprolactinemia. Recall that antipsychotic agents are dopamine antagonists and that hypothalamic dopamine is the major inhibitor of pituitary prolactin secretion, meaning the dopamine antagonism mediated by antipsychotic medications may indirectly result in increased serum prolactin levels.

8. What is the mechanistic basis for using bromocriptine in the treatment of a prolactinoma?
   Bromocriptine is a dopamine agonist that inhibits prolactin secretion by the anterior pituitary. This drug may even shrink the prolactinoma, making it easier to remove when surgery is performed.

9. How can head trauma with a severed pituitary stalk increase prolactin secretion (assuming the anterior pituitary itself was not damaged)?
   This can increase prolactin secretion by disrupting the tuberoinfundibular pathway, which runs from the hypothalamus through the pituitary stalk and is the source of dopamine. If the tuberoinfundibular pathway is damaged, dopamine is not able to reach the lactotrophs to inhibit prolactin secretion.
   Note: Plasma levels of all other anterior pituitary hormones (e.g., TSH, ACTH) will decrease with a severed pituitary stalk; prolactin is the only one that will increase because dopaminergic inhibition is lost.

STEP 1 SECRET

Be sure to understand the concept of tuberoinfundibular pathway disruption. It is especially important for you to know that the secretion of all anterior pituitary hormones (see Table 8.4) will decrease except for prolactin, which increases.

10. Why does hypothyroidism need to be considered in the evaluation of hyperprolactinemia?
    Hypothalamic TRH stimulates the secretion of both TSH and prolactin by the anterior pituitary. Because hypothyroidism causes elevated levels of TRH as a result of decreased negative feedback, it should be ruled out as a potential cause of hyperprolactinemia.

SUMMARY BOX: PROLACTINOMA AND HYPERPROLACTINEMIA

- Epidemiology: Prolactinomas are the most common type of pituitary tumor, usually occurring in women between 20 and 50 years old.
- Symptoms: Galactorrhea, decreased menstruation, and infertility as a result of inhibition of gonadotropin-releasing hormone (GnRH) secretion

- Pathophysiology: Prolactin-secreting pituitary adenoma
- Diagnosis: Magnetic resonance imaging (MRI) of the head and high levels of serum prolactin
- Treatment: Dopamine agonists (e.g., bromocriptine) for small adenomas; transsphenoidal resection of the pituitary adenoma for larger adenomas
- Complications: Bitemporal hemianopsia resulting from the compression of the optic chiasm; panhypopituitarism resulting from increased pressure on the normal pituitary gland; bone loss with reduced production of estrogen and testosterone; galactorrhea; reduced fertility

CASE 8.3

A 38-year-old man presents reporting fatigue from lack of sleep and joint pains in his hands and jaw. In the past 6 months, he has been involved in two car accidents despite previously never having been involved in an accident. He mentions that he "just didn't see the other car approaching." In addition, he reports of a constant headache but is unsure if it is related to the accidents. Given the suspected diagnosis, specialized testing is performed in which serum insulin-like growth factor 1 (IGF-1) levels are found to be elevated. To confirm the diagnosis, GH levels are measured following administration of an oral glucose load. No measurable decrease of GH is seen following the glucose load. Given the above results, an MRI scan of the brain is performed.

1. **What is the likely diagnosis?**
   Acromegaly (from the Greek roots *akros* [extremities] and *megalos* [large]: *large extremities*) is the most likely diagnosis, caused by a GH-secreting tumor of the anterior pituitary. Because the long bones have stopped growing due to closure of epiphyseal plates during puberty, GH is only able to stimulate cartilage and membranous bones to grow, resulting in gross deformities. The bones that are most commonly deformed include hands (metacarpals and phalanges), feet (metatarsals), and mandible (producing wide-spaced teeth). It most commonly affects middle-aged adults.
   Note: One good way to diagnose this disorder is to look at an old driver's license of the patient and compare it with the patient's current appearance. Because the physical changes progress subtly over decades, family members and friends often do not notice them. Also, patients will likely report tightening rings and that their shoes no longer fit because of the deformities of the hands and feet.

2. **What is likely to be seen on the MRI scan of the brain?**
   A mass is likely to be seen in the sella turcica (the space where the pituitary sits). This mass is a pituitary adenoma constitutively secreting GH.

3. **Why is hyperglycemia commonly associated with acromegaly?**
   GH promotes hepatic gluconeogenesis, resulting in increased serum glucose levels. This release in response to decreasing blood glucose concentration is one of the body's mechanisms for preventing hypoglycemia. The elevation of blood glucose can be significant enough in acromegaly that many of these patients will develop diabetes mellitus during their lifetime. In normal individuals, an oral glucose tolerance test will cause almost complete suppression of GH secretion, but it will *not* suppress GH secretion in patients with acromegaly.

4. **What are the normal physiologic functions of GH, and how is its secretion regulated?**
   GH secretion occurs primarily at night and in response to various stressors such as starvation and hypoglycemia. While fasting, GH is released and promotes lipolysis in adipocytes to release fats into the blood and increases gluconeogenesis in the liver to provide glucose to the brain. Within the liver, GH also promotes expression of IGF-1 via the Janus kinase/signal transducers and activators of transcription (JAK/STAT) signaling pathway. IGF-1 promotes bone, organ, and muscle growth. GH levels are often elevated after a protein-rich meal. The IGF-1 released from hepatocytes is important for cellular amino acid uptake.
   GH secretion is inhibited by somatostatin, high glucose levels, emotional stress, illness, malnutrition, obesity, glucocorticoids, and decreased thyroid hormone. Triiodothyronine (T_3) is required for normal function of GH.

5. **Given the normal physiology of GH, how can we explain this patient's presentation?**
   The enlarged mass in the sella turcica is explained by a pituitary adenoma composed of proliferating *somatotrophs*. This mass presses upon the optic chiasm, causing the patient's bitemporal hemianopsia and headache. Joint pain is due to tissue growth caused by the anabolic effect of GH. His fatigue may be due to macroglossia causing sleep apnea.
   Note: Most of the metabolic effects of GH are mediated through IGF-1. IGF-1 acts on bone to stimulate linear and lateral bone growth and also promotes the growth of cartilage and other soft tissues (Fig. 8.9).

6. **Why is octreotide useful in the treatment of acromegaly?**
   Octreotide is useful in the treatment of acromegaly because it is a somatostatin analog. Somatostatin is a peptide hormone secreted by the hypothalamus that inhibits GH secretion by the anterior pituitary.
   Note: Somatostatin is also synthesized by pancreatic islet cells (specifically the δ cells) and gastric mucosa. Somatostatin inhibits intestinal activity and gastrointestinal motility.

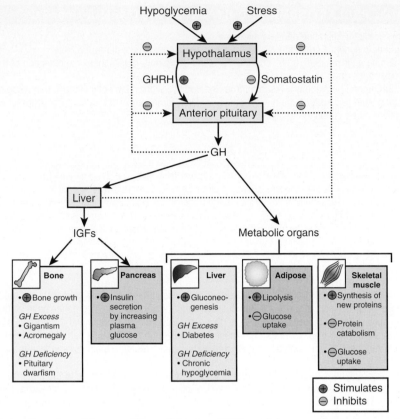

Figure 8.9. Physiologic actions of growth hormone. GH, growth hormone; GHRH, growth hormone–releasing hormone; IGFs, insulin-like growth factors. *(From Brown TA. Rapid Review Physiology. Philadelphia: Mosby; 2007.)*

7. **What is the difference between gigantism and acromegaly?**
   The fundamental difference between gigantism and acromegaly is whether the GH-secreting pituitary adenoma developed before or after puberty (i.e., closure of the epiphyseal growth plates). Excess GH stimulates uninhibited and proportional bone growth if the GH-secreting adenoma develops *before* the epiphyseal growth plates have fused, causing patients to grow to extreme heights known as *gigantism*. In contrast, acromegaly occurs when the GH-secreting adenoma develops *after* the epiphyseal growth plates have fused, leading to disproportionate changes in the hands, feet, brow, and jaw.

8. **What growth abnormality results from deficient secretion of GH during adolescence?**
   Short stature results from growth hormone deficiency (GHD).
   Note: The short stature caused by GHD is proportional (i.e., the limbs and trunk are of normal relative proportions), as opposed to the comparatively shorter limbs characteristic of short stature caused by *achondroplasia*. Of note, achondroplasia is most often caused by a spontaneous mutation of the fibroblast growth factor receptor gene 3 (*FGFR3*), which inhibits bone growth because cartilage is unable to develop into bone without FGFR3.

SUMMARY BOX: ACROMEGALY AND PHYSIOLOGY OF GROWTH HORMONE

- Epidemiology: Slow-growing tumor that is typically recognized in middle-aged patients
- Symptoms: Macrognathia (large jaw), macroglossia (large tongue), sleep apnea, coarsening of facial features, enlarged hands and skull, diabetes mellitus, and organomegaly
- Pathophysiology: Growth hormone (GH)-hypersecreting pituitary adenoma
- Diagnosis: Magnetic resonance image (MRI) of the brain showing mass in the sella turcica, elevated serum GH levels that are not suppressed by an oral glucose load, and elevated serum levels of insulin-like growth factor 1 (IGF-1)
- Laboratory tests: Serum IGF-1 level, oral glucose tolerance test, MRI of the brain
- Treatment: Transsphenoidal resection of the pituitary adenoma
- Complications: Arthralgias, diabetes mellitus, carpal tunnel syndrome, bitemporal hemianopsia, headache (due to mass effect), sleep apnea from macroglossia, hypertension, cardiomegaly

CASE 8.4

A 35-year-old woman has experienced fatigue, weakness, and hip pain for approximately 6 months. During this time, she has not had her menstrual cycle. She notes that her voice sounds deeper than usual. On physical examination, she appears moderately obese (with primarily a central distribution) and has a puffy face. No facial hair can be appreciated, but she does admit to shaving on a regular basis. Physical examination also reveals other notable findings such as a blood pressure of 165/100 mm Hg; darkening of the skin around her neck and axillae (i.e., acanthosis nigricans); purple striae over the breasts, abdomen, and thighs; and proximal muscle weakness. Laboratory tests show hyperglycemia and an elevated random serum cortisol level.

1. **What are the general causes of the hormonal abnormality most likely present in this woman?**
   This woman has hypercortisolism (Cushing syndrome), as indicated by her symptoms (muscle weakness, amenorrhea, deepening voice), classic examination findings (central obesity, abdominal striae, buffalo hump, acanthosis nigricans), and laboratory findings (hyperglycemia, elevated random serum cortisol). These sequelae can be explained by a pathologically elevated serum cortisol level.
   The most common cause of Cushing syndrome is the iatrogenic administration of glucocorticoids for inflammatory conditions. Other causes include a cortisol-hypersecreting adrenal adenoma (common) or carcinoma (rare), ACTH-secreting pituitary adenoma (i.e., Cushing disease), and ectopic paraneoplastic secretion by small cell carcinoma in the lung. The hirsutism and deepening voice in this patient are suggestive of an ACTH-dependent cause of Cushing syndrome, in which shunting of glucocorticoid precursors into the androgenic pathway causes imbalances in androgen and estrogen levels.
   A good way to distinguish Cushing syndrome from polycystic ovarian syndrome (PCOS) on the USMLE is to look for the mention of abdominal striae. This will most certainly be present on patients with Cushing syndrome but is unlikely to occur in a question stem describing a patient with PCOS.

CASE 8.4 CONTINUED:

Further workup shows elevated 11 p.m. salivary cortisol and plasma ACTH levels, both of which suppress moderately in response to the administration of high-dose dexamethasone.

2. **Why is the salivary cortisol level collected at nighttime?**
   Cortisol is naturally at its lowest level at nighttime, so elevated levels at night suggests that the etiology could be due to Cushing syndrome. The late evening cortisol is usually collected at 11 p.m. or midnight.

3. **What is the cause of the hypercortisolism in this patient?**
   Cushing *disease* is the elevation of cortisol by an ACTH-secreting pituitary adenoma. One would expect low serum ACTH levels if the adrenal glands were hypersecreting cortisol, as in Cushing *syndrome* (due to increased negative feedback actions of cortisol). Paraneoplastic ACTH secretion (i.e., small cell carcinoma) is suggested by an increased serum ACTH level, but ectopic ACTH secretion occurs independently of the HPA (hypothalamic-pituitary-adrenal) axis and therefore is *not* suppressed in response to glucocorticoids such as dexamethasone.
   In contrast, pituitary adenomas typically retain *some* feedback responsiveness to glucocorticoids. ACTH secretion may not suppress with low-dose dexamethasone, but it typically will with high-dose dexamethasone (Table 8.6).

Table 8.6. Features of Cushing Syndrome

	ACTH	CORTISOL	RESULTS OF DEXAMETHASONE SUPPRESSION TEST ON PLASMA CORTISOL
Cushing disease	High	High	High dose lowers cortisol
Ectopic ACTH production	High	High	No effect
Adrenal adenoma/carcinoma	Low	High	No effect
Iatrogenic	Low	High	No effect

ACTH, Adrenocorticotropic hormone.

4. **Why are the results of a dexamethasone suppression test read at a specific time of day?**
   Cortisol secretion has a wide circadian rhythm, with plasma levels varying several-fold throughout a 24-hour period (normal range 5–20 μg/dL) and peaking in the morning hours. The morning upsurge is preceded by an upsurge in ACTH before waking, so ACTH levels should also be measured at a specific time (usually 5 a.m.).

5. **Why has hirsutism developed in this woman?**
   Hirsutism is the presence of excess facial and body hair in women, especially in a male pattern. This typically indicates elevated androgens as a result of increased levels of ACTH, which in addition to stimulating cortisol synthesis also

promotes shunting of glucocorticoid precursors to the androgen pathway. Recall that cortisol is produced in the *zona fasciculata* of the adrenal glands, while androgens are produced in the *zona reticularis*.

6. **What is the mechanism behind this patient's acanthosis nigricans?**
   The precursor to ACTH is a protein called *POMC* (proopiomelanocortin). POMC is cleaved into ACTH, β-MSH (melanocyte-stimulating hormone), and β-endorphin. Along with the increase in ACTH, there is a concordant increase in β-MSH that stimulates the production of melanin, causing the darkening skin pigmentation that defines acanthosis nigricans.

7. **Why is hyperaldosteronism not typically seen in Cushing disease?**
   Although aldosterone is secreted by the adrenal cortex (specifically the *zona glomerulosa*), its synthesis and secretion are only minimally influenced by ACTH levels. Rather, the principal regulators of aldosterone secretion are angiotensin II (via the renin-angiotensin system) and serum potassium levels.

8. **What morphologic feature of the adrenal glands would you expect to see in this woman?**
   Bilateral adrenal *hyperplasia* (with widening of both the zona fasciculata and zona reticularis, specifically) is typically seen because ACTH is trophic (i.e., a stimulator for growth) for the adrenal glands. This feature is also present in ectopic production of ACTH.

9. **How is hypercortisolism contributing to hyperglycemia in this patient?**
   Cortisol promotes hyperglycemia by stimulating hepatic gluconeogenesis and inhibiting the peripheral utilization of glucose (similar to the actions of GH). The increase in gluconeogenesis is due to increased synthesis of gluconeogenic enzymes and greater mobilization of amino acids from skeletal muscle to the liver (hence this patient's muscle wasting). Recall that cortisol is the stress hormone that acts in the tissues to (1) promote gluconeogenesis to power the central nervous system (CNS) and erythrocytes and (2) increase lipolysis in adipocytes to meet the energy demand for other tissues (Fig. 8.10).

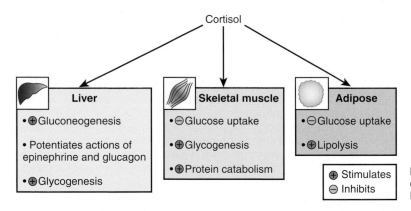

Figure 8.10. Metabolic actions of cortisol. *(From Brown TA.* Rapid Review Physiology. *Philadelphia: Mosby; 2007.)*

10. **How is hypercortisolism contributing to hypertension and hypokalemia in this patient?**
    At higher plasma levels, cortisol exerts mineralocorticoid effects similar to those of aldosterone. This causes sodium retention and plasma volume expansion, which contributes to hypertension. The sodium is retained in exchange for (and therefore at the expense of) serum potassium, which explains this patient's hypokalemia. Another contributing factor to this patient's hypertension is that cortisol stimulates the expression of α_1-adrenergic receptors in vascular smooth muscle, which function to constrict blood vessels and therefore increase intravascular pressure when stimulated.

11. **Why does not cortisol have mineralocorticoid actions in the normal physiologic setting?**
    Cortisol can bind mineralocorticoid receptors with an affinity similar to that of aldosterone, but cells in mineralocorticoid-sensitive tissues (e.g., kidneys, colon, salivary glands) produce *11β-hydroxysteroid dehydrogenase* (11β-HSD). 11β-HSD breaks cortisol down into cortisone, which cannot bind to the aldosterone receptor. When serum cortisol levels are significantly elevated, 11β-HSD becomes saturated, thereby allowing intracellular cortisol to exert its mineralocorticoid effects in these tissues. This explains the plasma volume expansion and hypertension discussed previously.
    Note: Licorice candy (if it contains licorice root from the licorice plant) also *increases* plasma cortisol levels by *decreasing* the activity of 11β-HSD, thereby potentially causing hypertension.

12. **What would an x-ray of this patient's bones likely reveal?**
    An x-ray of her bones would likely show a loss of bone density as a result of osteoporosis. Cortisol inhibits osteoblasts and stimulates osteoclasts, inducing bone resorption. Osteo**b**lasts "**b**uild" bone up, while osteo**c**lasts "**c**runch" bone down. Osteoporosis is an especially significant side effect in patients who are prescribed chronic steroid medications.

13. **What are the three layers of the adrenal cortex, and which one is responsible for the excess production of cortisol in this patient?**
Just think of the acronym for glomerular filtration rate (i.e., **GFR**) when remembering the three layers of the adrenal cortex—zona *g*lomerulosa, zona *f*asciculata, and zona *r*eticularis—which secrete mineralocorticoids (e.g., aldosterone), glucocorticoids (e.g., cortisol), and androgens (e.g., dehydroepiandrosterone [DHEA]), respectively (Fig. 8.11). Recall that the *adrenal medulla* contains neuroendocrine chromaffin cells that are responsible for the secretion of catecholamines (i.e., epinephrine and norepinephrine).
Glomerulosa—aldosterone
Fasciculata—cortisol
Reticularis—androgens (DHEA)

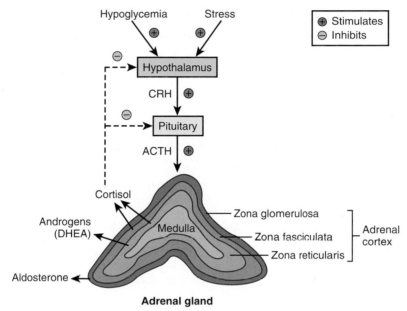

Figure 8.11. Hypothalamic-pituitary-adrenal (HPA) axis products and feedback loops. ACTH, adrenocorticotropic hormone; CRH, corticotropin-releasing hormone; DHEA, dehydroepiandrosterone. *(From Brown TA.* Rapid Review Physiology. *Philadelphia: Mosby; 2007.)*

14. **One treatment for Cushing syndrome is to remove both adrenal glands (i.e., bilateral adrenalectomy). What might happen to the pituitary gland following such a surgery?**
The removal of both adrenal glands will stop the production of cortisol, effectively removing its negative feedback on the anterior pituitary, resulting in the hypersecretion of ACTH. When ACTH production is increased, MSH production is also simultaneously increased, as discussed previously. The combination of rapid pituitary enlargement and MSH-induced hyperpigmentation that occurs following bilateral adrenalectomy is known as *Nelson syndrome.*

SUMMARY BOX: HYPERCORTISOLISM (CUSHING SYNDROME)

- Signs and symptoms
  - Central obesity: Cortisol stimulates protein breakdown in the extremities, but the hyperinsulinemia from the cortisol-induced hyperglycemia promotes central fat deposition.
  - Purple abdominal striae: Result of weight gain, weakened collagen, and capillary fragility or rupture from the effects of hypercortisolism. The presence of abdominal striae is one of the key distinguishing factors between Cushing syndrome and polycystic ovarian syndrome (PCOS), another favorite syndrome of the USMLE.
  - Hypertension: Due to mineralocorticoid actions of cortisol on the kidney and upregulation of α_1-adrenergic receptors on vascular smooth muscle
  - Hirsutism: Due to ACTH-induced shunting of glucocorticoid precursors to the androgenic pathway, causing increased production of androgens (i.e., DHEA)
  - Osteoporosis: Due to cortisol stimulation of osteoclasts and inhibition of osteoblasts
- Pathophysiology: The most common cause of Cushing *syndrome* is the iatrogenic administration of steroids. Hypercortisolism from an adrenocorticotropic hormone (ACTH)-secreting pituitary adenoma is termed *Cushing disease.*
- Diagnosis: Late evening cortisol level, dexamethasone suppression test, 24-hour urinary free cortisol level, computed tomography (CT) scan of the adrenal gland, and magnetic resonance image (MRI) of the pituitary gland

SUMMARY BOX: HYPERCORTISOLISM (CUSHING SYNDROME)—cont'd

- Treatment: For iatrogenic causes, carefully taper off the medication that is causing the symptoms. If an adrenal adenoma is present, it may be removed surgically.
- Complications of treatment: Bilateral adrenalectomy for Cushing syndrome can cause Nelson syndrome, which is characterized by pituitary enlargement (due to reduced negative feedback of cortisol on the anterior pituitary) with diffuse hyperpigmentation (due to increased melanocyte-stimulating hormone [MSH] production).

CASE 8.5

An 18-year-old man presents to the emergency department with dizziness and vomiting for the past 5 days. He reports that he has felt worsening fatigue over the past 6 months despite previously having an active lifestyle and playing school sports. Review of systems is significant for anorexia, nausea, and an unintentional 10-lb weight loss as a result of poor appetite. Blood pressure is 90/55 mm Hg. Physical examination reveals a man who looks pale and unwell, with darkening of his skin over various areas of his body. Laboratory workup reveals low sodium, high potassium, and low glucose levels. There is no fever, diarrhea, or abdominal pain.

1. **What do you suspect at this point?**
   This patient's vague symptoms of fatigue and weakness coupled with hypotension, changes in skin pigmentation, and the reported electrolyte disturbances are all concerning for adrenal insufficiency.
   Recall that aldosterone (and cortisol at extremely high levels) stimulates sodium retention and potassium excretion from the principal cells and H+ excretion from the intercalated cells of the kidneys. Cortisol and epinephrine also antagonize the actions of insulin. Given these physiologic functions, one can see how a *lack* of mineralocorticoid, glucocorticoid, and catecholamines can result in hypotension, hyponatremia, hypoglycemia, hyperkalemia, and metabolic acidosis.
   There are many causes of adrenal insufficiency, but the hyperpigmentation observed in this patient suggests elevated ACTH levels. POMC is the precursor released by corticotrophs in the anterior pituitary that is cleaved into multiple peptide hormones including ACTH and β-MSH, the latter of which can cause darkening skin pigmentation.
   Given these symptoms, we can deduce that the etiology of this patient's condition lies at the level of the adrenals (i.e., primary adrenal disorder). The resulting low cortisol levels decrease negative feedback on the anterior pituitary, leading to elevated ACTH levels. If this were secondary adrenal insufficiency, as seen in Sheehan syndrome, both ACTH and cortisol levels would be low.

2. **What are some general causes of primary adrenal insufficiency (also called *Addison disease*)?**
   Autoimmune destruction is the most common cause of Addison disease. Tubercular invasion of the adrenals in miliary (i.e., disseminated) tuberculosis is a common cause of Addison disease in developing countries. Metastatic invasion of the adrenals, which occurs frequently with lung cancer, is another cause. Other rarer causes include disseminated fungal infections (e.g., histoplasmosis), sarcoidosis, hemochromatosis, and lymphoma.

CASE 8.5 CONTINUED:

Further workup reveals an elevated morning plasma ACTH and low plasma cortisol levels. Injection of the ACTH analog cosyntropin elicits only a blunted increase in plasma cortisol. The patient is started on routine hydrocortisone and fludrocortisone.

3. **What is the cause of adrenal insufficiency in this patient?**
   All we can say with the given information is that this young man has primary adrenal insufficiency, which we can determine by noting the elevated ACTH and lack of response to cosyntropin. Because there are no clues to suggest malignancy or infection and we are not told that this patient is currently taking any medications, the likely cause of this patient's primary adrenal insufficiency is autoimmune destruction of the adrenals (i.e., autoimmune adrenalitis).

RELATED QUESTIONS

4. **What adrenal disease should be suspected in a young patient with bacterial meningitis as a result of *Neisseria meningitidis* who also becomes acutely hypotensive?**
   Waterhouse-Friderichsen syndrome typically causes bilateral adrenal hemorrhage, which can be rapidly fatal. The responsible bacterium is *Neisseria meningitidis*, a gram-negative diplococci. This association is a favorite of the USMLE exam.

STEP 1 SECRET

Waterhouse-Friderichsen syndrome is a high-yield diagnosis for clinical vignettes on the USMLE exam. Be on the lookout for symptoms of septicemia, disseminated intravascular coagulation (DIC), adrenal hemorrhage, and petechial rash.

5. How would we expect plasma aldosterone levels to be affected in a patient with secondary adrenal insufficiency (i.e., low ACTH secretion by the anterior pituitary)?

Aldosterone secretion is primarily stimulated by angiotensin II (via the renin-angiotensin-aldosterone system) and by elevated serum potassium levels. ACTH has little influence on aldosterone secretion, so aldosterone will not be significantly impacted by secondary adrenal insufficiency.

6. In general, why is it necessary to taper patients off steroid treatments such as hydrocortisone and fludrocortisone rather than abruptly stopping such treatments?

This is to protect the patient from acute primary adrenal insufficiency. When taking an exogenous source of cortisol, the HPA axis is blunted by negative feedback, causing little to no ACTH production. Abrupt withdrawal of exogenous cortisol before natural production of ACTH can be reestablished at normal levels can be physiologically catastrophic for the patient. By reducing exogenous cortisol levels over time (i.e., tapering), the HPA axis slowly regains its function, the adrenal glands gradually return to appropriate size, and only then will the adrenals become capable of naturally producing cortisol at appropriate levels in the absence of exogenous sources.

SUMMARY BOX: ADRENAL INSUFFICIENCY

- Symptoms: Primary adrenal insufficiency (PAI; Addison disease) can present with vague symptoms such as weakness and malaise, as well as with a specific constellation of metabolic abnormalities (e.g., hyponatremia, hyperkalemia, hypoglycemia, and metabolic acidosis). Hypotension as a result of vascular collapse is also common.
- Pathophysiology: Causes include autoimmune destruction, tubercular and metastatic invasion, fungal infections (e.g., disseminated histoplasmosis), and drugs (e.g., ketoconazole and metyrapone, which selectively inhibit the glucocorticoid pathway). The most common cause of adrenal insufficiency is the abrupt cessation of chronically administered steroids.
- Diagnosis: An elevated adrenocorticotropic hormone (ACTH) level suggests PAI, whereas a low ACTH level suggests a pituitary or, rarely, a hypothalamic etiology. Exogenous administration of an ACTH analog (i.e., cosyntropin) does not significantly increase serum cortisol levels in patients with PAI.
- The metyrapone stimulation test can distinguish between primary and secondary/tertiary insufficiency because metyrapone blocks the conversion of 11-deoxycortisol to cortisol. In primary insufficiency, ACTH is elevated, but 11-deoxycortisol levels stay low after administration of metyrapone. In secondary/tertiary insufficiency, however, both ACTH and 11-deoxycortisol levels will remain low.
- Treatment: Corticosteroid replacement therapy.
- Waterhouse-Friderichsen syndrome caused by *Neisseria meningitidis* can be rapidly fatal.

CASE 8.6

A 38-year-old man with a history of generalized anxiety disorder reports intermittent episodes of headache, palpitations, diaphoresis, and fear of "impending death." He was recently started on a beta-blocker for mild hypertension, but surprisingly, his hypertension has worsened. He denies any history of cocaine or amphetamine abuse.

1. What leading diagnosis do you suspect at this point?

Intermittent episodes of headache, palpitations, diaphoresis, and fear of "impending death" are classic for pheochromocytoma. The worsening of this patient's hypertension after the initiation of beta-blockers also suggests pheochromocytoma. The differential diagnosis includes panic attack (disorder), hypoglycemia, mastocytosis, and carcinoid syndrome.

2. Why does hypertension often worsen after starting a beta-blocker in patients with pheochromocytoma?

Plasma epinephrine, which is elevated in pheochromocytoma, has vasodilatory and vasoconstrictor effects depending on which adrenergic receptor (β or α) it activates. In the presence of a beta-blocker, epinephrine will primarily bind α_1-adrenergic receptors, resulting in *unopposed α_1-receptor–mediated vasoconstriction*, which leads to increased blood pressure. Recall that α_1-adrenergic receptors signal via the Gq pathway, resulting in increased intracellular calcium and subsequent vascular smooth muscle contraction.

CASE 8.6 CONTINUED:

A 24-hour urine collection reveals elevated levels of catecholamine metabolites, and a positron emission tomography (PET) scan shows what appears to be a highly vascular mass above the left kidney. The administration of clonidine does not suppress plasma catecholamine levels.

3. Based on this additional information, what is the most likely diagnosis?

Pheochromocytoma is the most likely diagnosis. Pheochromocytoma is a tumor that episodically releases large amounts of catecholamines, resulting in intermittent symptomatic episodes of hypertension, tachycardia, palpitations, chest pain, diaphoresis, anxiety, and headache. Pheochromocytomas generally arise from neural crest–derived chromaffin cells of the adrenal medulla. Tumors arising in paraganglia are termed *paragangliomas* or *extra-adrenal pheochromocytomas*.

Note: Remember the 5 P's of **p**heochromocytoma: **p**ain (headache), **p**erspiration, **p**alpitations, **p**allor, and **p**ressure (hypertension).

STEP 1 SECRET

You should know all of the derivatives of neural crest cells, as they are a commonly tested USMLE topic. These derivatives include chromaffin cells, parafollicular cells of the thyroid, Schwann cells, the autonomic nervous system (ANS), dorsal root and celiac ganglia, melanocytes, cranial nerves, pia and arachnoid mater, odontoblasts, skull bones, and the aorticopulmonary septum.

Knowing the embryologic derivatives of other tissue types is fair game for the USMLE Step 1 exam but is not nearly as high yield as neural crest derivatives.

---

4. **How can the administration of clonidine be used to distinguish pheochromocytoma from a chronically high-stress state such as general anxiety disorder?**
   Clonidine is a centrally acting α_2-agonist that inhibits sympathetic outflow from the CNS. Its administration will reduce natural catecholamine production by the CNS and adrenal medulla, but it does not reduce pathologic catecholamine production by an autonomously functioning pheochromocytoma.

5. **What is the "rule of 10s" for pheochromocytoma?**
   - 10% are familial
   - 10% are extra-adrenal in location
   - 10% are malignant
   - 10% occur in children
   - 10% are calcified
   - 10% affect the adrenals bilaterally

   Note: Most pheochromocytomas arise sporadically, but approximately 10% are associated with hereditary disorders such as multiple endocrine neoplasia (MEN) IIA or MEN IIB, von Hippel-Lindau (VHL) syndrome, or neurofibromatosis.

6. **What is the most feared complication in patients with a pheochromocytoma?**
   Pheo crisis is a serious life-threatening condition in which a large amount of epinephrine is released that can cause multiple system organ failure. This can lead to death, with mortality rates greater than 80%. Emotional stress, corticosteroids, tricyclic antidepressants (TCAs), and analgesics have all been associated with pheo crisis.

7. **What malignant tumor that most often occurs in children under 5 years of age also shows increased urinary levels of catecholamine metabolites?**
   Neuroblastoma, a neuroendocrine tumor arising from neural crest cells, is associated with increased urinary levels of catecholamine metabolites (e.g., homovanillic acid [HVA] and vanillylmandelic acid [VMA]). Children with neuroblastoma may present with hypertension and a palpable abdominal mass that *can* cross the midline (as opposed to a Wilms tumor, which typically *cannot*). Approximately 50% of cases are also associated with opsoclonus-myoclonus syndrome, in which patients exhibit chaotic eye movements. Neuroblastoma commonly metastasizes to skin, bone, and the posterior mediastinum. The tumor itself is associated with *N-myc* oncogene overexpression, bombesin (a commonly used tumor marker), and Homer-Wright rosettes histology (neuroblasts surrounding spaces filled with eosinophilic neuropil).

CASE 8.6 CONTINUED:

The patient is prescribed antihypertensive therapy that includes prazosin and propranolol and is informed that surgical correction can offer a cure.
   Note: First-line treatment for pheochromocytoma is surgical resection of the tumor.

---

8. **What types of receptors do norepinephrine and epinephrine bind to on the heart to increase the rate and force of cardiac contraction?**
   They bind to β_1-adrenergic receptors on nodal cells to increase the rate of cardiac contraction (positive *chronotropic* effect) and on cardiac myocytes to increase the force of cardiac contraction (positive *inotropic* effect). This is the reason that a beta-blocker (e.g., propranolol) is used as part of the management of hypertension in patients with pheochromocytoma. However, only give the beta-blocker *after* α blockade to prevent hypertensive crisis. This is an important concept not just for the USMLE exam, but also for the clinical wards and as a practicing physician. Prazosin is an α-receptor antagonist that is commonly used prior to β-blockers. Medications with the suffix "-zosin" (e.g., doxazosin, terazosin, and prazosin), are α_1-receptor antagonists; these receptors are located predominantly on vascular smooth muscle.

The initial administration of α_1-receptor antagonists (e.g., prazosin) will block all of the α_1-receptor activity, leaving only β_2-adrenergic receptors available for binding by subsequently released epinephrine. Stimulation of β_2-adrenergic receptors (via activation of G_S-protein coupled receptors) results in vasodilation (via nitrogen oxide and the endothelial nitric oxide synthase [eNOS] pathway), which lowers peripheral vascular resistance and ultimately reduces blood pressure.

STEP 1 SECRET

Concepts like these are USMLE favorites because they stress a broad conceptual understanding of physiology and pharmacology. Autonomic nervous system (ANS) hormones, receptors, and medications are five-star USMLE topics.

CASE 8.6 CONTINUED:

Blood pressure is normalized with phenoxybenzamine before surgery. Surgical resection of the affected adrenal gland is performed without complications.

9. Why was phenoxybenzamine given before surgery?

Phenoxybenzamine is an irreversible noncompetitive antagonist of α_1-adrenergic receptors. Because of its irreversible binding properties, it is preferred over other α_1-blockers for preoperative preparation because it minimizes the hypertensive effects of catecholamines that may be released during the surgery.

Note: *Phentolamine* is a reversible α_1-blocker while *phenoxybenzamine* is an irreversible α_1-blocker.

SUMMARY BOX: PHEOCHROMOCYTOMA

- Symptoms: Intermittent episodes of headache, palpitations, profuse sweating, and fear of "impending death" are classic for pheochromocytoma. Remember the 5 **P**'s of **p**heochromocytoma: **p**ain (headache), **p**erspiration, **p**alpitations, **p**allor, and **p**ressure (hypertension). Worsening hypertension after the administration of beta-blockers is also suggestive of pheochromocytoma.
- Diagnosis: Remember the "rule of 10s" for pheochromocytoma: 10% are familial, 10% are extra-adrenal in location, 10% are malignant, 10% occur in children, 10% are calcified, and 10% affect the adrenal glands bilaterally
- The increase of serum catecholamines (i.e., norepinephrine and epinephrine) that occurs with pheochromocytoma will result in the increased urinary excretion of catecholamine metabolites vanillylmandelic acid (VMA), homovanillic acid (HVA), and metanephrines, which can be measured to support the diagnosis.
- Treatment:
  - Clonidine is used to distinguish pheochromocytoma from increased sympathoadrenal outflow because of chronic stress or pain.
  - In pheochromocytoma, an α-blocker should be given *before* beta blockade to prevent unopposed α-blocker–mediated vasoconstriction. Phenoxybenzamine is an irreversible α_1-blocker that is preferred over other α_1-blockers during preoperative preparation because it minimizes the hypertensive effects of catecholamines released during surgery.
  - Neuroblastoma is a malignant tumor that typically manifests in young children as an abdominal mass that *can* cross the midline. Similar to pheochromocytoma, neuroblastoma will also cause increased urinary levels of catecholamine metabolites.

CASE 8.7

A 40-year-old woman presents to the clinic reporting of diarrhea, increasing anxiety, weakness, and palpitations for the last 8 months. During the past 2 months, she has been sleeping with fewer blankets than her husband. Also, she has unintentionally lost weight despite eating a lot more than she did 8 months ago.

1. What leading diagnosis do you suspect at this point?

There are only a few conditions associated with unintentional weight loss despite normal (or increased) food intake. These possibilities include diabetes mellitus, malabsorption syndromes, cancer, and hyperthyroidism. Both hyperthyroidism and malabsorption can cause diarrhea, but given this patient's heat intolerance and palpitations, hyperthyroidism seems most likely.

CASE 8.7 CONTINUED:

Physical examination is significant for a blood pressure of 165/75 mm Hg, a systolic ejection murmur, and tachycardia, as well as diffuse nontender enlargement of the thyroid gland, slight resting tremor, fine hair, separation of the fingernail plate from the nail bed (onycholysis), and brisk deep tendon reflexes. Laboratory tests reveal elevated free plasma thyroxine (T_4) and reduced TSH.

2. **What is the diagnosis?**
Based on the additional information provided, this patient can be diagnosed with hyperthyroidism, the most common cause of which is Graves disease. It affects women more than men and usually those in their 20s and 30s. Other causes of hyperthyroidism are listed in Table 8.7.

Table 8.7. Causes and Features of Hyperthyroidism

CAUSE	PATHOPHYSIOLOGY	PATTERN OF RADIOIODINE UPTAKE	CLASSIC PRESENTATION
Permanent Causes			
Graves disease (diffuse toxic goiter)	Activating antibodies to TSH receptor	Diffuse uptake throughout gland	Goiter, exophthalmos, dermopathy
Toxic multinodular goiter	Multiple hyperactive nodules, may have mutations in genes encoding TSH receptor or G proteins	Uptake in one or a few overly active "hot" nodules Uptake in remainder of thyroid is suppressed	History of nontoxic multinodular goiter in older adult May include cardiac complications such as atrial fibrillation or heart failure
Toxic adenoma (Plummer disease)	Hyperactive adenoma(s); may have mutations in genes encoding TSH receptor or G proteins	Uptake in one or a few "hot" nodules Uptake in remainder of thyroid is suppressed	History of a slowly growing "lump" in the neck in a younger adult
Pituitary adenoma	Hypersecretion of TSH	Diffuse uptake throughout thyroid	May include additional symptoms (e.g., headaches, bitemporal hemianopia, nausea and vomiting)
Transient Causes			
Autoimmune thyroiditis (e.g., Hashimoto disease)	Autoimmune destruction of thyroid	Suppressed uptake throughout thyroid	Hyperthyroidism initially, followed by hypothyroidism
Subacute thyroiditis (de Quervain thyroiditis)	Probably secondary to viral infection of thyroid Follows upper respiratory tract infection	Suppressed uptake throughout thyroid	Thyroid exquisitely painful to palpation
Iodine-induced (Jod-Basedow effect)	Iodine overload may stimulate autonomous nodules, which function independently of TSH stimulation, to hypersecrete thyroid hormone	Suppressed uptake throughout thyroid	Thyrotoxicosis in a patient with toxic multinodular goiter after administration of iodine-rich radiographic contrast media and iodinated drugs such as amiodarone
Thyrotoxicosis factitia	Inadvertent or intentional ingestion of large amounts of thyroid hormone	Suppressed uptake throughout thyroid	Ingestion of thyroid hormone to lose weight, typically by medical personnel
Struma ovarii	Thyroid tissue forms part of ovarian germ cell tumor (teratoma) and secretes excessive thyroid hormone	Suppressed uptake throughout thyroid	Hyperthyroidism in female
Trophoblastic tumors	Malignant trophoblastic tissue secretes hCG, which stimulates the TSH receptor	Diffuse uptake throughout thyroid	Hydatidiform moles, choriocarcinoma, metastatic embryonal carcinoma of the testis

hCG, Human chorionic gonadotropin; *TSH*, thyroid-stimulating hormone.

3. **Why has this woman experienced weight loss?**
The thyroid hormones increase the basal metabolic rate (BMR), principally by increasing the production and insertion of the Na^+/K^+-ATPase pumps in various cell types. Thyroid hormones also increase BMR via production of glycolytic enzymes. The increased metabolic rate results in weight loss and contributes to heat intolerance (Table 8.8).

Table 8.8. Intracellular and Physiologic Actions of T_3

SITE OF ACTION	INTRACELLULAR EFFECTS	PHYSIOLOGIC RESULTS
Cell membrane	Stimulates the Na^+/K^+-ATPase pump	Increased demand for metabolites, e.g., glucose
Mitochondria	Stimulates growth, replication, and activity; basal metabolic rate is raised	Increased heat production, oxygen demand, heart rate, and stroke volume
Nucleus	Increases expression of enzymes necessary for energy production	Lipolysis, glycolysis, and gluconeogenesis increased to raise blood metabolite levels and cellular metabolite use
Neonatal cells	Essential for cell division and maturation	Essential for normal development of central nervous system and skeleton

ATP, Adenosine triphosphate; T_3, triiodothyronine.
From Meszaros JG, Olson ER, Naugle JE, et al. *Crash Course: Endocrine and Reproductive Systems.* Philadelphia: Mosby; 2006.

4. What are the two thyroid hormones, and which is more potent?
T_4 and T_3 (triiodothyronine) are the two thyroid hormones. T_3 is much more potent than T_4 (≈ 5 times more so) and is primarily produced by the peripheral conversion of T_4 to T_3 (which is catalyzed by the intracellular enzyme 5′-deiodinase), although as much as 20% of T_3 can be secreted from the thyroid gland. Some authors prefer to call T_4 a *prohormone* because its activity is largely dependent on conversion to the more active T_3. However, T_4 is the main feedback regulator in the endocrine axis (Table 8.9).

Table 8.9. Comparison of T_3 and T_4

FEATURE	T_3	T_4
Proportion of secreted thyroid hormone	10%	90%
Percentage free in plasma	1%	0.1%
Relative activity	10	1
Half-life (days)	1	7

T_3, Triiodothyronine; T_4, thyroxine.
From Meszaros JG, Olson ER, Naugle JE, et al. *Crash Course: Endocrine and Reproductive Systems.* Philadelphia: Mosby; 2006.

5. How are the thyroid hormones synthesized?
Ultimately, four iodine residues are attached to two tyrosine residues to form T_4, or three iodine residues to form T_3.
The first step in the synthesis of either thyroid hormone is the uptake of iodide ion (I^-) via the Na^+/I^- symporter from plasma into follicular cells and eventually into the follicular lumen via the iodide pump pendrin. Within the lumen, the enzyme thyroid peroxidase then catalyzes the next two steps, in which iodide is oxidized to iodine (I_2) and iodine molecules are attached to tyrosine residues found on thyroglobulin (this is called the *organification step*). These iodinated tyrosine residues are then coupled together to form either T_4 or T_3. Endocytosis of this modified thyroglobulin protein into the follicular cells and its subsequent hydrolysis yields T_4 and T_3, which diffuse across the plasma membrane and back into circulation (Fig. 8.12).

6. Assuming the plasma levels of catecholamines are normal in this patient, what explains the tachycardia, tremors, palpitations, and increased pulse pressure?
Thyroid hormones increase the expression of adrenergic receptors in target tissues, resulting in increased sensitivity to normal levels of circulating catecholamines. Thyroid hormones also increase β-adrenergic receptor synthesis in the heart and have a direct stimulating effect (both inotropic and chronotropic) on the heart.
Pulse pressure increases because cardiac stroke volume increases (due to inotropic and chronotropic effects) while diastolic blood pressure decreases (due to widespread vasodilation caused by the metabolic demands of thyroid hormone–dependent tissue). Fig. 8.13 shows other potential clinical manifestations of hyperthyroidism.
Note: Beta-blockers (i.e., propranolol) are often given to alleviate the sympathomimetic effects (e.g., palpitations, tremor) of hyperthyroidism. Of note, untreated hyperthyroidism can predispose to osteoporosis and atrial fibrillation.

7. What is the difference between primary, secondary, and tertiary hyperthyroidism?
Primary hyperthyroidism results from excessive production of thyroid hormones by the thyroid gland itself, which in turn suppresses pituitary TSH production. In contrast, secondary hyperthyroidism results from excessive pituitary secretion of TSH. Tertiary hyperthyroidism is caused by increased hypothalamic secretion of TRH. As this patient most likely has Graves disease, TSH levels are expected to be decreased (Table 8.10).

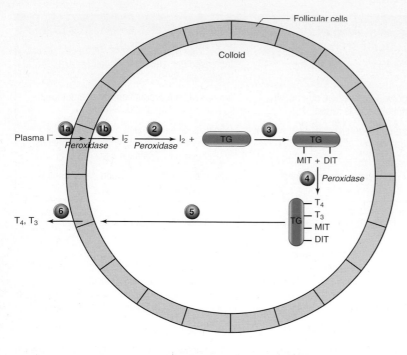

Figure 8.12. Thyroid hormone synthesis in the thyroid follicle. *DIT,* Diiodotyrosine; *I,* iodide ion; *I₂,* iodine; *MIT,* monoiodoty-rosine; *T₃,* triiodothyronine; *T₄,* thyroxine; *TG,* thyroglobulin. *(From Brown TA. Rapid Review Physiology. Philadelphia: Mosby; 2007.)*

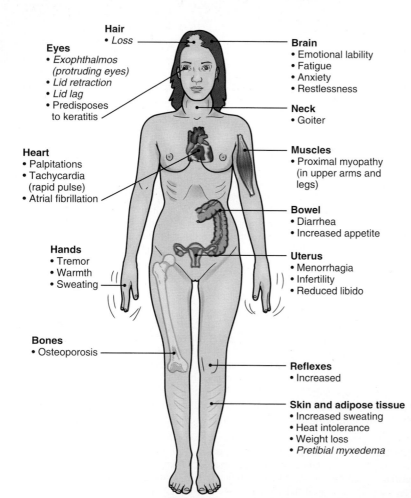

Figure 8.13. Symptoms and signs of thyrotoxicosis (hyperthyroidism). The features in *italics* are found only in Graves disease. *(From Meszaros JG, Olson ER, Naugle JE, et al. Crash Course: Endocrine and Reproductive Systems. Philadelphia: Mosby; 2006.)*

Table 8.10. Laboratory Values Associated With Each Type of Hyperthyroidism

TYPE	EXAMPLE	TRH	TSH	T$_4$
Primary hyperthyroidism	Graves disease	↓	↓	↑
Secondary hyperthyroidism	Pituitary adenoma	↓	↑	↑
Tertiary hyperthyroidism	Hypothalamic tumor	↑	↑	↑

T$_4$, Thyroxine; *TRH,* thyrotropin-releasing hormone; *TSH,* thyroid-stimulating hormone.

8. Based on your suspected diagnosis, what additional laboratory and physical findings might you expect?

   Graves disease is the most common cause of hyperthyroidism and is additionally characterized by exophthalmos, pretibial myxedema, and thyroid-stimulating immunoglobulins (TSI) that bind TSH receptors in the thyroid. The antibodies stimulate the thyroid in the same way TSH does. Notice that this woman had a diffusely enlarged thyroid gland, which is consistent with TSH receptor stimulation causing diffuse thyroid enlargement.

9. What type of hypersensitivity is caused by Graves disease?

   This is a type II hypersensitivity reaction to antibodies of the immunoglobulin M (IgM) or immunoglobulin G (IgG) isotype. Two other commonly tested type II hypersensitivity conditions include myasthenia gravis and pernicious anemia.

CASE 8.7 CONTINUED:

On further examination, you note the appearance of the skin of the lower extremities, as shown in Fig. 8.14.

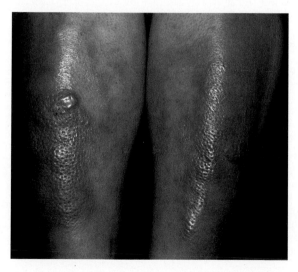

Figure 8.14. Appearance of lower extremities in the patient from Case 8.7.

10. What is the pathophysiology of this complication in Graves disease?

    Pretibial myxedema is a *nonpitting* edema caused by accumulation of interstitial glycosaminoglycans (GAGs) within the dermis. This is due to the TSI binding to TSH on the fibroblast cells of the skin. Paradoxically, pretibial myxedema can also be seen in severe hypothyroidism.

    Note: Graves disease has a unique triad associated with it: hyperthyroidism, exophthalmos, and pretibial myxedema.

11. What would a thyroid iodide-131 uptake scan likely reveal in this patient?

    Because iodide is used to synthesize thyroid hormone, Graves disease would show an increased diffuse uptake across the entire thyroid gland, corresponding to an increased synthesis of T$_3$ and T$_4$. When the gland is inactive due to exogenous thyroid hormone therapy or because of inflammation of the gland (e.g., thyroiditis), uptake would be low. See Figs. 8.15 and 8.16 for comparison.

12. What therapeutic options are available to this patient?

    Therapeutic options include medications such as thioamides and beta-blockers, surgery, radioactive iodine-131 ablation, and conservative treatment (watch and wait). Corticosteroids are indicated in patients with Graves ophthalmopathy in order to treat proptosis.

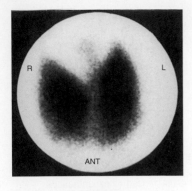

Figure 8.15. Graves disease, showing diffusely increased radiolabeled iodine uptake. *ANT,* Anterior; *L,* left; *R,* right. *(From Mettler FA Jr.* Essentials of Radiology. *2nd ed. Philadelphia: WB Saunders; 2005.)*

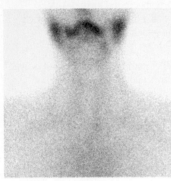

Figure 8.16. Thyroiditis, showing near absence of radiolabeled iodine uptake. *(From Rakel RE.* Conn's Current Therapy 2007. *59th ed. Philadelphia: WB Saunders; 2007.)*

13. **Why might a physician prescribe propylthiouracil or methimazole for this woman? How do these drugs work?**
Both propylthiouracil (PTU) and methimazole are largely concentrated in the thyroid and inhibit thyroid hormone synthesis via inhibition of thyroid peroxidase. To a small extent, PTU also acts by preventing the peripheral deiodination of T_4 to T_3.
   Note: PTU and methimazole both freely cross the placenta but can be used in pregnancy (though there are some risks, particularly with methimazole), whereas radioactive iodide is contraindicated in pregnancy. Methimazole is preferred to PTU except during the first trimester of pregnancy.

14. **What is thyroid storm? Why might PTU be used for this condition instead of methimazole?**
Thyroid storm (i.e., thyrotoxicosis) results from excessive levels of thyroid hormone, causing a substantial elevation in the BMR and extreme fever in which patients can seem to "burn up right in front of you." It is potentially fatal, and the beta-blocker propranolol is classically used to manage emergent cases. Both PTU and methimazole inhibit thyroid hormone synthesis, but because the thyroid has an abundant store of thyroid hormone, it may take weeks for this effect to manifest. However, at higher doses, PTU also inhibits the conversion of T_4 to T_3 in the peripheral tissues. Because T_3 is the more active form of thyroid hormone, PTU can have a fairly rapid effect.
   Note: Both PTU and methimazole can cause a fatal agranulocytosis, often preceded by a sore throat, so periodic monitoring is required.

15. **Why is iodide therapy generally initiated 2 weeks before thyroidectomy in hyperthyroid patients?**
By an unclear mechanism, administration of a large amount of iodide decreases the vascularity of the thyroid gland, which reduces bleeding complications during surgery. Excess iodide inhibits the uptake of more iodide, and as a result, thyroid hormone synthesis is reduced or stopped (via the Wolff-Chaikoff effect), which may be an intrinsic mechanism to protect against hyperthyroidism in a setting of iodine excess.

SOME DIFFERENTIAL DIAGNOSIS AND PHYSIOLOGY CONCEPTS

16. **How would a patient with hyperthyroidism secondary to de Quervain (i.e., subacute granulomatous) thyroiditis typically present clinically?**
Patients with this disease have an exquisitely tender thyroid gland and generally have a history of recent flu-like illness (e.g., fever, sore throat). Patients may have a hyperthyroid state initially and then transition to a hypothyroid state later in the course of this disease.

17. **How can a teratoma produce hyperthyroidism?**
A rare form of ovarian teratoma called *struma ovarii* is made up exclusively of functional thyroid tissue, which can produce enough thyroid hormone to cause clinical hyperthyroidism.

SUMMARY BOX: HYPERTHYROIDISM AND GRAVES DISEASE

- Hyperthyroidism classically presents with some combination of the following: heat intolerance, unintentional weight loss despite an excellent appetite, tremor, palpitations, anxiety, diarrhea, osteoporosis, hypercalcemia, atrial fibrillation, and high-output heart failure.
- Graves disease is the most common cause of hyperthyroidism and may be additionally characterized by exophthalmos, pretibial myxedema, and antibodies (IgG or IgM) to the thyroid-stimulating hormone (TSH) receptor in the thyroid. Toxic multinodular goiter is the second-most common cause of hyperthyroidism.
- Radiolabeled iodide uptake is diffusely increased across the thyroid in Graves disease but decreased in hyperthyroidism caused by exogenous thyroid hormone administration or in transient cases of hyperthyroidism because of thyroiditis.
- Thyroid hormones increase the basal metabolic rate (BMR) principally through increasing the production and insertion of the Na^+/K^+-ATPase pumps in various cell types, as well as by stimulating the production of glycolytic enzymes.
- Thyroxine (T_4) is a prohormone whose activity is largely dependent on peripheral conversion to the more active triiodothyronine (T_3).
- Mechanism of thyroid hormone synthesis: (1) uptake of iodide ion ($I-$) from plasma into follicular cells and the follicular lumen; (2) oxidation of iodide ion ($I-$) to iodine (I_2) and attachment of iodine to tyrosine on thyroglobulin, which are both catalyzed by thyroid peroxidase; (3) coupling of iodinated tyrosine molecules to form T_4 or T_3; and (4) endocytosis of modified thyroglobulin into follicular cells and hydrolysis to T_4 and T_3, which then diffuse across the plasma membrane and enter the circulation
- Thyroid hormones increase adrenergic receptor sensitivity to circulating catecholamines, contributing to tachycardia, tremor, and palpitations despite normal serum levels of catecholamines.
- Pretibial myxedema is a *nonpitting* edema caused by accumulation of interstitial glycosaminoglycans (GAGs) within the dermis.
- Treatment options for Graves disease include thioamides, surgery, radioactive iodine-131 ablation, beta-blockers, and a conservative "watch and wait" approach. Corticosteroids should be considered in patients with exophthalmos.
- Propylthiouracil (PTU) and methimazole are largely concentrated in the thyroid and inhibit thyroid hormone synthesis.
- Iodide therapy before surgery reduces the vascularity of the thyroid and therefore the bleeding complications of the surgery. Via the Wolff-Chaikoff effect, excess iodide also inhibits thyroid hormone synthesis, which may be an intrinsic mechanism to protect against hyperthyroidism in settings of iodine excess.

CASE 8.8

A 42-year-old woman presents to the clinic reporting recent weight gain despite a normal appetite, fatigue, and menorrhagia. On physical examination, she appears pale, speaks slowly, and has a diffusely enlarged nontender thyroid gland and a yellowish tinge to her skin.

1. What leading diagnosis do you suspect at this point?

   Weight gain, fatigue, and menorrhagia, as well as constipation and cold intolerance (which this patient does not report experiencing) are all classic symptoms of hypothyroidism. The pallor and psychomotor retardation also suggest hypothyroidism. However, other conditions such as depression and anemia must also be considered.

CASE 8.8 CONTINUED:

She denies any history of bipolar disorder or treatment with lithium.

2. Why would lithium use be relevant in the diagnostic workup of this patient?

   Lithium inhibits the uptake and organification of iodine by the thyroid gland and prevents the peripheral conversion of T_4 to T_3 by inhibiting 5′-monodeiodinase, thereby causing hypothyroidism. Amiodarone, an antiarrhythmic agent, is also known to cause hypothyroidism.

CASE 8.8 CONTINUED:

Laboratory results reveal elevated serum TSH and reduced serum T_4.

3. What is the diagnosis?

   This patient has hypothyroidism, the most common cause of which is Hashimoto (i.e., autoimmune) thyroiditis. Other causes of hypothyroidism include subacute granulomatous (de Quervain) thyroiditis, fibrous (Riedel) thyroiditis, iatrogenic causes (e.g., thyroidectomy, thyroid radiotherapy), endemic goiter, and medications (e.g., lithium, amiodarone).

For the USMLE Step 1 exam, you should be prepared to recognize the following associations regarding each potential etiology of hypothyroidism:
- *Hashimoto thyroiditis* is caused by autoimmune destruction of the thyroid gland.
- *Subacute granulomatous thyroiditis* typically develops after a viral upper respiratory tract infection and presents with an exquisitely *tender* thyroid gland.
- *Fibrous thyroiditis* is caused by fibrosis of the thyroid gland such that the thyroid gland may have a "wood-like" consistency on examination.
- *Endemic goiter* results from dietary iodide insufficiency in adulthood and is more common in developing countries.

4. **Does this patient have primary, secondary, or tertiary hypothyroidism?**
This woman has primary hypothyroidism. Reduced hormone production by the thyroid gland disinhibits the hypothalamic-pituitary axis, resulting in increased TRH and TSH. Secondary and tertiary hypothyroidism are caused by pituitary and hypothalamic dysfunction, respectively (Table 8.11). TSH levels would not be elevated in either of these cases.

Table 8.11. Laboratory Values Associated With Each Type of Hypothyroidism

CLINICAL FORM	T_4/T_3	TSH	TRH
Primary hypothyroidism	Low	High	High
Secondary hypothyroidism	Low	Low	High
Tertiary hypothyroidism	Low	Low	Low
Subclinical hypothyroidism	Normal	High	Normal

T_3, Triiodothyronine; T_4, thyroxine; *TRH,* thyrotropin-releasing hormone; *TSH,* thyroid-stimulating hormone.

5. **What diagnosis should you suspect in a hospitalized patient with abnormal thyroid hormone levels?**
Euthyroid sick syndrome refers to abnormalities in thyroid function that occur in ill patients without underlying thyroid or pituitary disease. Euthyroid sick syndrome may in part be caused by reduced peripheral conversion of T_4 to T_3. This condition commonly occurs following illness, nutritional deficiencies, and glucocorticoid administration. The exact cause of euthyroid sick syndrome is not known, but it is thought to be the body's attempt to conserve calories during states of caloric deficit or increased caloric need. Because of the prevalence of euthyroid sick syndrome and the difficulty in interpreting thyroid studies in sick patients, most endocrinologists do not recommend testing thyroid function in hospitalized patients.

CASE 8.8 CONTINUED:

Further workup reveals the presence of anti-TPO (antithyroid peroxidase) and anti-Tg (thyroglobulin) antibodies. A thyroid biopsy shows a diffuse lymphocytic infiltrate with Hurthle cell metaplasia.

6. **What is the diagnosis? Why might you also want to check serum vitamin B_{12} levels in this patient?**
Plasma anti-TPO and anti-Tg antibodies, biopsy showing lymphocytic infiltration, and Hurthle cell metaplasia of the thyroid gland are typical of Hashimoto (i.e., autoimmune) thyroiditis. *Hurthle cells* are epithelial cells with granular and eosinophilic cytoplasm. This disease is frequently associated with autoimmune conditions such as pernicious anemia, which is characterized by impaired absorption of vitamin B_{12} (Table 8.12). Therefore checking a vitamin B_{12} level would not be unreasonable. Also, this disease is associated with an increased risk of non-Hodgkin lymphoma, which is important to consider when answering questions about risk factors.

STEP 1 SECRET

Autoimmune conditions are most widely seen in young to middle-aged women. You are expected to know the antibodies associated with common autoimmune conditions and are likely to be asked at least one question from the information outlined in Table 8.12.

7. **Why has this patient experienced weight gain and yellowish skin?**
This patient's weight gain is due to her low metabolic state (i.e., low BMR) along with retention of salt and water. The retention of salt and water will put her at risk for congestive cardiomyopathy. The yellowing of her skin is due to the impaired conversion of β-carotenes into retinoic acid, which is normally driven by thyroid hormone.

Table 8.12. Commonly Tested Autoimmune Conditions

DISEASE	AUTOANTIBODY
Hashimoto thyroiditis	Antimicrosomal, antithyroglobulin
SLE	Antinuclear antibody (most sensitive, nonspecific) Anti-dsDNA (present with lupus-associated renal disease; indicates poor prognosis) Anti-Smith (very specific)
Drug-induced lupus	Antihistone
Scleroderma	Anticentromere (CREST) Anti-Scl-70/anti-topoisomerase (diffuse)
Graves disease	Anti-TSH
Myasthenia gravis	Anti-AChR
Pernicious anemia	Anti-intrinsic factor, antiparietal cell
Rheumatoid arthritis	Rheumatoid factor (anti-IgG)
Primary biliary cirrhosis	Antimitochondrial
Sjögren syndrome	Anti-Ro, anti-La
Celiac disease	Antigliadin, antiendomysial
Autoimmune hepatitis	Antismooth muscle
Goodpasture disease	Antibasement membrane
Granulomatosis with polyangiitis	c-ANCA (cytoplasmic)
Microscopic polyangiitis	p-ANCA (peripheral)
Pauci-immune crescentic glomerulonephritis	MPO-ANCA
Polymyositis Dermatomyositis	Anti-Jo-1
Diabetes type 1	Anti-glutamic acid decarboxylase

AChR, Acetylcholine receptor; *ANCA,* antineutrophil cytoplasmic antibodies; *CREST,* calcinosis, *R*aynaud syndrome, *e*sophageal dysmotility, *s*clerodactyly, *t*elangiectasia; *dsDNA,* double-stranded DNA; *IgG,* immunoglobulin G; *MPO,* myeloperoxidase; *SLE,* systemic lupus erythematosus; *TSH,* thyroid-stimulating hormone.

8. Given her history of menorrhagia, what hematologic disorder should we be worried about?
   Iron deficiency anemia is a concern as a result of her heavy periods, during which she loses blood and iron. The combination of pallor and fatigue also suggests this condition.

CASE 8.8 CONTINUED:

One year later, the patient is admitted to the emergency department (ED) with profound fatigue. Physical examination is significant for periorbital edema, blunted deep tendon reflexes, and sinus bradycardia. Laboratory workup shows a sodium level of 126 mEq/dL (normal range is 135–145 mEq/dL).

9. What is the diagnosis?
   This patient is experiencing *myxedema coma*, a complication of chronic hypothyroidism that can manifest as profound lethargy or coma, weakness, hypothermia, hypoventilation, hypoglycemia, and hyponatremia.

SOME DIFFERENTIAL DIAGNOSIS CONCEPTS

10. If this woman's history were significant for a recent upper respiratory infection and her thyroid were tender to palpation, what would be the most likely diagnosis?
    Those findings would suggest subacute granulomatous (de Quervain) thyroiditis. This disease starts out as *hyperthyroidism* as a result of inflammation causing release of stored thyroid hormones but then progresses to hypothyroidism once all of the stored hormone has been released. It is thought to involve viral infection of the thyroid gland, classically occurs following an upper respiratory infection, and usually resolves on its own.

Note: Subacute granulomatous thyroiditis is the only hypothyroid condition associated with a painful or tender thyroid on palpation.

11. **How can a thyroidectomy cause muscle cramps and paresthesias?**
Accidental removal of the parathyroid glands may occur during a thyroidectomy. The parathyroid glands are crucial for calcium homeostasis, and their accidental removal can lead to hypocalcemia, which may manifest with muscle cramps and paresthesias.
Signs of hypocalcemia include **C**hvostek sign (tap the patient's **C**heeks and see if facial muscles **C**ontract) and **T**rousseau sign (**T**ight blood pressure [BP] cuff causes hand **T**etany).

12. **What is the treatment option for hypothyroidism?**
Thyroid hormone replacement (i.e., levothyroxine) is needed, with a goal of normalizing TSH and relieving symptoms of hypothyroidism (Table 8.13).

Table 8.13. Manifestations of Hypothyroidism and Hyperthyroidism

FEATURE	HYPOTHYROIDISM	HYPERTHYROIDISM
Metabolic rate	Decreased	Increased
Body weight	Gain	Loss
Intestinal activity	Constipation	Diarrhea
Mental status	Memory loss/dementia	Psychosis, agitation
Body temperature	Cold intolerance	Heat intolerance
Deep tendon reflexes	Hypoactive	Hyperactive
Most severe complication	Myxedema coma	Thyroid storm

RELATED QUESTIONS

13. **How is it possible for a thyroid gland to develop at the back of the tongue?**
The thyroid begins its embryologic development at the back of the tongue and then migrates to its permanent position below the thyroid cartilage in the neck. Failure to migrate along the thyroglossal duct may result in a thyroid gland that is located at the back of the tongue. This is an important embryologic correlation to remember for the USMLE Step 1 exam.
Note: Persistence of the thyroglossal duct (the temporary passageway through which the thyroid migrates) can lead to a thyroglossal duct cyst.

14. **Why are thyroid hormone levels routinely evaluated in newborns?**
Congenital hypothyroidism is one of the preventable causes of intellectual disability. The most common etiology is due to thyroid dysgenesis during development. Newborns with congenital hypothyroidism will also present with macroglossia, hypotonia, umbilical hernia, and thickened facial features. If the hypothyroidism is left untreated during the first 2 to 3 years of life, permanent intellectual disability will develop.

SUMMARY BOX: HYPOTHYROIDISM

- Hypothyroidism classically presents with some combination of the following: weight gain, fatigue, cold intolerance, constipation, menorrhagia, and depression.
- The most common cause of hypothyroidism is Hashimoto thyroiditis, which is caused by autoimmune destruction of the thyroid gland. Hashimoto thyroiditis is often associated with other autoimmune conditions such as Addison disease, type 1 diabetes mellitus (T1DM), and pernicious anemia.
- Other causes of hypothyroidism include subacute granulomatous (de Quervain) thyroiditis, fibrous thyroiditis, iatrogenic thyroiditis (e.g., thyroidectomy or thyroid radiotherapy), cretinism, endemic goiter, and certain medications (e.g., lithium and amiodarone).
- *Euthyroid sick syndrome* refers to abnormalities in thyroid function that occur in ill patients without obvious thyroid or pituitary disease. It is common in hospitalized patients and may be related to reduced peripheral conversion of thyroxine (T_4) to triiodothyronine (T_3).
- Treatment for hypothyroidism is replacement therapy with thyroid hormone (i.e., levothyroxine), with a goal of normalizing serum levels of thyroid-stimulating hormone (TSH) and relieving symptoms.
- In the presence of a stressor such as infection, untreated hypothyroidism may progress to myxedema coma, which can manifest as profound lethargy or coma, weakness, hypothermia, hypoventilation, hypoglycemia, and hyponatremia.
- Congenital hypothyroidism is one of the preventable causes of intellectual disability.

CASE 8.9

A previously healthy 12-year-old boy presents to the clinic complaining of blurry vision, fatigue, and excessive thirst (polydipsia). His mother mentions that he has started to wet his bed at night again after many years of being toilet trained (secondary enuresis). His mother is also concerned because he has lost 10 lb despite an increasing appetite. A random (nonfasting) plasma glucose level is 220 mg/dL.

1. **What is the likely diagnosis?**
   The symptoms of polydipsia, enuresis, recent weight loss, and an elevated random plasma glucose in a young boy point to T1DM. You should also think about early-onset type 2 diabetes associated with sedentary lifestyle and obesity if the patient is overweight.

2. **Distinguish between type 1, type 2, and maturity-onset diabetes of youth.**
   T1DM is caused by autoimmune destruction of the pancreatic β cells. It classically occurs in children and adolescents. Patients are typically thin and their initial presentation may be one of diabetic ketoacidosis (DKA). The onset can be sudden, and insulin is always necessary for chronic management.
   Type 2 diabetes mellitus (T2DM) is caused by a combination of insulin resistance and pancreatic β cell dysfunction. It classically occurs in sedentary and overweight adults. Patients with type 2 diabetes are prone to hyperosmolar nonketotic syndrome and may occasionally experience DKA. There is more genetic predisposition for T2DM (90% in identical twins) than in T1DM (50% in identical twins).
   Maturity-onset diabetes of youth (MODY) is a group of dominantly inherited disorders caused by impaired insulin secretion. MODY mimics T1DM because of the impaired insulin secretion. There are currently six known types of MODY, with MODY2 and MODY3 being the most common. Patients with MODY typically do not experience DKA because they produce enough insulin for fatty acid uptake (Fig. 8.17).

CASE 8.9 CONTINUED:

An oral glucose tolerance test (OGTT) shows a plasma glucose level of 225 mg/dL 2 hours after the administration of a 75-g glucose load. Further workup reveals low levels of plasma insulin and C-peptide.

3. **Which type of diabetes does this boy have?**
   T1DM is associated with low levels of insulin and C-peptide as a result of autoimmune destruction of the pancreatic β cells. Recall that *C-peptide* is cosecreted (in equimolar amounts) with insulin because they share the same precursor molecule *proinsulin*. Proinsulin is cleaved into C-peptide and insulin at the Golgi organelles.

4. **How can measurements of plasma C-peptide be used to distinguish between factitious hypoglycemia and an insulinoma?**
   Because plasma C-peptide is cosecreted with endogenous insulin, serum levels of both C-peptide and insulin will be elevated in cases of an insulinoma. However, in factitious hypoglycemia, C-peptide levels will be low despite elevated insulin levels, as exogenous insulin administration does not lead to the production of C-peptide.

5. **Explain the mechanism by which the major metabolic pathways behave during insulin deficiency (i.e., explain why this patient has lost weight).**
   After consumption of a meal, insulin secretion is stimulated, which activates glycolysis, glycogenesis, fatty acid synthesis, and protein synthesis. In the setting of insulin deficiency, these pathways become less active and the opposing pathways (e.g., gluconeogenesis, glycogenolysis, and fatty acid catabolism) are stimulated; in essence, insulin deficiency causes a *hypercatabolic* state.

6. **What is the biochemical mechanism by which DKA develops in the setting of insulin deficiency?**
   Ordinarily, insulin stimulates fatty acid uptake by adipocytes by stimulating lipoprotein lipase. In the absence of insulin (or significant insulin deficiency), fewer fatty acids are taken up by the adipocytes. These fatty acids are in turn delivered to the liver where they are metabolized, resulting in the formation of ketoacids. Lack of insulin also promotes fatty acid catabolism, further exacerbating the problem. Finally, the acidosis is exacerbated because the corresponding hyperglycemia causes osmotic diuresis that leads to dehydration, making it more difficult for the kidneys to excrete acid.

7. **What is the short-term value of controlling the blood sugar in this boy?**
   Controlling this patient's blood sugar will prevent the symptoms of hyperglycemia (e.g., polyuria, polydipsia, and polyphagia), as well as prevent further unintentional weight loss. Additionally, in T1DM, the correction of insulin deficiency will prevent DKA.

8. **What is the long-term value of glycemic control in this boy?**
   Tight glycemic control has been proven to reduce the incidence of *microvascular* complications including retinopathy, neuropathy, and nephropathy. However, it has not yet been shown to reduce *macrovascular* events such as myocardial infarction and stroke, although future long-term studies may reveal such an effect as research continues.

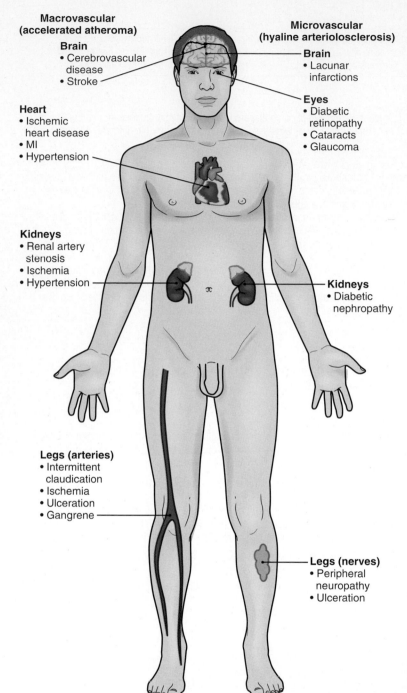

Macrovascular (accelerated atheroma)

Brain
- Cerebrovascular disease
- Stroke

Heart
- Ischemic heart disease
- MI
- Hypertension

Kidneys
- Renal artery stenosis
- Ischemia
- Hypertension

Legs (arteries)
- Intermittent claudication
- Ischemia
- Ulceration
- Gangrene

Microvascular (hyaline arteriolosclerosis)

Brain
- Lacunar infarctions

Eyes
- Diabetic retinopathy
- Cataracts
- Glaucoma

Kidneys
- Diabetic nephropathy

Legs (nerves)
- Peripheral neuropathy
- Ulceration

Figure 8.17. Chronic complications of diabetes mellitus. *MI,* Myocardial infarction. *(From Meszaros JG, Olson ER, Naugle JE, et al.* Crash Course: Endocrine and Reproductive Systems. *Philadelphia: Mosby; 2006.)*

9. What is the value of measuring the hemoglobin A_{1c} level routinely in this patient?
   The hemoglobin A_{1c} (HbA$_{1c}$) represents glycosylated hemoglobin, the levels of which are directly associated with levels of plasma glucose. It is an effective measure of long-term diabetes control because the life span of hemoglobin-laden red blood cells (RBCs) is approximately 120 days. Moreover, reduced HbA$_{1c}$ levels have been shown to correlate with better clinical outcomes.

10. Why should this patient's blood pressure be closely monitored as he ages and high blood pressure be treated aggressively with angiotensin-converting enzyme inhibitors if it develops?
    Blood pressure reduction substantially reduces the incidence of nephropathy and myocardial infarction in patients with diabetes. Angiotensin-converting enzyme (ACE) inhibitors are the most effective pharmacotherapy for preventing

nephropathy. Stroke is the number one killer in patients with diabetes, making it crucial to manage blood pressure to reduce the chances of a cerebrovascular infarct.

11. **Why are beta-blockers relatively contraindicated in diabetics?**

Beta-blockers are relatively contraindicated in patients with diabetes because they may mask the warning signs of pathologic hypoglycemia (e.g., tremors, shakes, and tachycardia). Additionally, by antagonizing hepatic β-receptors, beta-blockers make it more difficult for the liver to respond to epinephrine, a counterregulatory hormone that elevates blood glucose levels by stimulating glycogenolysis and gluconeogenesis. In T1DM, hypoglycemia is predominantly due to accidental insulin overdosing.

12. **What is the mechanism behind the boy's blurry vision?**

In a hyperglycemic state, there is a decreased glucose uptake by *insulin-dependent tissues* and increased uptake by *insulin-independent tissues*. In the eye, the enzyme aldose reductase converts excess intracellular glucose to sorbitol, an osmotically active molecule. The combination of glucose, sorbitol, and other metabolites increases osmotic pressure in the eyes and causes swelling of the lens. This causes the eyes' focal length to change, resulting in blurry vision.

CASE 8.9 CONTINUED:

The patient is diagnosed with type 1 diabetes mellitus and started on insulin therapy. One night, he inadvertently takes his nighttime insulin dose twice. He notices no ill effects that night, but the following morning his prebreakfast glucose value is substantially higher than normal.

13. **What has happened?**

Insulin-induced hypoglycemia during the night triggers release of stress hormones (e.g., cortisol, GH, glucagon, catecholamines) with counterregulatory functions that cause a compensatory increase in plasma glucose. If the patient is not educated about this, he may inappropriately increase the nighttime dose of insulin to reduce the morning blood sugar levels and potentially precipitate hypoglycemic coma or even death during the night.

SUMMARY BOX: TYPE 1 DIABETES MELLITUS

- Type 1 diabetes mellitus (T1DM) usually occurs in children and adolescents. Newly diagnosed patients are often thin and may present initially in diabetic ketoacidosis (DKA) or with a combination of polyuria, polydipsia, and polyphagia. The pathophysiology of T1DM is related to inadequate insulin secretion. The body behaves as if it is in a fasting state and, therefore, the processes of gluconeogenesis, glycogenolysis, and fatty-acid catabolism are all stimulated. Treatment for T1DM is insulin hormone replacement therapy.
- DKA occurs in the absence of insulin because fatty acids are delivered to the liver and metabolized to ketone bodies rather than being taken up by adipocytes. The hyperglycemia also causes an osmotic diuresis, which causes dehydration and exacerbates the metabolic derangements.
- Maturity-onset diabetes of the young (MODY) is an autosomal dominant inheritance disorder in which patients present with mild hyperglycemia from impaired glucose-induced release of insulin.
- Long-term tight glycemic control will delay the development of microvascular complications (i.e., retinopathy, neuropathy, nephropathy) and may also reduce the incidence of macrovascular complications (i.e., myocardial infarction, stroke, peripheral vascular disease).
- Hemoglobin A_{1c} (HbA_{1c}) levels reflect the percent of glycosylated hemoglobin at any given time. It is an effective measure of long-term diabetes control because the life span of hemoglobin-laden red blood cells (RBCs) is approximately 120 days. Reduced HbA_{1c} levels have been shown to correlate with better clinical outcomes.
- Beta-blockers are relatively contraindicated for diabetics, as they may mask the warning signs of pathologic hypoglycemia (e.g., tremors, shakes, and tachycardia).
- Taking too much nighttime insulin may result in an elevated morning plasma glucose level as a result of the pronounced counterregulatory response of catecholamines, glucagon, GH, and cortisol to the overnight hypoglycemia.

CASE 8.10

A middle-aged obese man being evaluated for a preemployment physical examination reports polydipsia and polyuria. His nonfasting (random) plasma glucose level is 275 mg/dL. Both of his parents were overweight, had "sugar problems," and died of cardiovascular complications.

1. **Is this patient more likely to have T1DM or T2DM?**

T2DM is commonly seen in overweight sedentary middle-aged adults with a strong family history of diabetes. Some of these patients are diagnosed after reporting increased thirst (polydipsia) and increased urinary frequency (polyuria). It has become more common for asymptomatic patients to be diagnosed during routine screening. Polyuria is caused by the osmotic diuresis of excess glucose in the blood, while polydipsia results from hypovolemia secondary to the polyuria.

2. **What is the pathogenesis of T2DM?**
   The early stage is characterized by impaired glucose tolerance, which leads to hyperinsulinemia in an attempt to compensate for peripheral insulin resistance. The later stages are characterized by pancreatic β cell dysfunction ("burnout"), which results in insulin deficiency.
   Either as the result of peripheral insulin resistance or insulin deficiency, hyperglycemia uniformly occurs in T2DM. Hyperglycemia results from increased lipolysis in adipose tissues (with glycerol acting as a gluconeogenic substrate in the liver). as well as reduced glucose uptake by skeletal muscle and adipose tissue.
   Note: The increased atherogenesis that occurs in diabetes may be explained *in part* by the increased plasma levels of free fatty acids.

3. **How does binding of insulin to the insulin receptor result in glucose uptake into cells?**
   It causes GLUT4 (insulin-dependent glucose transporter) to be incorporated into the membrane of cells in skeletal muscle and adipose tissue. Glucose is cotransported with potassium into the cell.

4. **What is the primary metabolic fuel in the fasting state?**
   Ketone bodies (β-hydroxybutyrate and acetoacetate) are the primary metabolic fuel in the fasting state. A notable exception to this is in the CNS, which relies exclusively on serum glucose in both the fed and fasting states. Only in periods of prolonged starvation will the CNS metabolize ketone bodies as well.

CASE 8.10 CONTINUED:

You take time to educate the patient about diabetes and plan a follow-up visit for 2 weeks. Fasting laboratory tests show plasma glucose of 180 mg/dL, total cholesterol of 250 mg/dL, low-density lipoprotein (LDL) cholesterol of 175 mg/dL, high-density lipoprotein (HDL) cholesterol of 30 mg/dL, and a urinalysis reveals microalbuminuria. The patient is told he has type 2 diabetes mellitus and is educated about the importance of diet and exercise. Pharmacotherapy is initiated with metformin. He returns to the clinic 3 months later, and his HbA$_{1c}$ has decreased from 8.5% to 7.5%.

5. **Why might therapy with a biguanide medication (e.g., metformin) make sense in this patient?**
   This patient has T2DM, is obese, and has dyslipidemia, all of which can be improved with metformin therapy.
   Metformin is widely considered to be the first-line medication for T2DM. It normalizes plasma glucose primarily by inhibiting hepatic glucose production and by stimulating peripheral uptake of glucose by adipose tissue and skeletal muscle. Furthermore, it has a beneficial effect on the lipid profile, it is very cheap (making it accessible to most patients), and it has an anorexic effect that may result in modest weight loss.
   Note: Metformin can very rarely cause a life-threatening lactic acidosis (though this side effect is commonly tested on USMLE exams). For this reason, metformin should be avoided in patients with congestive heart failure (CHF), liver disease, or renal disease and is usually held in hospitalized patients. In terms of cardiac risk stratification, diabetes is considered a coronary heart disease (CHD) risk equivalent, so a statin is indicated in the majority of patients with diabetes. Most patients with diabetes should be prescribed a statin, ACE inhibitor, and daily aspirin.

6. **What other classes of oral hypoglycemic agents are available to treat T2DM?**
   Sulfonylureas (e.g., *glipizide, glimepiride, glyburide*): Sulfonylurea increases insulin secretion by stimulating closure of the ATP-gated K$^+$ channel in pancreatic β cells. These drugs are associated with a risk of hypoglycemia in chronic kidney disease and may cause weight gain.
   Meglitinides (e.g., *repaglinide* and *nateglinide*): Meglitinides bind to the ATP-gated K$^+$ channel similar to sulfonylureas and increase insulin secretion by pancreatic β cells. These drugs have less of a risk of hypoglycemia than sulfonylureas, but are still associated with weight gain.
   α-Glucosidase inhibitors (e.g., *acarbose* and *miglitol*): These drugs prevent the breakdown of disaccharides into monosaccharides by brush border enzymes of the gut. This decreases the overall sugar level in the body.
   Dipeptidyl peptidase-4 inhibitors (e.g., *sitagliptin, saxagliptin, linagliptin*, and *alogliptin*): These drugs inhibit dipeptidyl peptidase-4 (DPP-4), which ordinarily functions to reduce incretin levels and increase glucagon production. Inhibiting DPP-4 will preserve (or increase) the plasma levels of insulin-stimulating incretins such as GLP-1.
   SGLT2 inhibitors (e.g., *canagliflozin, dapagliflozin, empagliflozin, ertugliflozin*): These agents promote the renal excretion of glucose by inhibiting SGLT2 in the proximal tubule of the kidney and must be used with caution in patients with reduced GFR, as a low GFR will reduce the efficacy of these agents. The resulting increased glucose load in the urine has a diuretic effect that is being studied for the treatment of heart failure.
   Thiazolidinediones (e.g., *pioglitazone* and *rosiglitazone*): These drugs are peroxisome proliferator-activating receptor γ (PPAR-γ) agonists. They increase insulin sensitivity in target tissues and decrease hepatic gluconeogenesis. These drugs are contraindicated in patients with heart failure, as they can exacerbate edema and weight gain.

7. **Why do the α-glucosidase inhibitors cause frequent gastrointestinal symptoms and annoying flatulence?**
   This class of drugs, which includes *acarbose* and *miglitol*, works by inhibiting intestinal α-glucosidases (e.g., sucrase, maltase, isomaltase), which break disaccharides down into monosaccharides that can be absorbed by the intestines. Following α-glucosidase inhibitor administration, the undigested sugars are metabolized by colonic bacteria, causing osmotic diarrhea and flatulence. These side effects are poorly tolerated by patients, and this drug class is therefore infrequently used.

Note: These drugs do not cause hypoglycemia, but if hypoglycemia occurs from a different oral hypoglycemic agent while the patient is taking an α-glucosidase inhibitor, oral glucose should be given because its intestinal absorption will not be impeded. Clearly, intravenous glucose would be given in a hospital setting.

8. Explain the mechanism of sulfonylureas in more detail.

   Sulfonylureas such as tolbutamide (first-generation agent) and glyburide (second-generation agent) act by stimulating insulin secretion. They accomplish this by increasing the potassium pump sensitivity to ATP: postprandial glucose uptake by the insulin-independent GLUT2 transporter results in more ATP production by the pancreatic β cell. Binding of ATP results in depolarization of the cell, which triggers the opening of voltage-gated calcium channels on the plasma membrane. The resultant influx of extracellular calcium stimulates insulin secretion, ultimately lowering plasma glucose levels.

   The mechanism of sulfonylureas relies on *intact pancreatic β cells.* If pancreatic β cells are already destroyed (e.g., in T1DM), sulfonylureas will *not* facilitate insulin release, and other drugs must be used to properly manage the patient's blood sugar levels.

9. What are some side effects of sulfonylureas?

   Improved glycemic control via increased insulin secretion may result in weight gain, because insulin stimulates fat synthesis. However, the more serious side effect of sulfonylureas is their propensity to precipitate hypoglycemia by causing excessive insulin secretion, particularly if a meal is skipped.

   Note: First-generation sulfonylureas (e.g., tolbutamide) can cause a disulfiram-like reaction and are now rarely used.

10. Besides the oral hypoglycemic agents, what other medications are available as an injection for the management of type 2 diabetes?

    GLP-1 analogs (incretin mimetics, e.g., *exenatide, lixisenatide, liraglutide, dulaglutide, semaglutide*): These medications stimulate pancreatic β cells to secrete insulin, inhibit glucagon secretion, and slow down gastric emptying. Notably, this drug class is associated with pancreatitis, but they may cause weight loss.

    Amylin analogs (e.g., *pramlintide*): Amylin is secreted alongside insulin. It slows down the gastric emptying time, regulates postprandial glucagon release, and decreases appetite.

    Insulin: See later for additional information about insulin.

11. Discuss the key pharmacologic timepoints (i.e., onset, peak, and duration) that distinguish rapid-acting, short-acting, intermediate-acting, and long-acting insulin preparations from one another.

    Rapid-acting (i.e., *lispro, aspart,* and *glulisine*): Rapid-acting insulin preparations have an onset of action within 30 minutes, peak in 1 to 2 hours, and last for no longer than 6 hours. These preparations induce the highest insulin peak of all the insulin preparation categories. They are administered subcutaneously and are typically administered prior to meals to control the postprandial glucose spike.

    Short-acting (i.e., *regular insulin*): Short-acting insulin preparations have an onset of action between 30 to 60 minutes, peak in 2 to 4 hours, and last no longer than 12 hours. These preparations are also administered subcutaneously.

    Intermediate-acting (i.e., *NPH insulin*): Intermediate-acting insulin preparations have an onset of action within 1 to 2 hours, peak in 4 to 6 hours, and last between 12 to 24 hours. These preparations are also administered subcutaneously.

    Long-acting (i.e., *detemir* and *glargine*): Long-acting insulin preparations have an onset of action within 1 to 4 hours, last for approximately 24 hours, and establish a stable plateau rather than a spiked peak during its course of action. These preparations are also administered subcutaneously and are often used to keep glucose levels regulated overnight or throughout fasting portions of the day (i.e., between meals).

    Note: Basal-bolus combinations are the recommended treatment for patients with poorly controlled diabetes, as this regimen includes the administration of a long-acting insulin earlier in the day along with a rapid-acting preparation prior to meals.

12. Why should this patient be educated about the importance of examining his feet periodically?

    Long-standing hyperglycemia in diabetes is associated with microvascular disease, as well as diabetic neuropathy. Microvascular disease causes poor perfusion of the feet (macrovascular disease can do this, too), leading to foot ulcers that do not heal well. In addition, diabetic neuropathy allows ulcers to fester without causing any noticeable pain.

    Note: Diabetic neuropathy is typically in a "stocking-glove" distribution, with the distal feet affected before the more distal aspects of the hands. This "stocking-glove" distribution is seen in other metabolic neuropathies as well, because longer axons are more susceptible to a metabolic abnormality.

CASE 8.10 CONTINUED:

The patient's creatinine gradually increased from 0.7 to 3.2 mg/dL over 2 years. A renal biopsy is as shown in Fig. 8.18.

13. What renal pathology should you suspect?

    Patients with diabetes are susceptible to nodular glomerulosclerosis and Kimmelstiel-Wilson nodules. The image in Fig. 8.18 shows nodular glomerulosclerosis with expansion of the mesangium by intensely periodic-acid Schiff (PAS)-positive material but without appreciable thickening of the glomerular capillary walls.

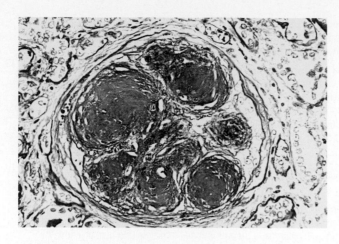

Figure 8.18. Light chain deposition disease. *(From Brenner BM. Brenner and Rector's The Kidney. 7th ed. Philadelphia: WB Saunders; 2004.)*

14. How can poor glycemic control cause this man to go into coma?

If he overdoses on sulfonylureas, he can go into a hypoglycemic coma. On the other hand, if his blood sugar runs too high, he can develop hyperglycemic hyperosmolar nonketosis. Finally, although patients with type 2 diabetes rarely go into DKA because of the presence of at least small amounts of insulin, if he becomes ill, DKA is another possibility.

SUMMARY BOX: TYPE 2 DIABETES MELLITUS

- Type 2 diabetes mellitus accounts for approximately 90% of cases of diabetes. Most patients with type 2 diabetes are overweight.
- The initial stage of type 2 diabetes is caused by peripheral insulin resistance and hyperinsulinemia. The later stage is caused by pancreatic β cell dysfunction and impaired insulin secretion.
- Clinical findings in type 2 diabetes include polyuria, polydipsia, vision problems (due to diabetic retinopathy), and diabetic neuropathy (in a stocking-glove distribution).
- Treatment for type 2 diabetes mellitus is exercise, diet control, and oral hypoglycemic agents. For the USMLE, you should be comfortable with the common diabetes drug classes and their side effects.

CASE 8.11

A 33-year-old pregnant woman with an unremarkable medical history is admitted to the hospital for her 24-week gestational screening. One hour after the administration of a 50-g glucose load, her plasma glucose is 166 mg/dL. She has no history of diabetes, and none of her family members have diabetes. She is asked to return 1 week later, and a 3-hour glucose tolerance test (100-g glucose drink) is administered. Her results are shown in Table 8.14.

Table 8.14. Results of Glucose Tolerance Test (Case 8.11)

TIME	SERUM GLUCOSE LEVEL	NORMAL RANGE
Fasting	95 mg/dL	95 mg/dL or below
At 1 hour	200 mg/dL	180 mg/dL or below
At 2 hours	181 mg/dL	155 mg/dL or below
At 3 hours	160 mg/dL	140 mg/dL or below

1. What is the diagnosis?

This patient has gestational diabetes. Gestational diabetes is defined as *new-onset* diabetes mellitus diagnosed during pregnancy but that begins *after a gestational age of 20 weeks*. If a pregnant patient has been diagnosed with diabetes mellitus prior to the pregnancy, she cannot be diagnosed with gestational diabetes as this would not be considered new onset. Similarly, if a pregnant patient has laboratory results indicating diabetes mellitus before week 20, that is *not* gestational diabetes. Gestational diabetes is associated with an increased risk for developing T2DM later in life.

All pregnant women should be screened between 24 and 28 weeks of gestation. In a 50-g glucose challenge test (GCT), a 1-hour postglucose challenge plasma glucose level of greater than 140 mg/dL is a positive finding. Confirmation of gestational diabetes is done using a 3-hour 100-g oral glucose tolerance test with a positive result having two or more values above the threshold value (after 1 hour > 180 mg/dL, after 2 hours > 155 mg/dL, and after 3 hours > 140 mg/dL).

2. **What is the cause of the relative maternal insulin resistance that develops during pregnancy, and how is this valuable to the fetus?**
   Maternal insulin resistance during pregnancy is thought to result from the placental secretion of human placental lactogen (hPL), a glycoprotein that lowers insulin sensitivity in the mother. Because glucose moves across the placenta by passive diffusion, this physiologic alteration is thought to facilitate delivery of glucose to the fetus.

3. **What is the most common undesired effect of maternal diabetes on fetal size, and why does this happen?**
   Fetal macrosomia (i.e., large fetus) is a complication of maternal diabetes and is problematic because of the increased risk of birth injury as an oversized fetus passes through the birth canal. Fetal size is increased because the maternal hyperglycemia stimulates fetal insulin secretion, which in turn stimulates fetal growth.

4. **Should hypoglycemia or hyperglycemia be expected in a baby born to a poorly controlled diabetic mother immediately following delivery? Explain.**
   Hypoglycemia is expected. While in utero, elevated fetal glucose levels (secondary to high maternal glucose levels) cause the fetal pancreas to secrete high amounts of insulin. Immediately following delivery, the fetal glucose levels drop because the glucose source from the mother disappears, but the fetus still produces a high amount of insulin. The treatment for this is to give the baby glucose after birth.

5. **What respiratory syndrome is the fetus at risk for at birth if the gestational diabetes is not corrected in the mother?**
   The fetus is at risk for respiratory distress syndrome (RDS) because surfactant production (by type II pneumocytes) is *decreased* by insulin and *increased* by cortisol and T_4. Mothers with gestational diabetes have higher-than-normal levels of insulin, increasing the risk of RDS in their newborn because of this lack of surfactant.

6. **What cardiac malformation is the fetus most at risk for when born to a diabetic mother?**
   Preexisting maternal diabetes is a risk factor for fetal transposition of the great vessels, where the aorta comes off of the right ventricle and the pulmonary arteries come off of the left ventricle. This is a cyanotic heart condition that requires an open ductus arteriosus for survival, to allow for the mixing of oxygenated and deoxygenated blood in the pulmonic and systemic circuits. In these cases, prostaglandins are given to the newborn to keep the ductus arteriosus patent; the definitive management is surgical.

SUMMARY BOX: GESTATIONAL DIABETES

- Gestational diabetes is defined as new-onset diabetes mellitus diagnosed during pregnancy but that begins after a gestational age of 20 weeks.
- All pregnant women should be screened with a glucose challenge test between 24 and 28 weeks of gestation. One hour after a 50-g glucose challenge test, blood glucose levels are taken, with a level greater than 140 mg/dL considered to be a positive screen. Confirmation can be made with a 3-hour glucose tolerance test.
- Gestational diabetes leads to an increased risk for diabetes later in life. It also predisposes newborns to macrosomia, hypoglycemia, and respiratory distress syndrome (RDS). Preexisting maternal diabetes can also lead to cardiac defects, such as transposition of the great vessels.

CASE 8.12

A 42-year-old registered nurse reports experiencing episodes of tremor, diaphoresis, and palpitations several hours after eating. She also notes similar symptoms when first waking in the morning. Symptoms are alleviated by eating. Her plasma glucose is low during symptomatic episodes, ranging from 30 to 60 mg/dL (she has access to a glucometer because her husband has diabetes). Review of systems is significant only for a 15-lb weight gain in recent months. Physical examination is unrevealing.

---

1. **What is the differential diagnosis for hypoglycemia in this woman?**
   Hypoglycemia can be reactive or due to insulin excess. Reactive (i.e., postprandial) hypoglycemia can occur under multiple circumstances, which are described later in this case. Excess insulin can be caused by an endogenous source (e.g., insulinoma, nesidioblastosis) or an exogenous source (e.g., factitious hypoglycemia).
   For the USMLE Step 1 exam, there is a correlation between patients with a significant psychiatric history or with access to prescription drugs (e.g., nurses, doctors) and exogenous insulin administration (i.e., factitious hypoglycemia).

2. **What is reactive (i.e., postprandial) hypoglycemia?**
   Reactive hypoglycemia can be categorized as functional, alimentary, or representing early (occult) diabetes.
   Functional hypoglycemia is the most common type. It occurs following meals and is associated with high-energy personalities. The mechanism of the hypoglycemia is unclear, but it is not thought to be related to excessive insulin secretion.

Alimentary hypoglycemia occurs in response to rapid glucose absorption. This is typically seen following gastric resections because gastric contents are delivered to the small bowel rapidly, resulting in a surge of insulin secretion and hypoglycemia. Symptoms will often respond to reduced carbohydrate intake, as well as smaller, more frequent meals.

Early or *occult* diabetes mellitus can also cause hypoglycemia. The mechanism is thought to be related to a delay in early insulin release from pancreatic βcells, resulting in hyperglycemia. An exaggerated late-phase insulin secretion then occurs in response to the hyperglycemia.

3. How can the C-peptide level help distinguish factitious from true hypoglycemia?

C-peptide and insulin are cleaved from the precursor hormone proinsulin. Therefore C-peptide is normally cosecreted from the pancreatic β cells with insulin in equivalent amounts. Exogenous insulin preparations do not contain C-peptide. Therefore patients self-administering insulin would be expected to have low levels of C-peptide, whereas patients with endogenous hyperinsulinism (e.g., insulinoma) will have high levels of C-peptide.

Note: It is important to recognize that sulfonylurea medications are an exception to this rule. Sulfonylureas act by stimulating pancreatic β cells to secrete proinsulin, which will increase serum levels of both insulin and C-peptide. Sulfonylurea ingestion can be very difficult to distinguish from an underlying insulinoma; therefore, obtaining a plasma sulfonylurea level can be helpful.

CASE 8.12 CONTINUED:

The patient returns the next day to the clinic, and blood work is performed. Fasting plasma glucose is low (35 mg/dL) and plasma insulin is markedly elevated. The patient is moderately symptomatic from her hypoglycemia. She is given some crackers and soda and her symptoms resolve.

4. Has the Whipple triad been satisfied by this patient?

Yes. The constellation of documented hypoglycemia, symptoms that can be reasonably attributed to hypoglycemia (e.g., confusion), and the resolution of these symptoms with eating (or the administration of glucose) is known as the *Whipple triad*. The Whipple triad is suggestive of, but not specific for, an insulinoma.

CASE 8.12 CONTINUED:

The patient is admitted for an observed 48-hour fast. A plasma sulfonylurea screen is negative. After 28 hours of observed fasting, the patient becomes confused and diaphoretic. Simultaneous measurements of glucose and insulin are again low and high, respectively. An MRI of the abdomen shows a small mass in the tail of the pancreas.

5. What is the most likely diagnosis?

Short of a definitive histologic diagnosis, we can be fairly certain that this patient has an insulinoma. Her insulin levels are inappropriately high in the presence of hypoglycemia. Furthermore, she does not appear to be abusing sulfonylureas, and the abdominal MRI is suggestive of a pancreatic insulinoma. The next step for this patient would be surgery.

SUMMARY BOX: HYPOGLYCEMIA AND INSULINOMA

- Hypoglycemia can manifest clinically as lethargy, tremor, and palpitations, which are due to stimulation of the sympathetic and parasympathetic arms of the autonomic nervous system.
- Hypoglycemia can be factitious in origin (as in a health care worker with access to insulin), reactive (i.e., postprandial), or secondary to endogenous hyperinsulinism (e.g., insulinoma).
- The diagnosis of an insulinoma requires demonstration of the Whipple triad—hypoglycemia, hypoglycemic symptoms, and resolution of symptoms with glucose.
- Proinsulin, when cleaved, produces two products: C-peptide and insulin.
- Another cause of hypoglycemia can be nesidioblastosis, or β islet cell hyperplasia. This is a rare hyperplasia disorder of the pancreatic β islet cells that results in excess insulin secretion, leading to a hypoglycemic state.
- Treatment of an insulinoma is surgical resection.

CASE 8.13

A 49-year-old man presents to the emergency department reporting left pelvic pain that radiates to the back for the past 2 weeks. A CT scan finds the presence of nephrolithiasis (renal stones) and a 5-cm mass at the head of the pancreas. On further questioning, the patient also reports visual problems and headache. An MRI of the head reveals a large mass located in the sella turcica.

1. **What do you suspect?**

   The presence of renal calculi suggests hyperparathyroidism, and the mass on the pancreas suggests a pancreatic adenoma. Visual deficits and the MRI finding are suggestive of a pituitary adenoma. The constellation of a pituitary adenoma, pancreatic neuroendocrine tumor, and hyperparathyroidism should make one think of MEN I. However, more information is needed to confirm this diagnosis.

CASE 8.13 CONTINUED:

Laboratory workup reveals elevated levels of gastrin, prolactin, and parathyroid hormone.

2. **What is the diagnosis?**

   The combination of hyperparathyroidism, hyperprolactinemia (likely due to a prolactinoma), and hypergastrinemia (likely from the pancreatic adenoma) confirm the diagnosis of MEN I. Hyperparathyroidism is the most common abnormality in MEN I, present in more than 90% of patients. It occurs 10 to 20 years earlier than the sporadic form of hyperparathyroidism and is much more aggressive. It typically involves all four parathyroid glands, meaning subtotal parathyroidectomy is rarely curative. MEN I is caused by mutations in the *MEN1* tumor suppressor gene. Hyperprolactinemia presents with amenorrhea and galactorrhea, while hypergastrinemia will commonly present with peptic ulcers.

   Note: The commonly tested constellation of symptoms that should make you think about hyperparathyroidism is described by the phrase "stones (i.e., nephrolithiasis), thrones (polyuria, constipation), bones and groans (bone pain as a result of cystic bone spaces with fibrous tissue), with psychiatric overtones (e.g., behavior changes, depression)." MEN I is described as having tumors in the 3 **P**'s: **p**ituitary, **p**arathyroid, and **p**ancreas.

3. **What is the danger of missing a diagnosis of MEN IIA?**

   MEN IIA is associated with medullary thyroid carcinoma, pheochromocytoma, and hyperplasia of the parathyroid glands. Cutaneous lichen amyloidosis has also been recently added. Medullary thyroid carcinoma, which can be life-threatening, has a frequency of almost 100% in patients with MEN IIA. This cancer forms from the parafollicular C cells in the thyroid and leads to increased calcitonin production, which can precipitate hypocalcemia. Pheochromocytoma has a frequency of around 40% to 50%, while hyperplasia of the parathyroid has a frequency of 10% to 20%. Therefore making the diagnosis and initiating early genetic screening are critical. MEN IIA is caused by mutations in the *RET* proto-oncogene.

4. **What is MEN IIB?**

   MEN IIB is very rare and is associated with medullary thyroid carcinoma and pheochromocytoma (as in MEN IIA), along with mucosal/acoustic neuromas and a marfanoid habitus. As with MEN IIA, medullary thyroid carcinoma is the most common component. However, unlike in MEN I and MEN IIA, hyperplasia of the parathyroid glands is not present. MEN IIB is also caused by mutations in the *RET* proto-oncogene, but this mutation is different from the mutation in MEN IIA.

5. **What is Zollinger-Ellison syndrome, and how is it related to MEN I?**

   Zollinger-Ellison syndrome is a disorder in which the hormone gastrin is produced in excess, directly causing the stomach to produce excess hydrochloric acid. This is usually due to a tumor that can arise in either the duodenum or pancreas. In this patient, a tumor of the pancreatic islet cells (gastrinoma) is causing the excessive gastrin production. Thirty percent of patients with gastrinoma of the pancreatic islet cells also have tumors of the parathyroid glands and the pituitary. These collective tumors are known as *MEN I*.

   Note: Other causes of hypergastrinemia include G cell hyperplasia, pernicious anemia, gastric outlet obstruction, renal failure, and chronic proton pump inhibitor use.

STEP 1 SECRET

Multiple endocrine neoplasia (MEN) syndromes are a USMLE favorite! You should know the tumors associated with all three types of MEN syndromes, as well as the constellation of symptoms that result from them. Exam questions on MEN syndromes are often straightforward but will most likely require you to identify the associated conditions without explicitly mentioning MEN syndrome, which can be tricky for some students. The best way to get good at this is to practice, practice, and practice some more.

SUMMARY BOX: MULTIPLE ENDOCRINE NEOPLASIA (MEN) SYNDROMES

- The constellation of a pituitary adenoma, pancreatic neuroendocrine tumor, and hyperparathyroidism should make one think of MEN I. Primary hyperparathyroidism is the most common abnormality in MEN I, present in more than 90% of patients. It occurs 10 to 20 years earlier than the sporadic form of primary hyperparathyroidism and is much more aggressive. It typically involves all four parathyroid glands, meaning subtotal parathyroidectomy is rarely curative. MEN I is caused by mutations in the MEN1 tumor suppressor gene, which codes for the protein menin.

SUMMARY BOX: MULTIPLE ENDOCRINE NEOPLASIA (MEN) SYNDROMES—cont'd

- MEN IIA is associated with medullary thyroid carcinoma, pheochromocytoma, and hyperplasia of the parathyroid. Cutaneous lichen amyloidosis has also been added.
- Medullary thyroid carcinoma, which can be life-threatening, has a frequency of nearly 100% in patients with MEN IIA. Therefore making the diagnosis and initiating early genetic screening are critical. MEN IIA is caused by mutations in the *RET* proto-oncogene.
- MEN IIB is rare and is associated with medullary thyroid carcinoma, pheochromocytoma, mucosal/acoustic neuromas, and a marfanoid habitus. As with MEN IIA, medullary thyroid carcinoma is the most common component and is also caused by mutations in the *RET* proto-oncogene. However, unlike in MEN I and MEN IIA, hyperplasia of the parathyroid is not present.
- Zollinger-Ellison syndrome is caused by a tumor in the duodenum or pancreas that secretes excessive amounts of gastrin. Approximately 30% of patients with a gastrinoma of the pancreatic islet cells have MEN I.

CASE 8.14

A 41-year-old woman with an unremarkable past medical history is noted to have asymptomatic hypercalcemia on routine screening. She takes no medications. Physical examination is unremarkable.

---

1. **What are some causes of hypercalcemia?**
   In healthy outpatients, primary hyperparathyroidism is the most common cause of hypercalcemia, while in hospitalized patients, hypercalcemia of malignancy is the most common cause. Together these two are responsible for approximately 90% of cases of hypercalcemia. However, there are many other causes of hypercalcemia to be considered. Primary hyperparathyroidism is associated with other endocrine disorders, such as the MEN I and IIA described previously in this chapter. Frequent use of calcium-containing antacids may lead to milk-alkali syndrome. Other medications (e.g., thiazide diuretics, lithium) can also cause hypercalcemia. Hypercalcemia can also be caused by either hyperthyroidism or Cushing syndrome. Paraneoplastic syndromes that produce parathyroid hormone–related peptide (PTHrP) can also cause hypercalcemia. A genetic disorder of the calcium-sensing receptor in familial hypocalciuric hypercalcemia (FHH) is yet another potential cause of hypercalcemia. Finally, excessive serum levels of vitamin D (which may occur due to toxic ingestion, lymphomas, or granulomatous diseases such as sarcoidosis) can also lead to hypercalcemia.

CASE 8.14 CONTINUED:

A review of this patient's medical records shows that she has had mild hypercalcemia since the age of 21. Upon questioning, it is discovered that her mother and an aunt both have mild hypercalcemia.

---

2. **How can this information be used to identify the most likely cause of her hypercalcemia?**
   Given the strong family history, this patient likely has either primary hyperparathyroidism (likely associated with a MEN syndrome) or FHH. Knowing if she has ever had nephrolithiasis can help us determine which of these two potential diagnoses should be our leading diagnosis.

CASE 8.14 CONTINUED:

She denies a personal or family history of nephrolithiasis. A 24-hour urine collection reveals low amounts of urinary calcium excretion. Polymerase chain reaction (PCR) testing shows a mutation in her calcium-sensing receptor (*CASR*) gene.

---

3. **What is the diagnosis?**
   Based on this additional information, our patient can be diagnosed with FHH, which is associated with hypercalcemia resulting in part from deficient renal calcium excretion. It is inherited in an autosomal dominant manner. In contrast with primary hyperparathyroidism (which is often associated with markedly elevated PTH, osteoporosis, and hypercalciuria causing calcium oxalate kidney stones), patients with FHH typically have only a modest elevation in PTH and rarely have kidney stones. Nonetheless, FHH is often confused with mild cases of primary hyperparathyroidism. The danger in misdiagnosing FHH for primary hyperparathyroidism is that these patients may unnecessarily undergo a parathyroidectomy.

4. **How does an inactivated calcium-sensing receptor gene in FHH cause hypercalcemia?**
   The *CASR* gene in the parathyroid glands mediates feedback inhibition of PTH secretion in response to high serum calcium. An inactivated CASR does not inhibit PTH secretion in response to hypercalcemia. This results

in a higher-than-normal serum calcium level required to inhibit PTH secretion, leading to mild hypercalcemia and a modest elevation in PTH. The degree of hypercalcemia depends on how severely the *CASR* gene is affected.

5. **What is the treatment for FHH?**
   FHH usually does not require treatment, and most affected persons are asymptomatic. However, for those who are symptomatic, thiazide diuretics may be given.

RELATED QUESTIONS

6. **What are the three hormones that regulate calcium levels in the blood and tissues and what is their origin of secretion?**
   PTH is secreted from the chief cells in the parathyroid glands. PTH is released in response to low serum calcium, and its purpose is to raise the serum calcium level. PTH is also nicknamed "**p**hosphate **t**rashing **h**ormone," as it also functions to lower serum phosphate levels. Notably, low magnesium levels (e.g., diarrhea, diuretics, alcohol) decrease PTH secretion, influencing serum calcium.

   Vitamin D is obtained from diet and synthesized from cholesterol with the help of ultraviolet (UV) light. Its purpose is to raise the serum calcium level.

   Calcitonin is produced by the parafollicular **C** cells in the thyroid gland. Calcitonin is secreted in response to high serum calcium and will lower the serum calcium level. It is also secreted in medullary thyroid cancer (e.g., MEN IIA and IIB).

7. **How does inactive vitamin D get converted to the active form?**
   See Fig. 8.19.

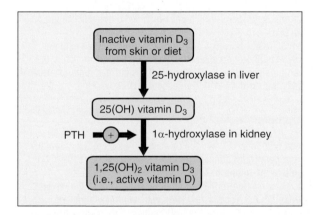

Figure 8.19. Activation of vitamin D. *OH,* Hydroxy; *PTH,* parathyroid hormone. *(From Meszaros JG, Olson ER, Naugle JE, et al. Crash Course: Endocrine and Reproductive Systems. Philadelphia: Mosby; 2006.)*

SUMMARY BOX: FAMILIAL HYPOCALCIURIC HYPERCALCEMIA

- Familial hypocalciuric hypercalcemia (FHH) is caused by autosomal dominant loss-of-function mutations in the calcium-sensing receptor (*CASR*) gene. Patients with FHH are typically asymptomatic and present with hypercalcemia, hypocalciuria, and normal or modestly elevated parathyroid hormone (PTH) levels revealed during routine lab testing.
- FHH can be diagnosed with genetic testing for *CASR* mutations, checking family history for hypercalcemia, and measuring 24-hour urine calcium excretion.
- Treatment for patients with FHH who are asymptomatic is simply observation. If the patient is symptomatic from the hypercalcemia, a thiazide diuretic is often enough to manage these symptoms.

CASE 8.15

A newborn baby presents with ambiguous external genitalia. The child seems to have an enlarged clitoris rather than a penis and has a scrotum-like structure that appears to be the result of labial fusion. Physical examination also reveals tachycardia, hypotension, irritability, and hyperpigmentation seen most readily in the areolae and genitalia. Laboratory tests show hypoglycemia, hyponatremia, and hyperkalemia. An ultrasound reveals normally developed ovaries, and the child's karyotype is found to be 46,XX.

1. **What is the most likely diagnosis?**
   This baby girl most likely has congenital adrenal hyperplasia (CAH), which is most commonly due to 21α-hydroxylase deficiency. All forms of CAH are characterized by deficient cortisol production, but depending on the specific enzyme that is deficient or defective, levels of other adrenal steroids will be either increased or decreased (Fig. 8.20). This

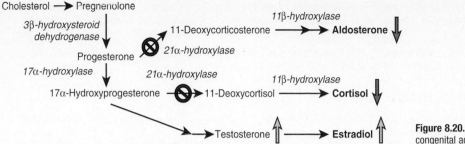

Figure 8.20. Pathophysiology of congenital adrenal hyperplasia.

information can be used to identify which particular enzyme is defective, and you should be comfortable recognizing these patterns on your USMLE exams.

21α-Hydroxylase deficiency accounts for about 90% of CAH cases, while 11β-hydroxylase deficiency accounts for most of the remaining 10%. Both 21α-hydroxylase and 11β-hydroxylase deficiency have decreased aldosterone and cortisol production and can be distinguished from one another by the presence of hypotension (21α-hydroxylase deficiency) or normal/mildly elevated blood pressure (11β-hydroxylase deficiency).

2. **How does 21α-hydroxylase deficiency cause virilization of females?**
The adrenal steroid biosynthetic pathways produce three major hormones: mineralocorticoids (e.g., aldosterone), glucocorticoids (e.g., cortisol), and sex hormones (e.g., androgens or estrogens). In CAH, 21α-hydroxylase deficiency will cause the production of aldosterone and cortisol to decrease, shunting the existing precursor ingredients into the only available biosynthesis pathway: sex hormones. This leads to an overproduction of steroid precursors (e.g., 17-hydroxyprogesterone) and excessive accumulation of adrenal androgens, which causes in utero masculinization of developing girls (i.e., virilization of a fetus with genotype 46,XX).

XY disorder of sex development (DSD) occurs when an individual is a 46,XY karyotype but has female external genitalia. The most common disorder that causes this condition is androgen insensitivity syndrome (AIS), which is the result of a defective androgen receptor. XX DSD occurs when an individual is a 46,XX karyotype but has male external genitalia and secondary sex characteristics. XX DSD is usually the result of CAH. Ovotesticular DSD, which is usually XX, presents with both testicular and ovarian tissues.

3. **Why does this patient exhibit hyperkalemia, hyponatremia, tachycardia, hypotension, and hypoglycemia?**
In CAH as a result of 21α-hydroxylase deficiency, aldosterone production is minimal or absent. Aldosterone is normally responsible for the maintenance of plasma volume and serum potassium concentration by promoting the reabsorption of sodium in exchange for potassium in the early distal tubule of the nephron. Aldosterone deficiency leads to hypovolemia, hyperkalemia, and, in the case of severe deficiency, hyponatremia from salt wasting. (Recall that sodium loss usually does not cause hyponatremia, but severe hypovolemia from sodium wasting will eventually stimulate antidiuretic hormone [ADH] release, which in turn may lead to hyponatremia as the ADH inadvertently dilutes the existing serum sodium while attempting to maintain fluid volume.)

Hypoglycemia is due to decreased cortisol activity, as cortisol typically serves a counterregulatory function against insulin.

Note: Cortisol deficiency is also a major contributor (if not the primary contributor) to hypotension in the setting of adrenal insufficiency. Cortisol upregulates α1-receptors on blood vessels to maintain cardiovascular tone and blood pressure. Acute cortisol deficiency can lead to severe hypotension that will be refractory to fluid resuscitation in the absence of glucocorticoid replacement. This is a common phenomenon in adult intensive care unit (ICU) patients, who may fail to adequately increase their cortisol secretion in response to the stress of critical illness (i.e., relative adrenal insufficiency). This is also common in surgery, as patients who have a blunted HPA axis (likely due to prescribed corticosteroid use) are unable to increase their cortisol secretion in response to stress to maintain blood pressure. It is important to give these patients extra doses of steroids prior to operating and to continuously monitor their status throughout the procedure.

These electrolyte and hemodynamic disturbances of cortisol deficiency make CAH and other forms of acute adrenal insufficiency rapidly fatal if left unrecognized. Once the condition is diagnosed, treatment is straightforward with replacement of cortisol. Often a synthetic mineralocorticoid (i.e., fludrocortisone) is also given, although because cortisol has some mineralocorticoid activity, some patients do well with cortisol replacement alone.

4. **Why might patients with CAH experience bilateral adrenal hyperplasia and hyperpigmentation?**
The low cortisol level reduces negative feedback on pituitary ACTH production, leading to dramatic increases in ACTH levels that stimulate bilateral adrenal glandular hyperplasia. Recall that ACTH also stimulates adrenal androgen synthesis, which further contributes to the virilization of females with CAH.

The hyperpigmentation is due to increased production of MSH. Remember that POMC is cleaved into ACTH, endorphins, and MSH. Any increase in ACTH production is accompanied by an increase in MSH, which stimulates melanin production and leads to hyperpigmentation.

Note: Except for the virilization, many of the disease manifestations of CAH are identical to those seen in adults with disorders of primary adrenal insufficiency, such as autoimmune adrenalitis (i.e., Addison disease). These features include hypotension, salt wasting with hypovolemia and hyponatremia, hyperkalemia, hypoglycemia, and hyperpigmentation.

RELATED QUESTIONS

5. How are the symptoms and laboratory results of 11β-hydroxylase deficiency different from those of 21α-hydroxylase deficiency?

   These two forms of CAH share the same presentation, except for one distinguishing factor. In 11β-hydroxylase deficiency, there is an accumulation of 11-deoxycorticosterone (11-DOC), which functions as a weak mineralocorticoid. This causes at least some salt and fluid retention, leading to preserved blood pressure (i.e., no hypotension), or even mild hypertension in some cases.

6. Why do males with 17α-hydroxylase deficiency present phenotypically as female?

   With regard to external genitalia, all fetuses are female by default; it is the production of androgens that masculinizes the external genitalia, and the presence of anti-Müllerian hormone (AMH) that prompts the development of internal male genital structures. However, with low levels of 17α-hydroxylase, insufficient levels of androgens are produced. In fetuses that are genetically male (i.e., 46,XY), this means the fetus will be unable to masculinize its external genitalia, resulting in male XY DSD.

   Note: Because estrogens are invariably synthesized from androgens (via aromatization), there is also low estrogen production in patients with 17α-hydroxylase deficiency. Thus girls with this rare form of CAH will usually present later in adolescence with delayed pubertal development or lack of menarche.

7. Why are patients with 17α-hydroxylase deficiency often hypertensive?

   17α-Hydroxylase deficiency blocks the androgen and cortisol biosynthesis pathways, increasing the flux of precursor ingredients through the aldosterone synthesis pathway. The resulting increase in aldosterone production causes increased salt and water retention, which may lead to hypervolemia and hypertension in this patient population.

8. Quick review: Cover the columns on the right side of Table 8.15 and list the signs and symptoms for the major congenital metabolic disorders within each metabolic pathway and their clinical manifestations.

SUMMARY BOX: CONGENITAL ADRENAL HYPERPLASIA (CAH)

- Congenital adrenal hyperplasia (CAH) is due to defects in glucocorticoid (i.e., cortisol) synthesis that result in hypoadrenalism and, depending on the specific enzyme involved, either increased or decreased levels of mineralocorticoids or sex steroids.
- 21α-Hydroxylase deficiency accounts for 90% of CAH. It results in deficiency of cortisol and aldosterone; excess adrenal androgens (resulting in ambiguous external genitalia in females); salt wasting with hypotension, tachycardia, hyponatremia, and hyperkalemia; hypoglycemia; and hyperpigmentation.
- 11β-Hydroxylase deficiency can lead to virilization of genetically female (i.e., 46,XX) fetuses, fluid retention, and hypertension due to excess 11-deoxycorticosterone production.
- 17α-Hydroxylase deficiency leads to excess aldosterone production, sex hormone deficiency, and disorder of sexual differentiation of genetically male (i.e., 46,XY) fetuses.

Table 8.15. Major Congenital Metabolic Disorders

METABOLIC PATHWAY	GENETIC DISEASES	PRIMARY CAUSE OF CLINICAL SYMPTOMS	MAJOR SIGNS/ SYMPTOMS
Glycogenolysis	Glucose-6-phosphatase deficiency (von Gierke disease)	Hypoglycemia	Hypoglycemic episodes, massive hepatomegaly
	Muscle glycogen phosphorylase deficiency (McArdle disease)	Inability of muscle to utilize glucose stored as glycogen	Muscle pain, exercise intolerance
Hexose monophosphate shunt (i.e., pentose phosphate pathway)	G6PD deficiency	RBC susceptibility to oxidative stress (e.g., sulfa or antimalarial drugs, infection)	Hemolytic anemia
Fatty acid oxidation	MCAD deficiency	Hypoglycemia	Hypoketotic hypoglycemia, hyperammonemia

Continued

Table 8.15. Major Congenital Metabolic Disorders—cont'd

Urea cycle	Various enzyme deficiencies	Hyperammonemia	Encephalopathy
Amino acid metabolism	PKU	Toxic accumulation of phenylalanine and phenylketone derivatives; lack of tyrosine	Mental retardation, light pigmentation, eczema, "mousy" odor
	Maple syrup urine disease	Toxic accumulation of branched-chain amino acids (especially leucine) and their ketoacid derivatives	Poor feeding, psychomotor retardation, maple syrup odor to urine
Heme synthesis	AIP and other acute porphyrias	Accumulation of porphyrin intermediates toxic to neurons	Neurovisceral symptoms (neuropathy, episodic abdominal pain)
	Porphyria cutanea tarda and other cutaneous porphyrias	Accumulation of photoreactive porphyrins within skin and/or RBCs	Photosensitive chronic blistering
	Hemolytic porphyrias		Hemolytic anemia
Adrenal corticosteroid synthesis	Congenital adrenal hyperplasia	Deficiency of cortisol and deficiency and/or excess of mineralocorticoids and sex steroids	*All forms*: adrenal insufficiency with glandular hyperplasia and hyperpigmentation
	21α-Hydroxylase deficiency	Low cortisol and mineralocorticoids; excess androgens	Virilization in females; salt wasting with hypotension, hyponatremia, hyperkalemia
	11β-Hydroxylase deficiency	Low cortisol, excess mineralocorticoids (11-DOC) and androgens	Virilization in females; hypertension and fluid overload

11-DOC, 11-Deoxycorticosterone; *AIP*, acute intermittent porphyria; *G6PD*, glucose-6-phosphate dehydrogenase; *MCAD*, medium-chain fatty acid decarboxylase; *PKU*, phenylketonuria; *RBCs*, red blood cells.

CHAPTER 9

MALE AND FEMALE REPRODUCTIVE SYSTEMS

Insider's Guide to Male and Female Reproductive Systems for the USMLE Step 1

Students tend to brush off reproductive physiology and pathology during their USMLE preparation, but this is a huge mistake in our opinion. This subject is incredibly straightforward (and bound to give you a lot of free points!) if you work hard at it. Reproductive physiology is tremendously important. You should have a thorough understanding of the menstrual cycle, hormonal regulation, and the factors controlling male and female sexual differentiation. This will be of enormous help when it comes to understanding pathology and pathophysiology. We have done our best to offer the most USMLE-like case presentations in this chapter. Whenever relevant, you should pay close attention to the laboratory findings associated with these diseases as they relate to disorders of the hypothalamic-pituitary-gonadal axis.

BASIC CONCEPTS

1. **What is the normal duration of the menstrual cycle? What are the two phases of the ovarian cycle and which occurs first?**

   The normal menstrual cycle is approximately 28 days. It can be subdivided into phases of either the uterine cycle or the ovarian cycle, both spanning the full length of the menstrual cycle simultaneously. The ovarian cycle describes the changes that occur within the ovary as the follicle matures, the ovum is released, and the corpus luteum develops. The ovarian cycle consists sequentially of the follicular and luteal phases. The first day of the menstrual cycle (and hence the follicular phase of the ovarian cycle) is defined as the day menstruation begins (Fig. 9.1). The uterine cycle, on the other hand, consists of menstrual flow, the proliferative phase, and the secretory phase. It describes the changes that occur to the endometrium (inner lining) of the uterus for implantation of a fertilized egg and shedding of that lining in the case of implantation failure.

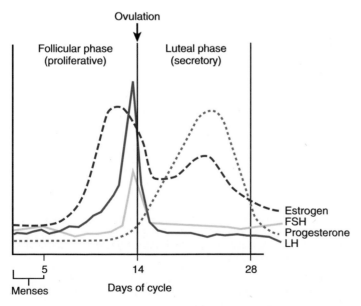

Figure 9.1. Menstrual cycle. *FSH,* Follicle-stimulating hormone; *LH,* luteinizing hormone. *(From Brown TA.* Rapid Review Physiology. *Philadelphia: Mosby; 2007.)*

2. **Which phase of the ovarian cycle is generally responsible for the cycle being longer or shorter?**

   The follicular phase is responsible for the cycle's length. For the USMLE, you should assume the luteal phase spans the latter 14 days of the menstrual cycle, as that is the case in the majority of females. Thus any differences in menstrual cycle length, whether longer or shorter than 28 days, can be accounted for by differences in follicular phase length.

3. During the follicular phase, what hormonal changes occur in the pituitary gland and the ovary?

Pituitary gland: If an egg is not fertilized by a sperm, the corpus luteum—the principal source of both estrogen and progesterone in the female reproductive system—involutes at the end of the luteal phase (see Fig. 9.1). This results in low estrogen and progesterone levels at the start of a new menstrual cycle (follicular phase). The reduction in estrogen's negative feedback on the anterior pituitary results in a rise in follicle-stimulating hormone (FSH), while the reduction in progesterone prompts menstruation, or shedding of the uterine endometrial lining.

Ovary: During the follicular phase, the rising FSH stimulates the development of several ovarian follicles, eventually provoking the emergence of a dominant follicle, which becomes a site of estrogen synthesis while the other follicles regress. The growing follicle secretes increasing amounts of estrogen, which has the effect of inhibiting pituitary FSH production, thereby gradually reducing serum FSH levels in the later part of the follicular phase. However, the dominant follicle becomes increasingly sensitive to circulating FSH, so plasma estrogen levels still continue to rise throughout the follicular phase.

Note: Inhibin is also secreted by the granulosa cells of the developing ovarian follicles and selectively inhibits FSH secretion without affecting luteinizing hormone (LH) secretion.

4. What occurs in the uterus during the follicular phase?

The estrogen secreted by the ovaries stimulates proliferation of the endometrial lining of the uterus throughout the follicular phase (i.e., the proliferative phase of the uterine cycle coincides with the follicular phase of the ovarian cycle).

5. What event triggers ovulation at the end of the follicular phase?

When plasma estrogen reaches a critical level, it switches from exerting negative feedback on the pituitary to exerting positive feedback by sensitizing gonadotropes to gonadotropin-releasing hormone (GnRH). This stimulates the pituitary to release a surge of LH and, to a lesser extent, FSH. The surge of LH, which remains elevated for approximately 24 hours, triggers ovulation, and causes rupture of the follicle and subsequent release of the ovum. This is an elegant design feature because high estrogen levels indicate to the pituitary gland that the ovarian follicle is sufficiently "mature" to be released.

6. What happens in the ovary and endometrium during the luteal phase?

After ovulation, the cells that lined the ruptured follicle (granulosa cells and theca interna cells) form the corpus luteum ("yellow body") under the influence of LH. The corpus luteum synthesizes both estrogen and a large amount of progesterone. The progesterone stimulates the endometrium to become more secretory and glandular in preparation for implantation. It also stimulates the spiral arteries to develop. These arteries empty into the intervillous space so that chorionic villi from the cytotrophoblast can extract oxygen if fertilization occurs. If fertilization does not occur, the corpus luteum degenerates, the levels of estrogen and progesterone fall, and the endometrium sloughs off in the form of menstrual flow.

You are expected to be able to differentiate between the histologic appearances of the endometrial lining during the follicular and luteal phases (Fig. 9.2). Notice the glandular hypertrophy, irregular shape of glands, and well-developed spiral arteries in the luteal (secretory) phase. In contrast, the glands in the follicular phase are smaller and straighter, and there is less vascularity in the stroma.

7. In females with amenorrhea (absence of menses), why does bleeding after the cessation of a brief course of progesterone indicate that the cause of amenorrhea is due to the lack of ovulation?

In order to answer this question, one has to have a thorough comprehension of the normal physiology of the menstrual cycle; hence, this is a good USMLE-style question.

The only source of endogenous progesterone is the corpus luteum, which forms as a result of ovulation. If there is no ovulation, there is no progesterone secretion, and no menses will ensue. However, if the administration and subsequent withdrawal of progesterone precipitates menses in an amenorrhoeic patient, it indicates the endometrium is capable of sufficient estrogen priming, yet no ovulation is taking place (anovulation).

The most common causes of anovulation are obesity, polycystic ovary syndrome, eating disorders (can result in decreased GnRH levels), premature ovarian failure, hyperprolactinemia (prolactin inhibits GnRH release), thyroid disorders (increased thyrotropin-releasing hormone [TRH] levels can stimulate prolactin release), adrenal insufficiency, and Asherman syndrome (multiple uterine intracavitary adhesions and loss of the proliferative layer of the endometrium commonly following overly aggressive dilation and curettage procedures).

8. How does fertilization prevent degeneration of the corpus luteum?

If the ovum is fertilized, the developing embryo will synthesize human chorionic gonadotropin (hCG), which acts similarly to LH and promotes maintenance of the corpus luteum during the first trimester.

9. How does the corpus luteum function in the maintenance of pregnancy?

During the first 6 weeks of pregnancy, the corpus luteum is the primary producer of estrogen and progesterone, hormones required for the continuation of pregnancy. After the sixth week of pregnancy, the placenta begins to take over as the principal site of steroidogenesis. After delivery and removal of the placenta, both estrogen and progesterone levels fall markedly.

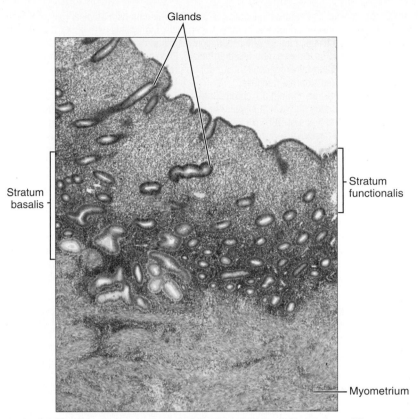

Figure 9.2. Low-magnification view of the uterine endometrium during the proliferative (follicular) phase of the reproductive cycle. Growing endometrial glands have straight profiles. *(From Telser A, Young J, Baldwin K.* Elsevier's Integrated Histology. *Philadelphia: Mosby; 2008.)*

10. What is the function of the *SRY* gene?

    The *SRY* gene is located on the Y chromosome and is responsible for testicular development (mediated by testis-determining factor). Testes contain two major cell types: Leydig cells and Sertoli cells. Leydig cells secrete testosterone, which stimulates the development of the mesonephric ducts. The mesonephric ducts develop into all of the male internal genitalia (epididymis, seminal vesicles, ejaculatory duct, and ductus deferens), with the exception of the prostate. Testosterone also is converted into dihydrotestosterone (DHT), which stimulates the development of the male external genitalia and prostate. Sertoli cells produce Müllerian-inhibiting factor (MIF), which permits the degeneration of the paramesonephric duct. If degeneration does not occur, the paramesonephric duct develops by default into the female internal genitalia (uterus, fallopian tubes, and upper third of the vagina).

11. What are the major functions of Sertoli cells?

    The major functions of Sertoli cells include support of spermatogenesis, formation of the blood-testis barrier, production of inhibin (inhibits FSH via negative feedback), production of MIF (represses paramesonephric ducts in utero), and production of androgen-binding protein (binds testosterone). Sertoli cells are activated by FSH. In contrast, Leydig cells produce testosterone in response to LH stimulation.

12. Describe the hormones associated with normal testicular descent.

    Normal testicular descent involves a transabdominal phase, which is mediated by MIF (a product of Sertoli cells), and a scrotal phase, which is mediated by androgens and β-hCG. The testes then descend into the scrotum via the gubernaculum. Cryptorchidism refers to incomplete descent of the testes into the scrotal sac. The most common location of undescended testes is in the inguinal canal. Generally, the condition is unilateral and resolves spontaneously by 3 months. If uncorrected, cryptorchidism can result in infertility secondary to arrested germ cell maturation. More specifically, the higher surrounding temperature of undescended testes in the abdomen, compared to descended testes in the scrotum, inhibits Sertoli cells from undergoing spermatogenesis and producing inhibin. In contrast, Leydig cells are typically unaffected. Failure to correct cryptorchidism also increases the risk of seminoma and testicular infarction secondary to torsion of the undescended testes.

13. What is a disorder of sex development?

    Ovotesticular disorder of sex development (DSD; note that there is some criticism of this term) refers to the presence of both male and female internal genitalia (ovotestes). This condition is very rare. An atypical genital appearance but not with both male and female gonads is more common; the term describes any person in whom there is discordance between the sex of the internal and external genitalia. 46,XX DSD presents with atypical genitalia and a 46,XX karyotype in the newborn period and is classic congenital adrenal hyperplasia. Individuals with 46,XX DSD do not have an *SRY* gene and thus do not develop testes. Lack of MIF production results in development of female internal genitalia from the paramesonephric duct (uterus, ovaries, and fallopian tubes). Exposure to excessive androgen concentrations during the early gestational period (either by exogenous intake during pregnancy or through congenital adrenal hyperplasia) stimulates production of virilized external genitalia.

Individuals with 46,XY DSD do contain a Y chromosome and thus develop testes. While the testes are usually undescended, they do still produce MIF, which inhibits the development of female internal genitalia. Yet, their external genitalia are feminized. Several types of DSD exist, including disorders of androgen synthesis (e.g., 17-β-hydroxysteroid dehydrogenase and 5-α-reductase deficiency), partial androgen insensitivity syndrome caused by androgen receptor gene mutations, and global defects in testicular function caused by mutations in genes involved in gonadal development. Other forms of DSD exist, but these are beyond the scope of the USMLE Step 1.

14. **What is 5α-reductase deficiency?**
This is one of the causes of 46,XY DSD. The enzyme 5α-reductase is responsible for converting testosterone into DHT. These patients have normal male testosterone levels, but the testosterone cannot be normally converted to DHT. Because DHT stimulates the production of male external genitalia and the prostate, lack of DHT at birth leads to ambiguous external genitalia in these males until puberty. At puberty, increased concentrations of testosterone promote masculinization and stimulate development of the male external genitalia (Table 9.1). Patients with this autosomal recessive condition are thus said to develop a "penis at 12." However, internal genitalia remain unaffected, as testicular development (and thus mesonephric duct development) is governed by the presence of the *SRY* gene on the Y chromosome.

Table 9.1. Conditions Affecting Development of the Genitalia

CONDITION	TESTOSTERONE	LH	EXPLANATION
Exogenous steroid use	↑	↓	The body perceives that there is too much testosterone, so it reduces production of LH and intratesticular testosterone, leading to testicular atrophy.
Androgen insensitivity syndrome	↑	↑	Although testosterone concentration is much higher than normal, LH production is not inhibited because the testosterone receptors on the pituitary that mediate feedback also are dysfunctional.
Primary hypogonadism	↓	↑	Problem with testosterone production; originates at the level of the testes.
Hypogonadotropic hypogonadism	↓	↓	Problem with production of GnRH or LH leads to decreased production of testosterone.

GnRH, Gonadotropin-releasing hormone; *LH*, luteinizing hormone.

STEP 1 SECRET

Disorders that influence the development of male and female genitalia are high yield for Step 1. Do not be surprised if you receive a question on your test that asks you to identify whether various hormone levels are increased/ decreased/normal in a patient with a genital development disorder. Use Table 9.1 as a guide.

CASE 9.1

A 29-year-old G2P2 (gravida 2 para 2) woman who just delivered her second baby wants to start birth control pills for contraception. She plans on breastfeeding her newborn.

1. **What important information should you find out before prescribing hormonal contraceptives?**
You should learn about tobacco use, breastfeeding, risk for sexually transmitted infections (STIs), past medical history, personal or family history of thromboembolism, and current medications. These factors may influence decisions about which type of contraceptive to prescribe.

CASE 9.1 CONTINUED:

You find out she has smoked one pack of cigarettes per day for the past 10 years. Her past medical history is significant for hypertension, for which she takes a beta-blocker. She has no personal history of breast or endometrial cancer, but her mother did have endometrial cancer.

2. **What are you concerned about in this woman's history with regard to hormonal contraception?**
Estrogen-containing hormonal contraceptives increase the risk for various thrombotic and thromboembolic phenomena, including stroke, myocardial infarction, deep venous thrombosis, and pulmonary embolism (PE). In females who smoke, such contraceptives increase this risk substantially (as does this woman's hypertension) and should therefore be used with caution. If this woman were over age 35, as well as a smoker, estrogen-containing contraceptives would be contraindicated.

3. **What are the absolute contraindications to using estrogen-containing contraceptives?**
Contraindications for estrogen-containing contraceptive use include being an active smoker older than age 35, a history of thromboembolic phenomena (e.g., PE, stroke), coronary artery disease, hepatic tumors (estrogens can make hepatic tumors grow and rupture), unexplained vaginal bleeding, impaired liver function, and personal history of estrogen-dependent cancers, such as endometrial carcinoma or breast carcinoma.

4. **What do oral contraceptives typically contain, and what is their mechanism of action?**
The two general types of oral contraceptives are combination pills (estrogen and progesterone) and progesterone-only pills. In the combination pills, the *constant* level of estrogen supplied continuously suppresses pituitary gonadotropin (LH and FSH) secretion, thereby removing the stimulus for ovulation. The progesterone in the combination pills serves two functions: first, it thickens the cervical mucous secretions, essentially making the vaginal/uterine environment less "receptive" to sperm; and second, it opposes the proliferative effects of estrogen, causing thinning of the uterine lining (which is important in reducing the risk of endometrial cancer from unopposed estrogen). The progesterone-only pills are only about 50% effective at inhibiting ovulation, but as mentioned, they also work by thickening the cervical mucus and altering the motility and secretions of the fallopian tubes, as well as thinning the endometrium.
 Important in this woman's history is that she wishes to breastfeed her baby. Combination hormonal contraceptives postpartum can interfere with milk production, so prescribing a progesterone-only contraceptive would be recommended for this patient.
 Other methods of hormonal contraception include the following:
- The transdermal patch and the vaginal ring are other forms of the combination estrogen and progesterone therapy.
- Injectable progesterone is an intramuscular form given every 3 months.
- Subdermal progestin implant
- Lactation amenorrhea occurs in females less than 6 months postpartum who are exclusively breastfeeding (see Case 9.4).
- Other types of contraception include the intrauterine device (IUD) with or without hormones, barrier methods (condoms, diaphragm, cervical cap), or tubal ligation/vasectomy.

5. **How can menstrual cycles be made regular by hormonal contraceptives?**
In order for menstruation to occur, there must first be estrogenic stimulation of endometrial proliferation, then progesterone must induce maturation and stimulate secretion by the endometrial glands. Menses begins following the decline in progesterone and estrogen levels near the end of the menstrual cycle. Estrogen and progesterone stimulation of the uterus can be provided artificially, which can mimic the natural menstrual period. Typically, to achieve this type of control, estrogen is given with progesterone for 21 days, and then placebo pills are given for 7 days to allow for menstruation secondary to the withdrawal of progesterone ("withdrawal bleed").

6. **Your patient asks if taking hormonal contraceptives will increase her risk for endometrial cancer. What should you tell her?**
Hormonal contraceptives (combined) actually decrease the risk of ovarian and endometrial cancer. The risk of breast cancer is controversial: Studies show either no effect or a slight increase in risk.

7. **How do ovarian cysts form, and how do oral contraceptives reduce their occurrence?**
The most common ovarian cysts are "functional cysts" that form when the normal follicular maturation and the corpus luteum formation process become somewhat aberrant. These are the follicular cysts and corpus lutein cysts, respectively. Follicular cysts develop after a mature ovarian follicle fails to rupture and be ovulated. Corpus lutein cysts are formed during the luteal phase and occur when the corpus luteum becomes abnormally large or hemorrhagic (corpus hemorrhagicum). Clearly, the inhibition of follicular maturation and ovulation by oral contraceptives should reduce the chance that these cysts will develop.

8. **Why may the drugs phenytoin, phenobarbital, and rifampin make oral contraceptives less effective at preventing pregnancy?**
These drugs all induce hepatic cytochrome P-450 enzymes, which can accelerate the rate of hepatic catabolism of estrogen and progesterone compounds, thus decreasing their effectiveness.

SUMMARY BOX: ORAL CONTRACEPTIVES

Hormonal contraceptives
- Increase risk for thromboembolic events
- Are contraindicated for smokers over age 35
- Can be progesterone-only or a combination of estrogen and progesterone
- Decrease risk of ovarian and endometrial cancer; effect on risk of breast cancer is unclear
- Cause normal menses with withdrawal of progesterone (not estrogen)

CASE 9.2

A 26-year-old woman has not had a period for approximately 2 months, whereas she was previously regular. She has also had several episodes of nausea and vomiting but has not otherwise felt ill.

1. Define primary and secondary amenorrhea. What are the differential diagnoses for primary and secondary amenorrhea?

    Primary amenorrhea is the failure of menarche to occur by 15 years of age. Secondary amenorrhea is the absence of menses for more than 3 months in females who previously had regular menstrual cycles and 6 months in females who had irregular menses.

    The differential diagnosis from *primary* amenorrhea includes hypothalamic or pituitary problems (e.g., eating disorders, excessive exercise, stress) and chromosomal or genetic abnormalities (e.g., Turner syndrome, androgen insensitivity syndrome).

    The differential diagnosis for *secondary* amenorrhea includes pregnancy (which is most common), tumor of ovary or adrenals, anatomic abnormalities (e.g., Asherman syndrome, in which intrauterine adhesions may occur following uterine surgery), ovarian failure or polycystic ovary syndrome (PCOS), hypothyroidism, hyperprolactinemia, and central nervous system (CNS) or hypothalamic disorders.

CASE 9.2 CONTINUED:

The patient is emphatic that she cannot be pregnant. Physical examination does not reveal any palpable abdominal or pelvic masses or tenderness.

2. What laboratory tests should you order?

    Even though the woman is emphatic that she cannot be pregnant, a serum β-hCG should always be done first to rule out pregnancy. If the β-HCG test is negative, one can proceed with further testing: thyroid-stimulating hormone (TSH), prolactin level, a progesterone-only challenge test, estrogen and progesterone challenge, FSH level, and LH level.

    If withdrawal bleeding is present with the progesterone-only challenge test, then the amenorrhea is secondary to anovulation (see question 7 under Basic Concepts section for further discussion). If withdrawal bleeding is absent with progesterone alone but present with estrogen and progesterone, then suspect inadequate endogenous estrogen and evaluate FSH and LH levels. Elevated LH and FSH are suggestive of ovarian failure and not a hypothalamic/pituitary process. If withdrawal bleeding is completely absent, an anatomic disorder such as Asherman syndrome may be present. Asherman syndrome refers to the removal of the stratum basalis owing to repeated curettage. Because the stratum basalis serves as the stem cell layer of the endometrium, destruction of this layer prevents regeneration of the functional endometrial tissue. Instead, endometrial fibrosis persists.

CASE 9.2 CONTINUED:

A serum β-hCG is done and is positive.

3. Does an elevated β-hCG level always indicate a developing embryo/fetus?

    It does not necessarily mean she is pregnant because gestational trophoblastic tumors (hydatidiform moles/invasive moles/choriocarcinoma), as well as several germ cell tumors of the ovary, also elaborate β-hCG. Note, however, that these are all rare entities such that an elevated β-hCG almost always indicates a pregnancy. You should confirm the presence of a developing embryo within the uterus by ultrasound.

4. What is β-hCG, and what is its normal function, aside from serving as a marker for pregnancy?

    The hormone β-hCG is similar in structure and activity to LH. It is secreted early in pregnancy by the placenta (specifically, the syncytiotrophoblast cells) and functions to maintain the corpus luteum, which is the principal site of ovarian steroidogenesis (estrogen and progesterone) during the luteal phase. Production begins approximately 1 week after conception and doubles in quantity every 2 days. The hormone is detectable in the blood by 8 days after conception and in the urine approximately 14 days after conception (around the time a woman would expect her next period). Plasma levels of β-hCG peak in the first trimester (by 10 weeks of gestation). Then, as the placenta begins to take over as the main site of maternal estrogen and progesterone secretion, β-hCG levels taper off (Fig. 9.3).

5. Relative to a normal pregnancy, how would the β-hCG level differ for an ectopic pregnancy?

    In ectopic pregnancy, there is poor placentation (there are fewer syncytiotrophoblast cells to produce β-hCG), and therefore the serum β-hCG is significantly lower than would be expected for normal pregnancy of the same gestational age. As a general rule of thumb, if β-hCG levels do not double appropriately and reach expected levels, you should suspect an abnormality with the pregnancy.

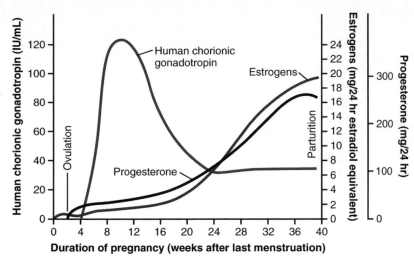

Figure 9.3. Human chorionic gonadotropin stimulates production of estrogen and progesterone by the corpus luteum. As the levels of this hormone drop, the placenta takes over as the major site of synthesis of ovarian steroids. *(From Hall JE. Guyton and Hall Textbook of Medical Physiology. 13th ed. Philadelphia: Elsevier; 2016: 1055-1069, Fig. 83-7.)*

6. Assuming the positive β-hCG test confirms a pregnancy in this woman, what was the approximate date of conception?
   Because ovulation occurs approximately 2 weeks after the onset of menses, and her last menses began 9 weeks ago, the approximate date of conception was 7 weeks ago.

7. What is the difference between the gestational age and the time since conception (developmental age)?
   The gestational age is the period that has elapsed since the first day of her last menstrual period. It is not the time since conception, a mistake commonly made by students. Because conception typically occurs 2 weeks later, the time since conception is 2 weeks shorter than the gestational age. Gestational age is the more commonly used term: She is 9 weeks by gestation.

8. At what time during development is the embryo/fetus most susceptible to teratogens?
   The third to eighth weeks (days 15–56, the "embryonic period") of the first trimester, when organogenesis occurs, is the window of greatest risk. Common teratogens include alcohol, cocaine, and a number of commonly prescribed drugs. While smoking exposure can result in low birth weight and numerous birth defects, whether nicotine should be classified as a teratogen remains controversial. Teratogenic medications to know for USMLE Step 1 are listed in Table 9.2.

Table 9.2. Teratogenic Medications

MEDICATION	SIDE EFFECT
ACE inhibitors	Renal dysplasia
Aminoglycosides	Ototoxicity (CN VIII)
Carbamazepine	Neural tube defects, fingernail hypoplasia, craniofacial defect, cardiovascular and urinary tract anomalies
DES	Vaginal clear cell adenocarcinoma (in daughter)
Lithium	Ebstein anomaly of the heart
Methotrexate	Neural tube defects
Phenytoin	Fetal hydantoin syndrome (microcephaly, craniofacial abnormalities, cardiac defects, IUGR, mental retardation) Neural tube defects
Tetracyclines	Discolored teeth, bone defects
Thalidomide (formerly used to treat nausea in pregnancy)	Limb defects
Valproic acid	Neural tube defects
Vitamin A/isotretinoin	Spontaneous abortion, cleft palate, cardiac abnormalities, hydrocephalus, microcephaly
Warfarin	Microcephaly, craniofacial and skeletal abnormalities, spontaneous abortion, fetal hemorrhage

ACE, Angiotensin-converting enzyme; *CN*, cranial nerve; *DES*, diethylstilbestrol; *IUGR*, intrauterine growth restriction.

9. What is fetal alcohol syndrome?
Fetal alcohol syndrome is the leading cause of congenital malformations in the United States and results from excessive alcohol intake during pregnancy. It is associated with a wide range of congenital defects, including intellectual disability, microcephaly, seizures, and motor disorders, all of which result from a disruption of neuroblast migration. Other defects include limb dislocation, heart abnormalities, and facial abnormalities (flat nasal bridge, upturned nose, "railroad track" ears, epicanthal folds, smooth philtrum, and small palpebral fissures) (Fig. 9.4).

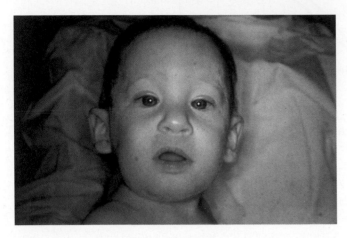

Figure 9.4. Infant with fetal alcohol syndrome. Note short palpebral fissures, mild ptosis, appearance of the nostrils, smooth philtral area, and narrow vermilion of the upper lip. *(From Gilbert-Barness E.* Potter's Pathology of the Fetus, Infant and Child. *2nd ed. Philadelphia: Mosby; 2007.)*

10. What are the effects of fetal exposure to cocaine, heroin, and nicotine?
See Table 9.3.

Clinical Pearl
Neonatal abstinence syndrome (NAS) is neonatal withdrawal from opiates that occurs after delivery and must be closely monitored by the pediatric team.

Table 9.3. Effects of Fetal Exposure to Cocaine, Heroin, and Nicotine

DRUG	FETAL EFFECT
Cocaine	Risk of placental abruption, stillbirth, fetal addiction
Nicotine	Preterm labor, intrauterine growth restriction (IUGR)
Heroin, methadone	Neonatal abstinence syndrome (NAS)

11. The risk of which fetal developmental abnormalities can be reduced by taking supplemental folic acid early during pregnancy?
Developmental abnormalities of the CNS and the spinal cord may cause neural tube defects such as spina bifida and anencephaly. Ideally, females of childbearing age with the possibility of pregnancy are taking prenatal vitamins *before* pregnancy, because significant neural development may occur before a woman's knowledge of her pregnancy.

12. Is the woman in Case 9.2 at high or low risk for having a baby with Down syndrome (trisomy 21)?
The incidence of Down syndrome increases significantly with maternal age (ova undergo more chromosomal divisions as they age, increasing their risk of a mutation), and because this woman is only 26, her risk is quite low. The risk increases with age from approximately 1 in 1500 for babies born to 16-year-old mothers versus approximately 1 in 25 babies born to 45-year-old mothers. Although this risk increases as females age, it is important to realize that the majority of babies with Down syndrome are born to younger mothers because of the higher birth rate in this population.

Clinical Pearl
Maternal serum α-fetoprotein (AFP) levels are often checked around the 16th week of pregnancy. High levels may indicate a neural tube defect, such as spina bifida, whereas low levels may indicate Down syndrome. Other laboratory findings associated with Down syndrome include decreased estriol and elevated β-hCG and inhibin A. This test is called the *quad screen.*

13. **What is polyhydramnios, and why does this commonly occur in patients carrying fetuses with Down syndrome? What is oligohydramnios?**
Polyhydramnios is defined as greater than 2000 mL of amniotic fluid. Amniotic fluid is normally produced by the fetal kidneys and is swallowed by the fetus to promote lung maturity. Down syndrome is associated with duodenal atresia (diagnosed by the "double-bubble" sign on radiograph or ultrasound); therefore, amniotic fluid cannot be swallowed and thus accumulates. Other common causes of polyhydramnios include tracheoesophageal fistula and gestational diabetes.
    Oligohydramnios is defined as less than 500 mL of amniotic fluid. Fetal causes include renal agenesis, polycystic kidney disease, and posterior urethral valves. Maternal causes include premature rupture of membranes (PROM) and uteroplacental insufficiency.
    Note: Potter syndrome (pulmonary hypoplasia, rocker-bottom feet, craniofacial abnormalities) may occur secondary to oligohydramnios. Be familiar with the description because it is high yield for USMLE Step 1.

14. **Why should ergot alkaloids (e.g., ergonovine), triptans (e.g., sumatriptan), and synthetic prostaglandins (e.g., misoprostol) all be stringently avoided during pregnancy?**
These agents all cause powerful uterine contractions that can result in abortion. The effects of ergot alkaloids and triptans are principally mediated through serotonin receptors. Misoprostol is a synthetic prostaglandin that causes contractions in an analogous fashion to endogenous prostaglandins. It is used in combination with mifepristone (progesterone blocker) to induce medical abortion.

SUMMARY BOX: SECONDARY AMENORRHEA

- Presentation: Postpubertal but premenopausal females with cessation of menses after menarche
  - Causes: Pregnancy is most common
  - Other causes include polycystic ovary syndrome (PCOS), hypothyroidism, and hyperprolactinemia
- Pathophysiology: May be attributed to anovulation, ovarian failure, or hypothalamic/pituitary deficiencies
- Diagnosis: β-human chorionic gonadotropin (hCG) serum levels
  - β-hCG levels peak at 10 weeks of gestation (approximately 100,000 mIU/mL). Levels usually double every 48 hours until this point.
  - Ectopic pregnancies have lower β-hCG levels and do not double appropriately.
  - Hormone levels, ultrasound, or karyotype may be considered in the secondary workup.
- Complications: Infertility

CASE 9.3

A 19-year-old G1P0 (gravida 1, para 0) woman who is 2 months pregnant by last menstrual period comes in for an urgent visit because of heavy vaginal bleeding.

---

1. **What is the differential diagnosis for first-trimester bleeding (<12–14 weeks)?**
The differential diagnosis is spontaneous abortion, ectopic pregnancy, molar pregnancy, and postcoital bleeding, as well as other nonpregnancy-related causes, such as vaginal laceration or trauma.

CASE 9.3 CONTINUED:

She has not been seen in clinic, but she knows she is pregnant by a positive urine pregnancy test. She has had severe nausea and vomiting but thinks that is normal "morning sickness." You are concerned about a spontaneous abortion and ectopic pregnancy. A pelvic ultrasound (Fig. 9.5) reveals a "snowstorm" pattern with no discernible fetus. Serum β-hCG levels are elevated far above what would be expected during pregnancy.

---

2. **What is the diagnosis?**
Molar pregnancy (hydatidiform mole) is likely. Molar pregnancy is one subtype of gestational trophoblastic disease (GTD).

3. **How can β-hCG levels differentiate between a normal pregnancy and a molar pregnancy (complete or incomplete mole)?**
Because these moles are made exclusively of trophoblastic (placental) tissue, the site of β-hCG synthesis, serum β-hCG levels are substantially elevated in comparison to a normal pregnancy of similar "gestational age." Other features that suggest a molar pregnancy include severe vaginal bleeding early in the pregnancy and vaginal passage of molar vesicles.
    Note: Another cause of elevated β-hCG is a multiple-gestation pregnancy.

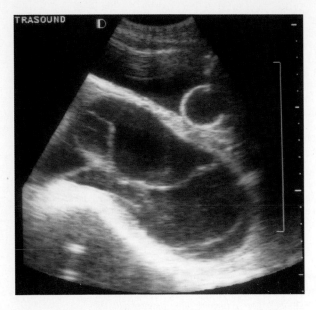

Figure 9.5. Pelvic ultrasound from patient in Case 9.3. *(From Ferri FF. Ferri's Clinical Advisor 2020. Philadelphia: Elsevier; 2020: 908-910.e2, Fig. 5.)*

4. **What is the difference between an invasive mole and choriocarcinoma, and from what does each generally arise?**
An invasive mole invades the myometrium but does not normally metastasize. A majority of them arise from benign molar pregnancies. Choriocarcinoma, on the other hand, is often metastatic and spreads hematogenously. Half of these develop from benign molar pregnancies; one-fourth after normal term pregnancy and one-fourth after miscarriage, abortion, or ectopic pregnancy. A key histologic distinction between invasive moles and choriocarcinomas is that choriocarcinomas are less differentiated and lack *a villous pattern*.

5. **What drug is used to treat GTDs including molar pregnancy and choriocarcinoma?**
Methotrexate is the initial drug of choice for GTDs.

6. **Cover the columns on the right side of Table 9.4 and try to identify the characteristics of the different GTDs.**
See Table 9.4 and Fig. 9.6.

Table 9.4. Gestational Trophoblastic Diseases

TYPE	SUBCLAS-SIFICATION	PERSISTENT MALIGNANT DISEASE	PATHOGENESIS	KARYO-TYPE	FETAL PARTS PRESENT
Molar pregnancy/ hydatidiform moles (80%)	Complete mole (90% of molar pregnancies)	Benign (in general)	15%–20%	Sperm fertilizes empty egg, then duplicates (rarely two sperm fertilize empty ovum)	Diploid (46,XX, rarely 46,XY)	No
	Incomplete/ partial mole	Benign (almost always)	1%-5%	Two sperm fertilize normal egg	Triploid (69,XXY or 69,XXX)	Yes
Invasive moles (10%–15%)		Malignant		Months to years after molar pregnancy (50%), normal pregnancy (25%), after abortion, ectopic (25%)	Diploid	No
Choriocarcinoma (2%–5%)		Malignant	Diploid	No		
Placental site trophoblastic tumor (rare)		Malignant	Diploid	No		

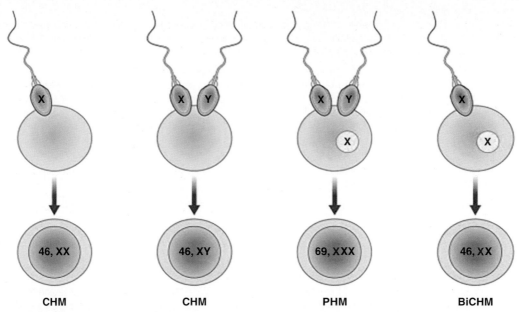

Figure 9.6. Patterns of fertilization to account for chromosomal origin of complete (CHM; 46,XX or 46,XY) and triploid partial moles (PHM; XXY). In a complete mole, one or two sperm fertilize an egg that has lost its chromosomes. Partial moles are due to fertilization of an egg by one diploid (46,XY) or two haploid sperm, depicted in this example as one 23,X and one 23,Y. *(From Mutter GL.* Pathology of the Female Reproductive Tract. *3rd ed. London: Churchill Livingstone Elsevier; 2014: 784-811, Fig. 34.7.)*

SUMMARY BOX: HYDATIDIFORM MOLES

- Presentation: Heavy vaginal bleeding, nausea, and vomiting during first trimester
- Genetics
  - Complete mole: Diploid (46,XX or 46,XY)
  - Incomplete/partial mole: Triploid (69,XXY or 69,XXX)
- Diagnosis
  - Increase in normal β-hCG levels
  - Ultrasound revealing "snowstorm" appearance of "grape-like vesicles" without a discernible fetus
- Complications: Choriocarcinoma, invasive mole, placental site trophoblastic tumor (PSTT)
- Treatment
  - Methotrexate

CASE 9.4

A 32-year-old G2P1 (gravida 2, para 1) woman at 12 weeks of gestation by last known menstrual period reports occasional palpitations, irritability, and heat intolerance.

1. **What is the differential diagnosis?**
   The differential diagnosis includes hyperthyroidism, normal pregnancy, anxiety, cardiac arrhythmia, and the always unlikely pheochromocytoma.

CASE 9.4 CONTINUED:

Except for a gravid abdomen, physical examination is unremarkable. Cardiac auscultation reveals a regular rate and rhythm without murmurs or gallops. An electrocardiogram (ECG) is normal.

2. **What would you like to do for further workup?**
   A thyroid panel to rule out hyperthyroidism.

CASE 9.4 CONTINUED:

The results reveal elevated levels of total and free thyroid hormones (triiodothyronine [T_3] and thyroxine [T_4]), as well as reduced levels of thyroid-stimulating hormone (TSH).

3. What is the diagnosis?

The diagnosis is gestational hyperthyroidism. In pregnancy, the total T_4 is usually elevated because estrogen increases the synthesis of thyroxine-binding globulin by the liver. Notice, however, that this woman had elevated free T_4 levels as well, and it is this elevated free T_4 (or free T_3) that causes hyperthyroidism.

4. How does the pregnant state predispose to hyperthyroidism?

This effect is due to the presence of β-hCG in the maternal circulation. β-hCG is a glycoprotein synthesized and secreted by the placenta in large amounts. Owing to its similarity in structure to TSH (TSH, FSH, LH, and β-hCG all share the same α-subunit), it often hyperstimulates the thyroid gland during pregnancy, resulting in gestational hyperthyroidism. This condition often spontaneously resolves following delivery of the fetus and placenta.

5. How are maternal levels of FSH and LH likely to be affected in this woman, given that she is pregnant?

They should be virtually undetectable because of significant negative feedback on the pituitary from the high levels of estrogen and progesterone.

6. Why is the decline in estrogen and progesterone after delivery beneficial for the beginning of lactation?

Both estrogen and progesterone inhibit lactation, and their withdrawal allows the elevated prolactin present at the time of delivery to facilitate milk letdown and lactation. Recall that the placenta is the major site of progesterone and estrogen secretion, so its expulsion after delivery will reduce the levels of these hormones.

7. How does breastfeeding act as a natural contraceptive?

Nipple suckling by the baby stimulates the release of prolactin by the anterior pituitary gland. Because one of the functions of prolactin is to inhibit the hypothalamic secretion of GnRH, this results in reduced FSH and LH secretion by the pituitary. Reduced levels of these gonadotropins *largely* inhibit ovulation in the nursing mother and act as a natural birth control pill. However, breastfeeding must be practiced continuously in order to be efficacious as a contraceptive method.

SUMMARY BOX: ENDOCRINOLOGY OF PREGNANCY

- In pregnancy the total thyroxine (T_4) is usually elevated because estrogen increases the synthesis of thyroxine-binding globulin by the liver.
- Increases in *free* T_4 and triiodothyronine (T_3) levels result in gestational hyperthyroidism.
- High levels of prolactin in a nursing mother inhibit hypothalamic secretion of gonadotropin-releasing hormone (GnRH), resulting in reduced gonadotropin secretion and suppression of ovulation.

CASE 9.5

A 28-year-old woman in her 33rd week of pregnancy reports increased fatigue and swelling of her hands and face. Urine dipstick testing shows 2+ proteinuria, and her blood pressure is elevated at 150/110 mm Hg (up from 130/90 mm Hg). Brisk deep tendon reflexes are also noted on examination.

1. What is the diagnosis?

The diagnosis is preeclampsia, which is defined by new-onset hypertension (>140/90 mm Hg) and proteinuria (>300 mg/day) occurring after 20 weeks of gestation. Although the definitive cause of preeclampsia is still unknown, the underlying cause is thought to be due to placental abnormalities that lead to generalized arterial constriction and vasospasm.

Note: The severity of preeclampsia is generally determined by the degree of proteinuria and blood pressure elevation.

2. How should this patient be managed?

This woman is classified as having mild preeclampsia. Because her pregnancy is not yet at term (<37 weeks), she should be recommended bed rest and medical therapy to control her blood pressure. She could also be given steroids, such as β-methasone, to enhance fetal lung maturity in the event that premature delivery is necessary.

CASE 9.5 CONTINUED:

The next week she develops right upper quadrant (RUQ) pain, her proteinuria worsens, and her blood pressure increases to 170/115 mm Hg.

3. What is your primary concern at this point?

The patient now has severe preeclampsia. Severe preeclampsia is defined by a blood pressure of at least 160/110 mm Hg with 5 g of protein in the urine or any signs of end organ damage. The RUQ pain is concerning for HELLP syndrome, which can be a complication of severe preeclampsia. The **HELLP** syndrome consists of **H**emolysis, **E**levated **L**iver enzymes, and **L**ow **P**latelets. About 10% of patients with severe preeclampsia develop HELLP syndrome.

4. What changes occur in the spiral arteries in patients with preeclampsia?

   Preeclampsia is associated with mechanical or functional obstruction of the spiral arteries. This is because abnormal trophoblastic tissue invades the spiral arteries. Additionally, patients demonstrate increased levels of vasoconstrictors and decreased levels of vasodilators along with increased concentrations of growth factors. The end result is placental hypoperfusion with spiral artery atherosclerosis. These placental abnormalities place the patient at increased risk for placental abruption.

CASE 9.5 CONTINUED:

Laboratory tests reveal anemia, thrombocytopenia, and elevated liver enzymes, and a peripheral blood smear shows the presence of schistocytes.

5. If this woman also develops seizures, how does that change the diagnosis?

   If this woman develops seizures, then, assuming she does not have a preexisting seizure disorder or metabolic abnormality, she has eclampsia, which is defined by the presence of seizures in a patient with preeclampsia and without other known causes of seizures.

6. What is the definitive treatment for preeclampsia, eclampsia, and HELLP syndrome?

   Delivery of the fetus is the only definitive treatment. Supportive management includes magnesium sulfate ($MgSO_4$) for seizure prophylaxis in eclamptic patients. In preeclamptic patients, $MgSO_4$ is also often given as seizure prophylaxis during labor and delivery. Although $MgSO_4$ is considered to be the first-line treatment for seizures in these patients, diazepam can also be given. Patients should be placed on salt-restricted diets. If the baby must be delivered prematurely for the health of the mother, steroids should be given to improve fetal lung maturity.

7. What are important symptoms of magnesium sulfate toxicity?

   Respiratory and CNS depression, pulmonary edema, acute kidney injury, and cardiac arrhythmias are important symptoms of $MgSO_4$ toxicity. Patients on continuous doses of $MgSO_4$ must be frequently evaluated for signs of $MgSO_4$ toxicity. This should include a thorough cardiopulmonary exam, deep tendon reflexes, and assessment of the urine output and vital signs.

8. Why are angiotensin-converting enzyme inhibitors or angiotensin receptor blockers not used to treat hypertension in preeclampsia?

   Angiotensin-converting enzyme (ACE) inhibitors and angiotensin receptor blockers (ARBs) should not be used to treat *any* pregnant woman because they carry the risk of causing fetal renal failure and even fetal death.

STEP 1 SECRET

Preeclampsia and eclampsia are high-yield subjects for boards. You should be able to recognize the findings associated with these diseases in pregnant patients and understand basic concepts regarding treatment.

SUMMARY BOX: PREECLAMPSIA

- Presentation: Fatigue, facial/hand swelling, and signs of hypertension in a pregnant woman at greater than 20 weeks of gestation
  - Patients with severe preeclampsia commonly present with right upper quadrant (RUQ) pain.
- Pathophysiology: Attributed to placental abnormalities that result in placental hypoperfusion and spinal artery atherosclerosis
- Diagnosis: Hypertension, proteinuria
- Complications: **HELLP** syndrome (**H**emolysis, **E**levated **L**iver enzymes, **L**ow **P**latelets), progression to eclampsia (preeclampsia with the addition of seizures), placental abruption
- Treatment: Delivery of the fetus, magnesium sulfate ($MgSO_4$) for seizure prophylaxis

CASE 9.6

A 26-year-old woman at 32 weeks of gestation presents to the hospital because she has been having contractions for the past 3 hours. Contractions are now occurring every 10 minutes. The diameter of her cervical canal is 2 cm. She is told she might be going into premature labor.

1. What pharmacologic agents can be used to suppress labor in this woman?

   Agents that inhibit uterine contractions are known as *tocolytics*. $MgSO_4$ is most widely used. Other classes of drugs include β_2-receptor agonists (usually terbutaline and ritodrine) and calcium channel blockers (nifedipine is most widely used). These latter two drug classes are smooth muscle relaxants. Additionally, indomethacin and other nonsteroidal anti-inflammatory drugs (NSAIDs) can decrease uterine contractions by inhibiting prostaglandin synthesis.

Note: After approximately 32 weeks of gestation, there is concern about NSAID use because of their potential to cause premature constriction of the ductus arteriosus. Remember that prostaglandins are vasodilatory and that NSAIDs inhibit prostaglandin synthesis.

2. **What is the main source of risk associated with premature delivery?**

The principal concern with premature delivery is immature fetal lungs, which can cause neonatal respiratory distress syndrome. Fetal lung maturity can be determined by the amount of surfactant present, which can be assessed with amniocentesis and evaluation of the lecithin-sphingomyelin ratio, which should be greater than 2 for mature lungs. Glucocorticoids can be given to the mother during or a few days prior to an anticipated preterm labor to increase the production of surfactant. Typically, surfactant production begins by 28 weeks and is complete by 36 weeks.

RELATED QUESTIONS ON LABOR AND DELIVERY

3. **If placenta previa were present at term (or when delivery is necessary), why would a cesarean section be mandatory?**

Placenta previa occurs when the placenta covers the internal cervical os. With a vaginal delivery, the placenta would have to rupture for the baby to pass through the cervix (a high-risk situation as a result of hemorrhage).

Note: Placenta previa classically presents as *painless* bleeding during any trimester. This is in contrast to placental abruption, placental detachment from the uterus, which is very *painful* and can present only in the third trimester.

4. **How can placenta accreta complicate the labor and delivery process?**

Placenta accreta occurs when the placenta has invaded into and attached firmly to the myometrium. In this situation, the placenta does not separate off the endometrial lining after delivery of the infant.

5. **What is oxytocin, and how is it used to augment or induce labor?**

Oxytocin is a peptide hormone produced naturally by the posterior pituitary and is a stimulant for uterine contractions. Exogenous oxytocin (Pitocin) enhances uterine contractions and accelerates the first stage of labor.

Note: During pregnancy, the number of oxytocin receptors on the uterus increases, which makes the uterus particularly sensitive to endogenous or exogenous oxytocin at the end of term.

6. **What pharmacologic agents could be used if delivery is complicated by postpartum hemorrhage?**

Several different pharmacologic agents, including the ergot alkaloids, oxytocin, and certain prostaglandins, cause uterine contractions, which reduce postpartum bleeding by clamping down on bleeding vessels. Two commonly tested pharmacologic agents include methylergometrine (ergot alkaloid) and carboprost (prostaglandin). Methylergometrine is contraindicated in patients with hypertension, and carboprost is contraindicated in patients with asthma.

SUMMARY BOX: LABOR AND DELIVERY

- Premature delivery
  - Primary risk is immature fetal lungs (neonatal respiratory distress syndrome).
  - Amniocentesis showing lecithin-sphingomyelin ratio greater than 2 suggests mature lungs.
  - Glucocorticoids can be given during or a few days prior to an anticipated preterm labor to increase surfactant production.
- Tocolytics: Used to suppress premature delivery. Classes of drugs include:
  - Magnesium sulfate ($MgSO_4$): most widely used
  - β_2-receptor agonists: for example, terbutaline and ritodrine
  - Calcium channel blockers: nifedipine most widely used
  - NSAIDs: contraindicated after 32 weeks of gestation because of their potential to cause premature closure of the ductus arteriosus
- Placenta previa
  - Placenta covers cervical os
  - Painless bleeding during any trimester
  - Cesarean delivery required
- Placenta accreta
  - Placenta invades and attaches to myometrium.
  - Placenta does not separate following delivery of the infant, potentially resulting in massive hemorrhaging, adult respiratory distress syndrome, disseminated intravascular coagulation (DIC), and death.
- Oxytocin
  - Stimulates uterine contractions
  - Exogenous oxytocin enhances uterine contractions and accelerates the first stage of labor.

CASE 9.7

A 26-year-old woman reports fever and pelvic pain, neither of which is related to her menstrual cycle.

1. **What is the differential diagnosis for pelvic pain?**
   There is a very broad differential diagnosis for pelvic pain, including gynecologic, urologic, gastrointestinal, musculoskeletal, or psychiatric causes. We need more information.

CASE 9.7 CONTINUED:

She has multiple sexual partners and rarely uses any form of barrier contraception. Cervical examination is significant for bilateral adnexal tenderness and a purulent cervical discharge.

2. **Based on the preceding additional information, what is the most likely diagnosis?**
   Pelvic inflammatory disease (PID) secondary to infection with *Chlamydia trachomatis*. *Neisseria gonorrhoeae* is another common cause of PID. PID typically presents with fever, lower abdominal pain, abnormal uterine bleeding, purulent vaginal discharge, and cervical motion tenderness.

CASE 9.7 CONTINUED:

Laboratory tests reveal a mild leukocytosis and a slightly elevated erythrocyte sedimentation rate (ESR). A quantitative β-hCG is negative, but a cervical smear is positive for *Chlamydia trachomatis*, confirming the diagnosis (Fig. 9.7).

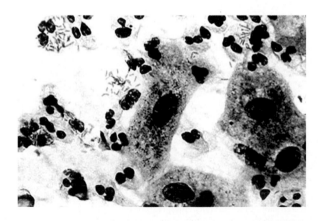

Figure 9.7. *Chlamydia trachomatis* cervicovaginal smear. Moth-eaten appearance and fine-walled intracytoplasmic vacuolated structures are characteristic. *(From Gupta PK, McGrath C.* Comprehensive Cytopathology. *4th ed. Philadelphia: Elsevier Saunders; 2015: 82-118.e3, Fig. 7-64.)*

3. **What long-term complications may possibly be prevented by treating this woman?**
   Tubal strictures can develop as a result of the inflammatory process, which can cause infertility or ectopic pregnancy. Tubes can also fill with pus, leading to hydrosalpinx. Adhesions between small bowel and pelvic structures can also develop, causing symptoms of bowel obstruction. An abscess can form around the tubes and ovaries (tubo-ovarian abscess), and their rupture can be a life-threatening event. Another potential complication of PID is Fitz-Hugh–Curtis syndrome, which is the spread of the infection into the peritoneum causing scar tissue formation on the surface of the liver. This manifests in the symptom of RUQ pain. Although treatment of PID cannot eliminate these complications, it can potentially reduce their frequency.

4. **How should this patient be treated?**
   She should be given antibiotics. A typical outpatient regimen for PID is doxycycline (to cover *C. trachomatis)* plus ceftriaxone (to cover *N. gonorrhoeae)* plus metronidazole (to cover anaerobic organisms).

5. **If someone presented with similar signs and symptoms but also had acute onset of right knee pain and swelling without any recent trauma to the joint, what infecting organism should you suspect?**
   N. gonorrhoeae, a gram-negative intracellular diplococcus, should be suspected. *N. gonorrhoeae* can also cause a septic arthritis if it disseminates.
   Note: You should suspect infection with *Actinomyces israelii* in a woman using an IUD who presents with symptoms of PID. This bacterium can be treated with penicillin.

SUMMARY BOX: PELVIC INFLAMMATORY DISEASE

- Presentation: Fever, pelvic pain, cervical discharge, abnormal uterine bleeding, lower abdominal pain, cervical motion tenderness
- Risk factors: Multiple sexual partners, unprotected sexual intercourse
- Pathophysiology: Infection with *Chlamydia trachomatis* or *Neisseria gonorrhoeae*
- Diagnosis: Leukocytosis, elevated ESR, cervical culture positive for *C. trachomatis* or *N. gonorrhoeae*
- Complications: Infertility, ectopic pregnancy, tubo-ovarian abscess, hydrosalpinx, bowel obstruction, Fitz-Hugh–Curtis syndrome, septic arthritis (with *N. gonorrhoeae* infection)
- Treatment: For outpatient therapy, doxycycline plus ceftriaxone to cover both organisms plus metronidazole to cover anaerobic organisms. Intravenous antibiotics may be necessary for sicker patients.

RELATED QUESTION ON GYNECOLOGIC INFECTIONS

6. What bacterium is responsible for maintaining the normal acidic pH of the vagina?
   Lactobacillus acidophilus (acid loving) maintains the vaginal pH at less than 4.5 (Table 9.5).

CASE 9.8

A 28-year-old woman who has never been pregnant with no history of prior surgeries reports chronic pelvic pain.

1. What is the differential diagnosis for pelvic pain?
   As mentioned in Case 9.7, question 1, the differential diagnosis is quite broad. The pain would need to be characterized to narrow the differential diagnosis.

CASE 9.8 CONTINUED:

The pain is particularly severe during her menstrual period (dysmenorrhea). She also reports significant pain during sexual intercourse (dyspareunia). Pelvic examination is significant for slight adnexal tenderness. Rectovaginal examination reveals fullness in the posterior cul-de-sac. Stains for *N. gonorrhoeae* and *C. trachomatis* are negative, and a β-hCG is also negative. A pelvic ultrasound does not reveal any cysts, fibroids, or structures suggestive of ovarian neoplasm.

2. Now what is the likely diagnosis, what is its etiology, and how do we confirm?
   The most likely diagnosis is endometriosis, given the history of severe pain during the menstrual period and negative workup for infectious and anatomic causes. Endometriosis is caused by the presence of endometrial tissue in ectopic (extrauterine) locations, such as the ovaries or uterine ligaments. Perhaps the most widely accepted theory to explain the presence of endometrial tissue in extrauterine sites is the phenomenon of retrograde menstruation through the fallopian tubes, a process that is thought to occur in most females. Unfortunately, such retrograde flow does not completely explain the presence of ectopic endometrial tissues in distant anatomic sites, such as the pleural cavity. An exploratory laparoscopy for direct visualization is the gold standard for diagnosis.

CASE 9.8 CONTINUED:

Laparoscopy is performed and reveals the presence of "chocolate" cysts on both ovaries.

3. What does the presence of these ovarian "chocolate" cysts indicate, and why do they appear black?
   Chocolate cysts are nonfunctional ovarian cysts (endometriomas) that develop from ectopic endometrial tissue present in advanced endometriosis. They appear dark brown to black because they contain a blood-filled cavity.

4. Why is pain worse during the menstrual period in this patient?
   Ectopic endometrial tissue undergoes the same cycle of proliferation and breakdown as the normal endometrial lining in response to estrogen and progesterone. The resulting bleeding causes inflammation and pain. Long term, this inflammation can lead to tissue damage, fibrosis, adhesions, and compression of adjacent structures, resulting in signs and symptoms such as chronic pelvic pain and infertility. Because of these effects, it is important to diagnose and treat endometriosis early in its development.
   Note: Although ectopic endometrial tissue is most frequently found in the pelvis, it can also be found in various other anatomic sites, such as the upper abdomen or thorax and the colon, leading to rectal bleeding. These sites can also become painful during menstrual cycling. If ectopic tissue deposits in the fallopian tubes, it can result in infertility.

Table 9.5. Infectious Causes of Vaginal Discharge

FEATURE	BACTERIAL VAGINOSIS	TRICHOMONIASIS	CANDIDIASIS
Chief concern	Malodorous discharge (fishy)	Thin, yellowish-greenish, foul-smelling, frothy discharge; "strawberry cervix"	White, cheesy exudate; itching
Pathogenesis	Overgrowth of normal vaginal flora (*Gardnerella vaginalis*)	STI	Yeast infection
Tests	Saline preparation shows "clue cells" (vaginal epithelial cells "studded" with adherent bacteria)[a] KOH whiff test produces a fishy odor pH 5–6	Motile protozoa on saline preparation smears[b] pH 6–7	KOH shows hyphae[b] pH $<$ 4.5
Treatment	Metronidazole or clindamycin	Metronidazole	Nystatin or fluconazole, clotrimazole or miconazole in pregnancy

[a] From Holmes KK: Lower genital tract infections in females: cystitis/urethritis, vulvo-vaginitis, and cervicitis. In: Holmes KK, Mardh PA, Sparling PF, et al., eds. *Sexually Transmitted Diseases*. New York: McGraw-Hill: 1984. Copyright © McGraw-Hill, Inc. Used by permission of McGraw-Hill Book Company.
[b] From Kaufman RH, Faro S, Brown D. *Benign Diseases of the Vulva and Vagina*. 5th ed. St. Louis: Mosby; 2004.
KOH, Potassium hydroxide; *STI,* sexually transmitted infection.

STEP 1 SECRET

Note that endometriosis results in **cyclic** *bleeding because the ectopic tissue is also governed by hormonal regulation. In general, it will be helpful for you to classify gynecologic diseases according to these types of patterns (e.g., Does the disease result in cyclic or noncyclic/anovulatory bleeding? Is the disease associated with menstrual pain?).*

5. What is first-line treatment for this 28-year-old woman?
   NSAIDs or hormonal contraceptives are good first-line agents for mild endometriosis. The choice will depend on the symptoms and whether she is trying to conceive.

6. What is the mechanism of action of leuprolide, a GnRH analog, in treating endometriosis?
   While the pituitary gland normally releases gonadotropins in response to the *pulsatile* secretion of GnRH from the hypothalamus, the *continual* presence of leuprolide (a GnRH receptor agonist) inhibits the pituitary release of LH and FSH. Suppression of FSH and LH secretion eliminates their stimulation of estrogen and progesterone production, essentially putting the woman in an artificial state of menopause. Without the estrogenic stimulation of the endometrial tissue for proliferation and the progesterone stimulation for maturation and eventual menses, there is no cycling with associated bleeding of ectopic endometrial tissue.
   Note 1: Because leuprolide causes a hypoestrogenic state, it is used for only brief periods of time because of the risks of osteoporosis, hot flashes, and other postmenopausal problems.
   Note 2: Danazol, a derivative of testosterone, which nonetheless has some progestational actions, is also used to treat endometriosis. It decreases pituitary FSH and LH secretion but has some unpleasant side effects (hirsutism, deepening of the voice) resulting from its androgenic actions.

7. Another option for treating this woman is total abdominal hysterectomy with bilateral salpingo-oophorectomy. What is the value of excising the ovaries, in terms of treating endometriosis, if there are no endometrial implants on the ovaries?
   The estrogens produced by the ovaries are responsible for stimulating the cycling of any ectopic endometrial tissue that is not removed with hysterectomy.

8. Another cause of dysmenorrhea is adenomyosis. What is this?
Adenomyosis is ingrowth of the endometrial glands into the myometrium. In addition to dysmenorrhea, it can also cause heavy menstrual bleeding (menorrhagia).

SUMMARY BOX: ENDOMETRIOSIS

- Presentation: Pelvic pain that worsens with menstrual periods and sexual intercourse
- Pathophysiology: Presence of ectopic endometrial tissue in extrauterine sites (e.g., the ovaries, uterine ligaments, or pleural cavity) that results in cyclic bleeding
- Diagnosis
  - Based on history, pelvic examination, and lack of positivity for sexually transmitted infections (STIs) or β-human chorionic gonadotropin (β-hCG)
  - Laparoscopy is the gold standard for diagnosis
- Complications: Ovarian "chocolate" cysts with advanced endometriosis
- Treatment: Total abdominal hysterectomy with bilateral removal of the ovaries, pharmacologic agents (nonsteroidal anti-inflammatory drugs [NSAIDs], hormonal contraceptives, gonadotropin-releasing hormone [GnRH] agonists, or androgen derivatives)

CASE 9.9

A 37-year-old African-American woman is being evaluated for abnormal uterine bleeding. She has regular periods, but they are heavy, and she also has some bleeding between her periods. Intercourse has become somewhat painful.

---

1. What is the differential diagnosis for abnormal uterine bleeding in a premenopausal woman?
The differential diagnosis for abnormal uterine bleeding in a premenopausal woman includes adenomyosis (invasion of the endometrium into the myometrium), endometriosis, endometrial polyps, uterine fibroids (leiomyomata), endometrial hyperplasia, and endometrial cancer.

CASE 9.9 CONTINUED:

Physical examination reveals the uterus to be enlarged and hardened, possibly with nodules. A pelvic ultrasound reveals an enlarged uterus with several tumorous growths within the myometrium (Fig. 9.8).

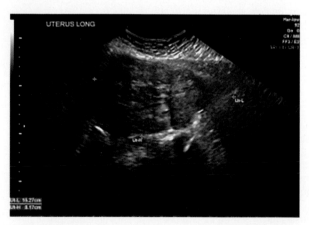

Figure 9.8. Pelvic ultrasound reveals an enlarged fibroid uterus. *(From Shwayder JM. Normal pelvic anatomy.* Obstetrics and Gynecology Clinics. *2019;46(4):563-580.)*

2. What is the probable diagnosis now?
Uterine leiomyomata (singular, *leiomyoma*), commonly referred to as *uterine fibroids,* is the probable diagnosis. These tumors are benign, local proliferations of smooth muscle cells of the uterus that occur in whorled patterns and are the most common of all tumor types in females. Uterine fibroids are the most common gynecologic tumor, and African-American females have a significantly greater risk of developing them. As shown in Fig. 9.9, uterine fibroids may be subserous, intramural, or submucosal depending on their location. Submucosal fibroids are a common cause of uterine bleeding.

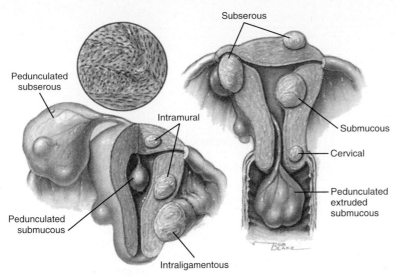

Figure 9.9. Histopathology of leiomyoma. Uterine fibroids are designated subserous, intramural, or submucosal depending on their location. Submucosal fibroids often cause abnormal uterine bleeding. *(From Sabiston D. Textbook of Surgery. 16th ed. Philadelphia: WB Saunders; 2000.)*

3. What are the common symptoms associated with leiomyoma?

Although the condition is asymptomatic in a sizable proportion of patients, others may experience menorrhagia (if the location is submucosal) because the smooth muscle cells cannot properly clamp down on the spiral arteries during menses. Other symptoms include infertility, dysmenorrhea, constipation secondary to pressure on the colon, and frequency and urgency secondary to pressure on the bladder.

4. How do oral contraceptives affect uterine fibroids?

Because these are estrogen-sensitive tumors, exogenous estrogens in oral contraceptives may make them grow. Additionally, the substantial increase in estrogen that occurs during pregnancy can make these tumors grow to significant proportions. After menopause, when estrogen levels fall off, these tumors often shrink in size and become asymptomatic.

Note: Pharmacologic agents that decrease plasma estrogen such as leuprolide, danazol, and progesterone can all be used to shrink uterine fibroids. Progesterone-containing IUDs may also be used depending on location of the fibroids.

5. Most fibroids are asymptomatic, but when is treatment with hysterectomy or myomectomy indicated?

If there is severe pain, rapid growth, very large or many leiomyomata, or urinary symptoms, hysterectomy may be indicated. Recurrent miscarriage is also a rare complication of fibroids, so if future fertility is desired, myomectomy can be performed to resect just the tumor, leaving a viable uterus.

6. What is uterine leiomyosarcoma?

Uterine leiomyosarcoma is a highly aggressive malignant tumor derived from smooth muscle cells of the uterus. It is not believed to arise from uterine fibroids. Uterine leiomyosarcomas are very rare but would be considered if there is very rapid growth of a mass in the uterus. Incidence is higher in African-American females than in White females.

SUMMARY BOX: UTERINE FIBROIDS (UTERINE LEIOMYOMATA)

- Presentation: Commonly asymptomatic but may be associated with abnormal uterine bleeding, menorrhagia, dysmenorrhea, constipation, and frequency/urgency
- Epidemiology: Most common tumor type in females, more common in African Americans
- Pathophysiology: Benign, local proliferation of uterine smooth muscle cells that are responsive to estrogen
- Diagnosis: History and pelvic ultrasound
- Complications: Infertility, recurrent miscarriage, progression to leiomyosarcoma
- Treatment
  - Hysterectomy is definitive treatment. Myomectomy is indicated if future fertility is desired.
  - Pharmacologic agents that decrease estrogen can be used to shrink fibroids.

CASE 9.10

A 49-year-old asymptomatic woman seen for a routine examination is noted to have enlarged ovaries bilaterally on pelvic examination.

1. What is the differential diagnosis for an ovarian mass?
   - PCOS, multiple cysts bilaterally
   - Ovarian cyst (functional, follicular and corpus luteum cyst, "chocolate" cysts)
   - Primary ovarian tumor
   - Epithelial mass (benign or malignant)
   - Germ cell tumor (benign teratoma = dermoid cyst, yolk sac, choriocarcinoma)
   - Sex cord stroma
   - Metastasis commonly from breast or gastrointestinal (GI) tract (Krukenberg tumor). Krukenberg tumors are usually bilateral.

2. What is polycystic ovary syndrome?
   PCOS occurs as a result of increased pituitary production of LH out of proportion to FSH (LH/FSH ratio >2) and hyperandrogenism secondary to unregulated synthesis by theca cells. Hyperandrogenism can result in hirsutism and virilization (male secondary sex characteristics and clitoromegaly), but androgens are also aromatized to estrogen in adipose tissue, thus increasing the risk of endometrial carcinoma. PCOS is associated with anovulation, obesity, and insulin resistance. The condition is often diagnosed at a younger age because symptoms generally appear at menarche. Polycystic ovaries have multiple 2- to 8-mm subcapsular cysts (Fig. 9.10A) that can be visualized on ultrasound (Fig. 9.10B). These cysts result in amenorrhea and infertility.

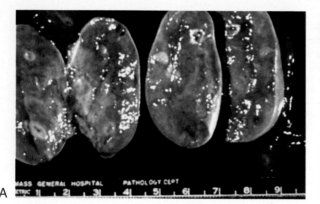

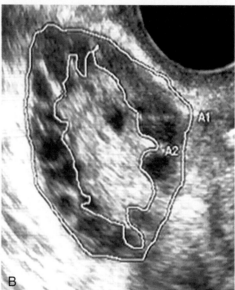

Figure 9.10. A, Sagittal section of polycystic ovaries illustrating a large number of follicular cysts and a thickened stroma. B, Ultrasound revealing ovarian cystic area (A1) and ovarian stromal area (A2). *(From Lobo RA. Comprehensive Gynecology. 7th ed. Philadelphia: Elsevier; 2017: 865-896. e3, Fig. 40.8 & 41.3.)*

Clinical Pearl
The Rotterdam Criteria are used to diagnose PCOS and require meeting two of the following three criteria: (1) anovulation, (2) hyperandrogenism, or (3) polycystic ovaries visualized on ultrasound.

STEP 1 SECRET

Expect to see a question on polycystic ovary syndrome (PCOS) on the USMLE Step 1.

CASE 9.10 CONTINUED:

Pelvic ultrasound shows a 10-cm cystic and solid mass with septations on the left and a 6-cm mass on the right. Given these ultrasound characteristics (>8 cm; solid, septations), it is thought to be highly suspicious for malignancy.

3. What is the most likely diagnosis in this patient?
Although 80% of ovarian tumors are benign, age is a risk factor for malignancy. Germ cell tumors are common in females under 20 years of age, whereas epithelial tumors are more common in those over 20 years of age. The highest incidence of ovarian cancer is in females who are 60 to 64 years of age.

4. What is the most common type of ovarian cancer?
Serous cystadenocarcinoma, an epithelial cell tumor, is the most common.

5. Is ovarian cancer hereditary?
About 90% of ovarian cancers are sporadic; 10% have a familial syndrome. Hereditary nonpolyposis colorectal cancer (HNPCC; Lynch II syndrome) is associated with a high rate of familial breast, ovarian, colon, and endometrial cancers. *BRCA1* and *BRCA2* mutations are also implicated in familial breast and ovarian cancers.

6. What are the major risk factors for ovarian cancer?
• Family history of ovarian cancer
• Long periods of uninterrupted ovulation (low parity)
• History of colon or breast cancer
  Remember: Hormonal contraceptives decrease risk of ovarian cancer because they suppress ovulation.

7. Are there any effective screening tests for ovarian cancer?
Not really. Cancer antigen 125 (CA-125) is a tumor marker in some ovarian cancers and is used to follow response to treatment, but it is *not* an appropriate screening tool for the general population because CA-125 is not specific for ovarian cancer.

8. What tumor markers are associated with different forms of ovarian cancer?
See Table 9.6.

Table 9.6. Ovarian Cancer Tumor Markers

TUMOR TYPE	TUMOR CLASS	TUMOR MARKER	HINT
Struma ovarii	Germ cell tumor	Thyroid hormone	Type of dermoid cyst that typically contains thyroid tissue
Dysgerminoma	Germ cell tumor	LDH, β-hCG	Similar to seminoma in males
Endodermal sinus tumor/yolk sac tumor	Germ cell tumor	AFP	Associated with Schiller-Duval bodies on histology
Choriocarcinoma	Germ cell tumor	β-hCG	Tumor composed of trophoblasts and syncytiotrophoblasts
Sertoli-Leydig cell tumor	Stromal tumor	Androgens	Associated with hirsutism and virilization
Granulosa-theca cell tumor	Stromal tumor	Estrogens	May cause precocious puberty, endometrial hyperplasia, or endometrial cancer Characterized by Call-Exner bodies, which are eosinophilic secretions
Serous, mucinous, clear cell, endometroid	Epithelial tumor	CA-125, CEA	65%–70% of all ovarian tumors

AFP, α-Fetoprotein; *β-hCG,* β-human chorionic gonadotropin; *CA-125,* cancer antigen 125; *CEA,* carcinoembryonic antigen; *LDH,* lactate dehydrogenase.

9. What is the prognosis for ovarian cancer?
The 5-year survival rate for ovarian carcinoma is 25% to 30%, typically because the disease is asymptomatic until advanced stages.

10. What lymph nodes are most likely to first show evidence of disease in patients with untreated ovarian cancer?
Para-aortic lymph nodes are the most likely to show evidence of disease related to ovarian cancer. These lymph nodes are responsible for drainage of ovaries in females and testicles in males. In contrast, the uterus, vagina, and scrotum are drained by the inguinal lymph nodes.

SUMMARY BOX: OVARIAN CANCER

- Polycystic ovary syndrome (PCOS) is characterized by anovulation, hyperandrogenism, multiple cysts on the ovaries, and elevated luteinizing hormone (LH).
- Krukenberg tumor is a metastasis to the ovary from another source: commonly gastrointestinal tract or breast. Hormonal contraceptives decrease the risk of ovarian cancer.
- Cancer antigen 125 (CA-125) is elevated in many ovarian cancers, but it is NOT a screening marker for ovarian cancer.

CASE 9.11

A 58-year-old postmenopausal woman presents with abnormal uterine/vaginal bleeding. She has been postmenopausal for 6 years and has never experienced this problem previously.

1. **What is generally assumed to be the cause of postmenopausal bleeding until proven otherwise?**
   Until proven otherwise, postmenopausal bleeding indicates endometrial cancer, which is the most common gynecologic cancer in the United States.

2. **What else should be considered in the differential diagnosis for postmenopausal bleeding?**
   Other uterine sources of bleeding should be considered, such as endometrial hyperplasia, as well as vaginal or cervical sources of bleeding such as vaginal atrophy/laceration, cervical polyps, or cervical cancer. Furthermore, postmenopausal females on hormone replacement therapy may experience bleeding, so this should be considered in the differential diagnosis as well.
   Note: Endometrial hyperplasia, which also commonly presents as postmenopausal bleeding, is a precursor to endometrial cancer. In fact, 40% of patients with atypical endometrial hyperplasia will progress to endometrial cancer.

CASE 9.11 CONTINUED:

A physical examination reveals the source of the bleeding to be the cervical os (i.e., uterine bleeding, not a vaginal source). There are no abnormal masses palpated on bimanual examination, and the uterus is of normal size and shape.

3. **What studies can be done to help with the diagnosis?**
   Pelvic ultrasound will show the anatomy—fibroids, polyps, or endometrial hyperplasia. Normally, a postmenopausal woman should have a very thin endometrial stripe because of lack of estrogen.

CASE 9.11 CONTINUED:

A pelvic ultrasound reveals a thickened endometrium, so an endometrial biopsy is done. The pathology report indicates malignancy.

4. **What is the most common type of endometrial cancer?**
   Adenocarcinoma (>80%) is the most common type of endometrial cancer.

5. **Why does endometrial cancer, once detected, generally have a much better prognosis than newly diagnosed ovarian cancer?**
   Endometrial cancer is usually detected at a much earlier stage than ovarian cancer thanks to the fact that abnormal uterine bleeding is an early warning sign. In contrast, there are few warning signs of early ovarian cancer.

6. **What are the risk factors for endometrial carcinoma?**
   Abnormally increased estrogen levels (e.g., PCOS, granulosa cell tumor) or use of estrogen without progesterone (e.g., hormone replacement therapy), obesity (adipose tissue can convert androgens into estrogens through the enzyme aromatase), hypertension, diabetes, early menarche, late menopause, and Lynch II syndrome are all risk factors.
   A commonly tested iatrogenic risk factor for endometrial carcinoma is tamoxifen use; look for this in patients with a history of breast cancer.

7. **In pathophysiologic terms, why does it make sense that the risk factors for endometrial cancer are similar to those for breast cancer?**
   The risk factors are similar because estrogen plays an important role in the etiology of both types of cancers. This is why obesity (increased peripheral production of estrogen), unopposed estrogens, nulliparity (increased exposure to *cycling* estrogens), and late menopause (increased estrogen exposure) are common risk factors for the development of breast cancer and endometrial cancer.

Remember: Hormonal contraceptives actually decrease risk of endometrial cancer because progesterone thins the uterine lining and prevents unopposed growth by estrogen.

8. **If this woman also has atrophic vaginitis, why should vaginal estrogen creams not be used to treat it?**
Endometrial cancer is estrogen-dependent; therefore, exogenous estrogens are contraindicated because of the risk of cancer progression.

SUMMARY BOX: ENDOMETRIAL CANCER

- Presentation: Abnormal uterine bleeding in a postmenopausal woman
- Epidemiology/risk factors
  - Most common gynecologic cancer in the United States
  - Risk factors include abnormally increased estrogen levels, obesity, unopposed estrogen use, nulliparity, and late menopause
- Pathophysiology: Atypical endometrial hyperplasia that progresses to endometrial cancer
- Diagnosis: Pelvic ultrasound revealing thickened endometrial stripe, confirmed with endometrial biopsy
- Treatment
  - Hysterectomy
- Prognosis: Excellent (frequently diagnosed at an early stage)

CASE 9.12

A 22-year-old woman is being evaluated for a breast mass she detected while showering. She has never had a mammogram and is wondering if she should get one.

---

1. **What is the differential diagnosis for a breast mass?**
   - Fibrocystic disease
   - Benign: fibroadenoma, cystosarcoma phyllodes, intraductal papilloma
   - Malignant carcinoma
2. **What characteristics of a breast mass are more consistent with benign versus malignant disease?**
   See Table 9.7 for these characteristics.

Table 9.7. Characteristics of Breast Masses

BENIGN: FIBROADENOMA	MALIGNANT: CARCINOMA
Soft	Firm
Tender	Nontender
Round, distinct borders	Irregular indistinct borders
Mobile	Fixed
Changes seen during cycle	No changes seen during cycle
Affects females 20–35 years of age	Affects females older than 35 years of age

---

CASE 9.12 CONTINUED:

The mass is round, mobile, rubbery, and nontender. There is no family history of breast or ovarian cancer.

---

3. **Should a mammogram be ordered to evaluate this breast mass? What other study can be done?**
   Mammogram can be used to further evaluate a suspicious mass, but ultrasound is useful if a palpable mass is questionable to determine if it is cystic or solid. A fluid-filled cyst can be drained with a needle in the office.

CASE 9.12 CONTINUED:

An ultrasound reveals the mass to be solid, not cystic, so an excisional biopsy is performed.

4. What is the most likely diagnosis?

Fibroadenoma is the most common breast tumor in premenopausal females; it is benign.

5. What is the difference between fibroadenoma and fibrocystic breast disease?

Both are benign processes, but fibroadenoma is an encapsulated tumor, whereas fibrocystic breast disease encompasses a wide spectrum of abnormalities, all to the result of an excessive stromal response to hormones and growth factors. These changes can include cyst formation, nodule formation, and epithelial hyperplasia.

Fibroadenoma is *not* a precursor to breast carcinoma. Fibrocystic disease usually does not increase risk of carcinoma except in cases of fibrocystic disease with atypical hyperplasia.

6. What is cystosarcoma phyllodes?

Phyllodes tumors are a variant of fibroadenoma and present as large bulky masses with rapid growth. Most are benign, but a few tumors do have malignant cells. These masses are often described as "leaf like" and commonly arise in females in their 60s.

7. If a female presents with bloody nipple discharge, what should be done, and what are the two diseases that can cause this?

The discharge should be sent for cytologic evaluation. A benign process, *intraductal papilloma*, which indicates local proliferation of the epithelial lining of the lactiferous ducts, is the most common possibility. The other possibility is *invasive papillary carcinoma*, a malignant process.

SUMMARY BOX: WORKUP OF PALPABLE BREAST MASS

- Soft, round, and mobile mass suggests benign disease. Firm, irregular, and immobile mass is concerning for malignancy.
- Ultrasound is used to determine if a mass is cystic or solid.
- Fibroadenoma is the most common benign tumor of the breast. It occurs in females 20 to 35 years of age. Cystosarcoma phyllodes is a variant of fibroadenoma with malignant potential.
- Intraductal papilloma is the most common cause of bloody nipple discharge, but invasive papillary carcinoma should be ruled out by sending discharge for cytologic evaluation.

CASE 9.13

A 59-year-old woman with a body mass index (BMI) of 31 is being evaluated for a breast mass she detected while showering. She is concerned about breast cancer because her mother was diagnosed with breast cancer at the age of 72.

1. Based solely on the family history and the known genetics of breast cancer, is this woman at high risk for developing a familial breast cancer?

No. The vast majority of breast cancers (≈90%) are sporadic. Because her mother was elderly when she developed breast cancer, it is highly unlikely that this patient had a familial predisposition (e.g., *BRCA1* or *BRCA2* mutations) to develop breast cancer. A first-degree relative family history is a risk factor for sporadic breast cancer, but postmenopausal breast cancer in a first-degree relative only slightly increases risk.

CASE 9.13 CONTINUED:

History is significant for a nontender mass that does not change in size or shape with her menstrual cycle and a single episode of bloody nipple discharge. Her menstrual cycles began at age 13 and she entered menopause at 55. She has no children and has never been pregnant.

2. What risk factors for breast cancer does she have?

- Female
- Age (postmenopausal)
- Late menopause
- Nulliparity
- Obesity

3. What is the significance of the age at menarche and age at menopause for the risk of developing breast cancer?
    The younger the age at menarche and the older the age at menopause are both correlated with a higher risk of breast cancer. These relationships are explained by increased cumulative exposure to estrogen.

CASE 9.13 CONTINUED:

On physical examination, her breasts are asymmetric: there is a firm, nontender, irregular mass in her right breast, with redness and dimpling of the skin, and her right nipple appears slightly retracted. All previous mammograms in this woman have been normal.

4. Based on the physical examination findings, does this woman likely have breast cancer?
    Yes, she has many of the classic signs: an irregular, firm breast mass causing retraction or dimpling of the skin or nipple (peau d'orange) and a bloody discharge.
    Remember: Intraductal papilloma, a benign process, is actually the most common cause of a bloody nipple discharge. Invasive papillary carcinoma is next.

CASE 9.13 CONTINUED:

A diagnostic mammogram is ordered, and she is referred to a surgeon for biopsy.

5. Which type of breast cancer is this woman most likely to have?
    Infiltrating (invasive) ductal carcinoma is the most common type of breast cancer and should be the presumed diagnosis pending a definitive pathology report. These tumors often present with an area of central necrosis on a histologic section (so-called *comedocarcinomas*).

6. If biopsy reveals estrogen receptor–positive and progesterone receptor–positive cells, why might treatment with tamoxifen or anastrozole be useful?
    Tamoxifen is a selective estrogen receptor modulator (SERM). It acts as an estrogen receptor agonist in certain tissues (e.g., bone, uterus) but as an estrogen antagonist in other tissues (e.g., breast). Anastrazole is an antiestrogen aromatase inhibitor that is also useful in estrogen receptor–positive (ER+) and progesterone receptor–positive (PR+) cancers. Because growth of ER+ and PR+ tumor cells is somewhat hormone-dependent, these cancers can be treated with agents such as tamoxifen or anastrozole. As previously mentioned, a commonly tested side effect of tamoxifen is the potential for endometrial proliferation and cancer resulting from its agonist effect on this tissue.

7. Another common receptor found in breast cancers is human epidermal growth factor receptor-2. What medication could be used for these tumors?
    A monoclonal antibody, trastuzumab, can be used for these tumors. This antibody targets the human epidermal growth factor receptor-2 (HER2) to inhibit activation of the receptor by the growth factor. A rare but serious side effect of this drug is dilated cardiomyopathy and subsequent development of congestive heart failure.

RELATED QUESTIONS

8. If an elderly woman presents with eczematous nipple changes, what should you suspect this is, what should you do, and why?
    Paget disease of the nipple should be suspected. Breast biopsy should be done because an underlying malignancy is found in the majority of patients with this disease.

9. If a woman has a unilateral inflamed breast and orange peel (dimpled) appearance to the skin of that breast, what disease process should you suspect, and what is the pathophysiology?
    She probably has inflammatory breast carcinoma, which can be attributed to the tumor embolizing into the dermal lymphatics. This in turn causes redness, swelling, and warmth. Because there has been tumor embolization, it is not surprising that there is axillary lymph node involvement. Distant metastases are frequent when this is found.

SUMMARY BOX: BREAST CANCER

- Presentation
  - Palpable breast mass or asymptomatic
- Epidemiology
  - Females older than 40 years of age
  - Risk factors include female gender, postmenopausal age, history of prior breast malignancy, nulliparity, early menarche, first-degree relative with breast cancer, obesity.

SUMMARY BOX: BREAST CANCER—cont'd

- Pathophysiology
  - Most cases are sporadic, but some females have genetic risk factors.
  - Tumors may be estrogen receptor (ER), progesterone receptor (PR), or human epidermal growth factor-2 receptor (HER2) positive.
- Diagnosis
  - Palpable breast mass on exam
  - Screening mammogram and biopsy of suspicious lesion
- Complications: Metastasis and death
- Treatment
  - Tamoxifen or aromatase inhibitors for ER+ tumors
  - Trastuzumab (an anti-HER2 monoclonal antibody) for HER2+ tumors

CASE 9.14

A 68-year-old man with a long-standing history of poorly controlled type 1 diabetes presents with difficulty maintaining an erection. He is embarrassed and concerned that he may never be intimate with his wife again.

1. **What is the diagnosis, and what is most likely etiology?**
   Erectile dysfunction (ED) is the diagnosis. Poor glycemic control can lead to vascular and neurologic damage to the penis. This affects 50% of men older than age 40. Other common causes of ED include peripheral vascular disease, trauma, history of prostate cancer (secondary to radiation or surgery), selective serotonin reuptake inhibitor (SSRI) antidepressants, and psychological causes.

2. **What is the normal physiology of the male sexual response including erection and ejaculation?**
   Erection is initiated by parasympathetic nerve stimulation of nitric oxide (NO) production from the vascular endothelium. NO promotes vasodilatation to increase blood flow to the penis and therefore causes an erection by stimulating an increase in cyclic guanosine monophosphate (cGMP), which stimulates the protein kinase G/myosin light chain kinase pathway. Emission is controlled by the sympathetic nervous system and delivers semen to the prostatic urethra. Ejaculation is controlled by sympathetic, parasympathetic, and somatic activity. The sympathetic nervous system closes the internal urethral sphincter, and the parasympathetic nervous system causes rhythmic contraction of the smooth muscle of the urethra. The somatic motor nerves (e.g., pudendal nerve) that innervate the bulbospongiosus (skeletal muscle) cause the final ejaculation.

3. **How is ED usually treated, and what is the mechanism of action of these drugs?**
   Oral phosphodiesterase-5 (PDE5) inhibitors (e.g., sildenafil, vardenafil, tadalafil, avanafil) are the mainstay of ED treatment. These drugs decrease degradation of cGMP and therefore an increase in the amount available to cause vasodilation. Other treatment options include penile self-injections with vasoactive drugs, intraurethral suppositories, vacuum erection devices, and penile prostheses, though these are beyond the scope of the USMLE Step 1 exam.

SUMMARY BOX: ERECTILE DYSFUNCTION

- Presentation: Classically seen in elderly men who report that they are unable to achieve or maintain an erection
- Epidemiology: Occurs in 50% of men who are above the age of 40
  - More common in patients with atherosclerotic risk factors such as diabetes mellitus, prostate cancer, and depression
- Pathophysiology
  - Vascular or peripheral nervous system dysfunction or damage secondary to hyperglycemia, atherosclerosis, or trauma
  - Psychological dysfunction or antidepressive medication
- Diagnosis: History
- Treatment
  - PDE5 inhibitors, such as sildenafil
  - Elimination of insulting agent such as a selective serotonin reuptake inhibitor (SSRI)
  - Psychological counseling

CASE 9.15

A 16-year-old boy visits the doctor because he worries that he has not yet gone through puberty. He has been unable to grow facial hair, and his voice has not become deep. Embarrassed, he admits that his genitals are smaller and less developed than what he thinks is normal for his age.

1. What is the differential diagnosis for delayed puberty?

   Because this case does not mention that the patient has ever had ambiguous or female external genitalia, for the purpose of the USMLE we can tentatively rule out disorders of sex development such as androgen insensitivity syndrome (AIS) and 5α-reductase deficiency (though as a general rule, you should never rule out a disease because the patient does not specifically mention something to you!). Consider constitutional delay, family history of delayed puberty, malnutrition, hypopituitarism, and Kallmann syndrome.

CASE 9.15 CONTINUED:

At birth, the patient presented with micropenis and cryptorchidism. He has also had a poor sense of smell for most of his life.

2. What is the most likely diagnosis in this patient?

   The most likely diagnosis is Kallmann syndrome, which is a genetic condition that leads to an absence of GnRH-producing neurons in the hypothalamus. This leads to lack of testosterone production and secondary sexual characteristics.

3. Why do these patients often present with anosmia?

   Kallmann syndrome can be associated with a lack of olfactory neurons in the brain as well. This results in a decreased or total loss of smell. Patients may also present with color blindness.

SUMMARY BOX: KALLMANN SYNDROME

- Presentation: Delayed puberty, hypogonadism, anosmia, color blindness
- Pathophysiology: Genetic deficiency in gonadotropin-releasing hormone (GnRH)-producing neurons in the hypothalamus
- Diagnosis: History

CASE 9.16

A 15-year-old girl is examined by an endocrinologist in the hospital. She has short stature, a webbed neck, and a broad shield-like chest with widely spaced nipples. Secondary sexual characteristics, such as breast development, are absent, and her external genitalia are infantile-appearing. She has never had a period. She has normal intellect and seems to be a happy, healthy person. A pelvic ultrasound reveals streak ovaries. The laboratory findings include a normal growth hormone level and an elevated FSH. Her karyotype is 45,XO. There is an absence of Barr bodies observed in cells from a buccal smear.

1. What disease do you suspect is responsible for this patient's amenorrhea?

   Turner syndrome, which occurs in 1 in every 2500 females, is most likely.

2. What causes the development of Turner syndrome?

   The presence of an incomplete sex genotype (45,XO) resulting from chromosomal nondisjunction (60%) or mosaicism (40%) is the cause. As a result, these females have decreased estrogen levels. About 80% of cases are caused by meiotic error in the father (i.e., the patient does not receive an X chromosome from her father).

   This disease is characterized by a number of physical abnormalities, including short stature, webbed neck, and broad chest. Young females with Turner syndrome also have ovarian dysgenesis. Instead of normal ovaries, they have "streaks" of connective tissue that do not produce normal quantities of estrogen or progesterone, hormones that are required for the development of secondary sexual characteristics. Because the ovaries are replaced by fibrous stroma and are devoid of oocytes by the age of 2, many of these females are infertile. However, a small percentage (5%–10%) has sufficient ovarian development to support fertility.

   Note: Turner syndrome is the most common cause of primary amenorrhea.

3. What phenomenon is responsible for this patient's webbed neck?

   This condition is called *cystic hygroma* and is a form of lymphangioma commonly found in the neck. Although the condition is benign, it can be quite disfiguring in some patients.

4. If this patient were to develop hypertension, what diagnostic test(s) should be performed?

   Patients with Turner syndrome are at increased risk for preductal coarctation of the aorta, which often results in hypertension limited to the upper extremities and cerebral vessels. In a manner analogous to renal artery stenosis, aortic coarctation causes hypertension because chronic underperfusion of the kidneys results in activation of the renin-angiotensin-aldosterone system and volume retention.

   The easiest initial diagnostic test is a comparison of upper and lower extremity blood pressures to assess for a significant discrepancy. Coarctation results in a lower femoral artery pressure and a delayed femoral pulse relative to the pressure and pulse of the brachial artery. A chest x-ray study will often show the classic "rib notching" as a result of increased collateral blood flow through the intercostal arteries, which bypass the coarctation. Imaging or often echocardiogram is usually performed to confirm the diagnosis.

5. **What are some other complications of Turner syndrome?**
Other complications include bicuspid aortic valve, horseshoe kidney, early osteoporosis, and hypothyroidism.

6. **How might this patient be managed pharmacologically to correct the lack of secondary sexual characteristics?**
Estrogen therapy for teenage girls with Turner syndrome can help promote development of secondary sexual characteristics.

7. **What is Klinefelter syndrome?**
The genotype of Klinefelter syndrome is 47,XXY (sometimes 48,XXXY). Because these individuals have a Y chromosome, they are males. The extra X chromosome becomes a Barr body (i.e., inactive). They undergo fibrosis of the seminiferous tubules, leading to azoospermia, infertility, and loss of Sertoli cells. Decreased inhibin production secondary to Sertoli cell loss leads to increased production of FSH. Patients with Klinefelter syndrome also exhibit abnormal Leydig cell function, which results in decreased production of testosterone and testicular atrophy. Because testosterone is unavailable to exert negative feedback upon the pituitary, LH concentrations become high. This stimulates the production of estrogens, leading to gynecomastia, eunuchoid body shape, and female hair distribution. These patients tend to be tall with long extremities because of delayed closure of the epiphyseal plates that results from decreased androgen concentrations.

STEP 1 SECRET

Turner and Klinefelter syndromes appear very frequently on the USMLE, so be sure that you can recognize their presentations.

8. **How does the presentation of the XXY Klinefelter phenotype differ from the XYY phenotype?**
XYY or double Y males are phenotypically normal with normal fertility. They tend to be taller than other males and often present with severe acne. They also have an increased risk of learning disabilities and behavioral problems.

9. **Besides Klinefelter syndrome, what other causes of gynecomastia can you identify?**
Gynecomastia is the enlargement of the male breast tissue secondary to estrogen exposure. Causes include cirrhosis (secondary to decreased estrogen metabolism by the liver), testosterone-secreting tumors, puberty (often resolves spontaneously), and iatrogenic causes (spironolactone, digitalis, cimetidine, alcohol, ketoconazole).

10. **What is trisomy X?**
Trisomy X refers to the genotype 47,XXX. These females often have no apparent abnormalities but may experience mild menstrual irregularities and exhibit mild intellectual disability. They are frequently taller than other females.

SUMMARY BOX: SEX CHROMOSOME DISORDERS

- Turner syndrome (45,XO) results in decreased estrogen levels and streaked ovaries. Patients typically present with short stature, webbed neck, and broadened chest. Turner syndrome is the most common cause of primary amenorrhea. It is associated with an increased risk of coarctation of the aorta.
- Coarctation of the aorta results in a discrepancy between upper and lower extremity blood pressures characterized by upper extremity hypertension. A chest x-ray will classically show rib notching. Other complications of Turner syndrome include bicuspid aortic valve, horseshoe kidney, and hypothyroidism.
- Klinefelter syndrome (47,XXY or 48,XXXY) results in decreased levels of testosterone and increased levels of estrogen. Patients typically present with infertility, gynecomastia, female hair distribution, eunuchoid body shape, tall stature, and long extremities.
- Trisomy X (47,XXX) females are typically normal but may experience mild menstrual irregularities or exhibit intellectual disability. They are generally tall.
- XYY individuals are phenotypically normal but may be taller with learning disabilities and/or behavioral problems.

CASE 9.17

A 16-year-old girl is concerned because she has not started having her period yet, whereas all of her friends have had periods for at least 2 years now. She additionally has no breast development. On physical examination, she has scant axillary and pubic hair, and the uterus is not palpable. On speculum examination, no cervix is visible (i.e., the vagina ends in a blind pouch). A pelvic ultrasound is performed, and she is found to have no uterus or ovaries but instead undescended testes. Consequently, a karyotype is performed, which comes back 46,XY.

1. **What is this patient's syndrome?**
This child likely has AIS, which is also known as *testicular feminization syndrome*. These patients are genetically and gonadally male but phenotypically female.

2. **What is the cause of this syndrome?**
    As mentioned in the Basic Concepts section of this chapter, genetic alterations in the androgen receptor make the tissues unresponsive to the androgenic effects of testosterone and other androgens. Testicles are present and functional (they produce testosterone), but the tissues do not respond.

3. **Why does this patient have a vaginal pouch?**
    In a normal male, the potent androgen DHT, which is produced from testosterone by the action of the enzyme 5α-reductase, acts upon the androgen receptor in the tissues of the urogenital fold to stimulate the formation of the external genitalia (i.e., penis, prostate, and scrotum) during development.

    In the absence of androgen activity, either in a normal female or in a male with androgen insensitivity, the urogenital fold defaults into a vaginal pouch.

    The effect of DHT on genital tissue has clinical relevance in the treatment of benign prostatic hyperplasia (BPH). Inhibitors of the enzyme 5α-reductase (e.g., finasteride) have been shown to reduce prostate size, often resulting in symptomatic improvement in men with BPH.

4. **Why does this patient have no pubic or axillary hair?**
    In both males and females, the initial development of secondary sexual characteristics, particularly pubic and axillary hair, adult body odor, and sebaceous gland activity, depends on adrenal androgen production. These changes usually occur before the hormonal changes of central puberty—that is, increased production of estrogen (specifically estradiol) in females and testosterone in males. In androgen insensitivity, lack of activity of adrenal or testicular androgens results in the lack of axillary and pubic hair.

    Recall that the major adrenal androgens include dehydroepiandrosterone (DHEA) and dehydroepiandrosterone sulfate (DHEA-S). In fact, DHEA-S is specific to the adrenal gland, and its levels will be increased in disorders of adrenal androgen overproduction, such as rare hormone-producing adrenal carcinomas and the virilizing forms of congenital adrenal hyperplasia.

5. **How can we explain the lack of uterus in this child?**
    Recall that the uterus is formed from the Müllerian duct. In males, these structures are dissolved by MIF, which is produced by the testes. Because there is no abnormality in the testes themselves in this disease, this substance will be secreted and the duct will dissolve, resulting in the absence of an internal female reproductive tract (i.e., fallopian tubes, uterus, and cervix).

    Recall that the internal male genital tract (i.e., the seminiferous tubules, the epididymis, and vas deferens) develops from the Wolffian duct, but this differentiation is not a default and requires the activity of testosterone.

    Thus, because the testes are normal and produce MIF in AIS, but the activity of testosterone is absent, neither a male nor a female internal genital tract develops.

6. **Would testosterone levels be low or high in this patient?**
    Testosterone levels would be high because the nonfunctional androgen receptors prevent negative feedback upon pituitary LH production. High LH levels in turn increase testosterone production by the testes. In other words, the lack of testosterone activity in the pituitary disinhibits LH release, which stimulates the testes to produce high levels of testosterone.

7. **Why should this patient's testicles be removed?**
    Undescended (or cryptorchid) testes from any cause, whether spontaneously undescended or undescended as part of a syndrome, are at increased risk for giving rise to testicular cancer. If an undescended testis fails to spontaneously descend within about a year or so of birth, it should be surgically replaced within the scrotum (i.e., orchiopexy) or surgically removed (i.e., orchiectomy).

SUMMARY BOX: ANDROGEN INSENSITIVITY SYNDROME

-   Presentation: Females with primary amenorrhea, scant axillary and pubic hair, and absence of other secondary sex characteristics
-   Pathophysiology
    -   Patients have a male karyotype (46,XY) and a defect in the androgen receptor.
    -   Their undescended testes produce Müllerian-inhibiting factor (MIF), which leads to degradation of the internal female reproductive tract.
    -   The defective receptor prevents development of the male reproductive tract in response to testicular testosterone.
    -   Male external genitalia cannot develop because they cannot respond to dihydrotestosterone (DHT).
    -   Secondary sexual characteristics such as adult body hair and odor normally develop in response to adrenal dehydroepiandrosterone sulfate (DHEA-S) in males and females; however, because of lack of androgen activity in patients with androgen insensitivity syndrome (AIS), they also lack these characteristics.
-   Diagnosis
    -   Physical exam/pelvic exam revealing lack of secondary sex characteristics and blind vaginal pouch
    -   Pelvic ultrasound showing absence of uterus or ovaries but presence of undescended testes
    -   Karyotype showing 46,XY
-   Complications: Testicular cancer secondary to cryptorchidism, infertility
-   Treatment: Surgical removal of the testes if they do not spontaneously descend within a year after birth

CHAPTER 10

ONCOLOGY

Insider's Guide to Oncology for the USMLE Step 1
It is no surprise that the USMLE Step 1 places heavy emphasis on oncology. As with pharmacology, almost every topic area has an oncology-related component. Yet before you can delve into these individual tumor types, you should develop a firm understanding of basic tumor biology. If you have the time to do so, we recommend that you read the "Neoplasia" chapter in *Robbins and Cotran Pathologic Basis of Disease*. Once you understand these concepts, you will see that every cancer type follows the same basic set of principles, and it will be much easier to focus on mastering specific facts. We also recommend focusing heavily on the mechanism of action and side effects of anticancer drugs. It is less important that you know the specific diseases for which they are used.

BASIC CONCEPTS—CELL BIOLOGY OF CANCER

1. What is the difference between an oncogene and a tumor suppressor gene?

   An oncogene is a mutated form of a normal gene called a *proto-oncogene*. Activating mutations convert proto-oncogenes into oncogenes and predispose an individual to neoplasia (uncontrolled, abnormal cell growth). Because only a single gene/allele needs to be mutated, oncogenes are seen as dominant mutations. An example of a proto-oncogene is a gene for a growth factor receptor that, when mutated, could lead to inappropriate activation of the receptor and uncontrolled cellular proliferation in the absence of excessive levels of that growth factor. Examples of important oncogenes and their associated cancers include *BCR-ABL*, a tyrosine kinase (chronic myeloid leukemia) and *c-MYC*, a transcription factor (Burkitt lymphoma).

   Tumor suppressor genes encode proteins that suppress cellular proliferation; therefore, if their function is lost (*disinhibited*), cancerous cells are permitted to survive. Mutations in tumor suppressor genes are said to be recessive because mutations must occur in both alleles in order to completely "knock out" the function of the gene (see question 3). Examples of important tumor suppressor genes and their associated cancers include *CDKN2A*, which encodes the p16 protein that regulates progression of the cell cycle from G_1 to S phase (pancreatic cancer, melanoma), and *APC*, which negatively regulates β-catenin concentrations (colorectal cancer).

2. Are tumor suppressor genes or oncogenes more commonly involved in familial cancer syndromes?

   Tumor suppressor genes are more commonly involved. This is because an embryo with one mutated copy of a tumor suppressor gene will likely develop normally, but acquisition of a second mutation later in life will predispose an individual to cancer (a mechanism known as *loss of heterozygosity;* a commonly seen example on USMLE Step 1 includes retinoblastoma and the two-hit hypothesis discussed subsequently). By contrast, an embryo is less likely to survive if it has inherited an oncogene because the effects of this dominant negative mutation are typically much more disruptive to development.

3. How does Knudson's "two-hit hypothesis" relate to tumor suppressor genes?

   Dr. Alfred Knudson studied a type of retinal cancer called *retinoblastoma,* which was later found to be caused by mutations of the retinoblastoma (*Rb*) tumor suppressor gene. At the time, he observed that in familial forms of *Rb*, tumors formed in patients at a much younger age than was typical for those arising in patients with no family history of the disease. He theorized that in familial cases, a germline mutation was inherited (the first hit) and that a second sporadic mutation occurred early in life (the second hit), thus deactivating both tumor suppressor genes and causing tumor formation. This theory was called the *two-hit hypothesis*. In nonfamilial cases, however, mutations of both tumor suppressor genes (both hits) had to occur sporadically and thus took much longer to manifest as tumor formation.

4. What are the phases of the cell cycle? Where is the restriction point?

   Most cells in the human body are quiescent (i.e., not actively dividing). Exceptions include cells of the hematopoietic system, the integument, and the intestinal mucosa. However, those cells that divide follow a well-defined cyclic pattern. Major challenges in cell replication include high-fidelity DNA duplication (in the S phase) and segregation of chromosomes into daughter cells (during mitosis or the M phase). Different phases and checkpoints help address these issues:
   - G0 phase: Resting phase; no division occurs
   - G1 phase: Gap period 1; cells increase in size
   - R: G1 restriction point

- S phase: DNA synthesis
- G2 phase: Gap period 2; continued cell growth and checkpoint for DNA damage
- M phase: Mitosis; orderly division of the cell

The restriction point occurs just before the S phase. It is important because once the restriction point is passed, a cell is committed to complete the cell cycle. Multiple cellular factors interact to allow a cell to pass the restriction point.

5. What is the function of cell cycle checkpoints (aka *cell cycle arrests*)?

The most important function of cell cycle arrest is to allow for the repair of cellular damage and DNA sequences. If improperly duplicated DNA is not repaired at cell cycle checkpoints, then DNA mutations quickly propagate, and the integrity of cellular homogeneity cannot be maintained. A cell may also arrest in the absence of proper nutrients, growth factors, or hormones.

Cyclins are proteins that regulate progression from one phase of the cell cycle to the next. Cyclins phosphorylate cyclin-dependent kinases (CDKs) to form cyclin-CDK complexes that must be in either an activated or inactivated state for various cell cycle stages to commence or terminate. CDKs are regulated by CDK inhibitors such as p16, p21, and p27. If these CDK inhibitors are mutated, the cell cycle becomes deregulated and cancer can result.

6. What is the importance of p53?

The p53 protein ("guardian of the genome") is a tumor suppressor gene protein responsible for regulating progression from the G_1 to S phase and promoting apoptosis (regulated cell death) in cells with excessive DNA mutations or cellular damage. p53 can activate DNA repair genes in response to DNA damage and initiate apoptosis in irreparable cells. p53 also activates the CDK inhibitor p21 to hypophosphorylate and activate Rb protein, preventing passage from G_1 to S phase. Loss of p53 can lead to loss of apoptotic regulation and thus uncontrolled cellular proliferation. The p53 gene, *TP53*, is the most commonly mutated gene in human cancers.

7. What is the function of the Rb protein?

Like p53, pRb is a tumor suppressor protein that functions to prevent cell cycle progression from the G_1 to S phase by binding to and inhibiting the transcription factor E2F. pRb is heavily regulated via p53 and cyclin-CDK complexes. When in a hypophosphorylated state (which is maintained by p53), pRb functions as a tumor suppressor and inhibits cell cycle progression until the cell is actively ready to divide. During the G_1 to S transition, increased levels of cyclins phosphorylate pRb and prevent its binding to E2F. E2F then activates additional proteins that push the cell cycle to the S phase. Loss-of-function mutations of *Rb* are present in several human cancers.

8. What is the difference between dysplasia and anaplasia?

Dysplasia refers to abnormal cell growth and is marked by loss of cell shape, orientation, and size compared to normal tissue. While dysplastic changes are regarded as precursors to neoplastic conditions, dysplasia is often reversible with cessation of the offending factor responsible for initiating the damaging mutations (e.g., ultraviolet radiation that predisposes an individual to skin cancer). In contrast, *anaplasia* is an irreversible condition that is marked by lack of cell differentiation. It is difficult to identify the tissue of origin in an anaplastic lesion.

Clinical Pearl

Dysplasia can be divided into different grades using a numeric scale (1–4) to distinguish the degree of cellular differentiation and mitotic activity. The grade is determined by the pathologist's analysis under the microscope. Low-grade dysplasia signifies a well-differentiated tumor that still bears histologic similarity to the tissue of origin. High-grade dysplasia signifies anaplasia, which carries a worse prognosis. The importance of prognosis based on the grade of dysplasia is the basis of cancer screening, so that physicians can detect low-grade dysplasia and appropriately treat the patient with a better overall prognosis rather than later detecting a high-grade dysplastic tumor with a worse prognosis. Examples of cancer screening for dysplastic changes include the Papanicolaou (Pap) test for cervical cancer (see Case 10.6).

---

9. How do carcinomas form?

A carcinoma is a cancer arising specifically in epithelial cells. Epithelial cells are among the most frequently mutated cells because of their high rate of replication. The epithelial cells that compose tissues are organized and grow on a basement membrane. Once a mutation is inherited, the epithelial cells will undergo hyperplasia (an increase in cell number) and dysplasia. This can progress to a preinvasive state called *carcinoma in situ,* where the epithelial cells appear cancerous but have not yet invaded the basement membrane. Once the cancerous cells manage to invade the basement membrane, the tumor is classified as an invasive carcinoma, which can metastasize (i.e., spread to a distant site through blood vessels or lymphatics) (Fig. 10.1).

10. What is the importance of angiogenesis in solid tumor growth?

It is thought that a solid tumor must form new blood vessels for a mass to grow larger than a few millimeters in diameter. Without this ability, a tumor would soon outstrip the physiologic blood supply and the tumor cells would die. Thus solid tumors must be able to allow for and encourage the formation of new blood vessels (angiogenesis) through expression of angiogenic growth factors (e.g., vascular endothelial growth factor [VEGF], fibroblast growth factor [FGF]) as the tumor mass expands. This concept has spurred the development of a drug class known as *angiogenesis inhibitors* (e.g., bevacizumab) for cancer treatment.

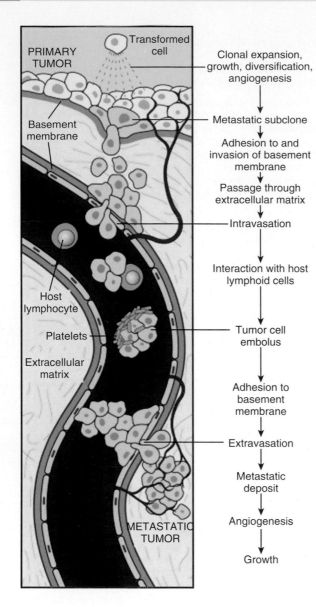

Figure 10.1 Sequential steps involved in the hematogenous spread of cancer from a primary to a distant site. Initially, there is clonal proliferation of a subset of primary tumor cells that have the capacity to metastasize. In order to invade from the primary site, the cancer cells must lose their cell-to-cell adhesion molecules such as E-cadherin, obtain the capacity to move through tissue, adhere to and degrade the basement membrane through metalloproteinases, pass through the extracellular matrix, and penetrate the vascular wall of a capillary (intravasation). In the bloodstream, the cancer cells encounter host defense cells (e.g., cytotoxic T cells, killer cells) and some are destroyed (type IV hypersensitivity reaction). Those that survive form tumor cell emboli that attach to the capillary endothelium of a distant organ (e.g., lung) and repeat the process of invasion of the capillary wall into the tissue of the distal organ, where it sets up a metastatic focus of tumor that will grow and continue to spread. *(From Kumar V, Fausto N, Abbas A, Aster J. Robbins and Cotran Pathologic Basis of Disease. 8th ed. Philadelphia: Saunders Elsevier; 2010: Fig. 7-36.)*

BASIC CONCEPTS—CANCER EPIDEMIOLOGY

1. What are the three leading causes of death in the United States?
   1. Heart disease
   2. Cancer
   3. Chronic lower respiratory disease

2. Aside from skin cancer, which cancers have the highest incidence in men and in women? Which cancers are the leading causes of death in men and in women?
   See Table 10.1. Note that *incidence* refers to the number of newly diagnosed cases of a particular disease. *Mortality* refers to the number of deaths resulting from that disease.

STEP 1 SECRET

Table 10.1 is considered to be very high yield for Step 1.

Table 10.1. Most Common Cancer Types by Gender

	MALE	FEMALE
Incidence	1. Prostate cancer 2. Lung cancer 3. Colorectal cancer	1. Breast cancer 2. Lung cancer 3. Colorectal cancer
Mortality	1. Lung cancer 2. Prostate cancer 3. Colorectal cancer	1. Lung cancer 2. Breast cancer 3. Colorectal cancer

BASIC CONCEPTS—CANCER CLASSIFICATION

1. What is the difference between *grade* and *stage* of a neoplasm?

    Grade: Tumor grade refers to its description under the microscope and is used to predict how rapidly the tumor is likely to grow and metastasize. The grade of a neoplasm is designated *pathologically* and requires tissue, usually from a biopsy. The pathologist analyzes the biopsy microscopically and assigns the grade based on cellular characteristics of the neoplasm, especially the degree of differentiation of the cells involved. Grades are reported numerically from 1 to 4, with the higher numbers representing more poorly differentiating cellular patterns.

    Stage: Tumor stage refers to the severity of the cancer and is used to predict the patient's prognosis and optimal treatment plan. The stage of a cancer is determined *clinically* by examining the site and size of the primary tumor and its spread to lymph nodes and distant organs through radiologic imaging (computed tomography [CT] scan, positron emission tomography [PET] scan, magnetic resonance imaging [MRI]). While the stage is determined through radiologic imaging, it often takes into account information provided by the pathologist (the grade). Stage is most frequently reported using the tumor-node-metastasis (TNM) system:
    - **T**: Tumor size. *T* refers to local growth measured by the size of the primary tumor.
    - **N**: Nodes. *N* refers to the involvement of regional lymph nodes and is an indication of the extent of tumor spread.
    - **M**: Metastases. *M* refers to the presence or absence of distant metastases. Presence of metastases typically confers a high stage.

    Staging is most helpful in determining prognosis. Higher stages indicate a poorer prognosis.

STEP 1 SECRET

While you will not be asked to determine the grade or stage of a cancer on USMLE Step 1, you will be expected to understand the aforementioned general concepts.

2. What is the difference between a benign tumor and a malignant tumor?

    The primary distinction is degree of invasiveness. Benign tumors remain localized to the tissue of origin and may be surrounded by a capsule (the exception to this rule is leiomyoma, which is a benign tumor that is not surrounded by a capsule). They grow slowly and in an organized pattern and do not metastasize unless they undergo malignant transformation (degeneration). With reference to tumor grade, these tumors tend to be well differentiated.

    Malignant tumors are characterized by their invasive properties. These tumors are not surrounded by a capsule, and tumor cells locally invade the surrounding tissues. They tend to grow rapidly and in a disorganized manner and may metastasize. Histologically, these tumors are typically poorly differentiated, indicating uncontrolled cellular proliferation.

    Even though malignant tumors generally have a worse prognosis than benign tumors, you should not be fooled into thinking that benign tumors are harmless. Depending on location, benign tumors can cause major obstruction that can severely compromise the function of that organ. Brain tumors are a great example of this principle.

3. How are cancers named according to the cell type they originate from?

    Because of their high rate of replication, epithelial cells are among the most commonly mutated cell type. Cancers may arise from glandular cells, squamous cells, or transitional cells. Benign epithelial tumors frequently end in the suffix *-oma.* Malignant tumors of epithelial origin are referred to as *carcinomas.* For example, a benign tumor of squamous cell origin is referred to as a *papilloma,* but when it becomes malignant, it is called a *squamous cell carcinoma.*

    Benign tumors can also arise from mesenchymal cells (also typically ending in *-oma*), but their malignant counterparts are called *sarcomas.* Thus a benign tumor originating from skeletal muscle is called a *rhabdomyoma,* whereas its malignant counterpart is called a *rhabdomyosarcoma.*

    Other cancers may originate from cell types that are not completely differentiated and may be able to give rise to other cell types (i.e., totipotent cells/germ cells). Leukemias and lymphomas are classified in this way and have a unique naming system. Many variations exist in the naming of cancers, but the rules mentioned here are helpful to remember.

CASE 10.1

A 50-year-old man is evaluated for a 6-month history of mild upper abdominal pain. The pain is associated with mild nausea and bloating and is unrelated to meals. He denies a retrosternal burning sensation. He reports early satiety and poor appetite. Over the past 3 months, he has unintentionally lost 10 lb. He is otherwise feeling well and does not take any medications.

1. **Given the limited information provided above, what is the differential diagnosis for this patient?**
   Overall, the most likely diagnosis for dyspepsia is gastrointestinal reflux disease (GERD); however, the patient's symptoms are not related to eating. We must include malignancy (with the clue of unintentional weight loss and early satiety). Because of the patient's age, we must consider cardiac ischemia (which can present with symptoms similar to dyspepsia). Less likely causes of dyspepsia include biliary tract disease such as cholelithiasis and choledocholithiasis, functional dyspepsia, and pancreatitis.

CASE 10.1 CONTINUED:

The patient is given a trial of omeprazole without relief of symptoms. He now notes worsening fatigue. Physical examination is unrevealing with the exception of the guaiac fecal occult test being positive for blood. There is no conjunctival pallor or lymphadenopathy in the left supraclavicular fossa.
   Laboratory workup reveals hemoglobin of 10.2 g/dL (normal value 14–17 g/dL) with a mean corpuscular volume (MCV) of 65 fL (normal value 80–100 fL).

2. **How does this information change your differential diagnosis?**
   The patient is bleeding into his gastrointestinal tract (as evidenced from his anemia and positive hemoccult test), most likely from peptic ulcer disease or a gastric adenocarcinoma. He needs to have an upper endoscopy performed as soon as possible.

STEP 1 SECRET

Whenever a patient has unintentional weight loss, particularly if appetite is suppressed, you should consider cancer as part of your differential diagnosis.

3. **How might you further characterize this patient's anemia?**
   This patient's anemia could be characterized as a microcytic anemia from iron deficiency secondary to ongoing blood loss in the gastrointestinal tract. Anemia of chronic disease is also possible but less likely in the setting of ongoing blood loss.

CASE 10.1 CONTINUED:

Upper endoscopy reveals an ulcer at the distal antrum of the stomach. It is not actively bleeding at the time of endoscopy. Biopsies are taken of the ulcer margin and the antrum.

4. **Why were biopsies taken at these sites?**
   Gastric ulcers are always biopsied on endoscopy because approximately 3% to 5% of ulcers, while often benign-appearing, are malignant. The antral biopsy is taken to test for *Helicobacter pylori* infection.

CASE 10.1 CONTINUED:

Biopsy of the ulcer margin shows gastric adenocarcinoma. Biopsy of the antrum is positive for *H. pylori*.

5. **What is the significance of the *H. pylori*–positive biopsy?**
   H. pylori is one of the two major etiologic agents for peptic ulcer disease (nonsteroidal anti-inflammatory drug [NSAID] use being the other), but it is also highly correlated with gastric adenocarcinoma. Chronic *H. pylori* gastritis of the distal stomach increases the relative risk for developing gastric adenocarcinoma 4- to 20-fold.

6. **What is the most common pathologic type of gastric cancer?**
   Adenocarcinoma accounts for 90% to 95% of the cases. Other types of gastric cancers include lymphoma, gastrointestinal stromal tumor, carcinoid, and squamous cell carcinoma.

7. **What are the two histologic distributions of gastric adenocarcinoma?**
Diffuse type: In this pattern, there is no cellular cohesion. Neoplastic cells invade the wall of the stomach diffusely without producing a distinct lesion. This type tends to occur in younger patients and has a poor prognosis. It is not commonly associated with *H. pylori* infection or intestinal metaplasia.
   Note: Diffuse gastric adenocarcinomas present with signet ring cells (Fig. 10.2).
   Intestinal type: In this pattern, cells cohere and form glandular structures that often have an ulcerative appearance. Lesions are most often found in the antrum and lesser curvature of the stomach. This type tends to occur in older patients and has a better prognosis than the diffuse type. It is associated with *H. pylori* infection, smoked foods (nitrosamines), smoking, achlorhydria, and intestinal metaplasia from chronic gastritis.

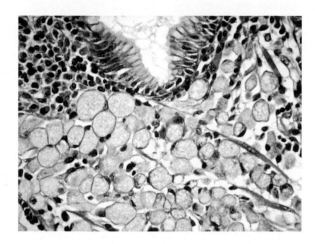

Figure 10.2. Diffuse type of gastric carcinoma with signet ring tumor cells. *(From Kumar V, Cotran RS, Robbins SL. Robbins Basic Pathology. 8th ed. Philadelphia: WB Saunders; 2007.)*

8. **What is linitis plastica?**
Linitis plastica ("leather bottle") is a morphologic variant of diffuse-type gastric cancer. The term is used to describe involvement of the submucosa throughout the stomach and suggests a rigid, atonic stomach. Grossly, the stomach appears thick and texturally similar to leather.

9. **What other signs of nontender lymphadenopathy might you appreciate on physical examination if this patient were to be examined at a much more advanced stage of his malignancy?**
   • Virchow node: Left supraclavicular lymphadenopathy
   • Sister Mary Joseph nodule: Umbilical nodule
   • Krukenberg tumor (in women): Ovarian tumors (often bilateral) that may be palpable on pelvic examination

10. **In retrospect, what aspects of this patient's presentation are most suspicious for gastric cancer?**
   • Onset of dyspepsia after age 40
   • Unintentional weight loss of 10 lb in 3 months
   • No response to proton pump inhibitor therapy
   • Development of early satiety
   • Iron-deficiency anemia from occult intestinal bleeding

SUMMARY BOX: GASTRIC ADENOCARCINOMA

• Presentation: Upper abdominal pain, nausea, vomiting, unintentional weight loss, early satiety, anemia
• Etiology: Comprises almost all gastric cancers
• Pathophysiology: 60% to 90% of cases of distal gastric adenocarcinoma attributed to chronic *Helicobacter pylori* infection
• Diagnosis: Upper endoscopy and biopsy

CASE 10.2

A 28-year-old woman is evaluated for a nontender lump in her left breast that she noticed while showering 2 days earlier. She is tearful and anxious. History is negative for pain or nipple discharge. Physical examination reveals a nontender, 2-cm mass in the left upper quadrant of the left breast. There are no skin changes in the area overlying the mass and no structural distortion of the breast. She has no lymphadenopathy.

1. **When examining a new breast lump, what findings may suggest breast cancer?**
Nontender, firm or hard masses with poorly delineated margins can suggest breast cancer. There may be skin or nipple retraction and slight asymmetry.

2. **What is the most common presentation of breast cancer, and where are most cancers found?**
Approximately 70% of new cases of breast cancer present with a new lump in the breast. About 90% of all lumps are found by the patient during self-examination, although the U.S. Preventive Services Task Force (USPSTF) recommends against teaching breast self-examinations (level D recommendation). Up to 60% of breast carcinomas are found in the upper outer quadrant of the involved breast.

3. **What do the following physical examination findings indicate?**
Bloody discharge from the nipple: This can be a sign of breast cancer but is more commonly found in intraductal papilloma (a small benign tumor of the milk duct) when the discharge is found to be coming from a single duct.

   Small erosions (1–2 mm) of the nipple epithelium: Dermatitis or Paget disease of the breast is possible. Although nipple erosions most frequently represent a dermatitis or bacterial infection, this sign may also indicate an underlying ductal carcinoma in situ (DCIS) extending to the skin surface. As pictured in Fig. 10.3, the neoplastic cells propagate toward the surface of the breast without violating the basement membrane. The presence of neoplastic cells violates the epithelial barrier, allowing extrusion of extracellular fluid onto the nipple surface.

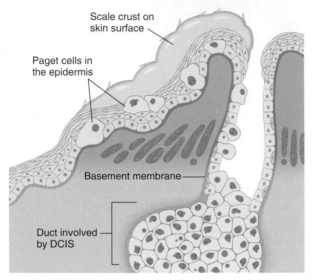

Scale crust on skin surface

Paget cells in the epidermis

Basement membrane

Duct involved by DCIS

Figure 10.3. Paget disease of the nipple. *DCIS,* Ductal carcinoma in situ. *(From Kumar V, Abbas AK, Aster JC.* Robbins and Cotran Pathologic Basis of Disease. *10th ed. Philadelphia: Elsevier; 2015.)*

   Rapidly growing breast with erythematous, edematous, and warm overlying skin: Inflammatory carcinoma should be a consideration. Invasion of the subdermal lymphatics by carcinoma can cause spreading erythema that can often be mistaken for infection. Resultant edema produces typical *peau d'*orange appearance (Fig. 10.4).

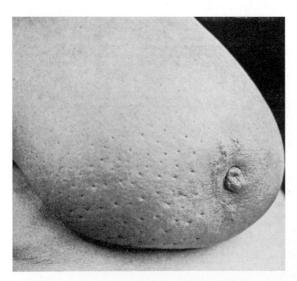

Figure 10.4. Peau d'orange ("skin of the orange") or edema of the skin of the breast. *(From Townsend CM, Beauchamp RD, Evers BM, et al.* Sabiston Textbook of Surgery. *17th ed. Philadelphia: WB Saunders; 2004.)*

4. **What is the most common cause of a dominant breast mass for a woman in her 20s?**
   Fibroadenomas are the most common cause. These are typically described as round, rubbery, discrete, and relatively mobile and measure 1 to 5 cm. They increase with size and tenderness in the presence of estrogen (as seen in menstruation and pregnancy) and do not confer an increased risk of breast cancer. No treatment is usually necessary. Diagnosis must be based on tissue biopsy or cytologic examination to avoid misdiagnosis of a malignancy.

CASE 10.2 CONTINUED:

During examination of the patient's right breast, a 1.5-cm discrete, nontender, mobile lump is found in the lower outer quadrant. The patient is very upset with the discovery of a lump in her right breast and reveals that her mother died of breast cancer at the age of 40 and that her older sister was diagnosed with breast cancer at the age of 27.

5. **What do bilateral breast lumps indicate with regard to a malignant or benign cause?**
   Bilateral breast lumps indicate fibroadenomas, which can occur at multiple sites in up to 10% to 15% of patients. Another possibility is fibrocystic disease, which does not typically increase the risk of carcinoma and is seen histologically as fluid-filled blue "domes" with ductal dilation. Simultaneous bilateral breast cancers can also occur, so a bilateral malignant process is also in the differential diagnosis.

6. **What disease is she at risk for with the finding of bilateral breast masses and a family history of two first-degree relatives?**
   She is at risk for hereditary breast cancer. Up to 45% of familial cases of breast cancer are associated with a germline mutation, and in these syndromes, presentation with simultaneous bilateral breast lumps is common. A family history of breast cancer in more than one first-degree relative, premenopausal diagnosis of breast cancer, and multiple breast tumors are highly suggestive of an inherited germline mutation.

7. **What specific genetic mutations confer a lifetime risk of 50% to 85% for developing breast cancer?**
   BRCA1 and *BRCA2* mutations confer a greater risk for developing breast cancer. These are tumor suppressor genes whose gene products inhibit tumor growth. A single mutation is inherited, and the second gene acquires a mutation (the "second hit") at some point in the patient's life. Multiple different inherited mutations to these genes have been identified. Though these genes have been well documented, they account for only approximately 25% of familial cases.

8. **If her tumor is found to be positive for *BRCA1*, for what other malignancy would this patient be at risk?**
   This patient would also be at risk for ovarian cancer.

CASE 10.2 CONTINUED:

The lump in her left breast is biopsied and is found to harbor ductal carcinoma. Surgical excision is planned.

9. **What are the common histologic types of breast cancers?**
   Carcinomas are divided into two broad categories: in situ and invasive carcinomas.
   Breast cancers are also classified as ductal or lobular based on where they arise: Ductal origin refers to cancers arising from the epithelial lining of the large or intermediate-sized ducts, and lobular origin refers to cancers arising from the epithelium of the terminal ducts of the lobules.
   - *In situ carcinoma* describes a neoplastic population of cells that has not penetrated the basement membrane of the affected duct or lobule (Fig. 10.5).
     - DCIS makes up 80% of in situ carcinomas. Approximately half of mammographically detected cancers are DCIS because they tend to present with calcifications. DCIS is thought to progress to invasive ductal carcinoma in most women.
     - Lobular carcinoma in situ (LCIS) never forms a density or calcifications and is therefore always an incidental finding on breast biopsy. It is found to be bilateral in 20% to 40% of women and turns into invasive cancer at a rate of approximately 1% per year; therefore, LCIS can be thought of as a risk factor for the development of invasive lobular carcinoma in either breast.
   - *Invasive carcinoma* is characterized by neoplastic cells that have penetrated the basement membrane and may significantly affect architectural distortion.
     - Ductal carcinoma accounts for up to 80% of invasive carcinomas. Most histologic types of invasive cancers (comedo, colloid, medullary, etc.) are subtypes of invasive ductal carcinoma.
     - Lobular carcinoma shows the classic histologic description of linear arrangements of cells (sometimes only one cell wide or in a "single file" pattern) invading surrounding tissue.
     - Medullary carcinoma is found in women with the *BRCA1* gene. Histology typically shows large, high-grade cells with sheet-like growth and prominent lymphoplasmacytic infiltrate. Up to 13% of cancers are of this type.

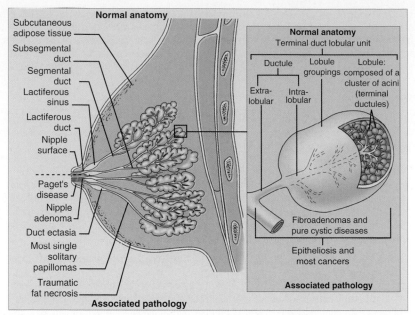

Figure 10.5. Anatomy of the breast. *(From Hayes D. Breast cancer. In Skarin AT, ed.* Atlas of Diagnostic Oncology. *Philadelphia: Lippincott; 1991.)*

10. **What are two important biomarkers of a breast cancer that help guide treatment?**
    1. Estrogen receptor (ER)/progesterone receptor (PR): If these receptors are present in the cytoplasm of cancer cells, then there is a better prognosis. After resection, patients are typically treated with tamoxifen (a selective estrogen receptor modulator [SERM]), which inhibits endogenous hormone stimulation of tumor cells. As a result, breast cancer is less likely to recur, and mortality rate may be decreased by as much as 25% among women with receptor-positive tumors. Anastrazole (an aromatase inhibitor) is used when the patient has contraindications to tamoxifen.
    2. HER-2/neu (also known as *ERBB2*): If a patient has a metastatic breast carcinoma that overexpresses this gene, trastuzumab may be used. Trastuzumab is a monoclonal antibody directed against the HER-2 receptor protein. When used with first-line chemotherapy following surgery, trastuzumab slows disease progression.

SUMMARY BOX: BREAST CANCER

- Presentation: Nontender, firm breast masses with poorly delineated margins are concerning for invasive breast cancer. Other findings concerning for breast cancer include nipple discharge, nipple scaling, breast asymmetry, nipple inversion, peau d'orange, erythema, and warmth.
- Epidemiology: The most common cause of a breast mass in a young woman is fibroadenoma.
- Diagnosis: Biopsy
- Pathophysiology:
  - *BRCA1* and *BRCA2* mutations predispose to the early development of breast cancer and account for approximately 25% of familial breast cancer syndromes.
  - Most breast cancers arise from the intermediate ducts and are invasive (invasive ductal carcinoma).
- Complications: *BRCA1* mutations confer increased risk for development of ovarian cancer.
- Treatment: Estrogen receptor/progesterone receptor (ER/PR) and *HER2/neu* (*ERBB2*) are important biomarkers. Their presence may guide adjuvant therapy for breast cancer following resection.

CASE 10.3

A 78-year-old retired postal worker is evaluated for a 2-month history of epigastric pain. He describes the pain as a vague pressure that occasionally radiates to his back. It does not reliably occur before or after meals. He has lost 20 lb in the past 2 months, which he attributes to his recent lack of appetite. NSAIDs have provided no relief. The pain occasionally subsides when he leans forward while sitting. He has a 60-pack-year history of smoking and drinks alcohol in moderation. Physical examination reveals scleral icterus and a nontender palpable gallbladder.

---

1. **What diagnosis is suggested by this presentation, and what are the key pieces of evidence?**
   Pancreatic carcinoma is the suggested diagnosis. Pain is present in over 70% of cases of pancreatic carcinoma and often radiates to the back. Weight loss is suggestive of underlying neoplasm but may also be related to depressive

symptoms often seen in pancreatic cancer. Scleral icterus suggests obstruction of the biliary ductal system. Courvoisier sign describes the finding of a nontender palpable gallbladder and painless jaundice and also indicates obstruction of the biliary ductal system. Courvoisier sign is more commonly seen in obstruction by a neoplasm, whereas scleral icterus results from obstruction by any mechanism.

2. **Where would a pancreatic mass most likely be located in order to cause biliary obstruction?**
A pancreatic mass would most likely be in the pancreatic head. Two-thirds of pancreatic cancers are located in the head of the pancreas, where they can easily obstruct the biliary ductal system. One-third of pancreatic cancers occur in the body or tail, which leads to a more insidious presentation and delayed diagnosis (see question 4).

3. **What are important acquired and hereditary risk factors for the development of pancreatic cancer?**
Acquired risk factors include age greater than 50 years, male gender, cigarette smoking (note that this patient was a smoker), industrial chemical exposure, diabetes mellitus, and chronic pancreatitis.

   Hereditary risk factors include a family history of pancreatic cancer (7%–8% of patients with pancreatic cancers have a first-degree relative with pancreatic cancer, vs. 0.6% of control subjects) and a familial form of chronic pancreatitis. The following familial cancer syndromes also confer an increased risk of developing pancreatic cancer:
   - Peutz-Jeghers syndrome
   - Ataxia-telangiectasia
   - Hereditary nonpolyposis colorectal cancer (HNPCC)
   - Familial breast cancer (*BRCA2*-positive)

4. **What is the prognosis for pancreatic adenocarcinoma?**
Prognosis is poor. Tumors located in the body or tail have an even poorer prognosis than those located in the head because they often do not produce signs and symptoms until they have invaded adjacent structures. Surgical resection (Whipple procedure) offers a median survival time of 18 months and a 5-year survival rate of approximately 20%. When tumors are not resectable and patients are treated with chemotherapy alone, the 5-year survival rate is less than 5%. Only 10% to 15% of all tumors are resectable at presentation.

CASE 10.3 CONTINUED:

CT of the abdomen reveals a mass at the pancreatic head. The splenic vein appears occluded by clot, and the tumor is compressing the superior mesenteric artery. No metastases are seen. The tumor is deemed unresectable, and he is offered palliative care.

5. **What serum cancer marker is likely to be elevated in this patient?**
Serum cancer marker CA 19-9 is likely to be elevated. However, CA 19-9 lacks sufficient sensitivity (50%–75%) and specificity (approximately 85%) to be used in the screening of asymptomatic individuals. However, there may be some utility in monitoring postresection levels to assess disease status. Carcinoembryonic antigen (CEA) can also be elevated in pancreatic cancer, but this is nonspecific.

   Please note that for screening purposes, the ideal screening test should have high sensitivity/low specificity during initial screening of the population, followed by testing the positive patients with a second test with low sensitivity/high specificity in order to identify the false positives as disease free.

6. **What is the most common histologic type of pancreatic cancer?**
The most common type of pancreatic cancer is pancreatic adenocarcinoma. In this presentation, neoplastic cells arise from ductal cells of the pancreas. Neoplastic cells will form ductules and may even secrete mucin.

   Other types of pancreatic cancers include neuroendocrine tumors and cystic tumors. These tumors are less aggressive than adenocarcinoma.

7. **Which genes are most frequently mutated in pancreatic cancer?**
The oncogene, *KRAS*, and the tumor suppressor genes, *CDKN2A* and *SMAD4* (*DPC4*), are the most frequently mutated in pancreatic cancer. The *KRAS* gene normally is involved in cellular signaling pathways through guanosine triphosphatase (GTPase). In pancreatic cancer (along with colon cancer and lung cancer), it is activated by a point mutation. These mutations cause a deactivation of the protein product's GTPase activity. As a result, the protein is constitutively active. The *CDKN2A* gene, which encodes the p16 protein, normally regulates the progression from G_1 to S phase. The *CDKN2A* gene is inactivated in 95% of pancreatic cancers. It also plays a role in melanoma.

CASE 10.3 CONTINUED:

The patient is evaluated 1 month later for right calf pain. A random glucose test (performed via finger stick) reveals a plasma glucose concentration of 180 mg/dL. The posterior right calf is tender, and the right calf diameter is enlarged relative to the left calf. A fasting glucose drawn 2 days later is 124 mg/dL.

8. **What two processes have developed in this patient?**

Glucose intolerance and deep vein thrombosis (DVT) have developed. Glucose intolerance and often frank diabetes can occur with pancreatic cancer, presumably as a result of the destruction of insulin-secreting β cells by the tumor.

This patient has likely also developed a DVT of the calf. Patients with cancer are at an increased risk for clotting because of the Virchow triad (hypercoagulability, endothelial damage, blood stasis) and frequently develop both deep and peripheral venous thromboses.

Clinical Pearl

When migratory peripheral venous thromboses are noted in a patient with pancreatic cancer, it is called *Trousseau syndrome*. DVT and pulmonary embolism are the most common thrombotic conditions in patients with cancer. Trousseau syndrome can be an early sign of pancreatic, lung, or gastric adenocarcinoma, as early as months to years before the tumor would otherwise be detected. Thus if this syndrome is observed, pancreatic, lung, and gastric adenocarcinoma should be included in the differential diagnosis and appropriately investigated.

Of interest, Dr. Armand Trousseau first described the finding of migratory venous thromboses in himself; he was subsequently found to have gastric cancer.

SUMMARY BOX: PANCREATIC CANCER

- Presentation: Epigastric pain radiating to the back, weight loss, scleral icterus, Courvoisier sign (nontender palpable gallbladder with painless jaundice)
- Epidemiology
  - General risk factors include age >50 years, male gender, cigarette smoking, diabetes mellitus, and chronic pancreatitis.
  - Hereditary risk factors include a family history of pancreatic cancer and a familial form of chronic pancreatitis.
- Diagnosis
  - History and physical exam (see Presentation)
  - Abdominal computed tomography (CT) scan or endoscopic ultrasound
  - Hyperbilirubinemia and abnormal γ-glutamyl transpeptidase and alkaline phosphatase levels
  - Elevated CA 19-9 levels
- Pathophysiology
  - Most common genetic mutations: *KRAS* (oncogene), *CDKN2A* (tumor suppressor gene), *SMAD4*, or *DPC4* (tumor suppressor gene)
- Complications
  - Glucose intolerance, diabetes
  - Hypercoagulability
  - Migratory thrombophlebitis (Trousseau syndrome)
- Treatment: Surgical resection (Whipple procedure), chemotherapy, radiation therapy
- Prognosis: Poor

CASE 10.4

A 63-year-old man with a history of chronic obstructive pulmonary disease (COPD) secondary to smoking is evaluated for a 1-week history of cough. In the past 2 to 3 days, he has noted that his sputum is blood tinged.

---

1. **What is the most common cause of hemoptysis?**

Acute bronchitis is the most common cause of hemoptysis. Other causes of hemoptysis include lung cancer, pulmonary infections such as tuberculosis and pneumonia, and sarcoidosis. Given this man's smoking history, lung cancer is a concern.

CASE 10.4 CONTINUED:

Chest x-ray film reveals a right hilar pulmonary nodule and right hilar lymphadenopathy. CT scan reveals a 2.2-cm intraluminal bronchial polypoid mass, multiple enlarged hilar lymph nodes, and no evidence of distant metastases.

---

2. **Aside from hemoptysis, how else might lung cancer clinically manifest?**

Change in character of a "smoker's cough," persistent upper respiratory infections or "post-obstructive" pneumonias, pleural or pericardial effusions, Horner syndrome, superior vena cava (SVC) syndrome, asymptomatic pulmonary nodule on routine chest x-ray, hoarseness, signs and symptoms of metastatic disease, or paraneoplastic syndrome might occur. Paraneoplastic syndromes include Cushing syndrome through adrenocorticotropic hormone (ACTH) secretion in small cell lung cancer (SCLC), syndrome of inappropriate antidiuretic hormone (SIADH) through antidiuretic hormone (ADH) secretion in SCLC, Lambert-Eaton myasthenic syndrome, and hypercalcemia through parathyroid hormone–related protein (PTHrP) secretion in squamous cell lung cancer.

3. What percentage of lung cancer occurs in patients with a significant smoking (or exposure) history?

Approximately 90% of lung cancer occurs in patients with a significant smoking history. There is also a direct association between the frequency of lung cancer and these smoking characteristics:

- Amount of daily smoking
- Duration of smoking
- Tendency to inhale

While cigarette smoking is an enormous risk factor for developing lung cancer, only 10% to 15% of people with high-risk smoking activity develop lung cancer. Of note, approximately 10% of lung cancers occur in nonsmokers or those with a very limited smoking history.

4. What are the four most common histologic types of lung cancers?

Squamous cell carcinoma, adenocarcinoma, small cell carcinoma, and large cell carcinoma comprise more than 90% of cases of primary lung cancer. For purposes of staging and treatment, these types of lung cancers are separated into two broad categories:

- SCLC
- Non–small cell lung cancer (NSCLC), which is more common than SCLC

SCLC is considered separately from NSCLC because it has a different natural history and is, therefore, treated differently.

The remaining 10% of lung cancers that are not accounted for by the four major categories mentioned here include bronchoalveolar carcinoma (this is often considered to be a type of adenocarcinoma and is associated with nondestructive growth of the tumor along the alveolar architecture) and bronchial carcinoid tumors. Malignant mesothelioma is another type of lung cancer popularly tested on the USMLE. This malignancy of the pleura occurs 25 to 40 years after exposure to asbestos and is associated with the formation of psammoma bodies (concentric calcium deposits).

5. How do SCLC and NSCLC behave differently in terms of aggressiveness, spread, treatment, and prognosis?

SCLC: Early hematogenous spread is typical. These cancers are rarely resectable or responsive to surgical therapy and are very aggressive, with a median untreated survival time of 6 to 18 weeks. Chemotherapy and radiation therapy are commonly administered.

NSCLC: This form tends to spread more slowly than SCLC and may even be cured if diagnosed in the early stages when local resection may be possible.

6. Which three types of lung cancer are most strongly associated with cigarette smoking?

Squamous cell carcinoma, small cell carcinoma, and large cell carcinoma are most strongly associated with cigarette smoking. Squamous and small cell carcinoma are located centrally within the lung, whereas large cell carcinoma is located peripherally. Adenocarcinoma is also peripherally located but can arise in nonsmokers.

7. Describe how the following symptoms or symptom complexes might be produced by local tumor invasion or regional metastases.

1. SVC syndrome

SVC syndrome (neck vein distention and facial swelling) is produced by compression of the SVC by an enlarging tumor. SVC syndrome is generally associated with SCLC and presents with puffiness and purple discoloration of the face, arms, and shoulder regions. Fatal complications of SVC syndrome include retinal hemorrhage and stroke as a result of increase in intracranial pressure. Treatment for SVC syndrome includes radiation therapy and stents to bypass sites of obstruction.

2. Horner syndrome

Horner syndrome (ptosis, miosis, anhidrosis) can be caused by invasion of the cervical sympathetic nerves and ganglia. This is most often associated with squamous cell carcinoma (in which the finding will be ipsilateral) and is referred to as a *Pancoast tumor*.

3. Diaphragmatic paralysis

Tumor invasion of the phrenic nerve can cause diaphragmatic paralysis.

4. Hoarseness

Tumor invasion of the recurrent laryngeal nerve, usually on the left, can cause hoarseness.

5. Tamponade, congestive heart failure (CHF)

Malignant pericardial effusion can produce these effects.

CASE 10.4 CONTINUED:

Sputum cytologic examination is performed. Results are shown in Fig. 10.6.

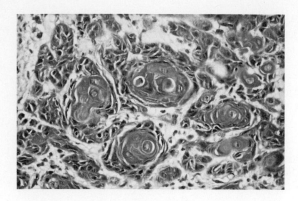

Figure 10.6. The many well-differentiated foci of eosinophilic-staining neoplastic cells produce keratin in layers (keratin pearls). *(From Forbes C, Jackson W. Color Atlas and Text of Clinical Medicine. 3rd ed. St. Louis: Mosby; 2003:211, Fig. 4-184.)*

8. What is the likely diagnosis?
   Squamous cell carcinoma is the likely diagnosis. This can always be differentiated from other types of lung cancers by the presence of keratin in layers (keratin pearls). Small cell carcinoma is also easy to recognize from the presence of small, blue neuroendocrine cells (Fig. 10.7). Adenocarcinoma is easily classified by the presence of mucinous glands.

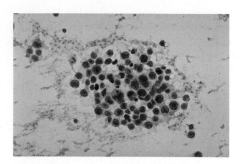

Figure 10.7. Small cell carcinoma, oat cell type. The characteristic features of oat cell carcinoma, including nuclear molding, hyperchromatic granular chromatin, and high nucleocytoplasmic ratios, are seen. Bronchial brushing (Papanicolaou). *(From Bibbo M, Wilbur D. Comprehensive Cytopathology. 3rd ed. Philadelphia: Saunders; 2009.)*

STEP 1 SECRET

USMLE test makers commonly include gross and histologic images of lung tumors on the examination.

CASE 10.4 CONTINUED:

A polypoid lesion is surgically resected. Adjuvant chemotherapy is started. The patient dies of complications of metastatic disease 6 months later.

9. To which distant sites does lung cancer commonly metastasize?
   Lung cancer commonly metastasizes to the brain, bone, liver, and adrenal glands.

SUMMARY BOX: LUNG CANCER

- Presentation: Change in cough, postobstructive pneumonia in an adult, persistent upper respiratory infection, hemoptysis, hoarseness, superior vena cava (SVC) syndrome, Horner syndrome, paraneoplastic syndromes
- Epidemiology
  - Lung cancer is the leading cause of cancer death. Lung cancer has a 16% incidence in men and a 13% incidence in women with a 33% mortality rate in men and 23% in women.
  - Percent occurring in smokers: 90% (squamous cell carcinoma, small cell carcinoma, and large cell carcinoma are most associated with smoking)
  - Percent occurring in nonsmokers: 10%
- Classification
  - By histology: squamous, small cell, adenocarcinoma
  - By size: small cell lung cancer (SCLC) and non–small cell lung cancer (NSCLC)

SUMMARY BOX: LUNG CANCER—cont'd

- Diagnosis
  - History: Change in cough, hoarseness, hemoptysis
  - Exam: Wheezing, signs of bronchial obstruction
  - Imaging: Chest x-ray, computed tomography (CT) scan
- Pathophysiology
  - Squamous cell carcinoma and small cell carcinoma are located centrally within the lung tissue and commonly result from cigarette smoke exposure. Large cell carcinoma is located peripherally and is also associated with smoking.
  - Adenocarcinoma is peripherally located and can arise in nonsmokers.
- Complications: Metastasis (typically to brain, bone, liver, and adrenal glands)
- Treatment: Surgical resection, chemotherapy, radiation therapy

---

CASE 10.5

A 50-year-old African American man with a history of well-controlled hypertension on hydrochlorothiazide is evaluated for his annual physical. Review of systems is unrevealing. Physical examination is likewise unrevealing, including a prostate examination. Screening labs reveal a prostate-specific antigen (PSA) of 5.4 ng/mL (normal <4.0 ng/mL).

---

1. **How is the anatomy of the prostate defined clinically (i.e., on digital rectal examination)?**
   On digital rectal examination, two lateral lobes separated by a central sulcus can be palpated. These lobes are felt for nodules and asymmetry. They make up the posterior portion of the posterior surface of the prostate gland, which is the only area accessible to digital rectal examination.

2. **What is the PSA, and what does it indicate?**
   PSA is produced in the cytoplasm of both benign and malignant cells of the prostate. It therefore correlates with the volume of prostatic tissue in a patient and is not specific for prostate cancer. PSA values increase normally with age, so men 40 to 49 years of age normally have values <2.5 ng/mL, whereas men 70 to 79 years old can have PSA values as high as 6.5 ng/mL and still be considered normal (due to age-related benign enlargement of the prostate). Nonetheless, a PSA value greater than 4.0 ng/mL is generally considered abnormal.

Clinical Pearl

The degree of prostate-specific antigen (PSA) elevation is important. Only 18% to 30% of men with an intermediate elevation in PSA (4.1–10.0 ng/mL) will be found to have prostate cancer. However, 50% to 70% of men with a PSA of >10.0 ng/mL will be found to have prostate cancer.

Because PSA indicates volume of prostatic tissue, it can be elevated in prostate cancer because of an increased volume of malignant prostatic cells or because of benign prostatic hypertrophy (BPH), in which the volume of benign prostatic cells is increased. It can also be elevated in cases of prostatitis.

Minor elevations in PSA values (4.1–10.0 ng/mL) can be associated with both BPH and prostate cancer. Always examine the values of free PSA. BPH is associated with elevations in free PSA values, but prostate cancer is not.

---

3. **What is a 50-year-old man's lifetime risk of developing prostate cancer and of dying from prostate cancer?**
   A 50-year-old man has a 40% chance of developing prostate cancer. However, he has only a 10% chance of developing clinical disease and only a 3% risk of dying from prostate cancer. Because such a small percentage of men with prostate cancer die from prostate cancer, the use of PSA as a screening tool remains rather controversial, and shared decision making is generally recommended.

CASE 10.5 CONTINUED:

The patient undergoes a transrectal ultrasound–guided prostate biopsy. A hyperechoic area in the peripheral zone of the prostate is visualized and needle biopsied.

---

4. **What is the most commonly found histologic type of prostate cancer?**
   Adenocarcinomas are the most commonly found histologic type of prostate cancer. This type arises from the glandular acini; however, the regions seen on biopsy are often heterogeneous (i.e., multiple patterns with varying degrees of differentiation can be seen). The Gleason grading system was developed to account for multiple patterns within a single biopsy. A score of 1 (most differentiated) to 5 (no glandular differentiation) is applied to the dominant histologic pattern.

A second score of 1 to 5 is applied to the second-most abundant histologic pattern. Adding the two scores together gives the Gleason score (2–10). This is the best marker, along with TNM staging, for predicting prognosis.

5. Why might a patient with prostate cancer present with urinary obstruction? With hematospermia?
Advanced local disease often presents with urinary obstruction as the tumor mass encroaches on the prostatic urethra. If the tumor invades the seminal vesicles, it can cause hematospermia or a decrease in ejaculate volume.

6. Where are the most common sites of metastasis? Which signs and symptoms might indicate metastases in this patient?
Bone and pelvic lymph nodes are the most common sites of metastasis. When affecting bone, prostate cancer most often metastasizes to the axial skeleton including the lumbar vertebral bodies. As a result, patients with advanced disease may present with lower back or pelvic pain. Osteoblastic metastases are virtually diagnostic for prostate cancer. An increase in serum alkaline phosphatase is also commonly observed. When affecting pelvic lymph nodes, metastases can cause unilateral lymphedema.

SUMMARY BOX: PROSTATE CANCER

- Presentations: Most cases of prostate cancer are asymptomatic and detected by abnormal findings on digital rectal examination or an elevated prostate-specific antigen (PSA) level. Prostate cancer spreads by local extension and metastases to bone (especially axial skeleton) and pelvic lymph nodes.
- Epidemiology: Common in men older than 50 years old; more common in Black men
- Diagnosis
  - Increased PSA and a needle core biopsy to determine Gleason score
- Pathogenesis
  - 70% of prostate cancer arises from the peripheral zone
- Prognosis
  - Only a small number of men who develop prostate cancer will die as a result of it.
  - Gleason score: Prognosis of prostate cancer is determined by Gleason score (2–10) and tumor staging (TNM system).

CASE 10.6

A 45-year-old woman who has not had regular medical care for years is evaluated for postcoital bleeding. Her vital signs are normal.

---

1. What is the differential diagnosis for this issue?
   - Carcinoma of the cervix: The most common presenting symptom for cervical cancer is irregular vaginal bleeding, particularly postcoital bleeding.
   - Endocervical polyp: These inflammatory polyps usually occur in the endocervical canal and may extrude from the external os and become visible. They occur in 2% to 5% of adult women and can also present with irregular vaginal bleeding.

2. Because postcoital bleeding in a woman who does not see a doctor regularly is a red flag for malignancy, what risk factors for cervical cancer do you want to ask her about?
   - Multiple sexual partners
   - Early age of onset of sexual activity
   - Tobacco use
   - Immunosuppression

   Note: In utero diethylstilbestrol (DES) exposure of a fetus is a risk factor for the development of a rare cancer type called *cervical* or *vaginal clear cell carcinoma*.

3. Why is a sexual history particularly important in this patient?
   Nearly all incidences of cervical cancer result from prior infection with human papillomavirus (HPV), which is transmitted sexually. HPV infection is very common and can be detected in more than 50% of sexually active women between the ages of 16 and 21. However, only a small percentage of these women develop cervical cancer because HPV infection is usually eradicated by the immune system. Cervical cancer is the result of persistent HPV infection.

CASE 10.6 CONTINUED:

Her history reveals that she has been sexually active since the age of 21 and has had two sexual partners. She has never been pregnant. She had a *Chlamydia* infection at age 29 that resolved with antibiotics. She does not smoke or take oral contraceptives. She has no family history of gynecologic cancer. Speculum examination reveals a fungating lesion near the external os of the cervix in the 3 o'clock position.

4. **What is the transformation zone of the cervix, and how is it relevant to the development of cervical cancer?**

The transformation zone is the area that is most susceptible to neoplastic change. The cervix is a 3- to 4-cm cylindrical, fibrous organ that contains an exocervix composed of squamous epithelium and an endocervix made up of columnar epithelium. The interface of these two types of epithelia is called the *squamocolumnar junction.* Until menarche, the squamocolumnar junction is on the surface of the cervix, meaning that the columnar cells extend out onto the exterior of the cervix. With age, columnar cells on the surface of the cervix begin to change into squamous cells in a metaplastic process. This results in a new squamocolumnar junction that migrates toward the endocervical canal. The area between the original squamocolumnar junction and new squamocolumnar junction is known as the *transformation zone,* and the cells within this zone are most susceptible to neoplastic changes. Thus squamous cell carcinoma of the cervix is most typically found here, and this is the area that Papanicolaou (Pap) tests attempt to screen (Fig. 10.8). Note that Pap tests screen for but cannot diagnose cancer; a tissue biopsy is required for this.

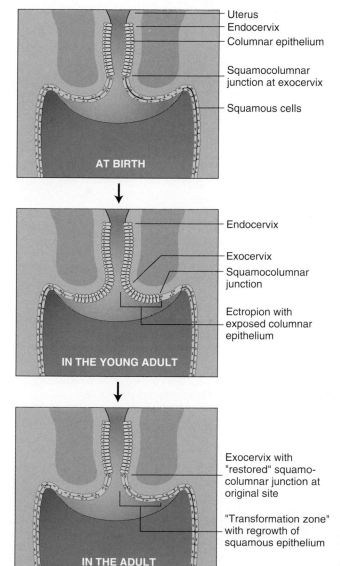

Figure 10.8. Schematic of the development of the cervical transformation zone. *(From Kumar V, Abbas AK, Fausto N, Mitchell RN. Robbins Basic Pathology. 8th ed. Philadelphia: Elsevier; 2007.)*

5. **Why is it important that this patient has not seen a physician in years?**

Since the advent of the Pap test, the incidence of invasive cervical cancer and related mortality risk has fallen by approximately 80%. Had this patient had regular medical care and Pap tests, it is likely that she would have had an abnormal Pap test before developing cervical cancer (the time from development of carcinoma in situ to invasion of the basement membrane is 10 to 20 years or more).

6. What are the current guidelines for cervical cancer screening?
   The USPSTF recommends that women have their first Pap test at age 21. Women ages 21 to age 29 should be screened with a Pap test every 3 years. Women ages 30 through 65 have the option of being screened every 5 years with a Pap test and HPV cotesting or every 3 years with a Pap test alone (another option is HPV testing alone every 5 years). HPV testing detects high-risk HPV types. Women who have had a hysterectomy to remove the uterus and cervix do not need to have cervical cancer screening unless the hysterectomy was done to treat a precancerous lesion or cervical cancer.

7. Which types of HPV are considered high risk for the development of cervical cancer? What types are associated with genital warts?
   High-risk HPV types are HPV 16 and 18. Other high-risk types that are not as prevalent include HPV 45, 31, and 33. Low-risk HPV types associated with condyloma acuminata (genital warts) are HPV 6 and 11. These subtypes do not increase risk of cervical cancer.
   Note: The other genital "wart," condyloma latum, is due to secondary syphilis.

8. What are the current recommendations regarding HPV vaccination?
   The Centers for Disease Control (CDC) recommends HPV vaccinations for males and females ages 11 to 26. The two types of vaccinations are Gardasil and Cervarix. Both vaccines protect against the high-risk serotypes (HPV 16 and 18). Gardasil also has additional protection against the low-risk strains HPV 6 and 11.

9. Why are Pap tests effective in preventing the development of cervical cancer?
   A Pap test is obtained by direct scraping of the cells in the transformation zone. If abnormal cells are seen, then the patient returns for colposcopy (visual examination of the vaginal and cervical mucosa using a lighted colposcope) and biopsy to determine whether the patient has cervical intraepithelial neoplasia (CIN). CIN refers to abnormal growth of cervical squamous cells (cervical dysplasia) and is categorized into grades CIN I, CIN II, and CIN III (Table 10.2).

Table 10.2. Cervical Intraepithelial Neoplasia (CIN) Grades

HISTOLOGY GRADE	CORRESPONDING CYTOLOGY	DESCRIPTION
CIN 1	LSIL (Low-grade intraepithelial lesion)	Mild dysplasia Confined to the basal one-third of the epithelium
CIN 2	HSIL (High-grade intraepithelial lesion)	Moderate dysplasia Confined to basal two-thirds of the epithelium
CIN 3	HSIL	Severe dysplasia Spans more than two-thirds of the epithelium but does not invade the basement membrane May sometimes be referred to as *cervical carcinoma in situ*

Even if this patient does have CIN, there are methods of treatment (e.g., excisional cone biopsy, loop electrosurgical excision procedure) that can excise the lesion and prevent the development of invasive cervical carcinoma.

The abnormal cells that we look for to detect cervical dysplasia are called *koilocytes*. Koilocytes are squamous epithelial cells that have undergone transformation secondary to papillomavirus infection. You should know how to recognize these cells for boards. They typically present with large, hyperchromatic nuclei with perinuclear halos (Fig. 10.9).

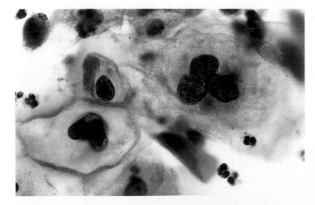

Figure 10.9. The cytologic appearance of cervical intraepithelial neoplasia as seen on the Papanicolaou smear. Normal cytoplasmic staining in superficial cells may be either red or blue. Image shows low-grade squamous intraepithelial lesion—koilocytes. *(From Kumar V, Abbas AK, Fausto N, Aster J. Robbins and Cotran Pathologic Basis of Disease. 8th ed. Philadelphia: Saunders; 2010. Courtesy Dr. Edmund S. Cibas, Brigham and Women's Hospital, Boston, MA.)*

10. Which HPV-associated oncogenes are responsible for causing cervical cancer?

Oncogenes E6 and E7 are responsible for causing cervical cancer. Protein products encoded by these genes interfere with functioning of the tumor suppressor proteins p53 and pRb. Specifically, the E6 protein binds p53 and increases its rate of proteolysis, which reduces levels of p53. The E7 protein prevents transcription of the *Rb* gene by binding and displacing bound transcription factors necessary for *Rb* transcription. This induces CIN, which progresses over time from CIN 1 to CIN 3.

CASE 10.6 CONTINUED:

The patient returns 1 week later for colposcopy and biopsy of the lesion. Pathologic examination shows squamous cell carcinoma, the most common histologic type of cervical cancer.

STEP 1 SECRET

Recall that if you are given an image of squamous cell carcinoma of the cervix, you will be able to spot keratin pearls (see Fig. 10.6).

11. Which symptoms are typically seen in a patient with cervical dysplasia or cervical carcinoma?

Many patients are asymptomatic, but some will present with vaginal bleeding (often postcoital), malodorous discharge, or dyspareunia. Advanced tumors can invade through the anterior uterine wall into the bladder and obstruct the ureters. Hydronephrosis and obstructive renal failure are the most common causes of death in patients with cervical carcinoma.

SUMMARY BOX: CERVICAL CANCER

- Presentation: Abnormal vaginal bleeding or postcoital spotting in a middle-aged female. Malodorous discharge and dyspareunia may also be present.
- Risk factors: More common in individuals with a history of multiple sexual partners, early age of onset of sexual activity, tobacco use, immunosuppression
- Pathophysiology: Caused by human papillomavirus (HPV); HPV 16 and HPV 18 are high-risk types.
  - HPV-associated viral oncogenes E6 and E7 interfere with the normal function of tumor suppressor proteins p53 and pRb, respectively.
- Diagnosis: Presence of koilocytes on Pap test followed by colposcopy and biopsy for confirmation of cervical intraepithelial neoplasia (CIN)
- Complications: Hydronephrosis and postrenal failure (most common causes of death)
- Treatment: Lesion excision

CASE 10.7

A 64-year-old man with a recent diagnosis of a right-sided glioblastoma multiforme is evaluated for sudden onset vision changes. Physical examination reveals a fixed and dilated right pupil.

1. Which cranial nerve is compressed that is leading to his right-sided fixed and dilated pupil?

Cranial nerve III (oculomotor nerve) is being compressed. This nerve has a somatic component and an autonomic component.

Somatic: Supplies four of the six extraocular muscles (superior rectus, inferior rectus, medial rectus, inferior oblique) and the levator palpebrae muscle

Autonomic: Parasympathetic innervation of the constrictor pupillae and ciliary muscles

Compression of cranial nerve III typically involves the autonomic, as well as the somatic limb. Removal of parasympathetic tone causes fixed dilation of the pupil unresponsive to light or accommodation. A fixed and dilated pupil could also be an early sign of uncal herniation secondary to increased intracranial pressure from the glioblastoma.

2. What are the three most common types of primary brain neoplasms in adults, and what are their respective cells of origin?

- Meningioma (most common)
- Glioblastoma
- Other astrocytomas

Meningiomas arise from arachnoid cells in the meninges (arachnoidal fibroblasts). They are benign in 90% of cases and are usually operable. However, malignant meningiomas can invade adjacent brain tissue. Gliomas include glioblastomas and astrocytomas and arise from the supportive cells (glial cells, astrocytes) of the central nervous system (CNS). The tumor cells invade the surrounding parenchyma and are often associated with areas of necrosis.

Note: You should keep in mind that the most common brain tumors are actually metastatic tumors (most commonly from lung and breast). Metastatic brain cancer typically presents with multiple, well-circumscribed tumors at the gray-white matter junction.

3. The World Health Organization system for grading astrocytomas is important for understanding the histologic patterns of this common brain tumor but is unlikely to be tested on the USMLE Step 1. How does glioblastoma multiforme fit into this grading system?

WHO grade I: Pilocytic tumors. Most are benign and are cured surgically. They are more common in children than adults.

WHO grade II: Diffuse astrocytomas. In these tumors, invading cells can be found in the brain parenchyma in areas distant from the expanding mass, and gray/white matter boundaries may be eliminated. Other features include low cellularity, low nuclear pleomorphism, no endothelial proliferation, and no necrosis.

WHO grade III: Anaplastic astrocytomas. These tumors are similar to grade II tumors except that there is much greater mitotic activity histologically. There is increased cellularity, nuclear pleomorphism, and mitotic activity.

WHO grade IV: Glioblastoma multiforme. These high-grade tumors are distinguished from anaplastic astrocytomas by the presence of endothelial proliferation or necrosis. Gross specimens show discoloration and cystic changes that result from hemorrhage and necrosis. Glioblastoma multiforme tumors infiltrate the brain quickly and extensively, contributing to their poor prognosis. They are usually found in the cerebral hemispheres and can cross the corpus callosum.

4. What does the histologic pattern of "pseudopalisading" represent?

In glioblastoma multiforme (Fig. 10.10), tumor cells can be seen to crowd around areas of necrosis, forming the appearance of palisades of cells surrounding acellular/necrotic areas.

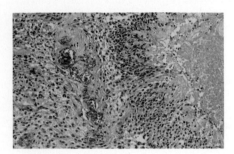

Figure 10.10. Glioblastoma with small, anaplastic tumor cells, vascular proliferation, and areas of necrosis with pseudopalisading of tumor cells. *(From Goetz CG. Textbook of Clinical Neurology. 3rd ed. Philadelphia: Saunders; 2008.)*

5. Different histologic stains can be used to highlight different types of CNS cells. What is the protein expressed in the cytoplasm of astrocytes that pathologists direct antibodies against to visualize cells of astrocytic origin?

Glial fibrillary acidic protein (GFAP) is expressed in the cytoplasm of astrocytes.

SUMMARY BOX: BRAIN CANCERS

- Epidemiology: Most commonly arise due to metastasis
- Complications: Cranial nerve compression, increased intracranial pressure, herniation syndromes

CASE 10.8

A 24-year-old man is evaluated for a small lump in his neck. He feels well but is concerned because his father, who died from a stroke at age 39 for unclear reasons, required neck surgery in the past. Physical examination reveals a 1-cm nodule in the right upper lobe of the thyroid gland. Laboratory workup reveals normal thyroid-stimulating hormone (TSH), moderately elevated calcium, and moderately reduced phosphate. Fine-needle aspiration of the nodule reveals cells suggestive of medullary thyroid carcinoma.

1. What is the cell of origin in the development of medullary thyroid carcinoma?

The parafollicular C cells are the cells of origin. This is a neuroendocrine tumor that secretes calcitonin, a hormone that lowers serum calcium levels by inhibiting intestinal and renal calcium absorption, decreasing bone resorption of calcium and increasing calcium excretion into the urine. As a result, measurement of calcitonin can be used in the diagnosis of this tumor and in postoperative follow-up if it is resected.

2. What are the major histologic categories of thyroid cancer?

See Table 10.3.

Table 10.3. Types of Thyroid Cancers

INCIDENCE	RISK FACTORS	HISTOLOGIC APPEARANCE	PROGNOSIS	OTHER CHARACTERISTICS
Papillary				
75%–80%	History of childhood head and neck radiation	Well-differentiated papillae lined by cells with "Orphan Annie eyes" with nuclear grooves Psammoma bodies Cervical lymph node metastasis is common	Good	Good prognosis Associated with a history of childhood exposure to radiation
Follicular				
10%–20%	Older age Diet low in iodine	Well differentiated Malignant proliferation of follicles that invade the surrounding fibrous capsule Distinguished from follicular adenoma by invasion of the fibrous capsule	Good	Must distinguish from follicular adenoma, which does not invade the fibrous capsule. This is performed via resection and pathologic evaluation, as fine-needle aspiration is unable to adequately assess the capsule. Unique in that it metastasizes hematogenously (as compared to most other carcinomas, which spread via lymphatics)
Medullary				
5%	Multiple endocrine neoplasia (MEN) type IIA and IIB (RET mutation)	Neuroendocrine tumor Parafollicular C cell hyperplasia Malignant cells in an amyloid stroma	Good	Secretes calcitonin, which can be used as a marker to diagnose and detect recurrence
Anaplastic				
<5%	Elderly age	Undifferentiated tumors of follicular epithelium	Very aggressive Poor prognosis: Mortality approaching 100%	Rapidly invasive neck mass, which can cause mass effect on local structures

3. **What test should be ordered to evaluate the hypercalcemia and hypophosphatemia?**
Parathyroid hormone (PTH) levels should be evaluated. Keep in mind that someone with medullary thyroid cancer would be expected to have decreased to normal serum calcium levels as a result of increased calcitonin, suggesting that a more complex process is occurring in this patient. PTH levels are often included in the workup of hypercalcemia and are especially important in the context of concurrent hypophosphatemia. Some cancers may even elaborate PTHrP, causing bone resorption. This is considered one of the paraneoplastic syndromes and is known as *humoral hypercalcemia of malignancy.* PTH levels are suppressed when PTHrP is causing hypercalcemia.

CASE 10.8 CONTINUED:

Serum PTH level is elevated at a follow-up visit 2 weeks later. The patient is still asymptomatic, and his physical examination findings are unchanged.

4. **What unifying diagnosis could explain his medullary thyroid carcinoma and primary hyperparathyroidism?**
Multiple endocrine neoplasia type IIA (MEN IIA) could be the unifying diagnosis.
- Medullary thyroid carcinoma is the most common manifestation of MEN IIA.
- Hyperparathyroidism also occurs in 15% to 20% of patients (due to parathyroid hyperplasia/adenomas).

5. **What other neoplastic process accompanies medullary thyroid carcinoma and hyperpara-thyroidism in MEN IIA?**
Pheochromocytoma is present in approximately 50% of patients with MEN IIA. Elaboration of epinephrine and norepinephrine causes hypertension, palpitations, nervousness, headaches, and flushing. These symptoms usually occur in episodes and can result in hypertensive emergencies such as hemorrhagic stroke or end-organ damage.

6. **How are the multiple endocrine neoplasia syndromes inherited? What mutations are associated with each subtype?**
All MEN syndromes are inherited in an autosomal dominant manner. Both MEN IIA and MEN IIB can be caused by mutations of the *RET* proto-oncogene that encodes a tyrosine kinase receptor. MEN I is caused by mutations in the *menin* tumor suppressor gene.

Because MEN IIA is inherited in an autosomal dominant manner, it is likely that his father also had MEN IIA and died of a stroke resulting from a hypertensive crisis.

7. **Which disorders are typically present in MEN IIB?**
    * Medullary thyroid carcinoma
    * Pheochromocytoma
    * Ganglioneuromatosis
    * Marfanoid habitus

8. **Which disorders are typically present in MEN I?**
    * Pituitary tumors (prolactin or growth hormone secreting)
    * Hyperparathyroidism
    * Pancreatic endocrine neoplasia (e.g., gastrinoma [Zollinger-Ellison syndrome], insulinoma, glucagonoma, VIPoma [Verner-Morrison syndrome or watery diarrhea, hypokalemia, achlorhydria, metabolic acidosis])

STEP 1 SECRET

You should expect to have at least one question on multiple endocrine neoplasia (MEN) syndromes on your examination. Know which disorders are associated with MEN I, MEN IIA, and MEN IIB.

SUMMARY BOX: THYROID CANCER

* Presentation: Thyroid nodule
    * Patients with multiple endocrine neoplasia (MEN) syndromes may present with additional symptoms (see previous discussion).
* Risk factors: Family history, head and neck radiation exposure (papillary subtype), dietary iodine (follicular)
* Pathophysiology: Medullary subtype involves mutations in parafollicular C cells; may be associated with MEN II syndromes.
* Diagnosis: Fine-needle aspiration and biopsy
    * Elevated calcitonin levels are associated with medullary thyroid carcinoma (MEN IIA and IIB).
    * Increased calcium and decreased phosphate levels are suggestive of hyperparathyroidism; MEN syndromes should be considered in these patients (technically MEN I can also cause hyperparathyroidism via parathyroid hyperplasia/adenomas, but only MEN II syndromes cause medullary thyroid cancer).

CASE 10.9

A 50-year-old man presents to his primary care physician (PCP) for his annual physical. He tells his physician that he is feeling well and has no concerns except intermittent constipation over the past few months. Sometimes he notices small amounts of streaked blood in his stool. His vital signs and physical examination are completely normal. On rectal examination, there are no masses. His fecal occult blood test is positive. He has no family history of colon cancer or inflammatory bowel disease and has not been diagnosed with diverticulitis in the past. The patient is scheduled for a colonoscopy (his first), as his doctor recommends that all of his patients get a colonoscopy once they reach 50 years of age, and he is particularly concerned because of the constipation and streaks of blood in the stool. The colonoscopy reveals a circumferential mass in the descending colon. Biopsies are taken.

1. **What is the predominant histologic type found in colon cancers?**
    * Adenocarcinoma: Approximately 98% of tumors in the large intestine
    * Carcinoid tumors
    * Approximately 2% of large intestine tumors but almost 50% of small intestine malignant tumors
    * Low-grade malignant proliferation of neuroendocrine cells that often secrete serotonin
    * Gastrointestinal lymphoma and mesenchymal tumors (gastrointestinal stromal tumors)

2. **In what part of the colon are most colon cancers found?**
(Listed in order from most to least common)
    * Rectosigmoid colon
    * Cecum/ascending colon

- Transverse colon
- Descending colon
- Other sites

Ninety-nine percent of colon cancers appear at one site (i.e., no synchronous tumor).

3. **How are left-sided (descending) and right-sided (ascending) colon carcinomas commonly differentiated?**

Left-sided colon carcinomas present as "napkin ring" or annular lesions that decrease the colon lumen caliber. Thus patients may report skinny stools or the classic "pencil-shaped stools." Patients may also report left lower quadrant pain and constipation, and some patients can even initially present with bowel obstruction. Bowel obstruction is more likely to occur on the left side of the colon because the stools are solid and formed and harder to pass through the smaller bowel lumen. Tumors of the descending colon will present as bright red blood either mixed with or coating the surface of the stool.

The right-sided colon is normally wider than the left-sided colon and will not usually present with constipation or bowel obstruction until the tumor has grown very large. The stools at the ascending colon are still liquid and easier to pass through the bowel. The tumors are typically raised lesions that ulcerate and slowly bleed into the colon. Therefore the majority of patients will initially present with occult bleeding and iron-deficiency anemia. Patients can also report melena or dark, tarry stools and vague pain. Other symptoms of colon carcinoma include nausea, vomiting, loss of appetite, bloating, abdominal fullness, and tenesmus or the feeling that the bowel has not completely emptied.

4. **What is the precursor lesion to adenocarcinoma of the colon?**

Adenoma is the precursor lesion to adenocarcinoma of the colon.

5. **What are the different types of gastric adenomas and their morphologic features?**

See Table 10.4.

Table 10.4. Gastric Adenomas and Their Morphologic Features

ADENOMA	MORPHOLOGY
Tubular adenomas >75% tubular architecture	Small and pedunculated Make up 90% of adenomas found in the colon
Villous adenomas >50% villous architecture	Large and sessile Make up 1% of adenomas found in the colon
Tubulovillous adenomas 25%–50% villous architecture	Varying morphology Make up 5%–10% of adenomas found in the colon

6. **What type of adenoma has the highest risk of turning into cancer?**

Cancer risk is highest with villous adenomas greater than 4 cm in diameter. Cancer risk is much lower with tubular adenomas less than 1 cm in diameter.

7. **Which genes are typically altered in the development of colorectal adenocarcinoma?**

The *APC, KRAS,* and *p53* genes are typically altered. The first step in carcinogenesis is thought to be mutation of the *APC* gene on chromosome 5q. Because *APC* is a tumor suppressor gene, a mutation must occur in both alleles in order to inactivate it. The second mutation is the so-called "second hit." After the second hit on *APC*, the sequence progresses with an activating mutation of the *KRAS* gene. Because *KRAS* is a proto-oncogene, only one allele needs to be activated for tumor progression (i.e., only one mutation needs to occur). The final step appears to involve loss of function in the *p53* tumor suppressor gene (Fig. 10.11).

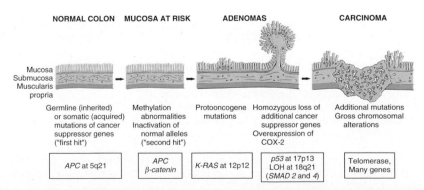

Figure 10.11. Schematic of the morphologic and molecular changes in the adenoma-carcinoma sequence. *COX-2,* Cyclooxygenase-2; *LOH,* loss of heterozygosity. *(From Kumar V, Abbas AK, Fausto N, Aster JC. Robbins and Cotran Pathologic Basis of Disease. 8th ed. Philadelphia: Saunders; 2010.)*

8. Without taking into account familial cancer syndromes, what is the importance of family history in the development of colorectal cancer?

A patient who has a first-degree family member diagnosed with colon cancer before 45 years of age has a relative risk 3.8 times that of the general population. This relative risk decreases to 2.2 if the family member was diagnosed at 45 to 59 years of age and 1.8 if the family member was diagnosed after 60 years of age. Hence, in patients with a family history of colorectal cancer, screening should start at 40 years of age or 10 years before the youngest-affected first degree relative was diagnosed, whichever is earlier.

9. What is the association of colon cancer with familial cancer syndromes?

HNPCC: Mutations in DNA mismatch repair genes (e.g., *MSH2, MLH1*) result in "microsatellite instability" and an 80% lifetime risk of developing colon cancer. Microsatellite nucleotide sequences are repeating sequences of noncoding DNA that are maintained during cell division. The integrity of the sequence is referred to as its *stability.* HNPCC tumors are predominantly right-sided. These patients are also at an increased risk of other tumors, including endometrial, ovarian, gastric, and skin cancers.

Familial adenomatous polyposis (FAP): Germline mutation of *APC* tumor suppressor leads to thousands of adenomatous polyps at a young age (i.e., the first hit is inherited). This confers a 100% lifetime risk of developing colon cancer. Other syndromes associated with FAP include Gardner syndrome (FAP, osteomas, and fibromatosis) and Turcot syndrome (FAP and CNS tumors).

10. What is the link between inflammatory bowel disease and colon cancer?

Though the link has been more firmly established between ulcerative colitis and colon cancer, it is now evident that both ulcerative colitis and Crohn disease confer an increased risk of colon cancer when compared to the general population. This risk begins to rise 7 to 10 years after disease onset and increases with duration of disease. Cancers tend to occur at a younger age than in the general population. There also has been an observed increased risk in small intestinal adenocarcinomas in patients with Crohn disease.

CASE 10.9 CONTINUED:

Biopsies from the colonoscopy reveal adenocarcinoma. As part of a surgical workup, a CT scan of chest, abdomen, and pelvis is performed and reveals metastases to the liver.

11. Why are colon cancers thought to metastasize to the liver? What are other common sites of metastasis?

Venous drainage of the colon and upper rectum is through the portal vein. Therefore metastases are often found in the liver of patients with colon cancer. Lymph nodes, lung, and peritoneal metastases are also seen.

SUMMARY BOX: COLON CANCER

- Presentation
  - Left-sided colon carcinomas: Decreased stool caliber, left lower quadrant pain, constipation, bowel obstruction, and blood-streaked stool
  - Right-sided carcinomas: Occult bleeding and iron-deficiency anemia
- Epidemiology: Adenocarcinoma is the most common type; the rectosigmoid colon is the most common location
- Pathophysiology: Mutation type is dependent on the subtype of colon cancer, but *APC, KRAS,* and *p53* are commonly involved genes.
- Diagnosis
  - Screening colonoscopy starts at the age of 50. If there is family history of colorectal cancer, screening starts at 40 years of age or 10 years before the youngest-affected first degree relative was diagnosed, whichever is earlier.
  - Biopsy is required if polyps are found
- Complications: Metastases to the liver

CASE 10.10

A 47-year-old man presents to his oncologist with persistent headaches for the past month. Six months prior, he had been treated with cisplatin and etoposide for limited-stage small-cell lung cancer (SCLC). He was told that his cancer had gone into remission and was asymptomatic until 1 month ago when he began developing headaches. His wife, who has accompanied him, says that he seems more confused lately. His vital signs are normal. On physical examination, he has no focal neurologic findings but does have trouble following some directions and seems confused.

1. **What is the most potentially serious explanation for this patient's headaches?**
   Metastatic disease to the brain is a potential explanation. The patient's cancer initially had been classified as limited-stage SCLC, yet it is assumed that micrometastases are present whenever SCLC is diagnosed. Although chemotherapy is quite successful in limited-stage disease (50%–70% complete response), remissions tend to last only 6 to 8 months. When cancer recurs, the median survival time is 3 to 4 months.

2. **Which cancers commonly metastasize to brain?**
   (Listed in order from most to least common)
   • Lung cancer
   • Melanoma
   • Renal cell carcinoma
   • Breast cancer
   • Colorectal cancer

CASE 10.10 CONTINUED:

The CT scan shows no brain metastases. The patient's laboratory tests reveal a serum sodium level of 124 mEq/L and a urine sodium level of 46 mEq/L. The patient is admitted to the hospital and is noted to have a blood pressure of 124/75 mm Hg that does not change significantly when taken lying down versus standing up. He has no edema. He says he drinks one to two glasses of water per day and stopped drinking alcohol 6 months ago when he was diagnosed with lung cancer.

3. **What basic electrolyte disturbance does this patient have?**
   This patient has hyponatremia.

4. **What is the likely cause of this patient's electrolyte disturbance?**
   SIADH secondary to SCLC is the likely cause. The patient has a euvolemic hyponatremia based on his lack of orthostatic hypotension. In the context of euvolemia, the kidneys' ability to excrete free water must be evaluated. The fact that this patient has a high urine sodium indicates that he is reabsorbing free water in the face of excess intravascular free water.

5. **What are the causes of SIADH?**
   ADH is normally secreted by the posterior pituitary gland, and SIADH may occur with CNS lesions (e.g., head trauma, stroke, subarachnoid hemorrhage, hydrocephalus). SIADH may also occur with lung lesions (tuberculosis, bacterial pneumonia, aspergillosis, etc.), but the pathophysiologic mechanism for this is unknown. It is also seen in many malignancies as a paraneoplastic syndrome, or it may be the result of drug effects.

6. **To what does the term *paraneoplastic syndrome* refer?**
   Paraneoplastic syndrome refers to a constellation of symptoms attributable to the ectopic secretion of peptides or antibodies by a neoplasm. The pathophysiology of paraneoplastic syndromes is incompletely understood.

7. **What paraneoplastic syndromes are particularly important in lung cancer?**
   Patients with SCLC can classically develop SIADH, and patients with squamous cell carcinoma can develop hypercalcemia as a result of PTHrP. Of note, most cases of hypercalcemia in cancer can be attributed to bone metastases leading to osteolysis as a result of PTHrP secretion. Other tumors associated with paraneoplastic syndromes are listed in Table 10.5.

STEP 1 SECRET

Paraneoplastic syndromes, especially those associated with various types of lung cancers, are among the highest-yield oncology topics for boards.

Table 10.5 Tumors Associated With Paraneoplastic Syndromes

PARANEOPLASTIC SYNDROME	ASSOCIATED CANCERS	ECTOPIC PEPTIDE OR ANTIBODY PRODUCED
Cushing syndrome	SCLC, renal cell carcinoma	ACTH or ACTH-like peptide
SIADH	SCLC, intracranial neoplasms	ADH
Polycythemia	Renal cell carcinoma, hemangioblastoma, hepatocellular carcinoma, pheochromocytoma, leiomyoma	Erythropoietin
Lambert-Eaton myasthenic syndrome	Thymoma, SCLC	Autoantibodies to presynaptic Ca^{2+} channels at neuromuscular junction
Carcinoid syndrome	Most common cancer is found in the appendix	Serotonin (5-HT) and bradykinin
Hypercalcemia	Squamous cell carcinoma (lung, head, and neck), breast carcinoma, ovarian carcinoma, renal cell carcinoma, bladder carcinoma	PTHrP
Zollinger-Ellison syndrome	Pancreatic, duodenal, stomach tumors	Gastrin

ACTH, Adrenocorticotropic hormone; *ADH*, antidiuretic hormone; *PTHrP*, parathyroid hormone–related peptide; *SCLC*, small cell lung cancer; *SIADH*, syndrome of inappropriate secretion of antidiuretic hormone.

8. **This patient was initially treated with cisplatin and etoposide. How do these chemotherapeutic agents work?**
Cisplatin is thought to have action similar to alkylating agents. It kills cells in all stages of the cell cycle by inhibiting DNA biosynthesis via intrastrand cross-links. Etoposide inhibits topoisomerase II, thereby resulting in DNA damage through strand breakage. It is specific to late S phase and G_2 phase of the cell cycle.

STEP 1 SECRET

Students always want to know how much they should learn about chemotherapeutic drugs for boards. First Aid has an excellent list of these drugs, but the various uses for these drugs are quite detailed. We recommend that you approach chemotherapeutic drugs in the following manner:
- Begin by learning the various drug classes (antimetabolites, alkylating agents, etc.) and their mechanisms of action. Classify each individual drug according to these groups.
- Learn the toxicity of each individual chemotherapeutic agent. "Chemo man," which is available on the Internet, is a terrific resource to help you undertake this task. Step 1 is fond of testing toxicities of chemotherapeutic drugs.
- Briefly study the drugs that can help neutralize the toxic effects of chemotherapeutic agents. By far the most important one to know is mesna, which can prevent hemorrhagic cystitis in patients receiving cyclophosphamide.
- Believe it or not, learning the clinical uses of chemotherapeutic agents is last on our list. You do not have to know which drugs are used for all types of cancers, but there are a few on which you should focus. For example, we recommend knowing the drugs that are useful for testicular cancer (etoposide, bleomycin, and cisplatin), choriocarcinoma (methotrexate), acute myelogenous leukemia (cytarabine), and brain tumors (nitrosoureas). You should also know that 5-fluorouracil can be given topically for actinic keratosis.

SUMMARY BOX: PARANEOPLASTIC SYNDROMES

- Presentation: Varies depending on tumor type (see Table 10.5)
- Pathophysiology: Ectopic secretion of peptides or antibodies by a neoplasm

CASE 10.11

A 45-year-old woman presents with questions regarding her risk of developing ovarian cancer. Her mother died at age 60 of ovarian cancer, and she has a sister who was recently diagnosed with breast cancer. She smokes two packs of cigarettes per day and drinks alcohol occasionally. She has three children and had an intrauterine device (IUD) inserted 5 years ago. The patient wants to know what her chances of developing ovarian cancer are.

1. **What is the risk of an American woman developing ovarian cancer in her lifetime? How is this risk altered if the woman has a first-degree relative with ovarian cancer?**
   Ovarian cancer is the fifth leading cause of cancer death among women in the United States and is the leading cause of death among gynecologic malignancies. A woman's lifetime chance of developing ovarian cancer is roughly 1.6% but increases to 5% with an affected first-degree relative.

2. **Older age and a family history of ovarian cancer in a first-degree relative are major risk factors for the development of ovarian cancer. What is the third major risk factor for the development of epithelial ovarian cancer, and how does it relate to theories regarding the pathogenesis of epithelial ovarian cancer?**
   Nulligravity is a major risk factor for developing epithelial ovarian cancer (EOC). The predominant theory is that repeated ovulation leads to minor trauma to the epithelial surfaces of the ovaries and that this repeated trauma predisposes the epithelium to malignant transformation. In women who have had children, there have been significant periods in their lives during which they were not ovulating; thus, the epithelial surfaces of their ovaries were not disturbed during this time.

3. **What are the protective factors against EOC?**
   Oral contraceptive pill use, multiparity, tubal ligation, and breastfeeding are protective against EOC. Any factors that inhibit ovulation are protective against EOC because there will be less repeated trauma to the epithelial surface of the ovaries that can potentially lead to malignant transformation. Breastfeeding inhibits ovulation by increasing prolactin levels that suppress the pulsatile release of GnRH.

4. **In a female patient with two first-degree relatives with diagnoses of ovarian and breast cancer, what genetic test is appropriate to determine her risk of developing ovarian or breast cancer?**
   BRCA gene testing. Germ-line mutation of the *BRCA* genes is one of the few identified genetic risk factors for ovarian cancer and is associated with both ovarian and breast cancer. Women with a *BRCA1* mutation have a 45% lifetime risk of developing ovarian cancer, and those with a *BRCA2* mutation have a 25% risk. Though it is usually inappropriate to use *BRCA* testing to screen for ovarian cancer risk, it is justified in this patient, who has two first-degree relatives with ovarian and breast cancer.

5. **What laboratory test might be used to follow an ovarian carcinoma once it has been diagnosed?**
   Cancer antigen 125 (CA-125). Annual CA-125 and transvaginal ultrasonography are not thought to be effective in screening the general population. However, CA-125 levels correlate well with disease progress and are frequently used to assess response to treatment and screen for recurrence.

STEP 1 SECRET

You should expect at least one question on tumor markers. These are listed in Table 10.6.

Table 10.6. Tumor Markers

MARKER	TUMORS/CONDITIONS MONITORED
CA-125	Ovarian cancer
CA-19-9	Pancreatic adenocarcinoma
PSA	Prostate cancer
α-Fetoprotein	Hepatocellular carcinoma Yolk sac tumor
CEA	Colorectal cancer Pancreatic cancer
β-hCG	Hydatidiform mole Choriocarcinoma
S-100	Schwannoma Melanoma
Chromogranin	Neuroendocrine tumors
Bence Jones proteins	Multiple myeloma Waldenström macroglobulinemia
TRAP	Hairy cell leukemia
Bombesin	Neuroblastoma

β-hCG, β-Human chorionic gonadotropin; *CEA,* carcinoembryonic antigen; *PSA,* prostate-specific antigen; *TRAP,* tartrate-resistant acid phosphatase.

CASE 10.11 CONTINUED:

The patient returns to the office to discuss results of the genetic testing that she requested. She is told that she has a *BRCA1* mutation and that, as a result, she has an 85% to 90% risk of developing breast cancer and a 45% chance of developing ovarian cancer in her lifetime. She decides to undergo prophylactic bilateral mastectomy and oophorectomy. On pathologic examination of the resected ovaries, she is found to have a 1-cm serous cystadenocarcinoma of the right ovary that had not been seen on preoperative ultrasonography.

6. **What are the three pathologic classifications of ovarian cancer?**
   EOCs: EOCs are seen as part of a spectrum of tumors that can arise from anywhere on the epithelial surface of the peritoneal cavity but tend to occur with the most frequency in the ovarian epithelium. The five major pathologic types of EOCs are as follows:
   • Serous
   • Mucinous
   • Endometrioid
   • Clear cell tumor
   • Brenner tumor
      Germ cell neoplasms: Germ cell neoplasms occur much less frequently and are typically found in younger patients. Common types are teratoma, dysgerminoma, endodermal sinus (yolk sac) tumor, and embryonal carcinoma. These tumors tend to behave aggressively and can often be cured with surgery and chemotherapy. There is much similarity between these tumors and male testicular cancers.
      Stromal tumors: Sex cords in the embryonic gonad eventually develop into the ovarian stroma in women. When undifferentiated, the sex cords can develop into either the specific cell types of men (Sertoli and Leydig cells) or women (granulosa and theca cells). Stromal tumors can also proliferate into granulosa-theca cell tumors and Sertoli-Leydig cell tumors. These neoplastic cells tend to produce the same estrogens or androgens that their precursor cells produce. As a result, feminizing or virilizing effects may be seen (Fig. 10.12).

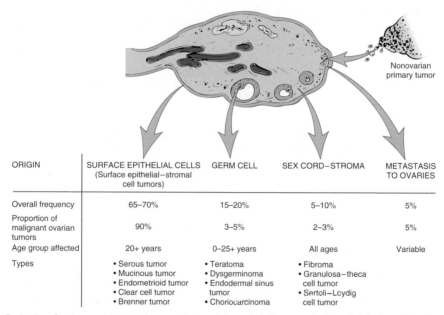

ORIGIN	SURFACE EPITHELIAL CELLS (Surface epithelial–stromal cell tumors)	GERM CELL	SEX CORD–STROMA	METASTASIS TO OVARIES
Overall frequency	65–70%	15–20%	5–10%	5%
Proportion of malignant ovarian tumors	90%	3–5%	2–3%	5%
Age group affected	20+ years	0–25+ years	All ages	Variable
Types	• Serous tumor • Mucinous tumor • Endometrioid tumor • Clear cell tumor • Brenner tumor	• Teratoma • Dysgerminoma • Endodermal sinus tumor • Choriocarcinoma	• Fibroma • Granulosa–theca cell tumor • Sertoli–Leydig cell tumor	

Figure 10.12. Derivation of various ovarian neoplasms and some data on their frequency and age distribution. *(From Kumar V, Abbas AK, Fausto N, Aster JC. Robbins and Cotran Pathologic Basis of Disease. 8th ed. Philadelphia: Saunders; 2010.)*

7. **What is a Brenner tumor?**
   A Brenner cell tumor is a transitional cell tumor mimicking the epithelium found in the bladder. These rare tumors make up only 2% of all EOCs and are mostly benign.

8. **In a patient with a granulosa cell tumor that secretes estrogen, for what other malignancy would she be at increased risk?**
   Such a patient would be at risk for endometrial carcinoma secondary to secretion of unopposed estrogen. Granulosa cell tumors are malignant sex cord stromal tumors and commonly produce estrogen. They can occur in women of all ages and typically present with symptoms of estrogen excess (e.g., precocious puberty, menorrhagia, postmenopausal bleeding).

9. **What is a Krukenberg tumor?**

Krukenberg tumor is the name for a mucin-secreting gastrointestinal cancer that metastasizes to the ovaries. This typically occurs bilaterally. Look for the presence of signet ring cells in the ovary on histology to confirm the diagnosis.

10. **What is the primary mode of spread in EOC?**

Neoplasms tend to form within cysts and eventually rupture through the surface of the ovary and spread along the peritoneal surfaces. Tumor cells may also spread through the lymphatics or hematogenously, though these tumors occur after peritoneal spread. Because an ovarian cancer tends to be asymptomatic until it has spread outside the affected ovary, most women are diagnosed in the advanced stages of ovarian cancer when they become symptomatic.

CASE 10.11 CONTINUED:

The patient has no signs of peritoneal spread of the tumor and makes an uneventful recovery.

SUMMARY BOX: OVARIAN CANCER

- Presentation: Patients tend to be asymptomatic until more advanced stages.
- Risk factors: More common in older women with a history of nulligravity, family history of ovarian cancer in a first-degree relative, obesity, and *BRCA* mutations. Less common in patients with a history of oral birth control use, multiparity, and breastfeeding.
- Pathophysiology: Repeated ovulation leads to minor trauma to the epithelial surfaces of the ovaries. The repeated trauma predisposes the epithelium to malignant transformation.
- Complications: Peritoneal metastatic spread, potential risk of breast and ovarian cancer development with *BRCA* mutations

CHAPTER 11

GENETIC AND METABOLIC DISEASE

Insider's Guide to Genetic and Metabolic Disease for the USMLE Step 1

Understanding biochemistry and genetics is crucial to achieving a good score on the USMLE Step 1. These subjects lay the foundation for many of the diseases that you are expected to know for boards. This is an intimidating thought for many students who think that they will be expected to memorize a bunch of pathways, enzymes, and intermediates, but this is not the case. Although you are not expected to memorize every step of every biochemical pathway, you should understand the implications of abnormalities in these pathways and how they result in various disease symptoms. Focus on the rate-limiting steps and key enzymes of the pathways that you learn, as well as reactions targeted by pharmacologic interventions. Pay attention to where the reactions take place (e.g., cytosol, mitochondrial membrane, mitochondrial matrix, or a combination of the aforementioned locations). More importantly, you should know how these pathways are regulated.

BASIC CONCEPTS

1. What is an enzymopathy, and how does it result in clinical symptoms?

    An enzymopathy is a genetic disease in which a deficiency in activity of an enzyme leads to a block in a metabolic pathway. The altered (usually reduced) enzymatic activity can be due to reduced cellular expression of the enzyme or to expression of a dysfunctional enzyme. The pathologic manifestations of the enzyme deficiency are a result of the accumulation of substrate (or its derivatives) before the blockage, a lack of the product(s), or a combination of both (Fig. 11.1).

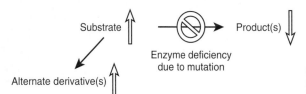

Figure 11.1. Mechanisms by which an enzymopathy produces clinical symptoms. ↑, Increased; ↓, decreased. *(From Brown TA, Brown D. USMLE Step 1 Secrets. Philadelphia: Hanley & Belfus; 2004.)*

2. What is the typical pattern of inheritance observed in enzymopathies?

    Almost all enzymes are produced in excess of minimal requirements. So, although heterozygous carriers of an enzyme deficiency typically have only 50% of normal enzyme activity levels, they are usually phenotypically normal. Thus almost all enzymopathies have an autosomal recessive pattern of inheritance, in which a phenotypic abnormality manifests only when there is nearly no enzyme activity. This generalization is extremely useful for the USMLE.

3. Explain why the pathologic consequences of X-linked enzymopathies are manifested almost exclusively in males.

    Again, enzyme deficiencies generally require a near-total loss of enzyme activity to result in phenotypic abnormalities. Because males have only a single X chromosome, inheritance of a single defective copy of an X-linked gene from the mother will result in the pathologic consequences of the enzyme deficiency/abnormality. Because females have two X chromosomes, female heterozygotes are often asymptomatic because the normal copy of a gene on one X chromosome masks the effect of the abnormal copy on the other X chromosome. Therefore females will generally exhibit the disease only if they are homozygous for the mutated alleles, which is far less likely. (For example, if the odds of a male inheriting a single defective gene is $1/p$, the odds of a female inheriting two defective copies will be approximately $1/p^2$.)

    Important examples of X-linked recessive enzymopathies include hemophilia A (factor VIII deficiency), hemophilia B (factor IX deficiency), glucose-6-phosphate dehydrogenase deficiency, Duchenne (and Becker) muscular dystrophy, and Lesch-Nyhan syndrome (LNS; hypoxanthine-guanine phosphoribosyltransferase [HGPRT] deficiency).

STEP 1 SECRET

The USMLE loves to ask students to calculate inheritance risk. This will require you to know the inheritance pattern of the disease in question and apply it to the Hardy-Weinberg principle. Recall that if a population is in Hardy-Weinberg equilibrium and p is the frequency of the normal allele while q is the frequency of the abnormal allele, disease prevalence = $p^2 + 2pq + q^2$, where p^2 and q^2 represent the prevalence of homozygosity and 2pq is heterozygosity prevalence (see Case 11.2, question 4).

4. **What is the process of lyonization, and how may it cause the manifestation of X-linked diseases in females?**
Because females have two X chromosomes, they would have twice the level of expression of genes located on the X chromosome were it not for the random inactivation of one X chromosome that occurs in each somatic cell early in embryogenesis. This process is called *lyonization* (named after the scientist Lyon, who was the first to propose it). One of the manifestations of lyonization is the Barr body (Fig. 11.2), a condensed, often drumstick-shaped body of DNA seen at the periphery of the nuclei of the cells of females, which corresponds to the inactivated X chromosome.

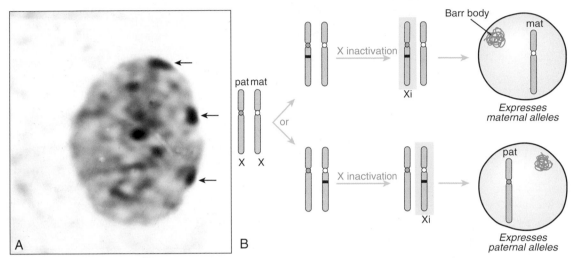

Figure 11.2. A, Three Barr bodies, indicating four X chromosomes. Three masses of densely staining chromatin material *(arrows)* are present at the periphery of the nucleus in this cytologic smear. The number of sex chromatin masses is one less than the actual number of X chromosomes. B, Random X chromosome inactivation early in female development. Shortly after conception of a female embryo, both the paternal *(pat)* and maternal *(mat)* X chromosomes are active. Within the first week of embryogenesis, one or the other X chromosome is chosen at random to become the future inactive X chromosome through a series of events involving the X inactivation center in Xq13.2 (*first black line* in the schematic). That X becomes the inactive X (Xi indicated by the *blue shading*) in that cell and its progeny, and it forms the Barr body in interphase nuclei. *(A from Mutter G, Pratt J.* Pathology of the Female Reproductive Tract. *3rd ed. Philadelphia: Churchill Livingstone; 2014, Fig. 2-25. B from Nussbaum R, McInnes R, Willard H.* Thompson & Thompson Genetics in Medicine. *7th ed. Philadelphia: Saunders Elsevier; 2007: 102, Fig. 6-13.)*

Owing to the normally random nature of the X chromosome inactivation, some females may happen to have a mutated X-linked allele on the active X chromosome of a large number of cells and, as a result, may exhibit some pathologic features. These rare individuals are termed *mosaics* or *manifesting heterozygotes*. For example, some female carriers of hemophilia A will have some degree of anemia if a large enough proportion of their bone marrow cells inactivate the X chromosome carrying the normal factor VIII allele.

5. **What is the significance of the autosomal dominant disease pattern of inheritance? What types of diseases are typically inherited in an autosomal dominant pattern?**
In autosomal dominant diseases, the disease manifests even though there is a normal copy of the gene remaining that produces 50% of the normal amount of gene product. Dominance of a defective gene can be attributed to one of the following reasons: more than 50% of normal gene product is needed for a nondiseased physiologic state; the defective protein adversely affects the normal gene product (a dominant negative effect); or the defective protein has acquired a novel, detrimental property.
Most diseases caused by mutations in nonenzymatic structural proteins (e.g., collagen, fibrillin) or in membrane receptors (e.g., low-density lipoprotein [LDL] receptor) are inherited in an autosomal dominant manner. This again is a useful generalization for the USMLE.

6. **What is the general relationship between the function of a protein and its pattern of inheritance?**
See Table 11.1.

7. **What are the following molecular biology diagnostic methods used for? Explain briefly how they work.**
1. Southern blotting
This technique involves detecting the presence of a specific DNA sequence within a mixture of DNA by using a sequence-specific strand of complementary DNA or messenger RNA (a "probe") that can hybridize to the targeted DNA. The specific steps include separating the mixture of DNA fragments by gel electrophoresis, denaturing the DNA (i.e., altering the DNA solution so that the double-stranded DNA separates into single strands), transferring (i.e., blotting) the DNA onto a membrane, and mixing the blotted DNA mixture with radioactively labeled probes to allow for hybridization.

Table 11.1. Proteins in Enzyme Deficiency

FUNCTIONAL CATEGORY[a]	INHERITANCE PATTERN	EXAMPLE DISEASE(S)	DEFECTIVE PROTEIN
Enzymes	Autosomal recessive	PKU	Phenylalanine hydroxylase
		Galactosemia	Galactose-1-phosphate uridyltransferase
		MCAD deficiency	MCAD
		Tay-Sachs disease	Hexosaminidase A
Transport proteins	Autosomal recessive	Thalassemias	α- or β-Hemoglobin
		Cystic fibrosis	Cystic fibrosis transmembrane conductance regulator
Structural proteins	Autosomal dominant	Osteogenesis imperfecta	Type I and type II collagen
		Marfan syndrome	Fibrillin
		Hereditary spherocytosis	Spectrin (found in the RBC membrane)
Developmental gene expression	Autosomal dominant	Achondroplasia	FGFR3
Metabolic receptors	Autosomal dominant	Familial hypercholesterolemia	LDL receptor or ApoB-100 protein

[a]The information presented conveys the general pattern, but a few exceptions can be found in each category.
FGFR3, Fibroblast growth factor receptor 3; *LDL,* low-density lipoprotein; *MCAD,* medium-chain acyl-CoA dehydrogenase; *PKU,* phenylketonuria; *RBC,* red blood cell.

In the laboratory, it is often used to detect the presence of large unique DNA sequences (e.g., a gene mutation) within a patient's genome.

2. Northern blotting

Northern blotting is very similar to Southern blotting, except that a specific sequence of RNA (rather than DNA) is detected using a nucleic acid probe. This technique is commonly used to measure expression of a gene in a patient, as determined by its production of messenger RNA (mRNA).

3. Polymerase chain reaction

Polymerase chain reaction (PCR) allows for detection of a specific DNA sequence (e.g., a mutant allele) by making billions of copies of that allele from as little as a single DNA molecule. This test is performed using two primers that are complementary to the DNA regions at the ends of the sequence of interest. There are three main steps in the process. First, the target DNA is denatured. Next, excess premade DNA primers hybridize (or anneal) to a specific sequence of DNA on each strand to be amplified. Finally, the DNA sequence following each primer is extended by a heat-stable DNA polymerase. These three steps are repeated over and over to amplify the amount of target DNA. The number of sequences created can be calculated as 2^n, where n = the number of rounds of PCR that have been completed.

4. Western blotting

This test is similar to Southern or Northern blotting, but rather than detecting a nucleic acid, it measures the level of a specific protein. First, the protein mixture is coated by a negatively charged detergent molecule that denatures the proteins (i.e., unfolds them and causes them to lose their structure) such that the proteins can be separated according to size using gel electrophoresis. Next, the proteins are blotted onto a membrane to which an antibody against the protein of interest (the primary antibody) is added. If the protein is present, the primary specific antibody will bind to the membrane and this binding, in turn, will be detected using a secondary antibody that is both directed against the first antibody and labeled in an assayable fashion. (For example, the primary antibody may be a specific sheep antibody, but the secondary antibody is an antisheep antibody linked to an enzyme that produces a colored product upon exposure to the reagents.) The size or intensity of the band produced is proportional to the amount of protein present, so Western blots are used clinically to measure the degree of protein expression of a gene. This is important because diseases can be caused by translational problems in which transcription of the gene into mRNA occurs normally but the translation of this mRNA is defective.

CASE 11.1

A 2-day-old infant boy tests positive for a relatively rare medical condition. The diagnosis is based on the presence of markedly elevated serum levels of an essential amino acid. A second positive test result is obtained at his 2-week checkup. His family history is remarkable for intellectual disability in a 45-year-old aunt.

1. **What is the most likely diagnosis in this baby, and how is it inherited?**
The most likely diagnosis is phenylketonuria (PKU), which, as with most enzymopathies, is inherited in an autosomal recessive manner.

2. **What is the major defect and underlying pathophysiology of this disorder?**
PKU is caused by the defective conversion of phenylalanine to tyrosine and results from mutations in the phenylalanine hydroxylase (PAH) gene (classic PKU). The PAH enzyme deficiency leads to both an accumulation of phenylalanine (substrate) and its phenyl ketone derivatives, including phenylacetate, phenyllactate, and phenylpyruvate. There is also a decrease in the levels of tyrosine (product) and its derivatives (e.g., DOPA and melanin). A rarer form of PKU, called *malignant PKU*, results from a deficiency in tetrahydrobiopterin cofactor (BH$_4$). During the process by which phenylalanine is oxidized to tyrosine, PAH must also oxidize BH$_4$ to dihydrobiopterin (BH$_2$). BH$_4$ not only serves as a cofactor for PAH but is also required for the synthesis of L-DOPA from tyrosine. L-DOPA is then converted to dopamine, which can be used to synthesize the catecholamines norepinephrine and epinephrine (Fig. 11.3).

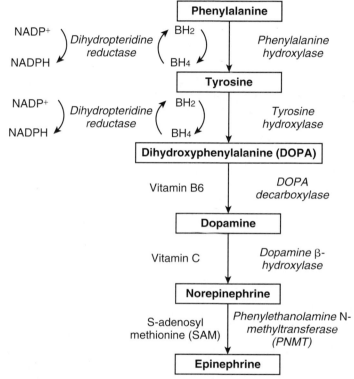

Figure 11.3. Biochemical pathway involved in conversion from phenylalanine to epinephrine. *BH$_2$,* Dihydrobiopterin; *BH$_4$,* tetrahydrobiopterin; *NADP$^+$,* nicotinamide adenine dinucleotide phosphate (oxidized form); *NADPH,* nicotinamide adenine dinucleotide phosphate.

In order to distinguish between classic and malignant PKU, one can examine levels of dopamine and prolactin. Recall that dopamine is a negative inhibitor of prolactin release. Classic PKU does not significantly affect dopamine synthesis, and prolactin levels are, therefore, relatively normal. BH$_4$ deficiency, on the other hand, will reduce dopamine synthesis. Thus prolactin levels will be elevated in these patients.

Regardless of cause, the pathology of PKU is primarily a result of substrate (phenylalanine) accumulation, which causes severe neuronal damage, intellectual disability, growth retardation, and motor dysfunction. The lack of neurotransmitter compounds derived from tyrosine (particularly the catecholamines dopamine, norepinephrine, and epinephrine) may also contribute to damage of the central nervous system (CNS). Other manifestations include a predisposition to eczema, a "musty" or "mousy" body odor (caused by phenyl ketone excretion into sweat), and fair skin coloring (due to tyrosine deficiency, which is precursor to melanin) (Fig. 11.4).

STEP 1 SECRET

The biochemical pathway affected in patients with phenylketonuria (PKU) shows up quite frequently on Step 1. Be familiar with the functions of phenylalanine hydroxylase and tetrahydrobiopterin and their relevance to this disease. You should also know every step of the catecholamine synthesis pathway—it is extremely high yield!

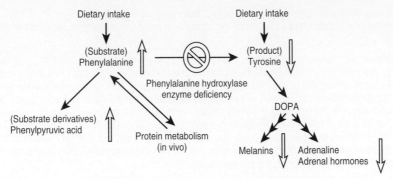

Figure 11.4. Pathologic mechanisms of phenylketonuria. *(From Brown TA, Brown D.* USMLE Step 1 Secrets. *Philadelphia: Hanley & Belfus; 2004.)*

3. How is phenylketonuria treated?

Patients with classic PKU need to follow a strict diet that restricts phenylalanine intake and is supplemented with tyrosine. If started within the first month of life, this diet is very effective in preventing intellectual disability. Because phenylalanine is found in breast milk, most babies with PKU must be placed on special phenylalanine-restricted formulas. Phenylalanine is also found in high concentrations in artificial sweeteners such as aspartame, which must be avoided.

Patients with malignant PKU often have additional neurologic problems that do not resolve with dietary phenylalanine restriction alone. This occurs because the BH_4 cofactor carries out additional roles such as the hydroxylation of tryptophan, a precursor of serotonin. Therefore individuals with a BH_4 deficiency generally require supplementation with a commercially available form of BH_4 and with neurotransmitter precursors such as L-DOPA.

4. Given the fact that PKU is a relatively rare condition (prevalence rates range from 1 in 2600 to 1 in 200,000 live births), why does it make sense to screen all neonates for this condition?

The screening test (Guthrie test) is inexpensive (as it simply involves measuring plasma phenylalanine levels), and PKU is easily prevented by dietary modifications. Furthermore, early screening detects the disease before irreparable damage (particularly to the CNS) has occurred (i.e., early intervention affects outcome). Screening should take place 2 to 3 days after birth because phenylalanine levels are often normal immediately following birth as a result of the presence of the maternal enzyme during fetal life.

5. If the parents have a female child with this disease, why is it crucial to advise the child about the risks to her baby if she becomes pregnant when she is older?

As patients generally tolerate more dietary phenylalanine with age, most women with PKU abandon the diet therapy by their early teens, well before they reach childbearing age. The termination of dietary therapy generally has limited ill effects on the women themselves at this age but will cause irreparable harm to a developing fetus should they become pregnant. Specifically, high levels of phenylalanine can diffuse across the placenta, causing brain damage in the developing fetus. So, although these babies will (virtually always) be heterozygous for the PAH mutation and are thus born without PKU, they can exhibit severe intellectual disability, microcephaly, growth retardation, and congenital heart defects, a condition termed *maternal PKU.*

RELATED QUESTION

6. Why is screening for congenital hypothyroidism, congenital adrenal hyperplasia, and galactosemia also routinely performed in newborns?

These diseases are similarly screened for because they are additional preventable causes of intellectual disability or death. In general, screening is performed on diseases for which treatment is available, for which a rapid and low-cost laboratory test is available, and that are frequent and serious enough to justify the screening cost.

SUMMARY BOX: PKU

- Epidemiology: Prevalence ranges from 1 in 2600 to 1 in 200,000 live births
- Presentation: Intellectual disability, growth retardation, motor dysfunction, eczema, a "musty" odor, and fair skin
- Pathophysiology: Defect in the phenylalanine hydroxylase gene (classic PKU) or deficiency in tetrahydrobiopterin (BH_4). Both instances result in accumulation of the phenylalanine substrate and its phenyl ketone derivatives, as well as the deficiency of the tyrosine product and its derivatives.
- Diagnosis: Guthrie screening test (measurement of plasma phenylalanine levels in neonate)
- Treatment: Low-phenylalanine, high-tyrosine diet; additional supplementation with L-DOPA or a tetrahydrobiopterin analog for malignant PKU. Women with a history of PKU who are pregnant or may become pregnant should strictly follow such a diet regardless of their personal symptoms because of the risk of fetal neurologic damage (maternal PKU) resulting from embryonic exposure to high phenylalanine levels.

CASE 11.2

A woman and her husband have a child who was recently diagnosed with cystic fibrosis (CF). Both the woman and her husband are in their 30s and are completely asymptomatic.

1. If the parents decide to have another child, what is the probability of that child having cystic fibrosis?

   Because cystic fibrosis (CF) is an autosomal recessive disease, the chance of the second child having CF remains at 25%. Each parent is a heterozygous carrier of the mutant allele such that each parent has a 50% chance of passing it on to their offspring, and the chance of the child receiving both mutant alleles is $0.5 \times 0.5 = 0.25$, or 25%.

   Note: Each birth is a completely independent event, such that the outcomes of prior pregnancies do not affect the odds of disease transmission in subsequent pregnancies.

STEP 1 SECRET

Students are frequently asked to calculate genetic probabilities on the USMLE.

2. Despite having mutations in the same gene, why do patients with CF exhibit significant variability in disease severity?

   The most common mutation in CF is the deletion of Phe508 from the *CFTR* gene. However, different patients may have different mutations of the same gene, with certain mutations causing less severe phenotypes. For example, mutations of the chloride channel gene that have a smaller detrimental effect on its function result in milder clinical manifestations. There are over a thousand mutations of *CFTR* that have been identified in patients with CF. This phenomenon of different mutations of the same allele resulting in differing disease manifestations is known as *allelic heterogeneity*. Interestingly, many patients with CF (>33%) are compound heterozygotes, with a different locus mutated on each copy of their *CFTR* genes.

   Second, even in patients with identical mutations, there is often some degree of clinical heterogeneity. This may be due to other genetic differences or to environmental variables that influence disease expression.

   Note: Many genetic diseases have allelic heterogeneity, leading to significant heterogeneity in clinical manifestations (e.g., thalassemias).

3. Assuming a cystic fibrosis prevalence rate of 1 in 2500, what is the carrier frequency for this disease?

   The carrier frequency for CF is 4%. Here, the Hardy-Weinberg law can be used to describe the genotypic distribution of an abnormal allele ($p + q = 1$) and the phenotypic distribution of the disorder:

   $$p^2 + 2pq + q^2 = 1$$

   p = frequency of normal allele
   q = frequency of abnormal allele ($1 - p$)
   p^2 = frequency of unaffected individuals
   $2pq$ = frequency of carriers (usually asymptomatic in autosomal recessive diseases)
   q^2 = frequency of disease

   Assuming a CF prevalence of 1 in 2500, $q^2 = 1/2500$ (0.0004) such that $q = 1/50$ (0.02). Because $p + q = 1$, p is 0.98. Therefore, the carrier frequency for CF is $2pq = 2 (0.98) (0.02) = 0.039$, or approximately 4% of the population. Thus in this example, 1 in every 25 individuals is a carrier. This is roughly the carrier frequency in Caucasians, whereas the mutation and the disease are less common in non-Caucasians.

   The Hardy-Weinberg law can be applied to alleles and populations that are in "genetic equilibrium" (i.e., populations in which the allele frequency is not undergoing rapid change). Genetic equilibrium exists when there are no mutations at the locus of interest, no selection for specific genotypes, no net migration of the population, population size is large, and mating is completely random. For the purposes of the USMLE, usually such equilibrium can be assumed.

SUMMARY BOX: POPULATION GENETICS AND PRENATAL GENETIC SCREENING

- Children born to two carriers of an autosomal recessive mutation have a 25% chance of inheriting the mutation, regardless of the outcome of prior pregnancies.
- The prevalence of various genotypes and phenotypes relating to an allele in genetic equilibrium in a population can be predicted using the Hardy-Weinberg equation.

CASE 11.3

A 9-month-old Jewish baby girl is brought to the hospital by her parents. The parents report that over the past 3 months, the baby has been having trouble feeding and has become lethargic and "floppy" appearing. They have also noticed that the child startles easily. More recently, the baby has developed worsening motor dysfunction, now with rigid and spastic movements. The parents are also concerned the baby girl is going blind. Fundoscopic examination results are shown in Fig. 11.5.

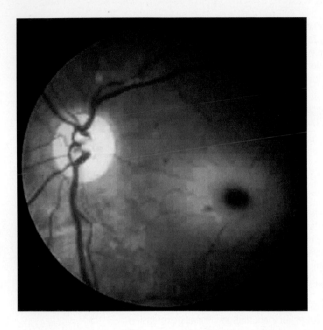

Figure 11.5. Ocular examination of patient in Case 11.3. *(From Martyn LJ. Neurometabolic disease affecting the eye. In: Tasman WJE, editor.* Duane's Ophthalmology. *Lippincott Williams & Wilkins: Philadelphia; 2010.*

1. **What two diagnoses are top considerations in the differential diagnosis at this point?**
   A child with progressive neurodegeneration and a funduscopic examination revealing a prominent red macular fovea centralis (sometimes called a *cherry-red spot*) should automatically make you think of Tay-Sachs disease (TSD) and Niemann-Pick disease (NPD). Both are autosomal recessive lysosomal storage diseases and, more specifically, sphingolipidoses. TSD is caused by a deficiency of hexosaminidase A, and NPD is caused by a deficiency in sphingomyelinase. The prevalence of both these diseases is higher in Ashkenazi Jews, who are primary descendants of a relatively small group of individuals that broke off from a larger population and bred among themselves (thus promoting the amplification of certain deleterious alleles within this population).
   Note: Many of the lysosomal storage diseases have multiple subtypes based on the underlying biochemical and molecular characteristics. The syndromes described here correspond to the most common subtype of each disorder.

CASE 11.3 CONTINUED:

Cells from this child are isolated and examined under the electron microscope, revealing "onion-skinning" of lysosomes.

2. **What is the most likely diagnosis?**
   This feature is associated with TSD but not NPD. On the other hand, "foamy histiocytes" (macrophages filled with sphingomyelin) are found in the tissues of patients with NPD (Fig. 11.6).
   The exaggerated startle reaction reported in the initial vignette is also particularly suggestive of TSD. The startle reaction is caused by hyperacusis and, because it does not occur in NPD, can be a major clue to the early diagnosis of TSD. The lack of hepatosplenomegaly on abdominal exam is another clue; sphingomyelin accumulation in hepatic and splenic macrophages can result in hepatosplenomegaly in NPD, but this is not usually the case in TSD.

3. **What is the pathogenesis of Tay-Sachs disease?**
   Hexosaminidase A is a lysosomal enzyme that cleaves a cerebral ganglioside (GM$_2$ ganglioside, a sphingolipid). Mutations make this enzyme less effective, leading to massive accumulation of GM$_2$ and its by-products within the lysosomes of neurons. These lysosomes become enormously enlarged such that they begin to interfere with normal cell function and ultimately cause neuronal death. Neuronal death that overlies the fovea centralis of the retina is responsible for the cherry-red spot seen on funduscopic examination. More specifically, ganglion cells in the retina fill

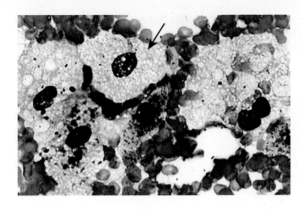

Figure 11.6. Macrophages in Niemann-Pick disease. *(From Goljan E. Rapid Review Pathology. 4th ed. Philadelphia: Elsevier; 2013, Fig. 14-15B.)*

with lipid, which imparts an opaque gray color to the retina. Because the optic disc does not contain ganglion cells, it remains red on a gray background, giving the look of a cherry-red spot (see Fig. 11.5). This is a common buzzword used by USMLE test makers.

The pathogenesis of other sphingolipidoses such as NPD or Gaucher disease is similarly due to accumulation of substrates of lysosomal enzymes. The differing disease manifestations of these sphingolipidoses depend upon the organs in which the sphingolipids accumulate and the underlying organ sensitivities. As mentioned previously, visceral sphingolipid accumulation and hepatosplenomegaly are prominent in NPD but not in TSD. TSD, in contrast, is characterized by relatively isolated CNS sensitivity to GM_2 accumulation.

Note that for both NPD and TSD, treatment options are limited and both disorders are usually fatal within the first few years of life.

4. What is the most common sphingolipidosis?

Gaucher disease is not only the most common sphingolipidosis but also the most common lysosomal storage disease (note that lysosomal storage diseases include both sphingolipidoses and mucopolysaccharidoses, which are discussed below). The disease is caused by deficiency of glucocerebrosidase and is characterized by the presence of glucocerebroside-laden Gaucher cells (Fig. 11.7), macrophages with characteristic "crumpled tissue paper" appearance and nuclei displaced by lipid. It is also more common among Ashkenazi Jews.

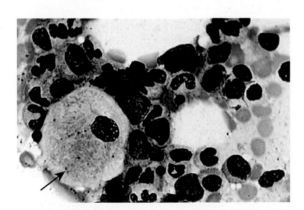

Figure 11.7. Gaucher cells. *(From Goljan E. Rapid Review Pathology. 4th ed. Philadelphia: Elsevier; 2013, Fig. 14-15A.)*

Unlike TSD and NPD, Gaucher disease usually spares neuronal tissue. Glucocerebroside instead accumulates in the reticuloendothelial system, namely the spleen and liver (causing hepatosplenomegaly), bone (causing bone pain, fractures, and avascular necrosis of the femoral head), and bone marrow (causing pancytopenia with particularly prominent thrombocytopenia). The two main contributors to thrombocytopenia are (1) decreased platelet production results from accumulation of Gaucher cells in the bone marrow and (2) entrapment of platelets in the spleen, which is overactive and enlarged with Gaucher cells.

Note: Despite the characteristic histologic or cytologic findings of many storage diseases, virtually all these disorders are diagnosed using genetic tests.

5. What are the mucopolysaccharidoses?

Mucopolysaccharidoses are a different type of lysosomal storage disease in which the substrates that accumulate in the lysosomes are extracellular matrix molecules called *glycosaminoglycans* (which were previously known as *mucopolysaccharides*). Like the sphingolipidoses, these diseases are caused by hereditary deficiency of lysosomal enzymes. The two main examples of this type of disease, Hurler syndrome and the similar but less severe Hunter syndrome, are both caused by accumulation of the glycosaminoglycans heparan sulfate and dermatan sulfate.

　　To keep these two disorders straight, think of a male HUNTER (X-linked) with aggressive behavior and great vision (no corneal clouding), whereas Hurler syndrome causes corneal clouding and has autosomal recessive inheritance. The only other commonly tested lysosomal storage disease that is X-linked recessive is Fabry disease (α-galactosidase A deficiency, resulting in accumulation of ceramide trihexoside or globotriaosylceramide). Look for peripheral neuropathy, angiokeratomas (dark red skin rash), and cardiovascular/renal involvement in a patient presenting with Fabry disease on the USMLE Step 1.

6. Quick review: Cover the three columns on the right side of Table 11.2, and attempt to describe the enzyme deficiency, accumulated substrate, inheritance pattern, pathophysiology, and any high-yield associations for the listed lysosomal storage disorders.

Table 11.2. Lysosomal Storage Diseases

LYSOSOMAL STORAGE DISEASE	ENZYME DEFICIENCY/ ACCUMULATED SUBSTRATE	INHERITANCE PATTERN	PATHOPHYSIOLOGY AND HIGH-YIELD ASSOCIATIONS
Sphingolipidoses			
Tay-Sachs disease	Hexosaminidase A/GM_2 ganglioside	Autosomal recessive	Accumulation of cerebral ganglioside causes progressive psychomotor deterioration, macular cherry-red spot, and lysosomes with onion-skinning.
Gaucher disease	Glucocerebrosidase/ glucocerebroside	Autosomal recessive	Gaucher cells (enlarged lipid-laden histiocytes with "wrinkled tissue paper" cytoplasm) accumulate in bone, marrow, liver, and spleen, causing bone pain and fractures (bone crises), osteonecrosis of the femoral head, massive HSM, and pancytopenia.
Niemann-Pick disease	Sphingomyelinase/ sphingomyelin	Autosomal recessive	Sphingomyelin accumulation in neurons and liver/spleen causes progressive psychomotor dysfunction, macular cherry-red spots, "foamy histiocytes," and HSM.
Fabry disease	α-Galactosidase A/ ceramide trihexoside	X-linked recessive	Angiokeratomas, peripheral neuropathy, stroke, renal and cardiovascular disease
Krabbe disease (globoid cell leukodystrophy)	Galactosylceramidase (i.e., galactocerebrosidase)/ ceramide galactoside (i.e., galactocerebroside)	Autosomal recessive	Demyelination and accumulation of globoid cells in CNS result in optic atrophy, peripheral neuropathy, and psychomotor retardation.
Metachromatic leukodystrophy	Arylsulfatase A/cerebroside sulfatides	Autosomal recessive	Central and peripheral demyelination result in ataxia and psychomotor degeneration and dementia in adults.
Mucopolysaccharidoses			
Hurler syndrome	α-L-Iduronidase/heparan sulfate and dermatan sulfate	Autosomal recessive	Coarse facial features (gargoylism), HSM, intellectual disability, joint and skeletal abnormalities, cardiac disease, and corneal clouding
Hunter syndrome	Iduronate-2-sulfatase/ heparan sulfate and dermatan sulfate	X-linked recessive	Same features as Hurler syndrome but with milder intellectual disability, aggressive behavior, and no corneal clouding

CNS, Central nervous system; *HSM,* hepatosplenomegaly.

SUMMARY BOX: TAY-SACHS DISEASE

- Epidemiology: Most common among Ashkenazi Jews
- Presentation: Floppy-appearing baby with lethargy, feeding trouble, visual defects, and signs of neurodegeneration/motor dysfunction; may be easily startled
- Pathophysiology: Mutation of hexosaminidase A gene, leading to accumulation of GM_2 ganglioside in neuronal lysosomes
- Diagnosis: Fundoscopic exam (macular cherry-red spot), abdominal exam (absence of hepatosplenomegaly, as opposed to Niemann-Pick disease), genetic testing, "onion-skinning" of lysosomes under electron microscopy
- Prognosis: Fatal in early childhood

CASE 11.4

A 2-year-old boy was brought to the clinic with choreoathetosis (constant and involuntary writhing movements of the legs and arms), spasticity (muscular hypertonicity with increased tendon reflexes), impaired cognitive development, and self-mutilation (compulsive biting of the fingers, lips, tongue, and inside of the mouth). The parents also observed the presence of orange "sand" in the child's diapers when the boy was a few months old.

1. What is the most likely diagnosis?

   The most likely diagnosis is LNS, a rare X-linked recessive disease that is caused by a defective HGPRT enzyme. The HGPRT enzyme is present in most cell types and is involved in the salvage pathway of purine metabolism. The most striking and characteristic neurologic symptom of this disease is self-mutilation.

   Recall that the purine bases are adenine and guanine and the respective nucleosides are adenosine and guanosine. A nitrogenous base linked to a sugar ribose or deoxyribose is referred to as a *nucleoside*, whereas a phosphorylated nucleoside is referred to as a *nucleotide*.

   The mnemonics "**PUR**e **A**s **G**old" and "**CUT** the **PY**" can be used to remember that **a**denine and **g**uanine are **pur**ine bases, whereas **c**ytosine, **u**racil, and **t**hymine are **py**rimidines.

2. What is the normal function of the purine "salvage" pathway?

   The purine salvage pathway functions to "salvage" purine metabolites such as hypoxanthine and guanine, preventing them from being unnecessarily degraded and then renally excreted as uric acid. (Hypoxanthine is another purine that is an intermediate in the synthesis or degradation of adenosine monophosphate [AMP] or guanosine monophosphate [GMP].) As shown in Fig. 11.8, the salvage pathway recycles these metabolites to replenish the purine bases, guanine and adenine, by the action of the HGPRT enzyme. Normally, the de novo pathway provides only about 10% of the daily purine requirement, whereas the salvage pathway provides the remaining 90%. The amount of net degradation to uric acid is always balanced with the amount of purines synthesized via the de novo pathway. It follows that the loss of the salvage pathway would result in a dramatic increase in de novo purine synthesis and a similarly dramatic increase in uric acid generation.

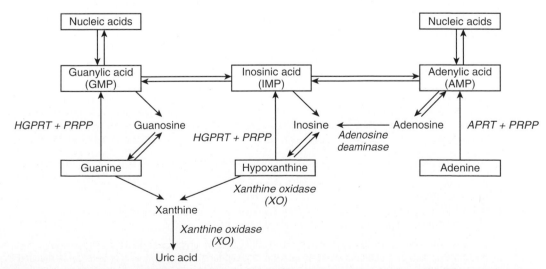

Figure 11.8. Purine metabolism. *APRT,* Adenine phosphoribosyltransferase; *HGPRT,* hypoxanthine-guanine phosphoribosyltransferase; *PRPP, 5'*-phosphoribosyl-1-pyrophosphate.

3. How do defects in the purine salvage pathway cause hyperuricemia?

In LNS, HGPRT activity is less than 1% of normal. Owing to the absence of HGPRT, the ability to reuse hypoxanthine and guanine to make the purine nucleotides inosine monophosphate (IMP) and GMP is lost, so these intermediates are degraded to uric acid. As explained in the preceding question, the purine requirements in this case must be met by increased de novo synthesis. Additionally, because of the reduced levels of IMP and GMP, the feedback inhibition normally exerted by IMP and GMP upon the de novo pathway is lost, further promoting the activity of the de novo synthesis pathway. Because purine synthesis via the de novo pathway must be balanced by purine degradation into uric acid, the dramatic increase in de novo synthesis results in severe hyperuricemia.

In other words, both excessive activation of the de novo pathway and insufficient HGPRT salvage of purine metabolites contribute to the hyperuricemia in LNS.

4. What was the orange "sand" in his diapers observed by his parents?

The sand represents uric acid crystals. Uric acid has limited solubility such that in conditions of extreme hyperuricemia, it will precipitate from urine, forming visible orange "sand." It can also precipitate from the plasma and accumulate in the joints, causing gouty arthritis. Interestingly, most patients with LNS do not develop gout, presumably because of the patients' short life spans (of about 20 years). However, patients with only a partial deficiency of HGPRT (with 1%–20% of normal activity) have a normal life span but are susceptible to developing severe tophaceous gout.

5. Why do patients with LNS typically present with renal dysfunction?

Patients with LNS develop kidney disease primarily from repeated uric acid kidney stones and urinary tract obstruction. In addition to nephrolithiasis, chronic hyperuricemia (from any cause) can result in renal insufficiency caused by urate deposition in the renal parenchyma, a process referred to as *urate nephropathy*.

Note: In contrast with the renal and joint disease, the cause of the neurologic symptoms in LNS is not well established.

6. How might this patient be managed pharmacologically?

Allopurinol is useful in the treatment of hyperuricemia of any cause. It works by preventing uric acid production by inhibiting the enzyme xanthine oxidase (XO). The xanthine and hypoxanthine that accumulate instead are more soluble and readily excreted than uric acid.

Other, more common uses of allopurinol include the treatment or (more commonly) the prevention of urate nephropathy, uric acid stones, gouty arthritis, and tumor lysis syndrome (which is caused by treatment of acute leukemias or disseminated lymphomas).

For patients with LNS who cannot tolerate allopurinol, a newer drug called *febuxostat* is a potential alternative. Febuxostat also works by inhibiting XO.

SUMMARY BOX: LESCH-NYHAN SYNDROME

- Epidemiology: Prevalent in males (X-linked disorder)
- Presentation: Intellectual disability, motor dysfunction (choreoathetosis and spasticity), self-mutilating behavior, presence of orange "sand" in diaper
- Pathophysiology: Defect in the purine salvage pathway (HGPRT enzyme), resulting in overactivity of the de novo purine synthesis pathway and excess generation of uric acid
- Treatment: Allopurinol or febuxostat (xanthine oxidase inhibitors) to reduce uric acid production
- Complications: Severe hyperuricemia can lead to tophaceous gout, uric acid kidney stones, and urate nephropathy
- Prognosis: Shortened life span (about 20 years)

CASE 11.5

A 4-year-old boy is evaluated for profound hypoglycemia and seizures. Physical examination is remarkable for nontender hepatomegaly. He has a history of multiple hospitalizations for seizures and hypoglycemia since he was 6 months old. His parents have noticed that he has never tolerated even short periods of fasting well. During his previous hospital stays, low blood sugar levels were consistently observed within a few hours after each feeding. He has also repeatedly had lactic acidosis, hyperlipidemia, and hyperuricemia. A liver biopsy indicates excessive accumulation of glycogen and fat.

---

1. What is the diagnosis?

The diagnosis is type 1 glycogen storage disease (or von Gierke disease), an autosomal recessive disorder, which is caused by deficiency of the enzyme glucose-6-phosphatase (G6Pase).

2. What type of enzymatic deficiency is present in all types of glycogen storage diseases?

These disorders are caused by a defect in either an enzyme required for glycogen synthesis or an enzyme required for glycogen catabolism (i.e., glycogenolysis). Glycogen storage diseases principally affect either the liver or skeletal muscle, the main sites where glycogen is stored. When they affect the liver, they can lead to hepatomegaly and predispose to hypoglycemia and its attendant complications (e.g., seizures and, with repeated episodes of hypoglycemia, neurologic impairment). When they affect the skeletal muscles, they can cause muscle pain and exercise intolerance, but they do not result in hypoglycemic episodes because skeletal muscle plays no role in maintaining plasma glucose. Recall that skeletal muscle lacks G6Pase, so it cannot deliver glucose to the bloodstream because glucose-6-phosphate (G6P) is unable to cross the plasma membrane.

3. **How is glycogen normally synthesized and degraded in the liver?**
Upon entry into a liver cell, glucose is phosphorylated to G6P, preventing it from diffusing out of the cell; this reaction is catalyzed by the enzyme glucokinase (this function is served by hexokinase in nonhepatic tissues). G6P is then converted into glucose-1-phosphate (G1P) by phosphoglucomutase. Next, G1P is converted to uridine diphosphoglucose (UDP-glucose) by UDP-glucose pyrophosphorylase, and UDP-glucose is attached to an existing glycogen molecule by the enzyme glycogen synthase. Glycogen synthase joins carbon 1 of UDP-glucose to carbon 4 of a glycogen molecule, creating α-(1,4) linkages between the molecules. Finally, there is a branching enzyme that breaks the α-(1,4) bonds and carries the broken glycogen chain to carbon 6, forming α-(1,6) bonds and giving glycogen its characteristic branched structure.

Glycogen degradation is primarily dependent on the activity of the enzyme glycogen phosphorylase, which catalyzes the breakdown of glycogen into G1P. However, glycogen phosphorylase only acts on nonreducing ends of a glycogen chain that are at least four glucoses away from a branch point. After this, another enzyme called the *debranching enzyme* transfers a trisaccharide from an α-(1,6) branch to an adjacent α-(1,4) branch. The remaining glucose molecule at the branch point is then released as free glucose. Therefore the two products of glycogen breakdown are G1P and glucose (Fig. 11.9).

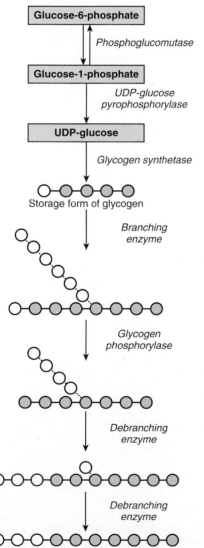

Figure 11.9. Glycogen synthesis and degradation. *UDP-glucose,* Uridine diphosphoglucose.

4. **How is glycogen breakdown regulated?**
Note that the regulation of glycogen breakdown is mediated by multiple substances, including epinephrine and glucagon. Both activate the enzyme adenylyl cyclase to generate cyclic adenosine monophosphate, which in turn activates protein kinase A. Protein kinase A converts an enzyme called *glycogen phosphorylase kinase* from the inactive to the active form. Glycogen phosphorylase kinase goes on to convert glycogen phosphorylase from the inactive to the active form, so glycogen breakdown can occur. Calcium and calmodulin in skeletal muscle also convert glycogen phosphorylase kinase to the active form, allowing glycogenolysis to be coordinated with muscle activity. It is important to note that insulin also modulates this pathway and has the opposite effect of epinephrine and glucagon; it activates protein phosphatases that convert glycogen phosphorylase kinase and glycogen phosphorylase to their inactive forms, thus preventing glycogen breakdown (Fig. 11.10).

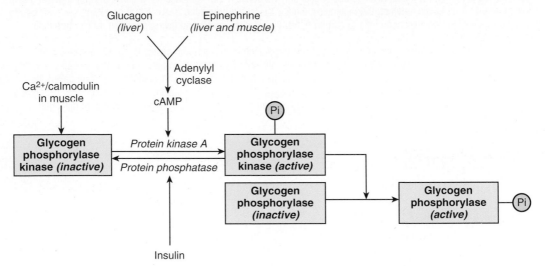

Figure 11.10. Regulation of glycogen degradation. *cAMP*, Cyclic adenosine monophosphate.

5. **Why is hepatomegaly seen on examination?**
The deficiency of G6Pase causes G6P to accumulate, which stimulates glycogen synthesis and, in turn, enlarges the liver.

6. **What is the explanation for this patient's severe fasting hypoglycemia and lactic acidosis?**
During short-term fasting, liver glycogenolysis is the major pathway that maintains blood glucose. When G6Pase is deficient, glycogenolysis is not effective at releasing glucose into the bloodstream, leading to hypoglycemia. In addition, the release of glucose made by gluconeogenesis during fasting is also impaired because this process is also dependent upon the enzyme G6Pase. This further contributes to hypoglycemia. Excessive accumulation of G6P greatly promotes glycolysis, resulting in high levels of pyruvate production. The pyruvate is then converted into lactate when the mitochondrial uptake of pyruvate is saturated, resulting in lactic acidosis.

For your own review, recall that the production of lactic acid from pyruvate does not cause any additional increase in production of adenosine triphosphate (ATP). The function of this pathway is to simply regenerate the electron carrier NAD^+ from NADH.

7. **Why is this patient susceptible to hypertriglyceridemia?**
Excessive accumulation of G6P overstimulates hepatic glycolysis, supplying substrate for downstream pathways. In addition to lactate synthesis, these pathways also include de novo fatty acid and triacylglycerol (i.e., triglyceride) synthesis. Because the hypoglycemia stimulates glucagon production over insulin release, lipolysis is promoted, providing abundant fatty acids to other tissues for energy production (i.e., β oxidation). A substantial portion of these fatty acids enters the mitochondria of various tissues to be oxidized, but the excess is repackaged in the liver to form triglyceride-rich, very-low-density lipoprotein (VLDL) particles to be released into the circulation. High insulin levels normally prevent formation and release of VLDL particles from triglycerides, but in states of profound hypoglycemia, this inhibitory signal is not present. Note that elevated blood lipid levels in patients with von Gierke disease occasionally cause them to develop xanthomas (accumulations of fat beneath the skin surface).

You should know how glucagon permits β oxidation to occur (Fig. 11.11). Note in Fig. 11.11 that glucagon stimulates activity of malonyl-CoA decarboxylase, which catalyzes the breakdown of malonyl-CoA into acetyl-CoA. Insulin, on the other hand, upregulates the enzyme acetyl CoA carboxylase, which stimulates the production of malonyl-CoA along the pathway of triglyceride synthesis. Malonyl-CoA provides an inhibitory signal to carnitine palmitoyltransferase I (CPTI) or carnitine acyltransferase I, a mitochondrial enzyme that shuttles long-chain fatty acids

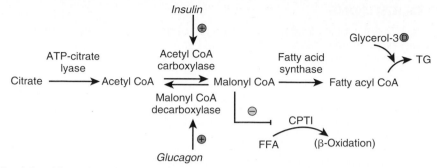

Figure 11.11. Regulation of fatty acid synthesis and breakdown by glucagon and insulin. *ATP,* Adenosine triphosphate; *CPTI,* carnitine palmitoyltransferase I; *FFA,* free fatty acid; *TG,* triglyceride.

into the mitochondrial matrix for β oxidation. Without CPTI activity, β oxidation cannot occur. It makes sense that insulin would prevent β oxidation from occurring, because it would be a waste of energy for the body to oxidize newly synthesized triglycerides in the fed state. At the same time, it would be advantageous to promote β oxidation when glucagon is present in the fasting state. See how important it is to know the biochemistry behind the diseases that you study?

STEP 1 SECRET

Notice that we did not suggest that you should memorize every step of the pathways that we depicted throughout the case. By simply understanding the major steps, key enzymes, and regulators of the pathways that you learn, you can better reason through disease findings. This is how the USMLE will expect you to think on the examination.

---

8. What causes the hyperuricemia in this patient?

As previously mentioned, a lack of G6Pase activity leads to an accumulation of G6P in the cell. G6P is shunted into the hexose monophosphate shunt (also known as the *pentose phosphate pathway*), leading to accumulation of both ribose 5-phosphate and PRPP (5′-phosphoribosyl-1-pyrophosphate). PRPP is the major allosteric activator of the rate-limiting enzyme (glutamine-PRPP amidotransferase) of the de novo purine synthetic pathway. As discussed in Case 11.4, an increase in de novo purine synthesis leads to an increase in purine degradation and, hence, increased uric acid production.

Hypoglycemia also makes cells less able to resynthesize the high-energy molecules adenosine triphosphate (ATP) and adenosine diphosphate (ADP) from AMP. The resulting increase in cytosolic AMP drives an increase in uric acid production.

Finally, the excess plasma lactate competes with uric acid for urinary excretion, further exacerbating the hyperuricemia. These patients can go on to develop gout as a result of the increase in circulating uric acid.

9. Quick review: Cover the columns on the right side of Table 11.3 and explain how glycogen storage diseases affect the activity of the rate-limiting enzyme in each pathway listed in the table.

Table 11.3. Metabolic Pathways in Glycogen Storage Diseases

PATHWAY	RATE-LIMITING ENZYME	EFFECT	BASIS OF EFFECT
Glycolysis	Phosphofructokinase-1	Increase	Increased substrate (G6P)
Glycogen synthesis	Glycogen synthase	Increase	Increased substrate (G6P)
Fatty acid synthesis	Acetyl-CoA carboxylase	Increase	Increased substrate (G6P is converted using pyruvate to acetyl-CoA) through exaggerated glycolysis
Hexose monophosphate shunt	G6P dehydrogenase	Increase	Increased substrate (G6P)
Triacylglycerol (triglyceride) synthesis		Increase	Increased substrate (glycerol and fatty acids from de novo synthesis or from lipolysis)

CoA, Coenzyme A; *G6P,* glucose-6-phosphate.

RELATED QUESTIONS

10. **Why does a deficiency of skeletal muscle glycogen phosphorylase (seen in type V glycogen storage disease or McArdle disease) not result in hypoglycemia?**

    Hypoglycemia does not occur because muscle does not contribute to maintenance of plasma glucose levels. Muscle glycogen phosphorylase is required for glycogenolysis (breakdown of glycogen into G6P) in muscle. There is a similar enzyme, encoded by a different gene, in the liver. However, unlike in the liver, there is no G6Pase present in muscle to dephosphorylate glucose. As such, glucose is unable to diffuse out of the muscle cell. Similarly, when glucose enters a muscle cell and is phosphorylated by hexokinase, it remains permanently trapped. In other words, glucose that enters a muscle cell cannot be released and instead must be consumed by that cell. For this reason, muscle normally makes no contribution to the maintenance of blood glucose.

    In McArdle disease, only muscle glycogen phosphorylase is lost. The corresponding liver enzyme is unaffected. The abnormal accumulation of G6P in muscle results in symptoms such as cramps and muscle fatigue, but there is no impairment in the maintenance of blood sugar. You may also see myoglobinuria (suggested by dark urine) associated with this condition as a result of muscle damage, particularly during strenuous exercise. Confirmation of this disease can be made with muscle biopsy, which will show an accumulation of glycogen and an absence of glycogen phosphorylase.

11. **Review the high-yield glycogen storage diseases.**

    See Table 11.4 for a summary of these diseases.

Table 11.4. Summary of High-Yield Glycogen Storage Diseases

GLYCOGEN STORAGE DISEASE	ENZYME DEFICIENCY	CLINICAL HALLMARKS
Type I (von Gierke disease)	Hepatic and renal glucose-6-phosphatase	Massive hepatomegaly and liver dysfunction, renal enlargement, severe hypoglycemia, growth failure
Type II (Pompe disease)	Lysosomal α-1,4-glucosidase	Cardiomegaly leading to cardiac failure; skeletal muscle weakness leading to respiratory muscle failure
Type III (Cori disease)	Debranching enzymes	Milder disease compared to von Gierke leading to stunted growth, hepatomegaly, and hypoglycemia
Type V (McArdle disease)	Muscle glycogen phosphorylase	Exercise-induced muscle cramps, myoglobinuria with strenuous exercise

Note: Although the liver accounts for the majority (about 90%) of gluconeogenesis and blood glucose maintenance, the kidney contributes about 10%. As such, type I disease can also result in less severe renal disease (with kidney enlargement, proteinuria, and renal insufficiency).

Also note that type II (Pompe) disease is both a glycogen storage disease and a lysosomal storage disease. Normally, a small percentage (about 2%) of cellular glycogen breakdown is carried out by lysosomal α-1,4-glucosidase. Because hepatic and renal glycogen phosphorylase are still functional, deficiency in the enzyme does not result in hypoglycemia but instead causes accumulation of glycogen within the lysosomes. This occurs most significantly in the cardiac and skeletal muscles.

SUMMARY BOX: GLYCOGEN STORAGE DISEASES

Type I Glycogen Storage Disease (Von Gierke Disease)
- Presentation: Seizures, poor growth, neurologic deficits, and low tolerance for fasting resulting from hypoglycemia
- Pathophysiology: Defect in glucose-6-phosphatase resulting in increased synthesis of glycogen, fatty acids, and triglycerides and increased activity of the hexose monophosphate shunt
- Diagnosis: Nontender hepatomegaly, lactic acidosis, hyperlipidemia, hyperuricemia, liver biopsy showing accumulation of glycogen and fat, low blood sugar levels within a few hours of fasting
- Complications: Xanthomas secondary to hyperlipidemia, gout secondary to hyperuricemia

Type V Glycogen Storage Disease (Mcardle Disease)
- Presentation: Cramps and muscle fatigue (particularly with strenuous exercise) in the absence of hypoglycemia
- Pathophysiology: Absence of muscle glycogen phosphorylase activity leading to abnormal accumulation of glycogen in muscle
- Diagnosis: History, myoglobinuria (dark urine), muscle biopsy showing glycogen accumulation
  Refer to Table 11.4 for a more detailed summary of the glycogen storage diseases.

CASE 11.6

An 8-month-old baby girl is brought to the emergency department by her parents. The baby has been vomiting and irritable over the past 2 days, and in the past 8 hours she has become very lethargic. On physical examination, her liver is mildly enlarged. Laboratory findings indicate hypoglycemia, moderate hyperammonemia, and abnormally low urine ketones (given the degree of hypoglycemia present). Analysis of the patient's urine reveals a mixture of organic acids ranging between 6 and 12 carbons long.

1. **What is the most likely diagnosis?**
   This baby likely has medium-chain fatty acyl-CoA dehydrogenase (MCAD) deficiency, the most common genetic disorder of fatty acid oxidation.

2. **What are the three length classifications of fatty acids?**
   Most edible fats contain a mixture of three types of fatty acids: short-chain, medium-chain (with 6–12 carbons), and long-chain. These fats (in fatty acyl-CoA form) are oxidized in the mitochondria of the peripheral cells by the enzymes LCAD (long-chain acyl-CoA dehydrogenase), MCAD (medium-chain AD), and SCAD (short-chain AD), respectively.

3. **What are the reasons for the clinical and laboratory findings exhibited by this patient?**
   Many tissues (especially heart and skeletal muscle) rely heavily on fatty acid oxidation as the primary fuel source for ATP production during fasting or during times of metabolic stress, such as exercise or illness, especially illness that results in decreased oral intake. In addition, a substantial amount of these fatty acids undergo β oxidation in the liver, which uses the resulting acetyl-CoA to produce ketone bodies that are released to provide energy for the brain (which is unable to directly oxidize fatty acids) (Fig. 11.12).

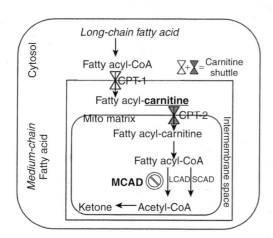

Figure 11.12. Summary of metabolism of fatty acids. *CoA,* Coenzyme A; *CPT,* carnitine palmitoyltransferase; *LCAD,* long-chain acyl-CoA dehydrogenase; *MCAD,* medium-chain acyl-CoA dehydrogenase; *SCAD,* short-chain acyl-CoA dehydrogenase. *(From Brown TA, Brown D.* USMLE Step 1 Secrets. *Philadelphia: Hanley & Belfus; 2004.)*

When MCAD is deficient, medium-chain fatty acyl-CoA molecules are unable to undergo β oxidation in these tissues. In addition, although long-chain fatty acyl-CoA compounds can be oxidized into medium-chain acyl-CoA molecules, β oxidation is arrested at the 12-carbon fatty acyl-CoA stage. As a result, medium-chain fatty acyl CoA molecules accumulate in the cytosol and mitochondrial matrix. Some of these medium-chain compounds are converted to the organic acid derivatives that can be detected in the urine. These derivatives may also be toxic to tissues that carry out β oxidation. In the liver, a substantial portion of these medium-chain fatty acyl CoA molecules is used in cytosolic resynthesis of triglycerides, resulting in liver enlargement from fatty infiltration.

MCAD deficiency also causes ATP production and ketogenesis to be greatly decreased. Without an adequate supply of energy, the rate of the urea cycle is decreased, leading to hyperammonemia. The rate of gluconeogenesis is similarly reduced, and the endogenous glucose supply (liver glycogen) is rapidly exhausted, resulting in hypoglycemia. Loss of MCAD function also results in decreased production of acetyl-CoA, which leads to decreased ketone production. This distinctive hypoketotic hypoglycemia pattern is characteristic of MCAD deficiency.

Other clinical features of MCAD deficiency reflect the involvement of organs that are (directly or indirectly) dependent on β oxidation. These findings include liver damage, neurologic impairment, and coma/sudden death. Interestingly, this constellation of features is similar to that seen in Reye syndrome (which occurs rarely in children after treatment of a viral illness with aspirin).

4. **How should this child be treated?**
   Avoidance of fasting and of medium-chain fatty acids in the diet is essential. By not allowing this child to rely on peripheral lipolysis and β oxidation for energy needs, hypoglycemia and accumulation of intermediates caused by the metabolic block will be minimized. Frequent small meals high in carbohydrates and protein and low in fat are

recommended. Patients with MCAD deficiency should take carnitine supplements to promote efficient long-chain fatty acyl-CoA transport into the mitochondria. Because the carnitine shuttle (i.e., mitochondrial uptake of long-chain fatty acids) is the rate-limiting step for long-chain fatty acid oxidation, promoting this pathway by supplementing carnitine may reduce the energy deficit caused by MCAD deficiency.

5. How are the pathways/cycles listed in Table 11.5 affected by MCAD deficiency?

Table 11.5. Medium-Chain Acyl-Coenzyme A (CoA) Dehydrogenase Deficiency

PATHWAY OR CYCLE	ACTIVITY OF PATHWAY	CAUSE
Hepatic gluconeogenesis	Decreased, causing hypoglycemia	Low ATP levels
Hepatic urea cycle	Decreased, causing hyperammonemia	Low ATP levels
β Oxidation of medium-chain fatty acids	Decreased	Enzyme deficiency
Hepatic ketogenesis	Decreased	Low acetyl-CoA production

ATP, Adenosine triphosphate; *CoA*, coenzyme A.

SUMMARY BOX: MEDIUM-CHAIN ACYL-COA DEHYDROGENASE DEFICIENCY

- Presentation: Vomiting, irritation, and lethargy in a young child
- Pathophysiology: Arrest of β oxidation at the 12-carbon stage resulting in hypoglycemia, hyperammonemia, increased triglyceride synthesis, impaired ketogenesis, and build-up of organic acids in the urine
- Diagnosis: Hypoketotic hypoglycemia, hepatomegaly, elevated muscle and liver enzymes
- Treatment: Dietary modification to avoid fasting and avoid intake of medium-chain fatty acids
- Complications: Liver damage, neurologic impairment, and coma/sudden death

CASE 11.7

A woman with acute intermittent porphyria (AIP) presents to her physician seeking advice on how to avoid exacerbations of her disease.

1. What are the porphyrias?
   The porphyrias are a series of disorders caused by enzymatic defects in heme biosynthesis. The enzymatic block leads to the accumulation of intermediates, porphyrins, in the heme biosynthetic pathway that have toxic effects when present at high serum levels. The various forms of porphyria can be diagnosed by detecting the presence of these porphyrin intermediates in the urine, serum, or stool. Each form of porphyria is associated with a particular pattern of porphyrin accumulation, with the pattern depending on the specific location of the block in the heme synthetic pathway.
   In contrast with a majority of enzymopathies, most of the porphyrias have an autosomal dominant mode of inheritance with reduced, but not altogether absent, heme synthesis. Complete absence of heme synthesis is presumably lethal.

2. What are the types of porphyrias?
   The three major types of porphyria are acute, chronic (hemolytic), and cutaneous. In acute porphyrias, patients usually experience disease exacerbations following specific triggers, which include certain drugs and chemicals (e.g., alcohol and barbiturates), hormones (i.e., estrogens and progestins), smoking, and various forms of stress (e.g., illness, fasting, infection, or surgery). The acute porphyrias tend to cause neurotoxicity, with prominent autonomic nervous system involvement, resulting in so-called *neurovisceral symptoms*, such as abdominal pain, vomiting, constipation, muscle weakness, and confusion. AIP, caused by a defect in porphobilinogen (PBG) deaminase, is the most common acute porphyria (and the most commonly tested porphyria on the USMLE Step 1).
   Defects in the later steps of heme biosynthesis cause accumulation of photoreactive intermediates, resulting in the photosensitivity characteristic of cutaneous porphyrias. Porphyria cutanea tarda (PCT) is both the most common cutaneous porphyria and the most common porphyria overall. PCT is caused by a defect in the enzyme uroporphyrinogen decarboxylase and results in chronic, blistering lesions of sun-exposed skin and, over time, scarring, pigment changes, and increased hair growth (hypertrichosis).
   The last (and least common) group of porphyrias is the hemolytic porphyrias. Significant heme synthesis occurs not only in the liver but also in red blood cell (RBC) precursors. In these disorders, RBCs are lysed when their accumulated photoreactive porphyrin intermediates are exposed to light as the RBCs pass through capillaries in the skin. This phenomenon can occur as the result of a deficiency in ferrochelatase, the final enzyme in the heme biosynthetic pathway. A diagram of diseases resulting from enzymatic defects in the heme biosynthesis pathway is shown in Fig. 11.13.

Intermediates	Enzymes	Diseases

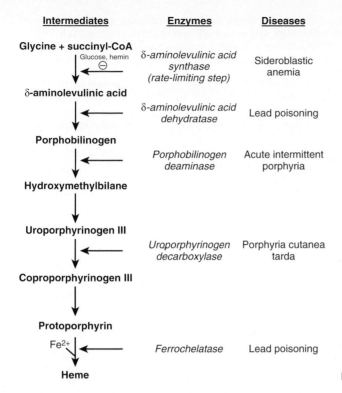

Figure 11.13. Heme biosynthesis pathway.

3. **Why may cigarette smoking or anticonvulsants such as phenytoin and phenobarbital trigger acute porphyrias?**

Cigarette smoke and many anticonvulsants are potent inducers of hepatic cytochrome P-450 enzymes. These P-450 enzymes contain heme and, consequently, their induction increases the demand for heme and increases its biosynthesis. In patients with AIP, a drug- or stress-induced increase in activity of the heme biosynthesis pathway results in an increased accumulation of the toxic porphyrin intermediates. In patients with AIP, acute attacks are often heralded by the development of red urine.

Interestingly, PCT is not triggered by P-450 inducers. However, it is strongly associated with various hepatotoxic agents such as alcohol, cigarette smoke, hepatitis C infection, and hemochromatosis, or iron overload. In women, it is also associated with estrogen exposure, both exogenous (e.g., oral contraceptives or hormone replacement) and endogenous (i.e., pregnancy).

4. **Why is hemin or glucose given to patients with acute porphyrias?**

Hemin, an oxidized form of heme, acts via negative feedback to decrease the synthesis of aminolevulinic acid (ALA) synthase, the rate-limiting enzyme of heme biosynthesis. This negative feedback mechanism is exploited therapeutically in the treatment of acute porphyrias as intravenous hemin is the most effective way of reducing porphyrin accumulation and the neurovisceral attacks. Glucose infusion (the opposite of fasting) can also be useful because glucose exerts a similar negative feedback upon ALA synthase.

PCT, interestingly, is effectively treated by phlebotomy. It is thought that blood loss decreases porphyrin production in the liver by decreasing total body and, most importantly, liver iron stores. Antimalarials such as chloroquine and hydroxychloroquine can also expedite removal of porphyrins from the liver by increasing their excretion.

Avoidance of triggers and treatment of exacerbating factors is important in the treatment of all forms of porphyrias.

RELATED QUESTIONS

5. **How does lead poisoning affect heme synthesis?**

Lead poisoning inhibits the heme synthesis enzymes, ALA dehydratase and ferrochelatase, resulting in anemia. For USMLE Step 1, know that RBCs on a peripheral blood smear in patients with lead poisoning will demonstrate basophilic stippling.

6. **What are the sideroblastic anemias?**

These anemias are due to defects in the heme biosynthesis pathway. Hereditary sideroblastic anemia is most commonly the result of an X-linked deficiency of ALA synthase, while acquired causes include alcoholism, lead poisoning, and vitamin B_6 deficiency (often a side effect of isoniazid treatment for tuberculosis). Unlike the porphyrias, the clinically apparent pathology results from insufficient heme production rather than the accumulation of toxic heme precursors.

Because a substantial amount of the body's iron is stored in heme, defects in heme synthesis can lead to abnormal iron accumulation. In the bone marrow of patients with sideroblastic anemia, iron will deposit within mitochondria to form "siderotic" granules in a ring pattern around the nucleus of some of the RBC precursors, so-called *ringed sideroblasts*. The treatment for sideroblastic anemias is pyridoxine, or vitamin B_6, which serves as a cofactor for ALA synthase.

SUMMARY BOX: ACUTE INTERMITTENT PORPHYRIA

- Epidemiology: Most common acute porphyria
- Presentation: Neurovisceral symptoms such as abdominal pain, vomiting, constipation, muscle weakness, and confusion following exposure to inducers of the P-450 enzyme system
- Pathophysiology: Autosomal dominant mutation that results in deficiency of porphobilinogen deaminase, leading to the accumulation of toxic porphyrin intermediates
- Diagnosis: Buildup of porphyrin intermediates in the urine, serum, or stool
- Treatment: Hemin or glucose, which inhibits aminolevulinic acid (ALA) synthase, the rate-limiting enzyme of heme biosynthesis

---

CASE 11.8

A 7-week old baby girl is brought to the office and presents with vomiting, diarrhea, poor feeding, and failure to thrive. The mother has recently noticed that the baby vomits or has diarrhea after nursing. Findings on physical examination include jaundice, dry skin, pallor, hepatomegaly, and poor tone. The laboratory findings include hypoglycemia, elevation in serum galactose and RBC galactose-1-phosphate (Gal-1-P), galactosuria, albuminuria, and indirect hyperbilirubinemia.

---

1. **What is the diagnosis?**

   This baby likely has galactosemia, which is a disease that can lead to severe intellectual disability if left untreated. It is due to defective galactose metabolism and elevated levels of serum galactose (recall that lactose, the sugar present in milk, is metabolized to glucose and galactose). Typically, disorders of galactose metabolism result from deficiencies in galactokinase, a condition called *galactokinase deficiency*, or galactose-1-phosphate (Gal-1-P) uridyltransferase (GALT), termed *classic galactosemia*. As demonstrated in Fig. 11.14, galactose is metabolized by galactokinase into Gal-1-P. If GALT is not present to metabolize Gal-1-P into glucose 1-phosphate, Gal-1-P can accumulate to toxic levels.

   Because both serum galactose and Gal-1-P were elevated this child, she likely has a deficiency of GALT, or classic galactosemia.

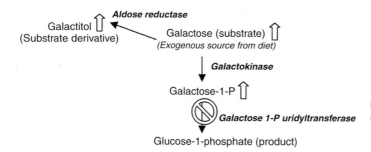

Figure 11.14. Pathophysiology of classic galactosemia. *UDP,* Uridine diphosphate. *(From Brown TA, Brown D. USMLE Step 1 Secrets. Philadelphia: Hanley & Belfus; 2004.)*

2. **Why does GALT deficiency manifest with jaundice?**

   As in other tissues such as nervous tissue, the lens, and the kidneys, pathologic manifestations of galactosemia in the liver and RBCs are due to the accumulation of Gal-1-P and galactitol. This accumulation results in the premature destruction of RBCs (i.e., hemolysis), which results, via the breakdown of hemoglobin, in increased release of unconjugated bilirubin into the circulation. Prehepatic jaundice develops because if the degree of hemolysis is significant enough, the liver will be incapable of conjugating the entire bilirubin load, leading to buildup of unconjugated bilirubin. The pathologic effect upon the liver can result in liver function test (LFT) abnormalities and liver dysfunction, further contributing to the hyperbilirubinemia.

   Recall that unconjugated bilirubin is indirect whereas conjugated bilirubin is direct. These terms reflect how conjugated bilirubin is water-soluble (i.e., charged) and can be measured directly, whereas in order to measure total bilirubin, a serum sample must be treated such that the water-insoluble (i.e., uncharged) unconjugated bilirubin is brought into solution.

3. **Why do infants with galactosemia tend to develop cataracts if left untreated?**

   When galactose (the substrate) accumulates as a result of the metabolic block, it enters an alternate reaction catalyzed by aldose reductase, leading to production of the sugar alcohol galactitol (the substrate derivative). Accumulation of galactitol in the lens leads to increased osmolarity, resulting in cataract formation as water is drawn into the lens tissue.

Note: The classic explanation for cataract formation in diabetes invokes the same mechanism of osmotic damage, with prolonged or repetitive hyperglycemia resulting in deposition of sorbitol (the sugar alcohol created by the activity of aldose reductase upon glucose) in the lens.

Any newborn with cataracts (especially if bilateral) should be evaluated for galactokinase deficiency, classic galactosemia, and other metabolic disorders. Other causes of neonatal cataracts include trisomies (i.e., Down, Edwards, and Patau syndromes) and other genetic disorders, as well as intrauterine infections (i.e., toxoplasmosis, rubella, cytomegalovirus, herpes simplex [TORCH]), particularly rubella.

4. What is the treatment for classic galactosemia?

The patient needs to follow a strict diet that eliminates all galactose-containing compounds, including lactose (milk and dairy products) and galactose-containing supplements. Recall that lactose is the disaccharide formed from galactose and glucose. Avoidance of dietary galactose intake quickly eliminates the risk of developing the complications of intellectual disability, poor growth, jaundice, anemia, liver disease, and cataracts and may help reverse any complications already present.

5. How does galactokinase deficiency manifest compared to classic galactosemia?

In general, the presentation of galactokinase deficiency is mild compared to that of GALT deficiency. Galactitol can accumulate if galactose is present in the diet, resulting in infantile cataracts. As a result, galactokinase deficiency may initially present as a failure to track objects or develop a social smile. Galactose also accumulates in the blood and urine. However, the more serious systemic symptoms of classic galactosemia, such as failure to thrive, jaundice, and hepatomegaly, are not present.

STEP 1 SECRET

Be able to recognize the signs and symptoms of classic galactosemia for the USMLE. These symptoms include infantile cataracts, jaundice, failure to thrive, hepatomegaly, and intellectual disability.

SUMMARY BOX: CLASSIC GALACTOSEMIA

- Presentation: Milk intolerance (vomiting and diarrhea), poor feeding, failure to thrive, jaundice, hypoglycemia, dry skin
- Pathophysiology: Defect in galactose-1-phosphate uridyltransferase (GALT), leading to accumulation of galactose derivatives (galactitol and galactose-1-phosphate) in neurons, kidneys, liver, and lenses
- Diagnosis: Physical exam (hepatomegaly, poor tone), elevated liver enzymes, total bilirubin, and serum galactose and galactose-1-phosphate levels
- Treatment: Dietary elimination of all galactose- and lactose-containing compounds
- Complications: Severe intellectual disability, liver disease, and infantile cataracts

CASE 11.9

A tall, slim 14-year-old boy is referred to the genetic disorders clinic by his ophthalmologist. He has ectopia lentis (detached lens), flat corneas, and hypoplastic irises. His mother, who was a tall, thin woman, died suddenly while jogging. An autopsy revealed aortic dissection to be her cause of death. On physical examination, the boy has an arm span–height ratio of 1.15 (normal <1.05), pectus excavatum (sunken chest), scoliosis, joint hypermobility, arachnodactyly (spider fingers), and stretch marks on his shoulders and thighs. He has positive thumb and wrist signs. An early diastolic decrescendo murmur heard best at the left sternal border is appreciated on cardiac examination.

1. What is the most likely diagnosis?

The patient likely has Marfan syndrome, an autosomal dominant disorder caused by mutations of the fibrillin (*FBN1*) gene. Fibrillin is a glycoprotein that serves as a scaffold for elastic fibers around connective tissue. The mutation shows no ethnic or geographic biases and affects males and females equally.

2. Why does this patient exhibit multiple pathologic presentations in the ocular, skeletal, and cardiovascular systems?

Fibrillin is a component of microfibrils, which are part of the extracellular matrix of eye tissue, aorta, skin, and periosteum. Microfibrils combine with elastin to form elastic fibers, which convey structural support and elasticity to many tissues. Detached or malpositioned lenses (ectopia lentis, typically upward and laterally), aortic dilation, and abnormally stretchy skin are all pathologic consequences of defective fibrillin. Progressive aortic dilation often results in separation of the leaflets of the aortic valve, resulting in aortic regurgitation and the corresponding diastolic murmur. Mitral valve prolapse is also associated with Marfan syndrome. The skeletal defects such as arachnodactyly (long, skinny, "spider-like" fingers and toes), tall stature, pectus excavatum, scoliosis, and joint hypermobility are caused by the periosteum's inability to provide the normal oppositional force to bone growth. Overgrowth of bone occurs when the periosteum has become too "flexible" as a result of defective fibrillin. The thumb and wrist signs are useful in demonstrating arachnodactyly. The thumb sign is positive when the thumb, when completely enclosed within a clenched fist, protrudes beyond the fist's ulnar border; the wrist sign is positive when the thumb and pinky overlap when wrapped around the opposite wrist.

3. **What are the major cause(s) of death in this disorder?**
The major causes of death in patients with Marfan syndrome are progressive heart failure from aortic regurgitation and sudden death from aortic dissection. The defect in fibrillin leads to cystic medial necrosis of the aorta, predisposing these patients to aortic incompetence and dissecting aortic aneurysms. Pregnancy or heavy exercise increases cardiac output greatly, thus elevating the risk of these major cardiovascular complications.

RELATED QUESTIONS

4. **What hereditary skeletal disease predisposes to bone fractures from minor stress? What structural protein defect underlies the disorder?**
Osteogenesis imperfecta (OI), caused by defects in type I collagen, is an inherited disorder of bone fragility. The most common form of the disorder (type I) is autosomal dominant, but interestingly, most cases are sporadic (i.e., due to a new mutation). Type I collagen is the predominant collagen type in the extracellular matrix of bone, but it is also found in other structures such as teeth, sclerae, ligaments, skin, and blood vessels. Type I OI is the least severe form, associated with fewer fractures and limited skeletal deformity. Distinct features of OI include blue sclerae, hearing loss (from involvement of middle ear ossicles), and abnormal teeth (i.e., dentinogenesis imperfecta, discolored teeth that wear easily). The reduced collagen content of the sclerae allows the dark choroid layer of the eye to show through the sclerae. Other, less specific features of OI include ligamentous laxity and joint hypermobility; kyphoscoliosis; smooth, thin, and lax skin; and easy bruising (from vessel fragility). Note that OI may be confused with child abuse in young patients who present with multiple fractures.

5. **What is the genetic defect in Ehlers-Danlos syndrome?**
Ehlers-Danlos syndrome can develop from multiple different genetic abnormalities in one of the collagen types. There are many types of Ehlers-Danlos syndrome, with the most common being autosomal dominant. Most forms are characterized by extreme skin hyperextensibility and joint hypermobility; tissue fragility; poor wound healing leading to thin, wide, atrophic scars; and easy bruising. The most common form or classical form is due to a defect in type V collagen. There is a vascular or ecchymotic form of the disorder, which is due to a defect in type III collagen, the major component of reticular fibers found in various organs and along the lining of blood vessels. This form of disease is important to diagnose because, in addition to ecchymoses, these patients are prone to catastrophic rupture of medium-sized arteries, bowel, or uterus (during pregnancy). These patients are predisposed to the development of berry and aortic aneurysms.

SUMMARY BOX: MARFAN SYNDROME

- Epidemiology: Affects males and females of all ethnicities and in all geographic locations
- Presentation: Tall and thin stature, arachnodactyly, pectus excavatum, scoliosis, joint hypermobility, stretchy skin, ectopia lentis (detached lens, usually upward and laterally)
- Pathophysiology: Inherited autosomal dominant defect in fibrillin, a component of the microfibrils found within elastic fibers
- Diagnosis: Family history, increased arm span-height ratio, positive wrist and thumb signs, diastolic heart murmur (aortic regurgitation), systolic heart murmur with midsystolic click (mitral valve prolapse)
- Complications: Rupture of berry aneurysms leading to subarachnoid hemorrhage, heart failure, sudden death from aortic dissection

---

CASE 11.10

A 6-year-old boy is brought to the hospital by his mother because of severe shortness of breath. He has fever and leukocytosis, and a chest x-ray study shows a right lower lobe infiltrate. His mother is worried because he has had pneumonia already three times as a child. A sputum culture grows *Pseudomonas aeruginosa*. A sweat test shows significantly elevated sodium and chloride.

1. **What is the most likely diagnosis?**
CF is the most likely diagnosis.

2. **What is the etiology of this disease?**
The defect underlying CF is found in the cystic fibrosis transmembrane regulator (*CFTR*) gene on chromosome 7, which codes for a chloride channel found in exocrine glands throughout the body. There are over 1500 mutations of *CFTR* that can result in CF, but the most common is deletion of phenylalanine 508. This mutation results in defective protein folding of the chloride channel so that it is degraded before it ever reaches the surface of the cell membrane. The

channel normally allows for active reabsorption of chloride from sweat and active secretion of chloride in the lungs, liver, and pancreas. As discussed in Case 11.2, CF is inherited in an autosomal recessive manner. It most commonly occurs in Caucasian individuals of northern European descent.

3. **How does the *CFTR* mutation lead to disease?**
The lack of active chloride secretion out of epithelial cells normally carried out by this channel prevents passive secretion of sodium and water into luminal secretions because water normally flows down its osmotic gradient. The consequence is abnormally thick secretions in the respiratory tract, pancreas, gastrointestinal (GI) tract, and biliary tree.

4. **Why does this child develop respiratory infections so easily?**
In CF, the abnormally viscous secretions of the tracheobronchial mucous glands impair mucociliary clearance of bacteria and debris, predisposing to recurrent pulmonary infections. In addition to increased susceptibility to the respiratory pathogens seen in normal hosts, patients with CF frequently become colonized and infected with organisms such as *Staphylococcus aureus*, gram-negative rods such as *P. aeruginosa*, and *Burkholderia cepacia*. Repeated pulmonary infections frequently lead to progressive lung disease, which is the major cause of CF-related death. Chronic infection and inflammation damage the airways, ultimately resulting in airway obstruction, air-trapping, and hyperinflation, which are physiologic changes similar to those seen in chronic obstructive pulmonary disease (COPD).

5. **Why might this child be susceptible to developing pancreatitis as he grows older?**
There is increased viscosity of pancreatic exocrine secretions, which impairs pancreatic secretion and predisposes to plugging and obstruction of the pancreatic ductules. Such plugging can cause pancreatitis and atrophy of pancreatic glands. Most common is pancreatic insufficiency, often resulting in failure to thrive in children, weight loss or poor weight gain, and fat malabsorption (with steatorrhea and flatulence). Fat malabsorption can lead to deficiencies in the fat-soluble vitamins A, D, E, and K.

Abnormal secretions occur in multiple organs and exocrine glands throughout the body. Other possible manifestations of this include high rates of meconium ileus at birth and poor intestinal motility in adults, as well as impaired bile secretion (which in some cases can lead to cholestatic liver disease or even obstructive cirrhosis). In the sweat glands, loss of *CFTR* function results in impaired reabsorption of chloride, allowing for the diagnosis of CF on the basis of elevated sweat chloride levels.

6. **What is bronchiectasis, and why does it commonly develop in CF?**
Ectasis or *ectasia* means dilation. Bronchiectasis is an irreversible dilation of one or more bronchi. The primary cause for the dilation is usually a combination of inflammation and obstruction (often subtotal obstruction) of the airways. In CF, repeated infection and poor mucous flow contribute to inflammation and airway obstruction.

Other clinical syndromes in which bronchiectasis occurs include obstructing tumors, mucous impaction, foreign body aspiration, necrotizing pulmonary infections (e.g., *Klebsiella*, *S. aureus*, or tuberculosis), or certain rheumatic and systemic diseases (e.g., rheumatoid arthritis). The dilated bronchi are easily collapsible, which causes or aggravates expiratory airflow obstruction and impaired secretion clearance, resulting in the clinical symptoms of dyspnea, cough (often severe), and occasionally hemoptysis.

STEP 1 SECRET

Expect to see at least one question on cystic fibrosis and its complications on the USMLE Step 1.

7. **Why is *N*-acetylcysteine used as a treatment for CF?**
N-acetylcysteine cleaves disulfide bonds in the glycoproteins that form mucus. This reduces the thickness of the mucus seen in patients with CF and loosens mucous plugs. *N*-acetylcysteine is also used as an antidote for acetaminophen toxicity.

RELATED QUESTION

8. **Why does primary ciliary dyskinesia produce clinical manifestations similar to those of CF?**
In primary ciliary dyskinesia (PCD; also known as *immotile cilia syndrome*), there is a primary disturbance in ciliary function and mucociliary clearance resulting from the dysfunction of the dynein arm of microtubules. Recall that microtubules are found within cilia of the upper respiratory epithelial cells and flagella of sperm. This defective mucociliary clearance compromises sputum expectoration, leading to repeated sinus and pulmonary infections. Patients often have chronic cough, and bronchiectasis can develop. It also leads to infertility as a result of sperm dysmotility and dysfunctional cilia in the fallopian tubes.

In CF, ciliary dysfunction is secondary to increased secretion viscosity, whereas in PCD it results from an intrinsic defect in the microtubules. In both diseases, there are recurrent sinopulmonary infections, as well as infertility in men. Note that the infertility that occurs in each disorder has a different cause. Infertility in CF is not due to abnormal secretions but instead is due to congenital absence of the vas deferens (presumably because the *CFTR* gene is involved in the embryonic development of the vas). Many women with CF have difficulties conceiving due to thickened cervical mucus. Malnutrition secondary to impaired fat absorption may also disrupt ovulation in these women.

Note: *Situs inversus* is observed in 50% of patients with PCD. The triad of sinusitis, bronchiectasis, and situs inversus is known as *Kartagener syndrome*. Situs inversus is characterized by complete left-to-right reversal of all organs and vessels of the body. For example, the heart would be on the right side of the thorax (i.e., dextrocardia), and the liver would be in the left upper quadrant of the abdomen. This is distinct from isolated dextrocardia, which can occur in the setting of congenital heart disease. It is felt that situs inversus occurs in ciliary dyskinesia because microtubules are involved in the normal polarization of the body that occurs early in embryogenesis. Without functional microtubules, the polarization of the body occurs randomly such that 50% of patients exhibit normal polarization and 50% exhibit complete reversal.

SUMMARY BOX: CYSTIC FIBROSIS

- Epidemiology: Most common in Caucasians of northern European descent
- Presentation: Meconium ileus at birth, recurrent respiratory infections, failure to thrive
- Pathophysiology: Inherited, autosomal recessive defect in the *CFTR* (cystic fibrosis transmembrane regulator) chloride channel, resulting in abnormally thick secretions of exocrine glands
- Diagnosis: Elevated sweat chloride level
- Treatment: *N*-acetylcysteine to loosen mucous plugs, chest physiotherapy, DNase, hypertonic saline (to promote mucus clearance), azithromycin (for antiinflammatory properties), pancreatic enzyme replacement
- Complications: Repeated respiratory infections leading to progressive, obstructive lung disease, bronchiectasis, and significant rates of morbidity and mortality; malnutrition secondary to impaired fat absorption; cholestatic liver disease; infertility later in life

CASE 11.11

While playing basketball over the weekend, a 35-year-old college professor experiences severe chest pain that radiates to his left jaw and left arm. He is taken by ambulance to the emergency department, where an electrocardiogram confirms that he has had a myocardial infarction (MI). Physical examination is significant for the presence of xanthelasma and several tendinous xanthomas. His family history is remarkable for coronary artery disease in two first-degree relatives diagnosed when they were in their mid-40s. Blood work reveals plasma total cholesterol of 420 mg/dL (Table 11.6), and a coronary angiogram reveals 90% occlusion of the right coronary artery and 50% occlusion of the left anterior descending artery. He responds well to coronary angioplasty and stenting and is discharged home after 3 days.

Table 11.6. Blood Workup for Case 11.11

	Measured Values	
LIPID	**PATIENT'S LEVEL (MG/DL)**	**REFERENCE RANGE (MG/DL)**
Triglycerides	150	60–160
Total cholesterol	420	<200
HDL cholesterol	31	≥35
VLDL cholesterol	30	20–40
LDL cholesterol	359	<100

HDL, High-density lipoprotein; *LDL,* low-density lipoprotein; *VLDL,* very-low-density lipoprotein.

1. **What is the most likely diagnosis based on this patient's family history and fasting lipid profile?**
   Familial hypercholesterolemia (FH) is the diagnosis. His MI at a young age, family history of premature cardiovascular disease, elevated total cholesterol almost entirely in the LDL fraction, normal triglyceride levels, and the presence of xanthelasma and tendinous xanthomas on examination are all consistent with FH. Xanthomas are pathologic depositions of lipids in nonvascular tissues. In heterozygous FH, xanthomas are often detectable as palpable nodules along tendons such as the Achilles or extensor tendons of the hand. Xanthelasmas are yellow-orange plaques on the eyelids and medial canthi that result from cholesterol deposition into these skinfolds around the eye. An additional ophthalmologic finding in patients with FH is corneal arcus, in which a grayish-white ring forms around the periphery of the cornea because of lipid infiltration of the corneal stroma.

   FH typically is caused by a defective or absent LDL receptor (and can also be caused by a defective ApoB-100 protein). This receptor is found on peripheral tissues that utilize lipids found in LDL particles and on the liver, which plays an important role in the clearance of cholesterol from the blood.

2. Based on his clinical presentations, is this patient likely to be heterozygous or homozygous for this deficiency?

This patient is likely a heterozygote. FH is usually inherited in an autosomal dominant fashion in which a single abnormal LDL receptor gene leads to disease. However, there is a gene dosage effect in that patients who are homozygous for the abnormal LDL receptor have more severe disease.

Homozygotes typically have their first MI before age 20, and their total cholesterol levels usually range between 500 and 1000 mg/dL. Prominent presence of cutaneous planar xanthomas is another telltale sign of homozygous FH. Heterozygotes typically have cholesterol levels between 300 and 500 mg/dL, and they do not have MIs until later in life. Occasionally, a few xanthomas can be found on the Achilles tendon in heterozygous FH.

3. What is the primary mechanism by which mutations in the LDL receptor impair LDL uptake from the plasma?

Physiologically, serum LDL is continually made from IDL (intermediate-density lipoprotein), which in turn is derived from VLDL degradation. About 75% of LDL is cleared via LDL receptor–mediated endocytosis, which occurs primarily in the liver and, to a lesser degree, in cholesterol-requiring tissues such as the adrenal cortex (where cholesterol is used as a substrate for steroid hormones). The remainder of LDL is cleared via poorly understood LDL receptor–independent mechanisms, which include, among others, endocytosis of oxidized LDL by macrophages.

Note: Five classes of mutations of the LDL receptor result in impairment of receptor-mediated uptake of LDL from the circulation. These mutations include (1) null mutations (which prevent LDL receptor protein synthesis); (2) defective transport mutations (which prevent normal insertion of the receptor into the plasma membrane); abnormal clathrin-mediated endocytosis resulting from (3) defective ligand receptor–binding mutations or (4) internalization mutations; and (5) defective recycling mutations (inability of the LDL receptor to be recycled back to the membrane).

4. What is the pathologic consequence of elevated plasma LDL?

The mechanism by which excess plasma LDL can result in atherosclerosis is briefly described next.

In the setting of a defective LDL receptor or excess serum LDL of any cause, plasma LDL clearance occurs via other mechanisms, including scavenger receptors on macrophages that "scavenge" (endocytose) modified (e.g., oxidized or glycosylated) LDL. Oxidized LDL levels are proportional to the levels of LDL and may be increased by other cardiac risk factors such as smoking or systemic inflammatory conditions. These macrophages then form foam cells and release the proinflammatory cytokines interleukin-1 (IL-1), IL-6, and tumor necrosis factor α (TNF-α). This, in turn, causes platelets and endothelial cells of the affected artery to release growth factors such as platelet-derived growth factor (PDGF), fibroblast growth factor (FGF), and transforming growth factor β (TGF-β), leading to migration of vascular smooth muscle cells from the tunica media to the tunica intima of the artery. The arterial smooth muscle cells proliferate at the site of cholesterol plaque formation. Initially, the smooth muscle cells produce enough extracellular matrix proteins to form a fibrous cap over the foam cells, forming a stable fibrous plaque. However, because the scavenger receptors are not downregulated by intracellular cholesterol concentration, the foam cells continue to endocytose oxidized LDL, accumulate in the vasculature, and release inflammatory mediators. In some cases, the inflammatory process erodes the fibrous cap, resulting in the formation of a thinly covered unstable plaque that can eventually rupture, resulting in acute thrombus formation. It is the process of unstable plaque rupture that underlies many strokes and most acute coronary syndromes (i.e., unstable angina and MI). Progressive luminal occlusion by growing stable fibrous plaques can result in chronic ischemic symptoms such as stable angina or claudication.

5. How might this patient be managed medically and pharmacologically to decrease his risk of future cardiovascular complications?

This patient should be managed the same as any other patient with cardiovascular disease and associated risk factors. He would be encouraged to undertake dietary and lifestyle modifications, such as increased exercise and smoking cessation, and would likely be treated pharmacologically with HMG-CoA (3-hydroxy-3-methylglutaryl coenzyme A) reductase inhibitors (i.e., statins), possibly in combination with other lipid-lowering drugs.

Along with statins, aspirin, beta-blockers, and angiotensin-converting enzyme (ACE) inhibitors or angiotensin II receptor blockers (ARBs) have also proven to be effective in the secondary prevention of MI (i.e., in patients with a history of MI, they decrease the risk of another MI).

RELATED QUESTION

6. How do HMG-CoA reductase inhibitors specifically reduce serum LDL levels?

HMG-CoA reductase is the rate-limiting enzyme in cholesterol synthesis. Statins lower serum LDL levels by decreasing intracellular levels of cholesterol within hepatocytes. Statins do so by decreasing de novo cholesterol synthesis. Hepatocytes and other tissues require free cytosolic cholesterol for synthesis of the plasma membrane, steroid hormones, and bile acids. The hepatocytes compensate for the decreased cytosolic cholesterol levels by increasing expression of their surface LDL receptors (the same receptors that are mutated in FH) in an attempt to take up more LDL from the bloodstream to replenish the cytosolic cholesterol supply.

Bile acid sequestrants such as cholestyramine, colesevelam, or colestipol act in a similar fashion. The loss of bile acids in the gut results in a compensatory increase in bile acid synthesis, which tends to consume cytosolic free cholesterol within hepatocytes. Again, this results in a compensatory increase in hepatocyte expression of surface LDL receptors.

SUMMARY BOX: FAMILIAL HYPERCHOLESTEROLEMIA

- Presentation: Personal or family history of premature atherosclerosis and coronary artery disease, signs of pathologic lipid deposition such as xanthelasmas and tendinous xanthomas; homozygotes have a more severe phenotype
- Pathophysiology: Absent or defective low-density lipoprotein (LDL) receptor leads to impaired uptake of LDL from the circulation. Excess plasma LDL is recognized by scavenger receptors on macrophages that take up oxidized LDL and turn into "foam cells," ultimately forming unstable atherosclerotic plaques that contribute to acute coronary syndromes.
- Diagnosis: Increased total cholesterol levels with elevated LDL but normal triglyceride levels
- Treatment: HMG-CoA reductase inhibitors (statins), bile acid sequestrants; dietary and lifestyle modifications; aspirin, beta-blockers, and angiotensin-converting enzyme (ACE) inhibitors or angiotensin II receptor blockers (ARBs) for secondary prevention of myocardial infarction (MI)

CASE 11.12

A 15-year-old boy is sent to a developmental pediatric clinic for evaluation of intellectual delay and hyperactivity. Physical examination is notable for an unusually long face with a prominent jaw, large ears, and large testes (macroorchidism). His 17-year-old sister was diagnosed with mild intellectual disability and a learning disability last year. His family history is also notable for learning disabilities in a maternal aunt diagnosed when she was young and a maternal great uncle. His mother and maternal grandfather, however, both had normal intellect. Neither his father nor any of his paternal relatives had learning disabilities or intellectual disabilities.

1. **What is the most likely diagnosis?**

   This child likely has fragile X syndrome, an X-linked dominant disorder. It is associated with intellectual disability and autism spectrum behaviors such as attention-deficit/hyperactivity disorder, perseveration, and social avoidance. The characteristic physical features such as long face, protruding jaw (prognathism), and large testes usually become apparent around puberty. There is also an increased incidence of mitral valve prolapse in these patients.

   Fragile X syndrome is the most common form of inherited intellectual disability. Among genetic disorders, it is the second-most common cause of intellectual disability (after Down syndrome, which can be inherited but usually is not).

2. **What is the pathogenesis of this disorder?**

   Fragile X is caused by expansion of a CGG trinucleotide repeat in the *FMR1* (familial mental retardation-1) gene. The *FMR1* gene normally contains a limited number of repeats (less than 40). However, patients with fragile X syndrome have an expanded number of repeats (usually over 200). The expansion results in a proportional decrease in expression of the fragile X mental retardation (FXMR) protein.

   The decreased expression occurs because the repeat region is a site of gene methylation. Recall that gene methylation is a normal regulatory mechanism for silencing gene expression. In this case, expansion of the repeat region results in hypermethylation of *FMR1* and abnormally low levels of expression.

   The disease pathogenesis is poorly understood. The FXMR protein is thought to play an important role in transporting nuclear mRNA from the nucleus into the cytoplasm before translation, but it is not clear how deficient levels of FXMR protein result in clinical disease. However, disease severity clearly correlates inversely with protein expression levels.

3. **Southern blot analysis indicates that his mother has 90 CGG trinucleotide repeats, whereas he has 350 CGG repeats. What accounts for this finding, and what is its clinical significance?**

   Fragile X syndrome and other trinucleotide repeat disorders exhibit genetic anticipation as a result of germline expansion of the trinucleotide repeat.

   The normal unexpanded *FMR1* gene is transmitted in a stable fashion. However, an expanded *FMR1* gene (with over 40 repeats) is unstable and is subject to further expansion. Furthermore, the longer the gene, the more unstable it is. However, in the case of the *FMR1* gene, this expansion occurs during oogenesis but not spermatogenesis. In other words, instability occurs only in meiosis in women. The result is that a female carrier of an expanded fragile X gene will often transmit an *FMR1* gene that is further expanded. As mentioned earlier, longer repeat regions result in more severe protein deficiency and more severe disease. As a result, subsequent generations experience more severe symptoms and earlier-onset disease, a phenomenon referred to as *genetic anticipation*. Genetic anticipation is uncommon in genetic disorders and usually results from expansion of trinucleotide repeats (Fig. 11.15).

   Note: Because the disorder is X-linked dominant, females with one normal *FMR1* gene and one mutated (expanded) gene will often have some disease features. However, the normal functioning *FMR1* gene usually attenuates the disease to some extent, such that females usually have mild intellectual impairment rather than severe impairment, even in the setting of a full mutation (i.e., >200 repeats).

   These two features, genetic anticipation and X-linked dominance, result in the significant but predictable variability of disease severity seen in families with fragile X syndrome.

90 repeats

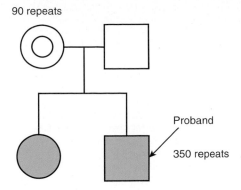

Proband

350 repeats

Figure 11.15. Anticipation caused by expansion of trinucleotide repeats (amplification). *(From Brown TA, Brown D.* USMLE Step 1 Secrets. *Philadelphia: Hanley & Belfus; 2004.)*

RELATED QUESTION

4. What other relatively common inherited disorder exhibits genetic anticipation?

Huntington disease is also due to a trinucleotide repeat expansion and exhibits genetic anticipation because of progressive expansion of the trinucleotide repeat in subsequent generations. It is caused by the expansion of a CAG repeat in the gene that codes for the huntingtin protein (located on chromosome 4). The disorder is characterized by the triad of motor dysfunction with choreoathetosis, behavior and personality changes (including aggression and depression), and dementia. Symptoms normally appear in individuals between the ages of 20 and 50. The disorder is often suspected on the basis of family history and findings from head computed tomography (CT) or magnetic resonance imaging (MRI), specifically prominent atrophy of the caudate nucleus and putamen. The diagnosis can be confirmed with genetic testing.

Huntington disease is the most common of a group of inherited neurodegenerative disorders (so-called *CAG repeat disorders*), which, similar to fragile X, all exhibit genetic anticipation as a result of the expansion of a trinucleotide repeat. However, unlike fragile X, they share autosomal dominant inheritance. Also, unlike fragile X, the germline expansion occurs in both males and females (i.e., in both oogenesis and spermatogenesis), as one might expect for autosomal disorders. In the case of Huntington disease, expansion of the CAG repeat results in an abnormally long huntingtin protein within neurons and other tissues. This elongated protein exhibits a toxic gain of function, such that a normal gene copy is unable to mask a mutated gene.

STEP 1 SECRET

The four most common trinucleotide repeat expansion diseases tested on the USMLE Step 1 are fragile X syndrome, Huntington disease, Friedreich ataxia, and myotonic dystrophy. Friedreich ataxia is caused by expansion of a GAA trinucleotide repeat in the FXN gene on chromosome 9, which codes for the frataxin protein. Myotonic dystrophy is caused by expansion of a CTG trinucleotide repeat in the myotonic dystrophy protein kinase (DMPK) gene.

SUMMARY BOX: TRINUCLEOTIDE REPEAT DISORDERS

Fragile X Syndrome

- Epidemiology: Affects males and females but is inherited in an X-linked dominant pattern, causing affected females to have a milder phenotype because of the presence of one normal X chromosome
- Presentation: Intellectual disability, autism spectrum-like behaviors (e.g., inattentiveness, hyperactivity, social avoidance), as well as characteristic physical features including prognathism (protruding jaw), long face, and macroorchidism (large testes) that appears around puberty
  - Most common inherited disorder of intellectual disability
- Pathophysiology: Expansion of a CGG trinucleotide repeat within the *FMR1* gene, leading to gene hypermethylation and abnormal silencing of gene expression
- Diagnosis: Presence of CGG trinucleotide repeat expansion on Southern blot

Huntington Disease

- Epidemiology: Affects males and females equally (autosomal dominant inheritance); symptoms appear between ages 20 and 50, although age of onset is earlier with each successive generation as a result of genetic anticipation
- Presentation: Triad of choreoathetosis, behavior and personality changes (including aggression and depression), and dementia
- Pathophysiology: Expansion of CAG trinucleotide repeat in the gene coding for the huntingtin protein, resulting in a toxic gain of function
- Diagnosis: Suggested by family history and prominent atrophy of the caudate nucleus and putamen on head computed tomography (CT) or magnetic resonance imaging (MRI)

CASE 11.13

A newborn boy, born to a 42-year-old woman, is evaluated by his pediatrician and is noted to have upslanting palpebral fissures, excess skin of the inner eyelid (epicanthal folds) and at the back of the neck, a flattened maxillary and malar region, and a single transverse palmar crease. The child also exhibits poor muscle tone. Cytologic testing reveals an abnormal karyotype.

1. What is the most likely diagnosis?

   The most likely diagnosis is Down syndrome, or trisomy 21, an aneuploid condition that leads to the most common genetic cause of intellectual disability. Aneuploidy refers to an abnormal chromosome number (that is not a multiple of 23), which is typically due to either a missing chromosome or an extra chromosome (i.e., monosomy or trisomy, respectively). Maternal age older than 35 (so-called *advanced maternal age*) greatly increases the incidence rate of Down syndrome and other chromosomal abnormalities. The chances of a child being born with Down syndrome increase from 1:1500 in women younger than 20 years old to 1:25 in women over 45 years of age.

   Note that although Down syndrome is the most common cause of congenital intellectual disability, it is not the most common hereditary cause of intellectual disability because 95% of cases of Down syndrome are due to meiotic nondisjunction (during meiosis I of oogenesis). Meiotic nondisjunction occurs when homologous chromosomes fail to separate and move to opposite ends of the dividing cell. As a result, one daughter cell ends up with two copies of the original chromosome while the remaining daughter cell has none. After fertilization, the first daughter cell receives another copy of the chromosome from the gamete of the other parent, becoming trisomic. The other daughter cell also acquires a chromosome copy from the other parent and becomes monosomic. Monosomy is incompatible with life, but the trisomic cell can survive to term. Less common causes of Down syndrome include Robertsonian translocation and mosaicism (see next question).

   Also note that although advanced maternal age is an important risk factor for Down syndrome, most children with Down syndrome are born to mothers younger than 35 years of age. On one hand, this may simply reflect the fact that women under 35 years of age become pregnant more often than women over the age of 35. On the other hand, it illustrates that errors of meiosis are fairly common in younger and older women alike. Nondisjunction events can result in viable states such as Down syndrome, but they often result in nonviable states. In fact, chromosomal abnormalities account for about half of all first-trimester spontaneous abortions.

2. What is a Robertsonian translocation, and how does a Robertsonian translocation in a parent result in Down syndrome in the offspring?

   A Robertsonian translocation is a rare subtype of chromosomal rearrangement that primarily involves acrocentric chromosomes (chromosomes with centromeres near their ends). When two acrocentric chromosomes break at their respective centromeres, they can rearrange to form a single chromosome with two long arms fused together. During meiosis, the long arm of chromosome 21 may attach to the long arm of another chromosome, usually chromosome 14 (with loss of the negligible short arms of both chromosomes). Despite this translocation, the individual will be phenotypically normal because he/she still has two copies of all chromosome arms. However, any progeny of this carrier may inherit the equivalent of trisomy 21, with two normal copies of chromosome 21 and an additional copy of chromosome 21 fused to chromosome 14. A second possible outcome is a balanced translocation, which results in a phenotypically normal individual who has a single normal copy of each of chromosomes 14 and 21, as well as the translocation product containing the fused long arms of chromosomes 14 and 21. Any patient with a Robertsonian translocation, regardless of whether that patient is affected by Down syndrome as a result of functional trisomy 21 or whether the patient appears normal because of the presence of a balanced translocation, has a chance of transmitting Down syndrome to offspring. Robertsonian translocations result in a familial form of Down syndrome that is unrelated to maternal age and accounts for 2% to 4% of all cases.

3. What is the mechanism that gives rise to mosaic Down syndrome, whereby only select tissues express the trisomy 21?

   Mosaic Down syndrome (which accounts for 1%–3% of cases) is caused by a mitotic nondisjunction event that occurs early in embryonic development. Thus mosaic Down syndrome is entirely independent of maternal events. This contrasts with the typical meiotic nondisjunction event responsible for most Down syndrome cases (and with the Robertsonian translocation, which is also due to an error in meiosis). As one would expect, the earlier during fetal life that the nondisjunction occurs, the more tissues that are affected and the greater the severity of disease.

4. How is Down syndrome diagnosed prenatally?

   Down syndrome may be suspected during the first trimester if increased nuchal translucency is present on first trimester ultrasound. When the fetus is affected with Down syndrome, results of the pregnancy quad screen performed on maternal serum during the second trimester show increased levels of β human chorionic gonadotropin (β-hCG) and inhibin A and decreased levels of α fetoprotein (AFP) and estriol. Newer, noninvasive diagnostic testing uses sequencing of cell-free fetal DNA collected from maternal plasma.

5. If the child fails to initiate proper feeding, what abnormality should be suspected?

   Children with Down syndrome are at risk for GI tract abnormalities such as congenital bowel obstruction caused by duodenal atresia. Duodenal atresia is caused by failure of normal recanalization of the GI tract during fetal development.

It can be suspected on the basis of the "double-bubble" sign on abdominal radiographs caused by gaseous distention of both the stomach and duodenum proximal to the atretic segment. Patients with Down syndrome are also at risk for other GI abnormalities such as imperforate anus or Hirschsprung disease (aganglionic megacolon). Annular pancreas is also more common in patients with Down syndrome.

6. What causes most of the deaths in infancy and in childhood in Down syndrome?
   Patients with Down syndrome are at increased risk for various congenital heart defects, which together represent the major cause of early death.

   The most common cardiac abnormalities are endocardial cushion defects, which include defects of the atrioventricular canal (i.e., atrioventricular valve abnormalities and atrial and ventricular septal defects). Patent ductus arteriosus and tetralogy of Fallot can also occur.

7. Which cancer types are associated with Down syndrome?
   Patients with Down syndrome are at substantially increased risk for developing acute leukemia (both acute lymphoblastic and, to a lesser extent, acute myelogenous leukemias).

8. What characteristic neuropathologic changes are seen in brains of older people (≥40 years of age) with Down syndrome?
   Almost all patients with Down syndrome in this age group develop the characteristic manifestations of Alzheimer disease, including neurofibrillary tangles and amyloid deposits in brain tissue. This predisposition to early-onset Alzheimer disease may relate to the fact that the gene for the protein found in the amyloid deposits (amyloid precursor protein [APP]) is found on chromosome 21. As a result, individuals with an extra copy of chromosome 21 may be predisposed to producing more APP, which can give rise to an increased number of amyloid plaques in the brain.

STEP 1 SECRET

The complications of Down syndrome are frequently tested on the USMLE Step 1.

RELATED QUESTIONS

9. What other two autosomal trisomies can sometimes produce live-born infants?
   Trisomy 18 (Edwards syndrome) and trisomy 13 (Patau syndrome) are both viable conditions. However, both trisomies produce more severe disease than in trisomy 21, causing death within the first few months or years of life. As with Down syndrome, most cases result from maternal nondisjunction during meiosis I of the respective chromosome pair.

   Both Edwards and Patau syndrome often result in rocker-bottom feet and cardiac defects. An important distinction is that Edwards syndrome often causes micrognathia (small lower jaw), whereas Patau syndrome results in microphthalmia (small eyes) and cleft lip and palate. In Edwards syndrome, the results of the second trimester pregnancy quad screen show decreased levels of AFP, β-hCG, and estriol with normal inhibin A levels. In Patau syndrome, the first-trimester pregnancy screen shows decreased levels of β-hCG and pregnancy-associated plasma protein A (PAPP-A).

10. What two diseases result from microdeletion of the same section of chromosome 15?
    Resulting diseases are Angelman syndrome and Prader-Willi syndrome.

11. Why is the parental source of the chromosome significant in the aforementioned microdeletion syndromes?
    It had once been a central dogma of genetics that phenotype is the same whether a given allele is from a paternal or a maternal source. Like most dogmas, however, this idea has not stood the test of time and it appears that the expression of a select number of genes depends on whether they are maternally derived or paternally derived. This phenomenon of gene expression based on parental origin is known as *genomic imprinting*. Genomic imprinting is felt to be due to differential methylation of chromosome regions in female and male gonads, resulting in different patterns of gene silencing depending on the parental source of the chromosomes.

    Angelman syndrome results from a microdeletion or mutation in the maternally derived chromosome 15, leading to a loss of function of many genes located in that region (Fig. 11.16). Patients with this disease often exhibit uncontrollable and inappropriate laughter ("happy puppet syndrome"), as well as intellectual disability, ataxia, and seizures.

    Prader-Willi syndrome is usually due to a microdeletion of the paternally derived chromosome 15. Patients often exhibit uncontrolled appetite (hyperphagia), frequently resulting in obesity, as well as intellectual disability, hypogonadism, hypotonia, and behavioral problems.

    Remember: Angel**M**an syndrome is due to loss of **m**aternal genes; **P**rader-Willi syndrome is due to loss of **p**aternal genes.

    Note that another (albeit less common) way for an individual to develop Angelman syndrome or Prader-Willi syndrome is through uniparental disomy, in which the offspring receives two copies of a chromosome from one parent and none from the other parent. This is typically more common in Prader-Willi than in Angelman syndrome.

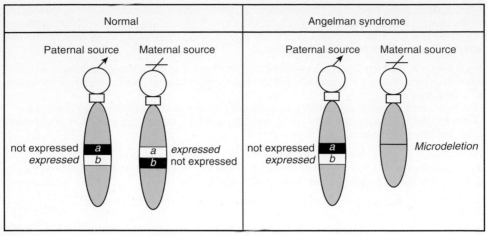

Figure 11.16. Maternal microdeletion in Angelman syndrome. *(From Brown TA, Brown D.* USMLE Step 1 Secrets. *Philadelphia: Hanley & Belfus; 2004.)*

SUMMARY BOX: DOWN SYNDROME

- Presentation: Intellectual disability and characteristic physical findings (upslanting palpebral fissures, exaggerated epicanthal folds, single transverse palmar crease, and hypotonia)
- Risk factors: Advanced maternal age
- Pathophysiology: Most commonly due to nondisjunction of chromosome 21 occurring during meiosis I of oogenesis; can also occur as a result of Robertsonian translocation t(14;21) or mosaicism
- Diagnosis: Postnatal karyotype or prenatal diagnosis with ultrasound (increased nuchal translucency) and pregnancy quad screen performed on maternal serum. Genomic analysis of cell-free fetal DNA collected from maternal plasma is a newer, noninvasive diagnostic technique.
- Complications: Gastrointestinal (GI) tract abnormalities (duodenal atresia, imperforate anus, Hirschsprung disease, annular pancreas), cardiac abnormalities (endocardial cushion defects, patent ductus arteriosus, tetralogy of Fallot), cancers (acute lymphoblastic and acute myeloblastic leukemias), early-onset Alzheimer disease

CASE 11.14

A 20-year-old woman comes to the office because of new-onset headaches and joint pain. She also notes that her hair has been falling out. Physical examination reveals dry, peeling skin and brittle nails. You believe that her signs and symptoms may be related to a new medication that she has been taking for severe acne.

1. What is the most likely diagnosis in this patient?

   Hypervitaminosis A (vitamin A toxicity) is likely. Because vitamin A is fat-soluble (along with vitamins D, E, and K), it can accumulate in adipose tissue and has the potential to reach toxic levels if consumed in excess. Isotretinoin, a drug used to treat severe acne, is a vitamin A derivative that can cause toxicity in patients who do not adhere to their doctor's instructions when taking this medication.

   Other potential sources of vitamin A toxicity include overconsumption of vitamin A–containing foods (e.g., egg yolk, butter, milk) or vitamin A/multivitamin megadoses.

2. What are the symptoms of vitamin A toxicity?

   Vitamin A toxicity results in **h**eadache, **a**rthralgias, **s**ore throat, **s**kin changes, **a**lopecia, **f**atigue, and **t**eratogenicity (cardiac problems, cleft palate, and spontaneous abortions). Owing to the high potential for teratogenicity that results from hypervitaminosis A, isotretinoin prescriptions require a negative pregnancy test and at least two forms of contraception.

   Remember: Vitamin A **HAS-SAF-T** (safety) issues.

3. What are the symptoms associated with vitamin A deficiency?

   Because vitamin A is an essential component of visual pigments (e.g., rhodopsin), deficiency results in night blindness. It is also required for differentiation of epithelial cells into specialized tissues and prevents squamous metaplasia. Deficiency can result in dry skin and squamous metaplasia of the conjunctiva (Bitot spots).

STEP 1 SECRET

Nutrition is an extremely important subject to understand for boards and when discussing health- and diet-related issues with patients. Most students will have at least one or two questions on this topic on their USMLE examination. Spend time learning the symptoms associated with deficiency (and toxicity, when relevant) of the different water-soluble and fat-soluble vitamins. The best resource for this information is your copy of First Aid.

SUMMARY BOX: HYPERVITAMINOSIS A

- Presentation: Headache, arthralgias, sore throat, skin changes, brittle nails, alopecia, fatigue. Risk factors include isotretinoin use for treatment of severe acne and overconsumption of vitamin A–rich foods.
- Pathophysiology: Accumulation of vitamin A in adipose tissue to toxic levels
- Complications: Severe teratogenicity (cardiac problems, cleft palate, and spontaneous abortions)

CASE 11.15

A 5-day-old boy is brought to the emergency department by his parents after a witnessed tonic-clonic seizure. He was born at full term after an uncomplicated pregnancy and had no issues until 2 days before presentation. During this time, the infant started becoming irritable and fed poorly. He was difficult to arouse before having the seizure this morning. Physical examination reveals tachypnea (80/min), scleral icterus, and poor muscle tone. Laboratory studies reveal the following:

Plasma ammonia, 310 μmol/L (normal = 10–40 μmol/L)
Blood urea nitrogen, 1.5 mg/dL (normal = 5–17 mg/dL)
Creatinine, 0.4 mg/dL (normal = 0.2–1.0 mg/dL)
  A plasma amino acid analysis reveals absence of citrulline. Urine amino acids reveal elevated orotic acid levels.

1. What is the most likely diagnosis in this patient?
   Ornithine transcarbamylase (OTC) deficiency is the most likely diagnosis. In the urea cycle, OTC combines carbamoyl phosphate and ornithine to create citrulline (Fig. 11.17). Recall that amino acid catabolism results in the formation of metabolites such as pyruvate and acetyl-CoA, which serve as metabolic fuels. The urea cycle functions to convert the excess nitrogen produced during this process to urea so it can be excreted by the kidneys. Deficiency of OTC interferes with the body's ability to excrete ammonia, resulting in hyperammonemia. This leads to complications such as intellectual disability, seizures, and, ultimately, death. In addition, excess carbamoyl phosphate that accumulates

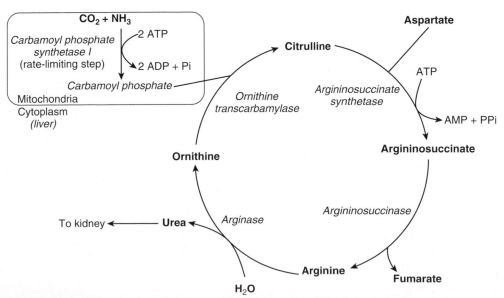

Figure 11.17. Urea cycle. *ADP,* Adenosine diphosphate; *AMP,* adenosine monophosphate; *ATP,* adenosine triphosphate; *Pi,* inorganic phosphate; *PPi,* pyrophosphate.

secondary to OTC deficiency gets shunted into the pyrimidine synthesis pathway and is converted to orotic acid, leading to increased orotic acid levels in the blood and urine. Patients often exhibit low blood urea nitrogen (BUN) levels as well, though this is not sufficient to make the diagnosis. Note that OTC deficiency is an X-linked recessive urea cycle disorder.

2. How is OTC deficiency treated?

Affected patients should consume a protein-free diet with compensatory increases in carbohydrates and lipids. Hemodialysis may be necessary in patients with severe hyperammonemia.

3. What other genetic disorder presents with increased orotic acid levels in the urine?

Orotic aciduria is an autosomal recessive disorder that results from a defect in uridine monophosphate (UMP) synthase, the enzyme that converts orotic acid to UMP in the de novo pyrimidine synthesis pathway. As a result, orotic acid accumulates in the urine. Another hallmark finding in orotic aciduria is megaloblastic anemia that results from the defect in pyrimidine synthesis but does not resolve with vitamin B_{12} or folate administration. A key finding that separates orotic aciduria from OTC deficiency is the absence of hyperammonemia. Orotic aciduria can be treated with oral uridine administration, which bypasses the need for UMP synthase.

4. Which genetic disorder results from blocked degradation of branched amino acids?

The resulting genetic disorder is branched chain ketoaciduria (maple syrup urine disease), an autosomal recessive disorder that results from a deficiency in α-ketoacid dehydrogenase, the enzyme necessary for the breakdown of branched amino acids (isoleucine, leucine, and valine). This condition leads to increased blood levels of branched amino acids, especially leucine. Elevated leucine levels can cause severe CNS defects, intellectual disability, and death. Symptoms classically present 4 to 7 days after birth and include poor feeding, vomiting, poor weight gain, and lethargy. In addition, accumulation of isoleucine causes the urine of these infants to smell like maple syrup or burnt sugar. Restricting amino acid intake is crucial in treatment, although a small percentage of cases respond well to vitamin B_1 (thiamine) supplementation because thiamine acts as a cofactor for α-ketoacid dehydrogenase.

SUMMARY BOX: DISORDERS OF AMINO ACID CATABOLISM

Ornithine Transcarbamylase (OTC) Deficiency

- Epidemiology: Most commonly affects males (X-linked recessive inheritance)
- Presentation: Poor feeding, irritability, seizures, intellectual disability
- Pathophysiology: Defect in OTC resulting in decreased ammonia excretion
- Diagnosis: Physical exam (tachypnea, scleral icterus, poor muscle tone), absence of plasma citrulline, hyperammonemia, increased orotic acid levels in blood and urine
  - Orotic aciduria also presents with increased orotic acid levels but is not associated with hyperammonemia. Patients with this disease will often have megaloblastic anemia that does not resolve with vitamin B_{12} or folate administration
- Treatment: Dietary protein restriction with compensatory increase in lipids and carbohydrates; hemodialysis for severe hyperammonemia
- Complications: Ultimately death

Branched Chain Ketoaciduria (Maple Syrup Urine Disease)

- Presentation: Vomiting, poor feeding, lethargy, and urine that smells like maple syrup during the first week of life
- Pathophysiology: Defect in the α-ketoacid dehydrogenase that degrades branched amino acids (isoleucine, leucine, and valine)
- Diagnosis: Increased blood levels of branched amino acids, especially leucine
- Treatment: Dietary amino acid restriction and thiamine supplementation in certain patients
- Complications: Leucine accumulation can lead to severe central nervous system (CNS) defects, intellectual disability, and even death

CHAPTER 12

ANEMIAS

Insider's Guide to Anemias for the USMLE Step 1

Hematology on the USMLE Step 1 is divided into three major subjects: anemias, bleeding disorders, and hematologic malignancies. We will be covering each of these subjects in a series of three chapters because of the sheer volume and immense importance of all these topics. Anemias are commonly tested on boards, and as you may have figured out, there are *many* different causes. The USMLE will expect you to reason through the cause of a patient's anemia based on clinical history and laboratory values. Images of blood smears will often be provided to aid you in your diagnosis. You should know the different cell morphologies associated with various types of anemia (e.g., sickled cells, bite cells, spherocytes, Heinz bodies) and what these cells look like on a blood smear. You should also know the various clinical tests and laboratory parameters used to classify and diagnose different anemias. These are discussed later in the chapter.

It will be of enormous benefit to you to group the causes of anemia according to their findings (e.g., intrinsic vs. extrinsic, hemolytic vs. nonhemolytic) as you study. If you develop a systematic approach to tackling anemias, you can make a complicated subject much simpler. We will attempt to demonstrate this practice within this chapter.

BASIC CONCEPTS

1. **What is the function of hemoglobin? What are the three main types of hemoglobin found within normal adult red blood cells?**

   Hemoglobin is an iron-containing protein found in red blood cells (RBCs) that carries and releases oxygen, which powers aerobic respiration in the majority of cells. The three primary types of hemoglobin in adult RBCs are hemoglobin A ($\alpha_2\beta_2$), hemoglobin A_2 ($\alpha_2\delta_2$), and fetal hemoglobin F (HbF) ($\alpha_2\gamma_2$). The vast majority (>95%) of hemoglobin in adult RBCs is normally of the hemoglobin A (HbA) type.

2. **What is anemia, and how is it defined?**

   Simply put, the term *anemia* is used to describe a reduction in the volume of RBCs in the circulation, which impairs the body's ability to oxygenate the tissues at optimal levels. Thus anemia results in a decrease in total oxygen content via a reduction in hemoglobin levels (note that O_2 saturation and Pao_2 are *not* affected). In practice, anemia is most commonly diagnosed via a decreased hematocrit level, which represents the ratio between volume of packed RBCs and total blood volume. However, in addition to quantitative anemia (decreased hemoglobin/RBC count), anemia may be qualitative (disordered cellular morphology or hemoglobin structure) or a combination of quantitative and qualitative. These abnormalities can be shown on a complete blood count (CBC), hemoglobin electrophoresis, peripheral blood smear, or, rarely, a bone marrow aspirate if necessary.

STEP 1 SECRET

Normal reference ranges for all important laboratory parameters (including hematologic parameters) will be provided to you, so do not waste time memorizing all of these numbers. Instead, focus on specific clues in the clinical presentation, laboratory tests, and histologic findings that are diagnostic for each particular condition and the major treatments and complications associated with each. Your designated question bank software should provide laboratory values in charts that closely resemble those you will find on the actual exam.

3. **What are reticulocytes?**

   Reticulocytes are RBC precursors with visible ribonucleic acid (RNA) filaments that will mature within 24 hours. Reticulocytes are produced by the bone marrow and released into the blood. In the setting of anemia, the bone marrow will attempt to increase the number of reticulocytes being produced to compensate for reduced RBC number or function. Therefore the number of reticulocytes present in the blood provides an indication of how effectively the bone marrow is producing RBCs and thus responding to an anemia.

   A normal reticulocyte count varies between approximately 0.5% and 1.5%. A low or normal reticulocyte count in a setting of anemia typically indicates an underproduction anemia (i.e., problem originates in the bone marrow). If reticulocytosis is occurring as expected, the source of anemia can be narrowed to outside of the bone marrow.

Calculation of the corrected reticulocyte count, which *corrects* for the degree of anemia, can help determine whether the marrow compensation is appropriate for the severity of the anemia. We typically expect the adjusted reticulocyte count to exceed 3% in cases of anemia. If the reticulocyte count is lower than expected, we can say that the bone marrow is unable to produce enough RBC precursors to ameliorate the anemia.

Clinical Pearl

Even though it is low yield for Step 1, it will be important for you to understand how to calculate a corrected reticulocyte count in your clinical years. The formula is as follows:

$$\text{Corrected reticulocyte count} = \text{absolute reticulocyte count (\%)} \times (\text{patient's hematocrit}/45)$$

In this case, 45% represents a normal hematocrit level and is used regardless of the patient's gender. As mentioned in the subsequent section, a corrected reticulocyte count of ≥3% represents a strong bone marrow response to the anemia, whereas a value lower than 3% demonstrates inadequate bone marrow compensation.

If polychromasia (presence of premature, bluish reticulocytes in the blood due to severe bone marrow stress) is observed, the corrected reticulocyte count must be further divided by 2 to obtain an accurate value. This is required because polychromatic RBCs have RNA filaments and will be falsely counted as reticulocytes.

4. What is the role of erythropoietin?

Erythropoietin (EPO) is a hormone synthesized by the kidney that stimulates division of erythroid stem cells in the bone marrow, leading to production of new RBCs. EPO is released in cases of hypoxemia and severe anemia. In the setting of end-stage renal disease (ESRD), anemia is principally caused by reduced production of EPO by the diseased kidneys. However, uremia from ESRD can also make the bone marrow less responsive to EPO. Anemia caused by ESRD typically responds well to exogenously administered EPO.

Note: Malignancy in the kidney (e.g., renal cell carcinoma) can be associated with ectopic EPO production, leading to overproduction of RBCs (polycythemia). Causes of reactive or secondary polycythemia include smoking and chronic hypoxemia (e.g., chronic obstructive pulmonary disease [COPD]), which stimulate compensatory increases in EPO levels. Contrast this with primary polycythemia (polycythemia vera), in which abnormal hyperproliferation of erythrocytes within the bone marrow leads to a reduction in EPO levels.

5. What are the three pathophysiologic mechanisms resulting in anemia?

The three pathophysiologic mechanisms are (1) decreased production of RBCs, (2) increased destruction of RBCs, and (3) loss of RBCs from circulation result in anemia. Decreased production of RBCs will result from any mechanism that hinders the bone marrow's ability to produce erythrocytes (e.g., decreased EPO, decreased iron, myelofibrosis). Increased destruction of RBCs is precipitated by factors that alter the structure or function of these cells (intrinsic defects; e.g., hereditary spherocytosis, sickle cell anemia) or may be attributed to causes outside of the RBC (extrinsic defects; e.g., autoimmune reactions, infections, drugs/toxins, mechanical shearing forces). Loss of RBCs from circulation is most commonly attributed to blood loss (e.g., acute hemorrhage, gastrointestinal [GI] bleed). Table 12.1 outlines the various causes of anemia that fall into these three general categories.

Table 12.1. Mechanisms Resulting in Anemia

DECREASED PRODUCTION OF RBCs	INCREASED DESTRUCTION OF RBCs	LOSS OF RBCs FROM CIRCULATION
Substrate Deficiency: Iron deficiency Folate/Vitamin B_{12} deficiency Anemia of chronic disease	Abnormal RBC Structure: Spherocytosis Sickle cell anemia	Chronic Blood Loss: Slow GI bleed Menstrual bleeding Endometriosis Fibroids Chronic NSAID use
Disorders of Heme Synthesis: Sideroblastic anemia Lead poisoning	Abnormal RBC Function: G6PD deficiency Pyruvate kinase deficiency Paroxysmal nocturnal hemoglobinuria	Acute Blood Loss: Hemorrhage
Disorders of Globin Synthesis: Thalassemias	Autoimmune: Warm agglutinin hemolytic anemia Cold agglutinin hemolytic anemia	

Table 12.1. Mechanisms Resulting in Anemia—cont'd

DECREASED PRODUCTION OF RBCs	INCREASED DESTRUCTION OF RBCs	LOSS OF RBCs FROM CIRCULATION
Impaired Marrow Responsiveness to EPO: Anemia of chronic disease	Drug Reactions: Cephalosporins Levodopa Methyldopa Levofloxacin Nitrofurantoin Penicillin	
Bone Marrow Infiltrative Conditions: Multiple myeloma Leukemias Lymphomas Myelofibrosis	Infections: Malaria Babesiosis	
Reduced EPO Production: Chronic kidney disease	Intravascular Damage: DIC TTP-HUS Prosthetic heart valves Aortic stenosis	
Failure/Destruction of Myeloid Precursors: Aplastic anemia		

DIC, Disseminated intravascular coagulation; *EPO,* erythropoietin; *GI,* gastrointestinal; *G6PD,* glucose-6-phosphate dehydrogenase; *NSAID,* nonsteroidal antiinflammatory drug; *RBC,* red blood cell; *TTP-HUS,* thrombotic thrombocytopenic purpura and hemolytic-uremic syndrome.

SECRETS FOR APPROACHING ANEMIAS ON THE USMLE STEP 1

Table 12.1 can be quite overwhelming if you do not spend some time organizing the causes of anemia in your head. On the other hand, having a systematic approach to cases of anemia will help ensure an inclusive and thorough differential diagnosis. Although there are many ways to classify anemias, we recommend that you group them according to two factors: (1) RBC size and (2) bone marrow compensation (e.g., reticulocyte count). This approach will help you drastically narrow down your differential diagnosis. RBC size is generally determined by mean corpuscular volume (MCV), which is calculated by dividing hematocrit (expressed as a percentage) by RBC count per liter. This value is nearly always provided for you on the USMLE Step 1 and thus will be an extremely useful way of ruling in or out various diagnoses. Normal reference range for MCV is 80 to 100 fL. All anemias can be grouped into three main categories based purely on MCV: microcytic (smaller than normal RBC size, <80 fL), normocytic (normal RBC size, 80–100 fL), and macrocytic (larger than normal RBC size, >100 fL).

Microcytic anemias are related to problems with hemoglobin production. Remember that this can result from impairments in heme synthesis (e.g., iron deficiency, lead poisoning, sideroblastic anemia) or globin synthesis (e.g., thalassemia).

Macrocytic anemias are divided into megaloblastic and nonmegaloblastic causes based on whether the macrocytosis is due to problems with DNA synthesis (megaloblastic) or another etiology (nonmegaloblastic). Only the megaloblastic anemias are high yield for the USMLE, but for the sake of completeness, advanced liver disease, hypersplenism, alcohol toxicity, and a robust reticulocytosis by the marrow in response to active bleeding or RBC hemolysis are all causes of nonmegaloblastic anemia. Megaloblastic anemias result from causes that impair DNA synthesis (e.g., vitamin B_{12} or folate deficiency), which inhibits the cell cycle from progressing through the stages of mitosis. Thus cells continue to grow without dividing, subsequently resulting in the formation of large, immature RBCs. It is important to keep in mind that impairments in DNA synthesis will affect all cells and not just RBCs. Thus megaloblastic anemias are commonly associated with the formation of large, immature, hypersegmented neutrophils on peripheral blood smear. This can be a helpful clue when diagnosing a megaloblastic anemia.

Normocytic anemias are the trickiest to diagnose and include the greatest number of potential causes, but they can be broken down according to the bone marrow's ability to compensate for the anemia (i.e., produce reticulocytes). Corrected reticulocyte counts <3% indicate problems within the bone marrow itself (e.g., aplastic anemia), stimulation of erythropoiesis (e.g., decreased EPO due to renal disease), or inadequate time for compensation (e.g., acute blood loss). Note that iron deficiency anemia and anemia of chronic disease, which are typically considered to be microcytic anemias, initially manifest as normocytic diseases until lack of adequate hemoglobin synthesis is severe enough to decrease RBC size. Corrected reticulocyte counts ≥3% indicate that the bone marrow is capable of responding to the anemia and has had enough time to compensate (i.e., chronic issue). As mentioned in question 5, these anemias can result from intrinsic RBC defects or from extrinsic defects not related to RBC structure.

Note: Many people prefer to classify normocytic anemias into hemolytic and nonhemolytic causes. Nonhemolytic anemias are usually the result of inadequate erythropoiesis. Once produced, the RBCs are normal but are simply too few in number. Hemolytic anemias are due to premature destruction of RBCs and can subsequently be divided into intrinsic and extrinsic causes, as mentioned previously. For board exam purposes, you should assume that all intrinsic RBC defects will promote some degree of hemolysis. Extrinsic hemolysis can occur as a result of infection, tumor, autoimmune disorder, medication side effects, etc.

The aforementioned classification scheme has been thoroughly broken down in Fig. 12.1. We recommend that you refer back to this figure while reading through the cases to help develop your differential diagnosis for each anemia.

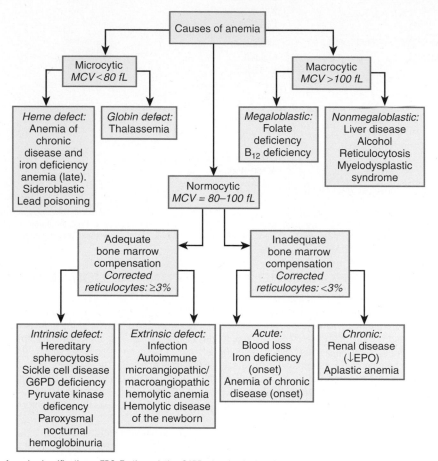

Figure 12.1. Anemia classifications. *EPO,* Erythropoietin; *G6PD,* glucose-6-phosphate dehydrogenase; *MCV,* mean corpuscular volume.

6. **Can a normocytic anemia present as a macrocytic anemia?**
   Yes. Reticulocytes are slightly larger than mature RBCs. Thus increased reticulocytosis secondary to bone marrow compensation may lead to an average MCV in the macrocytic range. However, if you were to exclude reticulocytes and only measure the size of mature RBCs in the blood, these cells would be normal in size. Variation in the size of the peripheral RBC pool is referred to as *anisocytosis* and will be reflected by an increased red blood cell distribution width (RDW). In other words, an increased RDW indicates that the RBC pool is not uniform in size. Acute iron deficiency anemia is a classic example of a disease in which RDW is increased; until hemoglobin synthesis is sufficiently impaired, half of the RBCs will be normocytic while the rest may be microcytic.

7. **Regarding hemolytic anemia, what is the difference between intravascular and extravascular hemolysis?**
   Intravascular hemolysis occurs when RBCs are directly lysed within blood vessels. Causative factors include complement-mediated hemolysis in paroxysmal nocturnal hemoglobinuria (PNH), destruction of RBCs by infectious agents, and mechanical fragmentation of RBCs by mechanical prosthetic valves as in macroangiopathic anemia or by fibrin clot products as in microangiopathic hemolytic anemias, which often occur in the setting of disseminated intravascular coagulation (DIC). Extravascular hemolysis, as the name implies, takes place outside the vasculature and inside the reticuloendothelial system. In extravascular hemolysis, splenic macrophages or Kupffer cells in the liver

destroy RBCs because of structural or morphologic abnormalities of the RBCs (e.g., hereditary spherocytosis, hypersplenism).

Note that the terms *intravascular* and *extravascular hemolytic anemia* are *not* equivalent to *intrinsic* and *extrinsic hemolytic anemia.* The latter refers to the cause of the anemia (is this a problem within the RBC?), whereas the former describes its location (is hemolysis occurring inside or outside of the vasculature?).

8. **Why is there a greater degree of hemoglobinemia and hemoglobinuria in intravascular hemolysis than in extravascular hemolysis?**
   In intravascular hemolysis, lysed RBCs spill their hemoglobin directly into the bloodstream (hemoglobinemia), which may then be filtered out into the urine (hemoglobinuria). In extravascular hemolysis, the hemoglobin in phagocytosed RBCs is metabolized intracellularly to bilirubin, reducing the amount of hemoglobin that ends up in the blood or urine (Table 12.2).

   Haptoglobin, a serum protein that binds free heme in the circulation, will attempt to reduce the free heme secondary to hemolysis regardless of etiology. For reasons previously explained, haptoglobin will be more greatly reduced in the setting of intravascular hemolysis than in extravascular hemolysis. You should keep this in mind for the USMLE!

Table 12.2. Characteristics of Hemolysis

HEMATOLOGIC FEATURE	INTRAVASCULAR HEMOLYSIS	EXTRAVASCULAR HEMOLYSIS
Hemoglobinemia	Yes	None or slight
Hemoglobinuria	Yes	None or slight
Plasma haptoglobin	Large decrease	Normal or slight decrease
Jaundice	Yes	Yes
Hepatosplenomegaly	No	Often
Example disorders	Microangiopathic hemolytic anemia, macroangiopathic hemolytic anemia, disseminated intravascular coagulation (DIC), thrombotic thrombocytopenic purpura (TTP), paroxysmal nocturnal hemoglobinuria (PNH)	Immune-mediated (ABO mismatch), hypersplenism, hereditary spherocytosis

9. **When does extramedullary hematopoiesis occur?**
   Extramedullary hematopoiesis refers to the production of hematopoietic cells (leukocytes, platelets, and RBCs) outside of the bone marrow. This occurs in the case of intrinsic bone marrow disease (e.g., myelofibrosis) or during times when accelerated erythropoiesis is necessary (e.g., during severe hemolysis). Common sites of extramedullary hematopoiesis include the spleen and liver; thus this process is typically associated with hepatosplenomegaly on physical examination.

CASE 12.1

An 8-year-old boy from Kenya is evaluated for several months of fatigue. Physical examination is significant only for a yellowish tinge to his sclera. Laboratory values are as follows:
   Hemoglobin 9.0 g/dL (normal: 12–15 g/dL)
   Hematocrit 27% (normal: 35%–42%)
   MCV 85 (normal: 80–100 fL)

1. **Based on this extremely limited information, what is the differential diagnosis for this patient?**
   This patient is anemic based on low hemoglobin and hematocrit levels. Normal MCV indicates that this patient has a normocytic anemia (see Fig. 12.1). His jaundiced appearance suggests that a hemolytic process is involved. Hemolytic conditions such as sickle cell disease and glucose-6-phosphate dehydrogenase (G6PD) deficiency are endemic to Kenya and other parts of Africa, so you should certainly have these in mind.

CASE 12.1 CONTINUED:

A peripheral blood smear is conducted and is shown in Fig. 12.2.

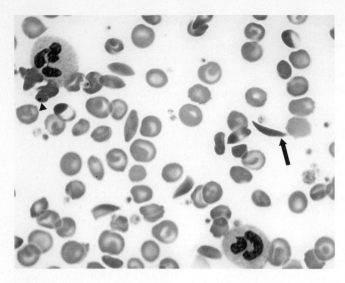

Figure 12.2. Peripheral blood smear in Case 12.1. *(Adapted from Hsi E.* Hematopathology: A Volume in the Series: Foundations in Diagnostic Pathology. *2nd ed. Philadelphia: Saunders; 2013.)*

2. What is the expected diagnosis now, and what is the confirmatory test?

The diagnosis now is sickle cell anemia, a hereditary hemoglobinopathy caused by a point mutation in position 6 of the β-globin chain that substitutes valine for glutamic acid. Note that the peripheral blood smear seen in Fig. 12.2 reveals sickled RBCs and Howell-Jolly bodies, two characteristic findings of this disease. Howell-Jolly bodies are dark-staining clusters of DNA in RBCs. Normally, they are removed by splenic macrophages. However, in patients who are asplenic or functionally asplenic, such as in sickle cell anemia, Howell-Jolly bodies persist and can be observed on peripheral smear.

Hemoglobin electrophoresis can provide definitive evidence to make a diagnosis of sickle cell anemia. In this test, RBCs are obtained from the patient, lysed to free up the hemoglobin proteins, and separated by size and charge on a gel. A banding pattern develops that corresponds with the size of the hemoglobin proteins. Each specific type of hemoglobin has an identical banding pattern based on the hemoglobin variant present. Therefore a patient with sickle cell anemia should show a hemoglobin electrophoresis banding pattern consistent with hemoglobin S (HbS), the sickle cell variant.

3. Is sickle cell disease likely in this patient if none of his immediate family members are affected?

Yes. Sickle cell anemia is inherited in an autosomal recessive pattern. In this case, both parents must be unaffected carriers of sickle cell trait to pass the trait on to their son. Approximately 25% of the offspring generated by two carriers will be affected with sickle cell disease. This patient's siblings may also be carriers of sickle cell trait, having received one copy of the mutation from one parent and a normal copy from the other, or they may be completely unaffected, having received normal copies of the gene from both parents.

CASE 12.1 CONTINUED:

Hemoglobin electrophoresis of the patient's blood shows the presence of abnormal HbS.

4. What causes "sickling" of red blood cells in this disease?

Because sickle cell anemia is caused by a substitution of the hydrophobic valine for the hydrophilic glutamic acid in the β-globin protein, there is deficient production of HbA with increased expression of abnormal HbS.

In its deoxygenated form, HbS is significantly less soluble than HbA and is therefore predisposed to precipitating from the cytoplasm under conditions that cause higher concentrations of deoxyhemoglobin. When these molecules aggregate, they polymerize into long, thin fibers within the RBC, giving these cells their characteristic shape.

5. Which conditions promote sickling of RBCs?

- Hypoxemia: Leads to decreased oxygen saturation of Hb (increases deoxyhemoglobin)
- Acidosis: Promotes oxygen release from hemoglobin (increases deoxyhemoglobin)
- Hyperosmolarity: Increases the concentration of Hb in the RBC by promoting fluid loss from the cell (increases the probability of HbS aggregation)
- Dehydration: Increases the concentration of Hb in the RBC due to low plasma volume (increases the probability of HbS aggregation)
- Inflammation: Promotes stagnation of RBCs within microvascular beds, resulting in extended exposure to low oxygen concentrations (increases deoxyhemoglobin)

Although the effects of hemoglobin precipitation are initially reversible, repeated bouts of hemoglobin precipitation lead to irreversible defects in structure and function of the RBC membrane, resulting in chronically sickled cells.

6. **How does the presence of HbS promote both hemolysis and microvascular occlusions?**
As HbS polymers form in the RBC, they puncture the RBC membrane. Damaged RBCs are rapidly phagocytosed by splenic macrophages, leading to extravascular hemolysis. Damaged RBCs are also mechanically fragile, promoting some degree of intravascular hemolysis as well.

Sickled RBCs inherently express more adhesion molecules than healthy RBCs, promoting occlusions within the vasculature. Occlusions are more prone to occur in locations where RBC transit time is slow, such as the microvasculature of the spleen and bone marrow. Inflammation (i.e., during infections) also promotes microvascular occlusions by enhancing the expression of adhesion molecules on endothelial cells, which can, in turn, slow transit of RBCs through the microvasculature. In addition, anything that promotes constriction of the vasculature (e.g., cold weather) can promote platelet aggregation and further occlude the vessels.

7. **If there is hemolysis producing the anemia, why is the spleen not palpable?**
By the age of 5 years, 94% of sickle cell patients will have experienced autoinfarction of the spleen as a result of sickled RBCs repeatedly occluding the tortuous circulation of the spleen. Lacking adequate oxygenation, the spleen becomes small, dense, and fibrotic. Calcification may be seen on abdominal x-ray films. Remember, autoinfarction of the spleen will result in the presence of Howell-Jolly bodies on peripheral smear.

Note: Before autoinfarction, splenomegaly may occur. Splenomegaly occurs when RBCs occlude the efferent splenic vessels, leading to accumulation of blood within the spleen and consequent engorgement of the organ. This can sometimes lead to a splenic sequestration crisis in which RBCs and platelets normally found within the general circulation pool become trapped in the enlarged spleen. Platelet counts and plasma levels of hemoglobin may fall below normal, causing hypovolemic shock and death.

Clinical Pearl

Parents of a child with sickle cell disease are often taught how to palpate the spleen whenever the child develop a febrile illness. Various infections can cause a "splenic sequestration crisis," in which the spleen enlarges acutely to aid in the immune response. This enlargement of the spleen results in compression of the splenic cords, which makes it more difficult for rigid sickled cells to pass through and can potentially cause massive RBC sequestration and hemolysis. Splenic sequestration can therefore cause a rapid drop in the hematocrit and symptoms of intravascular depletion and hypovolemic shock. If access to medical care (e.g., RBC transfusion) is not available, the mortality rate for these sequestration crises can approach 15%.

---

8. **Why should this boy receive vaccinations against encapsulated bacteria?**
He should receive vaccinations because of his asplenia. The polysaccharide capsule surrounding encapsulated organisms (e.g., *Streptococcus pneumoniae* and *Haemophilus influenzae*) prevents them from being easily attacked by immune cells. The spleen filters these encapsulated bacteria from the blood, where they are opsonized and phagocytosed by splenic macrophages. Recurrent vaso-occlusive crises in the spleen typically lead to fibrotic scarring of the spleen (referred to as *autosplenectomy*), which significantly increases susceptibility to infection by encapsulated bacteria.

CASE 12.1 CONTINUED:

Two weeks later, this patient's mother brings him in because of a significant increase in fatigue (evidenced by decreased desire to play), irritability, and a facial rash with a "slapped cheek" appearance.

---

9. **What infection do you suspect, and what serious complication should be considered?**
The slapped cheek appearance is characteristic of parvovirus B19 infection. Parvovirus is known to infect erythrocyte progenitor cells and cause aplastic crisis in sickle cell anemia. The combination of increased RBC hemolysis (sickled cells have a severely reduced life span) in sickle cell anemia and impaired erythropoiesis due to parvovirus B19 infection can precipitate a severe state of anemia.

CASE 12.1 CONTINUED:

Four months later, the patient is evaluated for a several-hour history of severe chest pain and dyspnea that started while he was playing basketball earlier in the day. Oxygen saturation is 84% on room air, and chest x-ray reveals perihilar infiltrates.

---

10. **What is the likely diagnosis, and why does it occur in sickle cell anemia?**
The likely diagnosis is acute chest syndrome, which is caused by occlusion of the pulmonary vasculature by sickled RBCs. This phenomenon is known as *vaso-occlusive crisis*, or, more commonly, *pain crisis*. Vaso-occlusive crisis results

in local lactic acidosis and pain secondary to tissue hypoxia. Any conditions that favor sickling (see question 5) can act as triggers. Locations commonly include the lungs (leading to acute chest syndrome), hands (leading to dactylitis), brain (leading to stroke), bone (leading to avascular necrosis), liver, spleen, and penis (leading to priapism). In this patient, development of acute chest syndrome may cause pulmonary edema and an elevated white blood cell (WBC) count and could thus be indistinguishable from pneumonia on chest x-ray. Treatment should include respiratory support, exchange transfusion, and empiric antibiotics for pneumonia due to fluid stasis in the lungs.

STEP 1 SECRET

A child experiencing chest pain during play is a commonly used clinical vignette on the USMLE. Whenever you see this, consider acute chest syndrome in a sickle cell patient. Additional medical history to support this diagnosis will be provided to you.

11. Why is this patient also at risk for papillary necrosis of the kidneys?
    The kidney is an additional location where vaso-occlusive complications may occur. In this case, conditions of hypoxemia, acidosis, and hyperosmolarity specifically present in the renal medulla (an area that is especially prone to hypoxia) increase sickling of RBCs, resulting in vaso-occlusion of the vasa recta in the renal papillae. This eventually leads to papillary necrosis. Of note, patients with sickle cell trait can also be affected by renal papillary necrosis.
    Note: Patients with sickle cell anemia may also present with microscopic hematuria due to medullary infarcts.

12. What two bone "diseases" are sickle cell patients predisposed to and why?
    As mentioned in question 10, vaso-occlusive phenomena in sickle cell anemia can cause avascular necrosis of bones, particularly avascular necrosis of the femoral head. These avascular areas of bone are then more susceptible to development of infection (osteomyelitis). *Salmonella* osteomyelitis is seen more frequently in sickle cell anemia. In contrast, *Staphylococcus aureus* is the most frequent cause of osteomyelitis in the general population.
    Note: *Salmonella* is an encapsulated organism. Patients with sickle cell crisis who undergo autosplenectomy are at risk for infection by encapsulated organisms. Therefore *Salmonella* osteomyelitis is more frequent in sickle cell anemia.

CASE 12.1 CONTINUED:

As his physician, you recommend prophylactic cholecystectomy once he is stable.

13. Why are patients with sickle cell disease at an increased risk for gallstones?
    About 70% of patients with sickle cell disease will get symptomatic cholelithiasis. Recall that these gallstones will be pigmented due to hyperbilirubinemia secondary to chronic hemolysis. Having a prophylactic cholecystectomy can also help distinguish gallbladder pain caused by cholelithiasis from abdominal pain caused by vaso-occlusive crises.

14. Some patients with sickle cell disease are treated with the chemotherapeutic drug hydroxyurea. What is the rationale for starting this patient on this treatment?
    Hydroxyurea is a chemotherapeutic drug that increases the production of HbF, which has a higher affinity for oxygen. This factor presumably decreases the amount of HbS expression and therefore decreases HbS polymerization and RBC sickling. However, the precise mechanism of action of hydroxyurea remains poorly understood. Some authors believe that its main mechanism of action is through stabilizing RBC membranes. Nevertheless, students should know that it is an important therapeutic agent for sickle cell disease.

15. How does sickle cell trait differ from sickle cell disease?
    The heterozygous carrier of the sickle cell mutation is said to have the sickle cell trait, genotypically referred to as *HbAS*. The hemoglobin alleles are codominant. Patients who have sickle cell trait produce both normal and abnormal hemoglobin. Approximately 90% of a patient's hemoglobin must be abnormal to produce symptoms of sickle cell anemia. Therefore patients with sickle cell trait are often asymptomatic and typically do not experience episodes of pain from vaso-occlusive crises.

16. What is the evolutionary pressure for sickle cell trait?
    The sickle cell mutation is more common in African Americans because, in its heterozygous form, it provides protection from infection with *Plasmodium falciparum*. In fact, in regions of Africa where malaria is common, up to 25% to 30% of the population is heterozygous for this mutation.

17. What is hemoglobin C?
    Hemoglobin C (HbC) is the product of an alternative mutation in position 6 of the β-globin gene in which lysine is substituted for glutamic acid. Similar to the sickle cell mutation, individuals heterozygous for the mutation often do not have any anemia, and homozygous individuals have a mild hemolytic anemia. Individuals with hemoglobin SC (HbSC) disease have a milder form of sickle cell disease than patients with hemoglobin S sickle cell (HbSS) disease.

SUMMARY BOX: SICKLE CELL DISEASE

- Presentation: Young patients with fatigue and jaundice
- Epidemiology: Common in individuals of African descent
  - Coincides with high prevalence of malaria in this region because the sickle cell mutation is protective against this disease
- Pathophysiology: Point mutation in β-globin gene that leads to replacement of a glutamate residue with valine
  - Results in production of hemoglobin S (HbS), which undergoes extensive polymerization when deoxygenated
- Diagnosis
  - Normocytic anemia
  - Sickled red blood cells (RBCs) and Howell-Jolly bodies on peripheral blood smear
  - Presence of HbS on hemoglobin electrophoresis
- Complications
  - Splenic sequestration crisis
  - Vaso-occlusive crisis (acute chest syndrome, renal papillary necrosis, stroke, aseptic necrosis of the femoral head, priapism, etc.)
  - Cholelithiasis
  - Infection with encapsulated organisms
  - Parvovirus infection (causes aplastic crisis)
- Treatment
  - Hydroxyurea

CASE 12.2

A 6-month-old boy of Greek descent is brought to the office by his parents because he has been sleeping much more than usual over the past 2 weeks. Physical examination reveals conjunctival pallor, scleral icterus, and hepatosplenomegaly. Concerned about a possible anemia, the pediatrician obtains an initial CBC to check for anemia and infection. The CBC reveals hemoglobin of 4.5 g/dL, MCV of 73 fL, and increased RDW.

1. **What is the differential diagnosis for a microcytic anemia?**
   Iron deficiency, anemia of chronic disease, thalassemia, sideroblastic anemia, and lead poisoning are considerations.

CASE 12.2 CONTINUED:

Serum iron, ferritin, and total iron-binding capacity (TIBC) are all normal. A peripheral smear shows many nucleated RBCs and target cells.

2. **How does this change your differential diagnosis?**
   This largely rules out the two most common causes of hypochromic, microcytic anemia—iron deficiency and anemia of chronic disease. Both conditions demonstrate decreased serum iron. Thalassemias, sideroblastic anemia, and lead poisoning move up to the top of the differential diagnosis.

CASE 12.2 CONTINUED:

Gel electrophoresis reveals elevated HbA$_2$ and HbF and the complete absence of β-globin subunits.

3. **What is the diagnosis?**
   β-Thalassemia major, also known as *Cooley anemia*, is the diagnosis. If there were partial expression of β-globin, then the diagnosis would be β-thalassemia minor, but this is usually either very mild or completely asymptomatic.

4. **What is the pathogenesis of thalassemia major?**
   Impaired synthesis of the β-subunit of hemoglobin due to a homozygous mutation is its pathogenesis. Normally, HbA is a tetramer made of two alpha chains and two beta chains. Impaired production of the beta chains leads to polymerization of the alpha chains within RBCs. These aggregates are insoluble and precipitate and damage the RBC membrane, causing premature hemolysis within the spleen and ineffective erythropoiesis in the bone marrow. The combination of the accelerated destruction and the impaired production of RBCs explains the severe anemia.

5. **Why did it not manifest until the age of 6 months?**
   For the first 6 months, this boy was asymptomatic because he still had large amounts of HbF, fetal hemoglobin, present in his circulation. Remember, HbF contains two alpha chains and two gamma chains and does not require β-globin

synthesis for proper functioning. As he transitioned to synthesis of adult hemoglobin (HbA contains two alpha and two beta chains), the symptoms began to manifest as he became reliant on HbA production.

CASE 12.2 CONTINUED:

Physical examination reveals conjunctival pallor, scleral icterus, and hepatosplenomegaly.

6. **Why are scleral icterus and organomegaly seen?**
   RBC hemolysis releases heme, which is degraded into bilirubin. The unconjugated bilirubin accumulates and deposits in the sclera, causing icterus. This eventually results in generalized jaundice.
   Hepatosplenomegaly occurs for two reasons. First, there is increased hemolysis of abnormal RBCs by macrophages in the spleen and liver. Second, there is extramedullary erythropoiesis in response to impaired bone marrow erythropoiesis. (However, this is no more effective than in the bone marrow because of the genetic defect in β-globin.)

STEP 1 SECRET

You may be given an x-ray film of a skull that demonstrates a "crew cut" appearance (Fig. 12.3). This is a sign of bone marrow expansion and is associated with β-thalassemia major and sickle cell disease.

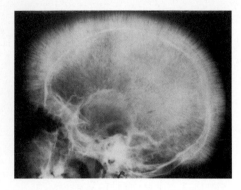

Figure 12.3. Thalassemia: X-ray film of the skull showing new bone formation on the outer table, producing perpendicular radiations resembling a crewcut. *(Courtesy Dr. Jack Reynolds, Department of Radiology, University of Texas Southwestern Medical School, Dallas, TX.)*

CASE 12.2 CONTINUED:

You tell the parents that their son will need frequent blood transfusions for the rest of his life. At the age of 4, the boy is seen in the emergency department because he is unable to walk after falling off his tricycle. X-ray films show a fracture of the right tibia.

7. **Why might this boy be more susceptible to fractures?**
   Ineffective erythropoiesis in the bone marrow results in markedly hyperplastic bone marrow and bone marrow expansion (see Fig. 12.3). This bone marrow expansion erodes away the cancellous and cortical bone, resulting in significant structural weakness.

CASE 12.2 CONTINUED:

This patient does well for many years, receiving frequent blood transfusions. At the age of 35, he is seen for a routine checkup and is found to have a fasting glucose level of 130 mg/dL. His skin is noted to be tanned, although he spends little time in the sun. An electrocardiogram (ECG) shows nonspecific ST-T wave changes.

8. **What is the diagnosis, and why did it occur in this patient?**
   Secondary (acquired) hemochromatosis is a common complication of repeated transfusions in patients with β-thalassemia major. Excess iron is delivered in the transfused RBCs and can deposit in organs such as the heart, pancreas, and skin, leading to complications such as restrictive cardiomyopathy and so-called bronze diabetes.
   Keep in mind that thalassemia is a disorder of globin chain deficiency, so iron studies will be completely normal. The board examination loves to test students on their understanding of various disorders, so you should expect to be asked conceptual questions like this on your examination.

The following type of question format commonly appears on boards:
    Example: Which of the following laboratory findings would be expected in a patient with β-thalassemia major who is receiving blood transfusions on a biweekly to monthly basis (compared with values for a normal patient)?

	β-Hemoglobin	Hemoglobin F	Serum Iron
A.	↓/Normal	↓	Normal
B.	↓/Normal	↓	↑
C.	↓/Normal	↑	↑
D.	↑	Normal	↓

The correct answer choice is C. Hematology, cardiology, nephrology, and pulmonology questions are especially suitable for this "↑/↓/normal" format. Thus when you study these subjects, you should be thinking along comparative terms. Purchasing question bank software will give you some additional practice with handling these types of questions.

9. **How could this secondary hemochromatosis have been prevented?**
Treatment with iron-chelating agents such as deferoxamine can reduce the incidence of hemochromatosis. Obviously, phlebotomy to reduce iron stores (the usual treatment for hereditary hemochromatosis) would be counterproductive for someone receiving transfusions for anemia.

10. **If this patient had presented in his early 20s with similar symptoms and blood tests, but β-globin is present on gel electrophoresis, what would be your diagnosis? What is the pathogenesis?**
α-Thalassemia is caused by impaired production of the α-subunit of hemoglobin. Gel electrophoresis will show β-globin chains but no bands corresponding to α-globin. There are two genes for the α-subunit on each chromosome, for a total of four genes. Unless someone is missing all four copies of the alpha chain gene, that person will still synthesize some alpha chains. For this reason, patients with α-thalassemia typically present later in life with milder symptoms than those with β-thalassemia. People missing one copy of the gene are asymptomatic because enough alpha chain is produced by the remaining three copies of the normal gene. Missing two copies (α-thalassemia minor) can cause a mild anemia that generally does not require treatment. Typically, this occurs in people of Asian or African descent. Those of African descent are more likely to have received one abnormal copy from each parent, leading to an α-/α- genotype. This is called *trans deletion*. Those of Asian descent are more likely to have gotten two abnormal copies from one parent, leading to an αα/— genotype, which is known as a *cis deletion*. Missing three copies results in a condition called *hemoglobin H* (HbH) disease, where excess β-chains form tetramers of HbH. The gel electrophoresis will show normal β-globin and decreased α-globin subunits.

11. **α-Thalassemia, in its most severe form, causes *hydrops fetalis* and can be fatal in utero. What is hydrops fetalis, and why is it fatal?**
Hydrops fetalis occurs when the fetus is missing all four copies of the α-globin gene. HbA, HbA₂, and HbF all require the alpha subunits to form, so in its complete absence, none of these can be made. The fetus instead produces hemoglobin consisting of four gamma chains (hemoglobin Barts). This form of hemoglobin has an extremely high affinity for oxygen and hinders the ability of RBCs to deliver this oxygen to tissues. Fetuses affected with this disease are born with profound anemia caused by tissue asphyxia and with congestive heart failure (CHF) from this asphyxia. This is often fatal in utero, as proper growth and development cannot occur in the setting of profound hypoxia. This is similar to the condition of babies afflicted with hemolytic disease of the newborn (Rh-positive babies born to Rh-negative sensitized mothers).

Pay close attention to age, racial, and ethnic clues provided in question stems. The USMLE will commonly present "textbook cases" in their clinical vignettes, so these clues may aid you in prioritizing the considerations in your differential diagnosis. For instance, α-thalassemia is most common in Africans and Asians, but β-thalassemia is most common in African and Mediterranean populations.

12. **Why is sickle cell disease less severe than normal in a patient who is a HbS/β-thalassemia heterozygote?**
Patients with β-thalassemia produce high levels of HbF, which decreases sickling of RBCs.

SUMMARY BOX: THALASSEMIAS

α-THALASSEMIA

- Caused by decreased α-globin synthesis
  - Africans: α-/α- (trans deletion)
  - Asians: $\alpha\alpha$/— (cis deletion)
- Symptoms based on the number of genes deleted
  - Asymptomatic
  - Mild anemia
  - Hemoglobin H (HbH) disease: Splenomegaly
  - Hb Barts: Hydrops fetalis—incompatible with life
- Diagnosis
  - Smear: Microcytic anemia, hypochromia, target cells
- Treatment: Blood transfusions

β-THALASSEMIA

- Caused by decreased β-globin synthesis
- Epidemiology: Mediterranean or African descent
- Symptoms
  - β-Thalassemia major: Anemia, jaundice, and splenomegaly at 6 months of age due to switch from fetal to adult hemoglobin
  - β-Thalassemia minor: Asymptomatic
- Diagnosis: Increased fetal hemoglobin (HbF) and hemoglobin A_2 (HbA_2) and decreased hemoglobin A (HbA) on gel electrophoresis
- Treatment
  - Transfusions + deferoxamine to increase iron excretion
  - Splenectomy
  - Possible bone marrow transplant

CASE 12.3

A 68-year-old woman with an unremarkable medical history is evaluated for several months of progressively worsening fatigue and shortness of breath with exertion. Laboratory values are as follows:

Hemoglobin: 8.3 g/dL (normal: male, 13.5–17.5 g/dL; female, 12.0–16.0 g/dL)

Hematocrit: 24.9% (normal: male, 41%–53%; female, 36%–46%)

MCV: 72 μm^3 (normal: 80–100 μm^3)

1. **What is the differential diagnosis for this patient?**

   A low hemoglobin and hematocrit in association with an MCV less than 80 μm^3 is diagnostic of microcytic anemia. The most likely cause of microcytic anemia in older individuals with absence of known renal disease or significant past medical history is iron deficiency anemia until proven otherwise. Iron deficiency anemia in this population is most commonly due to a chronic GI bleed, and colon cancer needs to be ruled out in all patients who present this with iron deficiency anemia. Other causes of iron deficiency anemia are possible, but they are lower on the differential. Anemia of chronic disease is a possibility, but this patient has no history of prior or chronic illness. Lead poisoning is possible but is more commonly seen in small children who ingest paint chips from old homes. Sideroblastic anemia and thalassemias are unlikely in this patient because we would expect these patients to have been diagnosed in childhood.

2. **Suppose this woman were 30 years old. What would be the most likely cause of her anemia?**

   In a woman of reproductive age, iron deficiency is usually caused by menorrhagia (heavy bleeding during menstruation) or pregnancy. In pregnancy, both the volume of RBCs and plasma expand, but the latter increases to a greater degree, resulting in a dilutional anemia. However, you would still want to rule out GI bleed through fecal occult stool testing to affirm that this underlying pathology is not missed.

3. **Suppose this woman were instead a 12-year-old boy who had recently emigrated from rural India. What would be the most likely cause of his anemia?**

   Hookworms (e.g., *Ancylostoma duodenale, Necator americanus*) are one of the leading causes of iron deficiency anemia internationally and should be considered in patients who have recently emigrated from developing countries where access to clean water and sanitation may be limited. Hookworms penetrate the skin from the soil and cause iron deficiency by attaching to the intestinal walls and feeding on the host's blood.

STEP 1 SECRET

The compulsive ingestion of nonfood substances, such as paper, clay, metal, chalk, soil, and sand, is called pica *and is frequently seen in patients with iron deficiency anemia. It is believed that mineral deficiency can trigger an individual to crave and ingest nonfood items to replete these minerals. On the Step 1 exam, pica is pathognomonic for iron deficiency anemia in patients without psychiatric illness or developmental delay.*

4. Suppose the patient in Case 12.3 presented with a burning sensation of the tongue, difficulty swallowing, and progressively worsening fatigue and shortness of breath on exertion. What syndrome associated with iron deficiency anemia would you be worried about?

   Plummer-Vinson syndrome, a clinically rare but high-yield syndrome, is characterized by the triad of iron deficiency anemia, esophageal webs, and atrophic glossitis. Patients typically present with a painful tongue, dysphagia, and odynophagia in addition to symptoms of iron deficiency anemia. On physical examination, a shiny, red tongue with an absence of papillae, inflammation of the lips (cheilitis), and spoon-shaped nails (koilonychias) are commonly appreciated. The cause of this syndrome is unknown but responds well to iron supplementation. However, patients with this condition are at an increased risk of squamous cell carcinoma of the esophagus.

5. How is dietary iron circulated throughout the body?

   Dietary iron is primarily absorbed in the proximal duodenum, where the acidic pH and presence of ferric reductase enzyme facilitate the conversion of ferric iron (Fe^{3+}) to ferrous iron (Fe^{2+}), which is more rapidly absorbed by enterocytes. Dietary iron is then transported out of the enterocyte and into circulation by the transmembrane protein ferroportin. Once outside the cell, ferrous iron (Fe^{2+}) is converted back to ferric iron (Fe^{3+}) and complexed to transferrin for intravascular transport. Transferrin is secreted by the liver and delivers iron to all cells of the body, particularly those in the liver, the bone marrow, and macrophages. Iron is then stored intracellularly complexed to the storage protein ferritin. This iron-storage complex (Fig. 12.4) is referred to as *hemosiderin*.

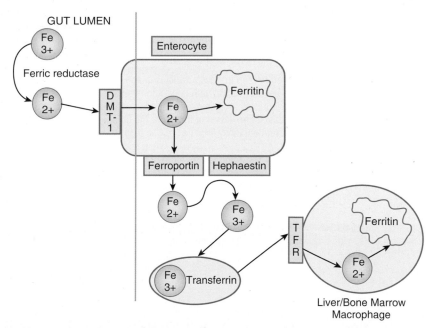

Figure 12.4. Iron absorption and storage process. *DMT-1,* Divalent metal transporter 1; *TFR,* transferrin receptor.

6. How is iron absorption regulated?

   Iron absorption is regulated by the protein hepcidin, which downregulates ferroportin expression on enterocytes and mononuclear phagocytes. When iron stores in the body are high, hepcidin expression increases, and release of iron into the circulation decreases secondary to ferroportin downregulation. When iron stores are low, hepcidin production is decreased. It is noteworthy to mention that hepcidin is increased by proinflammatory stimuli such as interleukin-6 (IL-6). This becomes important when distinguishing iron deficiency anemia from anemia of chronic disease, which will be discussed later in this chapter.

   Other factors that influence iron absorption are listed below. Most are not high yield for Step 1 but may be useful to know.

Increased absorption: organic iron, ferrous iron (Fe^{2+}), vitamin C, acids (e.g., citrate), low iron stores, high erythropoietin, pregnancy.

Decreased absorption: inorganic iron, ferric iron (Fe^{3+}), alkali (e.g., phosphates), high iron stores, low erythropoietin, infection, tannins (i.e., excessive tea drinking).

CASE 12.3 CONTINUED:

Iron study results are as follows:
  Serum iron decreased
  Ferritin decreased
  TIBC increased
  Corrected reticulocyte count 1.5% (decreased)
  Peripheral blood smear shows microcytic, hypochromic (pale) RBCs

7. **How does the peripheral blood smear and reticulocyte count support the diagnosis of iron deficiency anemia?**

   Microcytic, hypochromic (pale) RBCs are found in iron deficiency anemia. Because iron is required for hemoglobin synthesis, reduced cytoplasmic hemoglobin results in smaller (microcytic) cells. Additionally, the reddish hue of normal RBCs results from the binding of the iron found in heme to oxygen. If hemoglobin is low, there is less iron available to bind oxygen, resulting in what is described as a hypochromic RBC. These cells are also commonly described as having increased central pallor.

   The corrected reticulocyte count is low in this patient because low iron levels prevent the bone marrow from producing new RBC precursors. Remember that any anemia resulting from decreased erythropoiesis will result in a low reticulocyte count.

8. **What is the significance of the iron study results in this patient?**

   Decreased serum iron and ferritin, coupled with an increased TIBC, are consistent with a diagnosis of iron deficiency anemia. As expected, serum iron is low in this patient. Ferritin is the storage form of iron, particularly in the liver and bone marrow. Ferritin levels closely parallel the body stores of iron, such that in conditions of iron deficiency, ferritin is low, whereas in conditions of iron sequestration (e.g., anemia of chronic disease) or iron overload (e.g., hemochromatosis), ferritin is high.

   TIBC measures the capacity of the blood to bind iron with transferrin and correlates with serum transferrin levels. A helpful way to think about this value is to associate TIBC with how much the body wants or needs iron. In iron deficiency anemia, the low serum iron contributes to an increased proportion of unbound transferrin, and the liver is producing more transferrin to facilitate increased circulation of iron from the enterocytes to tissues (e.g., to the bone marrow to make more RBCs). Therefore in iron deficiency anemia, TIBC is high, and the body is trying to absorb as much iron as possible.

   Serum transferrin (measured indirectly by TIBC) and ferritin stores typically show an inverse relationship. High ferritin levels will reduce transferrin synthesis, whereas low ferritin levels will stimulate transferrin synthesis. Because ferritin levels are low in iron deficiency anemia, transferrin and TIBC will be high (Table 12.3).

Table 12.3. Comparison of Anemia of Chronic Disease and Iron Deficiency Anemia

	Characteristic Result	
STUDY	**ANEMIA OF CHRONIC DISEASE**	**IRON DEFICIENCY ANEMIA**
Serum iron	Low	Low
Total iron-binding capacity (TIBC)	Low to normal	High
Ferritin	Normal to high	Low
Percent transferrin saturation	Low	Low
Bone marrow iron stores	High	Low

CASE 12.3 CONTINUED:

Further history reveals small amounts of darkish blood in her stool for several months. Physical examination is negative for hemorrhoids, and fecal occult testing reveals blood in her stool. You order a colonoscopy, and a large necrotic mass is found and removed. Pathologic diagnosis is reported as adenocarcinoma.

9. What is the cause of her iron deficiency anemia?

The cause of this patient's iron deficiency anemia is chronic, slow blood loss from the intestinal tract secondary to malignancy of the colon. Remember that GI bleeds are the most common cause of iron deficiency anemia in middle-aged and older patients who are otherwise healthy; thus this diagnosis needs to be ruled out in all of these patients.

CASE 12.3 CONTINUED:

Suppose this woman had a history of *Helicobacter pylori* infection and came to the emergency department with a rapidly bleeding peptic ulcer. She is found to have a hemoglobin of 8.1 g/dL with an MCV of 81 fL.

10. How would the temporal course of an intestinal bleed affect whether the anemia will be normocytic or microcytic?

With acute, rapid GI bleeds, patients will initially present with a normocytic anemia. As the body ramps up RBC production to compensate for the loss of blood, RDW (see Basic Concepts question 6) will increase because of the release of large, immature reticulocytes into the circulation. When hemoglobin levels have dropped significantly, a microcytic anemia eventually develops as iron stores are drained to make new RBC precursors. RDW will remain elevated due to significant variation in RBC volume, though MCV (i.e., average RBC size) will decrease at this time.

SUMMARY BOX: IRON DEFICIENCY ANEMIA

- Presentation: Generalized fatigue and pallor
  - Plummer-Vinson Syndrome: Iron-deficiency anemia, esophageal web, and atrophic glossitis
- Epidemiology
  - Common in women of reproductive age who have heavy periods or are pregnant
  - Closely associated with malignancy of the colon in middle-aged and older individuals with no significant past medical history
- Pathophysiology: Decreased hemoglobin synthesis as a result of reduced iron stores; this can be caused by a multitude of reasons:
  - Poor intake of dietary iron
  - Iron loss through bleeding
  - Parasitic infection, especially hookworms
- Diagnosis
  - Decreased hemoglobin and decreased mean corpuscular volume (MCV) on complete blood count (CBC)
  - Microcytic, hypochromic red blood cells (RBCs) on peripheral blood smear
  - Low serum iron, low ferritin, and high total iron-binding capacity (TIBC) on iron study
- Complications: Fatigue, shortness of breath, pica (rarely)
- Treatment
  - Treatment of underlying pathology
  - Ferrous sulfate

CASE 12.4

A 42-year-old woman with rheumatoid arthritis (RA) comes into your office complaining of increasing fatigue and shortness of breath with exertion. Her CBC shows a microcytic anemia.

1. What is the differential diagnosis for microcytic anemia?

Iron deficiency anemia, sideroblastic anemia, lead poisoning, thalassemia, and anemia of chronic disease are all considerations.

CASE 12.4 CONTINUED:

Iron studies reveal low serum Fe, elevated serum ferritin, and reduced TIBC.

2. What is your diagnosis now?

Anemia of chronic disease secondary to RA typically presents as a mild hypochromic anemia, although it can also be normochromic and normocytic.

3. Explain the elevated ferritin and low iron in anemia of chronic disease.

The chronic inflammatory response results in large amounts of hepcidin, which sequesters iron, resulting in reduced levels of plasma iron. Bodily stores of iron are normal but unavailable for erythropoiesis. This is shown by the normal levels of ferritin, which is the intracellular storage form of iron. Ferritin levels closely parallel body stores of iron. Therefore ferritin levels are low in iron deficiency anemia but are normal to high in anemia of chronic disease. Ferritin levels may be elevated above normal in anemia of chronic disease because ferritin is an acute phase reactant secreted by the liver in inflammatory conditions.

Note: The postulated reason for iron sequestration in states of chronic inflammation is that this is the body's response to prevent microbes that have potentially invaded the host from acquiring iron required for their growth.

4. Why are transferrin saturation *and* TIBC reduced?

Transferrin is secreted by the liver and binds iron in the bloodstream. TIBC is a measure of transferrin that is not bound to iron. The mechanism of low TIBC in anemia of chronic disease is not actually known, but it is postulated that the chronic inflammatory response decreases transferrin production by the liver. In addition, the elevated levels of hepcidin sequester iron in the bloodstream, resulting in reduced transferrin saturation with iron. Recall from earlier that hepcidin downregulates cell surface expression of ferroportin and promotes internalization and degradation of ferroportin inhibiting intestinal iron absorption.

CASE 12.4 CONTINUED:

Further history reveals that her RA has been reasonably well controlled on methotrexate and nonsteroidal antiinflammatory drugs (NSAIDs).

5. Based on this additional information, what do you have to rule out as a cause for her anemia?

NSAIDs can cause gastric ulcers and upper intestinal bleeding. In a patient chronically on NSAIDs, you have to rule out bleeding and resultant iron deficiency as a cause for her anemia. This can be done with an occult blood test or upper endoscopy if suspicion is high enough. Methotrexate can suppress the bone marrow, resulting in a pancytopenia. This can be ruled out with a CBC by looking at all three cell lines (i.e., RBCs, WBCs, and platelets).

6. Why does her long-standing inflammatory condition predispose her to developing anemia?

Chronic inflammatory disorders with systemic involvement result in elevated plasma levels of many cytokines. These cytokines increase the phagocytic activity of immune cells, particularly in the spleen, resulting in increased phagocytic destruction of RBCs and a decrease in RBC life span. Additionally, these cytokines inhibit the secretion of erythropoietin, which normally stimulates erythropoiesis in the bone marrow. Another contributing factor is that hepcidin, which is released by inflammatory cells, binds serum iron and makes it unavailable for erythropoiesis. Patients with anemia of chronic disease typically respond well to exogenously administered erythropoietin.

7. Differentiate between anemia of chronic disease and iron deficiency anemia on the basis of plasma iron concentration, TIBC, ferritin, transferrin saturation, and bone marrow iron stores.

See Table 12.3, which compares the values of these tests for both types of anemia.

STEP 1 SECRET

The information listed in Table 12.3 is particularly high yield for the USMLE.

SUMMARY BOX: ANEMIA OF CHRONIC DISEASE

- Typically seen as mild anemia in patients with chronic inflammatory conditions including rheumatologic diseases, malignancy, and infections such as tuberculosis and endocarditis
- Characterized by a functional iron deficiency: Impairment of iron mobilization despite sufficient iron stores
- Symptoms: Fatigue, dyspnea on exertion, symptoms of the underlying condition
- Laboratory tests: Low serum iron and low total iron-binding capacity (TIBC), elevated ferritin
- Treatment: Treat the underlying condition. Severe anemia responds well to exogenous erythropoietin.

CASE 12.5

A 65-year-old man with a history of peptic ulcer disease who is otherwise healthy is evaluated for a 2-month history of mild fatigue and paresthesias in both of his feet. Laboratory values are as follows:

Hemoglobin: 10.3 g/dL (normal: male, 13.5–17.5 g/dL; female, 12.0–16.0 g/dL)

Hematocrit: 31.0% (normal: male, 41%–53%; female, 36%–46%)

MCV: 114 μm^3 (normal: 80–100 μm^3)

1. What is the differential diagnosis for this patient?

A low hemoglobin and hematocrit in combination with an MCV greater than 100 μm^3 is diagnostic of a macrocytic anemia. Recall from the Basic Concepts section of this chapter that macrocytic anemias can be further divided into megaloblastic (e.g., caused by impaired DNA synthesis) and nonmegaloblastic causes.

CASE 12.5 CONTINUED:

Further workup reveals the following:
    Corrected reticulocyte count 1%
Peripheral blood smear results are as shown in Fig. 12.5.

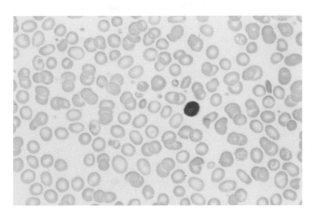

Figure 12.5. Peripheral blood smear in Case 12.5. *(From Goldman L, Schafer Al. Goldman-Cecil Medicine Volumes 1 & 2. 25th ed. Philadelphia: Elsevier: 2015.)*

2. Explain the peripheral blood smear results. How does this help narrow your differential diagnosis?

The peripheral blood smear reveals large, oval-shaped RBCs and hypersegmented neutrophils, both of which are characteristics of megaloblastic anemia (e.g., vitamin B_{12} or folate deficiency). Recall that vitamin B_{12} and folate are both required for nucleic acid synthesis via recycling of tetrahydrofolate (THF; discussed further in question 4 of Case 12.5). In the face of vitamin B_{12} or folate deficiency, DNA synthesis is impaired, but RNA and protein synthesis will remain unaffected. Thus cell cytoplasm will continue to expand but cellular division will not ensue, leading to the formation of megaloblasts (enlarged cells). Because impaired DNA synthesis will affect any rapidly dividing cell (e.g., neutrophils), these are among the first abnormal cells to appear on a peripheral blood smear, and they will appear large and hypersegmented (≥ 5 lobes) because of a lack of timely cell division.

Both vitamin B_{12} and folate deficiency are associated with the aforementioned peripheral blood smear findings, but vitamin B_{12} also plays a role in the synthesis of myelin and presents with neurologic symptoms (e.g., paresthesias), as seen in this patient. Thus this patient is most likely to have a vitamin B_{12} deficiency.

STEP 1 SECRET

Fig. 12.5 is particularly high yield for the USMLE. You should automatically associate hypersegmented neutrophils with vitamin B_{12} or folate deficiency.

3. Why is the reticulocyte count low in this patient?

Impaired DNA synthesis, such as that caused by folate or vitamin B_{12} deficiency, halts the development of reticulocytes in the bone marrow, leading to an insufficient response to the anemia.

4. What are the normal functions of vitamin B_{12}, and how do these functions relate to the clinical signs and symptoms of vitamin B_{12} deficiency?

Vitamin B_{12} is involved in two enzymatic reactions, one that catalyzes both the conversion of homocysteine to methionine and the recycling of methyltetrahydrofolate to THF and another that catalyzes the conversion of methylmalonyl coenzyme A to succinyl coenzyme A.

The anemia seen in vitamin B_{12} deficiency is believed to be due to reduced levels of THF, the form of folic acid involved in DNA synthesis.

The pathogenesis of the neuropathy seen in patients with a vitamin B_{12} deficiency is not entirely known. One popular hypothesis is that because vitamin B_{12} is required to convert methylmalonyl-CoA to succinyl-CoA, which is needed to properly myelinate nerves, a vitamin B_{12} deficiency would limit the production of succinyl-CoA and therefore limit nerve myelination. Another popular hypothesis attributes the neuropathy to the impaired methionine synthesis seen in vitamin B_{12} deficiency because methionine serves as a precursor for *S*-adenosylmethionine, which is needed to synthesize various myelin proteins and phospholipids.

Decreased myelination of the dorsal and lateral columns and spinocerebellar tracts (subacute combined degeneration) results in decreased vibration sense, decreased proprioception, gait apraxia, and paresthesias. Note that anemia always precedes neurologic symptoms in vitamin B_{12} deficiency (Fig. 12.6).

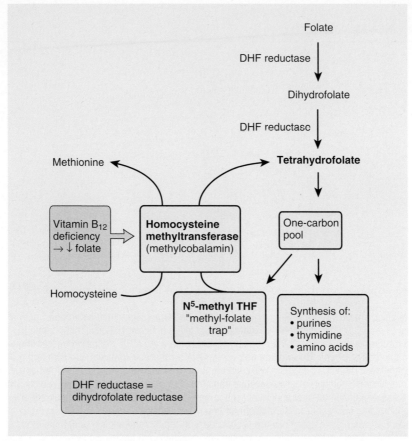

Figure 12.6. Role of folate and vitamin B_{12}. The only way to re-form tetrahydrofolate is via vitamin B_{12}–dependent synthesis of methionine, the methionine salvage pathway. *(From Clark A.* Crash Course: Metabolism and Nutrition. *Philadelphia: WB Saunders; 2005.)*

Clinical Pearl

Giving folate to a patient with a vitamin B_{12} deficiency can temporarily mask signs and symptoms of macrocytic anemia, although neurologic function will continue to worsen.

---

5. In addition to the fact that vitamin B_{12} deficiency presents with symptoms of neuropathy, how else might this condition be distinguished from folate deficiency?

Vitamin B_{12} deficiency can be distinguished from folate deficiency via blood work. This is especially useful in patients who have existing neurologic pathologies such as a patient with peripheral neuropathy secondary to diabetes. Vitamin B_{12} deficiency is associated with increased homocysteine and increased methylmalonic acid because both folate recycling and the succinyl-CoA myelination pathway are disrupted. Folate deficiency presents with increased homocysteine but normal methylmalonic acid because folate is not involved in the succinyl-CoA myelination pathway (Fig. 12.7).

CASE 12.5 CONTINUED:

An upper endoscopy and gastric biopsy show chronic inflammation of the mucosal lining of the gastric fundus.

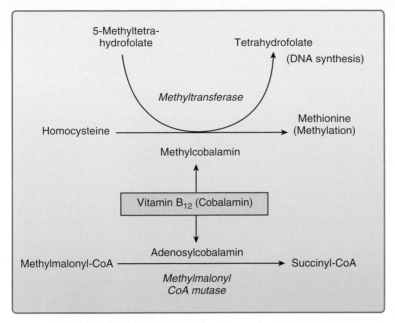

Figure 12.7. The biochemical role of cobalamin.

6. What is the pathogenesis of this man's vitamin B_{12} deficiency?

Chronic gastritis, either autoimmune or idiopathic in origin, results in destruction of gastric parietal cells that are found primarily in the fundus of the stomach (i.e., atrophic gastritis). When autoimmune destruction of parietal cells occurs, this is called *pernicious anemia*. Parietal cells normally produce intrinsic factor, which facilitates vitamin B_{12} absorption by the terminal ileum. Loss of parietal cells and intrinsic factor prevents adequate vitamin B_{12} absorption.

7. Explain how vitamin B_{12} is absorbed by the intestine.

Vitamin B_{12} absorption is defined by a complicated, stepwise digestive process where each step is dependent upon binding proteins synthesized in the previous step. Therefore proper vitamin B_{12} absorption requires working salivary glands, stomach, pancreas, and terminal ileum.

1. **Mouth:** Dietary B_{12} is initially coupled to animal protein when consumed. The protein is mechanically broken down, and R-factor is synthesized by the salivary glands.
2. **Stomach:** Vitamin B_{12} is separated from dietary protein by the enzyme pepsin, which is synthesized by the chief cells of the stomach. Free B_{12} is then complexed to R-factor to protect it from degradation by stomach acid. Intrinsic factor (IF) is secreted by the parietal cells of the gastric fundus in response to histamine, gastrin, and the presence of food.
3. **Duodenum:** Pancreatic proteases, such as trypsin and chymotrypsin, free B_{12} from R-factor. The freed B_{12} is now complexed to IF.
4. **Terminal ileum:** B_{12}-IF complexes are absorbed by enterocytes via receptors that are specific for these complexes. Note that enterocytes cannot absorb free B_{12}. IF also helps protect vitamin B_{12} from being broken down by intestinal bacteria.

8. What are the some of the other causes of vitamin B_{12} deficiency?

Vitamin B_{12} is primarily found in animal products, so strict vegans are at risk for this deficiency. It takes a very long time (at least several years) to deplete the body's stores of vitamin B_{12}, so deficiency due to nutritional issues is usually only seen in those whose diets have lacked animal products for many years. Additionally, malabsorption of vitamin B_{12} can be caused by ileal resection, gastric bypass surgery, bacterial overgrowth, celiac sprue, tropical sprue, Crohn disease, proton-pump inhibitors (PPIs), or *Diphyllobothrium latum* (fish tapeworm) infection.

CASE 12.5 CONTINUED:

You do a Schilling test, which confirms your diagnosis of pernicious anemia.

9. How does the Schilling test work?

The Schilling test is used to determine whether the cause of vitamin B_{12} deficiency can be attributed to pernicious anemia. It is performed in a stepwise fashion:

1. Unlabeled vitamin B_{12} is injected intramuscularly to temporarily saturate B_{12} receptors, particularly in the liver. This will prevent any additional B_{12} from binding to these receptors; if absorbed by the GI tract, this B_{12} will pass directly into the urine.

2. Radioactively labeled vitamin B_{12} is then administered orally. As mentioned, this B_{12} will be excreted into the urine, where it is measured. If less than 10% of the amount that was administered orally is found in the urine, this indicates poor absorption of vitamin B_{12} in the intestine (e.g., as seen in patients with pernicious anemia) because the vitamin B_{12} must be absorbed into the body via the small intestine to be later excreted by the kidney.

3. The test is repeated with the addition of exogenous IF. If pernicious anemia is the cause of vitamin B_{12} deficiency, IF will improve vitamin B_{12} absorption.

4. If pernicious anemia is not the culprit, the test may be repeated with the addition of antibiotics. If bacterial overgrowth is the cause of vitamin B_{12} deficiency, then antibiotics should improve vitamin B_{12} absorption.

5. The test may also be repeated with the addition of pancreatic enzymes. If pancreatitis or pancreatic insufficiency is the cause of vitamin B_{12} deficiency, then pancreatic enzymes will improve vitamin B_{12} absorption.

Note: The Schilling test is no longer widely used owing to concerns about use of radiation. However, this test nicely demonstrates the pathophysiology of vitamin B_{12} deficiency due to inadequate IF production.

10. What is the treatment for pernicious anemia?

Although high-dose oral therapy with vitamin B_{12} is sufficient in some patients, intramuscular injections of vitamin B_{12} are often required. Because vitamin B_{12} is water-soluble, overdose is not usually a concern in these patients. Remember, oral therapy is not effective for patients with autoimmune pernicious anemia because vitamin B_{12} cannot be absorbed without intrinsic factor!

11. What are some of the causes of folate deficiency?

Poor nutrition, increased folate requirement, and certain medications cause folate deficiency. Folate is primarily found in green leafy vegetables, and deficiency is commonly seen in those with poor diets (e.g., patients with alcohol use disorder) or those who tend to overcook their vegetables (such as the elderly, who may have problems chewing harder foods). Alcohol decreases the GI tract's ability to absorb folate, which results in increased folate excretion in the urine. Overcooking foods destroys folate altogether. Pregnant women and patients with hemolytic anemia also have an increased need for folate to support rapid cell turnover. Remember that maternal folate deficiency is associated with defects in neural tube closure during early fetal development and may present as spina bifida, myelomeningocele, or, rarely, anencephaly in the fetus. In addition, drugs such as methotrexate and phenytoin may interfere with folate-dependent biochemical pathways and can lead to folate deficiency.

SUMMARY BOX: VITAMIN B_{12} AND FOLATE DEFICIENCIES

VITAMIN B_{12} DEFICIENCY

- Presentation: Generalized fatigue and potential paresthesias in a strict vegan or an individual with gastrointestinal disease (e.g., pernicious anemia)
- Pathophysiology: Results in impaired DNA synthesis and cell division as well as impaired nerve myelination, causing macrocytic anemia and neurodegeneration
- Diagnosis
  - Decreased hemoglobin, increased mean corpuscular volume (MCV), and pancytopenia on complete blood cell (CBC) count
  - Macrocytic megaloblastic red blood cells (RBCs) and hypersegmented neutrophils on peripheral blood smear
  - Increased serum levels of lactate dehydrogenase (LDH), homocysteine, and methylmalonic acid
- Complications: Peripheral neuropathy, dorsal column degeneration (decreased vibration and proprioception), lateral corticospinal degeneration (upper and lower extremity weakness), spinocerebellar tract degeneration (ataxia), and dementia
- Treatment: Oral or intramuscular injections of vitamin B_{12} weekly until levels return to normal

FOLATE DEFICIENCY

- Presentation: Generalized fatigue in an elderly patient or patient with alcohol use disorder
- Pathophysiology: Leads to impaired DNA synthesis and cell division, resulting in macrocytic anemia
- Diagnosis
  - Decreased hemoglobin, increased MCV, and pancytopenia on CBC
  - Macrocytic, megaloblastic RBCs and hypersegmented neutrophils on peripheral blood smear
  - Increased serum levels of LDH and homocysteine with normal levels of methylmalonic acid
  - Decreased total RBC folate levels
- Complications: Neural tube defects in children born to mothers with folate deficiency during pregnancy
- Treatment: Oral folate supplementation

---

12. Cover each column of Table 12.4 and try to fill in the remaining information for yourself.

CASE 12.6

An 8-year-old boy is brought to your office by his mother for evaluation of several weeks of fatigue. Physical examination is significant for bilateral conjunctival pallor. CBC shows hemoglobin of 7.2 g/dL, MCV of 80 fL, and reticulocyte count of 11%. Total bilirubin is 2.0 mg/dL.

Table 12.4. Vitamin B$_{12}$ and Folate Deficiency

FEATURE	VITAMIN B$_{12}$	FOLATE
Food sources	Animal products	Vegetables
Stores	Long term, 2–12 years	Short term, 4–5 months
Water-soluble	Yes	Yes
Site and mechanism of absorption	Terminal ileum Absorbed with intrinsic factor	Duodenum and proximal jejunum
Function	Cofactor for enzymatic reactions important for DNA synthesis and myelination	1-carbon carrier
Dietary deficiency	Uncommon—occurs with vegan diet	Common—occurs in alcoholics; a leafy green salad will increase serum levels but not RBC folate, so testing for both is required
Neurologic damage	Yes	No

1. **What is the differential diagnosis for a normocytic anemia?**
   The differential diagnosis for normocytic anemia is categorized into hemolytic and nonhemolytic anemia. Refer to Fig. 12.1 for possible causes of normocytic anemia. The differential diagnosis includes hemoglobinopathies, enzyme deficiencies, aplastic anemia, anemia of chronic disease, chronic kidney disease, etc.

CASE 12.6 CONTINUED:

Patient history reveals that although both parents are healthy, the father did have his spleen removed years ago for "some type of blood problem."

2. **How does this change your differential diagnosis?**
   With a possible family history of anemia, you should focus your diagnosis on genetic causes of anemia. Hereditary spherocytosis, G6PD deficiency, sickle cell anemia, and pyruvate kinase deficiency are all options. Identifying the inheritance pattern of a hereditary anemia is very helpful in determining the cause of the anemia. G6PD deficiency is X-linked. (Remember, by definition, X-linked diseases are never passed from father to son!) Pyruvate kinase deficiency is autosomal recessive, so even though his father is "affected," his mother would also have to be a carrier of this rare condition. This seems unlikely, although not impossible. Sickle cell anemia, another autosomal recessive condition, presents similar genetic unlikelihood. Also, sickle cell anemia tends to occur in African Americans, making the diagnosis of sickle cell improbable. Hereditary spherocytosis, an autosomal dominant condition, would typically present with this pedigree of affected father and son. Also, this disease is quite common among individuals of Northern European descent.

STEP 1 SECRET

Inheritance patterns of genetic diseases and their associated epidemiology are very important (and high yield!) for Step 1. Taking the time to distinguish between diseases with similar presentations but different genetic pedigrees may often unlock a diagnosis for you. Pay special attention to diseases that affect particular ethnic, racial, or age groups. Although never an absolute, these demographic clues may also point you in the right direction of diagnosis.

CASE 12.6 CONTINUED:

A peripheral blood smear shows spherical RBCs that lack central pallor as well as Howell-Jolly bodies (Fig. 12.8). A laboratory test using test tubes filled with solutions of increasing salt concentration reveals an abnormally increased osmotic fragility of RBCs.

3. **What is the diagnosis?**
   Hereditary spherocytosis is the diagnosis.

4. **What is the etiology of this condition, and why do the RBCs assume a spherical conformation?**
   Most commonly, hereditary spherocytosis is caused by dysfunction of proteins involved in stabilizing the RBC membrane to the cytoskeleton. Normally, the protein spectrin provides stability to the RBC plasma membrane by interacting with

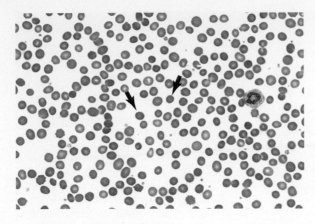

Figure 12.8. Peripheral blood smear shows numerous spherocytes, dark-staining red blood cells lacking central pallor (*arrows*). *(From Aster J, Pozdnyakova O, Kutok J. Hematopathology: A Volume in the High Yield Pathology Series. Philadelphia: Saunders; 2013.)*

cytoskeletal proteins such as ankyrin, protein 4.2, and band 3. Defects in any of these proteins can lead to the development of hereditary spherocytosis through destabilization of the RBC membrane. In the absence of the normal biconcave shape, the degree of central pallor created by hemoglobin displacement to the periphery (normally approximately one-third of the diameter of the RBC) is markedly reduced.

5. What is the osmotic fragility test, and how does it help diagnose hereditary spherocytosis?
   The osmotic fragility test involves placing a patient's RBCs in increasingly hypotonic salt solutions. In the hypotonic solution, water rushes into the RBC, causing it to swell and ultimately burst. As a result of the unstable membrane and decreased surface area to volume ratio in hereditary spherocytosis, the RBCs will burst at a less hypotonic solution concentration when compared with a normal RBC. This is the basis for the positive osmotic fragility test, which is diagnostic for hereditary spherocytosis.

CASE 12.6 CONTINUED:

Physical examination is notable for pallor, mild jaundice, and an enlarged nontender spleen. Both the direct and indirect Coombs tests are negative.

6. How do these Coombs tests work? Why are they both negative?
   Both Coombs tests are assays for antibodies in the plasma or antigens on the RBC surface that lead to an intravascular hemolysis due to antigen-antibody interaction. The direct Coombs test looks for antibodies *on* the patient's RBCs. The indirect Coombs test checks for antibodies to RBCs in the patient's serum. In hereditary spherocytosis, you would not expect an immune process to be a primary cause of RBC destruction. Instead, the abnormal RBCs are sequestered in the spleen because of their lack of distensibility and, as a result, are subject to extravascular hemolysis.
   More detailed information about direct and indirect Coombs tests can be found in Chapter 15.

7. What types of anemia will have a positive Coombs test?
   Autoimmune hemolytic anemias have positive Coombs tests. These disorders include warm and cold agglutinin and are idiopathic. In these disorders, the patient forms autoantibodies that bind to the RBC surface, resulting in destruction of the RBC. Warm agglutinin antibodies are immunoglobulin G (IgG), whereas cold agglutinin antibodies are immunoglobulin M (IgM).

8. Why is splenomegaly seen in this condition?
   During their normal course through the spleen, RBCs must undergo impressive conformational changes to exit the splenic cords (i.e., cords of Billroth) and enter the splenic sinusoids. Spherical RBCs are much less able to undergo this conformational change than are normal biconcave RBCs. As a result, spherocytes obstruct the splenic cords, resulting in splenomegaly. They are, ultimately, phagocytosed by the splenic macrophages at an abnormally high rate, leading to anemia.

9. Why might a splenectomy be reasonable for this patient?
   Although splenectomy does not fix the fundamental defect in these RBCs, it does prevent the anemia. Removing the spleen prevents the high rate of extravascular hemolysis that causes the anemia seen in this condition.

CASE 12.6 CONTINUED:

About 20 years later, this same patient is seen in a local emergency department with colicky right upper quadrant pain that increases after eating. He has a positive Murphy sign.

10. What is the most likely diagnosis? Why is this patient at increased risk for this condition?
Cholelithiasis is the diagnosis. Patients with hereditary spherocytosis are at increased risk for gallstones because of hemolysis and development of bilirubin (pigment) stones in the bile duct system. As expected, the incidence of bilirubin stone formation will be much lower if a splenectomy is performed to decrease the rate of hemolysis. However, given the relative fragility of spherocytes, postsplenectomy patients still have a moderately increased rate of hemolysis. Thus elevated indirect bilirubin can predispose to bilirubin (pigmented) gallstones.

SUMMARY BOX: HEREDITARY SPHEROCYTOSIS

- Defect in red blood cell (RBC) membrane protein (spectrin or ankyrin) causing abnormally shaped erythrocytes due to an unstable RBC membrane
- RBCs become sequestered in the spleen and are hemolyzed
- Inheritance pattern: Autosomal dominant
- Symptoms: Hemolysis (elevated bilirubin and decreased haptoglobin, jaundice), splenomegaly, gallstones
- Laboratory tests: Increased osmotic fragility, spherocytes on peripheral smear, reticulocytosis, hyperbilirubinemia
- Treatment: Splenectomy plus vaccination for *Streptococcus pneumoniae, Haemophilus influenzae, Neisseria meningitidis*

CASE 12.7

A 28-year-old African American man is planning to travel to India for work. He is given quinidine for antimalarial prophylaxis. Several days later, he becomes fatigued and has mild back pain and dark urine. He returns for evaluation and, at this time, appears jaundiced.
Laboratory values are as follows:
Hemoglobin: 11.5 g/dL (normal: male, 13.5–17.5 g/dL; female, 12.0–16.0 g/dL)
Hematocrit: 34.5% (normal: male, 41%–53%; female, 36%–46%)
MCV: 95 μm^3 (normal: 80–100 μm^3)

---

1. What is the differential diagnosis for this patient?
A low hemoglobin and hematocrit in combination with a normal MCV is diagnostic of a normocytic anemia. Recall from the Basic Concepts section that normocytic anemias can be associated with either normal or abnormal reticulocyte responses. Anemias that cause a low reticulocyte count, such as renal disease or aplastic anemia, are unlikely in a healthy young man with acute symptoms. (This may be helpful to keep in mind if a reticulocyte count is not specifically given to you on the Step 1 exam.) Normocytic anemias with an appropriate reticulocyte response can further be separated into anemias with an intrinsic or extrinsic defect, though this cannot be deciphered based on these laboratory values alone. In this patient, G6PD deficiency should top the differential diagnosis because this condition is commonly triggered by antimalarial therapy and is most commonly seen in African American men. Other possible causes of anemia in this patient include HbC defect, paroxysmal nocturnal hemoglobinuria, autoimmune hemolytic anemia, and RBC destruction secondary to infection. Hereditary spherocytosis, pyruvate kinase deficiency (hemolytic anemia of the newborn), and sickle cell anemia are usually diagnosed at birth or early in childhood and are unlikely etiologies in this patient. Microangiopathic anemia is unlikely in a patient without predisposing coagulopathy (e.g., DIC, thrombotic thrombocytopenic purpura [TTP], hemolytic uremic syndrome [HUS], systemic lupus erythematosus [SLE]), and macroangiopathic anemia is unlikely in a patient without a prosthetic heart valve.

CASE 12.7 CONTINUED:

The peripheral smear is shown in Fig. 12.9.

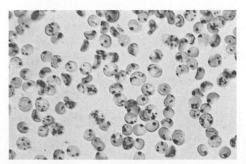

Figure 12.9. Peripheral blood smear in Case 12.7. *(From McPherson RA, Pincus MR. Henry's Clinical Diagnosis and Management by Laboratory Methods. 22nd ed. Philadelphia: Saunders; 2012.)*

2. What is the most likely diagnosis based on these findings?
   This peripheral smear is notable for Heinz bodies (RBC inclusions) and bite cells, both of which are consistent with a diagnosis of G6PD deficiency. G6PD deficiency is an X-linked recessive disorder that results in a defect in the G6PD enzyme; G6PD catalyzes the rate-limiting step in the hexose monophosphate pathway (pentose phosphate shunt; discussed further in subsequent question 3). Absence of G6PD results in oxidative damage to RBCs, leading to intravascular hemolysis. Oxidative stress also causes Hb to precipitate within the RBC, resulting in the formation of Heinz bodies. These inclusion bodies are removed by splenic macrophages as these RBCs pass through the splenic cords, producing so-called *bite cells* (Fig. 12.10).

   G6PD deficiency is the most common inherited hemolytic anemia and typically affects men of African and Mediterranean descent. As seen with sickle cell anemia, mutations in the G6PD gene are believed to be protective against *P. falciparum* malaria.

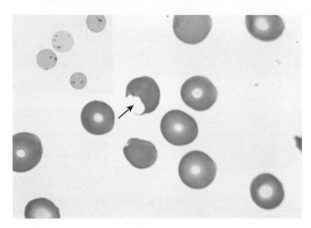

Figure 12.10. Peripheral blood smear in glucose-6-phosphate dehydrogenase deficiency. The *arrow* shows a bite cell with part of the red blood cell membrane removed. The *inset* shows a peripheral blood smear with a supravital stain visualizing punctate inclusions representing denatured hemoglobin (Heinz bodies). *(From Kumar V, Fausto N, Abbas A.* Robbins and Cotran Pathologic Basis of Disease. *7th ed. Philadelphia: WB Saunders; 2004; Fig. 13-8. Inset from Wickramasinghe SN, McCullough J.* Blood and Bone Marrow Pathology. *London: Churchill Livingstone; 2003.)*

3. What is the normal function of the hexose monophosphate shunt in red blood cells?
   In RBCs, the hexose monophosphate shunt (pentose phosphate pathway) is used primarily to generate the reduced form of nicotinamide adenine dinucleotide phosphate (NADPH). The NADPH generated recycles glutathione from its oxidized state to its active reduced state. Reduced glutathione is involved in combating oxidative damage by reactive oxygen species. A defect in the G6PD enzyme leads to a shortage of reduced glutathione, which decreases the ability of RBCs to handle increased oxidative stress and predisposes RBCs to intravascular hemolysis.

STEP 1 SECRET

Common precipitators of oxidative stress to look for on Step 1 include fava beans, infection, and certain medications such as sulfa drugs (e.g., trimethoprim-sulfamethoxazole [TMP-SMX]), dapsone, isoniazid, antimalarial drugs (e.g., primaquine, chloroquine, quinidine), fluoroquinolones (e.g., ciprofloxacin), nitrofurantoin, and nonsteroidal antiinflammatory drugs (e.g., ibuprofen, aspirin).

CASE 12.7 CONTINUED:

On physical examination, you note scleral icterus and splenomegaly. Total bilirubin is elevated. Urinalysis is notable for gross blood, high urine sodium, and muddy brown granular casts.

4. Is this man's hyperbilirubinemia most likely caused by conjugated or unconjugated bilirubin?
   This patient's hyperbilirubinemia is most likely caused by unconjugated bilirubin, also known as *indirect bilirubin*. Recall from Chapter 7 that bilirubin is a breakdown product of heme and that hyperbilirubinemia can be broken down into prehepatic, hepatic, or posthepatic causes. Hemolytic anemias, such as G6PD deficiency, result in the release of large amounts of hemoglobin during periods of intense RBC destruction, subsequently leading to elevated unconjugated bilirubin levels. This massive release of unconjugated bilirubin overwhelms the liver's ability to process it, leading to a backup of unconjugated bilirubin in the bloodstream. Deposition of excess bilirubin in the eyes and skin results in scleral icterus and jaundice, respectively.

5. Is this patient's haptoglobin level likely to be high or low?
   Haptoglobin level is likely to be low. Haptoglobin is a plasma protein that sequesters free heme in the circulation. Therefore levels of haptoglobin would be reduced as the haptoglobin gets consumed by the large amount of free heme generated via oxidative damage and intravascular hemolysis.

6. **What renal diagnosis does his urinalysis reveal, and why is this occurring? What is his prognosis?**
Acute tubular necrosis (ATN) is the diagnosis. Gross blood, high urine sodium, and muddy brown casts are red flags for damage to the renal architecture. Muddy brown casts on urinalysis (UA) are diagnostic for ATN. In ATN, the acute drop in hemoglobin due to hemolysis causes ischemia and necrosis of the epithelial lining of the renal tubules. Without the epithelial lining, gross blood escapes into the urinary space, and reabsorption of electrolytes is significantly decreased, leading to high urine sodium. The muddy brown casts are composed of the necrosed, sloughed-off tubular epithelial cells passed into the urine. Prognosis is very good as long as the tubular basement membrane is intact. His renal function would be expected to recover within 1 to 2 weeks as the epithelial lining regenerates.

7. **What caused the appearance of gross blood in the urine?**
Oxidative stress and resultant hemolytic anemia can manifest as hemoglobinuria in some patients with G6PD deficiency.

Clinical Pearl

Individuals with glucose-6-phosphate dehydrogenase (G6PD) deficiency must be closely monitored during infections, particularly urinary tract infections, as many of the commonly prescribed medications for *Escherichia coli* cystitis are contraindicated in these patients because of increased risk of hemolysis.

STEP 1 SECRET

The classic vignette on boards for glucose-6-phosphate dehydrogenase (G6PD) deficiency is an African American individual who serves as a missionary worker in a remote area and is treated for malaria before the appearance of hemolytic anemia. However, be on the lookout for other pharmacologic triggers of hemolysis in patients with G6PD deficiency.

8. **What is the treatment for this man's condition?**
For the USMLE (and in clinical practice), always consider the least invasive intervention first. In this case, the oxidant stressor (quinidine) must be immediately discontinued to prevent additional hemolysis. Depending on the degree of anemia and symptom severity, RBC transfusion may be indicated. The only long-term treatment for G6PD deficiency is avoidance of the triggering substance(s).

CASE 12.7 CONTINUED:

Two days later, this man's hemoglobin is still 9.7 g/dL, but his MCV is now 105 fL.

9. **Why might the MCV be slightly elevated in this patient, and how does this reflect the self-limited nature of this hemolytic anemia?**
A compensatory erythrocytosis in response to hemolysis produces increased numbers of circulating reticulocytes. Reticulocytes are premature RBCs that are much larger than mature RBCs, and their increased size explains the increased MCV. Furthermore, it turns out that G6PD activity in reticulocytes is much higher than in mature RBCs. A somewhat selective destruction of older RBCs therefore occurs in G6PD-deficient patients who are exposed to oxidative stress. This helps limit the nature of the hemolytic crisis, even if mild exposure to the oxidative stressor continues. Note that an acute crisis will typically resolve on its own in about one week's time as new erythrocytes are generated.

10. **Suppose this man presented with a similar episode but also complained of severe back and abdominal pain. What should you be concerned about in this case and why?**
Mesenteric ischemia and renal ischemia can often be complications of acute hemolytic crises in G6PD-deficient patients because their hemoglobin drops too rapidly for compensation to take place. Treatment is supportive unless signs of peritonitis develop, in which case the patient may require surgery to remove potentially necrotic bowel.

SUMMARY BOX: GLUCOSE-6-PHOSPHATE DEHYDROGENASE (G6PD) DEFICIENCY

- Presentation: Fatigue with acute-onset dark urine, jaundice, and/or scleral icterus in an otherwise healthy individual
- Epidemiology: Most commonly seen in men of African or Mediterranean descent (X-linked recessive disorder)
- Pathophysiology: Enzymatic defect in hexose monophosphate shunt decreases red blood cells' (RBCs') ability to handle oxidative stress and predisposes these cells to hemolysis.
- Diagnosis
  - Decreased hemoglobin with an appropriate reticulocyte response on complete blood count (CBC)
  - Heinz bodies and bite cells on peripheral blood smear
  - Low serum haptoglobin, elevated unconjugated/indirect bilirubin, and elevated lactate dehydrogenase (LDH)
  - Hemoglobinuria
- Complications: Acute tubular necrosis (ATN) and mesenteric ischemia
- Treatment: Avoidance of the triggering agent

CASE 12.8

A routine examination of a 1-day-old newborn reveals generalized jaundice, scleral icterus, conjunctival pallor, and possible hepatosplenomegaly. No bruising is obvious. Delivery was uneventful except for the finding that the placenta was moderately enlarged.

1. **What are some causes of jaundice in the neonate?**
   Infection, physiologic jaundice, intestinal obstruction, inborn errors of metabolism, and hemolytic disease of the newborn can cause jaundice. Whereas physiologic jaundice typically occurs within the first week, other diagnoses should be suspected if jaundice is seen on the first day.

2. **What is physiologic jaundice, and why does it develop?**
   Physiologic jaundice results from the increased destruction of RBCs with fetal hemoglobin during the newborn period. These cells are slowly being replaced by cells with adult hemoglobin over the first 6 months of life. Normal hemoglobin levels in the newborn range from 14 to 20 g/dL. Such high levels help compensate for the decreased partial pressure of O_2 available to fetal RBCs in utero. At birth, with the onset of respiration, erythropoiesis slows down as the relative hypoxemia is reduced. The fetal RBC also has a decreased life span compared with the adult RBC. Within the first 3 months, blood volume increases markedly. All of these factors lead to increased RBC destruction, a decreased hemoglobin concentration, and clinically visible jaundice that peaks on days 3 to 4 of life and starts to improve by days 4 to 5. It is thought that infants who develop physiologic jaundice do not yet have the hepatic capacity to clear the excess bilirubin that forms during this period. As the activity of uridine diphosphate (UDP) glucuronyltransferase increases over the first weeks of life, the jaundice usually becomes self-limited. Also note that though this is a clinical condition, almost every newborn will demonstrate a mild degree of physiologic jaundice. Phototherapy is indicated for those newborns who develop bilirubin levels >25 mg/dL in order to prevent kernicterus. Specific ultraviolet (UV) wavelength light directed at the skin of these newborns allows for a conformational change in the unconjugated bilirubin that allows it to be more water-soluble, effectively "skipping" the hepatic metabolism to allow for renal excretion of the bilirubin.

3. **What is the most serious complication of neonatal jaundice, and how does it develop?**
   Kernicterus is the deposition of insoluble unconjugated bilirubin in the brain, which can cause brain damage (particularly in the basal ganglia and hippocampus). Early signs include lethargy, poor feeding, vomiting, and hypotonia. Later symptoms include irritability, hypertonia, seizures, and deafness. Infants with their first case of jaundice are at highest risk for kernicterus. Risk factors include prematurity, sepsis, Asian ancestry, hemolytic disease, and high altitude.

CASE 12.8 CONTINUED:

Laboratory tests are significant for a hemoglobin of 12 g/dL (low for a newborn) and a marked reticulocytosis and elevated indirect bilirubin. A direct Coombs test is positive. Blood typing reveals that the mother is Rh-negative, the father is Rh-positive, and the baby is Rh-positive.

4. **What is the diagnosis?**
   Hemolytic disease of the newborn due to Rh incompatibility is the diagnosis. Parental heterozygosity allows an Rh-positive infant to be carried by an Rh-negative mother. Maternal blood comes into contact with fetal blood cells, and maternal antibodies are produced against the Rh antigen present on the fetal blood cell surface. During a subsequent pregnancy with an Rh-positive fetus, maternal IgG antibodies can cross the placenta and bind to fetal RBCs, leading to hemolysis via opsonization and complement-mediated destruction. Destruction of fetal RBCs causes increased unconjugated bilirubin in the fetal circulation, which is metabolized by the placenta while the fetus is still in utero. After delivery, however, the infant must process the unconjugated bilirubin in their own immature hepatocytes. Because the UDP glucuronosyltransferase activity is not yet mature at time of delivery, the infant is functionally incapable of handling the high bilirubin level created by the hemolytic anemia of Rh incompatibility. Severe anemia leads to extramedullary erythropoiesis, which results in hepatosplenomegaly that is potentially visible on prenatal ultrasound.

CASE 12.8 CONTINUED:

This patient's 3-year-old sister is also Rh-positive but was asymptomatic as a newborn.

5. **Why was the older sister unaffected?**
   The sister was the first child and probably sensitized the mother to the Rh antigen when there was mixing of maternal and fetal blood during delivery. Sensitization caused the mother to produce anti-Rh antibodies, which can cross the placenta. Before her first pregnancy, the mother did not make anti-Rh antibodies, so none could cross the placenta and cause hemolysis in the first child.

6. **What should have been given to the mother before delivery of her first child?**
    Anti-Rh immune globulin (RhoGAM) can be given to provide the mother with passive immunity against the Rh antigen. This antibody binds to any fetal Rh antigens that may enter the maternal circulation during delivery and prevents the mother's immune system from ever recognizing the Rh antigen. Without so-called sensitization of the immune system to the Rh antigen, no anti-Rh antibodies are ever synthesized. Thus there is no anti-Rh IgG available to cross the placenta and opsonize the fetal RBCs.

    Note: RhoGAM should be given to an Rh-negative woman in any situation in which there is potential for mixing of maternal and fetal blood, including spontaneous abortion, elective abortion, and abruptio placentae.

CASE 12.8 CONTINUED:

The baby is treated with phototherapy and exchange transfusions. Further testing reveals that the mother's blood type is O, the father's is A, and the baby's is A.

7. **Why is ABO incompatibility unlikely to be the cause of hemolytic disease of the newborn?**
    Anti-A and anti-B antibodies are predominantly IgM antibodies, which cannot cross the placenta. There are also multiple other cells that express the A and B antigens in the fetus, and these cells "mop up" most of any anti-A or anti-B antibodies that cross the placenta.

SUMMARY BOX: HEMOLYTIC DISEASE OF THE NEWBORN

- Erythroblastosis fetalis
- Caused by maternal sensitization to Rh antigens in an Rh-negative mother leading to the production of anti-Rh antibodies (IgG), which can cross the placenta and cause hemolysis of fetal red blood cells (RBCs) in an Rh-positive infant
- Sensitization: Requires previous exposure of the mother to Rh-positive blood from a prior pregnancy, abortion, placental abruption, or previous transfusion
- Symptoms: Large placenta, elevated indirect bilirubin, rapidly progressive jaundice after birth, hepatosplenomegaly, generalized edema (e.g., ascites, scalp fluid)
- Laboratory tests: Positive direct Coombs test, hyperbilirubinemia
- Treatment: Exchange transfusions for the infant
- Prophylaxis: Testing the mother's blood type early in pregnancy and administering RhoGAM during and immediately after delivery to prevent alloimmunization

---

CASE 12.9

A 2-year-old boy is brought to your office by his mother for recurrent abdominal pain that comes and goes but has been worsening over the past few weeks. Upon taking a full social history, you learn that the boy and his family recently moved into the area and are living with his grandmother in her old home. Because he is a new patient, you perform a full physical examination, including a CBC to rule out infection or inflammation. Pertinent findings include guaiac-negative stool.

Laboratory values are as follows:
Hemoglobin: 8.5 g/dL (normal [pediatric]: male and female, 11.0–14.0 g/dL)
Hematocrit: 25.5% (normal [pediatric]: 33%–42%)
MCV: 68 μm^3 (normal [pediatric]: 74–89 μm^3)

---

1. **What is the differential diagnosis for this patient?**
    A low hemoglobin and hematocrit in combination with a low MCV represents a microcytic anemia. As with adults, the most common cause of microcytic anemia in children is iron deficiency. However, lead poisoning must be ruled out in the workup of recurrent abdominal pain with anemia in a pediatric patient despite the fact that it typically causes a normocytic anemia. Other etiologies of microcytic anemia that should be considered (particularly in children) include thalassemia and congenital sideroblastic anemia.

CASE 12.9 CONTINUED:

The peripheral smear is shown in Fig. 12.11.

---

2. **What is the most likely diagnosis based on these findings?**
    The blood smear shows microcytic, hypochromic RBCs with basophilic stippling (small dots visible at the periphery of the RBCs), which is strongly suggestive of lead poisoning in a patient with a history of recurrent abdominal pain.

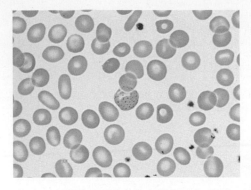

Figure 12.11. Peripheral blood smear of patient in Case 12.9. *(From McPherson RA, Pincus MR.* Henry's Clinical Diagnosis and Management by Laboratory Methods. *22nd ed. Philadelphia: Saunders; 2012.)*

Basophilic stippling results from accumulation of excess ribosomes in the RBC, as lead denatures many ribosomal degrading enzymes including ribonuclease.

3. What is the most likely source of lead toxicity in this child?
   Lead-based paint in his grandmother's home is the most likely source. Lead paint has a sweet taste and was frequently used in homes built before 1978. Paint chips from old homes are a common source of lead poisoning in children, particularly in developing toddlers who frequently put foreign substances into their mouths as a way of exploring the world.

4. Why does lead toxicity result in anemia?
   Lead binds to the sulfhydryl groups found on two of the enzymes involved in the heme synthesis pathway: δ-aminolevulinic acid dehydratase (ALA dehydratase) and ferrochelatase. This binding activity inhibits the formation of heme needed to make new RBCs, thus leading to anemia. Inhibition of ALA dehydratase and ferrochelatase results in the accumulation of their respective substrates, δ-ALA and protoporphyrin, in the blood and urine (a useful diagnostic tool for this disease).

CASE 12.9 CONTINUED:

The child started walking at 12 months but recently has become unsteady on his feet. His speech has also regressed. An x-ray film of his femur is shown in Fig. 12.12 and reveals thick transverse radiodense lines in the distal metaphysis and proximal tibias.

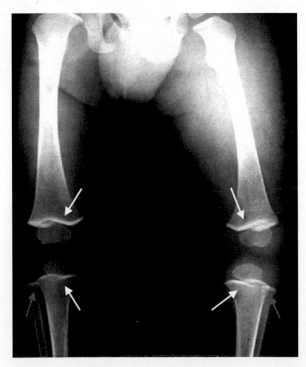

Figure 12.12. There are dense metaphyseal bands at the distal femurs and proximal tibias (*white arrows*). Note also there are similar dense bands at the heads of both fibulas (*darker arrows*). *(From Herring W.* Lead poisoning. *LearningRadiology.com. 2015. Accessed November 8, 2016. http://learningradiology.com/notes/bonenotes/leadpoisonpage.htm.)*

5. **What is the significance of the radiographic findings?**

The radiodense lines noted in the x-ray film are evidence of lead poisoning, and these are commonly referred to as *lead lines*. Excess lead accumulates in the metaphysis of long bones, where it competes with calcium for phosphate binding. Deposition of lead in bone leads to the formation of radiodense lead lines on x-ray film. Lead lines of a different type occur when lead deposits in the gums. These thin, grey lines (referred to as *Burton lines*) are a result of hyperpigmentation.

Clinical Pearl

Lead is also visible in the gastrointestinal tract on plain abdominal x-ray films.

---

6. **Why has this child recently developed an unsteady gait and regression of his speech?**

Lead poisoning causes acute encephalopathy through multiple mechanisms, as evidenced by unsteady gait and speech regression in this child. First, excess lead can accumulate around nerves and cause them to demyelinate and degenerate. Second, inhibition of the heme synthesis pathway leads to a buildup of the substrate δ-ALA, which is believed to be neurotoxic. Third, lead blocks *N*-methyl-d-aspartate (NMDA) receptors in the brain and therefore limits synaptic plasticity and memory. The effects of lead are particularly potent in the brains of children because lead interferes with normal neurologic development. Lead poisoning can also cause peripheral manifestations, such as foot drop and paresthesias.

7. **What is the treatment for lead toxicity?**

Chelation therapy using injections of ethylenediamine tetraacetic acid (EDTA), dimercaprol, or succimer, with the latter preferred in children. Treatment is most effective if lead poisoning is caught early. Unfortunately, neurologic symptoms are often irreversible, and children tend to have permanent intellectual and developmental disabilities.

STEP 1 SECRET

*Signs of lead poisoning can be remembered using the mnemonic **ABCDEFG**:*
  Anemia
  Basophilic stippling
  Colicky pain
  Diarrhea
  Encephalopathy
  Foot drop
  Gums (lead line)

SUMMARY BOX: LEAD POISONING

- Presentation: Fatigue, headache, and recurrent abdominal pain; sometimes accompanied by irritability, lethargy, and developmental regression or plateauing in children
- Epidemiology: Commonly seen in young children who live in houses built before 1978 or in individuals who are employed in mining, chemical processing, or factories that produce batteries or ammunition
- Pathophysiology: Excess lead inhibits the enzymes δ-aminolevulinic acid (ALA) dehydratase and ferrochelatase in the heme synthesis pathway, leading to a shortage of hemoglobin for new red blood cell (RBC) synthesis.
- Diagnosis
  - Burton lines on physical examination
  - Decreased hemoglobin and mean corpuscular volume (MCV) on complete blood count (CBC)
  - Microcytic and hypochromic RBCs with basophilic stippling on peripheral blood smear
  - Elevated serum lead levels, protoporphyrin, and δ-ALA
  - Lead lines in long bones on x-ray films
- Complications: Irreversible intellectual disability and neurologic damage
- Treatment: Chelation therapy

BLEEDING DISORDERS

BASIC CONCEPTS

1. Describe the antithrombotic properties of the endothelium.
   In the absence of injury, the intact endothelium prevents activation of platelets and the coagulation cascade through the production of antithrombotic substances (e.g., prostacyclin [PGI_2], nitric oxide [NO], adenosine diphosphatase, tissue plasminogen activator [tPA], and thrombomodulin). PGI_2 and NO are potent vasodilators that prevent platelet aggregation. Adenosine diphosphatase serves a similar function by degrading adenosine diphosphate (ADP), which normally activates platelets. tPA converts plasminogen to plasmin, which cleaves fibrin to prevent formation of platelet plugs (discussed subsequently). Thrombomodulin binds to thrombin to form a thrombin-thrombomodulin complex that activates protein C, an anticoagulant. Antithrombin III (produced by the liver) inactivates thrombin and other coagulation factors.

2. How does endothelial injury promote hemostasis?
   Hemostasis is the process used to stop bleeding or hemorrhage. It has two main components: vasoconstriction and temporary blockage with a platelet plug (a process known as *primary hemostasis*), and more permanent blockage with a fibrin clot (a process known as *coagulation* or *secondary hemostasis*). When the endothelium is injured, thrombogenic subendothelial collagen is exposed. Platelets adhere to this collagen, stimulating platelet activation. Endothelial injury also exposes tissue factor (TF; factor III), a prothrombotic molecule synthesized by the endothelium in response to acute-phase cytokine stimulation. TF acts in conjunction with factor VII to initiate the extrinsic pathway of the coagulation cascade, culminating in the generation of thrombin (discussed in more detail in question 5).

3. Differentiate between the processes of primary and secondary hemostasis.
   Primary and secondary hemostasis refer to platelet plugging and activation of the coagulation cascade, respectively. As mentioned previously, damage to endothelial cells results in exposure of the underlying thrombogenic collagen to circulating platelets. These platelets bind to the collagen via von Willebrand factor (vWF; see question 4). Adherence of platelets to collagen initiates platelet activation, which alters platelet shape and stimulates release of secretory granules containing ADP, Ca^{2+}, thromboxane A_2 (TXA_2), and fibrinogen. Release of these substances recruits additional platelets to the site of injury. Following adhesion, platelet aggregation occurs through binding of fibrinogen to their glycoprotein (GP) IIb/IIIa receptors. This action requires ADP, which promotes a conformational change in the GPIIb/IIIa receptors to allow fibrinogen binding. Fibrinogen bridges platelets together to form a platelet plug. This platelet plug is referred to as "temporary" because it is unstable at this stage (e.g., by nonlaminar blood flow, shear stress) unless fortified by secondary hemostasis (as shown in Fig. 13.1).

   Secondary hemostasis involves tissue-factor–mediated activation of the coagulation cascade and subsequent generation of thrombin. In association with ADP and TXA_2, thrombin binds to a protease-activated receptor (PAR) on the platelet surface, which induces platelet contraction and further aggregation. Platelet contraction creates an irreversibly fused mass that is difficult to disrupt. In addition, thrombin cleaves circulating fibrinogen into insoluble fibrin. This fibrin is then covalently cross-linked, resulting in enhanced stability of the irreversible platelet plug that prevents additional hemorrhage at the site of injury. Note that thrombin also recruits additional platelets to the site of injury and promotes their release of secretory granules (see Fig. 13.1).

   Note: Conditions affecting platelet plug formation (e.g., vWF deficiency, aspirin) will impair primary hemostasis, whereas disorders affecting the coagulation cascade (e.g., liver failure) will impair secondary hemostasis. Primary and secondary bleeding disorders can often be differentiated by their pattern and timing. Bleeding diatheses caused by

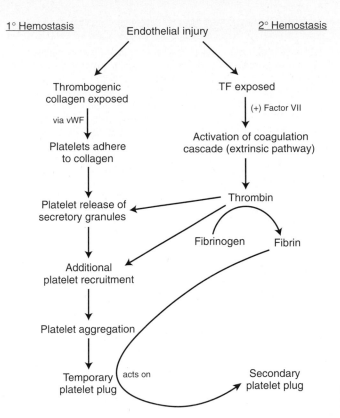

1° Hemostasis

2° Hemostasis

Figure 13.1. Mechanisms of primary and secondary hemostasis. *TF,* Tissue factor; *vWF,* von Willebrand factor.

impaired primary hemostasis typically present with bruising, petechiae, and mucosal bleeding (e.g., gingival bleeding, epistaxis, menorrhagia) or persistent bleeding after surgery or dental work. In contrast, bleeding diatheses caused by impaired secondary hemostasis typically present with delayed bleeding. The initial clot formed during primary hemostasis is able to prevent most of the immediate bleeding, but without the contribution of proper secondary hemostasis, it is highly unstable and often breaks down, resulting in slow, delayed bleeding after the initial injury. These bleeds involve deeper structures such as soft tissues, joints (hemarthrosis), and muscles (Table 13.1).

Table 13.1. Primary and Secondary Hemostasis

FEATURE	PRIMARY HEMOSTASIS	SECONDARY HEMOSTASIS
Definition	Temporary platelet plug	Permanent platelet plug
Example disease(s)	Immune thrombocytopenic purpura	Hemophilia A and B
Laboratory testing	Bleeding time, platelet aggregation studies	Prothrombin time (PT), partial thromboplastin time (PTT), international normalized ratio (INR)
Clinical manifestations of disease	Mucosal bleeding (e.g., menorrhagia, epistaxis), mucocutaneous petechiae	Bleeding into joint spaces (hemarthrosis)

4. **What molecule is responsible for the binding of platelets to collagen?**
   vWF, which is synthesized by the normal vascular endothelium, is responsible for binding platelets to collagen. Vessel injury results in the release of previously synthesized vWF. This extracellular vWF is responsible for binding to both subendothelial collagen and the platelet receptor GPIb, thus acting as a bridge between platelets and the injured vasculature.
   Of note, vWF also binds to factor VIII and protects it from degradation while in circulation. This is clinically important in conditions where levels of vWF are reduced because low vWF levels will decrease factor VIII levels as well (discussed in Case 13.3).

5. What constitutes the extrinsic, intrinsic, and common pathways in the coagulation cascade that result in formation of the fibrin clot (secondary hemostasis)?

Most clotting factors are formed in the liver and circulate in an inactive state. The cascade effect of activation allows for amplification of the end product (fibrin). The extrinsic and intrinsic pathways are separate biochemical pathways capable of activating the common coagulation cascade, which results in the formation of a fibrin clot (Fig. 13.2). These

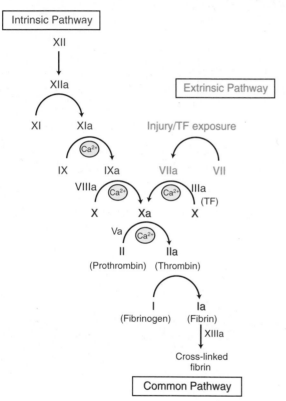

Figure 13.2. Intrinsic, extrinsic, and common pathways of the coagulation cascade. *TF,* Tissue factor.

distinctions are useful for understanding clotting tests but have physiologic limitations. The extrinsic pathway is referred to as "extrinsic" because the factor that activates it (TF) is normally *extrinsic* to the vascular space. It is exposed to the vascular space only when there is damage to the vascular endothelium. The extrinsic pathway includes TF (factor III) and factor VII. Factor VII is activated to factor VIIa when exposed to TF.

As the name implies, the intrinsic pathway does not require tissue damage and subsequent release of TF; all of the necessary components to activate this pathway are already present in the blood. In addition to clotting factors XII, XI, IX, and VIII, it requires two proteins (prekallikrein and high-molecular-weight kininogen) and calcium ions. The intrinsic pathway was long believed to be a laboratory phenomenon because it plays a minor role in normal physiologic homeostasis. However, it is now believed to play a role in many pathologic conditions where thrombosis occurs in the absence of tissue damage.

The intrinsic pathway is initiated by interaction of factor XII with negatively charged particles, which can be found on many substances including circulating lipoprotein particles (as seen in hyperlipidemia), bacteria, and homocysteine. This explains why high levels of these substances are associated with risk of thrombosis. When the primary hemostasis pathway is activated, platelets also release large, negatively charged molecules called *polyphosphates*, which further amplify the intrinsic pathway.

The common pathway is activated by either the extrinsic pathway or intrinsic pathway, and it eventuates in the formation of a fibrin clot. The common pathway includes factors X, V, II (prothrombin), and I (fibrinogen).

Note: Each reaction in the clotting cascade requires a substrate, enzyme, and cofactor. These components are assembled on phospholipid complexes that are upregulated on the surface of platelets following activation. The components are held together by calcium, which is secreted by platelets and binds to the phospholipid complexes. The presence of calcium is critical for progression of the coagulation cascade (see Fig. 13.2).

STEP 1 SECRET

Even though it may seem daunting to memorize the entire clotting cascade, it is important to know which factors are involved in the intrinsic versus extrinsic pathway so that you can understand anticoagulant pharmacology and interpret clotting tests. This is a commonly tested concept. Spend some time looking carefully at Fig. 13.2. We modify this figure throughout the chapter as we discuss pathophysiologic mechanisms of various bleeding disorders.

6. What information is provided by measuring the prothrombin time and partial thromboplastin time?

Measuring the prothrombin time (PT) and the partial thromboplastin time (PTT) provides information regarding the time it takes to form a fibrin clot upon the addition of specific reagents to the patient's blood. In other words, these tests screen for the activity of the clotting cascade and its associated factors. Prolongation of PT indicates a defect in the extrinsic pathway, whereas prolongation of the PTT indicates a problem in the intrinsic pathway. Note that calcium and phospholipids are required reagents in both tests because they are necessary for the proper function of the clotting cascade (see previous question 5).

The PT is measured by adding TF to the patient's blood sample, initiating the extrinsic pathway of clot formation. Deficiencies in clotting factors from either the extrinsic *or* common pathway can prolong the PT. The international normalized ratio (INR) is a modification of the PT, which accounts for the variability in potency of TF used in different laboratories.

The activated PTT is another assay that measures the time required to form a fibrin clot. In this test, a reagent containing a negatively charged activator (see subsequent Note) is used to robustly activate the intrinsic clotting factors. The PTT can be prolonged by clotting factor deficiencies in either the intrinsic or common pathway (Fig. 13.3).

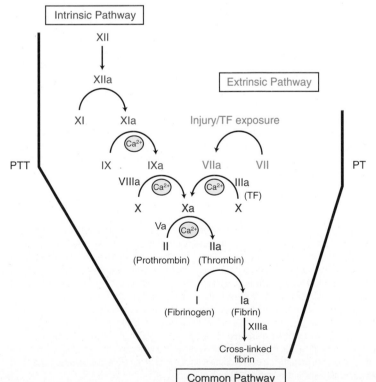

Figure 13.3. Prothrombin time (PT) and partial thromboplastin time (PTT). *TF,* Tissue factor.

Note: Although an excess of negatively charged phospholipids would be a more appropriate physiologic catalyst of the intrinsic pathway when measuring PTT, the laboratory test simply requires any negatively charged substance (e.g., silica).

7. **Define bleeding time. What is its clinical significance?**
Historically, bleeding time was measured by determining how long a person bleeds following introduction of a small incision. The amount of time it would take for the bleeding to stop directly correlated with the formation of a temporary platelet plug. Therefore bleeding time is an indicator of *platelet function*, whereas the PT and PTT are indicators of coagulation cascade function. Please note that even though the concept and clinical importance of bleeding time remain high yield for the USMLE, platelet function is more commonly assessed by in vitro platelet function assays rather than by measuring bleeding time.

Conditions marked by deficiencies in specific clotting factors (e.g., hemophilia) will show elevated PT/PTT values, but the apparent bleeding time will remain normal. Clinically, this is why diseases affecting secondary hemostasis are more likely to cause internal, slow bleeding (bruising, bleeding into joint spaces), whereas diseases affecting bleeding time will be more superficial (mucous membrane bleeding, increased bleeding with external trauma).

8. **What is the mechanism of action of the following drugs? How do they affect PT, PTT, and bleeding time?**
1. Aspirin
Aspirin inhibits platelet function by *irreversibly* inhibiting the enzymes cyclooxygenase-1 (COX-1) and cyclooxygenase-2 (COX-2), which function to synthesize TXA_2. TXA_2 stimulates platelet aggregation and vasoconstriction, both of which act to limit bleeding following vessel trauma. Consequently, inhibition of TXA_2 by aspirin results in a prolonged bleeding time.
Note: Because aspirin is an irreversible inhibitor of platelet COX, its effect on platelet function lasts as long as the affected platelets remain in circulation (~7 days). This is why patients who are about to undergo specific surgical procedures may be asked to avoid aspirin for 1 week before surgery.
2. Heparin
Heparin increases the activity of antithrombin III (ATIII), a potent inhibitor of thrombin (factor II), as well as factors XII, XI, X, IX, and VII (mostly involved in the intrinsic pathway). Because of this preferential inhibition of the intrinsic pathway, heparin can prolong the PTT but will do so only at high doses. Because it has no effect on platelet function, it normally does not alter the bleeding time, except in cases of heparin-induced thrombocytopenia (discussed more in Case 13.4).
Note: Excessive bleeding from heparin toxicity can be rapidly reversed by administering protamine sulfate, a positively charged peptide that binds and inactivates the negatively charged heparin molecule.
3. Warfarin
Warfarin inhibits the production of vitamin K–dependent clotting factors in the liver (factors II, VII, IX, and X) by antagonizing vitamin K epoxide reductase (decreases availability of active vitamin K). Recall that vitamin K is an important cofactor in gamma carboxylation, which is necessary for the activation of these clotting factors. Once vitamin K activates clotting factor precursors, it becomes biologically inactive and requires epoxide reductase to recycle it back to its active form. Because warfarin blocks this recycling by inhibiting epoxide reductase, warfarin administration will slowly deplete the availability of biologically active vitamin K, thus decreasing the production of active clotting factors (which typically takes a few days). For this reason, patients who require long-term anticoagulation are usually started on heparin and warfarin simultaneously; once the patient is sufficiently anticoagulated with warfarin, the heparin can be discontinued and the INR maintained within a therapeutic range (typically 2.0–3.0). INR is the preferred test for monitoring warfarin's effects, because although it affects factors from both the intrinsic and extrinsic pathways, factor VII of the extrinsic pathway has the shortest half-life. Therefore it is the first to decrease after starting warfarin. It is important to note that warfarin is contraindicated for use in pregnant women because it can cross the placental barrier.

Clinical Pearl

Although warfarin inhibits the activation of new vitamin K–dependent clotting factors, it takes 4 to 5 days to reach peak therapeutic effect because preexisting clotting factors need to be cleared from circulation. However, the effects of warfarin can be reversed quickly (in ~1 day) by administering excess vitamin K, which increases the levels of biologically active vitamin K and negates the need for vitamin K epoxide reductase recycling. This is the same reason why changes in dietary sources of vitamin K (e.g., leafy green vegetables) can interfere with a patient's INR values. For emergent surgical procedures, fresh frozen plasma (FFP) or prothrombin complex concentrate (PCC) can be given immediately to replace the deficient clotting factors. Warfarin also inhibits the production of protein C and protein S, vitamin K–dependent proteins secreted by the liver that exert *anti*coagulant effects through inactivation of factors Va and VIIIa. Note that the activation of protein C is dependent on thrombomodulin, whereas the activity of activated protein C is dependent on the cofactor protein S (Fig. 13.4). Both protein C and protein S have shorter half-lives compared to several of the vitamin K–dependent coagulation factors. Consequently, inhibition of protein C and protein S synthesis by warfarin can initially result in a hypercoagulable state (where the patient is prone to clotting). For this reason, "loading" doses of warfarin are not recommended. Instead, if the patient is believed to be at high risk for clotting, warfarin should be administered with heparin during the first week of therapy.

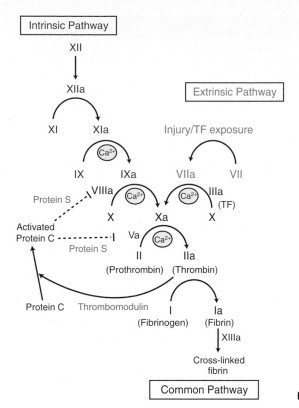

Figure 13.4. Mechanism of protein C activity. *TF,* Tissue factor.

Clinical Pearl

Warfarin can induce skin necrosis, a rare adverse effect often associated with administration of large loading doses. As mentioned previously, due to the short half-lives of proteins C and S, warfarin results in a transient hypercoagulable state initially. This is thought to be the cause of warfarin-induced skin necrosis. Patients with protein C or S deficiency are especially at high risk, and history of these disorders should be suspected if the clinical vignette mentions skin necrosis associated with warfarin administration.

Clinical Pearl

Neonates are born with a deficiency in vitamin K due to poor transplacental transfer of vitamin K, inadequate amounts of vitamin K in breast milk, and an immature enteric system not yet capable of producing vitamin K. Deficiency in vitamin K simulates an anticoagulated state and makes newborns more susceptible to spontaneous bleeding, especially intracranial hemorrhage. It is for these reasons that newborns are given a shot of vitamin K at the birth.

---

9. **What is the mechanism of action of tPA?**

As its name suggests, tPA is an enzyme that activates the plasma enzyme plasminogen, converting it into plasmin. Plasmin is an enzyme that proteolytically cleaves fibrin strands, thereby degrading fibrin clots that may obstruct vessels. In addition to tPA, streptokinase and urokinase also act by increasing plasmin levels and are collectively known as *fibrinolytics* or *thrombolytics*. Excessive bleeding that may result from these agents can be treated with plasmin inhibitors such as aminocaproic acid or tranexamic acid (Table 13.2).

Clinical Pearl

Tissue plasminogen activator (tPA), streptokinase, and urokinase are referred to as "clot-busting" drugs and can be administered to patients with ST elevation myocardial infarction or acute ischemic stroke.

CASE 13.1

A 7-year-old boy is evaluated for a swollen right knee. His mother states that this has happened in the absence of significant trauma several times over the past few years. Physical examination is positive for decreased range of motion, tenderness to palpation, pain with movement, and what appears to be a large subcutaneous hematoma. He is afebrile with a normal complete blood count (CBC). Both parents are healthy, although the mother says that her father (the boy's maternal grandfather) tended to bruise easily and had similar problems with his joints.

Table 13.2. Pharmacotherapy for Hemostasis

AGENT	MECHANISM OF ACTION	PREFERRED CLOTTING PROFILE TEST	NOTES
Aspirin	Irreversibly inhibits platelet function by inhibiting thromboxane A_2 synthesis (mediated by COX-1 and COX-2)	↑ bleeding time	Low-dose baby aspirin inhibits COX-1 and -2 in platelets with limited systemic effects. Irreversible effect that persists throughout the entire lifespan of the platelet (7 days)
Heparin	Stimulates ATIII, which primarily inhibits the intrinsic pathway	↑ PTT	Reversal: Protamine sulfate
Warfarin	Antagonizes vitamin K, thereby interfering with production of clotting factors II, VII, IX, and X, as well as the anticoagulant proteins C and S	↑ PT and ↑ INR. Note: Requires frequent monitoring because of small therapeutic window, significant risks of bleeding, and multiple drug/diet interactions	Reversal: Vitamin K, fresh frozen plasma, prothrombin complex concentrate. Must be "bridged" with heparin
tPA, rPA, TNK-tPA, streptokinase, urokinase	Stimulates production of plasmin, which degrades fibrin clot	↑ PT and ↑PTT	Reversal: Aminocaproic acid or tranexamic acid ± platelet transfusions, repletion of coagulation factors (e.g., cryoprecipitate, FFP, PCC)
Direct factor Xa inhibitors (apixaban, betrixaban, edoxaban, and rivaroxaban)	Inhibits factor Xa directly	↑ PT and ↑ PTT. Note: Does not require coagulation monitoring (unlike warfarin)	Reversal: Andexanet alfa
Direct thrombin inhibitor (argatroban, dabigatran)	Inhibit thrombin (factor IIa) directly	↑ PT and ↑ PTT	Reversal: Idarucizumab (for dabigatran)
Clopidogrel, prasugrel, ticagrelor	Prevents platelet aggregation by blocking the $P2Y_{12}$ component of ADP receptor signaling	↑ bleeding time	Used to prevent clotting after coronary stent placement or after MI/stroke
Abciximab, eptifibatide, tirofiban	Prevents platelet aggregation by blocking glycoprotein IIb/IIIa	↑ bleeding time	Used for unstable angina, non-ST elevation MI, and coronary angioplasty

ADP, Adenosine diphosphate; *ATIII,* antithrombin III; *COX,* cyclooxygenase; *FFP,* fresh frozen plasma; *MI,* myocardial infarction; *PCC,* prothrombin complex concentrate; *PT,* prothrombin time; *PTT,* partial thromboplastin time; *tPA,* tissue plasminogen activator; *rPA,* reteplase; *TNK-tPA,* tenecteplase.

1. What is the most likely diagnosis?

   Hemophilia is the most likely diagnosis. Hemophilia A and B are inherited disorders that typically present with spontaneous bleeding into joints (hemarthroses) and soft tissues or prolonged bleeding following dental procedures or minor surgery. Because hemophilia A is more common than hemophilia B, this boy most likely has hemophilia A.

2. What is the cause of this disorder, and how is it inherited?

   The cause of hemophilia A is hereditary deficiency of factor VIII, inherited in an X-linked recessive manner. Females are very rarely affected because they are likely to have at least one normal copy of the factor VIII gene on either of their two X chromosomes. In rare circumstances, females may be affected as a result of unequal inactivation (lyonization) of factor VIII or factor IX alleles (see Chapter 11, Genetic and Metabolic Disease, Basic Concepts, question 4, for more information).

   In this case study, in which the maternal grandfather was affected, the boy's mother is an asymptomatic female carrier who transmitted the abnormal X chromosome (from her symptomatic father) to her son.

   Note: Hemophilia B is an X-linked recessive disease in which factor IX is deficient.

3. **Which measure of coagulation will be abnormal in hemophilia A?**

PTT, which will be increased, will be abnormal in hemophilia A. A deficiency of factor VIII (hemophilia A) or factor IX (hemophilia B) impairs thrombin production by the factor IXa/factor VIIIa complex, resulting in dysfunction of the intrinsic pathway and prolonged bleeding (Fig. 13.5).

Note: PT remains normal because the extrinsic pathway is unaffected.

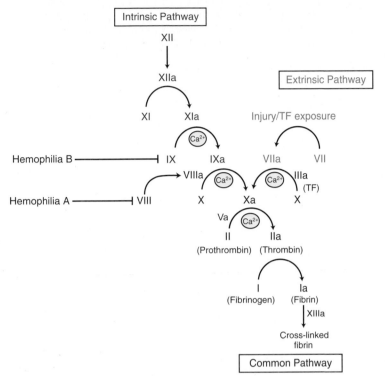

Figure 13.5. Mechanisms of hemophilia. *TF,* Tissue factor.

4. **What do you need to know about hemophilia C?**

Hemophilia C is relatively rare compared to hemophilia A and B. Hemophilia C is a disorder common among Ashkenazi Jews and is characterized by autosomal recessive deficiency of factor XI.

Clinical Pearl

The mainstay of medical treatment for this disease is infusion of a recombinant version of the missing factor (factor VIII for hemophilia A or factor IX for hemophilia B). Desmopressin is also used for treatment of hemophilia A and works by stimulating release of von Willebrand factor (vWF), which binds factor VIII in the circulation and increases its half-life.

SUMMARY BOX: HEMOPHILIA

- Presentation: Typically a male patient with easy bruising and joint pain
- Genetics: X-linked recessive disease
- Pathophysiology: Deficiency in either factor VIII (hemophilia A) or factor IX (hemophilia B)
- Diagnosis
  - Personal medical and family history (male gender, hemarthroses)
  - Confirmation with laboratory testing for prolonged partial thromboplastin time (PTT)
- Complications: Prolonged bleeding with trauma or minor surgery
- Treatment: Clotting factor replacement, desmopressin (for hemophilia A)

CASE 13.2

A 35-year-old woman experiences a missed abortion, in which a nonviable fetus is retained in the uterus. She subsequently develops petechiae on her skin and buccal mucosa, begins coughing up blood (hemoptysis), and observes blood in her stool. A CBC reveals anemia and thrombocytopenia. A peripheral smear reveals schistocytes. Additional laboratory results show an increased PT and PTT and elevated D-dimer level. Fresh frozen plasma and platelets are ordered.

1. **What is the most likely diagnosis?**
   Disseminated intravascular coagulation (DIC) is the most likely diagnosis. This disorder is characterized by thrombocytopenia, prolonged PT and PTT, and an elevated D-dimer level.

2. **What is the pathogenesis of disseminated intravascular coagulation?**
   The pathogenesis of DIC is an overwhelming release of prothrombotic substances into the blood. An inciting event (in this case, retention of the fetus), results in the release of procoagulant substances such as TF and fibrin throughout the circulation, activating the clotting cascade. This depletes clotting factors and platelets ("consumptive coagulopathy"), resulting in excessive bleeding. DIC is characterized by excessive clotting and bleeding *occurring simultaneously* throughout the body. Laboratory values will show decreased platelet count, decreased fibrinogen levels, and increased bleeding time in addition to prolonged PT/PTT (because clotting factors are being consumed). The main disease states in which DIC occurs are obstetric complications (missed abortion, abruptio placentae), gram-negative sepsis, trauma, and malignancies.

3. **What are schistocytes, and why do they form in DIC?**
   Schistocytes are red blood cells (RBCs) that have been mechanically fragmented. In DIC, widespread fibrin strands streak across blood vessels, shearing off part of the RBC membrane as they pass by (Fig. 13.6).
   Note: Schistocytes are a hallmark of *microangiopathic hemolytic anemias* (loss of RBCs due to mechanical destruction). This subtype is involved in DIC, thrombotic thrombocytopenic purpura (TTP), and hemolytic uremic syndrome (HUS). It can also be caused by autoimmunity, infections, drug use, or cancer.

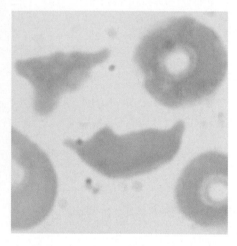

Figure 13.6. Schistocyte. Note that the schistocyte pattern shows red blood cells with refractile rings indicative of water artifact. *(From Young NS, Gerson SL, High KA. Clinical Hematology. Philadelphia: Mosby; 2005.)*

4. **How does the pathophysiology of TTP differ from that of DIC?**
   TTP involves *thrombosis, thrombocytopenia*, and abnormal bleeding as evidenced by *purpura* on examination. It is precipitated by widespread damage to the endothelium. TTP is usually marked by a deficiency of ADAMTS13, a metalloprotease that is responsible for the degradation of vWF multimers. Decreased ADAMTS13 prevents vWF breakdown, which subsequently leads to a hypercoagulable state. Mutations in the *ADAMTS13* gene or autoantibodies against ADAMTS13 are responsible for many cases of TPP, although the etiology may also involve reactions to drugs (e.g., quinine, clopidogrel, ticlopidine) or infection.
   Because platelets adhere to the exposed subendothelial collagen of damaged vessels, massive activation of platelet binding and aggregation can cause thrombocytopenia, resulting in bleeding (purpura) and prolonged bleeding time. However, clotting factors are not consumed as they are in DIC because this condition involves pathologic activation of only the primary hemostasis pathway. Thus PT and PTT are typically normal, contrary to DIC. Like DIC, TTP is an example of microangiopathic hemolytic anemia.

5. **What is the pentad of TTP, and how does this disorder differ from HUS?**
   The pentad of TTP is microangiopathic hemolytic anemia, thrombocytopenia, neurologic symptoms, fever, and renal dysfunction. Most of the manifestations are explained on the basis of clot formation, with fibrin strands causing the microangiopathic hemolytic anemia. Neurologic symptoms and renal dysfunction are due to clots and occlusion of the cerebral circulation and glomerular capillaries, respectively. HUS is very similar to TTP and involves most of the same symptoms and laboratory findings. The main distinction is that HUS does not involve neurologic manifestations. In addition, HUS is most classically seen in children with a history of diarrheal illness caused by enterohemorrhagic *Escherichia coli* O157:H7 or *Shigella*. Shiga-toxin can bind to and inactivate the ADAMTS13 metalloproteinase, resulting in a disease phenotype that resembles TTP.

6. Quick review: Cover the three columns on the right in Table 13.3 and try to differentiate the following bleeding disorders on the basis of pathogenesis, changes in blood elements, bleeding time, and changes in PT, activated PTT, and D-dimer levels.

Table 13.3 Thrombotic Thrombocytopenic Purpura, Hemolytic Uremic Syndrome, and Disseminated Intravascular Coagulation

	THROMBOTIC THROMBOCYTOPENIC PURPURA (TTP)	HEMOLYTIC UREMIC SYNDROME (HUS)	DISSEMINATED INTRAVASCULAR COAGULATION (DIC)
Pathogenesis	Abnormal platelet aggregation secondary to decreased vWF degradation	Endothelial damage secondary to bacterial toxins from diarrheal illness	Release of procoagulants or endothelial damage
Clinical picture	Autoimmune disorder most commonly affecting adult females	Diarrheal illness most commonly affecting children	Obstetric complications, sepsis, trauma, or malignancy
Changes in formed blood elements	Thrombocytopenia, schistocytes, microangiopathic hemolytic anemia	Thrombocytopenia, schistocytes, microangiopathic hemolytic anemia	Thrombocytopenia, schistocytes, microangiopathic hemolytic anemia
Bleeding time	Increased	Increased	Increased
PT	Normal	Normal	Increased
PTT	Normal	Normal	Increased
D-dimer	Normal	Normal	Increased

PT, Prothrombin time; *PTT,* partial thromboplastin time, *vWF,* von Willebrand factor.

STEP 1 SECRET

As mentioned in Chapter 12 (Anemias), hematology is a great subject for "↑/↓/normal" questions. We recommend that you thoroughly understand laboratory parameters for bleeding disorders. They are a favorite USMLE test topic because, as you may have guessed, they fit in very nicely with this popular, multiple-choice question format.

SUMMARY BOX: DIC, TTP, AND HUS

Disseminated intravascular coagulation (DIC)
- Presentation: Evidence of bleeding, petechiae on the skin/buccal mucosa
- Epidemiology: Associated with obstetric complications (missed abortion, abruptio placentae), gram-negative sepsis, trauma, and malignancy
- Pathophysiology: Overwhelming release of prothrombotic substances into the blood results in the release of procoagulant substances while simultaneously depleting clotting factors and platelets
- Diagnosis: Thrombocytopenia, prolonged prothrombin time (PT) and partial thromboplastin time (PTT), elevated D-dimer levels, decreased fibrinogen levels, and the presence of schistocytes on peripheral blood smear

Thrombotic thrombocytopenic purpura (TTP) and hemolytic uremic syndrome (HUS)
- Presentation: Fever, purpura, easy bleeding, altered mental status (for TTP)
- Epidemiology: HUS is associated with enterohemorrhagic *Escherichia coli* 0157:H7 and *Shigella*
- Pathophysiology:
  - TTP: Deficiency of ADAMTS13 prevents degradation of von Willebrand factor (vWF) multimers, leading to a hypercoagulable state with consumption of platelets and clotting factors
  - HUS: Endothelial damage secondary to bacterial toxins from diarrheal illness
- Diagnosis: Microangiopathic hemolytic anemia, thrombocytopenia
- Complications: Renal dysfunction, neurologic symptoms (TTP only)

CASE 13.3

A 27-year-old man is evaluated for persistent bleeding from the gums since a dental cleaning the prior afternoon. On physical examination, his gums appear to be bleeding profusely, and his mouth requires packing with gauze pads to limit the bleeding. He denies any history of abnormal bleeding or any family history of bleeding disorders. He is not taking aspirin or other nonsteroidal antiinflammatory drugs (NSAIDs). The clinician orders a PT and PTT, both of which are normal. However, bleeding time is prolonged at 15 minutes.

1. **What is the most likely diagnosis?**
The most likely diagnosis is vWD. Recall that the bleeding time measures platelet function. The prolonged bleeding time therefore indicates platelet dysfunction, whereas the normal PT and PTT argue against a coagulation cascade abnormality (e.g., hemophilia). vWD is the most commonly inherited coagulopathy and is therefore the most likely diagnosis.

   Note: Bleeding diatheses such as vWD (and others to be discussed), in which the coagulation cascades remain functional, are nonetheless referred to as *coagulopathies* because the ability of the blood to clot (coagulate) in these disorders is compromised.

2. **What is the pathogenesis of this man's disease?**
Recall that vWF binds to exposed subendothelial collagen, as well as the platelet GPIb receptor, forming a bridge that mediates platelet adhesion at the site of vascular injury (see Basic Concepts, question 4). A decrease in the amount (quantitative) or proper function (qualitative) of vWF results in vWD. Without adequate amounts of functional vWF, the formation of the temporary platelet plug after injury is delayed and inefficient, resulting in clinical symptoms of bruising, petechiae, mucosal bleeding (epistaxis, menorrhagia), and prolonged bleeding after surgery.

3. **Why may someone with vWD be mistakenly diagnosed with hemophilia A?**
Hemophilia A is caused by low levels of factor VIII. Because vWF acts as a carrier protein for factor VIII, patients with vWD can have low levels of factor VIII and an elevated PTT. A history of bleeding limited to the skin and mucous membranes along with normal PT and PTT largely rules out the possibility of hemophilia in this patient.

STEP 1 SECRET

Hemophilia and von Willebrand disease (vWD) may appear with similar clinical findings. Both may present with prolonged partial thromboplastin time (PTT), but hemophilia is often associated with deep bleeding and hemarthroses (unlike vWD). This is a good example of why it is important to read question stems carefully. The USMLE Step 1 exam often provides these giveaway details.

4. **What is the mechanism of action whereby administration of desmopressin acetate might help this man's symptoms?**
Desmopressin acetate (DDAVP), a synthetic analog of antidiuretic hormone (ADH), stimulates the release of vWF from endothelial cells, promoting formation of a temporary platelet plug. The released vWF will also increase factor VIII survival time in patients who demonstrate this complication.

   Because it stimulates vWF secretion and stabilizes factor VIII levels, DDAVP can also be used to treat mild hemophilia A and uremia-induced platelet dysfunction. DDAVP is not helpful for treating hemophilia B.

5. **If this man had normal levels of functional vWF and platelet function studies revealed a defect in platelet adherence to collagen, what rare disorder of platelet function might you suspect?**
One might suspect Bernard-Soulier syndrome. This disorder is caused by a lack of or abnormal function of the platelet GPIb receptor. The GPIb receptor on platelets allows adherence to vWF, linking them to the subendothelial collagen and facilitating formation of the platelet plug.

6. **If platelet function studies demonstrated platelets capable of adhering to collagen but unable to aggregate with other platelets, what other rare disorder of platelet function might you suspect?**
One might suspect Glanzmann thrombasthenia. This rare disease is caused by a lack of the GPIIb/IIIa receptor on platelets, which normally mediates platelet-to-platelet aggregation via fibrinogen bridges.

Clinical Pearl

von Willebrand disease (vWD), Bernard-Soulier disease, and Glanzmann thrombasthenia can all present with symptoms of primary hemostatic dysfunction (mucosal bleeding, postsurgical bleeding, and easy bruising), so the ristocetin assay is often used to differentiate among them. Although the exact mechanism is still unknown, ristocetin is an antibiotic thought to unwind one end of von Willebrand factor (vWF) so that both ends can bind to GPIb, allowing vWF to act as a platelet agglutinator (similar to GPIIb/IIIa). If there is a deficiency in vWF (as in vWD) or GPIb (Bernard-Soulier syndrome), the platelets will not agglutinate upon the addition of ristocetin, resulting in an abnormal test result. In contrast, if the patient has Glanzmann thrombasthenia, the addition of ristocetin will result in normal agglutination because both vWF and GPIb are still intact. These diseases can be further differentiated by partial thromboplastin time (PTT); vWD may affect PTT because vWF aids in carrying factor VIII in the blood, whereas Bernard-Soulier disease and Glanzmann thrombasthenia will not.

---

7. **Given the previously mentioned function of the GPIIb/IIIa receptor, why are drugs such as eptifibatide given to patients with acute coronary syndrome?**
These drugs prevent platelet aggregation by antagonizing the GPIIb/IIIa receptors on platelets; therefore they lower the risk for thromboembolic events in high-risk patients.

Clinical Pearl

Recall that acute coronary syndrome (ACS) encompasses unstable angina, non–ST elevation myocardial infarction (NSTEMI), and ST elevation myocardial infarction (STEMI) (see Chapter 1, Cardiology, for further details). To minimize the risk of cardiovascular mortality in ACS, patients are typically administered a GPIIb/IIIa inhibitor such as eptifibatide with aspirin and/or clopidogrel and heparin along with nitrates, beta-blockers, and opiates as indicated.

8. Why might you suspect prolonged bleeding time in this man if he suffered from diabetic nephropathy and osteoarthritis, for which he routinely takes NSAIDs?

Uremia and NSAIDs are common causes of acquired platelet dysfunction. In end-stage renal disease (ESRD), platelet dysfunction is hypothesized to result from a combination of toxic metabolites, increased nitric oxide (inhibiting platelet function), and vWF dysfunction (reducing platelet activation), resulting in reduced platelet aggregation and prolonged bleeding time. DDAVP can be used for treatment of platelet dysfunction secondary to uremia. NSAIDs cause platelet dysfunction by inhibiting the COX enzyme, preventing platelet production of TXA_2, a procoagulant molecule required for efficient clot formation.

9. Quick review: Cover the two columns on the right side of Table 13.4 and describe the mechanisms of action for the listed antiplatelet drugs.

Table 13.4 Antiplatelet Drugs

AGENT	MECHANISM OF ACTION	COMMENTS
Aspirin	Irreversible inhibition of COX-1 and COX-2 (inhibits thromboxane A_2 synthesis)	Most common cause of platelet dysfunction
Clopidogrel	Inhibits platelet ADP receptor activation	
Abciximab, eptifibatide Tirofiban	Platelet GPIIb/IIIa inhibitor	Mimics Glanzmann thrombasthenia
Dipyridamole	Prevents breakdown of cAMP, thus blocking platelet aggregation. Acts as a coronary vasodilator	Used in cardiac stress tests

ADP, Adenosine diphosphate; *cAMP*, cyclic adenosine monophosphate; *COX-1, -2*, cyclooxygenase-1, -2; *GP*, glycoprotein.

SUMMARY BOX: PLATELET DISORDERS

Von Willebrand disease
- Presentation: Easy bruising, prolonged bleeding after minor surgery, mucosal bleeding (menorrhagia, epistaxis)
- Epidemiology: Most commonly inherited disorder of platelet dysfunction
- Pathophysiology: Genetic deficiency in von Willebrand factor (vWF), which links platelets via the glycoprotein (GP) Ib receptor and is required for normal primary hemostasis
- Diagnosis: Low vWF levels, elevated or normal partial thromboplastin time (PTT), lack of platelet aggregation with ristocetin assay
- Treatment: Desmopressin acetate (DDAVP)

CASE 13.4

A previously healthy 35-year-old woman complains of easy bruising and occasional nosebleeds over the past few months. She does not take any medications. Physical examination reveals diffuse petechiae and ecchymoses (Fig. 13.7). A CBC yields the following results:

WBC 7200/μL (normal: 4500–10,000/μL)

PLT 5000/μL (normal: 140,000–400,000/μL)

RBC 4.6×10^6/μL (normal: $4.0–5.5 \times 10^6$/μL)

PT and PTT are normal, and peripheral blood smear is unrevealing. Specialized testing reveals the presence of antiplatelet antibodies.

1. What is the most likely diagnosis for this woman?

Immune thrombocytopenic purpura (ITP), also known as *immune thrombocytopenia* or *autoimmune thrombocytopenic purpura*, is the most likely diagnosis. However, it should be realized that ITP is a diagnosis of exclusion. Therefore other causes of thrombocytopenia (e.g., marrow-infiltrative processes [as can occur with malignancies], DIC, and TTP) must be considered.

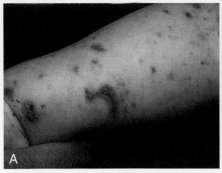 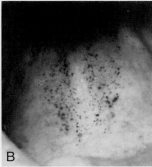

Figure 13.7. (A) Limb and (B) tongue of patient in Case 13.4. *(A from Singh SB. Petechial rash (case 55). In: Pediatrics: A Competency-Based Companion. Elsevier: Philadelphia; 2011:chap 98. B from Hoffbrand AV, Pettit JE, Vyas P, et al. Vascular and platelet bleeding disorders. In: Color Atlas of Clinical Hematology. Elsevier: Philadelphia; 2010:chap 24.)*

2. What is the etiology of immune thrombocytopenic purpura?
   Production of immunoglobulin G (IgG) autoantibodies against several platelet surface antigens, including the GPIb and GPIIb/IIIa receptors, is the etiology of ITP. When these antibodies bind to platelet receptors, it triggers opsonization and phagocytosis (see Chapter 15, Immunology) by macrophages within the liver and spleen, resulting in a massive decrease in circulating platelets. In children, ITP is often preceded by an upper respiratory tract infection for reasons that are unclear.

Clinical Pearl

In the absence of significant bleeding, treatment for immune thrombocytopenic purpura (ITP) is generally supportive, often even for platelet counts below 20,000/μL. Corticosteroids and intravenous immunoglobulin (IVIG) may be used with modest benefits. Platelet transfusion, the intuitive treatment, is generally unhelpful and is typically used only in cases of severe thrombocytopenia with significant bleeding. This is because the autoimmune condition that destroys the patient's platelets will also target the infused platelets. Splenectomy has shown to be of some benefit, although surgery in a setting of thrombocytopenia has obvious risks.

In recent years, it has become clear that some cases of ITP are, in part, due to deficient production of the platelet growth factor thrombopoietin (TPO). TPO receptor agonists (e.g., romiplostim, eltrombopag) are therefore under investigation as another treatment option for ITP.

3. What anticoagulant can also cause thrombocytopenia?
   Heparin can also cause thrombocytopenia. As many as 1% to 3% of patients receiving heparin may develop heparin-induced thrombocytopenia (HIT), which can present with either excessive bleeding or excessive thrombosis. Thrombocytopenia in HIT is thought to be caused by the production of IgG antibodies against immune complexes of heparin and a protein called *platelet factor 4* (PF4). Upon binding, the Fc region of the IgG antibody binds to an Fc receptor on the platelet surface, resulting in widespread platelet activation (prothrombotic state) and subsequent platelet depletion (i.e., thrombocytopenia).

4. Why is the absence of splenomegaly important and therefore helpful in determining the cause of thrombocytopenia?
   Splenomegaly/hypersplenism can result in increased platelet sequestration and subsequent thrombocytopenia. Splenomegaly most commonly results from congestion due to portal hypertension but may also result from leukemia, lymphoma, and several other disease processes. Splenomegaly is *not* typically seen in ITP, although it is occasionally seen in children with ITP following a viral infection.

5. If this woman were pregnant, would we need to be concerned about thrombocytopenia in the fetus?
   Yes. ITP can cause neonatal thrombocytopenia because the autoantibodies, predominantly IgG, are able to cross the placenta and attack fetal platelets. Physicians should strive to minimize bleeding during delivery and carefully monitor platelet count for a few days after birth.

6. What is the treatment strategy for ITP?
   Corticosteroid administration, which will suppress the immune destruction of platelets, is the treatment strategy. In patients with active bleeding, IVIG may be used to rapidly increase platelet count. IVIG infusion results in an excess of immunoglobulin that can bind and occupy immune cell receptors, preventing these cells from causing further destruction of platelets. Other agents with some efficacy include rituximab and thrombopoietin receptor agonists (e.g., romiplostim, eltrombopag). If necessary, a splenectomy may be required.

Clinical Pearl

Treatment of heparin-induced thrombocytopenia (HIT) includes withdrawal of heparin and continued anticoagulation therapy, usually with direct thrombin inhibitors (argatroban or bivalirudin).

SUMMARY BOX: IMMUNE THROMBOCYTOPENIC PURPURA

- Presentation: Easy bruising, frequent bleeding, diffuse petechiae in the setting of thrombocytopenia
- Epidemiology: Often preceded by upper respiratory infection in children
- Pathophysiology:
  - Caused by production of antibodies against platelet receptors, resulting in splenic destruction of circulating platelets
- Diagnosis: Diagnosis of exclusion
- Treatment: Corticosteroids, intravenous immunoglobulin (IVIG), immunosuppressants, splenectomy

CASE 13.5

A 58-year-old woman complains of a swollen and painful right leg since returning from a trip to Europe 2 days ago. Past medical history is significant for metastatic breast cancer, for which she is currently between chemotherapy regimens. On physical examination, her right calf is warm and tender to palpation and measures 20 cm in diameter, compared with her left calf, which is nontender to palpation and measures 16 cm in diameter. A venous ultrasound reveals a clot in the right femoral vein.

1. What is the diagnosis?

   Deep venous thrombosis (DVT) is the diagnosis. Risk factors for DVT include prolonged immobilization (e.g., recent surgery, long flight), malignancy, smoking, estrogen and oral contraceptives, obesity, and hereditary predisposition, with factor V Leiden thrombophilia being the most common hereditary type (see below).

   Clinical Pearl

   Less common risk factors for deep venous thrombosis (DVT) include prothrombin mutations, homocysteinemia, antiphospholipid syndrome, and heparin-induced thrombocytopenia (although this is common in hospitalized patients). Factor V Leiden thrombophilia involves the synthesis of a variant (mutated) factor V protein that cannot be "turned off" (inactivated) by activated protein C, thereby predisposing to clotting (see Fig. 13.4).

2. From what site do DVTs, which give rise to pulmonary emboli, typically arise?

   DVTs arise from the deep veins of the leg. Many originate in the calf veins but need to propagate into the deep veins of the proximal leg (popliteal, femoral, or iliac) to become large enough to cause clinically significant pulmonary emboli.

3. What is the Virchow triad, and how does it relate to this patient?

   The Virchow triad describes the three factors that contribute to the development of venous thrombosis, which are *abnormalities of the vessel wall* (as in vasculitis and atherosclerosis), *abnormalities of blood flow* (stasis), and *abnormalities of blood coagulability* (e.g., deficiencies of anticoagulants, presence of procoagulants). This patient had a recent history of immobilization from her long flight, which can cause hemostasis. Additionally, she is likely in a hypercoagulable state secondary to her malignancy.

4. How do deficiencies of proteins C and S and antithrombin III predispose to DVT?

   Protein C, protein S, and ATIII are all inhibitors of various clotting factors. Deficiencies therefore result in a hypercoagulable state. As previously discussed, protein C functions to degrade factors V and VIII. Patients with the factor V Leiden mutation synthesize a factor V that is resistant to degradation by activated protein C, resulting in a hypercoagulable state. Recall that protein S functions as a cofactor for activated protein C and promotes the degradation of factors V and VIII. Protein S deficiency therefore results in increased factor V and VIII levels, promoting a prothrombotic state. ATIII promotes the degradation of factor II and X and other coagulation factors. ATIII deficiency therefore results in increased levels of factors II and X, contributing to a prothrombotic state.

   Clinical Pearl

   Antithrombin III (ATIII) deficiency is associated with recurrent deep vein thrombosis (DVT), pulmonary embolism, and intrauterine fetal death (IUFD). In nephrotic syndrome, large amounts of ATIII are lost in the urine, resulting in a prothrombotic state due to increased levels of factors II and X. Treatment often involves administering anticoagulants.

5. What is antiphospholipid syndrome?

   Antiphospholipid syndrome (APLS) is an autoimmune coagulation disorder resulting from the production of antibodies to phospholipids. It has a high association with other autoimmune conditions (particularly systemic lupus erythematosus [SLE] and human immunodeficiency virus [HIV]) and predisposes patients to arterial and venous thrombosis syndromes.

You should consider this diagnosis in a woman with an autoimmune condition who experiences stroke, DVT, or hepatic vein thrombosis. In addition, the woman may have a history of early or repeated pregnancy loss, which may be due to placental thrombosis.

Clinical Pearl

Despite causing a prothrombotic state, antiphospholipid syndrome often presents with a prolonged partial thromboplastin time (PTT), a phenomenon known as *paradoxical anticoagulation.* This results from high affinity between the antiphospholipid autoantibodies and the phospholipids within the PTT reagent (in vitro), resulting in a false prolongation of the PTT.

SUMMARY BOX: DEEP VENOUS THROMBOSIS

- Presentation: Swelling and pain in the affected leg
- Epidemiology: Risk factors include prolonged immobilization, malignancy, estrogen and oral contraceptives, obesity, hereditary predisposition
- Pathophysiology: Vascular damage, clotting abnormalities, or venous stasis (e.g., long periods of immobility) resulting in clot formation in deep leg veins
- Complications: Pulmonary embolism

HEMATOLOGIC MALIGNANCIES

BASIC CONCEPTS

1. **What are the two principal lineages along which leukocytes differentiate?**

   The *lymphoid lineage* gives rise to B and T lymphocytes, as well as natural killer (NK) cells, and the *myeloid lineage* gives rise to mast cells, granulocytes (eosinophils, basophils, neutrophils), monocytes, megakaryocytes, and erythrocytes. Cells of the innate immune system derive from the myeloid lineage, but cells of the adaptive immune system derive from the lymphoid lineage. The exception to this rule is NK cells, which are considered players in the innate immune system (Fig. 14.1).

2. **What categories of hematologic malignancy arise from the lymphoid lineage?**

   - Lymphomas: Hodgkin lymphoma and the various types of non-Hodgkin lymphoma (NHL)
   - Lymphocytic leukemias: Acute lymphoblastic leukemia (ALL), chronic lymphocytic leukemia (CLL), hairy cell leukemia, adult T-cell lymphoma/leukemia, mycosis fungoides
   - Tumors of plasma cells (antibody-secreting B cells): Multiple myeloma, monoclonal gammopathy of undetermined significance (MGUS), and Waldenström macroglobulinemia (lymphoplasmacytic lymphoma)

     Note: All lymphoid neoplasms arise from a single transformed cell and are consequently phenotypically monoclonal.

3. **What is the general distinction between lymphoma and leukemia?**

   The terms *leukemia* and *lymphoma* are designated based on the normal tissue distribution of the neoplasm. *Leukemia* refers to an infiltration of neoplastic cells in bone marrow, which often leads to significant peripheral blood involvement. *Lymphoma* indicates a *mass* originating in the peripheral tissues (lymph nodes). However, this line is often blurred because lymphomas can evolve to infiltrate the marrow (a leukemic picture), and malignancies otherwise identical to leukemias may start out as peripheral tissue masses similar to lymphomas. A good example of how blurry this distinction can be occurs through comparison of small lymphocytic lymphoma (SLL) and B-cell chronic lymphocytic leukemia (B-CLL). Both SLL and B-CLL involve neoplasms of small, mature B lymphocytes, but SLL is confined to lymph nodes. Once the neoplastic B lymphocytes reach a threshold level in the blood, the disease is considered to be leukemic (B-CLL). Smudge cells are a characteristic feature of CLL on a peripheral smear (Fig. 14.2). These are cell remnants of fragile leukemic cells (note the lack of recognizable cytoplasm and nucleus).

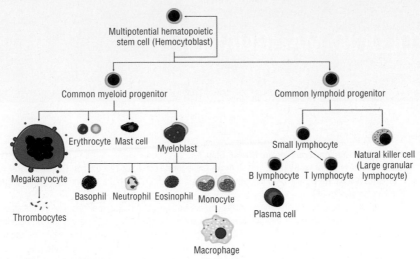

Figure 14.1. The lymphoid and myeloid lineages. *(From Lawrie C. Chapter 22, Converting Hematology Based Data into an Inferential Interpretation. In: Hematology - Science and Practice. London: IntechOpen; 2012.)*

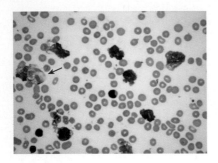

Figure 14.2. Smudge cells (*arrow*) on peripheral blood smear in patient with chronic lymphocytic leukemia (CLL). *(From Johansson P, et al. Percentage of smudge cells determined on routine blood smears is a novel prognostic factor in chronic lymphocytic leukemia. Leuk Res. 2010;34(7):892-898.)*

4. **When should a hematologic malignancy be suspected?**
   Leukemia/lymphoma should be on your differential in any patient who presents with a combination of the following symptoms:
   - History: Unexplained fever, night sweats, weight loss, fatigue, bone pain, frequent infections
   - Examination: Splenomegaly, petechial rash, ecchymoses, pallor
   - Laboratory values: Abnormal complete blood count (CBC) results (neutropenia, anemia, and/or thrombocytopenia), elevated serum lactate dehydrogenase (LDH) or uric acid, significantly elevated white blood cell (WBC) count

5. **What categories of hematologic neoplasms arise from the myeloid lineage?**
   - Acute myelogenous leukemia (AML)
     - Has multiple subclassifications
   - Chronic myelogenous leukemia (CML)
   - Myelodysplastic syndromes
     - Specific myeloid lineage replaces healthy bone marrow
     - Potential precursors of AML
   - Myeloproliferative disorders
     - Hyperproliferative myeloid lineage products (e.g., platelets, red blood cells [RBCs])
     All myeloid neoplasms arise from a transformed hematopoietic progenitor cell. Features of these neoplasms often overlap, confusing medical students and physicians alike. They may also infiltrate the bone marrow, resulting in anemia, thrombocytopenia, and leukopenia.

6. **Describe the distinction between acute and chronic leukemia.**
   As the names suggest, acute leukemias have a more sudden onset, whereas chronic leukemias are often insidious. There are additional distinguishing features that can help you differentiate between them.
   - Acute leukemias are neoplasms of *immature blast cells*. Because these cells remain in an immature state, they divide and accumulate rapidly, resulting in an acute onset. To make the diagnosis of acute leukemia, there must be greater than or equal to 20% leukemic blasts in the bone marrow at the time of biopsy. AML is subsequently

distinguished from ALL based on the lineage commitment of the blasts. Patients with acute leukemia typically have high serum LDH and uric acid secondary to increased cell turnover.
- Chronic leukemias are neoplasms of partially mature, dysfunctional cells. CLL is a lymphocytic leukemia, most commonly of mature B cells, whereas CML is caused by the proliferation of mature granulocytes (predominantly neutrophils). CML is the rarest of the four major leukemia subtypes.

STEP 1 SECRET

The most important form of acute myelogenous leukemia (AML) to know for boards is acute promyelocytic leukemia (APL) or the M3 subtype, which is characterized by circulating granulocytes and myeloblasts containing Auer rods. Auer rods are peroxidase-positive inclusion bodies in the cytoplasm of the neoplastic cells that are pathognomonic for this condition (Fig. 14.3). Release of these Auer rods can result in disseminated intravascular coagulation (DIC).

APL is marked by a characteristic t(15;17) translocation that involves the retinoic acid receptor, preventing the maturation of promyelocytes. Fortunately, this disease responds to treatment with all-trans-retinoic acid (ATRA).

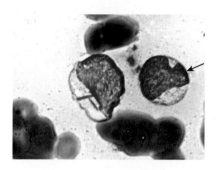

Figure 14.3. Auer rods (*arrow*) in acute myelogenous leukemia (AML). *(From McPherson RA, Pincus MR.* Henry's Clinical Diagnosis and Management by Laboratory Methods. *22nd ed. Philadelphia: Saunders, 2011: Fig. 33-25.)*

7. **Under what classification does hairy cell leukemia fall?**
   Hairy cell leukemia is a relatively uncommon subtype of B-CLL found predominantly in middle-aged Caucasian men. Most patients present with *massive splenomegaly* and abdominal discomfort because the spleen is the primary site for proliferation of neoplastic cells. Patients also present with symptoms suggesting pancytopenia. These include fatigue secondary to anemia, easy bleeding/bruising and petechiae secondary to thrombocytopenia, and frequent infections secondary to neutropenia. The characteristic finding on peripheral blood smear is cells with fine hair-like projections (hence the name "hairy cell leukemia"; Fig. 14.4). These cells stain positive for tartrate-resistant acid phosphatase (TRAP). The treatment of choice for this condition is cladribine, a purine analog.

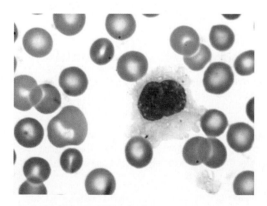

Figure 14.4. Hairy cell leukemia. *(From Ferry J.* Extranodal Lymphomas. *Philadelphia: Saunders; 2011: Fig. 13-06A.)*

8. **What is the distinctive feature of myelodysplastic syndromes?**
   In these diseases, a mutated myeloid stem cell that can give rise to *all* cell types of the myeloid lineage proliferates and populates the bone marrow, thus crowding out normal cells. However, this mutant stem cell produces cells of the myeloid lineage in an ineffective manner. Consequently, the peripheral blood shows one or more cytopenias (anemia, thrombocytopenia, and/or leukopenia) as a result of ineffective hematopoiesis and replacement of normal bone marrow cells. Moreover, the myelodysplastic syndromes are often premalignant and may evolve into AML if additional mutations are acquired.

Myelodysplastic syndromes are diagnosed when (1) a cytopenia is present that is otherwise unexplained or (2) a significant number of dysplastic cell changes are seen within a peripheral blood smear or bone marrow aspirate/biopsy. They usually occur in men who are 50 to 80 years of age. Dysplastic changes of myelodysplastic syndrome include Pelger-Huët cells with "aviator" nuclei (bilobed polymorphonuclear cells; Fig. 14.5), ringed sideroblasts (erythroid precursors with mitochondrial iron deposits; Fig. 14.6), and increased myeloblast cells (immature cells of the myeloid lineage).

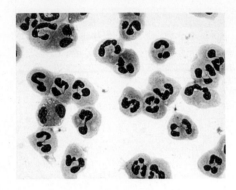

Figure 14.5. Bilobed polymorphonuclear cells. *(From Firestein G, Budd R, Gabriel SE, McInnes IB, O'Dell J. Kelley's Textbook of Rheumatology. 9th ed. Philadelphia: Saunders; 2013: Fig. 11-2.)*

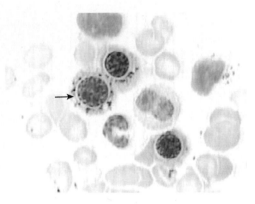

Figure 14.6. Ringed sideroblasts *(arrow). (From Kocjan G, Gray W, Levine T, Kardum-Skelin I, Vielh P. Diagnostic Cytopathology Essentials. Philadelphia: Churchill Livingstone; 2013: Fig. 7-091E.)*

Clinical Pearl

When the percentage of blast cells exceeds 20% of total cells on the smear, the diagnosis of acute myelogenous leukemia (AML) is made.

---

9. **What is the distinct feature of the myeloproliferative disorders?**

   In these diseases, a transformed hematopoietic progenitor cell causes a pathologically increased production of *one* of the final products of the myeloid lineage (granulocytes, erythrocytes, platelets). In other words, myeloproliferative disorders result from hyperproliferation of progenitor cells that retain their capacity for terminal differentiation (i.e., overproduction of *mature* cells). Examples include polycythemia vera (increased RBC production), essential thrombocytosis (increased platelet production), and CML, which results in an increased number of granulocytes.

   Myeloproliferative disorders are commonly associated with activating mutations in tyrosine kinases, which are commonly involved in mitogenesis. Polycythemia vera and essential thrombocytosis are associated with mutations in *JAK2*. CML is unique among the myeloproliferative disorders in that it has a characteristic genetic defect: a chromosomal translocation t(9;22), known as the *Philadelphia chromosome*. The classic treatment for CML is imatinib, a tyrosine kinase inhibitor.

10. **What is myelofibrosis, and why does it occur?**

    Myelofibrosis is fibrosis (collagen accumulation) of the bone marrow. It has multiple causes (e.g., radiation, drugs, and chemical exposure) but is most commonly idiopathic. It can also occur as a result of a myeloproliferative disorder. The fibrosis can result in a dry tap (or a failure to obtain bone marrow on bone marrow aspiration). Myelofibrosis is thought to result from excessive release of transforming growth factor β (TGF-β) and platelet-derived growth factor (PDGF) secondary to signaling from abnormal megakaryocytes. These molecules stimulate the proliferation of fibroblasts within the marrow. The resulting fibrosis can impair hematopoiesis, resulting in hypocellular bone marrow and pancytopenia. As a result, hematopoiesis is shifted from the marrow to peripheral sites (e.g., spleen and liver), resulting in massive splenomegaly and hepatomegaly (extramedullary hematopoiesis). Myelofibrosis is marked by dacrocytes (teardrop-shaped RBCs) on peripheral blood smear, which result from damage to the RBC structure as these cells try to escape the fibrotic bone marrow. If you see dacrocytes on a peripheral blood smear, you should immediately associate this finding with myelofibrosis (Fig. 14.7).

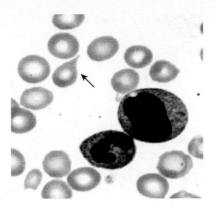

Figure 14.7. Peripheral blood smear showing tear-drop–shaped (*arrow*) red blood cells (dacrocyctes).

Clinical Pearl

Myelofibrosis is the most common cause of splenomegaly in the elderly.

---

11. **What are the histiocytoses?**

    A histiocyte is a phagocyte (macrophage or dendritic cell) found in tissue. The *histiocytoses* refer to disorders involving uncontrolled proliferation of histiocytes. For Step 1, students need only be familiar with Langerhans cell histiocytosis (LCH, also known as *histiocytosis X*), which, depending on age at presentation and clinical course, is classified as Letterer-Siwe disease, Hand-Schüller-Christian disease, or eosinophilic granuloma. Letterer-Siwe disease typically affects infants and presents with disseminated skin and bone involvement. Hand-Schüller-Christian affects children with osteolytic lesions, diabetes insipidus secondary to invasion of the posterior pituitary gland, and exophthalmos secondary to infiltration of the orbit. Eosinophilic granuloma affects preadolescents and adolescents with osteolytic lesions and often initially presents with a pathological fracture. A characteristic feature of LCH is *Birbeck granules* in the cytoplasm seen on electron microscopy, which you can easily recognize on Step 1 because they look like miniature intracellular tennis rackets (Fig. 14.8). In addition, LCH tumor cells are positive for S-100 and CD1a.

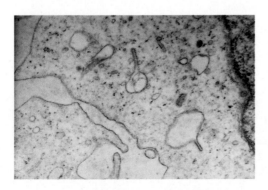

Figure 14.8. Langerhans cell histiocytosis (LCH; Birbeck granules). Electron micrograph demonstrates classic racquet-shaped Birbeck granules in the cytoplasm of an LCH cell. *(From Bolognia J, Jorizzo J, Schaffer J. Dermatology. 3rd ed. Philadelphia: Saunders; 2012: Fig. 91-5.)*

12. **How does the leukocyte alkaline phosphatase level help differentiate reactive leukocytosis from a true leukemia?**

    Reactive leukocytosis (leukemoid reaction or "left shift") is a pronounced increase in the WBC count with infection and is associated with high levels of leukocyte alkaline phosphatase (LAP). In contrast, the abnormally large increase in WBCs seen in leukemia is typically associated with low levels of LAP because the neoplastic cells cannot produce this enzyme. Moreover, the degree of leukocytosis in leukemia is often much higher (sometimes with leukocyte counts upwards of 100,000 cells/mm^3) than that seen in reactive leukocytosis.

13. **What are the two major classifications of lymphomas?**

    Lymphomas are generally classified as either Hodgkin or non-Hodgkin lymphomas. Both neoplasms arise in the lymphoid tissue and present with similar symptoms, but Hodgkin lymphoma is easily distinguishable from non-Hodgkin (a heterogeneous group of over 30 types of cancer) by the presence of neoplastic Reed-Sternberg cells (a must-know image for Step 1; Fig. 14.9). NHL is more common than Hodgkin lymphoma. Notably, the treatment and outcomes for these two cancer types can be radically different. Characteristics of NHL are presented in Table 14.1.

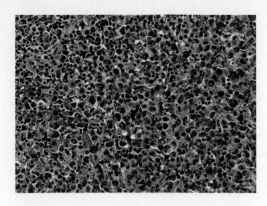

Figure 14.9. Classical Hodgkin lymphoma, lymphocyte-depleted type, lymph node biopsy. The biopsy shows a neoplastic infiltrate that consists predominantly of Reed-Sternberg cells and variants with a few admixed eosinophils and lymphocytes. *(From Aster J, Pozdnyakova O, Kutok J. Hematopathology: A Volume in the High Yield Pathology Series. Philadelphia: Saunders; 2013:198-199.)*

Table 14.1. Descriptions of Non-Hodgkin Lymphoma

NON-HODGKIN LYMPHOMA	GENETIC ALTERATION	DESCRIPTION	PATIENT PROFILE
Burkitt lymphoma	t(8;14); involves *c-Myc* activation on chromosome 8	Associated with EBV infection Endemic form in Africa, presents with jaw lesion Sporadic form is associated with pelvic and abdominal lesions Look for characteristic "starry sky" appearance on histology (sheets of neoplastic lymphocytes infiltrated with occasional macrophages) Fastest growing malignancy	Occurs in adolescents or young adults
Follicular lymphoma	t(14;18); leads to *BCL2* (antiapoptosis gene) overactivation	Associated with painless, generalized, waxing and waning lymphadenopathy and bone marrow involvement	Primarily in adults
Mantle cell lymphoma	t(11;14); increases cyclin D expression and promotes cell cycle progression	Clonal expansion of CD51 B cells within the mantle zone that surrounds germinal cell follicles Poor prognosis	Older males
Diffuse large B-cell lymphoma	Associated with *BCL6* and *BCL2* overexpression, which silences p53	Very aggressive lymphoma Can also be T cell in origin Can be primary in origin or evolve from CLL In immunocompromised individuals, the primary tumor can be located in the CNS Presents with waxing and waning symptoms Early stage is responsive to treatment	Older adults and children
Marginal zone lymphoma (MALToma)	Multiple translocations have been identified	Begins with reactive polyclonal B-cell proliferation, culminating in monoclonal B-cell neoplasm Associated with *Helicobacter pylori* infection, and may regress with treatment of *H. pylori*	Adults
Cutaneous T-cell lymphoma	HTLV-1 viral infection (ATLL only)	Caused by a T-cell dyscrasia (unlike most NHLs, which are B cell in origin) Examples include mycosis fungoides (primarily cutaneous lesions), Sézary syndrome (evolution to leukemia), and ATLL (skin lesions, hypercalcemia, osteolytic bone lesions)	ATLL associated with IV drug use and common in Japan, Caribbean region, West Africa, and southeastern United States

ATLL, Adult T-cell lymphoma; *CLL,* chronic lymphocytic leukemia; *CNS,* central nervous system; *EBV,* Epstein-Barr virus; *HTLV,* human T-cell lymphocytic virus; *IV,* intravenous; *NHL,* non-Hodgkin lymphoma.

STEP 1 SECRET

Reed-Sternberg cells are commonly presented in image format on Step 1. Reed-Sternberg cells are either multinucleated or have a bilobed nucleus, which give the cells an "owl-eye" appearance. You should be able to recognize these cells and distinguish them from the "owl's eye inclusion bodies" that are associated with cytomegalovirus (CMV).

14. Quick review with high-yield word associations. Cover the right column of Table 14.2 and attempt to list the associated diseases.

Table 14.2. High-Yield Word Associations

DESCRIPTION	DISEASE
>20% myeloid blasts in bone marrow	Acute myelogenous leukemia (AML)
>20% lymphoblasts in bone marrow	Acute lymphoblastic leukemia (ALL)
8;14 translocation (*c-Myc*)	Burkitt lymphoma
14;18 translocation (*BCL2*)	Follicular lymphoma
11;14 translocation (cyclin D)	Mantle cell lymphoma
Auer rods	Acute myelogenous leukemia
Bence Jones proteinuria	Multiple myeloma
Massive splenomegaly, B-cell proliferation, and presence of tartrate-resistant acid phosphatase in B cells	Hairy cell leukemia
Philadelphia chromosome, t(9;22)	Chronic myelogenous leukemia (CML)
Reed-Sternberg cells	Hodgkin lymphoma
Smudge cells on peripheral blood smear	Chronic lymphocytic leukemia (CLL)

15. Quick review. Cover the right column in Table 14.3 and attempt to list the cell type and pertinent high-yield facts regarding the hematologic malignancies in the left column.

Table 14.3. Leukemia and Lymphoma Lineages

DISORDER	CELL TYPE AFFECTED	COMMONLY OBSERVED FINDINGS
Lymphoid Lineage Acute lymphoblastic leukemia (ALL)	Lymphoblasts (Precursor B or T cells)	Peripheral blood and bone marrow display an increase in lymphoblasts T-cell ALL may present with a mediastinal mass
Chronic lymphocytic leukemia/small lymphocytic leukemia	B cells	Smudge cells on peripheral smear
Hairy cell leukemia	B cells	Peripheral smear shows cells with hair-like projections Positive tartrate-resistant acid phosphatase (TRAP) staining
Hodgkin lymphoma	B cells	Reed-Sternberg cells
Waldenström macroglobulinemia	Plasma cells	Monoclonal (M) spike is immunoglobulin M (IgM) Hyperviscosity symptoms
Multiple myeloma	Plasma cells	M spike is immunoglobulin G (IgG) or immunoglobulin A (IgA) Rouleaux formation Punched-out lytic bone lesions on x-ray film Anemia Primary amyloidosis

Continued

Table 14.3. Leukemia and Lymphoma Lineages—cont'd

DISORDER	CELL TYPE AFFECTED	COMMONLY OBSERVED FINDINGS
Non-Hodgkin lymphoma (NHL)	B or T cells	B-cell NHLs are classified according to the lymph node site they resemble T-cell NHLs involve cutaneous symptoms
Myeloid Lineage		
Acute myelogenous leukemia (AML)	Myeloblasts (early myeloid progenitors)	Auer rods (in M3 AML) Increased myeloblasts on bone marrow biopsy
Histiocytosis	Dendritic (Langerhans) cells	Birbeck granules on electron micrograph Lytic bone lesions
Myelodysplastic syndromes	Failure of hemopoietic stem cells to mature	Myeloid stem cell dysplasia Hypercellular bone marrow
Myeloproliferative syndromes	Abnormal proliferation of hematopoietic stem cells, resulting in excess numbers of one or more myeloid lineages	Chronic myelogenous leukemia (CML) = Philadelphia chromosome, proliferation of granulocytes Essential thrombocytosis (ET) = enlarged megakaryocytes, bleeding, thrombosis, *JAK2* mutation Polycythemia vera (PV) = hematocrit >55%, pruritus, *JAK2* mutation

CASE 14.1

A 65-year-old man is evaluated for recent onset of low back pain. There is no history of trauma or injury to the back. The pain is moderately severe and has been waking him at night. He also reports a 10-lb unintentional weight loss in recent months, as well as fatigue and recurrent sinus infections. Examination is significant only for focal tenderness to palpation at the level of the T12 vertebra.

1. **What is the differential diagnosis for back pain in an older patient?**
   The differential diagnosis includes musculoskeletal back pain (e.g., muscle strain, herniated disk), vertebral compression fracture, abdominal aortic aneurysm, and an infectious cause such as osteomyelitis, abscess, or tuberculosis (Pott disease). You should also have a high index of suspicion for malignancy (primary or metastatic), particularly in an older individual with constitutional complaints such as unintentional weight loss and fatigue, back pain that is waking the patient at night (one of the "alarm" symptoms of back pain), and recurrent infections. Malignancies to consider in an older man with back pain include metastatic prostate cancer and multiple myeloma.

CASE 14.1 CONTINUED:

An x-ray film of the skull is shown in Fig. 14.10. Serum protein electrophoresis reveals an M (monoclonal) spike. A urine dipstick test is negative for proteinuria, but a 24-hour urine protein collection reveals marked proteinuria.

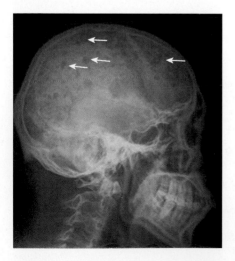

Figure 14.10. X-ray film of skull from patient in Case 14.1. White arrows point to "punched-out" lytic lesions within the skull. *(From Shi X, et al. Clinicopathologic analysis of POEMS syndrome and related diseases.* Clin Lymphoma Myeloma Leuk. *2015;15(1):e15-21.)*

2. What is the likely diagnosis?

Multiple myeloma is the likely diagnosis. The "punched-out" lytic lesions seen on x-ray film (shown by arrows in Fig. 14.10) are caused by cytokines released by the myeloma cells, which promote osteolysis. The M spike on serum protein electrophoresis indicates overproduction of a monoclonal antibody. The 24-hour urine collection showing increased protein represents the renal excretion of κ or λ light chains (Bence Jones proteins). Note that the urine dipstick test, which only detects negatively charged proteins such as albumin, will not show proteinuria, whereas a 24-hour urine protein collection will reveal marked proteinuria because of the detection of the positively charged light chains. Diagnosis can be confirmed by bone marrow biopsy showing >10% monoclonal plasma cells.

3. What blood abnormalities often present with multiple myeloma and why?

Anemia, increased creatinine ("renal insufficiency"), and hypercalcemia often present with multiple myeloma. The anemia occurs as a result of suppressed erythropoiesis. The reason for this is twofold: (1) cytokine secretion, particularly interleukin 6 (IL-6) by plasma cells, inhibits normal RBC production and (2) widespread marrow infiltration by the plasma cells inhibits RBC formation.

Renal insufficiency can occur for a variety of reasons, including significant hypercalcemia, but the primary cause is myeloma of the kidney. Light chains are directly toxic to the tubular epithelial cells of the nephron and can deposit within the tubular lumen (causing obstruction) and renal interstitium. In addition, myeloma patients are at increased risk of developing primary amyloidosis, which can further damage the kidneys.

The hypercalcemia can occur as a result of increased bone breakdown via two mechanisms: (1) bony metastasis and (2) elaboration of osteoclast-stimulating cytokines by tumor cells (primarily IL-1). This bone breakdown explains why myeloma patients are predisposed to pathologic fractures. Recall that symptoms of hypercalcemia include confusion, muscle weakness, polyuria, and constipation.

CASE 14.1 CONTINUED:

Blood work reveals the following:

Hematocrit: 29% (normal: 41%–53% in males)
Hemoglobin: 9.2 g/dL (normal: 13.5–17.5 g/dL in males)
Albumin: 2.2 g/dL (normal: 3.1–4.3 g/dL)
Total plasma protein: 8.6 g/dL (normal: 6.3–8.2 g/dL)
Blood urea nitrogen (BUN): 22 mg/dL (normal: 7–20 mg/dL)
Creatinine: 3.2 mg/dL (normal: 0.7–1.4 mg/dL)
Serum calcium: 12.4 mg/dL (normal: 8.5–10.5 mg/dL)
A bone marrow aspiration sample is shown in Fig. 14.11.

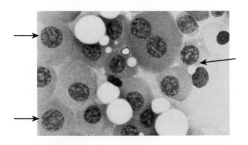

Figure 14.11. Bone marrow aspiration from patient in Case 14.1. Black arrows point to plasma cells. *(From Hoffman R, Benz EJ, Shattil SJ, et al. Hematology: Basic Principles and Practice. 4th ed. Philadelphia: Churchill Livingstone; 2005.)*

4. What cell type abnormally proliferates in multiple myeloma?

Plasma cells (shown by arrows in Fig. 14.11), which are terminally differentiated antibody-secreting B cells, abnormally proliferate in multiple myeloma. These malignant cells continuously secrete excessive amounts of a single monoclonal immunoglobulin (Ig), explaining the presence of the M spike seen on serum protein electrophoresis. This secretion of excessive amounts of a single immunoglobulin (typically IgG or IgA) is referred to as a *monoclonal gammopathy*. The resulting hypergammaglobulinemia explains the elevated total plasma protein levels commonly seen in multiple myeloma. Hypoalbuminemia is also typical of multiple myeloma, and it is thought to be secondary to elevated cytokine levels (e.g., IL-6) that reduce the hepatic synthesis of albumin.

5. What is the association between Bence Jones proteinuria and the previously mentioned monoclonal gammopathy?

Bence Jones proteins are immunoglobulin light chain subunits that are filtered by the kidney and excreted in the urine. The malignant plasma cells also secrete heavy chain immunoglobulin subunits, but these are of high enough molecular weight that they are not typically excreted in the urine.

6. What is amyloidosis, and why is this man at risk for developing it?
Amyloidosis is a clinical syndrome caused by the deposition of insoluble fibrillar protein in various tissues. In amyloidosis caused by multiple myeloma, the monoclonal gammopathy results in elevated levels of free light chains in the blood, which can undergo processing and be pathologically deposited in tissues throughout the body as amyloid. Histologic staining of involved tissues with Congo red will reveal the classic apple-green birefringence when visualized under polarized light.

7. How might the presence of elevated serum κ or λ light chains and amyloidosis affect kidney function in this patient?
They can seriously impair renal function. Renal failure is a major cause of death in multiple myeloma. Elevated serum light chain proteins get filtered and secreted by the kidney (Bence Jones protein). These proteins are toxic to renal tubular epithelial cells and may also combine with a urinary glycoprotein, the Tamm-Horsfall protein, to form casts that obstruct the tubules. Renal deposition of amyloid, which may occur in primary amyloidosis, can also seriously compromise renal function.

8. Explain why this man is at an increased risk for infection even though plasma levels of immunoglobulins are abnormally elevated?
Although total immunoglobulin levels are high, this is predominantly due to the presence of M protein. Recall that *M protein* ("myeloma protein") refers to the immunoglobulin light chain fragments that are produced in excess in the setting of multiple myeloma due to clonal expansion of plasma cells. The remaining immunoglobulins are low in number and diversity, predisposing the patient to infection.

9. This patient's anemia can be characterized as myelophthisis (or myelophthisic anemia). Why?
The suffix "-phthisis" refers to wasting away or atrophy of a body part. In this case, the myeloma has infiltrated into the bone marrow and caused it to waste away, thus reducing production of RBCs.

10. What is the characteristic finding on a peripheral blood smear, as shown in Fig. 14.12, and why does this occur?
Rouleaux formation (shown by arrows), in which RBCs are stacked on each other like a row of coins, occurs because of the agglutination of RBCs mediated by M protein.

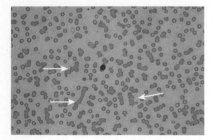

Figure 14.12. Peripheral blood smear of patient in Case 14.1. White arrows point to RBC's stacked upon each other resulting in Rouleaux formation. *(Courtesy Jean Shafer.)*

DIFFERENTIAL DIAGNOSIS

11. If workup reveals an IgM monoclonal gammopathy rather than an IgG or IgA gammopathy, what disease might you suspect?
Waldenström macroglobulinemia ("macro" for the large pentameric IgM molecule) might be suspected. It is most commonly due to lymphoplasmacytic lymphoma, a lymphocyte-plasma cell tumor (lymphoma cells have characteristics of both) that secretes IgM. The increased concentration of IgM increases plasma viscosity, which impairs blood flow and causes sludging in the retinal vessels and cerebral vasculature (and elsewhere), predisposing to visual disturbances and neurologic problems.

Although Waldenström macroglobulinemia is associated with an M spike and neoplastic cells, it differs from multiple myeloma in that there are no lytic bone lesions, hypercalcemia, renal insufficiency, Bence Jones proteinuria, or amyloid deposition.

SUMMARY BOX: MULTIPLE MYELOMA

- Presentation: Back pain, pathologic fractures, weight loss, fatigue, frequent infections, cytopenias, renal insufficiency, symptoms of hypercalcemia (confusion, muscle weakness, polyuria, and constipation)
- Epidemiology: Most common in older patients with a history of unexplained back pain or a pathologic fracture
- Pathophysiology: Abnormal clonal proliferation of antibody-secreting plasma cells, resulting in a monoclonal gammopathy
- Diagnosis: 24-hour protein collection, monoclonal (M) spike on protein electrophoresis, >10% malignant monoclonal plasma cells on bone marrow biopsy
- Complications: Amyloidosis, renal failure, infection

CASE 14.2

A 4-year-old girl is evaluated for fatigue, night sweats, anorexia, and a 10-lb weight loss over the past month. She also complains of pain in her lower back that she is unable to localize precisely. Because of this pain, she has started walking with a limp and, whenever possible, tries to avoid walking at all.

1. Her parents are worried she might have cancer. What is the most common cancer in children?
   ALL, caused by a malignant proliferation of immature precursor B or T lymphocytes (i.e., pre–B or pre–T cells), is most common in children younger than 15 years old. Of the two cell lines, pre-B ALL is more common overall.

Clinical Pearl

Children with trisomy 21 are at an increased risk for ALL.

CASE 14.2 CONTINUED:

Physical examination is significant for conjunctival pallor, hepatosplenomegaly, painless lymphadenopathy, and diffuse petechiae.

2. Why are fatigue, petechiae, and fever commonly seen in patients with ALL and myeloproliferative diseases?
   They are symptoms of pancytopenia. This occurs because of bone marrow replacement with neoplastic cells. Resulting anemia causes fatigue; thrombocytopenia causes petechiae and easy bruising and bleeding; and leukopenia (especially neutropenia) predisposes to infection and fever. Bone pain occurs as a result of massive bone marrow infiltration with malignant cells. Finally, hepatosplenomegaly results from extramedullary hematopoiesis, an attempt to compensate for bone marrow replacement by neoplastic cells.

3. How does lymphadenopathy from infection differ from lymphadenopathy due to malignancy?
   Infectious lymphadenopathy is often tender. Painless lymphadenopathy can be a warning sign for underlying malignancy, particularly when associated with constitutional symptoms such as fatigue, anorexia, weight loss, night sweats, and fever. Diffuse lymphadenopathy (spanning different lymph node groups), as well as fixed, immobile nodes also raise suspicion for underlying malignancy.

CASE 14.2 CONTINUED:

A CBC reveals marked lymphocytosis, thrombocytopenia, and anemia. A bone marrow biopsy is performed and reveals more than 50% lymphoblasts, karyotype analysis of which reveals multiple chromosomal translocations. Immunostaining of the abnormal marrow cells is positive for terminal deoxynucleotidyl transferase (TdT).

4. How does the preceding information affect the differential diagnosis?
   A diagnosis of ALL is now much more likely. TdT is a special DNA polymerase involved in the normal gene rearrangement and antigen specificity of *immature* lymphocytes (lymphoblasts). It is present in the vast majority of patients with ALL.

5. How does the presentation classically differ if the ALL is caused by a malignancy of pre–T cells rather than pre–B cells?
   ALL caused by pre–B cells has a peak age of incidence of 3 to 4 years. This type of ALL is primarily a leukemia, with predominant bone marrow and peripheral blood involvement. However, the less frequent ALL caused by pre–T cells typically occurs in adolescents and presents primarily as a lymphoma, with predominant involvement of the lymphatic system. This lymphomatous type of ALL may present with mediastinal masses, marked lymphadenopathy, splenomegaly, and thymic involvement. This is easy to keep straight if you simply recall that the thymus is the location of T-cell maturation.
   Because pre–B cells and pre–T cells can be difficult to distinguish morphologically, immunophenotyping based on cell surface markers is necessary to make a definitive diagnosis. Markers useful in distinguishing between types of ALL include B-cell markers (CD10, CD19, and CD20) and T-cell markers (CD2–CD8). In particular, T-cell lymphoblasts do not express CD10.

6. How is diagnosis of ALL differentiated from AML?
   ALL typically occurs in children under the age of 15 years, and AML occurs in older adults with a median age of onset of 65 years. Blood smears will show lymphoblasts in ALL and myeloblasts (perhaps with Auer rods) in AML. ALL may spread to the central nervous system and testes, so-called *sanctuary sites.* These sites are generally spared in AML.

7. **If she is started on high-dose chemotherapy and suddenly develops marked hyperuricemia, hyperkalemia, hyperphosphatemia, and hypocalcemia, what has happened?**

Tumor lysis syndrome, a metabolic emergency caused by massive destruction of tumor cells after initiation of high-dose chemotherapy, has occurred. The death of large numbers of tumor cells results in the metabolism of large amounts of DNA. This produces excessive amounts of uric acid, which can precipitate in the renal tubules and cause renal damage. Intracellular ions such as potassium and phosphate are also released in large amounts by dying tumor cells. The released potassium can cause marked hyperkalemia, potentially resulting in fatal arrhythmias. The hyperphosphatemia can precipitate with calcium within tubules, further contributing to renal damage.

   Tumor lysis syndrome can be treated with intravenous hydration to improve renal perfusion and glomerular filtration and to induce a high urine output state. In addition, allopurinol (a purine analog that blocks uric acid production) or rasburicase (a urate oxidase or uricase analog) can be given to either decrease formation of new uric acid (allopurinol) or convert uric acid into a more soluble form (rasburicase). Alkalization of urine to prevent uric acid precipitation is controversial because it may cause calcium precipitation.

8. **What are poor prognostic factors for ALL?**
   - B-cell ALL
   - WBC count greater than 100,000/μL at time of diagnosis
   - Presence of the Philadelphia chromosome t(9;22). This translocation is classically seen in CML but can be present in ALL as well.

SUMMARY BOX: ACUTE LYMPHOBLASTIC LEUKEMIA/LYMPHOMA

- Presentation: Night sweats, anorexia, weight loss/failure to thrive, symptoms of pancytopenia (fatigue, fever, easy bleeding/bruising, petechiae, recurrent infections), bone pain, conjunctival pallor
- Epidemiology: Classically presents in children under the age of 15
  - Increased risk in children with trisomy 21
- Pathophysiology: Malignant cells are nonfunctional lymphoblasts that replace the normal bone marrow.
- Diagnosis
  - Hepatosplenomegaly and painless lymphadenopathy on examination
  - Lymphocytosis, thrombocytopenia, and anemia on complete blood count (CBC)
  - Confirmation with bone marrow biopsy
- Complications: May spread to the central nervous system (CNS) and testes (sanctuary sites)
- Treatment: Chemotherapy
  - Tumor lysis syndrome can develop after initiation of chemotherapy.

CASE 14.3

A 35-year-old woman complains of fatigue for the past 3 weeks and recurrent spontaneous nosebleeds. Physical examination is significant for nontender lymphadenopathy, hepatosplenomegaly, truncal petechiae, and multiple ecchymoses. Peripheral blood smear shows the presence of numerous myeloblasts, cytogenetic analysis of which shows a translocation between chromosomes 9 and 22. CBC reveals a hematocrit of 25%, hemoglobin of 7.2 g/dL, WBC count of 22,000/μL, and platelet count of 30,000/μL.

---

1. **What is the likely diagnosis?**
   CML is the likely diagnosis. The presence of a translocation between chromosomes 9 and 22—the Philadelphia chromosome—is highly suggestive of CML.

2. **What is the pathogenesis of this disorder?**
   CML is a myeloproliferative disorder in which a transformed hematopoietic progenitor cell causes increased production of granulocytic cells in the bone marrow, causing a myeloid leukocytosis (predominantly neutrophils). Bone marrow biopsy in these patients will reveal an abnormally increased myeloid-erythroid ratio of approximately 15:1 to 20:1. The Philadelphia chromosome, present in a majority of CML patients, involves a translocation between the *BCR* gene on chromosome 9 and the *ABL* gene on chromosome 22. This translocation results in the formation of an overactive BCR-ABL tyrosine kinase that promotes abnormal cell division. A tyrosine kinase inhibitor, such as imatinib, is a classic drug of choice.

3. **What is the blast crisis that may occur in CML?**
   The blast crisis is an acute worsening of the disease, in which there is substantial medullary or extramedullary proliferation of myeloblastic cells. Blasts will often exceed 20% of marrow or blood cells. This is an ominous prognostic sign and suggests impending transformation to AML or ALL.

4. **Compare and contrast CLL and CML.**
   See Table 14.4.

Table 14.4. Chronic Lymphocytic Leukemia and Chronic Myelogenous Leukemia

FEATURE	B-CLL/SLL	CML
Evolution	Diffuse large B-cell lymphoma (Richter transformation) with progressive lymph node or spleen enlargement	Blast crisis with >20% blasts in the blood or bone marrow May indicate imminent transformation to AML or, more rarely, ALL
Immunophenotype and genetics	B-cell tumor that expresses B-cell antibodies and CD5, CD19, and CD20; varied chromosomal abnormalities	9;22 translocation (Philadelphia chromosome); *BCR-ABL* tyrosine kinase Treat with imatinib (*BCR-ABL* inhibitor)
Peripheral blood smear	Smudge cells	Mix of mature myelocytes
Typical age	Older adults >60 years old	Older adults with average age of onset of 64 years

ALL, Acute lymphoblastic leukemia; *AML,* acute myelogenous leukemia; *CLL,* chronic lymphocytic leukemia; *CML,* chronic myelogenous leukemia; *SLL,* small lymphocytic lymphoma.

SUMMARY BOX: CHRONIC MYELOGENOUS LEUKEMIA

- Presentation: Fatigue, weight loss, easy bleeding/bruising, petechiae, ecchymoses
- Epidemiology: Classically affects older adults with average age of onset of 64 years
- Pathophysiology: BCR/ABL fusion protein results in unregulated proliferation of granulocytes
- Diagnosis
  - Hepatosplenomegaly and nontender lymphadenopathy on examination
  - Marked leukocytosis, anemia, and thrombocytopenia on complete blood count (CBC)
  - Philadelphia chromosome, t(9;22)
- Treatment: Imatinib (tyrosine kinase inhibitor)
- Complications: Blasts exceeding 20% of marrow or blood cells suggest transformation to acute myelogenous leukemia (AML) or acute lymphoblastic leukemia (ALL)

CASE 14.4

A 22-year-old male track athlete at the local university presents with a 3-month history of fatigue. Upon questioning, he also admits to drenching night sweats and an unintentional 15-lb weight loss during this time. His past medical history is unremarkable.

---

1. Is this history concerning for a serious disease?

   Yes, it is suggestive of lymphoma. Lymphoma often presents with B symptoms, which include fever, unintentional loss of more than 10% of body weight, and night sweats. B-symptom staging is often used to distinguish symptomatic lymphoma patients from those without systemic symptoms. However, these symptoms are vague, and more information is needed to confirm the diagnosis (see question 2).

2. Other than malignancy, what else does the differential diagnosis include?

   In a 22-year-old, you want to consider and search the question stem for the following clues:
   - Infection: Human immunodeficiency virus (HIV) and tuberculosis can present with nonspecific symptoms like fever, night sweats, and weight loss.
   - Rheumatologic and autoimmune disease: Systemic lupus erythematosus (SLE), inflammatory bowel disease (IBD), and vasculitides can initially present with low-grade fevers and weight loss.
   - Other malignancy: Virtually any malignancy can present with intermittent fevers and weight loss.

CASE 14.4 CONTINUED:

On examination, nontender supraclavicular lymphadenopathy is noted along with a feeling of fullness in the left upper abdominal quadrant. A computed tomography (CT) scan of the chest reveals a mediastinal mass, and he is referred to oncology for further evaluation.

---

3. How does the location of the enlarged lymph nodes aid in the differential diagnosis?

   Cancer must always be ruled out in patients with enlarged supraclavicular nodes. In addition, remember that nontender lymphadenopathy is a red flag for malignancy. Mononucleosis or upper respiratory infections are often associated with tender, enlarged cervical nodes.

CASE 14.4 CONTINUED:

Biopsy of the enlarged supraclavicular node reveals the presence of large, binucleated cells amid normal-appearing lymphocytes, histiocytes, and granulocytes, as shown in Fig. 14.13.

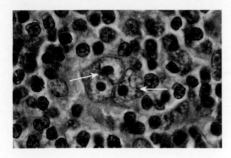

Figure 14.13. Histologic appearance of biopsy from patient in Case 14.4. White arrows point to B cells with bilobed nuclei called Reed-Sternberg cells. *(From Damjanov I, Linder J. Anderson's Pathology. 10th ed. St. Louis: Mosby; 1996:1145, Fig. 42-47A.)*

4. Name these cells and describe their lineage of origin and relation to this patient's diagnosis.
   These are Reed-Sternberg cells. They are CD301 and CD151 monoclonal B cells, the presence of which is pathognomonic for Hodgkin lymphoma. Lymphoma can be categorized into Hodgkin lymphoma and NHL, with the basic distinction that Hodgkin lymphoma is associated with Reed-Sternberg cells.

5. What are the main variants of Hodgkin lymphoma, and how do they relate to the prognosis?
   - Nodular sclerosis (60%–80% of patients): Lacunar variant of Reed-Sternberg cell with fibrotic collagen bands that divide the tumor into circumscribed nodules (excellent prognosis). Commonly presents with mediastinal mass and/or enlarged mediastinal or cervical lymph nodes. Peak incidence in young adulthood (15–34 years of age). Patients are predominantly female.
   - Mixed cellularity type (15%–30%): Heterogeneous (mixed) cellular infiltrate of lymph nodes (good prognosis). These patients are usually older. Seventy-five percent of patients are positive for Epstein-Barr virus (EBV).
   - Lymphocytic predominance: Predominantly lymphocytic infiltrate of lymph nodes with few Reed-Sternberg cells (excellent prognosis).
   - Lymphocyte-depleted: Predominantly Reed-Sternberg cells with scarce inflammatory cells. Typically affects older adults and HIV-positive patients (worst prognosis).
   In general, the more lymphocytes and the fewer Reed-Sternberg cells present on biopsy, the better the prognosis.

STEP 1 SECRET

Make sure to pay attention to patient demographics in the case of suspected malignancy. Hematologic malignancies often affect patients of a particular age or sex. This can be crucial in delineating between malignancies with similar clinical presentations. Refer to Table 14.5.

Table 14.5 Common Malignancy Demographics

DISORDER	DEMOGRAPHIC
Hodgkin lymphoma	Young adulthood *or* >55 years (bimodal) More common in men (except nodular sclerosis, which is slightly more common in women) Epstein-Barr virus (EBV) associated with 50% of cases
Non-Hodgkin lymphoma	Varies with subtype (refer to Table 14.1 for subtype specifics)
Multiple myeloma	Peak incidence in 60- to 70-year-old individuals More common in men
Acute lymphoblastic leukemia/lymphoma (ALL)	Less than 15 years of age Associated with Down syndrome
Small lymphocytic lymphoma/chronic lymphocytic leukemia	Greater than 60 years of age
Hairy cell leukemia	Largely occurs in adults

Table 14.5 Common Malignancy Demographics—cont'd

DISORDER	DEMOGRAPHIC
Acute myelogenous leukemia	Average age of onset is 65 years Associated with Down syndrome, radiation, chemotherapy, myeloproliferative disorders
Chronic myelogenous leukemia	Average age of onset is 64 years
Langerhans cell histiocytosis	Childhood

6. **What is the therapeutic value of distinguishing Hodgkin lymphoma from NHL?**
   Hodgkin lymphoma is often susceptible to more localized treatment with radiation. Unlike other lymphomas, it begins as a localized process and spreads in a consistent fashion to adjacent nodes. It commonly only affects a single set of axial nodes and rarely has extranodal involvement. NHLs frequently involve multiple peripheral nodes and extranodal sites, so they are less likely to respond to purely localized therapy.

SUMMARY BOX: HODGKIN LYMPHOMAS

- Presentation: "B symptoms" (fatigue, weight loss, night sweats, fever)
- Epidemiology: More common in men except for the nodular sclerosis variant
- Diagnosis
  - Painless lymphadenopathy on examination
  - Mediastinal mass on computed tomography (CT)
  - Reed-Sternberg cells on lymph node biopsy is confirmatory.
- Treatment: Radiation therapy
- Prognosis: More lymphocytes and fewer Reed-Sternberg cells on biopsy indicates better prognosis.

CASE 14.5

A 62-year-old woman with an unremarkable medical history is evaluated for a 4-week history of headaches, dizziness, and generalized itching, particularly after taking hot showers. She also complains of bouts of sudden-onset intense burning in her hands and feet with accompanied bluish discoloration of the surrounding skin, though she has found that aspirin brings rapid relief.

1. **What is the differential diagnosis?**
   Peripheral vascular disease, Raynaud phenomenon, or diabetic neuropathy can cause paresthesias and changes in skin color on the hands and feet. However, the pruritus, particularly after warm showers (aquagenic pruritus), is more suggestive of a myeloproliferative disorder such as polycythemia vera (PV) or essential thrombocytosis.

CASE 14.5 CONTINUED:

Physical examination is significant for elevated blood pressure and splenomegaly but is otherwise normal. Laboratory evaluation reveals the following:
   Hemoglobin: 19.6 g/dL
   Hematocrit: 60%
   WBC count: 15,800/μL
   Platelets: 500,000/μL

2. **What is the differential diagnosis of the erythrocytosis (elevated hematocrit)?**
   The differential diagnosis includes dehydration (decreased plasma volume leads to relative erythrocytosis), secondary polycythemia (physiologic conditions leading to the appropriate or inappropriate increase in RBC production; e.g., hypoxemia, renal tumors, exogenous erythropoietin, Cushing syndrome, and carboxyhemoglobinemia), and primary polycythemia (a pathologic increase in RBCs as seen in the myeloproliferative disorder).

CASE 14.5 CONTINUED:

Further blood work shows a low level of erythropoietin, normal oxygen saturation, and an elevated leukocyte alkaline phosphatase and uric acid. A peripheral smear is unremarkable, and a bone marrow aspirate shows hypercellularity with megakaryocytic hyperplasia and reduced iron stores.

3. **What is the likely diagnosis?**

PV is the likely diagnosis. Patients with this disorder often complain of pruritus after hot showers, which is due to enhanced mast cell degranulation and histamine release secondary to changes in skin temperature (note that this clue will commonly be provided to you in the question stem). The increased uric acid level is due to the high cell turnover associated with this condition. Patients also commonly present with a ruddy face, blurred vision, and headache, all secondary symptoms of vascular congestion.

Note: Enhanced mast cell degranulation in PV may also promote development of peptic ulcer disease because histamine can stimulate production of gastric acid.

4. **What is the pathophysiology of her symptoms of sudden-onset burning?**

This burning is a condition called *erythromelalgia* and is caused by microvascular thrombi in the extremities. It is seen in PV because this disorder also causes platelet dysfunction, resulting in increased "stickiness" that facilitates development of clots in small vessels. Aspirin is the most effective treatment to reduce pain. The combination of platelet dysfunction and markedly elevated blood viscosity and volume puts patients at an increased risk for other thrombotic events including myocardial infarction, deep venous thrombosis/pulmonary embolism (DVT/PE), splenic infarction, stroke, and Budd-Chiari syndrome.

Note: Erythromelalgia is also seen in essential thrombocytosis, another myeloproliferative disorder in which the increased platelet count results in clotting.

5. **What is the significance of low erythropoietin levels in diagnosing PV?**

During states of RBC overproduction such as PV, erythropoietin (EPO) levels are suppressed. EPO is produced by the kidneys when the body senses low RBC volume. This is an important clinical clue in distinguishing PV from other causes of *polycythemia*, which is a term used to describe any increase in RBC count. Appropriate polycythemia occurs in hypoxemic states that reactively trigger RBC production such as high altitude, pulmonary disease, and certain forms of heart disease. In these cases, oxygen saturation is decreased and EPO secretion is upregulated. In inappropriate absolute polycythemia, ectopic EPO secretion is responsible for increased RBC mass, such as in renal cell carcinoma. The final form of polycythemia that you should know for boards is relative polycythemia, which is marked by decreased plasma volume secondary to dehydration. Because plasma volume is reduced, RBC count (number of cells/plasma volume) appears to be elevated, but RBC mass (absolute number of RBCs) remains within normal limits. Blood oxygen levels are normal. You should know how to differentiate between these causes of polycythemia for Step 1 because this is another high-yield topic.

6. **How is PV managed?**

Nonpharmacologic approaches to PV include phlebotomy to reduce hyperviscosity of blood (attenuates risk of thrombotic events). Pharmacologic approaches include administration of hydroxyurea, ruxolitinib (*JAK1/2* inhibitor), or interferon-α.

7. **What is the classic presentation for essential thrombocytosis?**

The classic presentation for essential thrombocytosis includes thrombocytosis (thrombocythemia), bleeding, pruritus, and splenomegaly (i.e., many of the same symptoms seen in PV). Patients often have platelet counts greater than 600,000/μL and may have associated increases in RBCs and granulocytes. A peripheral smear classically shows large, hypogranular platelets. Bone marrow aspiration shows megakaryocytic hyperplasia but normal iron stores.

Note: A majority of PV cases and half of essential thrombocytosis cases occur secondary to mutations in *JAK2*, which is involved in hematopoietic growth factor signaling.

SUMMARY BOX: POLYCYTHEMIA VERA

- Presentation: Dizziness, generalized itching (especially after hot showers), intense burning in the hands and feet with bluish discoloration of the surrounding skin (erythromelalgia), symptoms of vascular congestion (ruddiness, blurred vision, headaches)
- Genetics: Associated with *JAK2* mutations
- Diagnosis: Elevated hematocrit, low erythropoietin (EPO) levels, normal oxygen saturation
- Bone marrow aspirate shows hypercellularity with megakaryocytic hyperplasia and reduced iron stores.
- Treatment: Phlebotomy, aspirin (pain management), hydroxyurea, ruxolitinib (*JAK1/2* inhibitor), and interferon-α
- Complications: Thromboembolic events, peptic ulcer disease

CASE 14.6

A 75-year-old man is evaluated for worsening fatigue and persistent fever. On physical examination, you notice many bruises on his arms and legs, which he admits is a relatively new phenomenon that he has attributed to "getting old." No lymphadenopathy or hepatosplenomegaly is noted.

1. **What is the differential diagnosis for a combination of fatigue, easy bruising, and recurring fever or infection in an older man?**

The differential diagnosis includes infection, malignancy, and vasculitis.

CASE 14.6 CONTINUED:

Blood work shows hemoglobin 9.5 mg/dL, hematocrit 35%, platelet count 62,000/μL, and WBC count 50,000/μL with 30% blast cells; a peripheral blood smear is shown in Fig. 14.14.

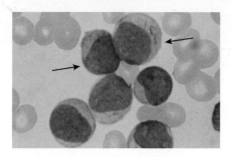

Figure 14.14. Peripheral blood smear from patient in Case 14.6. Black arrows point to myeloblasts with needle-like inclusions called Auer rods. *(From Goldman L, Schafer A. Goldman-Cecil Medicine. 25th ed. Philadelphia: Elsevier; 2016: Fig. 183-2.)*

2. What characteristics of the smear aid the diagnosis?

The smear in Fig. 14.14 shows circulating granular leukocytes known as *myeloblasts*, with eosinophilic needle-like inclusions called *Auer rods* (shown by arrows). Auer rods and peripheral blast cells are indicative of AML. Confirmation of the diagnosis requires a bone marrow biopsy demonstrating 20% or more myeloblasts.

STEP 1 SECRET

You should be able to recognize Auer rods on a peripheral blood smear. This is a high-yield image for the USMLE.

3. How do his laboratory values help explain his presenting symptoms?

Anemia explains his fatigue, and thrombocytopenia explains his easy bruising. Although he has an excess of WBCs due to AML, these cells are nonfunctional, causing a clinical neutropenia with consequent recurrent fevers/infections.

4. What is the distinctive feature of AML on bone marrow biopsy?

A substantial amount of bone marrow (≥20%) is replaced by relatively undifferentiated myeloblast cells that resemble one (or more) of the early precursors of myeloid differentiation. Consequently, there are multiple subclassifications of AML depending on which early cell type predominates (e.g., APL, acute myelomonocytic leukemia, acute megakaryocytic leukemia), of which the only subclassification that you will be responsible for is acute promyelocytic leukemia.

CASE 14.6 CONTINUED:

Bone marrow biopsy showed a predominance of promyelocytes with cytoplasmic Auer rods. Fluorescence in situ hybridization (FISH) reveals a translocation between chromosomes 15 and 17 in the affected cells. The translocation involves the retinoic acid receptor-α gene on chromosome 15. The patient is diagnosed with acute APL, also known as *AML subtype M3*.

5. What is the standard treatment for APL?

APL is unique in that traditional chemotherapy is combined with ATRA. The retinoic acid receptor (RAR) normally functions in the differentiation of promyelocytes into functional mature cells. In APL, the t(15;17) translocation causes a fusion of the *RAR* and *PML* genes, producing an abnormal protein that binds DNA and blocks transcription of differentiation genes, leading to an accumulation of immature granulocytes. ATRA binds to the retinoic acid receptor portion of the fusion protein, preventing its binding to DNA and allowing for differentiation and eventual cell death. Arsenic can be used for refractory cases.

SUMMARY BOX: ACUTE MYELOGENOUS LEUKEMIA (AML)

- Presentation: Fatigue, easy bruising, recurring fever or infection
- Epidemiology: Average onset occurs at age 65 years (see Table 14.5).
- Pathophysiology: Malignant cells are myeloblasts that replace the bone marrow.
  - A t(15;17) involving the retinoic acid receptor-α gene on chromosome 15 is unique to acute promyelocytic leukemia (APL).
- Diagnosis: Leukocytosis, anemia, and thrombocytopenia on complete blood count (CBC), Auer rods on peripheral blood smear (pathognomonic for AML)
  - Confirmation requires a bone marrow biopsy demonstrating ≥20% myeloblasts.
  - Subtyping requires fluorescence in situ hybridization (FISH).
- Treatment: All-trans-retinoic acid (ATRA) (for APL)

IMMUNOLOGY

BASIC CONCEPTS

1. Outline hematopoiesis, beginning with a pluripotent stem cell.
   See Fig. 15.1.

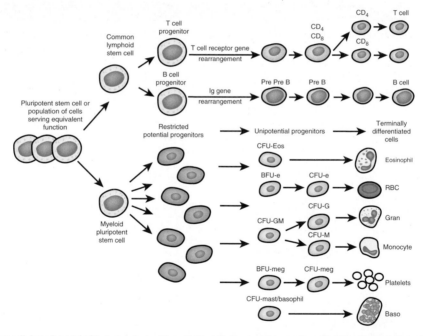

Figure 15.1. Stem cell–based model of hematopoiesis. *(From Noble J.* Textbook of Primary Care Medicine. *3rd ed. St. Louis: Mosby; 2001.)*

2. What are the major primary and secondary organs that make up the human lymphoid system?
   Lymphoid organs are classified as primary or secondary depending on whether they play a role in lymphocyte maturation or are involved in lymphocyte activation, respectively. Primary lymphoid organs include bone marrow, thymus, and fetal liver. Both precursor B and T lymphocytes are produced in the bone marrow, but only the B cells continue to mature there. T cells, on the other hand, leave the marrow to mature in the thymus. Maturation in these organs involves a stringent selection process that eliminates both poorly functioning and autoreactive lymphocytes. Secondary lymphoid organs include lymph nodes, spleen, and mucosa-associated lymphoid tissue (MALT). MALT ranges from poorly organized clusters of lymphoid cells to highly organized structures such as the appendix, tonsils, and Peyer patches. These secondary lymphoid organs provide a site for mature lymphocytes to respond to antigens presented on the surface of dendritic cells and other professional antigen presenting cells (APCs).

3. What is the function of the innate immune system?
   The innate immune system forms the first line of defense against pathogens and toxic compounds. Cells of the innate immune system are activated nonspecifically and contain various pattern recognition receptors (PRRs) that recognize a

diverse group of pathogen-associated molecular patterns (PAMPs) shared by different classes of microbes (e.g., lipopolysaccharides [LPS], flagellin, unmethylated CpG sites).

Epithelial surfaces provide the first line of defense to the host because intact epithelia (held together by tight junctions) provide a physical barrier between the internal and external world. Infectious agents must breach the epithelial barrier in order to colonize the host organism. Note that mucosal epithelial cells in the lungs and in the gut secrete mucus, which can provide an additional layer of protection and prevent bacterial cells from adhering to the epithelium. Additionally, epithelial surfaces may be covered with cilia (e.g., in the airways), which can clear foreign substances from the internal environment.

Most epithelial surfaces in the body are associated with commensal organisms that form the microbiome, a term that collectively refers to the collection of microorganisms present within the host. These microbial species form an additional first line of defense against pathogenic organisms through competition for resources and production of antimicrobial peptides. Antibiotic treatment may predispose the host to infection by killing "good" commensal bacterial species.

If pathogenic organisms breach the epithelial surfaces, they are met by a variety of leukocytes that form the second line of innate immune defense. Examples include phagocytes (neutrophils, dendritic cells, macrophages), granulocytes (eosinophils, basophils, mast cells), and natural killer (NK) cells. These cells perform a variety of protective functions that include production and release of free radicals, interferons, proinflammatory cytokines (e.g., interleukin 1 [IL-1], IL-6, and tumor necrosis factor [TNF]), pyrogenic substances, and iron-sequestering proteins (e.g., lactoferrin). They also augment the complement system and can be recruited to inflammatory sites through complement proteins and chemokine gradients. Neutrophils form the most abundant type of phagocyte and are first to reach the site of infection. Here, they engulf and destroy microbes. Pus is a viscous exudate that is composed of dead neutrophils at the infection site.

4. What is adaptive/acquired immunity?

Adaptive immunity involves the response of B and T cells following exposure to an antigen that they specifically recognize. A hallmark of adaptive immunity is cellular memory, which allows for a more intense immune response and efficient elimination of the offending agent upon repeat exposure to an antigen (Table 15.1). It is very important to recognize that stimulation of the adaptive immune response requires prior activation of the innate immune system. Dendritic cells (DCs) provide the bridge between the innate and adaptive immune systems because they present antigen to naive T cells (mainly in secondary lymphoid organs). Stimulation of PRRs on DCs triggers uptake of antigen. This antigen is then processed and presented on major histocompatibility complex (MHC) class I or class II to naive T cells via MHC–T-cell receptor (TCR) interactions. DCs also provide costimulatory and cytokine signals that help promote naive T-cell differentiation toward specific effector T-cell phenotypes (e.g., Th1, Th2).

Table 15.1. Characteristics of Innate and Acquired Immunity

	INNATE (NATURAL)	ACQUIRED (ADAPTIVE)
Effector cells	Neutrophils (polymorphonuclear neutrophils), macrophages, eosinophils, basophils, mast cells, natural killer (NK) cells	B cells and plasma cells, T helper cells (e.g., T_H1, T_H2 cells), cytotoxic T lymphocytes (CTLs)
Chemical mediators	Complement, lysosomal enzymes, cytokines, interferons, acute-phase proteins	Antibodies (immunoglobulins), cytokines, granzymes, perforin
Response characteristics	Rapid, nonspecific Same intensity against all antigens	Slow, antigen-specific Long-term memory generated after first exposure (e.g., more rapid and intense response upon repeat exposure)

Note: The primary and secondary immune responses refer to the activity of the adaptive immune system. The primary response is the activity of this system after first exposure to the pathogen, whereas the secondary response occurs after immunologic memory has been generated from a previous exposure. Thus the secondary response is more rapid and powerful.

5. What are the basic characteristics of cell-mediated and humoral immunity?

Cell-mediated immunity refers to immune responses that do not involve antibodies. Most commonly, cell-mediated immunity refers to activation of immune cells (particularly cytotoxic T lymphocytes [CTLs] and helper T cells [T_H cells]) and secretion of soluble mediators called cytokines.

When a bacterial or viral pathogen enters the body, nonspecific activation of DCs and macrophages through PRR engagement leads to secretion of IL-12, which stimulates naive T helper (T_H0) cells to differentiate into T_H1 cells. T_H1 cells secrete cytokines such as interferon gamma (IFN- γ) and IL-2. IFN-γ activates macrophages and enhances their microbicidal properties. IL-2 stimulates the proliferation of T_H and CTLs. CTLs have the ability to kill infected cells, neoplastic cells, and donor graft cells.

Humoral immunity refers to B-cell production of antibodies. Antibodies have a diverse set of roles, including neutralization of pathogens and toxins, opsonization of pathogens to facilitate phagocytosis, complement activation, stimulation of mast cell and basophil degranulation, and B-cell activation. Antibodies are grouped into five different isotypes (IgM, IgD, IgA, IgE, IgG) according to their constant domains. Production of IgA, IgE, and IgG requires B-cell interaction with T cells in a process known as *class switching* (see question 8).

Note: Both live and killed vaccines induce cellular and humoral immunity, but the relative contribution of various immune cell types in the protective response is dependent upon the nature of the vaccine. This distinction is responsible for the difference in the length of protection provided by different vaccines. A completed course of a live vaccine induces lifelong immunity by producing a strong T-cell memory response. Examples include measles, mumps, rubella, and Sabin polio vaccines. Due to the risk of conversion to a virulent form of the virus, live vaccines are avoided in pregnant women and patients with immunodeficiencies. Inactivated vaccines induce a strong B-cell or antibody-mediated immune response. Examples include influenza, hepatitis A and Salk polio vaccines. These vaccinations sometimes require a booster shot. Newer vaccines such as the vaccine against the severe acute respiratory syndrome coronavirus 2 (SARS-CoV-2) are mRNA-based, which use the patient's own ribosomes to make antigenic proteins that the immune system will create antibodies to.

6. Describe the difference between class I and class II major histocompatibility complex molecules.

T cells possess TCRs that interact with MHC molecules. MHC class I molecules are found on the surface of all nucleated cells, thus excluding only mature erythrocytes, and are encoded by *HLA-A, HLA-B,* and *HLA-C* genes. MHC class I molecules interact with the TCR of CD8$^+$ T cells (i.e., cytotoxic T lymphocytes). On the other hand, MHC class II molecules are primarily expressed on the surface of APCs (dendritic cells, macrophages, and memory B cells) and are encoded by *HLA-DR, HLA-DP,* and *HLA-DQ* genes. MHC class II interacts with the TCR of CD4$^+$ T cells (i.e., T$_H$ cells), with the CD4 molecule serving a necessary role for this interaction to occur. An easy way to remember which MHC molecule interacts with which T-cell type is to use the rule of 8:

$$\text{Class 1} \times \text{CD8} = 8$$

$$\text{Class 2} \times \text{CD4} = 8$$

For the purpose of boards, MHC class I displays endogenously synthesized peptides (including viral particles) to CD8$^+$ CTLs, and MHC class II displays exogenous peptides (obtained via phagocytosis or endocytosis) to CD4$^+$ T$_H$ cells. This is an important distinction. When MHC class I displays viral or non-self particles, it marks the cell for destruction by CTLs. CTLs release granules containing perforins and granzymes. This destruction is mediated by Fas-Fas ligand binding (leads to apoptosis), granzymes (proteases that initiate apoptosis), or perforin (creates a channel in the plasma membrane and mediates cytolysis), thus eliminating the infected cell. MHC class II binding leads to activation of the T$_H$ cells. T$_H$ activation induces cytokine production, resulting in subsequent macrophage activation, B-cell antibody production, and CTL activation.

7. Describe the general structure of an antibody.

Antibodies, also known as *immunoglobulins* (Ig), are Y-shaped proteins produced by B cells and plasma cells that recognize and bind to specific antigens. Each immunoglobin molecule consists of two identical light chains (classified as λ or κ by the constant region) and two identical heavy chains. The constant region of the heavy chain is called the Fc portion of the antibody. The Fc region is classified as α, δ, ε, γ, and μ and determines the antibody isotype (i.e., IgA, IgD, IgE, IgG, IgM). The variable region of the antibody, also known as the Fab region, is made up of two heavy chains and two light chain segments and determines its antigen specificity. Each antibody has two antigen binding sites (Fig. 15.2).

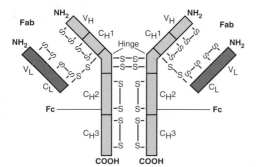

Figure 15.2. The structure of immunoglobulin (Ig) molecules. **Note:** The 12 complement-determining regions (CDRs) are the areas that most determine to which antigen the antibody will bind. *(From Mason RJ, Murray JF, Broaddus VC, et al. Murray & Nadel's Textbook of Respiratory Medicine. 4th ed. Philadelphia: WB Saunders; 2005.)*

8. What are the five classes (isotypes) of immunoglobulins? Describe their respective distributions in the body.

See Table 15.2.

Table 15.2. Immunoglobulin Isotypes

IMMUNOGLOBULIN ISOTYPE	LOCATION	FUNCTIONS
IgA	Dimeric IgA, joined by a J chain, is found in secretions Monomeric IgA is found in the blood	Found in mucosal secretions (e.g., tears, saliva, colostrum, gastrointestinal secretions); mediates mucosal immunity because it is produced in mucosal-associated lymphoid tissues (MALT) Poor activator of complement
IgD	Surface of mature B cells; some found in the blood	Unclear
IgE	Bound to FcεR1 receptors on the surface of tissue mast cells and blood basophils	Mediates type 1 hypersensitivity Mediates parasitic (e.g., helminthic) killing via ADCC (eosinophils possessing Fcε receptors are the effector cells and induce damage with major basic protein)
IgG	Found in the blood; crosses placenta Has the longest half-life of all isotopes and is thus used for passive immunization	Ligand for Fc receptors Activates classical complement pathway Involved in opsonization to mediate phagocytosis Most abundant immunoglobulin in secondary immune response Highest affinity for antigen (greatest strength of interaction between antigen and antibody)
IgM	Found in the blood, often in pentamers (joined by J chains) Monomeric form serves as a receptor on the surface of immature and mature B cells	Activates classical complement pathway Earliest antibody produced in any humoral response Most abundant immunoglobulin in primary immune response Highest avidity for antigen (greatest number of antigen-binding sites as a result of pentameric form)

ADCC, Antibody-dependent cellular cytotoxicity.

Note: In the T-cell–dependent response, B cells have the potential to produce any of the immunoglobulin classes. B cells present antigen to CD4$^+$ T cells via MHC II-TCR interactions (signal 1), and CD40L expressed on the activated T cell simultaneously binds to the constitutively expressed CD40 on the B cell (signal 2). These two signals are vital in facilitating the production of cytokines from the T cell. These cytokines can influence B-cell class switching via variable (V), joining (J), and sometimes (for the heavy chain) diversity (D) "V(D)J" recombination and subsequent production of IgG, IgE, and IgA. B cells capable of producing these antibodies are referred to as plasma cells.

In contrast, the T-cell–independent response consists almost exclusively of IgM. The T-cell–independent response generally occurs when the primary antigen is a polysaccharide (e.g., bacterial capsule, lipopolysaccharide on the gram-negative outer membrane) because these molecules are not processed by APCs in the same manner as peptide antigen. As a result, T$_H$ cells are not activated, and isotype switching cannot occur. This means that only IgM will be produced, and no secondary (memory) immune response will be established. Vaccines containing polysaccharide capsules (e.g., meningococcal vaccine, pneumococcal vaccine polyvalent, *Haemophilus influenzae* type B vaccine) are commonly conjugated to proteins to promote T$_H$-cell activation, class switching, and the formation of immunologic memory.

9. Most humans can produce 10^6 to 10^9 unique immunoglobulin molecules. However, the number of immunoglobulin genes is orders-of-magnitude less than this. How is this possible?
Antibody diversity is gained through several mechanisms: random combination of light and heavy chains, VDJ or VJ rearrangement, somatic hypermutation, and terminal deoxynucleotidyl transferase (TdT). Random combination of these two light and two heavy chains adds to antibody variability. Furthermore, each heavy and light chain contains a variable region, produced by V(D)J or VJ gene rearrangement, respectively. In this process, various gene segments in groups named V, D (heavy chains only), and J are first combined to form a unique code for the variable region and are then reconnected by *RAG1* and *RAG2* (recombination-activating genes) to the constant domain gene. This type of rearrangement is also seen in α and β chains of the TCR to achieve diversity in these molecules. Somatic hypermutation occurs after B-cell activation. When B cells proliferate, the enzyme activation–induced cytidine deaminase (AID) causes mutations in the antigen recognition portion of immunoglobulin, further increasing antibody diversity. Finally, the enzyme TdT is expressed during heavy chain rearrangement and increases variability by adding nucleotides to DNA during VDJ recombination. All these mechanisms contribute to the abundance of unique immunoglobin molecules.

10. **How do antibodies eliminate extracellular pathogens?**

    Extracellular pathogens (e.g., bacteria, free virions) commonly induce production of humoral antibodies. Extracellular pathogens that are coated with opsonizing antibodies (IgG or IgM) are efficiently phagocytized by macrophages and neutrophils via interactions between the phagocyte and the Fc region of the antibody. Following phagocytosis and processing of extracellular antigens, expression of antigenic peptides in association with MHC class II on the surface of APCs stimulates T cells, which further enhances the immune response. Keep in mind that IgG and IgM can activate the complement system that may lyse, neutralize, or opsonize extracellular pathogens.

11. **By what process can antibodies catalyze the elimination of intracellular pathogens?**

    Antibodies can catalyze the elimination of intracellular pathogens via antibody-dependent cellular cytotoxicity (ADCC). In ADCC, IgG antibodies coat the surface of target cells. Effector cells expressing Fcγ receptors can bind to the IgG through interactions with the Fc region of IgG. Binding and cross-linking of Fcγ receptors activate effector cells (monocytes, neutrophils, eosinophils, and NK cells), which mediate destruction of target cells through cytokine release and through cellular lysis.

12. **What are complement proteins, and how do they function in an immune response?**

    Complement proteins comprise a network of soluble plasma proteins that become activated as a cascade by IgM and IgG (classical pathway) or by surface molecules of microorganisms (alternative and lectin pathways). The complement proteins have many important biologic activities. The membrane attack complex mediates cell lysis, whereas other components participate in opsonization, chemotaxis, neutralization of pathogens, and clearance of immune complexes (Fig. 15.3 and Table 15.3).

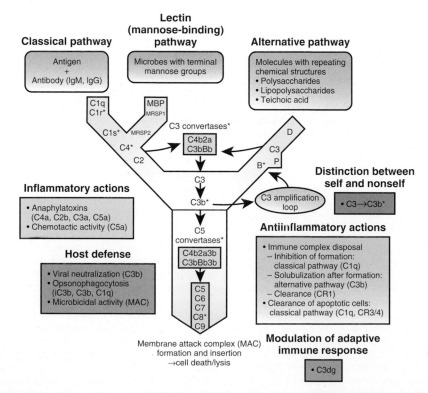

Figure 15.3. The complement cascade. *(From Mandell GL, Bennett JE, Dolin R. Principles and Practice of Infectious Disease. 6th ed. Philadelphia: Churchill Livingstone; 2005.)*

Table 15.3. Complement Pathway Components and Activity

BIOLOGIC ACTIVITY	COMPLEMENT COMPONENT(S)
Cell lysis	C5b-9 (membrane attack complex [MAC])
Degranulation of mast cells and basophils	C3a, C4a, C5a (anaphylatoxins)
Opsonization of particulate antigens	C3b, C4b, iC3b (opsonins)
Chemotaxis of leukocytes (mainly polymorphonuclear neutrophils)	C5a, C3a, C5b67 (chemotactic factors)
Viral neutralization	C3b, C5b-9
Solubilization and clearance of immune complexes	C3b

STEP 1 SECRET

There is no need to focus on learning every step of the complement cascade for the USMLE. Instead, focus on understanding the principles behind activation of different complement pathways, formation of the C3 and C5 convertases, and convergence on a final common pathway. The USMLE tests students on the roles of different complement proteins and consequences of complement factor deficiencies (see question 13). For example, you should know that patients with C5-C9 (membrane attack complex) complement deficiencies are highly susceptible to infection by Neisseria *species.*

13. Describe the ramifications of the most common complement protein deficiencies.
    See Table 15.4.
    Note: Because complement represents a set of proteins produced by the liver, generalized complement deficiencies can be seen in liver failure or in dietary deficiencies of certain essential amino acids.

Table 15.4. Complement Protein Deficiencies

COMPLEMENT PROTEIN(S)	DEFICIENCY
C1 esterase inhibitor	C1 esterase overactivity and overproduction of anaphylatoxins, leading to recurrent episodes of angioedema; this is also known as hereditary angioedema and is inherited in an autosomal dominant fashion. *Note:* C1 esterase inhibitor is inhibited directly by bradykinin, which explains the rare but life-threatening angioedema that may result as a side effect of angiotensin-converting enzyme (ACE) inhibitors (ACE is responsible for the degradation of bradykinin).
C2 or C4	These deficiencies often resemble autoimmune diseases (e.g., systemic lupus erythematosus, vasculitis) but frequently are asymptomatic. C2 deficiency is the most common complement deficiency and may be associated with septicemia (typically due to *Streptococcus pneumoniae*).
C3	Recurrent pyogenic infections as a consequence of decreased opsonization Red blood cells also recognize antigen-antibody-C3b complexes in circulation and transport them to the liver or spleen for phagocytic degradation. Decreased C3b levels in serum predispose patients to type III hypersensitivity reactions due to reduced immune complex clearance from circulation.
C5-C9	Increased risk of *Neisseria* infections *Note:* C5b-C9 forms the membrane attack complex (MAC), which can kill most unencapsulated gram-negative organisms.
Decay-accelerating factor (DAF) or CD55 and CD59	This protein is located on the surface of all human cells and destabilizes C3 convertase and C5 convertase, preventing MAC formation and thereby protecting human cells from lysis. Deficiency is manifested as an increase in complement-mediated lysis of red blood cells, clinically apparent as paroxysmal nocturnal hemoglobinuria (PNH). DAF deficiency is diagnosed with the Ham test, which checks to see whether the fragility of red blood cells increases when placed in a mildly acidic solution.

14. Which complement components and cytokines are required for neutrophil chemotaxis?

    IL-8, C5a (complement component), and LTB$_4$ (a leukotriene) are required for neutrophil chemotaxis. Leukotriene synthesis is dependent upon the enzyme lipoxygenase, which is inhibited by the drug zileuton.

15. As a review, list the effector functions of the major leukocyte classes.

    See Table 15.5.

Table 15.5. Leukocytes and Their Effector Functions

CELL	GENERAL DESCRIPTION	EFFECTOR MECHANISM
Monocyte	A phagocytic cell that constitutes 4%–10% of the WBCs in peripheral blood. Several hours after release from the bone marrow, monocytes will die or migrate into the tissue and differentiate into macrophages or dendritic cells.	Phagocytosis
Macrophage	This is a highly phagocytic, tissue-dwelling cell. Major functions include phagocytosis of particulate material, antigen presentation to T cells, and secretion of IL-1, TNF, IL-8, and IL-12. A special class of macrophages referred to as M2 cells is involved in wound healing and tissue repair.	Antimicrobial activity includes generation of both oxygen-dependent mediators (e.g., superoxide anion, hydrogen peroxide, hypochlorous acid) and oxygen-independent mediators (e.g., TNF-α, lysozyme, defensins, hydrolytic enzymes).
Dendritic cell	This potent APC forms an extensive web in tissues for trapping antigen (e.g., Langerhans cells in the epidermis) and activates naive T cells.	Phagocytosis
Neutrophil	This type of granulocyte makes up ~70% of WBCs in peripheral blood. Neutrophils are active phagocytes that are among the first cells to arrive at sites of inflammation.	Like macrophages, neutrophils employ both oxygen-dependent and oxygen-independent pathways to generate antimicrobial substances.
Eosinophil	This type of granulocyte makes up 2%–5% of the WBCs in peripheral blood. It is a phagocytic cell that migrates into the tissue spaces, where it plays a role in defense against parasitic organisms. Eosinophils have also been implicated in allergic processes.	Exocytosis of granules releases major basic protein, which is toxic to helminths and mammalian cells.
Basophil	This nonphagocytic granulocyte makes up 0.5%–1% of peripheral WBCs. Basophils play a major role in allergic responses.	Release of pharmacologically active substances (histamine and other vasoactive amines) from cytoplasmic granules upon cross-linking of surface-bound IgE by allergen
Mast cell	This tissue-dwelling cell plays a role in allergic responses similar to that of basophils. Mast cells have Fcε receptors (for IgE) and histamine-containing granules.	This cell releases pharmacologically active substances from cytoplasmic granules (histamine and other vasoactive amines) upon cross-linking of surface-bound IgE by allergen.
Helper T cell	This CD4$^+$ lymphocyte matures in the thymus and functions in cytokine production. Helper T cells play a central role in the immune response by regulating the function of cells such as CTLs, B cells, NK cells, and macrophages. Helper T cells are activated by foreign antigen in the context of MHC class II molecules.	T$_H$1 cells: IL-12 induces their differentiation (from T$_H$0 cells); secretes IFN-γ (which activates macrophages) and IL-2 (which activates CTLs and propagates the response) T$_H$2 cells: IL-4 induces their differentiation; synthesis of IL-4 and IL-5 promotes differentiation of B cells to plasma cells
Cytotoxic T cell	This CD8$^+$ lymphocyte matures in the thymus and functions in direct cell killing upon activation by foreign antigen presented by MHC class I molecules.	Perforins, granzymes, cytokines, and FasL
B cell	This CD19$^+$, CD20$^+$ lymphocyte has membrane-bound immunoglobulin. Upon activation by helper T cells, B cells may differentiate into plasma cells, which produce large volumes of antibodies. By presenting endocytosed antigen in the cleft of MHC class II, B cells also function as antigen-presenting cells in the activation of helper T cells.	Antibodies

Table 15.5. Leukocytes and Their Effector Functions—cont'd

CELL	GENERAL DESCRIPTION	EFFECTOR MECHANISM
NK cell	This is a large granular lymphocyte that has no markers in common with B or T cells and is not MHC-restricted. NK cells act to kill virally infected cells or neoplastic cells by recognition of the absence of MHC class I expression. They also kill via ADCC (surface CD16 binds Fc region of Ig attached to cells).	Perforins, granzymes, cytokines

ADCC, Antibody-dependent cellular cytotoxicity; *APC,* antigen presenting cell; *CTLs,* cytotoxic T lymphocytes; *FasL,* Fas ligand; *IFN-γ,* interferon-γ; IgE, immunoglobulin E; *IL,* interleukin; *MHC,* major histocompatibility complex; *NK,* natural killer; *TNF,* tumor necrosis factor; *WBCs,* white blood cells.

16. List the functions of the major cytokines secreted by various classes of immune cells.
    Secreted by all T cells
    - IL-2: T-cell proliferation
    - IL-3: Hematopoietic stem cell differentiation into myeloid progenitors
        Secreted by T_H1 cells
    - INF-γ: Activation of macrophages; suppression of T_H2 cells; promotes killing of intracellular pathogens
        Secreted by T_H2 cells
    - IL-4: T_H2 cell differentiation; promotes B-cell class switching to IgE and specific IgG subtypes
    - IL-5: Promotes eosinophil proliferation and chemotaxis; aids in B-cell class switching to IgA
    - IL-10: Antiinflammatory; inhibits T_H1 cells
        Secreted by macrophages
    - TNF-α: Acute-phase cytokine that activates adhesion molecule expression on endothelium; promotes vascular leak; responsible for septic shock and cachexia
    - IL-1: Acute-phase cytokine; activates adhesion molecule expression on endothelium and causes fever
    - IL-6: Acute-phase cytokine; promotes fever
    - IL-8: Neutrophil chemotaxis
    - IL-12: T_H1 cell differentiation; NK cell activation

17. List the major cell surface markers used to identify various classes of immune cells.
    See Table 15.6.

Table 15.6. Cell Surface Markers Used to Identify Classes of Immune Cells

T CELLS	B CELLS	MACROPHAGES	NK CELLS	RBCS/WBCS/ PLATELETS
CD2	Ig	CD14 (endotoxin receptor)	CD16	CD55 and CD59 (DAF; prevents complement-mediated damage)
CD3	CD19	CD16 (Fcγ receptor)	CD56	
CD4⁺ (helper T cells)	CD20	CD40		
CD8⁺ (CTLs)	CD21	B7		
CD28 (binds to B7)	CD40 (binds to CD40L)	MHC class II		
CD40L (binds to CD40)	B7 (binds to CD28)	CR1 (C3b receptor)		
TCR	MHC class II			

CD40L, CD40 ligand; *CTLs,* cytotoxic T lymphocytes; *DAF,* decay-accelerating factor; *Ig,* immunoglobulin; *MHC,* major histocompatibility complex; *NK,* natural killer; *RBCs,* red blood cells; *TCR,* T-cell receptor; *WBCs,* white blood cells.

CASE 15.1

A 2-year-old boy becomes acutely short of breath, has audible wheezing, and develops pruritic hives. He also has a bout of nausea and diarrhea. His mother takes him to the emergency department, where he is found to be hypotensive, with marked tachycardia and tachypnea.

1. What is the differential diagnosis for this presentation?
    Anaphylactic shock, asthma, bronchiolitis (inflammation of the small airways usually following a viral infection), foreign body aspiration, and toxin or allergen ingestion must be considered.

CASE 15.1 CONTINUED:

The mother is quickly questioned, and it is discovered that these symptoms developed shortly after the child took the first dose of a course of amoxicillin. The child is immediately given an intramuscular injection of epinephrine, as well as intravenous (IV) diphenhydramine and methyl-prednisolone. It is explained to the mother that this acute episode was most likely due to the amoxicillin, but she seems confused because he had taken amoxicillin previously to treat an ear infection and had no problems with it.

2. What is the most likely diagnosis?

Acute systemic anaphylaxis (anaphylactic shock) is the most likely diagnosis. The combination of bronchospasm, urticaria, and hypotension makes this diagnosis much more likely than the others. Anaphylaxis is the most serious consequence of a drug hypersensitivity reaction. The most common symptoms of drug hypersensitivity involve cutaneous manifestations, such as generalized flushing, urticaria (hives), or mild angioedema. Penicillins are the most common cause of medication-induced anaphylaxis, but this is still a very rare phenomenon with this class of antibiotics.

3. What type of hypersensitivity is anaphylaxis? What is its immunopathogenesis?

Anaphylaxis is the systemic form of the immediate hypersensitivity response (type I). During the host's first exposure to the antigen, APCs present antigen on MHC class II to naive CD4$^+$ T cells. The T cell may, in turn, convert into a T_H2 cell and produce cytokines (notably IL-4) that induce B-cell class switching toward IgE production (recall that the IgE antibodies produced are specific for the triggering antigen). Mast cells and basophils become "sensitized" when IgE produced by B cells binds to their surface Fcε receptors. Upon secondary exposure to antigen, the antigen binds to and cross-links IgE molecules on the surface of mast cells and basophils, triggering both release of granules containing preformed histamine, serotonin, tryptase, and heparin and the de novo synthesis and release of lipid mediators (e.g., leukotrienes, prostaglandins, platelet-activating factor [PAF], eosinophil chemotactic factor [ECF]). In the immediate phase (which occurs within minutes), preformed histamine induces a widespread increase in vascular permeability and smooth muscle contraction. In the late phase (>6 hours later), newly synthesized leukotrienes elicit prolonged bronchoconstriction, mucous secretion, and continued vascular permeability, while prostaglandin D_2 and PAF cause leukocyte migration and activation. Eosinophilia occurs along with the late-phase reaction due to release of ECF. Eosinophils release cationic granule proteins intended to destroy parasites, but in the absence of parasites, tissue damage and remodeling occur.

Table 15.7 summarizes the four major classifications of hypersensitivity reactions.

Table 15.7. Summary of Hypersensitivity Reactions

CLASSI-FICATION	DEFINITION	MEDIATOR	MECHANISM OF DESTRUCTION	CLINICAL PRESENTATIONS	DETECTION
Type I	IgE-mediated immediate hypersensitivity	IgE	Mast cell degranulation induced by allergen–cross-linked IgE	Systemic anaphylaxis, allergic rhinitis, bronchial asthma, atopic dermatitis, food allergies	Skin testing, RIST, RAST
Type II	Antibody-mediated cytotoxic hypersensitivity	IgM, IgG	Antibodies directed against cell-bound antigens induce destruction of cells or tissues.	Transfusion reactions, hemolytic disease of the newborn, autoimmune hemolytic anemia	Direct and indirect Coombs test
Type III	Immune complex–mediated hypersensitivity	Usually IgG	Antibodies directed against soluble serum antigen form circulating complexes that deposit in tissue nonspecifically; damage is complement mediated.	Serum sickness, glomerulonephritis, rheumatoid arthritis, SLE, hypersensitivity pneumonitis	WBC counts, total serum complement levels, serum C3 and C1q levels
Type IV	Cell-mediated delayed hypersensitivity	T_H1 cells	Antigen-specific T_H1 cells activate tissue macrophages and stimulate a local inflammatory response over 12–72 hours.	Contact dermatitis, tuberculin-type hypersensitivity, granulomatous hypersensitivity, acute tissue graft rejection	Patch test

IgE, IgG, IgM, Immunoglobulins E, G, M; *RAST,* radioallergosorbent test; *RIST,* radioimmunosorbent test; *SLE,* systemic lupus erythematosus; *WBC,* white blood cell.

4. Can free penicillin cause anaphylaxis?

No. Penicillin is univalent, meaning it is only large enough to bind to one arm of an antibody (i.e., the variable regions of only one heavy chain and one light chain). Penicillin is a hapten and therefore must be bound to a carrier protein to induce an immune response. When penicillin is bound to its carrier protein, it cross-links IgE molecules bound to Fc receptors on mast cells, leading to mast cell activation and release of inflammatory mediators.

5. What is the pathophysiologic explanation for the wheezing and diarrhea that developed?

Release of mast cell mediators such as histamine and leukotrienes causes an increase in vascular permeability and contraction of certain smooth muscle types in multiple organ systems. In the airways, this leads to laryngeal edema, bronchoconstriction, and mucous hypersecretion, resulting in wheezing. In the gastrointestinal (GI) tract, smooth muscle contraction and edema lead to nausea, vomiting, and diarrhea.

6. How does anaphylaxis result in the urticaria observed in this patient?

Urticaria, along with other atopic disorders such as eczema, asthma, and allergic rhinitis, are all symptoms of a type I hypersensitivity reaction. The systemic release of vasogenic amines allows fluid to leak from postcapillary venules into the superficial dermis, leading to edema and vasodilation. The latter, in turn, is responsible for erythema, which appears as wheals with a pale center encircled by a red flare.

7. Why did the child fail to have a reaction to amoxicillin when it was first administered for his previous ear infection?

Recall that anaphylaxis requires repeat antigen exposure (see question 3). His first exposure to amoxicillin led to mast cell sensitization (binding of IgE to surface Fc receptors), and secondary exposure resulted in manifestation of allergy symptoms.

8. What clinical testing can be performed to confirm that this immediate hypersensitivity reaction was caused by amoxicillin?

A few days after the attack, a skin test for amoxicillin and other common drug allergens can be performed. If the child is allergic, intradermal injections of amoxicillin will cause degranulation of local mast cells at the site of injection and wheals will develop within 30 minutes. This is why type I hypersensitivity reactions are also known as *immediate* hypersensitivity reactions.

9. Why was the child given epinephrine?

Epinephrine alleviates the symptoms of anaphylaxis through its adrenergic effects. Stimulation of β_2-receptors induces bronchial smooth muscle relaxation to open the airways. Stimulation of peripheral α_1-receptors constricts smooth muscle on small blood vessels to reduce vascular leakage and increase blood pressure.

10. Why was the child given diphenhydramine and methylprednisolone?

Diphenhydramine (Benadryl) is an H_1 receptor antagonist and will ameliorate the histamine-mediated components of anaphylaxis such as the urticaria. It will not reverse the life-threatening hypotension.

Methylprednisolone is a corticosteroid that acts synergistically with epinephrine by upregulating adrenergic receptors. It also promotes general downregulation of allergic inflammatory cascades, resulting in decreased eosinophil counts and inhibition of the enzyme phospholipase A_2. This latter action reduces production of prostaglandins and leukotrienes from arachidonic acid and thus decreases their release from mast cells.

Note: Although corticosteroids decrease plasma counts of many leukocyte subtypes, they can increase neutrophil counts on complete blood count (CBC) laboratory testing by reducing adhesion molecule synthesis and promoting detachment of neutrophils from endothelial walls/entrance into circulation. This is termed *neutrophil demargination* because those neutrophils previously were attached to the endothelium but now are mobilized.

RELATED QUESTIONS

11. What was the motivation for developing the second-generation H_1 receptor antagonists such as fexofenadine, cetirizine, and loratadine?

These agents are less lipophilic and do not cross the blood-brain barrier like the first-generation H_1 receptor antagonists. Therefore they reduce the side effect of drowsiness. They are generally used for allergic rhinitis.

12. List the common classes of drugs that are used to treat type I hypersensitivity disorders and their general mode of action.

See Table 15.8.

SUMMARY BOX: ANAPHYLACTIC SHOCK

- Presentation: Wheezing, shortness of breath, urticaria, hypotension, gastrointestinal (GI) problems
- Pathophysiology: Type I hypersensitivity reaction
  - Clinical manifestations result from widespread release of vasogenic amines such as histamine and leukotrienes
- Diagnosis: Clinical (based on history and examination)
- Treatment: Epinephrine, diphenhydramine, corticosteroids

Table 15.8. Drugs Used to Treat Type I Hypersensitivity Disorders and Their General Mode of Action

TYPE OF DRUG	MODE OF ACTION	CLINICAL INDICATION(S)	COMMENTS
Antihistamines	Block histamine (H_1 and H_2) receptors on target cells	Allergic rhinitis, atopic dermatitis, allergic conjunctivitis	Second-generation histamine receptor antagonists have fewer adverse side effects (e.g., they are nonsedating).
Mast cell stabilizers	Prophylactic inhibitors of mast cell mediator release	Allergic rhinitis and asthma	Include cromolyn sodium and nedocromil
Methylxanthines	Inhibition of phosphodiesterase, in addition to many other (debated) effects	Asthma, bronchospasm resistant to other modes of treatment	Include theophylline and aminophylline
Corticosteroids	Antiinflammatory; block production of inflammatory cytokines; multiple effects on several types of leukocytes	Allergic asthma, atopic dermatitis	Include prednisone, beclomethasone, triamcinolone, flunisolide
Sympathomimetics	Adrenergic effects	Asthma; epinephrine in anaphylaxis	Epinephrine has both α- and β-adrenergic effects; albuterol, salmeterol, and metaproterenol are selective β-adrenergic bronchodilators.
Monoclonal anti-IgE antibody	Binds to Fcε receptors, preventing IgE binding	Severe asthma, uncontrolled with corticosteroids	Includes omalizumab
Leukotriene pathway inhibitors	Prophylactic inhibitors of leukotriene synthesis or receptor antagonists	Asthma	Include cysteinyl leukotriene receptor antagonists (e.g., zafirlukast, montelukast) and 5-lipoxygenase inhibitors (e.g., zileuton)

IgE, Immunoglobulin E.

CASE 15.2

A 43-year-old man with uncomplicated pneumococcal pneumonia is prescribed a 10-day course of penicillin V. On the ninth day, he appears pale, mildly jaundiced, and his hematocrit has dropped significantly from when he was first seen. He denies any hemoptysis, hematemesis, melena, or hematochezia.

1. What is the differential diagnosis for this presentation?
   Hemolytic anemia, chronic liver disease (jaundice is common, as is a macrocytic anemia), occult hemorrhage, drug toxicity, tumor obstructing biliary tract (anemia is common in cancer, and biliary obstruction would lead to jaundice), and Gilbert syndrome (jaundice can occur if the stressor—anemia in this case —is severe enough to induce markedly reduced uridine diphosphate [UDP] glucuronyl transferase activity) are all considered.

2. What additional tests should be ordered to further analyze the anemia and jaundice?
   All patients with anemia should receive a CBC with erythrocyte indices (mean corpuscular volume [MCV], mean corpuscular hemoglobin [MCH], mean corpuscular hemoglobin concentration [MCHC], red blood cell (RBC) distribution width, and a reticulocyte count). The patient is also presenting with jaundice, necessitating liver function tests and direct (conjugated) and indirect (unconjugated) bilirubin levels.

CASE 15.2 CONTINUED:

The additional tests reveal a reticulocyte count of 7% (normal is <2.5%), an MCV of 90 fL (normal is 80–100 fL), and an elevated indirect bilirubin. With these results, you decide to order a direct Coombs test, which returns positive.

3. What is the most likely diagnosis?
   Drug-induced warm immune-mediated hemolytic anemia (IMHA) is the most likely diagnosis.

4. What is the significance of a positive direct Coombs test, and how does it support the diagnosis considered in this patient?

A Coombs test is an antiglobulin assay that detects both immunoglobulin that is attached to the surface of a patient's RBCs (direct test) and the presence of circulating immunoglobulin against RBCs (indirect test). A positive direct Coombs test supports, but does not prove, the presence of an immune antibody-mediated hemolytic process.

Note: Distinguishing between direct and indirect Coombs assays can be tricky, but it is important to understand the differences between the methodologies and uses for the two tests. The direct Coombs test is used to detect the presence of immunoglobulins directed against the patient's *own* RBCs (e.g., hemolytic disease of the newborn, drug-induced IMHA, transfusion reactions). Serum containing anti-Ig antibody is mixed with the patient's RBCs. If the RBCs are coated with immunoglobulin present in the patient's own blood, the addition of anti-Ig antibody will cause agglutination. In an indirect Coombs test, commercial RBCs bound with defined antigens are mixed with the patient's serum. If immunoglobulins directed against the RBCs are present in the patient's serum, agglutination will occur. Thus an indirect test determines the presence of immunoglobulins against *foreign blood products* that are not bound to the patient's own RBCs. This can be useful when screening for antibodies before blood transfusion, detecting Rh antibodies, etc.

5. How do medications such as penicillin cause IMHA?

Certain antibiotics (e.g., penicillin, cephalosporins, streptomycin, tetracycline) and other small molecules may nonspecifically adsorb to proteins on RBC surfaces. Recall that many of these drugs are generally too small to elicit an immune response by themselves; however, they can become immunogenic when combined with larger molecules such as membrane-associated proteins (i.e., they form a hapten-carrier complex). In certain individuals, this drug-protein complex can induce the formation of antibodies, which then bind to the adsorbed drug on RBCs and mediate RBC lysis.

6. What type of hypersensitivity does IMHA represent?

This is an example of a type II hypersensitivity reaction (cytotoxic hypersensitivity), in which IgM or IgG antibodies bind to cell surface antigens and mediate cellular destruction. Other examples of type II hypersensitivity include pernicious anemia, rheumatic fever, Goodpasture syndrome, bullous pemphigoid, pemphigus vulgaris, blood transfusion reactions, hyperacute rejection of organ transplants, and hemolytic disease of the newborn.

7. What is the mechanism by which hemolysis occurs in drug-induced IMHA?

IgG attached to RBC-bound antigens binds Fcγ receptors on effector cells (neutrophils, macrophages, and NK cells). The effector cells mediate destruction of the RBCs by phagocytosis or release of cytotoxic granules. Opsonization by either IgG or IgM can also induce complement-mediated lysis of RBCs, but this mode of destruction is less common in AIHA.

Note: In some individuals, the extended use of certain drugs, including methyldopa, levodopa, quinidine, and procainamide, can stimulate production of anti-RBC antibodies. The mechanism by which the autoantibodies are induced is unknown, and the antibodies do not cross-react with the drug that appears to elicit their production.

RELATED QUESTION

8. If this patient was infected with *Mycoplasma pneumoniae* instead of pneumococcus, what type of immune-mediated hemolytic anemia would have been considered?

Cold IMHA, in which anti-*M. pneumoniae* IgM cross-reacts with erythrocyte surface antigens, would have been considered. Optimal binding of IgM to erythrocytes occurs at 0°C to 5°C (compared with 37°C in warm IMHA), and IgM initiates complement-mediated hemolysis. This occurs intravascularly, whereas in warm IMHA, sequestration and hemolysis occur in the spleen (extravascular hemolysis).

SUMMARY BOX: IMMUNE-MEDIATED HEMOLYTIC ANEMIA

- Presentation: Pallor, jaundice
- Pathophysiology: Type II hypersensitivity reaction
  - Autoantibodies against red blood cell (RBC) surface antigens target cells for destruction by opsonization and phagocytosis
  - Can be induced by certain drugs (penicillin) acting as haptens
- Diagnosis: Low hemoglobin/hematocrit, elevated lactate dehydrogenase (LDH), reduced haptoglobin, positive Coombs test

CASE 15.3

A 12-year-old boy presents to the emergency department with puffy eyes, perioral swelling, a tight feeling in his throat, and widespread urticaria. A few hours after arrival, he develops a fever, enlarged lymph nodes, splenomegaly, and swollen, painful ankles. His mother reports that he stepped on a nail during vacation in Zimbabwe 1 week ago and was given horse anti-tetanus immune serum. His mother also states his urine appears foamy and discolored.

1. What is the differential diagnosis for this boy's presentation?

Nephrotic syndrome, serum sickness, infectious mononucleosis, glomerulonephritis, anaphylaxis, juvenile rheumatoid arthritis (acute febrile type), and upper respiratory tract infection should be considered.

CASE 15.3 CONTINUED:

Laboratory testing of the boy's blood reveals an elevated white blood cell (WBC) count, with primarily lymphocytosis. Plasma cells are detected in a peripheral blood smear. His total serum complement level, C1q, and C3 levels are decreased. Urinalysis reveals proteinuria and hematuria. The patient is started on prednisone, leading to progressive symptom improvement.

2. What is the most likely diagnosis?
   Serum sickness is the most likely diagnosis.

3. What is the pathogenesis of serum sickness?
   Type III hypersensitivity reaction is the pathogenesis of serum sickness. Serum sickness is caused by the formation of antibody-antigen immune complexes and their deposition in tissues, resulting in activation of the complement cascade. In this case, the immune complexes are composed of the patient's own IgG antibodies directed against horse serum proteins (most likely the Fc portion of the horse immunoglobulins). If large amounts of antigen and antibody are present, the mononuclear phagocyte system is overwhelmed and unable to clear all the immune complexes from circulation. As a result, the immune complexes deposit in tissues and result in local activation of the complement system, provoking an inflammatory response. Similarly, the Arthus reaction is also a classic type III hypersensitivity reaction. In the Arthus reaction, intradermal injection of foreign antigen induces antibody production and immune complex formation in the skin, leading to localized edema and necrosis from complement activation.

4. What is the reason for the delay from the serum administration to the onset of symptoms?
   The presence of antigen alone is insufficient to produce serum sickness. A time interval of 2 days to 2 weeks is generally necessary for antibody production to reach a level at which the number of antibody-antigen complexes exceeds their clearance threshold.
   Note: Symptoms generally resolve once the mononuclear phagocyte system "catches up" and is able to effectively clear the causative antigen.

STEP 1 SECRET

Be sure to pay close attention to time intervals on the USMLE exam because they can often provide significant clues to the type of hypersensitivity reaction taking place. Although serum sickness may cause urticaria similar to that associated with type I hypersensitivity, this reaction will occur days after antigen exposure in contrast with minutes after antigen exposure (seen with type I reactions).

5. What is the significance of decreased serum levels of complement?
   This signifies consumption of complement secondary to the activation of the classical pathway by immune complexes. Note that only IgG- and IgM-containing complexes can fix complement. IgM is generally more efficient than IgG at activating the complement cascade because it has more Fc regions to bind C1 protein.

6. What caused the hives and facial swelling in the patient?
   Activation of the complement cascade leads to the production of complement components C3a, C4a, and C5a (anaphylatoxins), which in turn elicit mediator release from mast cells. Histamine and leukotrienes cause vasodilation and increase vascular permeability, leading to urticaria and edema.

7. What is the significance of RBCs and protein in the urine?
   This suggests development of glomerulonephritis. One potential site of immune complex deposition in type III hypersensitivity is the renal glomeruli. Inflammation at the glomerulus leads to glomerulonephritis, which is hallmarked by hematuria and proteinuria. Note that most cases of glomerulonephritis are caused by a type III hypersensitivity reaction: postinfectious glomerulonephritis (mediated by complexes of IgG and *Streptococcus pyogenes* antigens) and systemic lupus erythematosus (SLE) nephritis (mediated by complexes of IgG and nuclear components). The antigen involved in IgA nephropathy is unclear, but the mesangial deposition of IgA and C3 suggests that this disease represents a rare instance of IgA fixing complement.

8. What is the cause of this boy's joint pain?
   Immune complex deposition in synovial tissue. This mechanism is identical to that seen in rheumatoid arthritis–associated joint pain.

9. Does a type III hypersensitivity reaction require previous exposure (sensitization) to antigen to occur?
   No. If enough exogenous antigen is given on first exposure, large numbers of immune complexes can form over time and activate the classical complement pathway. Nowadays, nonhuman antibodies are rarely administered to patients due to risk of serum sickness.

SUMMARY BOX: SERUM SICKNESS

- Presentation: Rash, fever, arthritis, facial and peripheral edema
- Diagnosis: Lymphocytosis, decreased serum complement levels, hematuria and proteinuria on urinalysis
- Pathophysiology: Type III hypersensitivity reaction
  - Immunoglobulin G (IgG) antibodies directed against horse serum proteins (or other nonhuman antigens) form immune complexes.
  - Immune complex deposition in tissue results in complement-mediated tissue destruction.

CASE 15.4

A 23-year-old woman comes to your office with a pruritic rash and no other symptoms. She is already wearing a gown when you enter the room, and you immediately notice large weepy, erythematous, crusted patches and plaques on her chest, face, and arms. As you move closer, you see clear and erythematous vesicles within these areas. She also has swollen eyelids.

1. What is the differential diagnosis for this woman's rash?

   Contact dermatitis (allergic type), contact dermatitis (irritant type), atopic dermatitis, varicella-zoster virus infection, and second-degree burn are considered.

2. How can allergic-type and irritant-type contact dermatitis be differentiated?

   Rash morphology and timing can help differentiate between these types of contact dermatitis. Allergic contact dermatitis (atopic dermatitis) is a rash that develops from skin-substance contact, after the patient has been immunologically sensitized (as seen with poison ivy). Irritant contact dermatitis is a rash that develops from repetitive skin irritation from chemical exposure or physical trauma (as seen with repetitive body washing, which is often a manifestation of obsessive-compulsive disorder).

   Additionally, atopic dermatitis and allergic contact dermatitis can be differentiated by rash characteristics and time of onset. Rashes of atopic dermatitis tend to show lichenification from chronic scratching and appear on the flexural body surfaces. Contact dermatitis tends to be erythematous, weepy, and sharply demarcated because it only appears in areas where direct contact occurred. It may appear as linear rashes if the patient brushed up against an allergen such as poison ivy. Atopic dermatitis (also known as eczema) is a type I, IgE-mediated hypersensitivity reaction and can be a chronic condition (similar to asthma and allergic rhinitis). However, symptoms can develop within minutes after exposure to the triggering allergen. Conversely, allergic contact dermatitis is a type IV, delayed-type hypersensitivity (DTH) reaction. In a previously sensitized patient, symptoms occur 12 to 72 hours after exposure to the allergen.

STEP 1 SECRET

Both atopic and contact dermatitis are high-yield topics for the USMLE Step 1 exam. It is important that you know how to differentiate them from one another.

CASE 15.4 CONTINUED:

You elicit the history from the patient and find that she recently began going to a tanning salon. About 1 week ago, she stayed in the light too long and acquired a sunburn covering her arms and upper chest. She used an aerosol spray of benzocaine and triclosan to relieve the pain of the sunburn. After 2 days, she developed a rash covering both of her arms, her chest, and her face. She took diphenhydramine to control the itching, but the rash did not improve. She denies fever, fatigue, or any other associated symptoms.

3. What is the diagnosis?

   Contact dermatitis (allergic type) is the diagnosis.

4. What is the causative agent and the mechanism by which it induced an immune response in the patient?

   Benzocaine is the causative agent. The active ingredients in topical drugs constitute a major cause of contact dermatitis. In DTH reactions, APCs in the skin called *Langerhans cells* internalize self-proteins that are bound to exogenous, haptenated molecules. These complexes are processed and displayed on MHC class II molecules, which bind to TCRs on $CD4^+$ T cells and induce differentiation into a T_H1 phenotype. T_H1 cells produce IFN-γ, which activates macrophages, and IL-2, which leads to expansion of $CD8^+$ CTLs. Release of lytic enzymes from activated macrophages and perforins and granzymes from CTLs results in epidermal damage, erythema, vesicle formation, and weeping rash.

Clinical Pearl

A positive tuberculin purified protein derivative (PPD) test and the granulomas found in tuberculosis are due to type IV delayed-type hypersensitivity (DTH) reactions.

5. Why did the patient have lesions in areas other than on her arms and upper chest (where she applied the spray)?

The topical drug can be transferred from the initial point of contact to other areas of the skin by the fingernails after scratching the itchy lesions at the primary site. Therefore unexpected sites can be affected (e.g., the eyelids and genitals). It is beneficial to cut fingernails short and thoroughly wash the skin to remove the drug and prevent further spread.

6. What is the treatment for allergic-type contact dermatitis?

Corticosteroids are the treatment. Topical corticosteroids are used for localized contact dermatitis. Widespread rashes require oral steroids. Oral diphenhydramine can help control itch.

7. Why is it important for the patient to avoid the use of benzocaine in the future?

When an individual is sensitized, each subsequent exposure not only produces the hypersensitivity reaction but also generates more effector and memory T cells. Thus the reaction becomes more severe with each subsequent exposure. Memory T cells can persist for the lifetime of an individual.

Note: The first contact with an allergen does not typically result in a type IV allergic response. Accordingly, contact hypersensitivity requires a sensitization stage in which a clonal population of memory T cells is produced and an elicitation stage whereby memory T cells become activated upon subsequent exposure to antigen. Additionally, an individual may be able to touch the allergen for many years without suffering an adverse reaction.

SUMMARY BOX: CONTACT DERMATITIS

- Presentation: Erythematous, weepy, well-demarcated pruritic rash
  - Hint: Classically seen with poison ivy exposure, resulting in linear rashes
- Pathophysiology: Type IV delayed type hypersensitivity reaction
  - T_H1 cells activate macrophages and cytotoxic T lymphocytes (CTLs), which mediate tissue damage
- Diagnosis: Clinical (history and physical examination)
- Treatment: Topical or oral corticosteroids, diphenhydramine for itch control, avoidance of exposure that caused the type IV delayed-type hypersensitivity reaction

---

CASE 15.5

A 4-month-old baby boy is brought to your office by his parents for evaluation of a runny nose and cough that have persisted for over a month. Examination reveals oral thrush, absence of tonsils and lymph nodes, and a fall from the 50th percentile in weight to the 10th percentile. A chest x-ray study is performed and demonstrates diffuse, symmetrical interstitial opacities. Laboratory tests reveal marked lymphopenia with slightly low numbers of CD20+ cells (B lymphocytes) and a severe deficiency of CD3+ cells (T lymphocytes).

---

1. What is the differential diagnosis?

Severe combined immunodeficiency (SCID), human immunodeficiency virus (HIV) infection (despite low risk in this patient), bare lymphocyte syndrome, ataxia-telangiectasia, and atypical DiGeorge syndrome (thymic aplasia) are considered.

CASE 15.5 CONTINUED:

Further specialized testing reveals lymphocytes are unresponsive to the B- and T-cell pokeweed mitogen (PWM). A diagnosis of *Pneumocystis jiroveci* (formerly *Pneumocystis carinii*) pneumonia is made, and the baby responds well to intravenous trimethoprim-sulfamethoxazole (TMP-SMX). HIV testing is negative.

---

2. What is the most likely diagnosis in this infant, given the fact that specialized testing revealed defects in both cellular and humoral function?

SCID is the most likely diagnosis. This condition is invariably fatal in infants unless recognized and treated by bone marrow transplantation. Before transplantation, SCID patients must avoid exposure to any microorganisms by residing in a sterile environment (e.g., "bubble boy"). Typically, infants with SCID become ill within the first 3 months of life and suffer from recurrent respiratory infections, pneumonia, thrush, diarrhea, and failure to thrive. Opportunistic infections with intracellular pathogens such as *Candida albicans*, *P. jiroveci*, *Cryptococcus neoformans*, cytomegalovirus (CMV), and mycobacteria are commonly observed in these infants.

3. Why might a bone marrow transplant from an appropriate donor cure this patient?

The pathogenesis of SCID involves abnormal production and function of mature B and T cells. Bone marrow transplant will reconstitute this infant's immune system with normal lymphocyte progenitors that can differentiate into mature, functional B and T lymphocytes.

4. What is the significance of the marked lymphopenia and complete lack of CD3⁺ cells?

SCID is a family of primary immune disorders that is characterized by low numbers of circulating *lymphocytes*. The most common form of SCID is X-linked and caused by a mutation in common gamma chain (γ_c), which is an integral component of several interleukin receptors (IL-2, IL-4, IL-7, IL-9, IL-15, IL-21) important in T- and B-cell development and differentiation. Within the lymphocyte population, T-cell numbers are typically low to absent, B-cell numbers can range from fairly normal to absent (although these B cells are typically nonfunctional), and NK cell numbers can be low to normal. Thus there is failure to mount both humoral and cell-mediated immune responses. It is the lack of cell-mediated immunity that makes patients with SCID highly susceptible to opportunistic infections with intracellular organisms, the hallmark of this disease. The other forms of SCID are autosomal recessive, the most common being adenosine deaminase (ADA) deficiency. In ADA deficiency, accumulation of adenosine is thought to be toxic to lymphocytes.

Note: SCID may look very similar to DiGeorge syndrome, in which failure to develop the third and fourth pharyngeal pouches results in an absent thymus and a resultant complete lack of T cells. Both SCID and DiGeorge syndromes can produce an absent thymic shadow on chest x-ray films. (The USMLE may show you an x-ray film and have you identify the thymus; look for the sail sign.) However, DiGeorge syndrome does not affect B cells, is generally associated with congenital heart defects, and often produces symptoms of hypocalcemia due to absent parathyroid glands. Lymph node biopsy of SCID patients will reveal lack of germinal centers due to B-cell dysfunction.

5. Why are B-cell defects not evident in many babies when they are first diagnosed with severe combined immunodeficiency?

Infants have circulating maternal antibodies that are passively obtained from transplacental circulation (IgG) and breast milk (IgA). As these antibodies are cleared over time, the infant is unable to synthesize its own immunoglobin, and levels will be low to absent.

RELATED QUESTIONS: B-CELL DISORDERS

6. Which primary immunodeficiency should be suspected in a child with normal cell-mediated immunity but almost complete absence of plasma immunoglobulins?

X-linked Bruton agammaglobulinemia should be suspected. Affected boys have few B cells in blood and lymphoid tissue and have very low levels of circulating immunoglobulins. The defect involves Bruton tyrosine kinase, which is crucial for the maturation of pre–B cells. Patients present with recurrent bacterial and enteroviral infections after 6 months of age, when maternal immunoglobin drops. Lack of CD19⁺ B cells supports the diagnosis.

STEP 1 SECRET

X-linked immunodeficiencies can be remembered using the mnemonic Missing WBCs, which stands for hyper-IgM syndrome, Wiskott-Aldrich syndrome, Bruton agammaglobulinemia, Chronic granulomatous disease, and SCID (severe combined immunodeficiency; most common type).

7. A patient with a history of recurrent sinopulmonary infections receives a blood transfusion after a motor vehicle accident. The patient subsequently develops anaphylaxis. Which disorder does this patient likely suffer from?

The patient is likely suffering from IgA deficiency, the most common primary immunodeficiency. Many patients are asymptomatic, but symptomatic patients often have recurrent sinopulmonary infections, persistent giardiasis, diarrhea, allergies, and asthma. Transfusion of blood products containing IgA can result in life-threatening anaphylaxis due to the presence of antibodies against IgA molecules in the patient's serum. IgA deficiency is also associated with celiac disease and can cause a false negative anti-tissue transglutaminase antibody, because this is an IgA antibody.

STEP 1 SECRET

The scenario of an anaphylactic reaction following blood transfusion is a favorite on the Step 1 exam. Consider this whenever a patient has an anaphylactic reaction after blood transfusion.

8. Can you name some other primary immunodeficiencies?

See Table 15.9.

Table 15.9. Summary of Primary Immunodeficiencies

CLASSIFICATION	EXAMPLE(S) OF IMMUNODEFICIENCY SYNDROMES	IMMUNE DEFECT	SUSCEPTIBILITY
B-cell deficiencies	Bruton agammaglobulinemia (X-linked hypogammaglobulinemia)	Few to no B cells (<1% of CD19+ cells confirms defect); all isotypes of Ig decreased	Recurrent pyogenic infections appear after age of 6 months (when maternal IgG is diminished)
	X-linked hyper-IgM syndrome	No B cell class switching from IgM to other isotypes (due to a defect in CD40 ligand)	Recurrent pyogenic infections; poor response to immunizations; opportunistic infections with *Pneumocystis*, *Cryptosporidium*, and CMV
	IgA deficiency	B cells fail to produce IgA	Recurrent sinus, respiratory, and gastrointestinal infections; anaphylactic transfusion reactions
	Common variable immunodeficiency	Late-onset (ages 20–35 years) agammaglobulinemia that has acquired and inherited characteristics; commonly follows viral infection	Recurrent pyogenic infections; increased risk of various autoimmune diseases and lymphoma
T-cell deficiencies	DiGeorge syndrome	T-cell deficit resulting from thymic aplasia (pharyngeal pouch maldevelopment)	Opportunistic infections: viral and fungal infections
	Chronic mucocutaneous candidiasis	T-cell dysfunction specific to *Candida albicans*	Recurrent skin and mucous membrane *C. albicans* infections
	Hyper IgE syndrome (Job syndrome)	STAT3 defect leads to T_H17 cell deficiency and impaired neutrophil recruitment to infection sites; T-cell defect leads to decreased IFN-γ and excess IgE	Cold noninflamed *Staphylococcus aureus* abscesses; patients often have fair skin, red hair, eczema, retained primary teeth, and coarse "leonine facies."
Combined deficiencies	Severe combined immunodeficiency (SCID)	Deficit of both B and T cells	Opportunistic infections from viruses, bacteria, fungi, and protozoa
	Ataxia-telangiectasia	Defect in *ATM* gene, which codes for a DNA repair enzyme, IgA deficiency, cerebellar degeneration, and skin and conjunctiva telangiectasia	Recurrent infections, increased risk of lymphoma
	Wiskott-Aldrich syndrome	X-linked F-actin assembly defect in T cells and platelets; normal IgG, decreased IgM, and increased IgA and IgE	Infections with encapsulated bacteria; atopic dermatitis; thrombocytopenia
	Bare lymphocyte syndrome	Defective or absent MHC class I and/or II molecules	Recurrent infections, commonly viral
Complement deficiencies	See Table 15.4		
Phagocyte deficiencies	Chronic granulomatous disease (CGD)	Defective phagocytic respiratory burst, resulting from mutations in the NADPH oxidase gene	Increased susceptibility to certain bacteria and fungi; widespread granuloma formation

Table 15.9. Summary of Primary Immunodeficiencies—cont'd

CLASSIFICATION	EXAMPLE(S) OF IMMUNODEFICIENCY SYNDROMES	IMMUNE DEFECT	SUSCEPTIBILITY
	Chédiak-Higashi syndrome	Microtubule dysfunction leads to defective neutrophil phagosome-lysosomal fusion	Recurrent staphylococcal and streptococcal infections
	Leukocyte adhesion deficiency	Defective neutrophil integrin (LFA-1: mediates adhesion), resulting in defective migration and chemotaxis	Recurrent pyogenic infections of skin and mucosa; impaired neutrophil chemotaxis causes neutrophilia; delayed umbilical cord separation
	IL-12 receptor deficiency	Defective IL-12 receptor prevents differentiation of T_H1 phenotype with subsequent impact on IFN-γ production	Disseminated, severe mycobacterial infections
	IFN-γ receptor deficiency	Defective IFN-γ receptor prevents macrophage activation and the killing of intracellular pathogens	Disseminated, severe mycobacterial infections
	Cyclic neutropenia	Autosomal dominant; irregular production of G-CSF leads to neutropenia for 3–6 days approximately every 21 days	Severe bacterial infections during neutropenic phase only

CMV, Cytomegalovirus; *G-CSF,* granulocyte colony-stimulating factor; *IFN-γ,* interferon-γ; *IgA, IgE, IgG, IgM,* immunoglobulins A, E, G, M; *IL,* interleukin; *LFA-1,* lymphocyte function–associated antigen-1; *MHC,* major histocompatibility complex; *NADPH,* nicotinamide adenine dinucleotide phosphate (reduced).

SUMMARY BOX: SEVERE COMBINED IMMUNODEFICIENCY

- Presentation: Infants with failure to thrive and oral thrush; recurrent bacterial, viral, fungal, and protozoal infections
- Epidemiology: 50% of cases are X-linked and therefore more common in boys
- Diagnosis: Lymphopenia, hypogammaglobulinemia, absence of thymic shadow on chest x-ray film
- Pathophysiology: Represents a family of diseases resulting in both T- and B-cell defects
  - Common gamma chain mutation results in various defects in interleukin receptors (X-linked)
  - Adenosine deaminase deficiency (autosomal recessive)
- Treatment: Bone marrow transplant

CASE 15.6

A 5-year-old boy presents to the emergency department with severe shortness of breath, a persistent cough, and chest pain. Chest x-ray reveals the presence of multiple large, fuzzy opacities in both lung fields. Laboratory tests reveal a normal WBC count with normal proportions of neutrophils, lymphocytes, and monocytes. A brief review of the boy's medical history shows multiple infections with organisms in the genera *Staphylococcus* and *Burkholderia*. Laboratory tests from 1 month ago showed a similar WBC profile along with serum antibody levels in the high normal range and normal levels of complement proteins.

1. **What is the differential diagnosis for this boy's apparent immunodeficiency?**
   The differential diagnosis includes chronic granulomatous disease (CGD), Chédiak-Higashi syndrome (CHS), and leukocyte adhesion deficiency (LAD). Complement deficiencies and B-cell disorders can also cause recurrent bacterial infections, though these generally involve encapsulated organisms (e.g., *Streptococcus pneumoniae, H. influenzae, Neisseria meningitidis, Salmonella* spp.). The presence of recurrent *Staphylococcus aureus* and *Burkholderia* (catalase-positive gram-negative rods) infections is strongly suggestive of a phagocyte deficiency.

CASE 15.6 CONTINUED:

In a WBC function test, the boy's monocytes and neutrophils fail to reduce nitroblue tetrazolium (NBT), a test of the adequacy of the oxidative respiratory burst. Sputum cultures grow *Aspergillus fumigatus*. The patient is promptly started on IV liposomal amphotericin B. He slowly improves over a 2-month period, but during this time in the hospital he contracts two bacterial respiratory infections. Upon discharge, he is started on IFN-γ injections and given daily prophylactic TMP-SMX.

2. What is the diagnosis?

   CGD, a genetic disorder that results from nicotinamide adenine dinucleotide phosphate (NADPH) oxidase deficiency (65% of cases are X-linked recessive and 35% are autosomal recessive), is the diagnosis. It is important to understand the basis of the NBT test. The color of NBT is changed from yellow to deep blue in the presence of reactive oxygen species generated from respiratory burst. Absent color change indicates lack of functional NADPH oxidase.

3. What are the two mechanisms that a macrophage can employ to kill bacteria following phagocytosis?

   Oxygen-dependent respiratory burst and oxygen-independent mechanisms can be employed. During phagocytosis, macrophages and neutrophils are capable of performing the respiratory burst. This process is dependent upon the activity of NADPH oxidase, which catalyzes the production of superoxide (O_2^-) from oxygen. Superoxide dismutase (SOD) converts superoxide to hydrogen peroxide (H_2O_2), which is converted to hypochlorite ($HOCl^-$) by myeloperoxidase (MPO). $HOCl^-$ (the active ingredient in bleach) is responsible for killing bacteria. Hydrogen peroxide (H_2O_2) that leaks out of the phagolysosome is potentially harmful to tissues and is neutralized to water by catalase, whose activity requires the conversion of reduced glutathione (GSH) into its oxidized form, glutathione disulfide (GSSG) (Fig. 15.4).

   Macrophages also kill ingested pathogens through oxygen-independent mechanisms via the action of lysozyme, hydrolytic enzymes, and cytotoxic peptides.

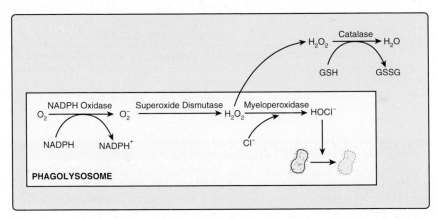

Figure 15.4. Respiratory burst. *GSSG*, Glutathione disulfide; *GSH*, glutathione; *NADPH*, nicotinamide adenine dinucleotide phosphate.

4. What is the basis for widespread granuloma formation in chronic granulomatous disease?

   A deficiency in NADPH oxidase results in an inability of phagocytes to kill many types of phagocytosed pathogens. Therefore these microorganisms persist, leading to the formation of granulomas in an attempt to sequester pathogens. Widespread granulomas can be found in patients with CGD even in the absence of active infection.

5. What are the contents of a granuloma, and why is it formed?

   A granuloma is a collection of epithelioid histiocytes and giant cells surrounded by a fibrous capsule. Epithelioid histiocytes are modified macrophages that form epithelial-like configurations. Giant cells are formed from macrophage fusion, generating large, multinucleated cells. These cells are maintained by continued secretion of IFN-γ by local T_H1 cells (Figs. 15.5 and 15.6). Generally, a granuloma forms to contain an intracellular pathogen that has been resistant to elimination, but sterile granulomas are common in CGD.

STEP 1 SECRET

It is important to be able to recognize images of granulomas and their major constituents for the purpose of the USMLE.

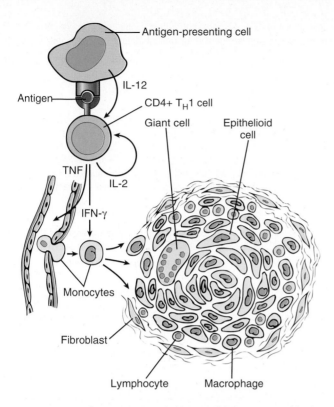

Figure 15.5. Schematic illustration of granuloma formation. *IL-2, -12,* Interleukin-2, -12; *IFN-γ,* interferon-γ; *TNF,* tumor necrosis factor. *(From Kumar V, Abbas AK, Fausto N.* Robbins & Cotran Pathologic Basis of Disease. *7th ed. Philadelphia: WB Saunders; 2005.)*

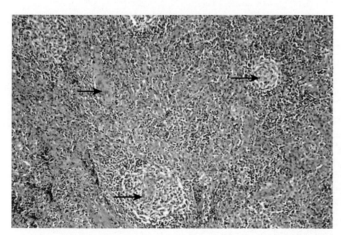

Figure 15.6. Lobectomy of left lower lobe with dense acute inflammatory infiltrate and granulomas (*arrows*). In chronic granulomatous disease of childhood, neutrophil function is defective, leading to an inability to kill a variety of infectious organisms. Hematoxylin-eosin (H&E) stain, ×100 magnification. *(From Love GL.* Hyalohyphomycoses. In: Pathology of Infectious Diseases. *Philadelphia: Elsevier; 2015:chap 23.)*

6. Patients with chronic granulomatous disease often experience recurrent staphylococcal infections, but streptococcal infections are rare. Why?
Organisms in the genus *Streptococcus* are catalase negative. As mentioned earlier, catalase catalyzes the degradation of hydrogen peroxide ($2H_2O_2 \rightarrow 2H_2O + O_2$). In the absence of catalase, hydrogen peroxide is not degraded and can be "stolen" by the phagocyte and converted to hypochlorite by myeloperoxidase. This allows for killing of the organism in the absence of functional NADPH oxidase.
   Conversely, catalase-positive organisms quickly eliminate all hydrogen peroxide that they produce and cannot be killed via respiratory burst in hosts lacking functional NADPH oxidase. Common catalase-positive infecting organisms in CGD include *S. aureus, Serratia, B. cepacia, Aspergillus, Nocardia,* and *Candida*. Note that *Neisseria*, although catalase positive, rarely causes infections in CGD because phagocytes have a propensity to kill this organism by oxygen-independent mechanisms (see question 3).

7. What is the mechanism of action of amphotericin B?
The polyene family, including amphotericin B and nystatin, act by binding to ergosterol in the plasma membrane of fungal cells and creating pores in the membrane. This results in leakage of intracellular components, precipitating cell

death. Amphotericin B possesses broad antifungal coverage, but its undesirable side effect profile (chills, fever, nephrotoxicity, arrhythmias, hypotension) can be prohibitive. Nystatin is reserved for topical (diaper rash, vaginal candidiasis) and oral (oral candidiasis) use.

RELATED QUESTIONS: PHAGOCYTE DISORDERS

8. How does CHS differ from CGD?

CHS is a primary immunodeficiency of the myeloid lineage. It is an autosomal recessive disorder characterized by microtubule (MT) dysfunction, resulting in failure of the phagolysosome to form. The presence of giant intracytoplasmic granules in polymorphonuclear leukocytes (PMNs) and monocytes supports CHS. Recurrent infections with *S. aureus*, as well as *Streptococcus* and *Pseudomonas,* are seen in CHS. In addition to a failure of phagosome-lysosome fusion, MT defects affect trafficking in melanocytes, nerve cells, and platelets. This can manifest as peripheral neuropathy, partial albinism, and bleeding diathesis. In contrast with CGD, CHS yields a normal NBT or dichlorofluorescein test because NADPH oxidase is functional.

SUMMARY BOX: CHRONIC GRANULOMATOUS DISEASE

- Presentation: Recurrent infections from catalase-positive organisms such as *Staphylococcus aureus, Burkholderia, Nocardia, Serratia, Aspergillus,* and *Candida*
- Epidemiology: More common in boys (65% of cases are X-linked recessive and 35% are autosomal recessive)
- Diagnosis: Failed nitroblue tetrazolium (NBT) test
- Pathophysiology: Nicotinamide adenine dinucleotide phosphate (NADPH) oxidase mutation results in defective respiratory burst
- Treatment: Antibacterial prophylaxis and treatment of infections

---

CASE 15.7

A 5-day-old girl is brought to you by her mother for evaluation of "repeated muscle seizures" that began 3 days ago. She is afebrile. Physical examination reveals several facial abnormalities, including low-set ears, a prominent nose, wide-set eyes (hypertelorism), and an undersized jaw (micrognathia). Laboratory tests are remarkable for hypocalcemia and lymphopenia. Chest x-ray reveals a boot-shaped heart, decreased pulmonary vasculature markings, and the absence of a thymic shadow.

---

1. What is the likely diagnosis in this infant, and what is the pathophysiology of her disorder?

DiGeorge syndrome (thymic parathyroid aplasia) is the likely diagnosis. This genetic disorder is caused by microdeletions on chromosome 22q, resulting in dysmorphogenesis of the third and fourth pharyngeal pouches during embryologic development. The thymus originates from the ventral wing of the third pharyngeal pouch, the superior parathyroid glands arise from the dorsal wing of the fourth pouch, and the inferior parathyroid glands arise from the dorsal wing of the third pouch. These structures are therefore absent in DiGeorge syndrome (Fig. 15.7). For similar embryologic reasons, the heart and aorta are often affected. DiGeorge syndrome is typically detected in the first week of life after evaluation of infants with hypocalcemia-induced tetany as a result of hypoparathyroidism. Tetany can be mistaken for seizures in infants.

2. Joseph Heller might ask, "What tried and true medical school mnemonic can be used to remember the classic manifestations of DiGeorge syndrome?"

Just remember **CATCH 22**:

Congenital heart abnormalities (commonly truncus arteriosus or tetralogy of Fallot)
Abnormal facial features
Thymic aplasia
Cleft palate
Hypocalcemia from hypoparathyroidism
22q deletion

3. To what types of infections might this child be vulnerable, given that thymic development is abnormal?

This child might be vulnerable to viral, bacterial, and fungal infections. The thymus is a primary lymphoid organ that is responsible for the maturation of progenitor T cells. When the thymus is underdeveloped or lacking, there is a dramatic decrease in all populations of T cells and a corresponding lack of cell-mediated immunity. Patients with DiGeorge syndrome who survive the immediate neonatal period are susceptible to recurrent or chronic fungal and viral infections that would normally be eradicated by CTLs. Additionally, because T_H cells and their cytokines (e.g., IL-2, IL-4, IL-5) are critical for the proliferation and differentiation of B cells, deterioration of humoral immunity will occur as maternal

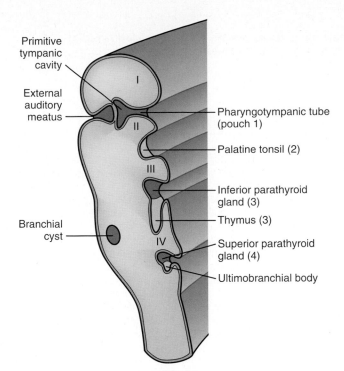

Primitive
tympanic
cavity

I

External
auditory
meatus

II

Pharyngotympanic tube
(pouch 1)

Palatine tonsil (2)

III

Inferior parathyroid
gland (3)

Thymus (3)

Branchial
cyst

IV

Superior parathyroid
gland (4)

Ultimobranchial body

Figure 15.7. Maturation of the pharyngeal pouches.
(From Cummings CW, Flint PW, Haughey BH.
Otolaryngology: Head & Neck Surgery. *4th ed.*
Philadelphia: Mosby; 2005.)

antibodies are degraded in the infant. Thus the patient will also become susceptible to infection with extracellular
pathogens such as bacteria, which are normally warded off by the humoral immune system.

4. **What might a lymph node biopsy in this infant reveal?**
Thymic absence or hypoplasia in DiGeorge syndrome results in inadequate production of functionally mature T cells.
Histologic analysis of lymph nodes would therefore reveal near complete absence of T cells in T-cell–dependent zones.

RELATED QUESTION

5. **What does the process of thymic education involve?**
The education of thymocytes involves both positive and negative selection and ensures that mature T cells will be MHC-
restricted and self-tolerant, respectively. T-cell precursors enter the thymus as double positive cells that express both
CD4 and CD8 molecules. During positive selection in the cortex, T cells that bind MHC molecules are selected to survive
whereas T cells unable to bind MHC undergo apoptosis. Cells that interact with MHC class I become CD8+ single
positive cells. Cells that interact with MHC class II become CD4+ single positive cells. Negative selection occurs in the
medulla and involves apoptosis of T cells that avidly bind self-peptide in association with MHC molecules (potentially
self-reactive T cells). Less than 5% of thymocytes survive these selection processes.

SUMMARY BOX: DIGEORGE SYNDROME

- Presentation: Abnormal facial features (low-set ears, wide-set eyes, prominent nose, micrognathia, cleft palate) in a
young child with a history of recurrent viral and fungal infections, tetany, and cardiac complications
- Pathophysiology: Deletion in chromosome 22q results in failure of structures to develop from third and fourth
pharyngeal pouches (affects the thymus, parathyroid glands, heart, and aorta).
  - Results in lack of T-cell maturation and susceptibility to infections
- Diagnosis: Low parathyroid hormone (PTH), hypocalcemia, lymphopenia (absent T cells and normal B cells), absence
of thymic shadow on chest x-ray

CASE 15.8

A 25-year-old man comes to your office, for the first time in many years, with complaints of general fatigue, a headache, muscle aches, and a mild
fever. He states that this has persisted for "4 or 5 days" and that he "just wants to get my energy back." He takes no medications. He appears
tired. Physical examination is notable for scattered lymphadenopathy and a small patchy nonspecific rash on the neck.

1. **What is the differential diagnosis?**
   Infectious mononucleosis, hypothyroidism, influenza, occult infection, anemia, depression, acute HIV infection, malnutrition, adrenal insufficiency, non-Hodgkin lymphoma, and dermatomyositis should be considered.

CASE 15.8 CONTINUED:

You write orders for a battery of standard tests and give the patient directions to the laboratory. As you are about the leave the room, the patient stops you and asks, "A few months ago, I started using intravenous heroin. Do you think that might be related to these problems?"

2. **What must be suspected? What tests are used to diagnose this disease after the acute stage?**
   HIV infection, which can be spread through blood, semen, vaginal fluid, and breast milk, must be suspected. Intravenous heroin use with an HIV-contaminated needle is the most likely cause of disease in this patient.

   Current Centers for Disease Control and Prevention (CDC) guidelines indicate initial testing for HIV should be a laboratory-based immunoassay that detects HIV-1 p24 antigen and HIV-1 and HIV-2 antibodies. Specimens that are positive should be tested with a confirmatory HIV-1/HIV-2 antibody differentiation immunoassay. If these studies are indeterminate, HIV RNA PCR (polymerase chain reaction) testing is performed.

   Before 2014, the preferred screening test for the detection of HIV was by enzyme-linked immunosorbent assay (ELISA; high sensitivity), and if positive, followed by confirmatory Western blot analysis (high specificity). A Western blot must be positive for antibodies to at least two important HIV antigens (e.g., gp120, gp41, p24). If only one antibody is positive, the result is indeterminate; the test must be repeated after a few months, or an HIV RNA PCR assay must be performed. Because it takes several weeks for antibodies to develop after acute HIV infection, the CDC recommends the revised testing strategy described previously. Note that ELISA and Western blots may be falsely positive in newborns born to HIV-infected mothers because these antibodies can cross the placenta.

STEP 1 SECRET

Step 1 questions are not always updated to reflect the most current guidelines. It is important to understand the previous human immunodeficiency virus (HIV) testing strategy of using enzyme-linked immunosorbent assay (ELISA) and Western blot but to also be aware of current recommendations.

3. **Describe the enzyme-linked immunosorbent assay test.**
   An ELISA test is performed to detect and quantify a specific protein of interest. First, known antigens (HIV-1 proteins, in this instance) are fixed to the bottom of a well. Next, the patient's serum is incubated in the well. If antibodies directed against the known antigen are present in the patient's serum, they will bind to the fixed antigen. Wells are typically washed before the addition of a detection antibody to remove any unbound (nonspecific) antibodies. The detection antibody is specific for human IgG and can thus bind to any antigen-antibody complexes that remain present in the well after the wash step. The detection antibody is typically conjugated to an enzyme that facilitates a colorimetric reaction when substrate is (next) added. Addition of substrate and subsequent color change indicate that the secondary antibody has bound to the antigen-antibody complex. Thus the amount of color change can be directly used to quantify (via spectrophotometry) the presence of antibodies in the patient's serum directed against the fixed antigen. The highest dilution of the patient's serum in which color change is detected represents the antibody titer.

CASE 15.8 CONTINUED:

The results of his HIV ELISA and Western blot test are positive. You continue to follow up with him regularly. Five years later he comes for another regularly scheduled appointment with a few questions. You note in his chart that he has been on highly active antiretroviral therapy (HAART) for a few years now. He states that he has been reading about the stages of HIV and asks, "Which stage am I in?" Additionally, he said he heard about "something called *P. jirovecii* pneumonia (PCP) that can happen when your CD4$^+$ T-cell count gets below 200" and requests more information on this topic.

4. **Briefly describe HIV and its life cycle.**
   HIV is an enveloped retrovirus composed of two positive-strand RNA molecules. The viral surface glycoprotein gp120 binds to the CD4 receptor on T cells. A conformational change allows gp120 to interact with a coreceptor on the cell, *CXCR4* or *CCR5*. GP41, another viral protein, initiates virus-cell membrane fusion and entry into the cell. Macrophages, dendritic cells, and microglial cells may also be infected by HIV. Upon cell entry, the virus copies its RNA genome into double-stranded DNA using viral reverse transcriptase. Viral integrase incorporates viral DNA into the host genome. Host machinery translates viral polyproteins. Functional proteins are expressed when viral protease cleaves the polyproteins into smaller mature proteins (Fig. 15.8).

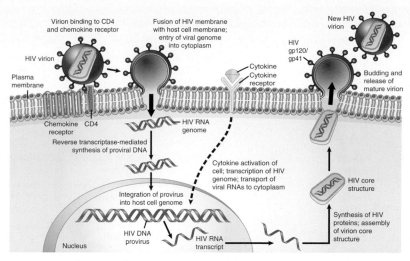

Figure 15.8. The life cycle of human immunodeficiency virus (HIV). *CTLs,* Cytotoxic T lymphocytes. *(From Kumar V, Abbas AK, Fausto N. Robbins & Cotran Pathologic Basis of Disease. 7th ed. Philadelphia: WB Saunders; 2005.)*

5. **Define the four major stages of HIV infection.**

   With *acute HIV infection,* the individual may remain asymptomatic or develop an acute illness that resembles influenza or infectious mononucleosis; symptoms usually develop within 2 to 6 weeks after infection (as seen in this patient). During the acute stage, antibodies to HIV are generally undetectable. Seroconversion usually occurs during *clinical latency,* an asymptomatic period that lasts approximately 7 to 10 years in an untreated patient. Persistent low-level replication of HIV causes a gradual decrease in CD4$^+$ T cells, and minor opportunistic infections may occur. During the *crisis* phase, escalation of viral replication leads to a more rapid T cell decline (Fig. 15.9). This is clinically apparent as weight loss, fever, fatigue, and lymphadenopathy. Acquired immunodeficiency syndrome (AIDS) is diagnosed when an HIV-positive individual has a CD4$^+$ T-cell count below 200 μL^{-1} or contracts an AIDS-defining illness (see question 9).

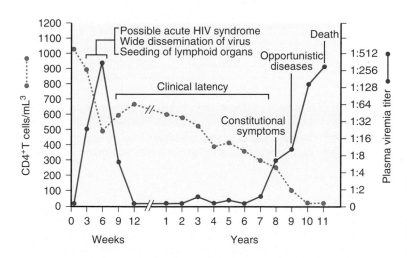

Figure 15.9. Typical course of human immunodeficiency virus (HIV) infection. *(From Kumar V, Abbas AK, Fausto N. Robbins & Cotran Pathologic Basis of Disease. 7th ed. Philadelphia: WB Saunders; 2005.)*

6. **What are the classes of drugs used in HAART?**

   The first class of antiretroviral drugs includes two types of reverse transcriptase inhibitors. Nucleoside analog reverse transcriptase inhibitors (NRTIs) are incorporated by reverse transcriptase (RT) into replicating DNA and terminate strand extension, thereby inhibiting viral replication. They require phosphorylation by thymidine kinase to become active and incorporated into DNA. Nonnucleoside reverse transcriptase inhibitors (NNRTIs) do not require activation by thymidine kinase and inhibit reverse transcriptase by binding to a site outside the catalytic domain. A second class of drugs called *protease inhibitors* (PIs) inhibits viral protease, an enzyme necessary for viral maturation and replication. HAART refers only to combinations of two NRTIs plus either one NNRTI or one PI. Table 15.10 lists some anti-HIV drugs (common names) that are in clinical use.

Table 15.10. Drugs in Clinical Use for Treatment of Human Immunodeficiency Virus (HIV) Infection

CATEGORY	DRUG NAMES	MECHANISM OF ACTION	SIDE EFFECTS
Protease inhibitors (end in "navir")	Atazanavir Darunavir Fosamprenavir Indinavir Lopinavir Ritonavir Saquinavir	Inhibit viral protease, which cleaves HIV polyproteins to mature functional proteins Resistance develops via mutations in *pol* gene.	Hyperglycemia, nausea, vomiting, diarrhea, central adiposity, insulin resistance
Nucleoside reverse transcriptase inhibitors (NRTIs)	Abacavir Didanosine Emtricitabine Lamivudine Stavudine Tenofovir Zidovudine *Note:* Lamivudine is also used for treatment of hepatitis B. Zidovudine is used to decrease vertical transmission of HIV.	Prodrugs that become activated by nonspecific kinases Become incorporated into DNA by reverse transcriptase (RT) and cause chain termination due to lack of 3′OH Resistance develops via mutations in RT.	Bone marrow suppression, lactic acidosis, rash, pancreatitis (didanosine), peripheral neuropathy (stavudine)
Nonnucleoside reverse transcriptase inhibitors (NNRTIs)	Efavirenz Nevirapine Delavirdine *Note:* Nevirapine reduces vertical transmission.	Not prodrugs like NRTIs Bind to and inhibit RT	Rash (Steven-Johnson syndrome [SJS]), hepatotoxicity, insomnia, and dysphoria (efavirenz)
Integrase inhibitors	Raltegravir	Inhibits viral integrase and prevents incorporation of viral cDNA into host genome	Generally well tolerated Occasional nausea, headache, diarrhea, myositis (rare)
Fusion inhibitors	Enfuvirtide Maraviroc	Enfuvirtide prevents viral gp41 from initiating viral membrane fusion with CD4$^+$ cells. Maraviroc prevents viral fusion by inhibiting viral gp120 from interacting with *CCR5*.	Enfuvirtide can cause injection site hypersensitivity reactions.

STEP 1 SECRET

Learning the various human immunodeficiency virus (HIV) drugs can be a difficult task, but they are commonly tested on the USMLE. It is important to recognize both the mechanism of action and potential side effects for all HIV drugs mentioned in Table 15.10.

7. Suboptimal compliance with HAART rapidly leads to resistance. Why?
   Any allowance of continued viral replication (e.g., from missed doses) is dangerous because HIV reverse transcriptase mutates quickly because of its error-prone nature. This promotes rapid development of drug resistance. In general, NRTI resistance occurs through mutations that prevent nucleoside analog incorporation or create a mechanism of adenosine triphosphate (ATP)–mediated nucleoside analog removal. Resistance to NNRTIs and PIs usually occurs through mutations that alter the binding sites for these drugs.

8. What are the most important determinants of the progression of HIV infection?
   CD4$^+$ T-cell count indicates the severity of damage that has occurred to the immune system. High CD4$^+$ counts are desirable. Normal count ranges from 500 to 1500 μL^{-1}. Viral load is an indication of the pace at which the disease is progressing. Undetectable viral load is an indication of effective drug therapy.

9. What is PCP pneumonia, and what other opportunistic infections and malignancies might befall an AIDS patient?
   PCP refers pneumonia caused by the fungus *P. jirovecii* (formerly *P. carinii*). *P. jirovecii* pneumonia is the most common significant opportunistic infection in HIV patients and typically occurs in patients with a CD4$^+$ count below 200. Therefore

patients with CD4$^+$ counts 200 or lower are started on prophylactic TMP-SMX. Patients with *Pneumocystis* pneumonia often have a chest x-ray film revealing a bilateral "ground-glass" appearance of the lungs. Other opportunistic pathogens and malignancies that are a major cause of death in AIDS are listed in Table 15.11.

Table 15.11. Opportunistic Pathogens and Malignancies With Major Mortality Risk in Acquired Immunodeficiency Syndrome

PARASITES	BACTERIA	FUNGI	VIRUSES	MALIGNANCIES
Toxoplasma spp.	*Mycobacterium tuberculosis*	*Pneumocystis jiroveci*	Herpes simplex virus	Kaposi sarcoma
Cryptosporidium spp.	*Mycobacterium avium* complex	*Cryptococcus neoformans*	Cytomegalovirus Varicella-zoster virus	Burkitt lymphoma
Leishmania spp.		*Candida* spp.		
Microsporidium spp.	*Salmonella* spp.	*Histoplasma capsulatum*		Non-Hodgkin lymphoma
		Coccidioides immitis		

High-yield opportunistic infections to know for the USMLE Step 1 include *Toxoplasma* encephalitis at CD4+ counts less than 100/μL (ring-enhancing lesions on computed tomography [CT] scan), cryptococcal meningitis at less than 100/μL (budding yeast in cerebral spinal fluid [CSF] by India ink stain), *Mycobacterium avium* complex at less than 50/μL (tuberculosis-like disease), and cytomegalovirus retinitis at less than 50/μL (cotton wool spots on fundoscopic exam). CMV retinitis is treated with ganciclovir, a competitive guanosine analog. In the event that ganciclovir fails, foscarnet (viral DNA polymerase inhibitor) is used.

10. Explain why certain individuals remain infected with HIV for longer than 10 years with no symptoms.
The clinical latency stage is variable and tends to run longer in patients with low viral load or who possess a mutant HIV strain with partially defective replication machinery. In these individuals, CTLs are able to control the virus without destroying large numbers of CD4$^+$ T cells, thus delaying the onset of opportunistic infections. Additionally, certain genetic polymorphisms in the *CXCR4* and *CCR5* genes prevent interaction with gp120 and have been shown to delay disease progression. Individuals homozygous for *CCR5* mutations are resistant to HIV infection.

SUMMARY BOX: HUMAN IMMUNODEFICIENCY VIRUS

- Presentation
  - Acute human immunodeficiency virus (HIV) infection resembles the flu or mononucleosis.
  - Clinical latency involves an asymptomatic period of several years.
  - Progresses to acquired immunodeficiency syndrome (AIDS) when CD4 count drops below 200/μL or patient contracts AIDS-defining illness
- Risk factors: Intravenous drug use, unprotected sex with an infected individual
- Diagnosis
  - New guidelines: Immunoassay detecting HIV-1 p24 antigen and HIV-1/HIV-2 antibodies; confirmatory HIV-1/HIV-2 antibody differentiation immunoassay
  - Before 2014: Enzyme-linked immunosorbent assay (ELISA) testing and confirmatory Western blot
  - Acute infection requires HIV RNA polymerase chain reaction (PCR) testing.
- Pathophysiology
  - RNA retrovirus infects CD4$^+$ T cells.
  - Viral gp120 and gp41 initiate infection of CD4$^+$ T cells via interactions with *CXCR4* and *CCR5*.
  - Progressive decline in CD4$^+$ T cells results in disease progression to AIDS.
- Treatment: Highly active antiretroviral therapy (HAART)—two nucleoside reverse transcriptase inhibitors (NRTIs) plus either one nonnucleoside reverse transcriptase inhibitor (NNRTI) or one protease inhibitor (PI)
  - If CD4 count is less than 200/μL, treat with trimethoprim-sulfamethoxazole (TMP-SMX) for *Pneumocystis jirovecii* pneumonia prophylaxis.
  - If CD4 count is less than 50/μL, treat with azithromycin for *Mycobacterium avium* prophylaxis.

CASE 15.9

A 55-year-old woman developed end-stage renal disease as a result of poorly controlled type 1 diabetes mellitus. She underwent hemodialysis twice a week for 6 months while waiting for a kidney transplant. Because she had no living blood relatives, she was in need of a cadaveric donor. A cadaveric kidney was found from a 28-year-old woman who was fatally injured in a car accident. The donor was blood type B, Rh-positive (matching the patient's blood) with one matched HLA-A allele. Before the transplantation, a final crossmatch was performed in which the recipient was shown to be nonreactive. Immunosuppressive therapy following the transplant procedure consisted of azathioprine, cyclosporine, methylprednisolone, and antithymocyte globulin (ATG). Two weeks following the procedure, the patient was discharged from the hospital on azathioprine, cyclosporine, and prednisone. Her blood pressure was normal, and serum creatinine was 1 mg/dL.

She now presents to your office for her 2-week follow-up visit. She complains of decreased urine output, and her blood pressure is 155/95 mm Hg. On physical examination, the region of the graft is enlarged and tender to the touch. You order standard laboratory tests, and the chemistry panel is notable for a serum creatinine of 4 mg/dL.

STEP 1 SECRET

You should know that a fair number of vignettes presented on the USMLE Step 1 will be long and detailed like the one presented in Case 15.9. This is especially important to keep in mind if you consider yourself a slow reader. Some students find it helpful to read the question before the vignette to know what to focus on in the history. Using the highlighter tool to mark salient information such as pertinent clinical findings, abnormal laboratory values, or medications can also help organize your thinking for the longer clinical vignettes.

1. What two diagnoses immediately rise to the top of your differential diagnosis list?

   Transplant rejection and cyclosporine toxicity are two possible diagnoses. In view of her recent surgical history, transplant rejection (acute, given the timing of the progression of the variables in the case) must be considered. Cyclosporine toxicity is also possible given that its two most common adverse effects are nephrotoxicity and hypertension.

2. What is the mechanism of action of cyclosporine?

   It is an immunosuppressive drug that inhibits calcineurin. Cyclosporine forms a complex with the immunophilin cyclophilin to inhibit the activity of calcineurin. Inhibition of calcineurin blocks dephosphorylation and nuclear translocation of the transcription factor NFAT (nuclear factor of activated T cells), thus leading to decreased transcription and production of IL-2. IL-2 is essential for differentiation, activation, and clonal expansion of T cells. Suppression of T-cell response is advantageous in prevention of transplant rejection (Fig. 15.10).

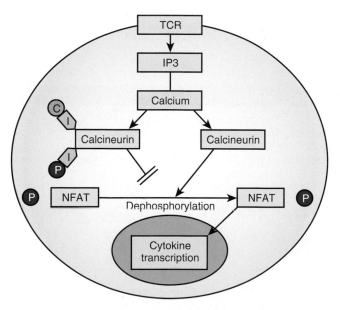

Figure 15.10. Mechanism of action of cyclosporine and tacrolimus. *C,* Cyclosporine; *I,* immunophilins; *IP3,* inositol 1,4,5-trisphosphate; *NFAT,* nuclear factor of activated T cells; *TCR,* T-cell receptor. *(From Adkinson NF Jr, Yunginger JW, Busse WW. Middleton's Allergy: Principles and Practice. 6th ed. Philadelphia: Mosby; 2003.)*

CASE 15.9 CONTINUED:

A renal biopsy is performed and shows the presence of many lymphocytes in the transplant, indicating that the kidney is undergoing acute rejection. She is given high-dose methylprednisolone and OKT3/muromonab (anti-CD3). This immunosuppressive regimen proves successful. Within a year of the transplant, she is doing well. She continues to take low doses of azathioprine, prednisone, and cyclosporine.

3. Discuss the genetics of the major histocompatibility complex molecules and the role of classes I and II in histocompatibility.

Every human has a set of MHC glycoproteins that are referred to as human leukocyte antigens (HLAs). Class I glycoproteins are known as HLA-A, -B, and -C antigens and appear on the surface of nearly all *nucleated* cells. Class II glycoproteins are known as HLA-DR, -DP, -DQ antigens and appear only on antigen-presenting cells (e.g., dendritic cells, B cells, macrophages, Langerhans cells). There are multiple alleles that code for each of the class I and class II glycoproteins. Each person receives one set of genes (a haplotype) encoding all six of these antigens from each parent. The HLAs are codominantly expressed on all cells and are antigenic among different individuals. Because of these molecular differences, transplanted tissues between genetically different members of the same species (allogeneic) are likely to be antigenically different and therefore stimulate an immune response.

Note: Even when a tissue is transplanted between genetically different individuals with a perfect ABO blood group match and a perfect MHC match, rejection can occur because of differences at various minor histocompatibility loci. Although the rejection is usually less aggressive, successful transplantation between MHC-matched individuals still requires some immunosuppression.

4. What types of rejections may occur in transplant recipients?

Hyperacute rejection is mediated by preformed serum antibodies in the recipient that are usually directed against ABO antigens on graft endothelial surfaces or mismatched HLA antigens. It generally occurs within minutes of transplantation. Immunoglobulin and complement deposition lead to endothelial injury and widespread thrombosis of the graft vasculature. This, in turn, can result in ischemia and necrosis. Hyperacute rejection is untreatable and the organ must be removed. It often presents in multiparous women who have antibodies to paternal HLA antigens shed by the fetus or in patients with prior transfusions.

Hyperacute rejection of transplanted tissue is a type II hypersensitivity response. *Acute* rejection can be cell mediated or humorally mediated. Acute cellular rejection occurs when CTLs become activated against donor MHC and attack graft parenchymal cells, leading to a dense interstitial infiltrate in the donor organ. Acute humoral rejection develops when the host produces antibodies against donor MHC, leading to ADCC and complement-mediated graft vasculitis. These reactions develop over a period of weeks to months. Acute rejection is treatable with immunosuppressive drugs.

Chronic rejection generally occurs months to years after transplantation. Recipient T cells interact with donor APCs in the graft and become sensitized to (foreign) donor antigens. This leads to irreversible T-cell–mediated and antibody-mediated damage to the graft. Chronic rejection leads to specific changes depending on the organ involved: atherosclerosis of the heart, obliterative bronchiolitis and atherosclerosis of pulmonary vessels in the lungs, destruction of bile ducts in the liver and vascular fibrosis, glomerular loss, intimal smooth muscle hypertrophy, and shrinkage of renal parenchyma in the kidney. Chronic rejection is untreatable.

STEP 1 SECRET

The typical question stem of an individual with chronic rejection is a patient with a history of kidney transplant presenting with a progressive rise in serum creatinine over 4 to 6 months, increasing proteinuria, and worsening hypertension.

5. What is the significance of the patient having no living blood relatives?

It is much easier to identify good HLA matches in blood relatives. Identical twins have the same histocompatibility type (HLA identical). The probability is approximately 0.25 that two siblings with the same parents are HLA identical at a given locus and approximately 0.50 that they are one-half HLA-matched (haploidentical) at a given locus. Furthermore, parents and children are almost always haploidentical across all loci. Because the patient had no living relatives, a cadaveric donor was her only option. A cadaveric donor that is blood group–compatible is often considered even with a poor MHC match.

6. What does a nonreactive final crossmatch indicate?

It indicates that the recipient has no antibodies against the WBCs of the potential donor. Sensitizing events, including blood transfusions, pregnancies, and previously failed transplants, may elicit the production of anti-HLA antibodies in the recipient. A positive crossmatch indicates the presence of preformed antibodies and puts the patient at risk of hyperacute graft rejection.

7. How does azathioprine work as an immunosuppressive agent? Antithymocyte globulin? OKT3? Methylprednisolone?

Azathioprine, metabolized to 6-mercaptopurine, is a purine analog that interferes with purine synthesis/metabolism and can be incorporated into DNA to inhibit replication. It is most effective in interfering with rapidly dividing cells, such as activated lymphocytes.

ATGs are antibodies directed against human T cells that are produced in animals (heterologous antibodies). They are used to deplete the T-cell pool in transplant recipients.

OKT3/muromonab is a murine monoclonal antibody that is specific for CD3 on the surface of T cells. It not only has the ability to inhibit T cell recognition of alloantigens but also reduces T-cell counts. It is quite effective in management of acute rejection.

Methylprednisolone is a glucocorticoid antiinflammatory agent that functions to reduce the number of circulating lymphocytes and to diminish the ability of lymphocytes to activate and proliferate. Glucocorticoids inhibit NF-κB (nuclear factor kappa light chain enhancer of activated B cells), which is a transcription factor responsible for the synthesis of many inflammatory cytokines and protein mediators. Glucocorticoids also decrease the number of leukocytes in sites of inflammation by reducing chemotaxis (Table 15.12).

Note: The major goal of transplant-related immunosuppression is to decrease the generation and activation of helper T cells and CTLs, which mediate acute rejection.

Table 15.12. Transplantation-Related Immunosuppressive Drugs

AGENT(S)	MODE OF ACTION	COMMENTS
Cyclosporine and tacrolimus (FK-506)	Calcineurin inhibitors; block IL-2 synthesis, thereby preventing T-cell activation	Cyclosporine is nephrotoxic; FK-506 can be administered at lower doses and has fewer side effects than with cyclosporine.
Rapamycin and sirolimus	TOR inhibitors, block IL-2–dependent activation of T cells	Rapamycin can be administered at lower doses and has fewer side effects than with cyclosporine.
Cyclophosphamide	One metabolite is alkylating agent (cross-links DNA); suppresses B cells more than T cells	Acrolein (another metabolite) causes hemorrhagic cystitis (treated with mesna).
Azathioprine and mycophenolate mofetil (MMF)	Mitotic inhibitors (interfere with purine synthesis and metabolism), target proliferating lymphocytes	MMF has greater lymphocytic selectivity and therefore fewer side effects than those associated with its predecessors, azathioprine and cyclophosphamide.
Corticosteroids	Block cytokine production by macrophages (TNF, IL-1); decrease number of circulating lymphocytes	Side effects include hypertension, osteoporosis, muscle wasting, acne, hyperglycemia, and cataracts.
Antilymphocyte globulin (ALG)/antithymocyte globulin (ATG)	Decrease lymphocyte numbers and T-cell numbers, respectively	Are heterologous sera (from another species), so adverse reactions include serum sickness, immune complex-induced glomerulonephritis, and anaphylactic reactions
OKT3/muromonab (anti-CD3)	Murine monoclonal antibody against CD3 that functions to eliminate T cells	Is a nonhuman antibody, so side effects in humans include serum sickness and immune complex-induced glomerulonephritis
Basiliximab and daclizumab (anti-CD25)	Monoclonal antibody against IL-2 receptor (CD25), blocks IL-2 binding, preventing T-cell activation	Chimeric murine-human monoclonal antibodies; thus side effects less severe/frequent than with pure murine form

CTLS, Cytotoxic T lymphocytes; *IL-1, -2,* interleukin 1, 2; *TNF,* tumor necrosis factor.

SUMMARY BOX: TRANSPLANT REJECTION

- Presentation: Ischemic/thrombotic complications in a patient with a history of organ transplant
- Pathophysiology
- Hyperacute rejection
  - Occurs within minutes of transplant
  - Preformed antibodies induce injury to graft vessels
- Acute rejection
  - Occurs within days to weeks
  - Cytotoxic T lymphocytes (CTL)–dependent or antibody-dependent cellular cytotoxicity (ADCC)-mediated tissue destruction
- Chronic rejection
  - Occurs months to years later
  - Precipitated by interactions between recipient T cells and donor antigen-presenting cells (APCs)
- Treatment: Immunosuppressive drugs

CASE 15.10

A 52-year-old man received a bone marrow transplant from his HLA-matched brother in an attempt to cure multiple myeloma. The patient was admitted to the hospital and given a course of busulfan and cyclophosphamide to eradicate his lymphocytes. He was then intravenously administered bone marrow removed from the donor's iliac crest. His hospital recovery went smoothly, and he was sent home, only to return 4 weeks after the transplant. He now presents to you with complaints of an itchy rash on his chest and upper extremities and severe bloody diarrhea, abdominal pain, nausea, and vomiting. Physical examination reveals a maculopapular rash with fine excoriations in the aforementioned distribution, mild jaundice, and mild hepatomegaly. His liver aminotransferases are significantly elevated. The patient is started on tacrolimus (FK506), methotrexate, and topical corticosteroids. The rash fades, but the intestinal symptoms persist. After initiation of weekly injections of a monoclonal antibody to CD2, the diarrhea finally resolves.

1. **What caused the adverse reaction in this patient 4 weeks after transplantation?**
   Graft-versus-host (GVH) disease caused the adverse reaction. This is considered to be acute GVD because the signs and symptoms began within 100 days of transplantation.
   Note: Diagnosis is typically confirmed via biopsy of the affected organ.

2. **What is the pathogenesis of GVH disease?**
   GVH disease occurs when immunocompetent cells are transplanted into an immunocompromised host. It is frequently encountered in bone marrow transplants but can also occur in specific organ transplants (e.g., liver) because of the large number of lymphocytes in these organs. Transplanted immunocompetent donor T cells recognize host HLA antigens as foreign and thus attack host cells. Donor T cells release cytokines that promote host tissue damage. However, the majority of destruction is primarily mediated by $CD8^+$ CTLs. Acute GVH disease classically involves the skin, liver, and intestines and produces rash, hepatic dysfunction, and diarrhea.

Clinical Pearl

The graft-versus-host (GVH) reaction can be beneficial in patients with leukemia. Transplanted allogeneic T cells are used to control leukemic cells in the host. This is the called the *graft-versus-leukemia effect*.

---

3. **Why did the donor's cells react against the recipient's when they were HLA-matched?**
   Individuals who are HLA-matched share the same MHC haplotypes. In other words, they have MHC class I and class II molecules that are genetically and antigenically identical. However, even in HLA-matched individuals, disparities in minor histocompatibility antigens exist. These allogeneic molecules, which are likely to vary in all donor-recipient pairs other than identical twins, have the potential to activate mature T cells of the donor.
   Note: Unlike MHC antigens, which are recognized directly by T cells, minor histocompatibility antigens are recognized only when presented by self-MHC molecules. Thus tissue rejection due to minor histocompatibility differences takes longer to develop (several weeks) and is often less vigorous.

4. **Why are the skin and the intestinal tract the major sites of GVH disease?**
   Recall that the epidermal barriers of the skin and the GI tract are two of the major portals of attempted entry for microorganisms. The immunologic protection at these two sites is robust, and MHC antigens are expressed at high levels. In GVH disease, such expression increases the probability and severity of attack at these two sites.

5. **How do monoclonal antibodies against CD2 help treat GVH disease?**
   CD2 is an antigen found on thymocytes and mature T cells. Giving antibody against CD2 is effective at decreasing T-cell numbers by eliciting their clearance by the reticuloendothelial system (i.e., splenic macrophages). ATG would have a similar effect.

6. **What is the mechanism of action of busulfan?**
   Busulfan is an alkylating agent that cross-links DNA. It is toxic to myeloid cells and lymphocytes at low doses and hematopoietic stem cells at high doses. When given in combination with cyclophosphamide, high-dose busulfan can be used to eradicate a patient's leukocytes in preparation for bone marrow transplantation. Commonly tested side effects of busulfan are pulmonary fibrosis and dysplasia (so-called *busulfan lung*). Other side effects include myelosuppression and hyperpigmentation.

7. **What is the mechanism of action of methotrexate?**
   Methotrexate is a folic acid analog that inhibits dihydrofolate (DHF) reductase. This prevents recycling of DHF to tetrahydrofolate (THF) and depletes nucleotide precursors needed for DNA synthesis. The cytotoxic effect is most pronounced in rapidly dividing cells, such as proliferating T cells in GVH disease. Notable adverse effects of methotrexate include myelosuppression, steatosis of the liver, mucositis, and stomatitis.

SUMMARY BOX: GRAFT-VERSUS-HOST DISEASE

- Presentation: Rash, diarrhea, abdominal pain, nausea, vomiting, and jaundice in a patient with a history of organ transplant
- Epidemiology: Most frequently encountered in patients who receive bone marrow transplants but can also occur in specific organ transplants
- Diagnosis: History and clinical evaluation, biopsy for confirmation
- Pathophysiology: Transplanted immunocompetent $CD8^+$ T cells attack immunosuppressed host cells secondary to major and minor histocompatibility mismatches.
- Treatment: Immunosuppressive agents (e.g., monoclonal antibodies against CD2)

CASE 15.11

A 26-year-old man comes to your office with a chief complaint of new-onset pain in his right knee and left ankle after returning from a trip to northern New England 2 weeks ago. He also mentioned the onset of fatigue, a mild fever, and an "eye problem" to the medical assistant. Before seeing him, you briefly review his medical history and see only a history of psoriasis and a laboratory test result showing that he is HLA-B27 positive.

---

1. His presentation, coupled with his HLA-B27 status, brings what three diagnoses into consideration?
   The seronegative spondyloarthropathies— ankylosing spondylitis, reactive arthritis (previously known as Reiter syndrome) and psoriatic arthritis —are considered.

2. Complete the initial differential diagnosis.
   Trauma must be considered in a potentially active patient. Also, until the sexual history is known, gonococcal arthritis cannot be ruled out. Lyme disease should be considered as well, given his travel history, and the time course and symptoms would be suggestive of stage 2. Other possibilities include rheumatoid arthritis, SLE, substance/drug-induced arthritis, septic arthritis, and viral arthritis depending on his history.

CASE 15.11 CONTINUED:

You interview the patient, and he recounts the following story about his joint pain: "First it was my right knee, then it was my left ankle, and now I think my right ankle might be hurting a little too." He also remembers that he had multiple episodes of dysuria 2 weeks ago, and this symptom has now returned. Upon discussion of his social history, the patient discloses that he had sexual intercourse with a partner he met for the first time on his trip. Physical examination reveals that the right knee and left ankle are tender and immobile, with moderate effusions. Ophthalmologic examination reveals anterior uveitis of the left eye. Examination of the genitals is unremarkable.

---

3. What is the most likely cause of the patient's clinical picture?
   Reactive arthritis is the most likely cause.

4. What organisms are most commonly associated with reactive arthritis?
   Chlamydia trachomatis, *Campylobacter jejuni*, *Yersinia*, *Salmonella*, and *Shigella* are classically associated with reactive arthritis.

5. What should be done next?
   Perform arthrocentesis to rule out septic joint. Owing to the high likelihood that his reactive arthritis is related to *Chlamydia*, he should have a urine test for this organism and for *Neisseria gonorrhoeae*. It would be advisable to initiate presumptive treatment for *Chlamydia* with azithromycin or doxycycline at this time. Consider additional testing for sexually transmitted infections, such as HIV and syphilis. In terms of his reactive arthritis, the symptoms are best treated with nonsteroidal antiinflammatory drugs (NSAIDs).

6. Describe the pathogenesis of reactive arthritis.
   Though still debated, reactive arthritis is likely due to an immune-mediated reaction that develops from bacterial antigen molecular mimicry. When bacterial antigens that have a composition similar to proteins found in joints, genitourinary tract, and the eye are introduced to the host, an immune response can ensue against both bacterial *and* self-antigens, resulting in arthritis, urethritis, conjunctivitis, and uveitis.

7. The cardiac manifestations of rheumatic fever represent one of the best examples of molecular mimicry. Discuss the cross-reacting proteins.
   The M protein of *S. pyogenes* is the organism's primary antiphagocytic factor. Certain types of the M protein closely resemble myocardial myosin. If an *S. pyogenes* infection is not treated in under 9 days, some patients will produce cross-reactive antibodies, leading to myocardial damage. M protein molecular mimicry is thought to play a role in the

other symptoms of rheumatic fever (polyarthritis, cardiac valvular disease, skin nodules, skin rash, and Sydenham chorea) as well.

8. **In addition to molecular mimicry, what are the two other proposed major mechanisms of autoimmunity?**
   Alteration of self-proteins: Binding of a substance to self-proteins causes the latter to appear foreign to the immune system. Examples include penicillin-induced IMHA (see Case 15.2) and drug-induced lupus. A similar scenario occurs when certain viruses infect a cell and alter select surface proteins.
   Compromise of immunologically privileged sites: Certain tissues are never exposed to the immune system, and thus tolerance toward them is never developed. Examples include the blood-testis barrier (sperm protected by Sertoli cells), the blood-brain barrier (central nervous system protected by endothelial cells), and certain parts of the eye. If the barrier is compromised, proteins that were previously unseen by the immune system are released into circulation. These proteins become immune-activating antigens, and immunologic attack on the source tissue ensues. Similarly, the immune system usually does not develop tolerance to intracellular proteins such as those associated with the nucleus (e.g., DNA, histones). Therefore cellular damage and release of these antigens (as might be seen with a lytic virus) are thought to play a role in the development of immune-mediated diseases such as SLE.

RELATED QUESTIONS: MECHANISMS OF TOLERANCE

9. **T-cell tolerance in the thymus (central tolerance) was discussed in Case 15.7, question 5. Discuss the important principles of peripheral T-cell tolerance.**
   All T_H cells require three things to become activated: (1) the interaction of the TCR and CD4 with MHC class II presenting antigen, (2) costimulatory signals, and (3) cytokine signals. If the first interaction is present but one of the vital costimulatory signals is absent and/or cytokine signals include antiinflammatory molecules (e.g., IL-10), the T cell becomes anergic (nonreactive). The most commonly cited costimulatory signal is the binding of B7 on APCs to CD28 on the T cell. The interaction of these two molecules can be prevented by downregulation of APC B7 expression. A major inducer of peripheral tolerance is regulatory T cells (Tregs). Tregs express CTLA-4, which competes with CD28 for B7 binding on APCs. CTLA-4 and B7 interactions lead to downregulation of B7 on the APC so that it is unavailable for binding to CD28. Tregs are often identified by the unique expression of the transcription factor forkhead box P3 (FOXP3) and produce antiinflammatory cytokines such as IL-10. These antiinflammatory cytokines can broadly dampen the immune response through a variety of mechanisms that are unimportant to know for Step 1.

10. **Describe B-cell tolerance.**
    B-cell tolerance is not as well characterized as T-cell tolerance. Central tolerance occurs in the bone marrow, but in contrast with thymic education, the approach is single-pronged: only self-reactive B cells are deleted (negative selection). Peripheral tolerance is also important and likely is directed to a large degree by suppressor T cells.

SUMMARY BOX: REACTIVE ARTHRITIS

- Presentation: Fatigue, mild fever, joint pain, symptoms of urethritis, ophthalmologic issues.
- Diagnosis: Positive HLA-B27 testing, elevated acute phase reactants, confirmation of infection (i.e., positive urine *Chlamydia* testing).
- Pathophysiology: Bacterial molecular mimicry induces autoantibody production, which cross-react against self-antigens in joints, eyes, and the genitourinary tract.
  - Common culprits: *Chlamydia trachomatis*, *Campylobacter*, *Yersinia*, *Salmonella*, and *Shigella*
- Treatment: Treat genitourinary infections and administer nonsteroidal antiinflammatory drugs (NSAIDs) for arthritis.

Insider's Guide to Psychiatry for the USMLE Step 1

Psychiatry is a straightforward subject on the USMLE if studied for correctly. Focus on learning the diagnostic criteria for the diseases covered in First Aid. Also, make sure to pay special attention to specific details (e.g., duration of symptoms) that help differentiate one disease from another distinct but closely related one. Popularly tested subjects include personality disorders, defense mechanisms, delirium versus dementia, eating disorders, panic disorder, drug abuse and withdrawal, and depression. Take time to learn the antipsychotic drugs and their side effects. They are commonly tested on Step 1.

As a preface to the field of psychiatry, we refer to the *Diagnostic and Statistical Manual of Mental Disorders, Fifth Edition* (*DSM-5*). Paramount to the study and practice of psychiatry, the *DSM* serves as the universally accepted guide to classifying, diagnosing, and treating psychiatric illness in the United States. Updated in 2013, the current fifth edition is slightly different from the previous version. These changes are minor (including the use of an Arabic numeral instead of a Roman numeral to identify the edition number), and it is not essential for you to be aware of them for Step 1. It is unlikely that you will be tested on *DSM-5*–specific criteria; at this point, testable concepts are common to both *DSM-IV* and *DSM-5*. However, for your general knowledge, the following items highlight the major changes of the *DSM-5*. Note that some of these changes have faced substantial criticism for a multitude of reasons.

- The overall organization has been modified. Perhaps most substantially, the current edition has abandoned its previous "multiaxial system," choosing instead to integrate the previous five "axes" into one section.
- The fifth edition also introduces dimensional assessments, allowing for severity ratings to be used rather than just the presence or absence of individual symptoms.
- Other notable changes include incorporation of Asperger syndrome into the more general "autism spectrum" classification, removing schizophrenia classification subtypes, etc.
- In many cases, definitions and names have been modified slightly. For example, *intellectual disability* has replaced the term *mental retardation*, and *dysthymia* is now referred to as *persistent depressive disorder*.
- Additional changes to the new edition, although not important to memorize, are noted in the specific sections that follow.

CASE 16.1

A 20-year-old college student has been doing poorly for the past 8 months. He has become socially withdrawn and apathetic, and his grades, previously good, have been suffering. He reports to the campus physician that he has been hearing voices, asserting that the TV news anchor has been giving him secret messages that instruct him to infiltrate a terrorist organization and thwart their assassination attempt on the President. He also wants to go into hiding because he believes that the CIA is after him. An extensive workup to identify organic causes of his symptoms (thyroid function tests, drug screening, head computed tomography [CT], and magnetic resonance imaging [MRI]) is negative.

1. What is the most likely diagnosis?
   Schizophrenia, a psychotic disorder characterized by impaired perception, abnormal behavior, and emotional instability, is the most likely diagnosis. Schizophrenia has an overall prevalence of 1%, and initial onset of symptoms in those afflicted typically occurs during young adulthood. The differential diagnosis also includes schizoaffective disorder, mood disorder with psychotic features, and psychosis secondary to a general medical condition or substance abuse.
   Note: The typical age at onset of schizophrenia is 18 to 24 years in men and 26 to 34 years in women.

2. According to the *Diagnostic and Statistical Manual of Mental Disorders* (*DSM-5*), what criteria must be met to make the diagnosis of schizophrenia?
   The diagnosis requires symptoms to be present for at least 6 months with a 1-month period of active symptoms. Typically, symptoms will have had a negative impact on major areas of functioning such as work or school, interpersonal relations, or self-care.
   Active symptoms include (two or more required to make the diagnosis, one or more must be from symptoms 1–3):
   1. Delusions (substantially irrational beliefs, e.g., a belief that you are the reincarnation of George Washington)
   2. Hallucinations (false perception of auditory, visual, or tactile stimuli, e.g., hearing voices that only you can hear)
      Note: The primary cause of auditory hallucinations in a psychotic patient is schizophrenia. You should make this association for the USMLE.
   3. Disorganized speech (e.g., incoherence)
   4. Grossly disorganized or catatonic behavior
   5. Negative symptoms (e.g., social withdrawal, flat affect, lack of motivation, diminished speech or thought)

3. **What are the differences between positive and negative symptoms experienced in schizophrenia?**
Positive symptoms are symptoms whose presence is abnormal. These include (as was just mentioned in question 2) thought disturbances, delusions, and auditory and visual hallucinations. These symptoms are mediated by increased levels of dopamine in the mesolimbic pathway and can be treated with typical antipsychotic drugs. Negative symptoms are thoughts and behaviors normally present among the general population whose absence often indicates a psychiatric disorder. They can include social withdrawal and isolation, anhedonia, and apathy. Negative symptoms are the result of decreased activity of mesocortical dopaminergic projections. They can be exacerbated by use of typical antipsychotics.

4. **What would be the diagnosis if this man had these symptoms for only the past 3 months rather than for 8 months (with a negative workup for other causes)?**
The diagnosis would be schizophreniform disorder, which is diagnosed in a patient displaying symptoms of schizophrenia for a period of more than 1 month but no longer than 6 months. If the symptoms existed for less than 1 month, then the diagnosis would be considered brief psychotic disorder.

STEP 1 SECRET

Many psychiatric disorders are associated with time intervals that are required to make a definitive diagnosis of the disease. The USMLE will expect you to know these time intervals (e.g., schizophreniform disorder and schizophrenia both present with the same symptoms, but schizophrenia is diagnosed only in patients who are symptomatic for at least 6 months).

5. **What would be the likely diagnosis if this man presented with these symptoms and later developed depressive, manic, or mixed features (both depression and mania)?**
Schizoaffective disorder would be the likely diagnosis. Schizoaffective disorder is similar to the distinct "major depression with psychotic features," but schizoaffective disorder requires a period of at least 2 weeks with psychotic symptoms in the presence of a stable mood (in addition to a major depressive and/or manic episode at some point in the past). In other words, it is a primary psychotic disorder with mood features. Conversely, major depressive disorder (or bipolar disorder) with psychotic features is a primary mood disorder with psychotic features. The USMLE likes to test the distinction between these two types of disorders.

6. **What would be your diagnosis if this man had symptoms of schizophrenia following a severe stressor and these symptoms resolved within 1 month?**
Brief psychotic disorder would be the diagnosis. In this case, it would be a reactive psychosis because it is associated with marked stressors. A brief psychotic disorder is characterized by temporary psychosis that is usually (but not always) stress-related, lasting at least 1 day but less than 1 month. It cannot be due to a general medical condition, associated with a mood disorder, or caused by substance use. If a brief period of psychosis had followed or had been attributed to a medical illness, it would be diagnosed as psychosis secondary to a general medical condition. Postpartum psychosis describes a particular manifestation having peripartum onset (during pregnancy or within 4 weeks following delivery).

7. **What neurotransmitter abnormality is thought to play the primary role in this man's disorder?**
The current theory is that an abnormality of dopamine activity in certain regions of the brain is the cause of schizophrenia. Increased dopamine signaling in the *mesolimbic* pathway has been associated with the positive symptoms of schizophrenia, whereas the negative symptoms are thought to be linked to decreased dopamine signaling in the *mesocortical* pathway. Patients with schizophrenia who are treated with dopamine receptor antagonists (the typical antipsychotics) show a beneficial response. These drugs treat the positive symptoms of schizophrenia but have little effect on negative symptoms. Alternatively, the atypical antipsychotics, which have a more varied and less well understood mechanism, are capable of treating positive and negative symptoms. It is worth noting that drugs with dopaminergic effects will aggravate existing psychosis and, in some patients (e.g., Parkinson disease), can result in new-onset psychosis.

STEP 1 SECRET

It is important that you remember which neurotransmitters are affected in different psychiatric and neurologic disorders. Table 16.1 provides a summary of the ones worth memorizing.

8. **What is the relationship between schizophrenia and suicide?**
People with schizophrenia are at greatly increased risk for attempting suicide, and between 10% and 15% of schizophrenic patients will ultimately die by suicide.

Table 16.1. Neurotransmitters Affected in Different Psychiatric and Neurologic Disorders

	NOREPINEPHRINE	DOPAMINE	SEROTONIN	ACETYLCHOLINE	GABA
Anxiety	↑		↓		↓
Depression	↓	↓	↓		
Schizophrenia		↑			
ADHD	↓	↓			
Alzheimer dementia				↓	
Parkinson disease		↓	↑	↑	
Huntington disease		↑		↓	↓

ADHD, Attention deficit/hyperactivity disorder; *GABA,* gamma-aminobutyric acid.

9. When initiating therapy for patients like this college student, it is important to keep potential side effects in mind and to educate the patient about them. What types of side effects are more commonly seen with high-potency typical antipsychotics such as haloperidol and fluphenazine than with other antipsychotics?

Extrapyramidal side effects (EPS) such as acute dystonia, parkinsonism, akathisia, and tardive dyskinesia (TD) are commonly seen. Acute dystonia results in excessive muscle tone and muscle spasms (e.g., torticollis, laryngospasm) after only short-term exposure (typically within hours). Parkinsonism is characterized by shuffling gait, cogwheel rigidity, bradykinesia, and resting tremor. Onset is usually on the order of weeks. Akathisia is a subjective sensation of inner restlessness or desire to move. Individuals with this condition may appear anxious or agitated and may move about and pace because they are unable to sit still. TD presents with involuntary movements of the tongue, lips, face, trunk, and extremities (generally irreversible) and occurs in patients treated with long-term dopaminergic antagonist medications (months to years). The risk of developing TD is about 3% per year with typical agents.

10. What is the treatment for the previously mentioned extrapyramidal side effects?

Both dystonia and drug-induced parkinsonian syndrome are best treated with an anticholinergic agent such as benztropine or diphenhydramine. If there is acute airway obstruction due to laryngeal spasms in acute dystonia, intravenous diphenhydramine should be administered immediately. Akathisia typically requires administration of a beta-blocker such as propranolol, as well as reduction of drug dosage or substitution of medications. Oftentimes, TD does not improve or resolve despite discontinuation of the drug. This irreversible complication is thought to be the consequence of compensatory sensitization of dopamine receptors after long-term dopamine-blocking therapy.

11. Why might this man develop the following symptoms if he is being treated with low-potency typical antipsychotics such as chlorpromazine or thioridazine?

1. Urinary retention

The term *low-potency* refers to the fact that a greater dose is required to reach the same dopaminergic effect, thus limiting the drugs' ability to induce EPS effects. Therefore these low-potency antipsychotics do not typically cause extrapyramidal side effects. However, the low-potency typical antipsychotics, in addition to blocking D_2 receptors, also have antihistamine, anticholinergic, and anti–α_1-adrenergic effects. Urinary retention can result from muscarinic (cholinergic) blockade, which affects the bladder's detrusor muscle.

Note: The muscarinic antagonism also causes the common anticholinergic side effects of dry mouth, loss of visual accommodation leading to blurry vision, and constipation.

2. Orthostatic hypotension

Orthostatic hypotension can be caused by alpha blockade.

3. Sedation

Antihistamine H_1 blockade can produce a sedative effect. Administration of the drug at bedtime may reduce daytime sedation.

12. Perhaps the most feared complication of antipsychotics is an idiosyncratic reaction characterized by severe muscle rigidity, myoglobinuria and elevated plasma creatine kinase, fever, autonomic instability, and altered mental status. What is the name of this lethal side effect, and what is the treatment?

Neuroleptic malignant syndrome (NMS) may occur with any antipsychotic but is much more commonly seen with the typical agents. If this occurs, the offending drug should be discontinued immediately. In addition, NMS can be treated with a dopamine agonist such as bromocriptine or with dantrolene, which decreases muscle contractions by preventing release of calcium from the sarcoplasmic reticulum.

13. **How do typical and atypical antipsychotics differ with respect to their mode of action and to their effect on positive and negative symptoms?**

    Atypical antipsychotics (e.g., clozapine) are "atypical" in that they are more effective against the negative symptoms of schizophrenia, while still treating the positive symptoms. They are also much less likely to cause extrapyramidal side effects (e.g., acute dystonia, TD) than are the typical antipsychotics. In addition to dopamine receptor blockade, atypical antipsychotics block the serotonin receptor of the 5-HT_2 subtype; this is thought to offer some protection against EPS. Atypical antipsychotics are believed to be effective in mesolimbic blockade of dopamine (hyperactive in schizophrenia) without significantly blocking the mesocortical dopaminergic circuit (hypoactive in schizophrenia). Specific atypical antipsychotics also appear to have additional dopamine receptor actions. For example, clozapine is a very effective D_4 antagonist, and aripiprazole is a dopamine autoreceptor agonist and a D_2 partial agonist.

14. **What are the four major dopamine pathways of the brain, and how are they involved in the pathophysiology and/or pharmacology of schizophrenia?**

    1. The tuberoinfundibular pathway

       The tuberoinfundibular pathway involves projections of dopaminergic neurons in the arcuate nucleus to the median eminence, below the hypothalamus. Dopamine released here inhibits prolactin secretion from the anterior pituitary. Some antipsychotics inhibit this dopamine release, leading to increased prolactin levels, which can then in turn inhibit gonadotropin-releasing hormone (GnRH). This inhibition of GnRH can cause gynecomastia, galactorrhea, and menstrual dysfunction, which are known side effects of many antipsychotics (particularly risperidone).

    2. The mesolimbic pathway

       The mesolimbic pathway involves projections of dopaminergic neurons in the ventral tegmentum to the nucleus accumbens. Hyperactivity of this pathway due to increased dopamine output here is thought to be responsible for the positive symptoms seen in schizophrenia, such as hallucinations, delusions, and agitation.

    3. The mesocortical pathway

       The mesocortical pathway involves projection of dopaminergic neurons in the ventral tegmentum to the frontal lobes. Hypoactivity of this pathway due to decreased dopamine output here may be implicated in the negative symptoms of schizophrenia, such as social withdrawal and flat affect.

    4. The nigrostriatal pathway

       The nigrostriatal pathway involves a neural circuit connecting the substantia nigra with the striatum. Loss of neurons in this pathway is responsible for the symptoms of Parkinson disease, so the blockade of dopamine here will cause parkinsonism (bradykinesia, rigidity, masked facies, resting tremor, shuffling gait). These symptoms are reversible with discontinuation of antipsychotics.

15. **Recent studies have suggested that there is not a large difference in effectiveness and tolerability between the typical and atypical drugs, with the exception of clozapine. Although the typical antipsychotics have significant side effects, the atypical antipsychotics also come with their fair share of problems. Which atypical antipsychotics are most strongly correlated with the following side effects?**

    1. Gynecomastia, galactorrhea, and menstrual dysfunction

       Recall from question 14 that many antipsychotics can cause these side effects, but risperidone in particular has been associated with these symptoms. Risperidone is similar to typical antipsychotics in that it is a very potent blocker of the D_2 receptor. D_2 receptor blockade of the tuberoinfundibular pathway leads to hyperprolactinemia, which causes gynecomastia, galactorrhea, and menstrual dysfunction.

2. Hyperlipidemia, glucose intolerance, and weight gain
   Olanzapine and clozapine appear to carry the greatest risk, followed by risperidone and quetiapine, for these side effects. However, in 2003, the U.S. Food and Drug Administration (FDA) requested manufacturers of *all* atypical antipsychotics to include product label warnings about the potential for an increased risk of hyperglycemia and diabetes.
3. Increasing the QT interval
   Of the atypical drugs, ziprasidone has the greatest effect on QT prolongation and should therefore be avoided in patients with increased QT intervals or known heart disease.
4. Agranulocytosis
   Clozapine (see subsequent text) is associated with agranulocytosis.

16. **Why is clozapine recommended for use only in schizophrenia refractory to other antipsychotics?**
    Clozapine is an atypical antipsychotic that often works in patients who have been refractory to other antipsychotics. The big drawback of using clozapine is that in 1% of patients it can precipitate agranulocytosis, which can be fatal. Weekly blood test monitoring is required for the first 6 months of treatment, followed by less frequent but still regular blood testing to ensure adequate white blood cell (WBC) counts. Other drugs that can cause agranulocytosis include carbamazepine, colchicine, propylthiouracil, methimazole, and dapsone. The USMLE loves to ask questions on this concept! Look for a patient on treatment for schizophrenia who presents with high fevers and a sore throat.

SUMMARY BOX: PSYCHOTIC DISORDERS

Schizophrenia
   Diagnosis: Presence of two active symptoms for at least 1 month (delusions, hallucinations, disorganized speech, disorganized or catatonic behavior, negative symptoms) and signs of illness for at least 6 months
   Duration of 1 to 6 months: Schizophreniform disorder
   Duration of 1 day to 1 month: Brief psychotic disorder
   Schizoaffective disorder meets criteria for schizophrenia and criteria for major depressive episode, manic episode, or mixed episode
• Accompanied by delusions and hallucinations for 2 weeks *without* mood symptoms to differentiate it from major depressive disorder with psychotic features
Antipsychotics
• Atypical preferred over typical antipsychotics because they are more effective against the negative symptoms of schizophrenia and are much less likely to cause extrapyramidal side effects
• Low-potency typical agents: High incidence of anticholinergic side effects, sedation, and orthostatic hypotension
• High-potency typical agents: High incidence of extrapyramidal side effects
• Atypical agents: Metabolic syndrome, hyperprolactinemia

CASE 16.2

A 22-year-old college man reports problems with his mood and is referred to a psychiatrist by the campus physician for further evaluation. He states that for the past week he has been incredibly productive because he has required very little sleep. During the interview, the physician notes pressured speech, distractibility, euphoric mood, and psychomotor hyperactivity. The patient denies any history of auditory or visual hallucinations or use of alcohol or other drugs. Just before this period, however, he experienced a 2-month period characterized by hypersomnia, anhedonia, decreased appetite, and psychomotor retardation. Physical examination is noncontributory, and laboratory tests indicate normal thyroid activity.

---

1. **What is the diagnosis?**
   He has bipolar disorder—specifically, bipolar type I. Bipolar I is characterized by manic episodes (must last at least 1 week), whereas the milder form of the disorder, bipolar type II, requires only a hypomanic episode lasting at least 4 days in addition to a depressive episode for diagnosis. The major difference between a manic episode and a hypomanic episode is that hypomania does not involve psychotic symptoms or lead to social or occupational dysfunction or hospitalization. Manic episodes consist of abnormal mood with hospitalization or three or more of the following symptoms present for at least 1 week:
   • **B**efuddled/distracted
   • **I**deas upon ideas (racing thoughts)
   • **G**randiosity
   • **S**leep decrease
   • **H**ypersexuality
   • **I**rresponsible actions
   • **F**ocused activity
   • **T**alkative or pressured speech
   (Note the mnemonic **BIG SHIFT** to help you remember these symptoms.)

STEP 1 SECRET

You can easily recall the symptoms of manic episodes by remembering that manic episodes cause a **BIG SHIFT** *in mood.*

2. Was the previous depressive episode required to make the diagnosis of bipolar in this patient?
   No, only a single manic episode is required. All patients who have experienced a manic episode are considered bipolar (specifically bipolar type I), regardless of whether they have also had a depressive episode. This can be confusing because the term bipolar implies manic and depressive features. However, most patients with a history of manic episodes will ultimately experience a depressive episode, even if they have not at the time of their manic presentation.
   Note: Unlike bipolar I, bipolar II does require at least one major depressive episode. There is also a milder form of the disorder called *cyclothymia,* which requires a minimum 2-year history of both hypomanic and depressive episodes, but the depressive episodes should not fulfill requirements for major depression. In addition, the patient must not be symptom-free for more than 2 months.

3. The physician prescribes lithium and informs the patient that he needs to have his blood levels of lithium monitored regularly. Why is this necessary?
   Lithium has a very narrow therapeutic window, meaning that there is only a small difference between the therapeutically effective and toxic concentrations of lithium. This makes it a relatively dangerous drug to give. Lithium toxicity presents with coarse tremor (fine tremor is a common side effect of lithium), stupor, ataxia, vomiting, diarrhea, and cardiac arrhythmias. Since lithium (Li^+) is a monovalent cation like sodium (Na^+), any mechanism where increased sodium reuptake in the kidney occurs or decreased renal clearance would occur can cause lithium toxicity even without dosage changes (e.g., hydrochlorothiazide, nonsteroidal antiinflammatory drugs [NSAIDs], angiotensin-converting enzyme [ACE] inhibitors).

4. After taking lithium for an extended period of time, the patient develops polyuria and polydipsia. The urine has a low osmolarity, and administration of antidiuretic hormone (vasopressin) does not have a significant effect on either the polyuria or the low urine osmolarity. What is happening?
   A distinctive but rare side effect of lithium is nephrogenic diabetes insipidus. This occurs when the kidneys do not respond effectively to antidiuretic hormone (ADH) and so do not conserve water or concentrate the urine effectively, hence the polyuria and polydipsia.

5. True or false: Treatment of this lithium-induced nephrogenic diabetes insipidus with diuretics may be effective in decreasing the symptoms of polyuria.
   True. Although this effect is seemingly counterintuitive, loop diuretics and thiazide diuretics will actually decrease polyuria in nephrogenic diabetes insipidus because they promote proximal tubular reabsorption. However, extracellular fluid depletion can also increase the risk of lithium intoxication by enhancing lithium reabsorption at the proximal tubule, so careful monitoring is required to avoid lithium toxicity. Amiloride is perhaps the best choice of a diuretic because it is least likely to increase lithium levels.

6. The patient also mentions that he has become rather depressed after being on lithium for a while, is having memory problems, and seems to be cold all the time. Rather than putting this patient on an antidepressant, the physician orders thyroid-stimulating hormone and thyroxine levels first. Why?
   Another side effect of lithium is hypothyroidism, which can cause the previously mentioned symptoms.
   Note: Although the issue is not pertinent to this patient, lithium can also lead to congenital problems in offspring if lithium is taken by pregnant women. A well-established complication of lithium is Ebstein anomaly, which is a congenital malformation of the heart characterized by apical displacement of the tricuspid valve leaflets.

7. Because the patient is not tolerating lithium well, his physician decides to substitute a drug that is effective not only for bipolar disorder but also for several seizure disorders. What is this drug, and what regular monitoring should be done?
   The drug is valproic acid. Because valproic acid has lower toxicity and fewer side effects than lithium, this drug is often prescribed as the first-line mood stabilizer. It is also effective in treatment of absence seizures, partial seizures, and generalized seizures. Valproic acid is also more effective than lithium in rapid-cycling and mixed-state episode bipolar disorder. Very rare but potentially fatal side effects of valproic acid therapy include necrotizing hepatitis (children are at increased risk) and agranulocytosis. Periodic monitoring of liver enzymes and blood counts is therefore indicated in patients on long-term valproic acid therapy. Administration of valproic acid in pregnant women can also cause neural tube defects in the fetus because of decreased intestinal absorption of folate. It is therefore contraindicated in pregnant women or in women who may become pregnant.

8. At his next visit, the patient's symptoms seem to be well controlled with valproic acid, but his liver enzymes are markedly elevated. The valproic acid is discontinued, and he is prescribed another anticonvulsant that may also cause leukopenia or agranulocytosis but is not hepatotoxic. What drug was he likely given?

He was likely given carbamazepine. Although this drug is only effective in acute manic episodes, it is known to produce persistent leukopenia and possible hyponatremia. Therefore regular monitoring of laboratory values is required. Another possible severe side effect of carbamazepine is Stevens-Johnson syndrome, a dermatologic complication consisting of fever and malaise, which is rapidly followed by an erythematous, macular rash, eventually progressing to toxic epidermal necrosis and skin sloughing.

9. Why should valproic acid be used with extreme caution in patients also taking phenobarbital?

Valproic acid inhibits the hepatic metabolism of phenobarbital and displaces phenobarbital from plasma proteins. These effects result in elevated levels of free plasma phenobarbital, which puts the patient at risk for barbiturate-induced coma.

10. In someone with a seizure disorder that is well controlled with phenytoin, why may the addition of carbamazepine cause seizures to occur again?

Carbamazepine induces hepatic enzymes of the cytochrome P-450 system, which increase the metabolism of phenytoin and can reduce its plasma level to subtherapeutic levels. Thus a patient taking phenytoin to prevent seizures would be at increased risk of breakthrough seizures due to relatively insufficient dosing of the phenytoin.

SUMMARY BOX: BIPOLAR DISORDER

Bipolar I disorder
- Defined as one or more manic or mixed episodes (major depressive episode is not required, although it commonly occurs as well in these patients)

Bipolar II disorder
- Consists of one or more major depressive episodes and at least one hypomanic episode

Cyclothymia
- A milder, longer-lasting form of bipolar disorder characterized by multiple episodes of depression and hypomania occurring over at least a 2-year period

Treatments
- Lithium
  - Mood stabilizer
  - Narrow therapeutic index
  - Major side effects: Nephrogenic diabetes insipidus and hypothyroidism
- Valproic acid
  - More favorable side effect profile and lower toxicity compared with lithium
  - More effective than lithium in rapid-cycling and mixed-state episode bipolar disorder

CASE 16.3

A 48-year-old man reports poor appetite, insomnia, decreased interest in activities that he used to enjoy, difficulty concentrating, and loss of energy for much of the past year. He has lost 20 lb in the past 6 months. He denies illicit drug use or alcohol abuse and is not taking any medications. Physical examination is unremarkable. Laboratory evaluation reveals normal thyroid-stimulating hormone (TSH) and thyroxine (T_4) levels.

1. What is the most likely diagnosis?

Major depressive disorder is the most likely diagnosis. However, the differential diagnosis for depression includes hypothyroidism, bipolar disorder, schizophrenia, Parkinson disease, chronic renal failure, anemia, dementia, substance withdrawal, and anxiety.

2. According to the *DSM*-5, what criteria must be met to make the diagnosis of major depressive disorder?

Major depressive disorder can be diagnosed when at least five of the following symptoms are present on an almost daily basis for at least the past 2 weeks and when at least one of the symptoms is either depressed mood or loss of interest or pleasure in activities that were previously enjoyable (anhedonia):
1. Depressed mood
2. Anhedonia
3. Significant change in appetite or weight
4. Insomnia or hypersomnia
5. Psychomotor agitation or retardation
6. Fatigue or loss of energy
7. Feelings of worthlessness or excessive/inappropriate guilt
8. Diminished ability to think or concentrate
9. Recurrent thoughts of death, suicidal ideation with or without a plan, or a suicide attempt

A commonly used mnemonic for recalling these symptoms is **SIGECAPS**: **S**leep changes, lack of **I**nterest, **G**uilt, lack of **E**nergy, lack of **C**oncentration, **A**ppetite changes, **P**sychomotor retardation, **S**uicidality.

In addition, these symptoms must cause significant impairment in social, occupational, or other important areas of functioning. These symptoms cannot be better explained by a general medical condition (e.g., hypothyroidism), substance abuse, or other organic cause. The *DSM-IV* used to exclude this diagnosis in the case of bereavement (e.g., loss of a loved one), but the updated *DSM-5* does not allow for this exclusion.

3. What does the monoamine deficiency theory propose with respect to the etiology of depression?
   A deficiency in any one (or combination) of the monoamine neurotransmitters norepinephrine, dopamine, or serotonin can result in depression. There is accumulating pharmacologic evidence in support of this theory because therapeutically increasing central activity of serotonin, norepinephrine, and dopamine, either individually or in combination, has been shown to be beneficial in the treatment of depression. Drugs that inhibit monoamine oxidase, the enzyme responsible for breaking down these neurotransmitters, were one of the first recognized treatments used in this disorder. These so-called monoamine oxidase inhibitors (MAOIs) are still used today, but because of side effects, they are typically reserved for refractory cases of depression.

STEP 1 SECRET

For Step 1 and *for your clinical years, it will be important to remember which neurotransmitter levels are altered in various psychologic and neurologic diseases because treatment is generally aimed at correcting these abnormalities (see Table 16.1). You can remember which neurotransmitters are affected in depression by considering our poor friend Ned. **NeD'S DOWN** because he has depression. The acronym, **Ne** (norepinephrine), **D** (dopamine), **S** (serotonin), and **DOWN,** refers to decreased levels of all three of these neurotransmitters in depressed patients.*

4. Why does hypothyroidism have to be ruled out in this patient?
   Hypothyroidism can produce symptoms similar to those of depression.

5. What pharmacologic therapies are available to treat depression?
   • Selective serotonin reuptake inhibitors (SSRIs) (e.g., fluoxetine, paroxetine, sertraline) are typically first-line treatment.
   • Tricyclic antidepressants (TCAs) (e.g., amitriptyline, nortriptyline)
   • Monoamine oxidase inhibitors (MAOIs) (e.g., phenelzine, tranylcypromine)
   • Serotonin/norepinephrine reuptake inhibitors (SNRIs) (e.g., venlafaxine, duloxetine)
   • Mixed serotonin reuptake inhibitor–serotonin receptor antagonist (e.g., nefazodone, mirtazapine)
      Note: Electroconvulsive therapy (ECT) and psychotherapy are other options. ECT is a very safe and effective treatment for depression and is the therapy of choice when there is a high risk of suicide, the patient has been refractory to pharmacotherapy, or there is insufficient time for a trial of medication. ECT has a response rate of 90% compared with 70% for pharmacotherapy; the main side effect is anterograde amnesia (which usually resolves within 6 months). After ECT, combined pharmacotherapy and psychotherapy is the most effective treatment. Of the psychotherapies, cognitive behavioral therapy has the best results for depression.

6. On review of systems, the patient expresses concern about a history of premature ejaculation. What class of antidepressant may help address this concern?
   SSRIs commonly produce sexual dysfunction (e.g., delayed orgasm or anorgasmia) as well as diminished libido. In a patient with premature ejaculation, however, the effects of delaying ejaculation might be considered desirable.

7. Why have the SSRIs become first-line treatments for depression over the tricyclic antidepressants?
   SSRIs have become a first-line treatment because of fewer and more benign side effects and because they present less danger in overdose relative to the TCAs. TCAs cause anticholinergic, orthostatic hypotensive, and sedative side effects; in overdose, they can cause cardiac arrhythmias, convulsions, and even coma or death. Although SSRIs can cause sexual dysfunction, this is a relatively benign side effect compared with the side effect profile of the TCAs. When treating severe depression with TCAs, one must also consider that they are quite lethal in overdose. A patient with a suicide plan may save up the medication and overdose on it. The toxic potential of TCAs makes this a potential risk, whereas SSRIs are quite safe, even if ingested in large quantities.
      If you suspect that a patient may be considering suicide, a useful mnemonic to assess suicide risk is: **SAD PERSONS**: **S**ex (males at greater risk), **A**ge (teenagers and elderly), **D**epression, **P**rior attempt, **E**thanol or drug use, loss of **R**ational thinking, **S**ickness (medical illness and/or taking 3+ medications), **O**rganized plan, **N**o spouse, lacking **S**ocial support.

8. Why might you want to avoid administering SSRIs and other antidepressants to this patient if his history is also significant for manic episodes?
   He may have bipolar disorder, and antidepressants could precipitate a manic episode. This may happen in approximately 3% to 5% of bipolar patients. In patients with bipolar depression, atypical antipsychotics such as lurasidone may be considered.

9. What class of antidepressant was this man likely started on if he experienced symptoms of dry mouth, blurred vision, constipation, orthostatic (postural) hypotension, urinary retention, and memory impairment?

TCAs have strong anticholinergic side effects (e.g., dry mouth, blurred vision, urinary retention), antihistaminergic side effects (e.g., drowsiness and sedation), and antiadrenergic side effects (e.g., orthostatic hypotension). TCAs should be used with caution in elderly patients because the orthostatic effects may increase the risk for falling with the potential for a hip fracture. Nortriptyline and desipramine have the least sedative, orthostatic, and anticholinergic side effects of the TCAs.

Note: The anticholinergic effects of the TCAs (urinary retention) make them effective for treating enuresis (bed wetting). Imipramine is used for this (in children and adolescents). Clomipramine is commonly used in cases of comorbid obsessive-compulsive disorder (OCD), and amoxapine is useful in patients with psychosis in addition to major depression because of its ability to also block dopamine.

10. Assume that this patient responded well to some form of antidepressant therapy but then presented to the emergency department 3 weeks later with priapism. What antidepressant was he likely given?

Trazodone can cause this rare but rather serious complication in men. Trazodone and nefazodone are both mixed serotonin reuptake inhibitors–serotonin receptor antagonists; remember these two drugs as being in the z-group because they both have zs, and the patient gets very sleepy (i.e., they are very sedating) from taking them. Accordingly, these drugs are especially helpful in patients with depression and insomnia.

11. If this man is addicted to red wine with cheese, what class of antidepressant should be avoided and why?

MAOIs, such as phenelzine and tranylcypromine, should be avoided. The tyramine present in wine and cheese is ordinarily degraded by monoamine oxidase in the gastrointestinal (GI) tract. Inhibition of MAO in the GI tract and liver can increase levels of tyramine in the blood. Massive displacement of norepinephrine by tyramine from adrenergic storage sites can then lead to hypertensive crisis.

When discontinuing MAOIs from a patient's treatment plan, it is recommended that the physician wait at least 2 weeks before administration of a new antidepressant medication to avoid hypertensive crisis that may occur with excess monoamine levels.

12. How do MAOIs work, and what are the two classes of MAOIs?

MAOIs work by inhibiting the oxidative degradation of monoamines (dopamine, norepinephrine, and serotonin) in presynaptic neurons. Nonselective MAOIs (e.g., tranylcypromine, phenelzine, and isocarboxazid) inhibit both monoamine oxidase A and monoamine oxidase B, resulting in an overall reduction in the breakdown of norepinephrine and serotonin, and are therefore useful in treating depression.

Note: Selective monoamine oxidase B inhibitors (e.g., selegiline, rasagiline) primarily reduce the breakdown of dopamine and are therefore useful in treating Parkinson disease.

13. What is the main danger of prescribing both an SSRI and an MAOI?

The combination of an MAOI and an SSRI or TCA can cause pathologically elevated levels of serotonin, resulting in the serotonin syndrome (SS). The SS is characterized by mental status changes, autonomic hyperactivity, and neuromuscular abnormalities. It can be very difficult to distinguish from NMS if the patient has received both antipsychotics and drugs that can produce SS. Tachycardia, diaphoresis, fever, and agitation can be seen in both syndromes, but hyperreflexia and clonus (including horizontal ocular clonus) are more likely to occur in SS than in NMS. Symptoms can progress to hallucinations, hyperthermia, widespread rigidity, spontaneous clonus, rhabdomyolysis, delirium, and even death. Suspected cases of SS can be treated with the 5-HT$_2$ receptor antagonist cyproheptadine.

A useful mnemonic for recalling the symptoms of SS is **HARMED**: **H**yperthermia, **A**utonomic instability, **R**igidity, **M**yoclonus, **E**ncephalopathy, and **D**iaphoresis.

Note: The street drug "ecstasy" (3,4-methylenedioxymethamphetamine [MDMA]) is known for producing very severe cases of SS. Amphetamines and cocaine can also contribute to SS. It is important to keep in mind that any process that will elevate serotonin levels may contribute to the syndrome (e.g., increased synthesis from tyramine; decreased breakdown from MAOIs; decreased serotonin reuptake from meperidine, TCAs, and SSRIs; and serotonin receptor agonism from lysergic acid diethylamide [LSD]).

A helpful mnemonic for recalling key drugs that can contribute to the SS is the following phrase: **S**inners **S**ell **D**rugs **T**hat **M**ake **ME TRIP**: **S**t. John's wort, an over-the-counter (OTC) herbal treatment for depression; **S**SRIs; **D**extromethorphan, ingredient in OTC cough syrup (can be abused); **T**CAs; **M**AOIs; **ME**peridine; **TRIP**tans (e.g., sumatriptan, a serotonin agonist used to treat migraines). Step 1 likes to test on this concept. Look for a patient on an SSRI or TCA given meperidine for pain or a triptan for migraines.

14. If this patient has depression and is additionally a smoker who is trying to quit, which drug might be effective?

Bupropion would be an excellent choice for this patient. It has been shown to be effective in smoking cessation, especially when used with nicotine replacement therapy. Although its exact mechanism of action is not completely understood, it is believed to be a nicotinic receptor agonist and has the ability to inhibit the reuptake of both dopamine and norepinephrine, thereby enhancing both dopaminergic and noradrenergic transmission. Bupropion is a nice alternative to the SSRIs because it lacks their adverse sexual side effects.

Note: One major concern with this drug is that it lowers the threshold for seizure development, particularly in women with an underlying eating disorder such as anorexia or bulimia, which can cause electrolyte imbalances.

15. **If this man experienced much milder symptoms of depression for longer than 2 years, what would be his probable diagnosis?**
Persistent depressive disorder would be a probable diagnosis.
    Note: Persistent depressive disorder used to be called *dysthymic disorder* in the *DSM-IV*.

16. **How might your diagnosis change if this man had been divorced 2 months ago and his symptoms of depression were milder?**
This man would have an adjustment disorder with depressed mood. The appearance of emotional or behavioral symptoms that are the response to an identifiable stressor within 3 months of the appearance of symptoms is the hallmark of adjustment disorder. These symptoms must either cause a person significant distress over what would be expected in that situation or cause significant social or occupational dysfunction in order to be considered an adjustment disorder. Upon removal of the stressor, the symptoms should resolve within 6 months. If the patient were experiencing loss of a loved one, then it would more appropriately be classified as bereavement, which, according to the revised *DSM-5*, would not exclude the diagnosis of major depressive disorder. The adjustment disorder should be classified as chronic or acute and may be further classified as with depressed mood, with anxiety, with mixed anxiety and depressed mood, with disturbance of conduct, with mixed disturbance of emotions and conduct, or unspecified.

17. **If this man's spouse died 1 year ago and he was still experiencing these symptoms, what would his probable diagnosis be?**
Major depressive disorder would be the probable diagnosis. Normal grieving, which can mimic depression, is largely resolved within 6 months. Regardless, normal grieving does not necessarily rule out depressive disorder. If the **SIGECAPS** symptoms are present in a grieving individual, the diagnosis is major depressive disorder, not bereavement or adjustment disorder.

SUMMARY BOX: DEPRESSION

Categories of depression
- Major depressive disorder: Requires one or more major depressive episode(s)
- Persistent depressive disorder (previously, dysthymic disorder): Mildly depressed mood for at least 2 years
- Adjustment disorder with depressed mood: Upon removal of the stressor, the symptoms should resolve within 6 months.
Treatments
- Selective serotonin reuptake inhibitors (SSRIs)
  - Treatment of choice for depression
  - Very effective and have much more tolerable side effect profiles than other treatment options
- Tricyclic antidepressants (TCAs)
  - Cause anticholinergic, orthostatic hypotensive, and sedative side effects
  - Overdose can cause cardiac arrhythmias, convulsions, and even coma or death
- Electroconvulsive therapy (ECT)
  - Response rate of 90% compared with 70% for pharmacotherapy
- Combination of a monoamine oxidase inhibitor (MAOI) and an SSRI or TCA (as well as other drugs) can cause pathologically elevated levels of serotonin, resulting in serotonin syndrome

CASE 16.4

A 12-year-old boy's twin brother is killed in a car accident. The surviving twin has depressed mood, feelings of guilt, and frequent emotional outbursts. He has begun to wear only his brother's clothing. He has been writing his thoughts in a diary since the accident. He has also begun to treat his other younger brother badly, talking to him harshly and even physically abusing him.

1. **Instead of speaking to his deceased brother, which this patient believes would be viewed as unacceptable, he begins to keep a diary, which he believes is a more acceptable outlet for his emotions. What is the defense mechanism used by this boy?**
This patient is using the defense mechanism of *sublimation,* which involves altering a socially unacceptable impulse or idealization into an acceptable one. By channeling the desire to communicate with his brother into writing his thoughts in a diary, the patient uses sublimation to express his inner thoughts and feelings.

2. **Why does this young man begin to wear his brother's clothing? What term is used to describe this type of activity?**
This activity is described as *identification,* a process in which an individual subconsciously adopts the patterns or behaviors of another. By wearing his deceased brother's clothing, he feels like part of his brother is still with him, and he does not have to face the loss of his brother.

3. The patient feels angry at his parents for being responsible for the car accident that killed his twin brother. He instead takes out his frustrations on his younger brother by verbally abusing him. What defense mechanism is being described?

This patient is using *displacement*, which involves the expression of an emotion felt from one situation onto another. A common example is frustrations at work being taken out at home by starting an argument or being difficult. He is displacing his anger about his parents onto a more vulnerable subject, his younger brother.

4. What are the categories of defense mechanisms, and what are some examples of each type?
   - *Mature defenses* include altruism, humor, sublimation, and suppression.
   - *Neurotic defenses* include repression, intellectualization, identification, rationalization, displacement, and regression.
   - *Immature defenses* include acting out, fantasy, hypochondriasis, and projection.
   - *Psychotic defenses* include denial and distortion.

STEP 1 SECRET

There is some disagreement in the literature as to which ego defenses fall under which categories, so this is less important. However, the specific nature of each of the various defenses is a favorite topic on the boards, so spend sufficient time learning this.

CASE 16.5

A 42-year-old married businessman with six children is diagnosed with Huntington disease after being seen by a specialist in movement disorders. The patient is told that there is no cure for his disease and that he will progressively decline physically and mentally before dying within 10 years. To make matters worse, he is told that several of his six children may have the disease. He comes home from his appointment and, for the first time in his life, he is physically abusive to his spouse.

1. What are the five stages of grief this man will likely experience?

Denial, anger, bargaining, acceptance, and *sadness* are the five stages of grief according to the Kübler-Ross model. The grieving person may not experience all of these stages and may pass through a stage quite rapidly, appearing not to experience it at all.

2. What term is used to describe taking his frustration out about his diagnosis by abusing his spouse?

His behavior can be described as *displacement*, where he takes his emotions about his diagnosis out on another entity (his spouse).

3. What defense mechanism would this patient be using if he ignored the doctor's visit and went on with his life without acknowledging his diagnosis?

The patient would be using *denial,* which involves subconscious refusal to acknowledge that there is a problem. There is cognitive and emotional unawareness of the truth. The person does not believe what they have been told, and it does not register emotionally.

4. What term would be used to describe his behavior if while hospitalized he begins crying for his mother and demanding that other people feed him and take care of things he is fully capable of doing?

He would be exhibiting *regression.* This term is used to describe an attempt to return to an earlier phase of functioning to avoid conflict. It is quite common in the medical setting.

5. Cover the left column of Table 16.2 and attempt to name the defense mechanisms described in the middle column.

SUMMARY BOX: EGO DEFENSES

Sublimation
- Involves altering a socially objectionable aim or object into an acceptable one

Identification
- Involves seeing oneself as being like the other person

Acting out
- Involves the expression of an impulse through action to avoid dealing with what the feelings mean

Denial
- Involves unconsciously refusing to acknowledge that there is a problem

Regression
- Attempting to return to an earlier phase of functioning to avoid conflict

See Table 16.2 for descriptions and examples of other ego defenses.

Table 16.2. Defense Mechanisms

DEFENSE MECHANISM	DESCRIPTION	EXAMPLE
Splitting	Categorization of things into good or bad ("everything is black or white," no gray); associated with borderline personality disorder	A patient describes you as "the best doctor," whereas her last physician is a "quack."
Altruism	The act of giving or serving, not for feeling of obligation or recognition, merely for the sake of doing good	A wealthy widow donates half of her husband's estate to benefit the local children's hospital.
Reaction formation	Turning a strong impulse that is unacceptable into the opposite to "undo" the feeling	A boy is angry with his mother for grounding him, and he wishes she would die. Feeling guilty, he runs downstairs, hugs her, and tells her how much he loves her.
Suppression	Consciously or semiconsciously postponing attention to a conscious impulse; discomfort is minimized but still acknowledged	A woman tries to avoid thinking about her husband, who recently died by suicide, by removing his clothing from their shared closet.
Repression	Withholding an idea or feeling from consciousness; impulses are consciously inhibited to the point of losing, not just postponing, goals	A woman tries to avoid thinking about her husband, who recently died by suicide, by burning all his clothing and removing all his photos from the wall.

All ego defenses are unconscious, with the exception of suppression.

CASE 16.6

An 8-year-old boy is brought to the physician by his mother for behavioral problems. The mother says that for as long as she can remember he has been much more "difficult" than his other brothers and sisters. She is also concerned because he has been doing poorly in the first grade, and his teacher has complained to her several times about his disruptive behaviors in class. In the physician's office, the boy appears distracted and fidgety; when asked by the doctor to respond to five questions on a questionnaire, the boy answers only two of the questions. When addressed by the physician, he seems distracted and does not appear to be listening.

1. What are the considerations in the differential diagnosis?

Attention-deficit/hyperactivity disorder (ADHD), oppositional defiant disorder (ODD), conduct disorder, learning disorders, and even normal behavior are all considered.

CASE 16.6 CONTINUED:

The boy does not argue with adults, defy or refuse to comply with requests, or deliberately annoy people. He also does not display aggression to people and animals or destruction of property.

2. What is this patient's likely diagnosis?

ADHD, a disorder characterized by a pattern of hyperactivity, impulsiveness, inattention, and distractibility, is likely. It is divided into inattentive type, hyperactive type, and mixed type. The diagnosis requires that the symptoms be present in at least two settings (i.e., in school and at home), and the onset of these symptoms must occur before 7 years of age. Sometimes it can be difficult to properly assess a child's behavior in the situation if they behave differently in the office. In this case, the physician must rely on second-hand information from parents and teachers. Rating scales can be beneficial in accomplishing this objective.

Note: ODD involves a pattern of negative, hostile, and deviant behavior lasting at least 6 months. Affected patients show at least four of the following behaviors: argue with adults, lose their temper, defy or refuse to comply with requests, deliberately annoy people, blame others for their mistakes, are angry and resentful, or are spiteful and vindictive.

Conduct disorder is a pattern of behavior in which other peoples' basic rights are violated or societal rules or norms are broken, demonstrated by at least three of the following in the past 12 months and at least one in the past 6 months: aggression to people and animals, destruction of property, deceitfulness and theft, or a serious violation of rules. The onset of this disorder is in childhood, and diagnosis requires that the individual is under the age of 18. These individuals typically meet the criteria for antisocial disorder after the age of 18.

3. Using the *DSM-5* criteria, how would ADHD be classified?

ADHD is classified as a neurodevelopmental disorder in the *DSM-5*. Recall that the previous version of the *DSM* (*DSM-IV*) was organized into five "axes," but this is no longer used; instead, all disorders are included within Section II of the *DSM-5*.

4. What class of drugs is the primary treatment for ADHD?
First-line treatment of ADHD includes the use of amphetamine derivatives (e.g., methylphenidate, dextroamphetamine), which results in increased attention, decreased motor activity, and improvement in learning tasks. Treatment of ADHD is associated with better psychosocial outcomes including better grades, less likelihood of going to prison, and lower likelihood of unplanned pregnancy.

5. What is the most common side effect of amphetamines?
Amphetamines suppress appetite, so patients may lose weight.

6. What psychiatric symptoms might be evident in an individual following an overdose of amphetamines?
Psychotic features may appear and are presumably related to increased dopamine. This also illustrates the importance of ruling out substance abuse as a cause before making a diagnosis of schizophrenia in a psychotic patient.

SUMMARY BOX: BEHAVIORAL CHILDHOOD DISORDERS

Attention-deficit/hyperactivity disorder (ADHD)
- Pattern of hyperactivity, impulsiveness, inattention, and distractibility; symptoms must be present in at least two settings and must occur before 7 years of age
- Treat with amphetamine derivatives

Oppositional defiant disorder (ODD)
- A pattern of negative, hostile, and deviant behavior lasting at least 6 months

Conduct disorder
- Violation of other peoples' basic rights or societal rules or norms are broken, demonstrated by at least three of the following in the past 12 months and at least one in the past 6 months:
  - Aggression to people and animals
  - Destruction of property
  - Deceitfulness and theft or a serious violation of rules

CASE 16.7

A 4-year-old boy is brought to the pediatrician by his mother because he is having trouble "fitting in" with his peers at preschool. His teacher says he is a fine student academically but does not like to play with others during free time, only plays with the red blocks, and refuses to leave the room until all books are stacked perfectly. Yesterday, he showed no interest in show-and-tell. He can speak in four-word sentences, hop and skip, dress himself, and use a fork and a spoon. His mother says he has never been an emotional boy and has always been content spending time alone. In the office he does not make eye contact when spoken to and instead focuses on tapping his right thumb repetitively.

---

1. What is the differential diagnosis?
Autism spectrum disorder, learning disorder, intellectual disability, sensory impairment (e.g., difficulties with hearing or vision), genetic disorders, and normal behavior should be considered.

2. What are the criteria for autism spectrum disorder (ASD)?
ASD is characterized by deficits in social communication and interaction (deficits in social-emotional reciprocity, nonverbal communicative behaviors, and sustaining interpersonal relationships) and restricted, repetitive patterns of behavior, interests, or activities (at least two of the following: stereotyped or repetitive movements, use of objects, or speech; insistence on sameness or rigid adherence to routines; abnormally intense fixation on an interest or object; hyper- or hyporeactivity to sensory stimuli).
   Note: Asperger syndrome and autistic disorder were distinct in the *DSM-IV* but are now both considered ASD, so these older terms are no longer used.

3. What is known about the etiology of ASD?
Heritability estimates are around 92%, but no specific genes have been identified. Factors that have been linked to ASD include genetics, maternal grandmother smoking, perinatal infections (e.g., rubella), obstetric complications, perinatal toxin exposure, medications (e.g., SSRIs), and parental age. Some parents refuse vaccinations for their children because they believe vaccinations such as measles, mumps, and rubella (MMR) can contribute to autism risk. Note that there has been no evidence to support this association, and numerous large studies have repeatedly disproven such claims.

4. What if the patient was not doing well academically and these behaviors and social impairments were manifested only at school?
The diagnosis might be a learning disorder because cognitive or academic difficulties are often associated with disruptive behavior in children.

5. What should the workup include?
Intelligence quotient (IQ) testing and standardized tests for math, reading, and writing should be performed.

6. **What would be the diagnosis if the patient scored 70 or below on IQ testing?**

The diagnosis would be *intellectual disability* (formerly mental retardation). It presents before age 18 and is characterized by an IQ below 70 and limitations in two behavioral areas including communication, activities of daily living (ADLs), problem solving, and interpersonal skills.

It is further classified by subtype depending upon the score on IQ testing:

- 50 to 69: Mild
- 35 to 49: Moderate
- 20 to 34: Severe
- <20: Profound

An IQ between 70 and 84 is considered borderline intellectual functioning. These patients typically have trouble with abstraction.

SUMMARY BOX: COGNITIVE CHILDHOOD DISORDERS

- Learning disorder
  - Specific difficulty in mathematics, reading, or writing can present with disruptive behavior
- Intellectual disability
  - Intellectual and multiple behavioral difficulties
  - Intelligence quotient (IQ) <70
- Autism
  - Multiple deficits in social interaction and impairment in communication. The previously distinct Asperger syndrome has been incorporated into the classification of autism spectrum disorder.

CASE 16.8

A 14-year-old boy is brought to see a psychiatrist by his parents. The mother reports three different episodes of walking into his room while he was masturbating, and she is worried that he has some kind of "problem."

---

1. **If the psychiatrist explains this boy's developmental maturation in terms of psychosexual development, what psychologist are they referring to, and what are these stages of development?**

Sigmund Freud identified five stages of psychosexual development:

- *Oral stage*: Birth to 18 months
- *Anal stage*: 18 months to 3 years
- *Phallic stage*: 3 to 6 years
- *Latency stage*: 6 years to puberty
- *Genital stage*: Puberty to young adulthood

2. **Freud discusses the id, ego, and superego. How do these concepts relate to this patient?**

The *id* represents the instinctual drives with which people are born. The id operates in the subconscious mind and lacks the ability to delay or change the drives with which one is born.

The *ego* spans both the conscious and unconscious. Consciously, logical and abstract thinking and verbal expression are handled by the ego. Unconsciously, defense mechanisms are used by the ego. The ego uses external reality to harness instinctual drive of the id and substitutes realities for pleasure.

The *superego* serves to monitor a person's behavior, thoughts, and feelings according to a strict set of morals and values internalized from that of the parents; it makes comparison to these standards and offers approval or disapproval. For example, the superego deems it inappropriate for the boy to keep masturbating and causes him to feel guilty about it. The id represents the pleasure he receives from masturbation. The ego processes the inputs from the id, the superego, and the external reality. The ego compromises by giving in sometimes and masturbating, but other times it substitutes other pleasurable activity, such as playing a board game, for masturbating.

3. **If the psychiatrist discusses the boy's development in terms of stages of cognitive development, what psychologist are they referring to, and what are these stages of cognitive development?**

Piaget identified four stages of cognitive development:

Sensory-motor: Between the time of birth and about 2 years of age, babies begin to develop an understanding of object permanence. No longer do they fear that "mommy is gone" when she covers her face with her hands. "Peek-a-boo" begins to lose its charm. They develop the ability to control movement and observe their surroundings via their developing senses.

Preoperational: As the child ages from about 2 to 7 years, they begin to associate events with external happenings, leading to a belief of phenomenalistic causality. For example, a negative thought directed toward someone who falls and breaks a leg causes the child to believe the fall was caused by the inappropriate thought. They also tend to operate in an egocentric fashion. These children are unable to process how their behavior or an outside event affects other people.

Concrete operational: From ages 7 to 11, children begin to understand conservation of objects. They develop the ability to understand that a small cup full of juice is "less" than a big cup that is half full, but they still might have trouble understanding a nickel is less money than a dime ("it's bigger") because they have not mastered abstract thought. Children in this stage may become strict rule followers; obsessive traits may begin to emerge.

Formal operations: From age 11 until the end of adolescence, teens begin to develop the ability to understand abstract thought and reason. They begin to be able to process ideas and concepts lacking a concrete basis.

4. If the psychiatrist explains this boy's development in terms of development of the ego, what psychologist are they referring to, and what are the stages of ego development?

Erikson theorized that a person must overcome certain basic conflicts in eight stages of life in the process of development. These stages are as follows:

- *Trust versus mistrust* (birth–1 year): The child learns whether their basic needs will be met and whether their care providers can be relied upon.
- *Autonomy versus shame* (1–3 years): Toddlers begin to show mastery over excretory functions such as urination and defecation.
- *Initiative versus guilt* (3–5 years): Children are allowed to initiate behavior and interests; their conscience is established.
- *Industry versus inferiority* (6–11 years): Children learn that they are able to master and complete tasks; inadequacy may develop if their social environment is unsupportive.
- *Identity versus role confusion* (11–21 years): Young people develop a sense of who they are and where they are going.
- *Intimacy versus isolation* (21–40 years): People establish sexual relationships, deep friendships, and deep associations, as long as there is no underlying identity confusion.
- *Generativity versus stagnation* (40–65 years): People's main interest is in guiding and establishing future generations or improving society.
- *Integrity versus despair* (over 65 years): Satisfaction is sensed if people feel that their life has been productively lived.

Failure to meet each of these conflicts results in stagnation of development, but successfully resolving each conflict allows progression to the next stage of development.

SUMMARY BOX: PSYCHOLOGY

- Freud identified five stages of psychosexual development
  - Oral, anal, phallic, latent, and genital
- Freud discussed three structures of the mind
  - Id, ego, and superego
- Piaget identified four stages of cognitive development
  - Sensory-motor, preoperational, concrete operational, and formal operational
- Erikson identified eight stages of life in the process of development
  - Trust versus mistrust (birth–1 year)
  - Autonomy versus shame (1–3 years)
  - Initiative versus guilt (3–5 years)
  - Industry versus inferiority (6–11 years)
  - Identity versus role confusion (11–21 years)
  - Intimacy versus isolation (21–40 years)
  - Generativity versus stagnation (40–65 years)
  - Integrity versus despair (over 65 years)

CASE 16.9

A 75-year-old man presents to the emergency department with severe midepigastric pain radiating to the back, malabsorption, steatorrhea, and polyuria. An abdominal x-ray film shows pancreatic calcifications.

1. What is the most likely diagnosis?

Chronic pancreatitis is the most likely diagnosis.

2. What is the most likely etiology?

Pancreatitis describes the autodigestion of the pancreas by its own digestive enzymes. Chronic pancreatitis is generally a complication of recurrent bouts of acute pancreatitis that are most commonly related to chronic alcohol use. Acute pancreatitis can be caused by many things, which can be remembered using the mnemonic **GET SMASHED**: **G**allstones, **E**thanol abuse, **T**rauma, **S**teroids, **M**umps, **A**utoimmune disease, **S**corpion sting, **H**ypercalcemia/hypertriglyceridemia, **E**ndoscopic retrograde cholangiopancreatography (ERCP), **D**rugs (e.g., sulfa drugs).

The patient is promptly admitted to the medicine service. He admits his heavy alcohol use to the intake team.

3. **What concern does this man's alcohol use pose to the medicine team?**
This man's chronic pancreatitis is more than likely due to his alcohol use disorder. If he is not treated appropriately for alcohol use, all that can be expected for his pancreatitis is symptomatic control of his periodic exacerbations. Additionally, patients who consume large quantities of alcohol (or have regular consumption of smaller quantities) are at risk for symptoms of withdrawal.

4. **What are the expected symptoms of withdrawal, and how are they managed?**
Withdrawal is displayed in two stages. Early symptoms of withdrawal might include tachycardia, tremors, nausea, vomiting, or hypertension. These initial symptoms are usually controlled with lorazepam, a benzodiazepine. The later, more life-threatening concern is the appearance of delirium tremens (DTs). Usually presenting after about 48 hours of abstinence, these severe tremors may be accompanied by hallucinations (generally these are tactile hallucinations, e.g., experiencing "bugs crawling on one's skin"), delirium, and mild fever. DTs are often preceded by seizures, which rarely lead to status epilepticus. Seizures can be managed by intravenous benzodiazepines. Phenobarbital is also being used more routinely in acute withdrawal and DTs prevention and treatment. The DTs can be managed with benzodiazepines and supportive care. The affected patient may need intensive care, especially in the case of autonomic instability. These symptoms typically last for ~3 days but may persist for weeks.
    Note: Alcohol is one of few drugs that are cleared from the body through zero-order kinetics. In zero-order kinetics, a constant *amount* of the drug is cleared from the body per unit time, compared with first-order kinetics in which a constant *fraction* of the drug is cleared per unit time. Phenytoin, aspirin, and heparin are other examples of drugs with zero-order kinetics.

5. **What is the mechanism by which the administration of benzodiazepines is able to control the DTs?**
Alcohol potentiates the γ-aminobutyric acid (GABA) receptor, as do the benzodiazepines. Recall that GABA is an *inhibitory* neurotransmitter. Gradual tapering, rather than abrupt termination, of this agonistic effect allows the central nervous system to acclimate to the increased stimulation experienced as alcohol is removed.

6. **Another class of drugs acts as agonists of the GABA receptor at a different site. What is the name of this group of drugs, and how do the pharmacokinetic effects differ from those of benzodiazepines?**
Barbiturates such as phenobarbital also agonize the GABA receptor at a site distinct from that of the benzodiazepines. The benzodiazepines eventually reach a maximal effect, whereas barbiturates continue to increase their effect as dosage is increased. The result is that barbiturates are much more likely to cause a fatal respiratory depression than benzodiazepines (although this is still a concern).
    Note: Benzodiazepines work by increasing the frequency of chloride channel opening, and barbiturates increase the duration that the chloride channel is open.

7. **What are the criteria for a substance use disorder?**
A substance use disorder is diagnosed when two of the following have occurred over the past 12 months: using more than intended; having a persistent but unsuccessful desire to cut down or quit; spending lots of time acquiring, using, or recovering from use; craving; inability to fulfil roles at work/home/school due to use; continued using despite consequences; giving up hobbies in order to use; using in hazardous situations; recurrent using despite knowing that a physical or psychological problem is due to use; tolerance; and withdrawal. Severity is based on how many criteria are met and is graded as mild (2–3), moderate (4–5), or severe (6+).

SUMMARY BOX: ALCOHOL

- Alcohol, benzodiazepines, and barbiturates all act at the γ-aminobutyric acid (GABA) receptor.
- Barbiturates are much more likely to cause a fatal respiratory depression than benzodiazepines.
- Substance use disorder is characterized by meeting two of the following in a 12-month period:
  - using more than intended
  - having a persistent but unsuccessful desire to cut down or quit
  - spending lots of time acquiring, using, or recovering from use
  - craving
  - inability to fulfill roles at work/home/school due to use
  - continued using despite consequences
  - giving up hobbies in order to use
  - using in hazardous situations
  - recurrent using despite knowing that a physical or psychological problem is due to use
  - tolerance
  - withdrawal

CASE 16.10

Law enforcement officials bring a 27-year-old man to the emergency department. He is combative and disoriented and is screaming that bugs are crawling on his skin. His blood pressure, pulse, and respiratory rate are all elevated. He appears to be sweating profusely. On examination of the head, you notice some dried blood around one of his nostrils and see that his pupils are dilated. Once he settles down and begins talking with you, he reports that he feels lightheaded and his chest hurts.

1. Abuse involving which class of drugs should be expected in this man?
   This patient is suffering from intoxication of a stimulant, which in this case is cocaine. Tactile hallucinations, impaired judgment, transient psychosis, and agitation are commonly seen in stimulant intoxication. Other characteristic symptoms include tachycardia or bradycardia, dilated pupils, hyper- or hypotension, chills or fever, nausea and emesis, and confusion. Amphetamine intoxication could present in a similar fashion.
   Note: Formication (bugs crawling on skin) is often called "cocaine bugs" because it so often is caused by cocaine intoxication. However, it is also seen in DTs and in amphetamine psychosis.

2. Would you be surprised if this man's electrocardiogram revealed myocardial ischemia?
   It should not be surprising if this man's cardiac tissue has become ischemic. The cocaine he has been using can cause vasospasm, which can reduce cardiac perfusion leading to ischemia. He may also have "demand ischemia" from his agitation where his activity outpaces his ability to deliver oxygen to his myocardium. Other drugs that can cause vasospasm include amphetamine and sumatriptan.

3. What is the correct treatment of acute sympathomimetic toxicity-induced agitation?
   Intravenous benzodiazepines are indicated.
   Note: Do not give a beta-blocker for patients acutely on cocaine because that will lead to (theoretical) unopposed alpha-receptor stimulation by the cocaine, resulting in further vasospasm and hypertension.

4. What are typical symptoms experienced by a person who is withdrawing from use of cocaine?
   These patients experience severe psychological craving for the drug, extreme fatigue, hunger, headaches, cramps, and perspiration. These symptoms peak in 48 to 96 hours. These patients do not require inpatient management unless needed for the intense craving because withdrawal is otherwise self-limited. Clonidine, an α_2-adrenergic agonist, may be helpful in reducing the craving.

5. A favorite on boards is to provide an emergency department presentation of somebody with a drug overdose and ask you to determine the drug responsible for the patient's symptoms. The question will provide enough information to narrow the choices down to a single drug and therefore will rely upon the use of trigger words. Try to memorize the trigger words in Table 16.3. Be sure to learn drug withdrawal symptoms as well. These symptoms are often the opposite of those seen with drug toxicity.

Table 16.3. Drug Intoxications

DRUG INTOXICATION	TRIGGER WORDS	WITHDRAWAL
Opioids	Pupils constricted, ↓ RR	Flu-like symptoms, rhinorrhea, anxiety, piloerection
Amphetamine	Pupils dilated, delusions, ↑ HR, ↑ BP	Hunger, hypersomnolence
PCP	Nystagmus (especially vertical), ataxia, ↑ BP, clenching/grinding of the teeth (bruxism), random acts of violence and belligerence, hyperthermia	Depression
LSD	Flashbacks, pupillary dilation, depression, hallucinations	
Marijuana	Increased appetite, conjunctival irritation, paranoia, increased appetite, hallucinations	Irritability, depression, nausea, decreased appetite
MDMA ("ecstasy")	Hyperthermia, bruxism	
Anticholinergics—TCAs, pesticides[a]	Dry skin, flushing, fever, urinary retention, dilated pupils, delirium, cardiac conduction delays, thirst, ↑ HR	
Benzodiazepines, barbiturates ("benzos," "barbs")	History of anxiety, ataxia, somnolence, life-threatening respiratory depression with barbiturates	Anxiety, insomnia, seizures
Cholinergic poisoning—organophosphates, anticholinesterases	Salivation, ↓ HR, vomiting, urination, defecation, pupil constriction	

[a]You should know the antidotes for TCA and pesticide overdose: For TCA toxicity, administer sodium bicarbonate ($NaHCO_3$) to alkalize the serum. Organophosphate pesticides cause irreversible inhibition of acetylcholinesterase; overdose requires administration of atropine and pralidoxime (to regenerate acetylcholinesterase). Organophosphate poisoning is a commonly asked Step 1 concept.
BP, Blood pressure; *HR*, heart rate; *LSD*, lysergic acid diethylamide; *MDMA*, 3,4-methylenedioxymethamphetamine; *PCP*, phencyclidine; *RR*, respiratory rate; *TCA*, tricyclic antidepressant.

SUMMARY BOX: DRUG INTOXICATION

- Cocaine intoxication
  - Dilated pupils, formication, transient psychosis, agitation, tachycardia, hypertension
- Know the signs of drug intoxication and withdrawal.

CASE 16.11

A 72-year-old woman with early-stage Alzheimer disease is admitted to the hospital for extreme dyspnea and is diagnosed with pneumonia. Intravenous fluids and antibiotics are started. Upon admission, she is alert and oriented to person and time but not to place. She is able to score 26/30 on a Mini-Mental Status Examination administered to her shortly after her admission. The following morning, she is found to be febrile. The attending physician believes that she is not responding as expected and changes her antibiotic. A few hours later, this woman has become confused and aggressive and believes that the hospital staff has been trying to kill her.

1. Would this woman's current state be best described as dementia or delirium?
   This is an important distinction that must be made when there are acute mental status changes. This woman is suffering from delirium. Although she may have an underlying dementia, she has clearly become acutely delirious.
   Note: One caveat applies if this patient has been misdiagnosed with Alzheimer disease and in fact has Lewy body dementia (LBD), now thought to be the second most common cause of degenerative dementia. Along with dementia, the three core features of LBD are fluctuating cognition, visual hallucinations, and parkinsonism. Of note, one of the features of LBD is that it tends to worsen with neuroleptic agents.

2. What is the most likely cause of this woman's delirium?
   The two most common causes of a delirious state, especially in the elderly, are prescribed drugs and acute infections. This woman's pneumonia or the antibiotics being used to treat her pneumonia are most likely the cause of her delirious state. Other causes that should be investigated include drug or alcohol withdrawal, metabolic derangement, head trauma, epilepsy, and cerebral hypoperfusion. In addition to pneumonia, urinary tract infections (UTIs) are also a common cause of delirium in the elderly.

3. Distinguish dementia from delirium regarding onset, course, level of consciousness, and presence of delusions and hallucinations.
   Dementia typically has a gradual, insidious onset. It often goes unnoticed by family members who see the person every day. The course tends to be a gradually progressive decline in cognitive function, especially in short-term memory, without any changes in level of consciousness. In early stages, patients can be quite oriented with a normal level of consciousness. Later stages involve behavioral alterations and impaired judgment. Delusions or hallucinations may or may not be seen in a patient with dementia.
   Delirium typically has an acute to subacute onset. It often has an abrupt onset, typically within hours to days. It is characterized as a waxing and waning of the sensorium. Electroencephalogram (EEG) results are abnormal. Short-term memory and poor attention span are common cognitive defects. It is a sudden impairment in the level of consciousness, and patients can rapidly fluctuate. Delusions are typically fleeting, often persecutory, and may be related to the disorientation. Hallucinations are common; visual hallucinations strongly suggest delirium.

SUMMARY BOX: COGNITIVE DISORDERS

Dementia
- Memory impairment plus one of the following:
  - Aphasia
  - Apraxia
  - Agnosia
  - Disturbance in executive functioning
Delirium
- Disturbance in consciousness that develops over a shorter period of time and fluctuates throughout the day

CASE 16.12

A 32-year-old previously healthy businesswoman presents to the emergency department with a recent onset of chest pain, shortness of breath, dizziness, and an intense fear that she is dying. Her symptoms came on "out of the blue" while she was working in her office on a presentation she was scheduled to give in a few days. She has a strong family history of cardiovascular disease and is convinced she is having a heart attack. An extensive workup including an electrocardiogram, chest x-ray, and serial cardiac enzymes is negative for a myocardial infarction. After a short while in the emergency department, her symptoms appear to resolve.

1. **What is the most likely diagnosis in this woman?**
   This woman most likely had a panic attack, which is frequently misinterpreted as a heart attack by patients. *Panic attacks* consist of a discrete period of intense fear or discomfort during which the symptoms develop abruptly and usually peak within 10 minutes. These symptoms often mimic those of a heart attack and can include perspiration, palpitations, chest pain, shaking, sensation of choking, nausea, dizziness, chills, fear of dying, fear of losing control, or a feeling of derealization. *Panic disorder* is characterized by recurrent, unexpected panic attacks. For at least 1 month, people with panic disorder have had concerns about further attacks, fear the consequences of these attacks, or significantly altered their behaviors because of the panic attacks.

2. **If this woman subsequently developed a fear of leaving the house, what term should be used to describe her condition?**
   Agoraphobia is intense anxiety felt about being in situations from which escape is difficult (or embarrassing) or where help may not be available in the event that a panic attack occurs. If the avoidance is limited to specific situations, specific phobias, social phobia, or OCD should be considered. Patients who have panic disorder may or may not experience agoraphobia.

3. **What are the considerations in the differential diagnosis for panic disorder?**
   Generalized anxiety disorder, substance-induced anxiety disorder, and anxiety due to a general medical condition may resemble panic disorder.

4. **Why might an outpatient physician want to check this woman's blood levels of thyroid hormone and urinary vanillylmandelic acid (VMA) and 5-hydroxyindoleacetic acid (5-HIAA)?**
   Multiple organic conditions can mimic a panic attack, including hyperthyroidism (or "thyroid storm"), pheochromocytoma (elevated VMA), and carcinoid syndrome (elevated 5-HIAA). These conditions can be ruled out by a laboratory workup.

5. **How can this woman's panic disorder be treated?**
   SSRIs are first-line drugs for the treatment of panic disorder. Additionally, benzodiazepines can be used to decrease the anxiety associated with panic attacks in the first few weeks of treatment with an SSRI or when other therapies have failed. Beta-blockers can also be used to limit the physiologic effects of anxiety experienced in specific phobias, such as performance anxiety, when a person is certain to be exposed to that situation.

SUMMARY BOX: PANIC DISORDER

- Panic disorder
  - Recurrent unexpected panic attacks followed by at least 1 month of persistent concern about having another, worry about the implications, or a significant change in behavior related to the attacks
  - Can occur with or without agoraphobia
- Treatment
  - Selective serotonin reuptake inhibitors (SSRIs) are first-line treatment

CASE 16.13

A 16-year-old girl is admitted to a tertiary psychiatric referral center. For several months she has been having severe emotional outbursts and fits of anger. She has had trouble falling asleep and has been having recurrent nightmares when she does sleep. She has a history of sexual and physical abuse by her father before he left the family when she was 10. Her nightmares often revolve around these episodes of abuse.

1. **What is the most likely diagnosis in this girl?**
   She has posttraumatic stress disorder (PTSD) with delayed onset because the symptoms appeared more than 1 month after the stressor and persist for at least 1 month. If symptoms last between 2 days and 1 month, the condition is termed *acute stress disorder.*

2. **What are the requirements needed to make this diagnosis?**
   To make the diagnosis of PTSD, the patient has to have witnessed or been exposed or subjected to a traumatic event in which either (1) actual or threatened death or injury or (2) a threat to the physical integrity of self or others has

occurred. In addition, there must be a reexperiencing of the event, manifested through distressing dreams, acting out, or intrusive recollections of the event. The person also avoids thoughts, feelings, and activities associated with the event; such patients may avoid activities, feel detached, and stop expressing their feelings. There is also an increase in arousal. The person may have trouble falling asleep, become irritable or have anger outbursts, have trouble concentrating, or show an exaggerated startle response. Once again, these symptoms must persist longer than 1 month. Remember that it is crucial to pay attention to time intervals on boards!

3. **Is this condition very disabling to patients, and how is it best managed?**
PTSD can be very disabling to patients and can be a lifelong impairment. Group therapy has been very successfully used in the treatment of PTSD. In group therapy, patients are encouraged to talk about their trauma with other patients who have lived through similar experiences. Pharmacologic therapy for PTSD involves use of the SSRIs. Typically, a combination of group therapy and SSRIs is implemented for patients with PTSD.

SUMMARY BOX: POSTTRAUMATIC STRESS DISORDER

Posttraumatic stress disorder (PTSD)
- At least 1 month duration of the following symptoms after a traumatic event:
  - Persistent reexperiencing of the event(s)
  - Amnesia or emotional numbing
  - Increased arousal, causing impairment in social or occupational functioning
If symptom duration is less than 1 month, then it is called *acute stress disorder.*
  Treatment
- Selective serotonin reuptake inhibitors (SSRIs) are first-line treatment

CASE 16.14

A thin, frail-looking 17-year-old girl comes into your office for a physical examination before joining the cheerleading team at school. When you ask her the date of her last menstrual period, she tells you she cannot remember but knows she has not bought tampons in months.

1. **What conditions are considered in the differential diagnosis for this patient?**
Anorexia nervosa, pregnancy, Turner syndrome, hypothalamic-pituitary-ovarian (HPO) axis abnormalities, Asherman syndrome, stress, adrenal insufficiency, and thyroid disorders are all considered.
   Note: You must gather from this history that this girl has stopped having periods, making primary amenorrhea an unlikely cause. She is also thin, which makes obesity and polycystic ovary syndrome far less likely causes of her amenorrhea.

CASE 16.14 CONTINUED:

To confirm your suspicions of this patient's diagnosis, you look at the charts that the nurse has filled out and see that the patient is 5'4" and weighs 98 lb (body mass index (BMI) = 16.8).

2. **What is this patient's likely diagnosis?**
The likely diagnosis is anorexia nervosa, which is an eating disorder associated with intense fear of weight gain and significantly low body weight. A history of amenorrhea is common but not required for diagnosis in women.

3. **Why does anorexia lead to amenorrhea?**
Anorexia nervosa is associated with a decrease in GnRH production by the hypothalamus, which decreases estrogen production, leading to amenorrhea.

4. **What other conditions are associated with anorexia nervosa?**
   - *Depression:* Depression commonly coexists with anorexia but is not required for diagnosis.
   - *Stress fractures* (particularly metatarsal stress fractures): Decreased GnRH levels lead to a decrease in estrogen levels, which reduces bone density and promotes bone fracture.
   - *Lanugo:* Fine, soft body hair.
   - *Anemia:* Decreased food intake leads to inadequate levels of iron, vitamin B_{12}, and folate. If anorexia becomes severe, bone marrow will respond with pancytopenia.
   - *Dental cavities:* Decreased food intake leads to inadequate salivary gland stimulation. Since saliva plays a role in the prevention of dental caries, this can be a common problem in anorexic patients. Along similar lines, anorexic patients are also prone to halitosis.

- *Electrolyte disturbances and heart rhythm abnormalities:* Electrolyte disturbances are often secondary to vomiting, which induces metabolic alkalosis. The body responds to this by shifting potassium into cells in exchange for hydrogen out of cells (to restore blood pH). This results in a hypokalemic state, which can lead to ventricular arrhythmias. In addition, dehydration if present induces the renin-angiotensin-aldosterone system and further propagates hypokalemia. As mentioned in Chapter 5 (Acid-Base Balance), metabolic alkalosis also results in a compensatory respiratory acidosis with increased carbon dioxide (CO_2) levels.

5. **Compare the diagnoses of anorexia nervosa and bulimia nervosa.**

   A common misconception among students is that bulimia nervosa is marked by purging whereas anorexia is not. This, however, is not true. Purging behaviors may be present in both disorders, and neither disorder requires purging to make a diagnosis. Binge eating/purging type or restricting type is specified for anorexia. The major difference between the two conditions is that bulimic patients maintain normal (or obese) body weight whereas anorexic patients have abnormally low weight. Bulimia can lead to many of the same conditions as anorexia but is not generally associated with abnormal GnRH levels. It can, however, be marked by conditions that arise from excessive vomiting, such as parotitis, enamel erosion, Mallory-Weiss syndrome, Boerhaave syndrome, and Russell sign (calluses on the knuckles or back of the hand from repetitive induction of vomiting).

6. **How should this patient be managed?**

   Unfortunately, anorexia nervosa is not an easy condition to manage. Treatment may involve antidepressants such as SSRIs and mirtazapine. Mirtazapine is especially beneficial for anorexic patients with depression because it has a side effect of weight gain. However, the majority of treatment programs for anorexia nervosa are geared toward weight stabilization and individual and family therapy.

SUMMARY BOX: EATING DISORDERS

- Anorexia nervosa
  - An eating disorder marked by fear of gaining weight and severe, self-inflicted starvation
  - The patient has low body weight.
  - Patients with bulimia nervosa are often of normal or obese weight.
- History of amenorrhea is common in anorexia nervosa.
- Common symptoms of anorexia nervosa include:
  - Depression, stress fractures, anemia, lanugo, dental cavities, electrolyte disturbances, and heart abnormalities.
- Treatment
  - Anorexia nervosa is a difficult condition to manage clinically.
  - Antidepressants may help in some cases, but treatment primarily involves weight stabilization and individual/family counseling.

CASE 16.15

A 35-year-old surgeon is 2 hours late for an appointment with his physician and is told by the secretary that he will need to reschedule his appointment. He loudly demands to be seen immediately by the physician and states that his time is just as important as this physician's. While waiting to be worked in, he paces across the waiting room, muttering about how this university-affiliated clinic is not good enough for the leading surgeon in his field. Finally, when seen by the physician, he challenges the doctor's understanding of his condition and argues against the recommended therapy.

---

1. **What type of personality disorder does this man likely have?**

   This man is most likely has narcissistic personality disorder. These individuals have an exaggerated sense of self-importance, have a sense of entitlement, require excessive admiration from others, are arrogant, lack empathy, and take advantage of others to achieve their own ends.

CASE 16.16

A 22-year-old woman has a long history of unstable relationships and has had multiple suicide attempts and episodes of self-mutilation. After being seen by a particular physician for the first time, the woman tells the physician that he is the most amazing doctor she has ever seen. At the next appointment, he begins to discuss lifestyle changes to help her with her irregular sleep patterns. At this, she becomes enraged, yelling, "You are such a quack! I am going to see Dr. Jones. He knows how to treat insomnia!" She then storms out of the office.

---

1. What type of personality disorder does this woman likely have?

It is likely that she has borderline personality disorder. These patients have unstable relationships, a poor self-image, labile affect, and poor impulse control, and they commonly use splitting (see Table 16.2) as a defense mechanism. Psychotherapy, specifically dialectic behavioral therapy, is the treatment of choice.

CASE 16.17

A 42-year-old woman often appears preoccupied with herself and is inconsiderate and demanding of others. When seen by a male physician, she is flirtatious and makes inappropriate sexual comments. When the nurse enters the room, she fakes fainting just so the physician has to catch her. She has threatened suicide many times in the past, but her physician is convinced that these threats are not genuine and that the patient is manipulating him.

1. What type of personality disorder does this woman likely have?

Histrionic personality disorder is a likely diagnosis. These patients display excessive emotionality and sexual provocativeness and are very attention-seeking.

CASE 16.18

A 28-year-old man has spent the past 5 years in prison after being convicted for assault and robbery. His behavior has always been characterized by utter disregard for the feelings of others. As a child, he was sexually abused by his father, and he frequently tortured animals for entertainment. He appears to have no conscience and lies whenever it is convenient. His father and grandfather have alcohol use disorder, and he has a long history of alcohol abuse.

1. What type of personality disorder does this man likely have?

He has from antisocial personality disorder because he displays a general disregard for people and willingly violates the rights of others. This personality disorder parallels conduct disorder except that antisocial personality disorder is diagnosed in individuals 18 years of age or older, whereas minors are diagnosed with conduct disorder. In many ways antisocial personality disorder can be thought of as a continuation or progression of conduct disorder into adulthood.

Note: The four personality disorders just mentioned (narcissistic, borderline, histrionic, and antisocial) are all considered "cluster B" personality disorders. As a group, they are considered to be the "wild" personality disorders and have been associated with substance abuse and mood disorders.

CASE 16.19

A physician frequently has calls from a 38-year-old female patient for very minor health concerns, such as common colds and minor cuts and scratches. When soliciting the physician's advice regarding her health care at regularly scheduled appointments, the woman invariably responds that she will do whatever he thinks is best and that her opinion does not matter in the slightest. At home, she defers almost all decision making to her husband, on whom she is very reliant.

1. What type of personality disorder does this woman likely have?

It is likely that she has dependent personality disorder. These individuals are submissive, have low self-confidence, and rely heavily on the support of others.

CASE 16.20

A 52-year-old man has worked in the same position in a large factory for 30 years. He is an excellent worker but has always turned down offers of promotion. He explains this by saying he loves his current job, but secretly he fears criticism of his job performance. He does not go out for dinner with his colleagues or attend the annual Christmas party because he becomes anxious in these situations.

1. What type of personality disorder does this man likely have?

He demonstrates avoidant personality disorder. Even though patients with avoidant personality disorder also crave acceptance and fear criticism, they generally will not reach out to others and risk rejection and humiliation to get their needs met.

CASE 16.21

A 19-year-old college student normally receives excellent grades in school, but sometimes her grades suffer because of handing in a "perfect" paper past the deadline. She is wonderfully reliable to her friends but causes them some frustration because of her insistence on maintaining a fixed rigid schedule and her moralistic and sometimes judgmental views. She pays excruciatingly close attention to minor details and is very sensitive to any criticism.

1. What type of personality disorder does this young woman likely have?

   Obsessive-compulsive personality disorder (OCPD) is likely. Do not confuse this with OCD. Patients with OCPD *do not* have obsessions or compulsions that mark the diagnosis of OCD. Rather, they are preoccupied with general perfectionism, order, and control and are unable to change their routines. Patients with OCPD exhibit behaviors consistent with their own beliefs (ego-*syntonic*). This contrasts with patients who have OCD; these patients dislike performing their compulsive behaviors but exhibit little control over their actions (ego-*dystonic*).

   Note: The three personality disorders just mentioned (dependent, avoidant, and obsessive compulsive) are all considered "cluster C" personality disorders. As a group, they are considered to be the "worried" personality disorders and have been associated with anxiety disorders.

CASE 16.22

A 38-year-old woman has no close friends and "prefers to do things on my own." She has never had a boyfriend and is unperturbed by the frequent criticism of her parents regarding her unmarried status. Although she is a highly successful professional, she is indifferent to the praise of her coworkers and peers. She appears cold and unemotional but is not confrontational.

1. What type of personality disorder does this woman likely have?

   Schizoid personality disorder is demonstrated by a detachment from social relationships and restricted affect. Common manifestations include lack of desire to socialize or be part of groups or family, little interest in sexual relations or other pleasurable activities, detachment and emotional coldness, and indifference to the praise or criticism of others.

2. In addition to the previously mentioned personality characteristics, she states that she often sees her soul float away from her body and feels that after this happens, she is able to predict the future. She adds that other people know of her abilities, and she feels they are "out to get her." What personality disorder might you diagnose in this woman?

   Schizotypal personality disorder is a pattern of social and emotional deficits in addition to some cognitive or perceptual eccentricities. Persons who have schizotypal personalities often have odd beliefs, superstitions, or magical thinking. They may have inappropriate affect, odd speech patterns, and a paucity of close friends or confidants. Unlike those with schizoid personality disorder, patients with schizotypal personality disorder do not attempt to avoid people but may have difficulty maintaining interpersonal relationships.

3. What personality disorder would you diagnose if she were reclusive but really did yearn for social contact?

   A likely diagnosis would be avoidant personality disorder, which is seen in people who have a fear of being ridiculed and view themselves as inept and inadequate. They desire social interaction, but the anxiety felt over being placed in social situations keeps them in the shadows. They are reluctant to take personal risks or engage in new activities for fear of being embarrassed.

   Note: Schizoid personality disorder, schizotypal personality disorder, and paranoid personality disorder are considered "cluster A" personality disorders. As a group, they are considered to be the "weird" personality disorders and have been associated with schizophrenia. Avoidant personality disorder is an important distinction from schizoid personality disorder in that the schizoid label implies voluntary social withdrawal as opposed to the desire to form relationships characteristic of the avoidant personality.

SUMMARY BOX: PERSONALITY DISORDERS

- Personality disorders are life-long by definition
- Paranoid personality disorder
  - Mistrust of others without justification
- Schizoid personality disorder
  - Socially and emotionally detached individuals
- Schizotypal personality disorder
  - Similar to schizoid but with ideas of reference, odd beliefs, or magical thinking
- Antisocial personality disorder
  - Repetitive disregard for society at large and basic rights of others (narcissistic patients also lack empathy and use people to get what they want, but they are not as aggressive as antisocial patients)
- Borderline personality disorder
  - Unstable relationships, poor self-image, labile affect, and poor impulse control
- Histrionic personality disorder
  - Excessive emotionality and high need for attention
- Narcissistic personality disorder
  - Requires constant admiration, displays envy, lack of empathy, and grandiose thinking
- Avoidant personality disorder
  - Social inhibition, feelings of inadequacy, and fear of criticism
- Dependent personality disorder
  - Excessive need to be taken care of
- Obsessive-compulsive personality disorder
  - Orderliness, perfectionism and control without flexibility, and efficiency; no obsessions or compulsions

CHAPTER 17

NEUROLOGY

Insider's Guide to Neurology for the USMLE Step 1

Neurology is one of the toughest subjects on boards because of the broad range of information that must be mastered. Unfortunately, there is no way to comprehensively cover all of the information that you must know for neurology in this chapter or any single board review book. The best prepared students use a mix of review sources to study for neurology. You might consider having a proper neurology textbook nearby so that you can refer to some diagrams included in it as well.

High-yield neurology topics include neurodegenerative disorders, Alzheimer disease, spinal cord syndromes, and the consequences of central nervous system (CNS) lesions to upper and lower motor neurons. For strokes or demyelinating processes, it is important to understand not only the general functional and deficits that you would expect to find in the patient but also the side of the body that will be affected based on the site of the lesion. Practice, practice, and practice while studying, and you will sharpen your intuition and minimize your efforts on test day.

Neuroanatomy is also high yield for boards. You will be expected to recognize anatomic structures present at various levels of the brain or spinal cord and make clinical correlations to diseases that affect these structures. This will require you to know which section of the CNS you are looking at when presented with an image. We recommend using *High-Yield Neuroanatomy* of the High-Yield Series. This book covers the depth of information that you need to breeze through neuroanatomy on boards, and users also are quite impressed with its brevity.

BASIC CONCEPTS

1. **What is a motor unit? Will most alpha motor neurons innervate few or many muscle fibers in a large muscle such as the gluteus maximus?**

   A motor unit is a group of muscle fibers that is innervated by a single alpha motor neuron. In the large muscles, alpha motor neurons will innervate many muscle fibers, which is why fine control of muscle movement (contraction) is limited. On the other hand, in the smaller muscles (e.g., extraocular muscles or muscles of the hand), a given alpha motor neuron will innervate only a few muscle fibers, resulting in much finer control of movement. In both types of muscles, increasing the strength of muscle contraction occurs primarily by *recruitment* of additional motor units.

2. **How do upper motor neurons differ from lower motor neurons?**

   Motor neurons, as the name implies, are neurons involved in stimulating movement. The axons of alpha motor neurons project directly to skeletal muscle (extrafusal) fibers, whereas gamma motor neurons project to muscle spindles (intrafusal) fibers, contraction of which do not result in movement but play an important role in muscle tone and proprioception. Alpha and gamma motor neurons are examples of lower motor neurons (LMNs). Upper motor neuron (UMN) cell bodies are located in the cerebral cortex (corticospinal tract) and brainstem and have no direct contact with skeletal muscle (Fig. 17.1). The axons of UMNs synapse either directly or indirectly, via interneurons, on LMNs located in the ventral horn of the spinal cord or brainstem motor nuclei (e.g., facial nerve motor nucleus).

STEP 1 SECRET

Upper motor neuron (UMN) lesions produce a different set of symptoms than lower motor neuron (LMN) lesions that you should recognize for boards. Whereas LMN lesions result in flaccid paralysis and weakened reflexes because of decreased contractions from denervated muscles, UMN lesions result in spastic paralysis, clonus (oscillatory contractions and relaxations of muscles in response to muscle stretching), and heightened reflexes due to loss of inhibition of gamma motor neurons by UMNs and hypersensitivity to group I and II sensory afferents from the muscle spindle. LMN lesions result in fasciculations (random twitches of denervated motor units) and muscle atrophy. UMN lesions are associated with a positive Babinski sign (toes extend upward with plantar stimulation), but LMN lesions are not. UMN and LMN symptoms are explored further in Case 17.1.

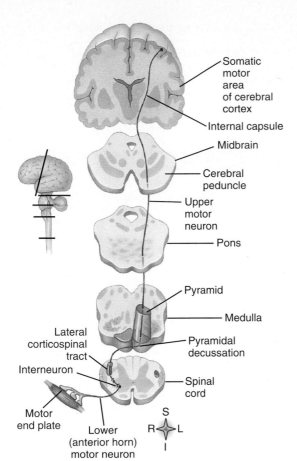

Somatic
motor
area
of cerebral
cortex

Internal capsule

Midbrain

Cerebral
peduncle

Upper
motor
neuron

Pons

Pyramid

Medulla

Lateral
corticospinal
tract

Pyramidal
decussation

Interneuron

Spinal
cord

Motor
end plate

Lower
(anterior horn)
motor neuron

S
R ✦ L
I

Figure 17.1. Examples of somatic motor pathways. R, Right; L, Left; S, Superior; I, Inferior. *(From Thibodeau G, Patton K.* Anatomy & Physiology. *6th ed. St. Louis: Mosby; 2006.)*

3. **What is the primary function of the cerebellum in movement?**
   The cerebellum finely tunes movement. It does this by comparing commands sent by the motor cortex to the muscular system with proprioceptive feedback it receives about the movement that *actually* occurred. The cerebellum receives this feedback through the spinocerebellar tracts. When differences in the planned movement and the actual movement occur, the cerebellum uses this feedback to correct errors and influence future output of the motor cortex.

4. **Why do cerebellar lesions classically produce ipsilateral symptoms?**
   The cerebellar hemispheres influence motor activity by their projections to the contralateral motor cortices (via the motor thalamus) and to the contralateral red nuclei. In turn, both the corticospinal tract and the rubrospinal tract arising from these structures cross back over en route to their target motor neurons, thereby producing symptoms on the same side of the body as the lesion. Remember: Cerebellar lesions double-cross their more cerebral friends.

5. **What are the two ascending sensory pathways, and what information does each convey?**
   1. The *anterolateral system*, also referred to as the *spinothalamic tract*, conveys sensations of pain, temperature, and crude (nondiscriminative) touch.
   2. The *dorsal column–medial lemniscus pathway* conveys the sensations of fine touch, vibration, pressure, and conscious proprioception.
      Note: Unconscious proprioception is transmitted by the spinocerebellar pathways.

6. **What are the two anatomic divisions of the dorsal columns, and from which anatomic structures do these respective divisions relay sensory information?**
   1. The *fasciculus gracilis*, which relays information from the lower extremities and from the lower thorax (level T7 and below), is located most medially in the dorsal columns, just as the gracilis muscle is the most medial muscle of the thigh.
   2. The *fasciculus cuneatus*, which relays information from the upper thorax and the upper extremities (levels C2–T6; recall that the C1 spinal nerve provides motor innervation to the muscles of the occipital region), is immediately lateral to the fasciculus gracilis (Fig. 17.2).
      Note: Both fasciculi carry fibers that synapse on their respective nuclei in the medulla, the nucleus gracilis, and nucleus cuneatus.

7. At what neuroanatomic locations do projections in the corticospinal tract, dorsal columns, and anterolateral system (spinothalamic system) cross over?

The corticospinal tract crosses over (i.e., decussates) as it descends along the inferior aspect of the medulla through the medullary pyramids. The dorsal columns' (ascending) projections cross over between their nuclei in the brainstem and the thalamus, via the internal arcuate fibers of the medial lemniscus, which are located in the caudal medulla. The axons of the anterolateral system cross over almost immediately after their first-order neurons synapse in the dorsal horn of the spinal cord.

STEP 1 SECRET

Memorize the corticospinal tract, spinothalamic tract, and dorsal column–medial lemniscus pathways. You must know these three common tracts, because they are the most clinically relevant in determining the location of a lesion. Memorize where they decussate because this will determine the side on which a patient experiences symptoms if one of the neurons in the aforementioned pathways is damaged. Remember, the USMLE is most interested in clinically relevant information! It will be far more valuable for you to practice pinpointing the site of a patient's lesion based on common sets of symptoms than to memorize a dozen different tracts.

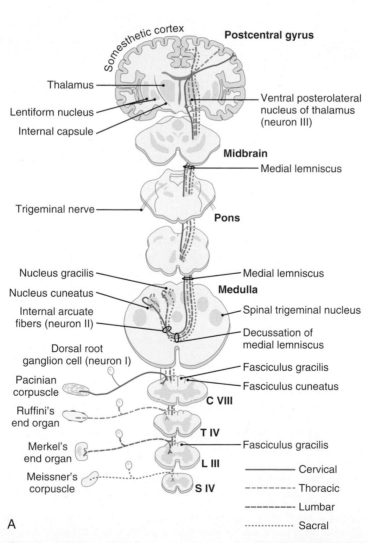

A

Figure 17.2. A, The formation and course of the posterior columns in the spinal cord and the medial lemniscus in the brainstem. B, Divisions of the ascending sensory pathways. *(A, Modified from Carpenter MB. Human Neuroanatomy. Baltimore: Williams & Wilkins; 1983. B, From Lindsay KW, Bone I, Callander R. Neurology and Neurosurgery Illustrated. 3rd ed. Edinburgh: Churchill Livingstone; 2002.)*

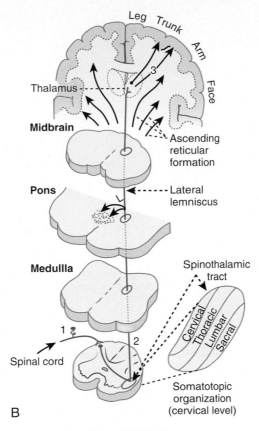

Figure 17.2. Cont'd

8. Because you know where the major motor and sensory pathways cross over, identify and explain the neurologic deficits that occur in the Brown-Séquard syndrome.

Brown-Séquard syndrome is caused by a lateral hemisection of the spinal cord. The motor loss will be on the same side as that of the lesion because the corticospinal tract has already crossed superior to the lesion (in the medulla), and in the spinal cord it innervates only motor neurons on the same side as it courses. Loss of LMNs in the anterior horn will result in ipsilateral symptoms of hyporeflexia and flaccid paralysis at the level of the lesion. However, ipsilateral UMN signs will also be present because UMNs synapse with LMNs at all levels of the spinal cord.

The loss of fine touch, vibration, and proprioception (modalities of the dorsal columns) will be on the same side as that of the lesion. This is because the sensory information of the dorsal columns does not cross over until a more superior location (between the brainstem nuclei and the thalamus). The loss of pain and temperature sensation (anterolateral system), however, will be contralateral to the side of the lesion because the fibers of the anterolateral system ascend and cross over shortly after entering the spinal cord (Fig. 17.3).

Note: There may be some loss of all modalities at the level at which the lesion occurs.

9. Where will the motor and sensory deficit manifest (below the head) if there is a lesion of the internal capsule?

The corticospinal tract, dorsal columns, and anterolateral system all travel to or from the cerebral cortex through the posterior limb of the internal capsule. Because all these tracts either originated from, or will eventually cross over to, the contralateral side, there will be a contralateral hemiplegia from effects on the corticospinal tract, along with a contralateral sensory loss from both ascending sensory systems.

STEP 1 SECRET

Clinically the only two places you can get pure motor strokes are in the posterior limb of the internal capsule and the pons. The only place for pure sensory strokes is the thalamus.

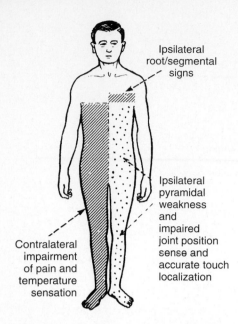

Ipsilateral root/segmental signs

Ipsilateral pyramidal weakness and impaired joint position sense and accurate touch localization

Contralateral impairment of pain and temperature sensation

Figure 17.3. Brown-Séquard syndrome. *(From Lindsay KW, Bone I, Callander R, eds.* Neurology and Neurosurgery Illustrated. *3rd ed. Edinburgh: Churchill Livingstone; 2002.)*

HOW TO APPROACH CASES

Determine whether the problem is central or peripheral. Central lesions will present as asymmetric symptoms, whereas peripheral lesions will present as symmetric.
1. If central, what is the level? It could be in the cerebrum (cortical vs. subcortical), brainstem, or spinal cord. Brainstem will usually have cranial nerve findings, whereas spinal cord lesions will have no facial symptoms.
2. If it is peripheral, is it in the peripheral nerve, neuromuscular junction, or muscle?

CASE 17.1

A 45-year-old man presents with a 6-month history of generalized muscle weakness, trouble swallowing (dysphagia), and difficulty speaking (dysarthria). When reaching above his head to reshelve heavy board review books, he experiences arm weakness, accompanied by shoulder muscle cramps and neck cramps. His dysphagia and dysarthria manifest as difficulty swallowing liquids and solids and a slow, strained speech pattern.

1. How might we approach a case of suspected motor neuron disease?
   Consider that a lesion causing muscle weakness could occur at the level of the motor neuron, neuromuscular junction, or muscle. For example, the differential diagnosis for muscle weakness, dysarthria, and dysphagia may include amyotrophic lateral sclerosis (a disease of motor neurons), myasthenia gravis (an autoimmune attack at the neuromuscular junction), or polymyositis (an inflammatory disease of muscle). Suspected motor neuron disease can then be investigated for UMN or LMN signs.

CASE 17.1 CONTINUED:

Neurologic examination reveals a strange combination of flaccid and spastic paralysis, as well as hypo- and hyperreflexia. Diffuse muscle wasting and fasciculations are visible on the lateral aspects of the tongue. Sensation is intact to all modalities in all areas tested. A Mini–Mental State Examination is within normal limits for the patient's age and cultural background, although he does have difficulty articulating.

2. What UMN signs are present in this patient?
   UMN signs include spastic paralysis (the muscles have an increased resistance to passive movement or manipulation), hyperreflexia (hyperactivity of deep tendon reflexes [DTRs]), and clonus (alternating contraction and relaxation of a muscle in rapid succession in response to sudden stretching of the muscle). Notice this patient has spastic paralysis and hyperreflexia.

3. Why are the signs of hyperreflexia, spastic paralysis, and clonus seen with an UMN lesion?
   The most widely accepted theory is that UMNs are tonically inhibitory to LMNs, such that disruption of UMNs will *disinhibit* (i.e., allow activation of) LMNs. This makes the motor component of the DTRs more active and increases baseline muscle tone, which increases resistance to passive movement.

4. **What LMN signs are present in this patient?**
   When an LMN is damaged, the muscle it innervates is no longer tonically stimulated, resulting in muscle atrophy and reduced tone (*hypotonia*). The denervated muscle also exhibits *flaccid paralysis* (the muscles have decreased resistance to passive movement or manipulation), and the efferent part of the DTRs is blunted, so the DTRs are weak or absent (*hyporeflexia*). *Fasciculations* are also observed.
   Note: LMN function can be evaluated by electromyography (EMG) and nerve conduction studies.

CASE 17.1 CONTINUED:

Serum analysis is negative for antibodies to the acetylcholine (ACh) receptor. Cerebrospinal fluid (CSF) analysis is negative for oligoclonal bands (of immunoglobulins), elevated protein, or white blood cells (WBCs). Magnetic resonance imaging (MRI) of the brain and spinal cord appears normal.

5. **What is the most likely diagnosis?**
   Amyotrophic lateral sclerosis (ALS), or Lou Gehrig disease, is a chronic neurodegenerative disease of both UMNs and LMNs resulting in progressively worsening muscle weakness, which causes disability and ultimately death within 3 to 5 years. Causes of death typically include respiratory failure, aspiration pneumonia resulting from respiratory muscle weakness, skin ulcers from weakness-induced immobility causing systemic infection, and deep vein thrombosis due to weakness-induced immobility causing pulmonary thromboembolism.
   Note: *Myotrophic* means "muscle enlargement." *Amyotrophia* means "muscle atrophy." *Lateral sclerosis* refers to palpable hardness (sclerosis) of the lateral corticospinal tracts of the spinal cord at autopsy.

6. **Why are the MRI and CSF findings notable?**
   The absence of periventricular plaques on MRI and oligoclonal bands in CSF makes the diagnosis of multiple sclerosis (MS) much less likely because most MS patients have these findings. Another important distinction between MS and ALS is that ALS affects only the motor system, whereas MS affects both motor and sensory systems. The distinction between these diseases is important: Although both are incurable, ALS is relentlessly progressive, whereas MS has a more variable course.

CASE 17.1 CONTINUED:

A muscle biopsy for this patient is shown in Fig. 17.4.

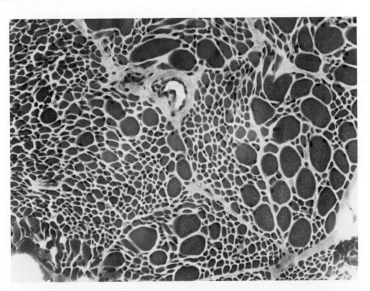

Figure 17.4. Muscle biopsy from a patient with spinal muscular atrophy type I demonstrating denervation atrophy with residual hypertrophic fibers (magnification ×300). *(From Samuels MA, Feske SK. Office Practice of Neurology. 2nd ed. Philadelphia: Churchill Livingstone, 2003.)*

7. **What process leads to the findings seen in this biopsy specimen stained with hematoxylin-eosin?**
   The atrophied and angulated fibers reflect denervation due to the death of the innervating motor neurons. This death of an entire group of neighboring muscle fibers (of the same type, because they are innervated by the same motor neuron) is called *group atrophy*. It occurs with disease progression.

8. **What would myosin adenosine triphosphatase staining of this specimen show?**

This histologic stain would distinguish type I (slow twitch) from type II (fast twitch) muscle fibers. Normally, these different types of muscle fibers will be intermingled in a checkerboard-like pattern, owing to the innervation of adjacent muscle fibers by different anterior horn motor neurons. However, when muscle fibers lose their motor innervation as a result of the death of anterior horn cells, the axons that innervate neighboring muscle fibers will sprout new axons and take over the denervated fibers. This leads to *type grouping*, in which muscle fibers of the same type are grouped together, with loss of the checkerboard pattern.

9. **What are the principal pathologic findings in ALS? What is the prognosis? Are there any treatments available for ALS?**

Loss of pyramidal cells in the motor cortex and fibrosis of the lateral corticospinal tracts are the pathologic findings in ALS. Affected muscles show denervation atrophy with (muscle) fiber type grouping upon reinnervation. There is typically sparing of sensory tracts and cognitive function, which explains why this patient's mental status and sensory function are both completely normal. Of note, the physicist Stephen Hawking had a rare slowly progressive form of this disease. Extraocular muscles also are often spared, leaving some patients with severe disease progression no means of communication other than eye movements (Fig. 17.5).

Patients with ALS have a very poor prognosis, and the disease is fatal within a few years of diagnosis. Riluzole, an antagonist of presynaptic glutamate release, is the only approved pharmacologic treatment and increases survival by a few months at best. Patients with ALS typically die from respiratory failure or aspiration pneumonia.

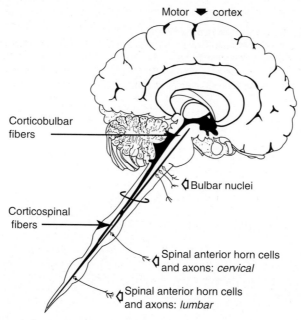

Figure 17.5. Sites of the lesions in amyotrophic lateral sclerosis (ALS). *(From Pryse-Phillips WM, Murray TJ.* Essential Neurology: A Concise Textbook. *New York: Medical Examination Publishing; 1992.)*

10. **What might you expect EMG and nerve conduction studies to show in this patient?**

EMG could indicate LMN involvement by revealing signs of denervation (fibrillation potentials). *Fibrillations* are invisible contractions of single muscle fibers, seen on EMG only. *Fasciculations* are involuntary contractions of one or more muscle units (which are often visible) and may also be present in LMN lesions. Notice this patient had fasciculations, often visible on the tongue.

In contrast to myasthenia gravis, where nerve conduction studies are grossly abnormal at disease onset, ALS patients typically have normal nerve conduction studies in the early stages of disease. However, later in disease course the studies resemble myasthenia gravis, with LMNs showing reduced response to repetitive stimulation. Sensory nerves are usually entirely preserved in both diseases.

11. **Is ALS more commonly inherited or acquired?**

ALS is more commonly acquired, although the precise causes of the acquired form(s) remain unknown. Interestingly, soccer players are at increased risk, suggesting the possible role of head trauma triggering the neurodegenerative process. Of note, one of the familial forms has been associated with mutations in the zinc/copper superoxide dismutase 1 gene (SOD1), which plays an important role in scavenging free radicals in metabolically active cells such as neurons.

12. **Why is ALS often confused with syringomyelia and vice versa?**

ALS is often confused with syringomyelia and vice versa because both conditions typically present with progressive weakness of the muscles. Syringomyelia is a disease marked by enlargement of the central canal of the cervical spinal cord, often by a mass. This leads to destruction of the anterior horn cells in the upper levels of the spinal cord, resulting in atrophy of intrinsic hand muscles. Because atrophy and weakness of hand muscles are early signs of both ALS and syringomyelia, the disease presentations are often confused. However, enlargement of the central canal in syringomyelia also affects the decussating fibers of the anterolateral spinothalamic tract, resulting in bilateral loss of pain and temperature sensation in the upper extremities. ALS, on the other hand, has no sensory changes!

SUMMARY BOX: AMYOTROPHIC LATERAL SCLEROSIS

- Clinical presentation is one of chronic degeneration of upper and lower motor neurons, generally without sensory or cognitive involvement.
- Pathologic examination shows degeneration of pyramidal cells in the motor cortex and fibrosis of the lateral corticospinal tract.
- Muscle biopsy shows type grouping and group atrophy of muscle fibers.
- Most cases are acquired; one familial form is associated with superoxide dismutase 1 mutations.
- Amyotrophic lateral sclerosis (ALS) and syringomyelia both result in hand muscle atrophy. Syringomyelia also results in bilateral loss of pain and temperature sensation, while ALS is not associated with sensory changes.
- ALS is a unique neurodegenerative disease in which patients experience both upper motor neuron (UMN) and lower motor neuron (LMN) symptoms.

CASE 17.2

A 70-year-old man presents with a tremor in one hand that causes him to appear to be rolling something between his fingers.

1. **With what actions is this tremor most likely to appear?**

This patient's pill-rolling tremor is likely a resting tremor, which is most prominent when the arms are relaxed and the patient is not paying attention to his position or action.

2. **Differentiate resting tremor, intention tremor, and postural tremor.**

Resting tremor occurs when the patient is not moving (*resting*) and typically decreases with voluntary activity. Intention tremor, which typically has cerebellar origins, appears as the patient moves a limb toward a target, and is often irregular in amplitude and trajectory. Postural tremor, the most common cause of which is essential tremor (a common, benign condition often associated with aging), appears as the patient actively holds the limbs in a position against gravity.

CASE 17.2 CONTINUED:

During the interview, you note that the tremor occurs at rest and disappears when the patient either extends his arms parallel to the floor or reaches for a pen. However, he has difficulty initiating movements (akinesia), finally doing so successfully, albeit slowly (bradykinesia). You also note an expressionless face, decreased spontaneous blink rate, and forward stooped posture. On physical examination, the patient maintains this posture and walks with a slow, narrow-based, festinating gait. Motor examination shows that his muscles demonstrate a cogwheel rigidity, in which muscle rigidity gives way to passive stretching in a series of successive jerks.

3. **In light of these signs, what is the most likely diagnosis?**

Parkinson disease (PD) is the most likely diagnosis. PD is characterized by resting tremor, hypokinesia/bradykinesia, muscle rigidity, and postural instability. The etiology of PD involves neurodegeneration of the substantia nigra causing loss of dopamine production.

4. **Why should we determine whether this patient is taking medications such as haloperidol or metoclopramide?**

Recall that PD is caused by insufficient dopaminergic output by the substantia nigra. Certain antipsychotic and antiemetic agents that act as central dopamine receptor antagonists can therefore cause or exacerbate parkinsonian symptoms such as rigidity, bradykinesia, and resting tremor. This is commonly tested on Step 1 as a diabetic patient who is started on metoclopramide (a dopamine antagonist) for gastroparesis and who subsequently develops parkinsonism. When making the diagnosis, it is critical for physicians to distinguish Parkinson disease from parkinsonism, which can present with a similar symptomatology and may be drug-induced, postencephalitic, or neurodegenerative but with different anatomic lesions from those in PD.

Note: *Parkinsonism* refers to clinical features of PD (i.e., bradykinesia, rigidity, resting tremor) from any cause (PD, mediations, PD-like conditions such as progressive supranuclear palsy).

5. **What cerebral structures are affected in Parkinson disease, and how does this play into the observed bradykinesia and akinesia?**

   In PD, the dopaminergic, neuromelanin-containing neurons in the substantia nigra selectively degenerate over time. These neurons normally project to the basal ganglia via the nigrostriatal tract. The basal ganglia then influence execution of learned motor plans by modulating signals between the (motor) thalamus and motor cortex. Within the basal ganglia, there are two pathways leading to output to the thalamus: the direct and indirect pathways. Activation of the direct pathway facilitates desired movement by stimulating the thalamus via inhibition of the globus pallidus internus and substantia nigra pars reticularis (both of which normally inhibit the thalamus), whereas activation of the indirect pathway inhibits unwanted movement by inhibiting the thalamus. Nigrostriatal dopaminergic inputs activate the direct pathway and inhibit the indirect pathway, thus stimulating motion. Decreased dopamine levels in PD manifest with a net decrease in motor activity. However, this model does not yet account for the patient's tremor. Because dopamine decreases release of acetylcholine (ACh), a decrease in dopamine levels leads to a relative excess of striatal ACh in patients with PD. ACh opposes the actions of dopamine and activates the indirect pathway, which disinhibits suppression of unwanted movements and results in the pill-rolling tremor that is characteristic of the disease. It is important that you understand the imbalance of dopamine and ACh levels in PD patients because dopamine agonists and anticholinergics are useful in treating this disease (Fig. 17.6).

   Note: The striatum consists of the caudate nucleus and putamen, both of which are part of the basal ganglia. You should be able to identify the basal ganglia on an anatomic section. The caudate and thalamus lie medial to the internal capsule, and the globus pallidus and putamen lie lateral.

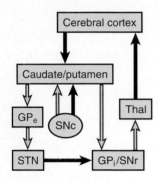

Figure 17.6. Schema of anatomic nuclei and pathways involving the basal ganglia. *Black arrows* represent excitation, and *shaded arrows* represent inhibition. *GP_e*, Globus pallidus, external segment; *GP_i*, globus pallidus, internal segment; *SNc*, pars compacta of the substantia nigra; SNr, pars reticularis of the substantia nigra; *STN*, subthalamic nucleus; *Thal*, thalamus. *(From Goetz CG. Textbook of Clinical Neurology. 2nd ed. Philadelphia: WB Saunders; 2003.)*

CASE 17.2 CONTINUED:

When you see the patient in clinic 6 months later, you note marked improvement of his bradykinesia and resting tremor. You attribute this success to the patient's current treatment.

6. **What medication did you start the patient on, and why is it, rather than dopamine, used to treat Parkinson disease?**

   Dopamine cannot cross the blood-brain barrier. However, levodopa (L-dopa), a lipid-soluble precursor to dopamine, can cross the blood-brain barrier and increases CNS dopamine levels once converted by dopa decarboxylase. In fact, parkinsonian syndromes are often initially misdiagnosed as Parkinson disease, and the diagnosis is later corrected when the patient does not respond to L-dopa.

7. **Why is levodopa typically administered with carbidopa?**

   Carbidopa is a dopa decarboxylase inhibitor that cannot cross the blood-brain barrier, so it inhibits the peripheral metabolism of L-dopa to dopamine. This both increases the delivery of L-dopa to the brain and minimizes the side effects of peripheral L-dopa/dopamine. These side effects include autonomic symptoms such as orthostatic hypotension, nausea/vomiting, confusion, hallucinations, and infrequently, arrhythmias. Long-term side effects include dyskinesia, particularly choreoathetosis of the face and distal extremities. CNS symptoms (confusion and hallucinations) are last to disappear.

8. **Drugs such as bromocriptine and pergolide are also used to treat Parkinson disease. How do they exert their effects?**

   These drugs are dopamine receptor agonists and increase central dopaminergic activity without increasing dopamine levels, which of course is beneficial in PD.

9. **What is the mechanism of action of selegiline, a drug used in treating Parkinson disease?**

   Selegiline selectively inhibits monoamine oxidase B (MAO-B), an enzyme that degrades dopamine. Selegiline can cross the blood-brain barrier, so it can be used without L-dopa.

10. **Why is it preferable to selectively inhibit MAO-B, rather than both MAO-A and MAO-B, in Parkinson disease?**

Monoamine oxidase A (MAO-A) principally degrades norepinephrine and serotonin, whereas MAO-B is more selective for dopamine degradation. Because MAO-A inhibitors increase serotonin and norepinephrine levels, they have been used for treating depression, but they are not expected to be as effective in treating the motor symptoms of PD.

11. **Why are anticholinergic drugs useful in the treatment of Parkinson disease?**

Benztropine is an anticholinergic drug (like atropine) that crosses the blood-brain barrier and is commonly used in the treatment of PD. Recall that there is a *relative* excess of striatal ACh in PD because of the deficiency of dopamine. Thus anticholinergics that can enter the CNS are also useful in treating the bradykinesia and akinesia of PD.

12. **Which antiviral medication is also effective in treating Parkinson disease?**

Amantadine, which is effective against influenza A, was incidentally discovered to be effective in PD. Though its mechanism is not fully understood, amantadine has anticholinergic and antiglutamatergic effects and acts by increasing dopamine output from the substantia nigra.

13. **How does the drug MPTP (1-methyl-4-phenyl-1,2,3,6-tetrahydropyridine) cause parkinsonism, and is this a reversible or irreversible process?**

MPTP is an analog of the opioid meperidine and is occasionally present as a contaminant in certain illicit drugs. It causes irreversible parkinsonism by selectively destroying neurons in the substantia nigra. In fact, the clinical and pathologic consequences of MPTP toxicity mimic those of PD so well that MPTP is often used in animal models to study PD.

14. **Why should you be suspicious of a diagnosis of Parkinson disease in a patient being treated for schizophrenia?**

Antipsychotic drugs that block dopamine receptors in the mesolimbic system to achieve their effect can also block dopaminergic activity in the nigrostriatal tract and cause symptoms similar to those of PD (pseudoparkinsonism, which is often reversible with discontinuation of the antipsychotics). However, the choreoathetoid motor disorders that develop after prolonged use of antipsychotics (e.g., tardive dyskinesia) may prove to be irreversible.

15. **What would a pathologist look for to establish the diagnosis of Parkinson disease in evaluation of the brain at autopsy?**

A pathologist would look for bilateral depigmentation of the midbrain substantia nigra, due to loss of dopaminergic, neuromelanin-containing neurons.

SUMMARY BOX: PARKINSON DISEASE

- Hypokinetic movement disorder presenting with pill-rolling tremor, bradykinesia, festinating gait, stooped posture, and masked facies
- Characterized by relatively too little dopamine and too much acetylcholine, respectively, in the basal ganglia
- Depigmentation of substantia nigra on autopsy due to loss of neuromelanin-containing dopaminergic cells
- Pharmacologic treatment targeted at increasing levels of dopamine in the brain, as well as decreasing acetylcholine activity in the central nervous system

---

CASE 17.3

A 40-year-old man has become notably demented and has developed involuntary movements, such as facial grimaces and a dance-like gait in which his legs move in sudden, rapid, jerky movements. During the interview, you note that the patient makes continuous jerky movements with his arm, which he seems to complete as purposeful movements to smooth his hair. The patient also complains that his mind does not feel as sharp as it used to be.

---

1. **What term describes the patient's movements, and what conditions may cause these movements?**

Chorea (from the Greek for dance) describes involuntary, sudden, rapid movements of a body part. Choreic movements often appear on a spectrum with athetosis, which are involuntary movements of the trunk and extremities (especially the fingers) that may give a writhing, snake-like, or dancing appearance to the patient's movements. The differential diagnosis of chorea is broad but includes Huntington disease, Sydenham chorea (poststreptococcal immune-mediated, and often accompanied by rheumatic fever), Wilson disease (abnormal copper accumulation), cerebrovascular accidents, and senile-related chorea.

2. **Why might medications such as haloperidol and L-dopa cause chorea?**

Neuroleptics such as haloperidol block dopamine receptors. Although the goal of drugs such as haloperidol is to block dopamine receptors in the mesolimbic-mesocortical pathway and reduce psychotic behavior, long-term antagonism of dopamine receptors in the nigrostriatal pathway can cause choreoathetoid movements. This side effect is called *tardive dyskinesia,* which as the name implies, develops slowly after medication is started and may persist after the medication is discontinued. A variety of dyskinesias are often seen in patients who have been taking L-dopa for long periods of time. The most common presentation is choreoathetosis of the face and distal extremities.

CASE 17.3 CONTINUED:

While you are talking with the patient and his wife, the wife tells you that the patient saw a psychiatrist a few years ago because of some gradual changes in his mood.

3. **What sorts of psychiatric changes might the patient's wife be referring to?**
   She might describe a gradual development of emotional lability, increased aggression and irritability, hypersexuality, or depression. Such behavioral changes are often initially misdiagnosed as psychiatric disease.

4. **If a Mini-Mental State Examination shows the patient to be mildly demented, with deficits in organization, concentration, and short-term memory, what is the most likely diagnosis?**
   The classic clinical triad of dementia, behavioral changes such as aggression and depression, and chorea points toward Huntington disease. This diagnosis is often supported by the family history, as this is an autosomal dominant genetic disorder characterized by trinucleotide repeats.

5. **What pathologic lesion would be visible on imaging?**
   MRI of the head is notable for significant atrophy of the basal ganglia, especially the caudate nucleus. In fact, Huntington disease is caused by degeneration of γ-aminobutyric acid (GABA) neurons belonging to the indirect pathway in the caudate nucleus. This is significant because the striatal nuclei are the main inhibitors of undesirable movement. The ventricular enlargement that is often apparent on autopsy (Fig. 17.7, right) is due to loss of neurons in the basal ganglia.

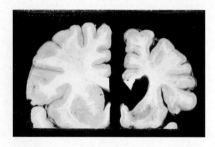

Figure 17.7. Huntington disease (HD). Normal hemisphere on the left compared with the HD hemisphere on the right showing atrophy of the striatum and ventricular dilation. *(Courtesy Dr. J.P. Vonsattel, Columbia University, New York, NY.)*

CASE 17.3 CONTINUED:

After discussions of your initial diagnosis, the patient reveals that he has known for a while that this was going to happen to him because he had tested positive for the gene that caused his father to have similar problems. However, the patient is upset because the disease has developed several years earlier in his life than in his father's.

6. **What neurotransmitter is reduced in the basal ganglia in Huntington disease, and how does this relate to the hyperkinetic motor abnormalities seen in the disease?**
   GABA, the major inhibitory neurotransmitter of the CNS, is reduced. In Huntington disease, loss of inhibitory signals within the basal ganglia results in *disinhibition* of the motor thalamus, explaining the hyperkinetic motor abnormalities seen in this disease. Note that the deficiency of GABA within the basal ganglia has the opposite effect (i.e., hyperkinesia) from that seen with the deficiency of dopamine associated with Parkinson disease (i.e., hypokinesia). The loss of GABA leads to an increase in glutamate signaling, which is thought to worsen neurologic damage due to increased stimulation of *N*-methyl-D-aspartate (NMDA) receptors and excitotoxicity.

7. **What does the term *penetrance* imply with respect to genetic diseases and is the penetrance of Huntington disease high or low?**
   Penetrance is the frequency with which a pathologic phenotype is observed in the presence of the disease genotype. In Huntington disease, which has a penetrance of 100%, every individual with the gene defect will eventually develop the disease. This is why this patient knew he was going to get the disease. Fortunately, most genetic diseases have incomplete penetrance.

8. **What types of gene mutation give rise to Huntington disease?**
   Huntington disease results from the accumulation of trinucleotide repeats (CAG) in the huntingtin gene on chromosome 4. This region of the genome contains many CAG repeats, even in normal individuals, but when the number of repeats is too great, then the huntingtin protein becomes unstable and causes disease. It is not known whether Huntington disease results from a loss of function (such as neuroprotection) or a gain of function (such as neurotoxicity) of the gene product.

This CAG repeat expansion occurs during gametogenesis and is due to the tendency of DNA polymerase to "misread" these highly repetitive regions and get "stuck," inserting extra repeats. This results in an expansion of the region across generations in affected families, a process that geneticists refer to as "anticipation." Individuals who inherit these lengthy repeats will go on to develop Huntington disease later in life and will pass it on to their children even in the absence of further repeat expansion.

9. Why might it make sense to measure levels of serum ceruloplasmin in patients who present with similar motor abnormalities and a similar family history?

Serum ceruloplasmin is a screening test for Wilson disease (hepatolenticular degeneration), which is also hereditary and causes movement abnormalities. In this autosomal recessive disease, a genetic mutation in copper transport (*ATP7B* gene on chromosome 13) results in impaired excretion of copper into the bile. This buildup of copper in the body leads to decreased levels of ceruloplasmin, the serum carrier protein for copper and elevated serum copper, causing hemolytic anemia. As a result of chronically high copper levels, copper also begins to deposit in peripheral tissues such as the brain, liver, cornea, kidneys, and joints. All symptoms of Wilson disease are directly caused by toxic buildup of copper in these tissues, especially the lenticular nuclei (globus pallidus and putamen), leading to ataxia, dyskinesia, slurred speech, dementia, and personality changes, which can be confused with Huntington disease.

STEP 1 SECRET

On the boards, any time you see a patient with both liver and neurologic abnormalities, immediately think Wilson disease. One high-yield pathognomonic finding that clinches the diagnosis is the presence of Kayser-Fleischer rings in the cornea, which are gold-brown copper deposits forming a ring around the iris.

What makes this such a high-yield point is that unlike Huntington disease, Wilson disease is easily treatable with penicillamine, a copper chelating agent that clears the blood of free copper. Untreated Wilson disease increases the risk of hepatocellular carcinoma.

SUMMARY BOX: HUNTINGTON DISEASE

- Classic clinical triad: dementia, behavioral changes, choreoathetosis
- Inherited in autosomal dominant manner with 100% penetrance
- Caused by pathologic expansion of CAG repeats in the huntingtin gene resulting in insertion of a polyglutamine tract and dysfunction of the huntingtin protein
- Typically presents in middle-aged patients, but because of genetic anticipation in which the number of CAG repeats increases, it presents at younger ages with successive generations.

CASE 17.4

A 30-year-old woman complains of a long history of double vision (diplopia) and some difficulty swallowing solid foods (dysphagia). Her physical appearance is remarkable only for drooping of her upper eyelids (ptosis) and slight atrophy of facial muscles. While thinking about whether her motor symptoms reflect abnormality of motor neurons, the neuromuscular junction, or muscle, you perform a cranial nerve examination.

1. Given her diplopia, which cranial nerves should you examine particularly carefully?

Diplopia may reflect asymmetric pathology of the extraocular muscles (EOMs), which would be detected during the test of cranial nerves CN IV (innervating the superior oblique), CN VI (innervating the lateral rectus), and CN III (innervating all other EOMs). Diplopia may also be due to lesions of the medial longitudinal fasciculus, a midbrain circuit that coordinates the EOMs of the left and right eyes to move both eyes in a given direction, or of the optic nerves, both of which can be affected in MS. Diplopia may reflect pathology of the globes (e.g., trauma, Graves disease) or brain (e.g., stroke). Finally, diplopia can occur from ischemic damage to one of the cranial nerves controlling eye movement (mononeuropathy), as can occasionally be seen in diabetes.

Note: Diplopia and other ocular pathologic conditions are discussed in further detail in Chapter 18 (Ophthalmology).

CASE 17.4 CONTINUED:

After a complete physical examination, you notice that her ptosis seems more pronounced than it was 30 minutes ago. When asked to look upward for 1 minute without closing her eyes, she closes her eyes after only 15 seconds due to muscle weakness. She then admits that she has been feeling fatigued lately; after mild exercise, her arms and legs feel weak, though not painful. All of these symptoms seem worse in the evening.

2. **Why would an edrophonium chloride (Tensilon) test help determine whether the symptoms are of nerve, neuromuscular junction, or muscle origin?**

The Tensilon test involves the administration of edrophonium, a short-acting cholinesterase inhibitor. The function of cholinesterase is to degrade synaptic ACh. By antagonizing cholinesterase, edrophonium increases the concentration of ACh in the synaptic cleft. This helps overcome a deficiency of available ACh receptors by activating a higher percentage of the ACh receptors that are present. Thus a positive test (one where muscle strength improves in response to edrophonium) reflects deficiency of ACh action at the neuromuscular junction, possibly because of reduced availability of ACh receptors. This occurs in myasthenia gravis, in which the serum of affected patients contains autoantibodies to postsynaptic ACh receptors.

3. **If computed tomography (CT) and MRI scans of the chest were ordered, what diagnosis would be supported by finding a thymoma?**

Myasthenia gravis is often associated with thymoma or thymic hyperplasia, and a thymectomy frequently helps reverse the symptoms.

STEP 1 SECRET

You may be expected to identify a thymoma on chest x-ray study and will be expected to use this finding to aid your diagnosis of myasthenia gravis.

4. **What is the pathophysiology of the motor weakness in myasthenia gravis?**

As mentioned previously, myasthenia gravis is an immune-mediated disorder characterized by the production of autoantibodies to proteins involved in signaling at the neuromuscular junction. The antibodies are most commonly directed against postsynaptic nicotinic ACh receptors present on skeletal muscle fibers. These antibodies reduce the number of ACh receptors on the motor end plate, making the motor end plate less responsive to ACh. Less frequently, autoantibodies are directed against a muscle-specific tyrosine kinase involved in ACh receptor clustering.

Reduced binding of ACh to its receptor at the neuromuscular junction results in the compensatory release of more ACh, which can result in depletion of presynaptic ACh with repeated muscle contractions and subsequent striated muscle weakness. The muscles of the eye are particularly prone to weakness due to their relatively high frequency of contraction. Common initial findings in patients with myasthenia gravis include diplopia, ptosis, dysphagia to solids and liquids (due to esophageal striated muscle weakness), and proximal muscle weakness.

5. **What is the normal mechanism by which an action potential is generated in skeletal muscle cells?**

Recall that nicotinic ACh receptors are ligand-gated sodium channels and that binding of ACh to ACh receptors produces an end plate potential in skeletal muscle cells. This end plate potential has to be above a certain threshold value for activation of fast voltage-gated sodium channels and generation of an action potential, which causes muscle contraction by triggering release of calcium from the sarcoplasmic reticulum. In myasthenia gravis, there are not enough ACh receptors to respond to the synaptic ACh and depolarize the cell to reach the threshold for action potential formation.

6. **Why is edrophonium not used to treat myasthenia gravis, and what are other treatment options?**

Edrophonium is a *short-acting* cholinesterase inhibitor. For long-term management of myasthenia gravis, the long-acting cholinesterase inhibitors pyridostigmine and neostigmine are used.

7. **If someone being treated for myasthenia gravis overdosed on one of the cholinesterase inhibitors, what side effects might occur?**

A side effect profile with an overdose of cholinesterase inhibitors would mimic excessive stimulation of the parasympathetic nervous system (i.e., excessive cholinergic activity), resulting in diarrhea, miosis, bronchospasm, excessive urination, bradycardia, salivation, and lacrimation. Additionally, because the sympathetic nervous system stimulates sweating via the release of ACh from postganglionic sympathetic fibers, excessive sweating may also occur. All these side effects occur as a result of ACh activity at *muscarinic* ACh receptors at end organs. *Nicotinic* ACh receptors exist at the neuromuscular junction and at sympathetic ganglia.

Note: If someone is poisoned with organophosphates (e.g., parathion), which are *irreversible* cholinesterase inhibitors, treatment is aimed at reducing total cholinergic activity. This is accomplished with pralidoxime, which regenerates active cholinesterase, and with the anticholinergic atropine.

STEP 1 SECRET

Autonomic nervous system (ANS) pharmacology is one of the highest yield topics to know for boards. This topic is further explored in Chapter 23 (Pharmacology and Toxicology).

8. **What is the mechanism of action of the nondepolarizing neuromuscular blockers, and why are these drugs more potent in patients with myasthenia gravis?**

These agents are analogs or derivatives of curare (e.g., rocuronium) and work by antagonizing the nicotinic ACh receptor at the neuromuscular junction. They are often used as an adjunct in surgical anesthesia to achieve muscle relaxation. Nondepolarizing neuromuscular blockers would be more potent given that patients have fewer receptors. Similarly, depolarizing neuromuscular blocking agents such as succinylcholine a would need much higher doses because it continually stimulates ACh receptors to cause temporary paralysis; in myasthenia gravis there are fewer functional receptors to do so.

9. **Myasthenia gravis and Lambert-Eaton myasthenic syndrome (LEMS) can have very similar clinical presentations. How is LEMS similar, and what causes this disease?**

LEMS is an immune-mediated disease caused by the abnormal production of self-reactive antibodies to voltage-gated calcium channels located in the terminal bouton of presynaptic neurons, which results in insufficient neurotransmitter (ACh) release. Thus muscle strength increases with continued effort (contraction) and buildup of released ACh, a phenomenon called *facilitation*. This distinguishes LEMS from myasthenia gravis, in which continued effort at contraction depletes ACh and leads to (1) a subsequent decrease in strength and (2) increased muscle fatigue, as seen in our patient, a phenomenon called *fatiguability*.

Note: LEMS is often associated with paraneoplastic syndromes, particularly small cell carcinoma of the lung.

SUMMARY BOX: MYASTHENIA GRAVIS

- Autoimmune attack on neuromuscular junction; antibodies usually are directed against acetylcholine (ACh) receptors.
- Causes motor weakness, often of extraocular, bulbar, and facial muscles; weakness and fatigue increase with increased use of muscles.
- Diagnose with edrophonium (short-acting cholinesterase inhibitor).
- Associated with thymoma; removal of thymus often resolves symptoms.
- Treat with pyridostigmine and neostigmine (long-acting cholinesterase inhibitors).
- Contrast with Lambert-Eaton myasthenic syndrome: autoimmune attack on presynaptic calcium channels, often paraneoplastic, increased strength with increased effort.

CASE 17.5

A 35-year-old man presents with bilateral loss of pain and temperature sensation in the arms and upper thorax and with several painless ulcers on his fingers from burning his hands repeatedly while cooking. Fine touch, vibration, and proprioception remain intact in all areas, although pain and temperature sensation are severely compromised in both arms and the upper thorax. MRI reveals a fluid-filled cavity within the spinal cord (Fig. 17.8).

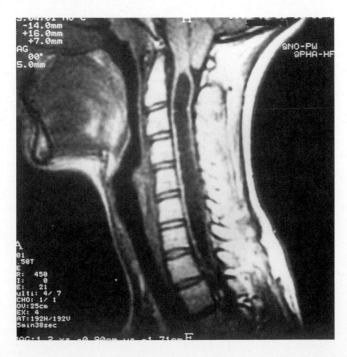

Figure 17.8. Magnetic resonance image demonstrates a large syringomyelic cavity in the cervical cord. *(From Bradley WG, Daroff RB, Fenichel GM, et al. Neurology in Clinical Practice. 4th ed. Philadelphia: Butterworth-Heinemann; 2004.)*

1. What is the diagnosis, and which ascending sensory system is affected in this man?

This patient has syringomyelia, which is caused by an expanded fluid-filled cavity (a syrinx) in the central canal of the spinal cord. The anterolateral system is affected because of compression from the syrinx on the anterior white commissure, which is located just ventral to the central canal and contains the decussating fibers of second-order neurons in the spinothalamic system. The anterolateral system, also called the *spinothalamic system*, conveys modalities of pain, temperature, and crude touch. Thus the sensory deficit will occur in areas supplied by fibers that decussate at the level of the fluid-filled cavity. Recall that tactile information (which includes fine touch, pressure, and vibration) and proprioception are conveyed by the dorsal column–medial lemniscus pathway.

Note: Syringobulbia is a variant of syringomyelia in which fluid-filled, slit-like cavities are located in the medulla. Remember, *myelo* = spinal cord and *bulbar* = brainstem.

2. At what general level in the cord is syringomyelia most commonly found?

Syringomyelia most commonly occurs in the cervical spinal cord, as shown in the MRI in Fig. 17.8. In the image shown, the syrinx extends into the thoracic spinal cord as well.

3. If the patient also had the cerebellar anomaly shown in Fig. 17.8, what diagnosis should be suspected?

Fig. 17.8 shows herniation of the cerebellar tonsils into the foramen magnum. This anatomic anomaly in association with syringomyelia is typical of type I Arnold-Chiari malformations.

4. Why is the sensory loss caused by syringomyelia typically called "suspended-dissociated" loss?

The loss of pain and temperature sensation caused by syringomyelia is generally limited to the dermatomes innervated by the spinal nerves affected by the spinal level of the syrinx. Sensation above and below the syrinx is expected to be intact. Thus the body area of sensory loss is "suspended" between two areas of normal sensation. The sensory loss is said to be "dissociated" because only the modalities of pain and temperature (and crude touch) are affected; tactile and proprioceptive senses are intact because the dorsal column–medial lemniscal pathway is not affected (Fig. 17.9). Another frequently used descriptor of the sensory loss is "cape-like."

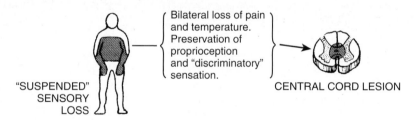

Figure 17.9. Syringomyelia. *(From Lindsay KW, Bone I, Callander R, eds.* Neurology and Neurosurgery Illustrated. *3rd ed. Edinburgh: Churchill Livingstone; 2002.)*

5. How can this disease progress to cause atrophy of the muscles of the hands and hypoactive reflexes of the upper extremities?

The syrinx can expand to compress the ventral horns of the spinal cord, thereby producing the LMN signs of muscle atrophy and hyporeflexia.

Note: If the interossei and lumbrical muscles of the hand are primarily affected, suspect involvement of the C8–T1 segments.

6. From what area of the body does pain and temperature sensation travel to the cerebral cortex via the medial lemniscus?

Recall that the anterolateral system carries pain and temperature sensation for most of the body, except the areas innervated by the trigeminal nerve. Though we generally think of the trigeminal nerve as innervating the face, remember that it does not innervate the angle of the jaw and does not stop at the anterior hairline. The trigeminal nerve can more accurately be thought of as innervating the anterior two-thirds of the head (Fig. 17.10). This innervation includes the modalities of fine touch, pressure, vibration, proprioception (for the muscles of mastication), pain, temperature, and crude touch. In this trigeminal mechanosensory pathway, pseudounipolar neurons in the trigeminal ganglion synapse with second-order neurons in one of three nuclei in the trigeminal brainstem complex. The axons of these second-order neurons decussate in the pons before ascending in the medial lemniscus on their way to the ventral posteromedial nucleus of the thalamus.

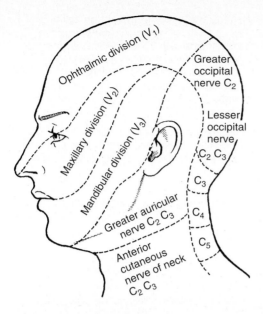

Figure 17.10. Divisions of the trigeminal nerve. *(From Lindsay KW, Bone I, Callander R, eds.* Neurology and Neurosurgery Illustrated. *3rd ed. Edinburgh: Churchill Livingstone; 2002.)*

SUMMARY BOX: SYRINGOMYELIA

- Syringomyelia refers to a fluid-filled expansion of the central canal of the spinal cord. A similar syrinx can occur in the brainstem and is called *syringobulbia.*
- This often occurs in the cervical spinal cord but can extend into the thoracic spinal cord.
- Compression of the anterior white commissure of the anterolateral (spinothalamic) system causes suspended-dissociated "cape-like" loss of pain and temperature sensation.
- Compression of the ventral horn motor neurons can cause atrophy of muscles innervated by the spinal nerves arising from the level of the syrinx.

CASE 17.6

A 65-year-old woman complains of intermittent episodes of lancinating pain in her right lower jaw. She is occasionally wakened at night from this pain. She mentions that she read about something called trigeminal neuralgia on the Internet and wonders if this might be related. An extensive workup does not reveal any dental disease, and an MRI does not reveal any mass lesions in the posterior fossa.

1. In following up on her suggestion of trigeminal neuralgia, about what aspects of history should you inquire?
   Trigeminal neuralgia (tic douloureux) is diagnosed based on the medical history. Classic presentation includes pain of a sudden, shooting quality that involves one or more branches of the trigeminal nerve unilaterally and lasts seconds to minutes. The pain may be accompanied by brief facial spasms or tics. It is essential that trigeminal neuralgia be differentiated from cluster headaches, which similarly present with attacks of severe, periorbital pain but are much longer in duration (15 minutes or more) and may be associated with autonomic symptoms.

2. What is the value of imaging the posterior fossa in this woman?
   The trigeminal nerve courses from its nuclei in the pons through the posterior fossa and exits the cranium via the superior orbital fissure (V_1), foramen rotundum (V_2), or foramen ovale (V_3). Compression or meningeal inflammation anywhere along this pathway may cause similar symptoms.

3. In thinking about associated neurologic problems, what disorder might trigeminal neuralgia be associated with in a younger patient?
   Trigeminal neuralgia in a young patient might suggest MS, especially if bilateral. Trigeminal neuralgia in an older patient is more often idiopathic.

4. Which division of the trigeminal nerve is affected in this woman? What is the anatomic distribution of the other divisions?
   In this woman it is the mandibular division (or V_3), which innervates the lower jaw *but does not extend to the angle of the jaw.* The maxillary division (V_2) innervates the upper jaw and cheek, and the ophthalmic division (V_1) innervates the region of the nose, eyes, and forehead, *extending posterior to the hairline* (see Fig. 17.10).

5. If surgical sectioning of the involved branch were performed in this woman, what modalities of sensation would we expect to be impaired?

All modalities of sensation would be lost in the distribution of the mandibular division in this woman because the trigeminal nerve conveys all sensory information from the face (i.e., pain, temperature, fine touch, vibration, and proprioception). These trigeminal nerve afferents then synapse in the appropriate subdivision of the trigeminal brainstem complex: the principal sensory nucleus for tactile sensation, the spinal nucleus for pain and temperature, and the mesencephalic nucleus for proprioceptive information from the muscles of mastication. (The trigeminal brainstem complex is extensive, spanning from the midbrain to upper cervical spinal cord.)

6. Why might therapy with carbamazepine (Tegretol) make sense for this woman?

Carbamazepine is an anticonvulsant medication that is also used for trigeminal neuralgia and is prescribed for treating neuropathic pain of almost any etiology. It acts by reducing the rate of nerve transmission by inhibiting voltage-gated sodium channels in neurons.

SUMMARY BOX: TRIGEMINAL NEURALGIA

- Diagnose by history: Attacks of sharp pain, often unilaterally, involve one division of the trigeminal nerve and are accompanied by facial spasm or tic.
- Trigeminal nerve anatomy: Pseudounipolar neurons in the trigeminal ganglion provide motor innervation to muscles of mastication and sensory innervation to the anterior two-thirds of the head. Three sensory divisions exit the cranium through different foramina.
- First-line therapy for trigeminal neuralgia is with carbamazepine, an anticonvulsant that inhibits voltage-gated sodium channels.

CASE 17.7

A 45-year-old woman with a history of macrocytic (megaloblastic) anemia and who is on folic acid supplements is evaluated for a several-month history of mild depression and paresthesias in her hands and feet.

Examination is notable for the absence of papillae over much of the surface of the tongue (atrophic glossitis), positive Romberg sign, and bilateral Babinski signs. Fasting plasma glucose and glycated hemoglobin (HbA_{1c}) are both normal.

1. What should you reflexively think of when you see "megaloblastic anemia" on boards?

Try to make a quick association with vitamin B_{12} or folate deficiency. There are several ways to become deficient in vitamin B_{12} or folate, such as malnutrition, chronic alcohol use, or malabsorption, but the initial association will help you focus. Because we know the patient is taking folic acid, vitamin B_{12} deficiency seems likely. Folate deficiency is also not associated with neurologic deficits.

2. What findings might you see on a peripheral blood smear from a patient deficient in folate or vitamin B_{12}?

If you are given a blood smear, you likely will see large, immature, oval red blood cells (RBCs) (remember, you can use a lymphocyte as a scale for judging RBC size) and hypersegmented (five or more visible segments of the nucleus) polymorphonuclear neutrophils (PMNs).

3. Why would both vitamin B_{12} and folate deficiency cause a preponderance of large, immature red blood cells (macro-ovalocytes) on a blood smear?

Vitamin B_{12} and folate are needed for production of the nucleotide precursors of deoxyribonucleic acid (DNA), specifically, the conversion of dUMP → dTMP (deoxyuridine monophosphate to thymidine monophosphate) and of homocysteine → methionine. When DNA synthesis is impaired by vitamin B_{12} or folate deficiency, cell division is blocked, while ribonucleic acid (RNA) and protein synthesis continue. The expanding cytoplasmic volume and prevention of mitosis lead to large, immature RBCs (see Chapter 14 for more information).

4. How is a positive Romberg sign elicited on examination? Why might vitamin B_{12} deficiency give rise to a positive Romberg sign?

To elicit the sign, ask the patient to stand with her feet close together. If she is steady and not swaying when her eyes are open but sways or falls when you ask her to close her eyes, this is a positive Romberg sign. A positive sign indicates proprioceptive sensory loss that can be compensated for by visual input but becomes apparent when visual input is removed. In this case, the proprioceptive loss is due to demyelination of the dorsal columns. Recall that vitamin B_{12} deficiency leads to a buildup of propionyl-coenzyme A (CoA), which prevents normal myelination from occurring.

Note: It is a common misconception that a positive Romberg sign indicates cerebellar dysfunction, but this is not the case. This is a test for *sensory* ataxia. Patients with cerebellar dysfunction will have ataxia regardless of whether their eyes are open or closed.

5. Given the atrophic glossitis and neurologic symptoms, what is the likely diagnosis?
This patient most likely has a vitamin B_{12} deficiency neuropathy (subacute combined degeneration). Vitamin B_{12} deficiency can cause a megaloblastic anemia, which can be corrected with folic acid supplementation. However, folic acid supplementation does not prevent the neurologic manifestations of vitamin B_{12} deficiency. Therefore in a patient with megaloblastic anemia, both serum folate and vitamin B_{12} levels should be tested, and both vitamins should be supplemented. Should the patient become pregnant, adequate folate supplementation also helps prevent neural tube defects in the fetus. However, note that *folate deficiency does not cause neurologic dysfunction.*

STEP 1 SECRET

It is very high yield to know that supplementation of a B_{12}-deficient patient with folate will reverse the megaloblastic anemia but will not correct the neurologic symptoms. Why? Excess folate supplementation will normalize DNA synthesis, but myelin synthesis will still be defective because B_{12} is required for the conversion of homocysteine to methionine, a precursor of myelin.

6. What is a positive Babinski sign, and what does it indicate?
As was mentioned in the Basic Concepts section of this chapter, a positive Babinski sign refers to spontaneous dorsiflexion of the big toe upon stroking the lateral plantar surface of the foot from the heel toward the big toe. It indicates a UMN lesion and likely represents demyelination of the corticospinal tracts in this patient.
Note: Positive Babinski signs are normal in infants (up to 12 months) because of inadequate myelination at this time in life. Suppression of the Babinski reflex by higher brain centers is a prerequisite for learning to walk.

7. What is the value of obtaining a fasting plasma glucose level in this patient?
Diabetic neuropathy has paresthesias and sensory loss similar to those seen with vitamin B_{12} deficiency and generally presents in a "stocking and glove" pattern (meaning that the symptoms commonly appear initially in the feet and lower legs and then in the hands, both bilaterally).

8. What is the value of obtaining a methylmalonic acid level?

$$\text{Propionyl CoA} \rightarrow \text{Methylmalonyl CoA} \rightarrow \text{Succinyl CoA} \qquad [17.1]$$

In the fatty acid metabolic pathway shown in Eq. 17.1, vitamin B_{12} is a cofactor for the conversion of methylmalonyl CoA to succinyl CoA. Thus vitamin B_{12} deficiency causes a buildup in propionyl CoA and methylmalonyl CoA. A serum methylmalonic acid level is the *most sensitive test* for vitamin B_{12} deficiency. Methylmalonic acid levels will be normal in folate deficiency.

9. Given the paresthesias and positive Romberg and Babinski signs, where is the anatomic lesion?
Vitamin B_{12} neuropathy, also called *subacute combined degeneration*, can cause degeneration of both the lateral corticospinal tract and the dorsal columns (hence, *combined*). Lesions of the latter lead to paresthesias; UMN loss in the corticospinal tract leads to a positive Babinski sign and spasticity. Lesions within the dorsal columns lead to proprioceptive dysfunction.
It is very high yield to know that tabes dorsalis (tertiary syphilis) also results in degeneration of the dorsal columns, leading to a positive Romberg sign and sensory ataxia. Tabes dorsalis can be differentiated from subacute combined degeneration by the presence of an Argyll Robertson pupil (a pupil that can accommodate but does not react to light). Argyll Robertson pupil previously was referred to as *prostitute's pupil* ("because it accommodates but does not react"), but this nomenclature is discouraged because it is pejorative. Furthermore, patients will present with Charcot joints (flat feet) and areflexia due to nerve root involvement. Lancinating pains are also seen in tabes dorsalis.
Vitamin B_{12} deficiency is commonly seen in pernicious anemia (autoimmune gastritis) and in patients who have had surgical resection of the terminal ileum (e.g., patients with Crohn disease).

SUMMARY BOX: VITAMIN B_{12} (COBALAMIN) DEFICIENCY

- This deficiency can present as some combination of paresthesias, proprioceptive dysfunction, cognitive changes, and corticospinal tract dysfunction.
- Vitamin B_{12} is important for deoxyribonucleic acid (DNA) synthesis. Deficiency can cause megaloblastic anemia, with macro-ovalocytes and hypersegmented polymorphonuclear neutrophils (PMNs) (as can folate deficiency).
- Folate acid supplementation will treat the anemia but *not* the neurologic symptoms.
- The way to differentiate B_{12} from folate deficiency is by the accompaniment of neurologic symptoms in B_{12} deficiency.
- An increased serum methylmalonic acid level is highly sensitive for vitamin B_{12} deficiency.

CASE 17.8

A 32-year-old woman is evaluated for a several-week history of left-hand paresthesias. Fundoscopic and neurologic examinations are normal. She asks you whether she might have multiple sclerosis.

1. Why is it impossible to make a definite diagnosis of multiple sclerosis (MS) at this time?
   A hallmark of MS is its variability over time. To make a definite diagnosis of this disease, one needs to see a larger picture of recurrent attacks of neurologic dysfunction. One episode, especially one that presents as classically as it does here (and as it will on boards)—a young adult woman with optic neuritis or paresthesias or weakness—may raise a suspicion of MS, but it is insufficient to make a diagnosis.

STEP 1 SECRET

The USMLE loves to test students on multiple sclerosis. Be sure to pay close attention to the details of this case.

CASE 17.8 CONTINUED:

The patient returns 1 year later and describes episodes of sudden-onset clumsiness due to weakness of her left leg, slight tremor with movement, frequent bladder incontinence, and numbness and tingling sensations in her right arm. The episodes were occasionally accompanied by double vision. She has experienced three such episodes over the past year, each lasting about 2 weeks. Ocular examination demonstrates intact convergence. However, when she is asked to look left, her left eye abducts while her right eye stays at midline, and when she is asked to look right, her right eye abducts while her left eye stays at midline. There is also bilateral nystagmus of the abducting eye.

2. Where is the lesion underlying her oculomotor abnormalities?
   The lesion is likely in the medial longitudinal fasciculus (MLF). The MLF is a white matter tract in the brainstem that connects the abducens cranial nerve (CN VI) nucleus with the contralateral oculomotor (CN III) nucleus, allowing for conjugate gaze. Lesions of the MLF can cause *internuclear ophthalmoplegia* that manifests as diplopia, as seen here. The pathology of MLF syndrome is further described in Chapter 18 (Ophthalmology).
   Note: Bilateral internuclear ophthalmoplegia is pathognomonic for MS.

CASE 17.8 CONTINUED:

Given the constellation of episodes and symptoms, you order some studies. MRI of the brain reveals multiple white matter periventricular plaques. CSF analysis reveals the presence of oligoclonal immunoglobulin bands (absent in the serum), and elevated levels of immunoglobulin G (IgG) and myelin basic protein.

3. What is the diagnosis?
   MS is the diagnosis. The patient's time course of relapsing and remitting symptoms, MRI, and CSF findings are definitive for diagnosis of MS, an immune-mediated disease that involves demyelination of various white matter areas of the CNS. This occurs secondary to T-cell recognition of myelin basic protein as an antigen, which results in T-cell activation, cytokine production, and subsequent activation of macrophages and B cells. This sequence of events further destroys myelin sheaths and oligodendrocytes (myelin-producing cells of the CNS) in a type IV hypersensitivity reaction. In addition, MS may involve production of autoantibodies against the myelin sheath and oligodendrocytes.
   MS can have a relapsing and remitting course (as in this patient) or a chronically progressive course. The various neurologic manifestations that develop are due to inflammation and demyelination at different sites within the CNS.
   MRI classically shows multiple plaques in different areas of white matter, most notably in the periventricular areas. Oligoclonal immunoglobulin bands on electrophoresis of CSF are a sign of demyelination.

4. What cell type is attacked and destroyed in MS?
   As mentioned in the preceding discussion, oligodendrocytes are attacked by CD8$^+$ T cells. In contrast, Schwann cells, which provide myelination in the peripheral nervous system, are spared in MS; however, Schwann cells are attacked in Guillain-Barré syndrome (GBS, or acute inflammatory demyelination polyradiculopathy), another demyelinating disease that can be confused for MS.
   Note: One oligodendrocyte can myelinate many neurons, but one Schwann cell can myelinate only one neuron.

5. Is there any reason to consider the diagnosis of Guillain-Barré syndrome in this patient?
   Yes, although GBS would be unlikely. GBS classically presents with fatigue, distal limb paresthesias, and often an ascending weakness or even paralysis. GBS typically follows an acute infectious process and is most commonly associated with *Campylobacter jejuni* infection due to immune-mediated attack of peripheral myelin, which resembles

Campylobacter proteins (molecular mimicry). On the boards, this may be indicated on patient history as a recent diarrheal illness followed by ascending paralysis. GBS can rarely occur following vaccination with the influenza vaccine.

Although GBS is similar to MS in being an *inflammatory demyelinating disease*, it does not involve alterations in the CNS (i.e., demyelinated plaques in the brain and spinal cord). Rather, it is due to segmental demyelination of the peripheral nerves secondary to endoneurial inflammatory infiltrates. CSF analysis typically shows increased protein with a normal cell count (albuminocytologic dissociation). Papilledema may result secondary to increased CSF oncotic pressure. In addition, patients may present with severe irregularities in autonomic system function. Finally, you should remember that GBS is an acute illness and thus does not relapse and remit as MS does. Treatment for GBS includes respiratory support because the diaphragm can become paralyzed should the inflammation ascend sufficiently and, in some cases, patients may require plasmapheresis and IV immunoglobulins. A chronic form of GBS also exists called *chronic inflammatory demyelination polyradiculopathy*.

6. Would electromyography reveal slow, fast, or normal peripheral nerve conduction velocity in this woman who has multiple sclerosis?

Normal conduction velocity would be shown. Although myelinated nerve fibers conduct impulses faster than unmyelinated nerve fibers, the peripheral nerves are *not* subject to demyelination in MS. However, in GBS, there may be a reduction in nerve conduction velocity due to peripheral nerve demyelination.

7. Would you expect patients with multiple sclerosis to show signs of upper or lower motor neuron lesions?

UMN signs would be characteristic of patients with MS, because MS involves white matter in the brain and spinal cord and does not affect LMNs.

8. Given the inflammatory basis of the disease, what treatment might be considered?

There are several drugs that can greatly increase quality of life, reduce the frequency of exacerbations/relapses, and manage symptoms. Interferon beta has long been considered first-line therapy and has been shown to decrease the rate of relapse. Immunosuppressive drugs such as corticosteroids also are used to treat acute exacerbations of MS. Natalizumab, a vascular cell adhesion molecule (VCAM) inhibitor, may serve to reduce CNS inflammation by blocking extravasation of leukocytes across the blood-brain barrier and has been shown to be effective in reducing the frequency of exacerbations (but has the severe side effect of reactivating latent John Cunningham [JC] virus causing progressive multifocal leukoencephalopathy). Other disease-modifying drugs include glatiramer, dimethyl fumarate, and fingolimod. Symptomatic treatment for neurogenic bladder (muscarinic antagonists), spasticity (baclofen, a GABA receptor agonist), and pain (gabapentin, opioids if severe) may also be indicated.

SUMMARY BOX: MULTIPLE SCLEROSIS

- The classic patient is a young woman presenting with multiple episodes of neurologic dysfunction, such as limb paresthesias, motor weakness, and visual impairment due to optic neuritis or internuclear ophthalmoplegia. Other symptoms of multiple sclerosis (MS) include bladder/bowel incontinence, intention tremor, and sensory deficits on one side of the body.
- Other specific key history findings and buzzwords include symptoms exacerbated in the heat (Uhthoff phenomenon), an electric shock-like sensation induced by flexion of the neck (Lhermitte phenomenon), and a band of paresthesia around the chest or torso ("MS hug").
- The pathogenesis involves an immune-mediated attack on oligodendrocytes, leading to inflammation and demyelination in the central nervous system (CNS) (*not* the peripheral nervous system).
- Laboratory findings include an elevated immunoglobulin G (IgG) level and myelin basic protein in cerebrospinal fluid (CSF) and oligoclonal bands on CSF electrophoresis. Brain magnetic resonance imaging (MRI) classically reveals diffuse periventricular white matter plaques.
- Gross findings are demyelinating plaques in brain and spinal cord white matter, especially in periventricular regions.

CASE 17.9

A 70-year-old man with a history of moderately well-controlled hypertension and dyslipidemia and a 40-pack-year history of smoking is evaluated for sudden-onset left-sided hemiparesis and left leg anesthesia.

1. What is the likely diagnosis?

Stroke (cerebrovascular accident [CVA]) or transient ischemic attack (TIA) is the likely diagnosis. The patient's age and symptom severity should raise immediate suspicion for a stroke. There are two major kinds of strokes: ischemic and hemorrhagic. In the absence of other information, you should reason that ischemic stroke is more likely than hemorrhagic stroke, simply because ischemic stroke is the more common of the two types of strokes. Note that TIA should also be considered, particularly if his symptoms resolved quickly (<24 hours) and no lesions were found on imaging.

CASE 17.9 CONTINUED:

Noncontrast CT of the brain is unrevealing. MRI is subsequently performed, and a site of arterial occlusion is identified. The patient is examined and questioned for contraindications to treatment with tissue plasminogen activator (tPA) (i.e., severe hypertension, recent gastrointestinal [GI] bleeding, intracranial bleeding, recent surgery, or stroke onset more than 4.5 hours ago) and is cleared for thrombolytic therapy.

2. **Why is the lack of intracranial bleeding on CT important?**
   Before administering tPA, it is important to rule out intracranial hemorrhage using CT because any thrombolytic therapy could exacerbate active or recent bleeding. This is why thrombolytic therapy is contraindicated in hemorrhagic stroke. Remember that a head CT will appear normal in ischemic stroke until at least 12 to 24 hours after the event; therefore if there are any early findings on CT, you can rule out ischemic stroke for the purpose of board exams. If you do see abnormalities on CT, know that hemorrhagic stroke will appear as a hyperdense mass due to the iron content of blood, while ischemic stroke will appear normal or hypodense at later time points because of the edema associated with postischemic inflammation.

3. **What are the three primary types of intracranial hemorrhage?**
   Epidural, subdural, and subarachnoid hemorrhages are the primary types of intracranial hemorrhage.
   There are four main categories of intracranial hemorrhage that you must know for boards. Epidural hemorrhage is due to rupture of the middle meningeal artery, which is most commonly attributed to temporoparietal bone fracture (e.g., blow to the head). This type of hemorrhage often presents with a lucid interval in which the patient briefly loses consciousness, appears asymptomatic for a bit, and then deteriorates again. Expansion of the bleed can cause a transtentorial herniation and subsequent CN III palsy. On CT scan, look for the presence of a biconvex disk that does not cross suture lines (but may cross the falx cerebri and tentorium).
   Subdural hemorrhage is attributed to rupture of the bridging veins that extend between the dura and the arachnoid layers. This is generally due to blunt/generalized trauma or anticoagulation. The elderly are particularly susceptible to subdural hemorrhage because cerebral atrophy leads to stretched bridging veins, making them more susceptible to injury. Shaken baby syndrome also may cause subdural hemorrhage. Look for the presence of a crescent sign that is capable of crossing suture lines accompanied by a midline shift on CT scan.
   Subarachnoid hemorrhage is generally attributed a ruptured aneurysm (less commonly due to an arteriovenous malformation). Suspect subarachnoid hemorrhage in patients who report a sudden-onset "worse headache of my life" headache. Examiners often like to use subarachnoid hemorrhage to test your knowledge of connective tissue disorders such as adult polycystic kidney disease (ADPKD), Marfan syndrome, and Ehlers-Danlos syndrome, which can predispose patients to berry aneurysms in the circle of Willis. Look for a star-shaped area of hemorrhage on CT scan known as the *crab of death*.
   For completeness' sake, note that a fourth type of intracranial bleed exists, a parenchymal hematoma, which results from vessel rupture secondary to hypertension or amyloid angiopathy (associated with aging and Alzheimer disease). This is not high yield for Step 1.

STEP 1 SECRET

You should expect to have at least one question on causes of intracranial hemorrhage. We consider this topic in greater detail later in the chapter.

4. **Why is the patient's history of hypertension, hyperlipidemia, and smoking important to the etiology of ischemic stroke?**
   Ischemic strokes result predominantly from atherosclerosis and subsequent thromboembolic phenomena either intra- or extracranially. Hypertension, hyperlipidemia, and smoking all increase the risk of ischemic stroke by contributing to a state of vascular endothelial damage, hypercoagulability, and inflammation.

5. **How does atrial fibrillation predispose to stroke?**
   Atrial fibrillation makes it easier for blood to pool and clot within the atria, and the clots can then embolize to the brain. This is why patients with atrial fibrillation are routinely put on anticoagulation. If a patient presents with bilateral infarcts, your index of suspicion for a cardioembolic stroke should be extremely high.

6. **How does myocardial infarction predispose to stroke?**
   Similar in concept to atrial fibrillation, inefficient ventricular ejection after myocardial infarction can lead to clotting and subsequent embolus. For this reason, patients with a left ventricular thrombus require anticoagulation.

7. **Where does intracerebral vessel rupture due to hypertension occur most often?**
   Branches of the lenticulostriate vessels, which supply the basal ganglia, often develop aneurysms that may rupture. These are referred to as *Charcot-Bouchard microaneurysms* and most commonly affect the thalamus and basal ganglia. Note that these regions of the brain are especially prone to ischemia. It is important to distinguish these microaneurysms from hypertensive arteriolar sclerosis, which is a common cause of small lacunar strokes and occurs in patients with

chronic hypertension in the same anatomic distribution as microaneurysms. Sclerosis will differ from aneurysms histologically by the presence of lipohyalinosis and microatheromas. It is important to note that the strokes that they do cause will not be visible initially on CT because they are ischemic rather than hemorrhagic in nature.

8. Given the patient's loss of sensation in his left leg, what artery was probably occluded in this patient?

The right anterior cerebral artery or its downstream branches were likely occluded because this artery serves the motor and sensory cortices devoted to the contralateral (left) leg (Fig. 17.11).

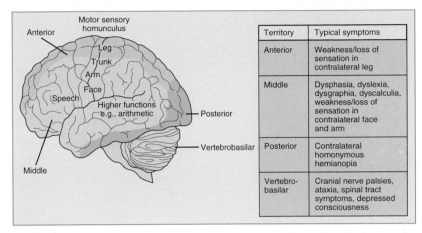

Figure 17.11. Cerebral artery territories and symptoms of strokes in those areas. *(From Mihailoff GA. Crash Course: Nervous System. Philadelphia: Mosby; 2005.)*

9. What motor and sensory abnormalities might develop from occlusion of the middle cerebral artery or its branches?

The middle cerebral artery supplies the motor and sensory cortex for the contralateral upper extremity, head, neck, and face, so occlusion can cause abnormalities in this distribution.

10. If someone suddenly developed difficulty understanding or articulating speech as the result of an ischemic stroke, branches of which major cerebral artery are most likely occluded?

The middle cerebral artery on the dominant (typically the left) side of the brain, which controls speech, is likely occluded. Difficulty understanding speech (*receptive aphasia*) results from lesions in Wernicke area of the *temporal lobe* and is called *Wernicke aphasia.* Although people with this lesion can articulate, their speech is devoid of semantic structure and often amounts to what is called a "word salad." Difficulty articulating speech (*expressive aphasia*), without impaired comprehension, is due to a lesion in Broca area of the *frontal lobe* and is called *Broca aphasia.* Global aphasia impairs both Wernicke and Broca areas, such that patients have difficulty articulating words and have impaired comprehension. On the other hand, conduction aphasia, which affects the arcuate fasciculus that connects Broca and Wernicke areas, impairs neither speech nor comprehension (Fig. 17.12). These patients have trouble with speech repetition.

11. How might occlusion of the right posterior cerebral artery or its branches cause loss of the left visual field of each eye (left homonymous hemianopia)?

The posterior cerebral artery supplies the visual cortex in the occipital lobe. The visual cortex on the right receives sensory input from the nasal retina of the left eye and the temporal retina of the right eye, each of which receives sensory information from the left visual field.

A branch of each posterior cerebral artery also supplies the lateral geniculate nucleus on the same side, which is the major relay center from the optic tract to the visual cortex.

12. Why does occlusion of the most proximal segment of the anterior cerebral artery typically not result in stroke symptoms?

If the occlusion is proximal to the anterior communicating artery, collateral blood flow from the contralateral anterior cerebral artery through the communicating artery can prevent a perfusion deficit.

STEP 1 SECRET

It is important to know the arrangement of blood vessels that supply the brain and spinal cord. The USMLE will commonly ask second- or third-order questions for which the answer depends on the student's ability to correctly identify cerebral blood vessels on an angiogram.

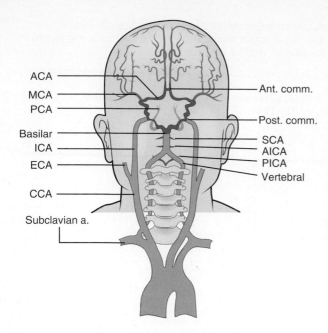

Figure 17.12. Coronal view of the extracranial and intracranial arterial supply to the brain. *ACA,* Anterior cerebral artery; *AICA,* anterior inferior cerebellar artery; *Ant. comm.,* anterior communicating artery; *CCA,* common carotid artery; *ECA,* external carotid artery; *ICA,* internal carotid artery; *MCA,* middle cerebral artery; *PCA,* posterior cerebral artery; *PICA,* posterior inferior cerebral artery; *Post. comm.,* posterior communicating artery; *SCA,* superior cerebellar artery; *Subclavian a.,* subclavian artery. *(From Andreoli TE. Cecil Essentials of Medicine. 5th ed. Philadelphia: WB Saunders; 2001.)*

13. In a sudden hypotensive episode, what regions of cerebral circulation are particularly susceptible to infarction and why?

Watershed areas, or the bordering zones between regions of the brain that require simultaneous perfusion two cerebral arteries, are particularly susceptible. A reduction in perfusion in either cerebral artery puts watershed areas at risk for ischemia and/or infarction. Bilateral upper leg and arm weakness and defects in higher order visual processing are common in patients with severe, sudden-onset hypotension.

14. What mechanism exists to protect the brain tissue from inadequate perfusion during systemic hypotension?

Cerebral autoregulation allows for adequate cerebral perfusion despite widely fluctuating systemic arterial pressures. Such perfusion is critical because neurons of the CNS have a high metabolic rate and are especially sensitive to ischemic and hypoxic insults. Similar to the mechanisms used in other tissues, particularly the kidneys, cerebral autoregulation primarily occurs via arterial and arteriolar constriction and dilation.

Cerebral perfusion is largely controlled by Pco_2 levels, with higher levels causing verebral vasodilation and thus increasing cerebral perfusion. Therefore, therapeutic hyperventilation can effectively decrease intracranial pressure in cases of cerebral edema by artificially decreasing Pco_2, which reduces cerebral blood flow.

15. Describe the gross pathologic findings in stroke.

Classic findings include a wedge-shaped area of pale (in ischemic stroke) or hemorrhagic infarction that develops first at the periphery of the cerebral cortex. The brain undergoes liquefactive necrosis with potentially dangerous swelling. Then, myelin will break down, causing loss of demarcation between the gray and white matter. Astrocytes will proliferate near the infarct as a reaction to injury, and microglia (resident tissue macrophages of the CNS) will remove debris from liquefactive necrosis. After many days to weeks, cystic areas may develop.

SUMMARY BOX: CEREBROVASCULAR ACCIDENTS

- The two types of cerebrovascular accidents, or strokes, are ischemic and hemorrhagic. Hemorrhagic strokes must be ruled out with a noncontrast computed tomography (CT) scan to determine whether the patient is potentially eligible for thrombolytic therapy.
- Major risk factors are hypertension, smoking, hyperlipidemia, atherosclerosis, and atrial fibrillation.
- Recent surgery, recent gastrointestinal (GI) bleeding, intracranial bleeding, and severe hypertension are contraindications to thrombolytic therapy.

CASE 17.10

A 37-year-old man is evaluated for a 2-hour history of a headache that came on abruptly. He describes the headache as the "worst headache of my life." He has vomited twice in the past hour, and the ceiling lights are bothersome to him. He is afebrile.

1. What is the classic cause of the "worst headache of one's life," especially in association with the other symptoms presented here?

Subarachnoid hemorrhage (SAH) is the classic cause. Though atypical presentations are common clinically, Step 1 boards will use this classic presentation.

2. What is the first step that should be taken to diagnose this patient?

A noncontrast CT scan should be performed first, because it can be done quickly. If performed within 6 hours of onset of symptoms, the sensitivity is very high for detection of SAH. As time progresses, the blood dissipates in the CSF and sensitivity decreases. If this is nondiagnostic, the next step is either a lumbar puncture (to detect blood and xanthochromia) or a CT angiogram (to detect an aneurysm).

CASE 17.10 CONTINUED:

A CT scan is performed and shows blood in the basal cisternae (areas of expansion of the subarachnoid space, located rostral to the pons and between the temporal lobes). Subsequently, cerebral angiography is performed and localizes the site of bleeding. (To view this image, please refer to LearningRadiology.com: http://learningradiology.com/archives2007/COW%20266-Subarachnoid%20hemorrhage/subarachnoidcorrect.html.)

3. If CT scanning did not reveal any characteristic bleeding into the subarachnoid space, what other diagnostic test can be done to establish the diagnosis of subarachnoid hemorrhage?

A lumbar puncture should be performed if the CT scan is negative or equivocal but suspicion for SAH is high. Blood found in the CSF, which is sampled from the subarachnoid space, supports a diagnosis of SAH. An alternative modality is CT angiography that, if normal, also results in a low pretest probability of SAH (if there is no aneurysm or arteriovenous malformation [AVM] detected).

Note: Because the spinal cord terminates at the level of L1–L2 in adults, lumbar punctures are performed at the level of the L3–L4 or L4–L5 interspace. An external landmark to use to locate the L4 spinous process is the iliac crest.

4. Why does subarachnoid hemorrhage cause headache, nuchal rigidity, photophobia, and nausea/vomiting?

The headache, photophobia, and nuchal rigidity are caused by meningeal irritation; blood is very irritating to the meninges. Nausea and vomiting are due to increased intracranial pressure and meningeal irritation.

5. What are some common causes of subarachnoid hemorrhage?

As mentioned in Case 17.9, common causes of SAH include ruptured berry aneurysm, ruptured arteriovenous malformation, and head trauma. Ruptured aneurysm is the most common cause of SAH, though head trauma is also a common cause. Berry aneurysms can be congenital or acquired.

6. What are some major risk factors for acquired berry aneurysms?

Hypertension and cigarette smoking are major modifiable risk factors. Family history and connective tissue disorders are also risk factors for SAH.

7. Where do berry aneurysms typically develop and why?

They often develop in the circle of Willis, at the junction of communicating arteries with main cerebral arteries. This is because these junctions lack an internal elastic lamina and have an attenuated tunica media. The most common site is the junction containing the anterior cerebral artery (Fig. 17.13).

SUMMARY BOX: SUBARACHNOID HEMORRHAGE

- Subarachnoid hemorrhage (SAH) classically presents with severe ("the worst of my life") headache, photophobia, meningeal irritation, and nausea/vomiting.
- Initial diagnostic study is a noncontrast computed tomography (CT). If performed within 6 hours of symptom onset, a negative head CT has a strong negative predictive value for ruling out SAH. If performed after 6 hours, the patient requires either a lumbar puncture (for blood or xanthochromia) or CT angiogram (for detection of aneurysm or arteriovenous malformation [AVM]).
- The most frequent cause is ruptured aneurysm.
- Hypertension, such as in the setting of polycystic kidney disease, predisposes one to develop berry aneurysms.
- Berry aneurysms frequently occur at the junctional points of the circle of Willis, especially in the anterior circulation.

CASE 17.11

After some heroic neurosurgical procedures involving clipping the ruptured aneurysm, the patient in the previous vignette managed to survive the SAH. However, several days later he develops severe headaches and difficulty walking. Additionally, his wife now complains that his memory has become very poor and that he has difficulty paying attention to anything.

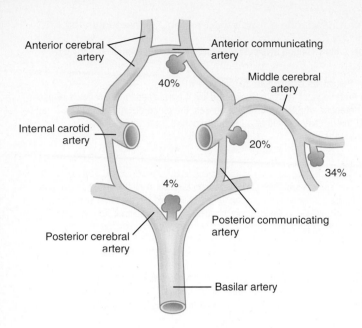

Figure 17.13. Frequency of aneurysmal sites. *(From Cotran RS, Kumar V, Collins T. Robbins Pathologic Basis of Disease. 6th ed. Philadelphia: WB Saunders; 1999.)*

1. **What are some potential complications of SAH?**
   The most worrisome acute complication is rebleeding, for which the risk is highest within a few days after the SAH presents. Other complications include hydrocephalus and delayed ischemia due to vasospasm at the site of a subarachnoid blood clot.

CASE 17.11 CONTINUED:

Ophthalmic examination shows papilledema, and a CT scan of the brain is as shown in Fig. 17.14.

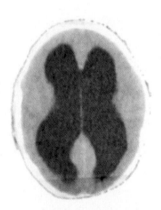

Figure 17.14. Massively dilated lateral ventricles. *(From Lindsay KW, Bone I, Callander R. Neurology and Neurosurgery Illustrated. 3rd ed. Edinburgh: Churchill Livingstone; 2002.)*

2. **What is the diagnosis?**
   The patient has hydrocephalus, most likely secondary to his SAH.
   Note: About a third of hydrocephalus cases in adults are idiopathic, and the remaining two-thirds develop following meningitis, SAH, intracranial surgery, head injury, intracranial tumor, or congenital aqueductal stenosis. For example, an ependymoma is a tumor derived from the cells that line walls of the ventricular system, so its growth can easily obstruct CSF flow by compressing the cerebral aqueduct.

3. **How is CSF produced, and what is its function?**
   CSF is produced via an active secretory process (rather than mere filtration of plasma) by the choroid plexus of the lateral ventricles, third ventricle, and fourth ventricle. Its function is to cushion and suspend the brain and spinal cord, protecting these soft tissues from the compressing forces of gravity and their own weight.

4. What is the pathway of CSF flow?

CSF flows from the lateral ventricles into the third ventricle via the (intraventricular) foramen of Monro. From the third ventricle, it flows through the cerebral aqueduct (of Sylvius) into the fourth ventricle. From the fourth ventricle it then flows into the subarachnoid space via the *l*ateral foramina of *L*uschka and the *m*edial foramen of *M*agendie (Fig. 17.15).

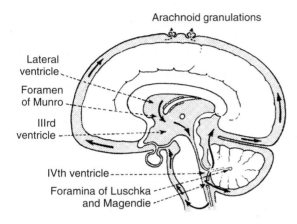

Arachnoid granulations

Lateral ventricle

Foramen of Munro

IIIrd ventricle

IVth ventricle

Foramina of Luschka and Magendie

Figure 17.15. Pathway of cerebrospinal fluid flow. *(From Lindsay KW, Bone I, Callander R, eds.* Neurology and Neurosurgery Illustrated. *3rd ed. Edinburgh: Churchill Livingstone; 2002.)*

5. How is CSF reabsorbed?

CSF empties from the subarachnoid space into the dural venous sinuses via the arachnoid granulations. To be more specific, arachnoid granulations protrude into the superior sagittal sinus, which eventually drains into the internal jugular vein.

6. What happens if the cerebral aqueduct is blocked?

This creates a backup of CSF in the ventricles, thereby enlarging the ventricles, compressing the brain, and possibly leading to headache and neurologic dysfunction. This type of hydrocephalus is called *noncommunicating* because the communication between the ventricular system and subarachnoid space is blocked. On CT scan or MRI, the lateral and third ventricles are enlarged, but the fourth ventricle is normal in size because its outflow is not obstructed.

7. In contrast with noncommunicating hydrocephalus, what is communicating hydrocephalus?

In communicating hydrocephalus, the communication between the ventricular system and subarachnoid space is preserved. In this case, hydrocephalus may be caused by excess production of CSF (which is rare) or by defective absorption of CSF (more common; may be caused by scarring of the arachnoid layer after meningitis). The overall increase in CSF leads to elevated intracranial pressure, which can result in bilateral papilledema and herniation. If not properly managed, papilledema can result in vision loss.

Two high-yield variations of communicating hydrocephalus are normal pressure hydrocephalus and hydrocephalus *ex vacuo.* Unlike classic communicating hydrocephalus, normal intracranial pressure (no papilledema or herniation) is seen in both of these special variations. The root cause of normal pressure hydrocephalus is unknown, but it is very high yield to know that enlargement of the lateral ventricles pushes on a white matter structure called the *corona radiata,* resulting a classic clinical triad of ataxia, urinary incontinence, and cognitive dysfunction (wobbly, wet, and wacky). Hydrocephalus *ex vacuo* is a relative increase in CSF due to a decrease in overall brain mass, commonly due to neurodegenerative conditions causing cerebral atrophy such as Huntington disease, Alzheimer disease, alcoholism, or Pick disease. Because the ventricles are expanding at the same rate as the parenchyma is shrinking, you do not see any symptoms related to white matter compression in hydrocephalus *ex vacuo.*

SUMMARY BOX: HYDROCEPHALUS

- Cerebrospinal fluid (CSF) is secreted by the choroid plexus lining the ventricular system. CSF flow is as follows: lateral ventricles → foramen of Monro → third ventricle → cerebral aqueduct → fourth ventricle → foramina of Luschka and Magendie → subarachnoid space → arachnoid granulations → dural venous sinuses.
- Excess volume of CSF can cause expansion of the ventricular system and compression of the brain.
- Symptoms include headaches, ataxia, and neurologic deficits such as dementia. Nausea/vomiting, incontinence, and visual disturbances are also possible.
- Hydrocephalus can be communicating or noncommunicating, depending on whether communication between the ventricular system and subarachnoid space is open.
- Hydrocephalus is a potential complication of subarachnoid hemorrhage.

CASE 17.12

A boy playing baseball gets hit on the left side of his head by a pitch and falls unconscious.

1. **What types of bleeds can result from blunt trauma to the head?**
   The major types of bleeds resulting from trauma to the head are epidural (extradural) or subdural in location. Epidural and subdural hemorrhage differ in the vessels involved, clinical presentation, and imaging findings. However, both can cause increased intracranial pressure, leading to herniation and death.

CASE 17.12 CONTINUED:

The boy quickly recovers consciousness and refuses to be taken to the hospital but agrees to sit out the rest of the game. After a few minutes, he appears to act confused, lethargic, and disoriented, and an ambulance is called to take him to the hospital. Examination at the hospital shows a dilated left pupil. CT scan shows the presence of a rapidly expanding biconcave disk-shaped mass between the dura and the skull.

2. **What type of injury did this boy most likely sustain?**
   This is likely an epidural hematoma, which is the result of intracranial bleeding that dissects the periosteal layer of dura away from the cranium. The *lucid interval* (a period of clear consciousness between the initial blow and later changes in consciousness) seen here is classic for epidural hematoma.

3. **What are the three different layers of the meninges?**
   The outermost layer is the dura mater (*dura* means "tough or durable") and is made of a fibrous connective tissue. The next layer is the arachnoid layer, which contains the subarachnoid space that CSF flows through and that blood vessels course through. The innermost layer is the pia mater, which is attached directly to the brain parenchyma.
   Note: Recall that the dura mater comprises two layers: a periosteal layer, adherent to bone, and a meningeal layer, continuous with the arachnoid mater. Because these two layers are normally also adherent to each other, no true space exists on either side of the dura under normal circumstances.

4. **What vascular structures are typically involved in an epidural hematoma?**
   An epidural hematoma occurs when there is a rupture of a blood vessel, usually an artery, between the outermost membrane covering of the brain (the dura mater) and the skull. The middle meningeal artery is most commonly involved, and the rupture is associated with fracture of the temporoparietal bone overlying it.

5. **What vascular structures are typically involved in a subdural hematoma?**
   The bridging veins that connect the subarachnoid space, and the dural venous sinuses are severed. Subdural hematomas are more common in elderly people whose brains have atrophied. Because the atrophied brain can move around more in the skull, mild trauma such as a fall can tear these bridging veins more easily (Fig. 17.16). Subdural hematoma may also occur in shaken baby syndrome.

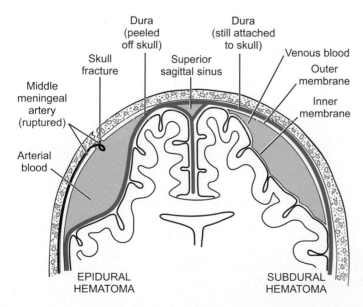

Figure 17.16. Vascular structures typically involved in a subdural hematoma. (*From Kumar V, Abbas AK, Fausto N:* Robbins and Cotran Pathologic Basis of Disease. *7th ed. Philadelphia: WB Saunders; 2005.*)

6. Why do the symptoms of subdural hematomas typically develop slowly?
   Because these hematomas result from tearing of the low-pressure bridging veins, it takes more time for blood to accumulate and cause compressive symptoms.

7. How does the radiographic appearance of a subdural hematoma differ from the biconcave disk shape of an epidural hematoma?
   A subdural hematoma is crescent-shaped, following the contours of the skull, because flow of the hemorrhaged blood is not limited by the strong attachment points of the dura mater to the cranium at the cranial suture lines.

8. Would cerebrospinal fluid analysis in this patient show multiple red blood cells?
   No. Blood from an epidural bleed does not reach the subarachnoid space, where the CSF is located.

SUMMARY BOX: EPIDURAL AND SUBDURAL HEMATOMAS

- Epidural bleeding results from rupture of a high-pressure artery, most often the middle meningeal artery after temporal bone fracture.
- Epidural hematoma is associated with a lucid interval.
- Subdural hematomas are more common in the elderly and result from rupture of low-pressure bridging veins. The slow oozing of blood here implies that symptoms develop slowly.
- Epidural hematoma is a biconcave disk limited by suture lines. Subdural hematoma is crescent-shaped and not limited by suture lines.
- Both hematomas can eventually cause an altered level of consciousness, herniation, and death.

CASE 17.13

Upon awakening one morning, a 50-year-old neurologist realizes she cannot smile or grimace on her right side. Her initial worry is that she may have suffered a small stroke.

---

1. Lesion of what cranial nerve might cause these symptoms?
   Damage to the facial nerve (CN VII), which provides motor innervation to muscles of facial expression such as the orbicularis oris and platysma, can cause such symptoms.

2. Assuming a stroke has caused these symptoms, where would the lesion be located?
   She would have a lesion of the contralateral facial area of the motor cortex or its associated corticobulbar tract (i.e., a UMN lesion). The UMNs of the facial motor cortex send fibers through the corticobulbar tract down to the facial motor nucleus. For UMNs controlling the *upper face* (muscles such as orbicularis oculi and frontalis, necessary for blinking and frowning, respectively), there is *bilateral* innervation from both cerebral hemispheres. For UMNs controlling the *lower face*, there is only *contralateral* innervation. Thus unilateral disruption of the motor cortex or corticobulbar tract will cause paralysis of the lower face, but the other hemisphere can still provide adequate innervation and motor control to the upper face.

CASE 17.13 CONTINUED:

This neurologist then realizes that she cannot blink her right eye. While talking with her husband, she realizes that his voice seems louder than usual and is somewhat painful to listen to (hyperacusis). Her husband then takes her to the emergency department, where the examining physician detects an absent corneal reflex on the right and a lack of taste sensation in the anterior two-thirds of the right side of her tongue.

---

3. Given these findings, what is the likely diagnosis and best treatment option?
   This patient likely has Bell palsy (facial paralysis), also known as *idiopathic facial nerve palsy*. Regardless of the underlying cause, symptoms are typically due to inflammation of the facial nerve and often resolve acutely with corticosteroid administration. Severe cases likely also benefit from valacyclovir administration.

4. What is causing hyperacusis in this patient?
   This is due to paralysis of the stapedius muscle, which functions to dampen the oscillations of the stapes footplate against the oval window. The facial nerve innervates the stapedius.

5. Why is the corneal reflex absent in this woman?
   The corneal reflex causes blinking of the eye when the cornea is touched. Touch sensation from the cornea is carried by the ophthalmic division (V_1) of the trigeminal nerve (afferent loop of the reflex). The efferent part of the reflex is carried by the facial nerve and causes contraction of orbicularis oculi. Because the facial nerve is paralyzed in this patient, the efferent part of the reflex is defective.

6. Why is taste sensation absent from the anterior two-thirds of the right side of this woman's tongue?

A branch of the facial nerve called the *chorda tympani* joins the lingual nerve (a division of the mandibular part of the trigeminal nerve). This path allows the chorda tympani to provide taste sensation to this part of the tongue.

STEP 1 SECRET

Innervation of the tongue is rather complicated, and it may be for that reason that the USMLE loves to ask questions about it. Touch sensation from the anterior two-thirds of the tongue is mediated by CN V, whereas taste from the anterior two-thirds of the tongue is mediated by CN VII. Touch and taste sensation of the posterior one-third of the tongue is innervated by CN IX. The muscles of the tongue are innervated by CN XII.

7. Why do the following produce symptoms similar to those seen in Bell palsy?

Mumps infection: The parotid gland, through which the facial nerve travels, becomes inflamed (parotitis) in mumps. Note that other viral infections such as herpes simplex virus 1 (HSV-1) and varicella zoster are also potential causative agents of parotitis.

Acoustic neuroma (schwannoma): Acoustic neuromas (tumors of the Schwann cells of the eighth cranial nerve) commonly arise adjacent to where the facial nerve exits the pons. These tumors can compress the facial nerve at this location and should be suspected if a patient also presents with hearing loss or difficulties with balance.

8. If this patient reported the recent development of palpitations, as well as a long-time passion for hiking, what diagnosis should be suspected?

When a cause of facial nerve palsy is identified, it is very high yield to know that it is often a manifestation of stage 2 Lyme disease (caused by the spirochete *Borrelia burgdorferi*, transmitted by the *Ixodes scapularis* tick). On the boards, a near-pathognomonic finding of *B. burgdorferi* infection is erythema chronicum migrans, a spreading, target-shaped ring of erythema around the site of inoculation. Other clues include flu-like symptoms (stage 1), cardiac block (stage 2), and delayed migratory polyarthritis and encephalopathy characterized by memory impairment, irritability, and somnolence (stage 3). Bilateral Bell palsy is more likely due to Lyme disease.

Whether the palsy is idiopathic (a true Bell palsy) or a result of Lyme disease or other identifiable cause, the pathogenesis is nearly always related to inflammation within the facial canal. As such, it makes sense that symptoms would resolve with corticosteroid administration. If she were to subsequently test positive for *Borrelia*, it is very high yield to know that she would additionally need doxycycline to treat the underlying infection.

SUMMARY BOX: BELL PALSY

- Inflammation or compression of the facial nerve causes paralysis of the muscles of facial expression, loss of innervation to the stapedius, and loss of taste sensation in the anterior two-thirds of the tongue.
- Potential causes include viral infections, acoustic neuroma, and Lyme disease.
- Upper motor neurons in the facial nerve nucleus provide bilateral cortical innervation for upper facial muscles and contralateral (unilateral) cortical innervation for lower facial muscles.
- Facial nerve paralysis can be distinguished from stroke by identifying whether there is paralysis of upper facial muscles.

CASE 17.14

An 8-year-old boy is brought to the neurologist by his concerned mother. His mother tells the neurologist that he occasionally experiences episodes during which he appears to lose consciousness and wets his pants. In addition, his whole body seems to become rigid. After a minute, his seemingly rigid body undergoes rhythmic jerks, and he simultaneously begins frothing at the mouth. After he stops seizing, his mother notes that he appears to be confused and lethargic for about an hour (postictal state).

1. What kind of seizure does this patient seem to experience?

A generalized tonic-clonic seizure (previously referred to as *grand mal seizures*) is likely. Patients who undergo this type of seizure typically experience loss of consciousness and whole-body rigidity (tonic phase) followed by whole-body jerks (clonic phase).

2. If whole-body rigidity is described as tonic, what happens in an atonic seizure?

Atonic seizures, or "drop" seizures, are associated with sudden loss of muscle tone.

3. What is the principal difference between a partial and a generalized seizure?

A partial seizure begins focally within one cerebral hemisphere (although it may *secondarily* become generalized, it begins in one hemisphere). In contrast, a generalized seizure has its focus of onset diffusely throughout both hemispheres.

4. **What is the difference between a simple and a complex seizure?**
   In a simple seizure, there is no alteration in consciousness. A complex seizure, by definition, implies alteration in consciousness.

5. **Differentiate the seizure types listed in Table 17.1 in terms of their origin in the brain and any alteration in consciousness.**
   See Table 17.1 for these comparisons.

Table 17.1. Seizure Types

SEIZURE TYPE	SEIZURE ORIGIN	ALTERATION IN CONSCIOUSNESS
Partial	Focal (one cerebral hemisphere)	Yes *or* No
Simple partial	Focal	No
Complex partial	Focal	Yes
Generalized	Diffuse (both hemispheres)	Yes
Absence seizure	Diffuse	Yes
Tonic-clonic	Diffuse	Yes

6. **What effects do most anticonvulsants have on neuronal firing?**
   They decrease the frequency of neuronal firing by increasing the threshold required for neuronal depolarization (i.e., they stabilize neuronal membranes). For most anticonvulsants, this is achieved by blocking sodium or calcium channels, but the benzodiazepines (e.g., diazepam) and barbiturates (e.g., phenobarbital) facilitate the inhibitory action of GABA by increasing chloride channel activity.

7. **In Table 17.2, cover the right column and, looking at the side effects listed on the left, name the anticonvulsants best known for causing them.**
   Note: Ethosuximide is first-line therapy for absence seizures and blocks T-type calcium channels. Benzodiazepines are used as first-line agents for acute seizure activity. Because the brain is in a constant state of hyperactivity, it can result in widespread neuronal death and be extremely damaging to the brain, ultimately resulting in permanent neurologic damage and/or coma.

Table 17.2. Anticonvulsants and Their Side Effects

SIDE EFFECT(S)	SEIZURE MEDICATION(S)
Agranulocytosis	Carbamazepine
Gingival hyperplasia, nystagmus, ataxia, cytochrome P-450 induction	Phenytoin
Hepatotoxicity	Valproic acid
Respiratory depression	Phenobarbital, diazepam
Stevens-Johnson syndrome	Lamotrigine, ethosuximide
Tremor	Gabapentin

STEP 1 SECRET

You should know key mechanisms and side effects for the anticonvulsant drugs, as well as which drugs are first-line agents for various seizure types.

8. **If this were the first seizure that this patient experienced, can he be diagnosed with epilepsy?**
   No. Epilepsy describes the presence of *recurrent, unprovoked seizures.* Unprovoked seizures are seizures that occur spontaneously, such that they are not secondary to infection (meningitis), toxic conditions (uremia), drug withdrawal (delirium tremors), fever (febrile seizures), head trauma, hyperventilation, or sleep deprivation. A diagnosis of epilepsy can be made only after a patient experiences another seizure and all possible other causes of seizure have been ruled out.

CASE 17.15

An 80-year-old woman has become increasingly demented over the past 10 years. She has difficulty remembering recent things (like where she put her keys) and recent conversations but has a good memory of her earlier years. Her son, who accompanies her on her visit to the office, says that when relating events that have happened to her recently, she makes things up to fill in gaps in her memory but seems unaware that she is doing so (confabulation). Past medical history is negative for stroke, and there are no focal neurologic deficits on physical examination. A Mini-Mental State Examination reveals that she is moderately demented.

1. **Assuming this woman is victim to the most common cause of dementia, what specific pathologic microscopic findings are characteristic of this disease at autopsy?**
   Neurofibrillary tangles and neuritic senile plaques are characteristic of Alzheimer disease, the most common cause of dementia in the elderly. The plaques are extracellular aggregates of beta-amyloid protein (a cleavage product of amyloid precursor protein), and the neurofibrillary tangles are cytoplasmic tangles of hyperphosphorylated tau protein. These changes are toxic to neurons.

2. **Why might this patient be at higher risk for intracerebral hemorrhage?**
   Deposition of beta-amyloid protein in intracranial vessels (amyloid angiopathy) causes weakening of the vessel walls and may lead to intracranial hemorrhage.

3. **What is the second most common cause of dementia in the elderly, and how does it arise?**
   Multi-infarct (vascular) dementia occurs because of the cumulative effect of multiple small or large infarcts. It often presents with focal neurologic deficits because of the infarcts, which helps to differentiate it from Alzheimer disease clinically. It also tends to have a stepwise progression of disease.

4. **How would the pattern of cortical atrophy differ if this woman had Pick disease rather than Alzheimer disease?**
   Pick disease (frontotemporal dementia) is characterized by selective atrophy of the frontal and temporal lobes, as opposed to the diffuse cerebral atrophy of Alzheimer disease. In addition to dementia, symptoms of Pick disease include parkinsonian aspects and personality changes. Intracellular tau protein aggregates called *Pick bodies* can be found at autopsy.

5. **What is the pathophysiologic rationale for treating Alzheimer disease patients with cholinesterase inhibitors?**
   In Alzheimer disease, there is a selective destruction of cholinergic neurons (though other transmitter systems are variably affected). Cholinesterase inhibitors are believed to compensate for this to some degree by increasing the concentration and prolonging the action of acetylcholine in the synaptic cleft.
   Note: Donepezil is a relatively new anticholinesterase used in Alzheimer disease that does not have the hepatotoxic effects that the older drug tacrine does.

6. **If this woman also suffered from depression, as many Alzheimer disease patients do, why should we avoid prescribing tricyclic antidepressants?**
   Tricyclic antidepressants have powerful anticholinergic side effects that could exacerbate her cognitive decline due to Alzheimer disease. The newer selective serotonin reuptake inhibitors (SSRIs) would therefore be a better choice for treating her depression.

7. **Based on what you know about the brain regions that are selectively destroyed in Alzheimer disease, why would you expect long-term potentiation to be affected in these patients?**
   Long-term potentiation, which occurs in the hippocampus (among other locations), is currently believed to be the mechanism by which neurons form "memories" of previous synaptic inputs of importance. The hippocampus is an early site of degeneration in Alzheimer disease, and this degeneration is believed to be one of the causes of the memory loss in these patients.

8. **Our patient's son worries that if his mother in fact does have Alzheimer disease, he and his siblings might also get Alzheimer disease. Is this likely to happen?**
   No. Most cases of Alzheimer disease are sporadic. About 10% of cases have a known genetic basis, usually associated with genes on chromosome 1, 14, 19, or 21. However, genetics are a common cause of presenile (early onset) Alzheimer disease, which often strikes before the age of 40.

9. **What important gene related to Alzheimer disease is on chromosome 21? On chromosome 19?**
The gene encoding amyloid precursor protein (APP) is located on chromosome 21. APP is cleaved into Aβ-amyloid by β/γ-secretases. Extracellular Aβ-amyloid protein is responsible for the formation of senile plaques. Because Down syndrome patients have three copies of this chromosome and thereby increased levels of APP, they are at high risk for early-onset (before age 40) Alzheimer disease.

Chromosome 19 contains the apolipoprotein E gene. The E4 allele confers increased risk for late-onset Alzheimer disease and thus accounts for some familial forms.

Note: Phosphorylated tau protein (insoluble cytoskeletal components) forms the neurofibrillary tangles that are also seen in Alzheimer patients. These tangles accumulate intracellularly and correlate directly with the degree of dementia that the patient has.

SUMMARY BOX: ALZHEIMER DISEASE

- Alzheimer disease is the most common cause of dementia in the elderly; the second most common cause is multi-infarct (vascular) dementia.
- Alzheimer disease is clinically distinguished by the presence/absence of focal neurologic deficits.
- Pathology involves defective degradation of amyloid precursor protein, leading to β-amyloid plaques, and hyper-phosphorylated tau protein, leading to neurofibrillary tangles.
- Cholinesterase inhibitors are a potential treatment.
- This differs from Pick disease in frontotemporal versus diffuse cortical atrophy.
- Amyloid can deposit in and weaken vessel walls, causing hemorrhage (amyloid angiopathy).
- Most forms are sporadic. Amyloid precursor protein (APP) and apolipoprotein E4 (*APOE4*) genes are important in familial forms.
- Down syndrome patients are at high risk for early-onset Alzheimer disease.

CASE 17.16

A homeless man with a long history of alcohol abuse tries to gain admission to the hospital to get something to eat. He enters the emergency department and uses his usual trick of complaining about "pain all over." However, he also honestly admits that his memory is getting increasingly worse, and he has difficulty standing up when sober. After sitting in the emergency department for a few hours, he appears to be confused and irritable and complains of a headache. A quick blood glucose test reveals hypoglycemia.

---

1. **This patient was given intravenous glucose to relieve his hypoglycemic condition. Why should thiamine be administered before administering glucose to this patient?**
Thiamine (vitamin B_1) deficiency is commonly observed in alcohol abuse. Thiamine is a necessary cofactor for pyruvate dehydrogenase, which catalyzes the conversion of pyruvate (from glucose breakdown) to acetyl CoA. In the absence of thiamine, pyruvate (from glucose metabolism) is converted to lactic acid by lactate dehydrogenase, causing lactic acidosis within the CNS, which is detrimental to neuronal cells.

2. **What syndrome is most often caused by thiamine deficiency? What does each part of the syndrome's name refer to?**
Wernicke-Korsakoff syndrome is often found in chronic alcohol abuse. Acute CNS changes due to thiamine deficiency are called *Wernicke encephalopathy.* The triad of ataxia, nystagmus, and ophthalmoplegia is *reversible.* However, chronic, *irreversible* CNS changes due to thiamine deficiency such as retrograde (as this patient complains of) and anterograde memory impairment, as well as confabulation, are called *Korsakoff psychosis.*

3. **What brain regions are typically affected in Wernicke-Korsakoff syndrome?**
Petechial hemorrhage and infarction often are seen in the mammillary bodies, thalamus, and periaqueductal gray matter (Fig. 17.17). The limbic system is also affected in Korsakoff psychosis.

4. **While our malingering patient is in the hospital, he becomes agitated and develops anxiety, muscle cramps, tremors, delusions, and hallucinations. What is happening and what drugs could have been used to prevent/relieve these symptoms?**
He is going through alcohol withdrawal, the most severe manifestations of which are termed *delirium tremens* (DTs). Long-acting benzodiazepines or barbiturates prevent DTs.

5. **Explain why benzodiazepines and barbiturates are useful in treating alcoholic withdrawal.**
Alcohol, benzodiazepines, and barbiturates all bind to and activate the same receptor, $GABA_A$. When activated, this receptor opens a chloride channel, resulting in neuronal hyperpolarization. The net effect of this hyperpolarization is reduced neuronal excitability. However, if given for prolonged times or in large doses, any of these pharmacologic agents can cause downregulation of the GABAergic system. If these substances are then acutely withdrawn, the CNS loses inhibitory signals and becomes hyperexcitable. This causes manifestations similar to what this patient experienced. Consequently, the benzodiazepines and barbiturates are effective in treating withdrawal because they are essentially alcohol substitutes.

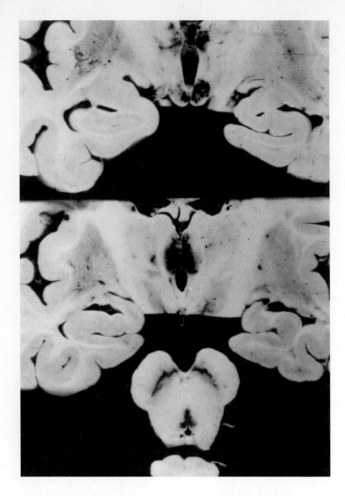

Figure 17.17. Wernicke's encephalopathy. Gross appearance of the brain characterized by petechial hemorrhages in the typical locations. *(Reprinted with permission from Okazaki H. Fundamentals of Neuropathology. 2nd ed. New York: Igaku Shoin; 1989.)*

Note: The longer-acting benzodiazepines and barbiturates cause significantly milder withdrawal symptoms than the short-acting agents. The benzodiazepine competitive antagonist flumazenil can be used for iatrogenic overdoses of benzodiazepines but is not used for overdoses in patients who chronically use benzodiazepines as it can precipitate seizure activity.

6. How do the mechanisms of action of benzodiazepines and barbiturates differ?
   Benzodiazepines increase the *frequency* of chloride channel opening, whereas barbiturates increase the *duration* of chloride channel opening.

7. Why do chronic alcohol users often require a larger dose of benzodiazepines than nonusers to achieve the same pharmacologic effect?
   Chronic alcohol use can lead to *cross-tolerance* to other $GABA_A$ agonists. Alcohol consumption causes downregulation of the $GABA_A$ receptor, which makes $GABA_A$ agonists such as the benzodiazepines and barbiturates less effective.

8. Why is it dangerous to discharge this patient with a benzodiazepine or barbiturate prescription?
   Because this person is at high risk of continuing to abuse alcohol, the interactions of the benzodiazepines or barbiturates with alcohol can lead to respiratory depression and possibly even respiratory failure and death. Both drug classes also have a potential for dependence.

SUMMARY BOX: ALCOHOL AND RELATED DRUGS

- Thiamine (vitamin B_1) is an important cofactor for the production of adenosine triphosphate (ATP) from glucose.
- Thiamine deficiency, as seen in alcoholics, can cause Wernicke-Korsakoff syndrome, characterized by confusion (including confabulation), ataxia, ophthalmoplegia, and memory loss.
- Pathologically, the mammillary bodies, thalamus, and limbic system are affected in Wernicke-Korsakoff syndrome.
- Alcohol withdrawal can be treated acutely with benzodiazepines or barbiturates, which act as $GABA_A$ agonists and affect chloride channels.

CASE 17.17

A 48-year-old woman presents complaining of a new-onset headache that is worse in the morning. She additionally complains of being nauseated and has vomited several times in the past few weeks. Funduscopic examination reveals papilledema.

1. What does the clinical finding of papilledema in this woman represent?
   It represents edema of the optic disk, which is most commonly due to increased intracranial pressure, malignant hypertension, or central retinal vein occlusion.

2. Why might a brain tumor present with these symptoms?
   Brain tumors often present with mass effects, meaning that the symptoms are related to the effect of a mass compressing the brain and raising the pressure within the restricted space of the skull. Mass effects include hydrocephalus, papilledema, nausea/vomiting, headache, and mental status changes. Tumors may also present with seizures, focal neurologic signs, or dementia.

3. Given that our patient is an adult, what is the most likely location of a primary brain tumor? What about in a pediatric patient?
   Adult: Supratentorial, meaning that the tumor is located above the tentorium cerebelli (where the dura mater folds on itself, between the cerebrum and cerebellum).
      Child: Infratentorial, meaning that the tumor is located below the tentorium cerebelli.

CASE 17.17 CONTINUED:

The neurologic examination reveals focal deficits with strength and sensory loss in her left arm. An MRI reveals a brain mass in the right cerebral hemisphere. An extensive workup does not reveal any primary tumor outside the CNS. A biopsy is then performed and reveals the diagnosis of astrocytoma.

4. Prior to biopsy, why is a presumptive diagnosis of astrocytoma reasonable?
   Astrocytoma is the most common *primary* brain tumor in adults, although metastases are the most common sources of brain tumor *overall.* Metastatic brain cancer commonly presents with multiple lesions of varying size. However, when possible, biopsy must be done to distinguish between these two possibilities.

5. What type of astrocytoma has the worst prognosis?
   Glioblastoma multiforme (grade IV astrocytoma) is the most common primary brain tumor overall and carries the worst prognosis, with life expectancy under a year. Other lower grades of astrocytoma, such as juvenile pilocytic astrocytoma or anaplastic astrocytoma, may evolve into a glioblastoma multiforme.
      Note: Microscopically, glioblastoma multiforme has a characteristic *pseudopalisading arrangement* of pleomorphic tumor cells bordering central areas of necrosis and endothelial proliferation with hemorrhage. Grossly, the tumor often crosses over into both hemispheres (butterfly glioma).

STEP 1 SECRET

When studying primary brain tumors, it will be helpful to focus on unique histologic characteristics of the tumor cells themselves.

6. If our patient's CT scan had shown calcifications in the intracranial mass, what tumor types might we suspect?
   Meningiomas and oligodendrogliomas can both calcify, and both often arise in the frontal lobe. Microscopically, meningiomas have a whorled pattern with psammoma bodies; oligodendrogliomas have a "fried egg" appearance.

7. What is the second most common primary brain tumor in adults? In children?
   Adults: Meningioma, a benign tumor of arachnoid cells of the meninges, is second most common in adults. Because meningiomas are external to the brain (extra-axial), they can typically be resected easily during surgery. Meningiomas, however, have a propensity to recur.
      Children: Medulloblastoma, a malignant tumor of the cerebellum, is second most common in children. The most common type in children is astrocytoma.

8. What pharmacologic property of drugs such as lomustine and carmustine makes them more suitable for treatment of brain tumors?
   These drugs belong to a class of alkylating agents called *nitrosoureas* and can effectively penetrate the blood-brain barrier.

9. **What biophysical properties allow a drug to cross the blood-brain barrier?**
Generally, small, lipid-soluble, nonpolar molecules cross most easily.

SUMMARY BOX: BRAIN TUMORS

- Tumors in the brain often present with mass effect, seizures, focal neurologic signs, or personality changes.
- Most brain malignancies are metastases from tumors in other organs rather than primary brain tumors.
- Most primary brain tumors are located above the tentorium in adults and below the tentorium in children.
- The most common type of brain tumor is astrocytoma.
- The second most common type of brain tumor is meningioma in adults and medulloblastoma in children.
- Drugs that are small, nonpolar, and lipid-soluble penetrate the blood-brain barrier most easily.

CASE 17.18

You are examining a 6-year-old child with a history of epilepsy, intellectual impairment, and a heart murmur that was initially present at birth but resolved shortly thereafter. On physical examination, you note the presence of multiple, ovate, hypopigmented macules and a rough skin patch on the lower back.

1. **What is the most likely diagnosis in this child?**
Tuberous sclerosis, which is a rare, autosomal dominant neurocutaneous disorder that is marked by the presence of epileptogenic subependymal tubers, is the most likely diagnosis. Patients with tuberous sclerosis commonly experience seizures and some degree of cognitive impairment. The dermatologic findings in this patient (hypopigmented ash-leaf spots and the shagreen patch on his back) strengthen our confidence in this the diagnosis.

2. **Patients with neurocutaneous disorders are generally at risk for several different types of tumors. What tumors are most commonly associated with tuberous sclerosis?**
Renal angiomyolipoma, cardiac rhabdomyoma, CNS hamartomas (including retinal glial hamartomas), and subependymal giant cell astrocytomas are associated with tuberous sclerosis. The history of a cardiac murmur at birth that eventually resolved is good evidence that this child most likely had a cardiac rhabdomyoma, which often regresses spontaneously in these patients. Patients with tuberous sclerosis should be monitored regularly for evidence of these tumor types.

3. **If the patient in this case presented with hyperpigmented macules, pigmented nodules on the iris, and multiple neurofibromas covering the skin, what neurocutaneous disorder would you expect?**
This is a classic description of neurofibromatosis type I, which is characterized by café au lait spots, Lisch nodules, and multiple neurofibromas (Fig. 17.18). It is an autosomal dominant disorder that results from a mutation on chromosome 17. In contrast, neurofibromatosis type II results from a mutation on chromosome 22 and presents with tinnitus and sensorineural deafness due to the presence of bilateral schwannomas (this tumor type often localizes to and impinges on CN VIII).

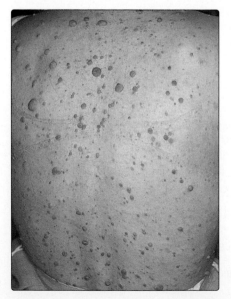

Figure 17.18. Multiple cutaneous neurofibromas. *(From Gawkrodger DJ, Ardern-Jones MR. Dermatology: An Illustrated Colour Text. 6th ed. London: Elsevier; 2017.)*

SUMMARY BOX: NEUROCUTANEOUS DISORDERS

- Symptoms of tuberous sclerosis result from the presence of subependymal tumors and include epilepsy, intellectual impairment, ash-leaf spots, and shagreen patches. Associated tumors include cardiac rhabdomyoma, renal angiomyolipoma, central nervous system (CNS) hamartomas, and giant cell astrocytoma.
- Neurofibromatosis I presents with neurofibromas, café au lait spots, and Lisch nodules on the iris.
- Neurofibromatosis II presents with tinnitus and sensorineural deafness due to the formation of bilateral schwannomas that impinge on CN VIII.

CASE 17.19

A 43-year-old woman is taken to the emergency department by ambulance following a minor motor vehicle accident. She complains of headache, neck pain on the sides of the neck, and lower back tightness on the sides of the back but appears otherwise normal on physical examination.

1. What is the most likely cause of this patient's symptoms?

   The patient appears to have experienced a minor cervical strain (whiplash) caused by rapid acceleration and deceleration, which can cause hyperextension of the neck and compression of soft tissues surrounding the spinal cord. Symptoms of cervical strain can be immediate or appear days later. They generally result from local inflammation around the spinal cord and include headache, neck/back pain, and tightness.

CASE 17.19 CONTINUED:

Her daughter picks her up from the emergency department, where she was discharged with a prescription for ibuprofen. Later that evening she begins experiencing intermittent dizziness and a "pulling sensation" to the right when she gets up from the couch to use the bathroom. She attributes it to the stress of the day and tries to sleep it off.

2. What is vertigo? Name some common causes of central and peripheral vertigo.

   Vertigo is a term describing the symptom of illusory movement, like the transient spinning sensation you experience after twirling around a few times. Approximately 80% of vertigo cases are peripheral in etiology; on boards this is most commonly tested as benign paroxysmal positional vertigo (BPPV), vestibular neuritis, or Meniere disease. BPPV is typically attributed to calcium deposits in the posterior semicircular canal. Vestibular neuritis is caused by inflammation of the vestibular nerve, possibly due to a viral infection, and is easily treated with corticosteroids. Meniere disease is particularly high yield for boards and results from an idiopathic increase in endolymphatic fluid pressure.

   Central vertigo typically involves the vestibular nuclei in the brainstem but can also involve the cerebellum. Damage to these nuclei commonly occurs with various patterns of brainstem ischemia, multiple sclerosis, cerebellar infarction, or the presence of a Chiari I malformation. It is important to note that central vertigo never occurs in isolation and will always be accompanied by other neurologic deficits.

3. Damage to what brainstem structure could cause her difficulty with balance?

   The patient appears to be experiencing lateropulsion, which is a pulling sensation to one side. This is commonly a result of damage to the ipsilateral vestibulocerebellar system, such as the inferior cerebellar peduncle, and is distinct from muscle weakness or vertigo.

CASE 17.19 CONTINUED:

The next day she is extremely dizzy when she wakes up. She struggles to sit up without falling to her right side. She calls in sick to work and stays in bed that morning. Her daughter brings her breakfast, which she refuses to eat, complaining that the food tastes funny and is sticking in her throat, causing her to gag. She also complains of double vision and decreased pain and temperature sensation of her right face and her left trunk/extremities. She appears clumsy and struggles to take her ibuprofen. Her daughter, who is now very concerned, brings her back to the emergency department for further evaluation.

4. Which brainstem structures are involved in pain and temperature sensation to the face and body, respectively? What is the significance of crossed findings?

   The spinal trigeminal nucleus sits in the lateral medulla and is responsible for relaying pain and temperature information from the ipsilateral face to higher brainstem regions. The spinothalamic tract carries pain and temperature information through the lateral medulla from the contralateral body, crossing through the gray matter of the spinal cord a few levels above the entry point of the corresponding peripheral nerve fibers. Crossed findings are highly suggestive of a brainstem lesion because this is the only anatomic location where information from different sides of the face and body are transmitted in close proximity to each other.

5. **Damage to which brainstem structures could cause diplopia?**
   Eye movements are controlled by the third, fourth, and sixth cranial nerves. Damage to any of these nerves or their associated brainstem nuclei will lead to diplopia.

6. **Which brainstem structure is important in swallowing and speech production? Taste sensation?**
   The nucleus ambiguus in the lateral medulla is responsible for the motor innervation of the ipsilateral palate, pharynx, and larynx (CN IX, X, and XI). Lesion of this nucleus would result in hoarseness and dysphagia due to paralysis of the oropharyngeal muscles. On physical examination, you would expect to see ipsilateral vocal cord paralysis and uvular deviation *away* from the affected side on phonation, as the lesion would result in an inability to elevate the ipsilateral palate.
   The nucleus solitarius is important for taste sensation and is present in the lateral medulla.

CASE 17.19 CONTINUED:

On further examination, the attending physician notes that her right pupil is 2 mm bigger than her left pupil. He also notes some drooping (ptosis) and dryness (anhidrosis) of the right eye. He also observes nystagmus, dysmetria, uvular deviation to the left side, and marked ataxia in the neurologic examination.

7. **What classic triad of ocular symptoms is this patient exhibiting? How is it related to her other symptoms?**
   The patient is exhibiting Horner syndrome, which is caused by a loss of sympathetic input to the face. The oculosympathetic pathway begins in the hypothalamus and is comprised of three neurons. The first-order neuron projects ipsilaterally from the hypothalamus to the lateral horn of T1 spinal cord, traveling down the intermediolateral column of the spinal cord. The second-order neuron then projects up the sympathetic chain to the superior cervical ganglion. Finally, the third-order neuron branches to follow the external and internal carotid arteries, innervating the sweat glands of the face, as well as the smooth muscle of the eyelid and pupil. Any interruption of this pathway results in *ipsilateral* Horner syndrome, a triad of unilateral ptosis, miosis, and anhidrosis. Common causes of Horner syndrome include damage to the lateral medulla, a lesion of the spinal cord above T1 (Brown-Séquard syndrome, Pancoast tumor, syringomyelia), and carotid dissection.

8. **What is the most likely cause of her symptoms?**
   The combination of vertigo, Horner syndrome, ataxia, dysmetria, dysphagia, hoarseness, taste change, and lack of pain and temperature sensation on opposite sides of the face and body all point to lateral medullary syndrome (Wallenberg syndrome). Wallenberg syndrome is a cluster of symptoms caused by occlusion of the posterior inferior cerebellar artery (PICA), which results in the infarction of brainstem nuclei involved in these functions normally and subsequent neurologic deficits.

CASE 17.19 CONTINUED:

The physician suspects a brainstem stroke and orders an MRI of her neck, which reveals hyperintensity of the right vertebral artery, which is highly suggestive of arterial dissection. She is started on aspirin and clopidogrel (antiplatelet therapy) and is admitted to the neurology unit for observation and supportive care. Her condition slowly improves, and she is discharged from the hospital a few weeks later. She is eventually able to return to her normal routine with no residual deficits, but she remains on her new drug regimen.

9. **How did this injury likely occur? How can arterial dissection cause a clot?**
   The PICA is a branch of the vertebral artery, and damage to the vertebral artery is the most common cause of Wallenberg syndrome. The region of the vertebral artery that lies along C1 is most vulnerable to damage and is commonly affected by major trauma to the neck as can occur in a motor vehicle accident. Trauma can cause the artery to tear, exposing the tunica media and externa to blood flow. Tissue factor then initiates the occurrence of secondary hemostasis, resulting in blood clot formation. Eventually the clot can occlude the vessel entirely or throw off an embolus, which then gets lodged in smaller blood vessels, causing ischemia in the surrounding tissue.
   Note: Dissection is the most common cause of stroke in younger patients (Fig. 17.19).

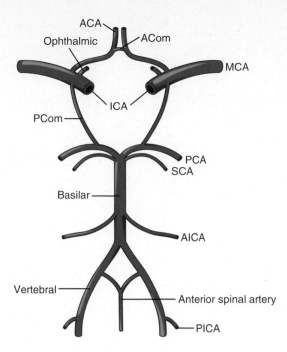

Figure 17.19. Circle of Willis, major supply and distributing vessels. Supply vessels include the left and right internal carotid arteries (*ICA*) and the left and right vertebral arteries. The major distributing vessels include the anterior cerebral arteries (*ACA*), middle cerebral arteries (*MCA*), and posterior cerebral arteries (*PCA*). The anterior and posterior communicating arteries (*ACom, PCom*) complete this vascular loop and allow for collateral blood flow between vascular territories. The major branches of the vertebrobasilar system are also labeled. *AICA,* Anterior inferior cerebellar artery; *PICA,* posterior inferior cerebellar artery; *SCA,* superior cerebellar artery. *(From Hemmings Jr HC, Egan TD.* Pharmacology and Physiology for Anesthesia. *Philadelphia: Elsevier; 2013.)*

OPHTHALMOLOGY

BASIC CONCEPTS

1. Describe the course of visual information arriving from the left and right visual fields.
    1. Light from the left visual field encounters the right half of each retina, nasally in the left and temporally in the right eye (Fig. 18.1).
    2. Fibers from the temporal retina of the right eye travel in the right optic nerve and pass along the outside of the optic chiasm without crossing.
    3. Fibers from the nasal retina of the left eye travel in the left optic nerve to the optic chiasm, where they cross over and join the temporal fibers from the right eye to form the right optic tract (Fig. 18.2).
    4. The right optic tract synapses primarily in the right lateral geniculate nucleus (LGN; located in the thalamus) and in the Edinger-Westphal nucleus for pupillary reactions (located in the midbrain).
    5. Projections from the right LGN divide. The left upper visual field information travels through the temporal lobe, and the left lower visual field information travels through the parietal lobe.
    6. These optic projections synapse in the right visual cortex within the occipital lobe.
        The visual information coming from the right visual field follows the same concepts as described for the left visual field but encounters the left half of each retina. The input from the right visual field of the two eyes is combined at the chiasm and travels to the left side of the brain.

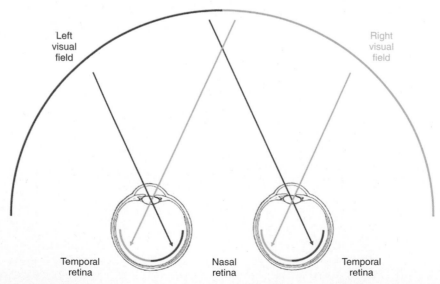

Figure. 18.1. The temporal visual field information is received by the nasal retina, and the nasal visual field is received by the temporal retina. *(Courtesy Katie Carsky.)*

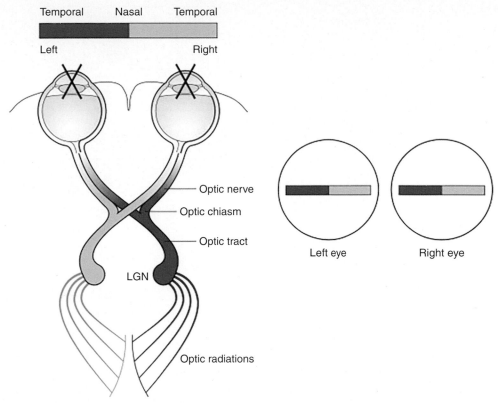

Figure. 18.2. The red path shows the course of sensory information from the left visual field. The gray path shows the course of sensory information from the right visual field. *LGN*, lateral geniculate nucleus. *(From Kaufman DM, Geyer HL, Milstein MJ.* Kaufman's Clinical Neurology for Psychiatrists, *8th ed. Philadelphia: Elsevier; 2017: 27–54, Fig. 4.1.)*

2. What visual field defect results from midline sectioning of the optic chiasm?

   Bitemporal hemianopia, which is a loss of the temporal (lateral) fields of vision in both eyes that results in "tunnel vision," is the resulting defect. Recall that the optic chiasm contains fibers from the left and right nasal retinas as they cross over. The left nasal retina receives visual input from the left temporal visual field, while the right nasal retina receives visual input from the right temporal visual field. These fibers travel through their respective optic nerves and cross at the optic chiasm, where they then join the temporal fibers from the opposite eye to form the optic tract. Thus, a lesion in the optic chiasm will result in an inability to see the temporal fields bilaterally, resulting in a constricted visual field.

   One of the most common causes of bitemporal hemianopia tested on the boards is a pituitary tumor compressing the optic chiasm. Pituitary tumors to be aware of include craniopharyngiomas, which are embryologic derivatives of the Rathke pouch that commonly occur in children, and prolactinomas, which commonly occur in adults and can present with galactorrhea, amenorrhea, and hypogonadism. Fig. 18.3 shows the visual field deficits resulting from lesions at various points in optic pathways. Take the time now to think about why all of these occur to ensure that you fully understand the course of visual information. We will continue to practice throughout the rest of this chapter.

STEP 1 SECRET

Boards may not openly make the diagnosis of bitemporal hemianopia for you when, for instance, describing a patient with a pituitary tumor. You will often have to arrive at this conclusion for yourself in the context of patient history. Be on the lookout for clues such as a patient's inability to see traffic on the left and the right (i.e., peripheral vision defect) when driving.

3. What visual field deficit will occur with sectioning of the left optic tract and why?

   Right homonymous hemianopia results from the loss of the right field of vision in both eyes. The left optic tract receives input from the right nasal retina and left temporal retina, both of which receive information from the right visual space (see Figs. 18.1, 18.2, and 18.3).

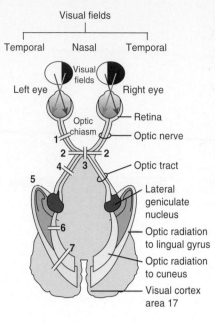

Lesion	Visual defect
1. Optic nerve	Ipsilateral blindness
Optic chiasm 2. Bilateral lateral compression	Binasal hemianopia
3. Midsagittal transection/ pressure	Bitemporal hemianopia
4. Optic tract (left)	Right hemianopia
Optic radiation (left) 5. Lower division	Right upper quandrantanopia
6. Upper division	Right lower quandrantanopia
7. Both divisions	Right hemianopia with macular sparing

Figure. 18.3. The visual pathways, showing the consequences of lesions at various points. *(From Brown TA.* Rapid Review Physiology. *Philadelphia: Mosby; 2007.)*

4. **What visual field deficit is likely with a tumor in the right temporal lobe?**
   Left superior homonymous quadrantanopia, loss of left upper quadrant of the visual field in both eyes ("pie in the sky"), would result. Temporal radiations from the right LGN travel through the temporal lobe as the Meyer loop on their way to the visual cortex. A tumor in this area will damage these fibers, causing loss of the contralateral superior quarter of the visual field from each eye. These patients might also experience seizures or olfactory hallucinations.

STEP 1 SECRET

Visual field defects that result from damage to the optic nerve, optic chiasm, optic tract, lateral geniculate body, or occipital cortex are favorites on boards. Be sure to pay special attention to the side (left or right) on which the damage occurs. Do not hesitate to diagram these pathways on your marker board if you encounter one of these problems on test day. Being able to localize a lesion in this pathway is the single most important skill you can learn from this chapter.

5. **A physician shines a light into a patient's right eye and notes bilateral constriction of both pupils (normal response). Describe the pupillary light reflex.**
   The pupillary light reflex consists of an afferent limb, conducted by the optic nerve (CN II), and an efferent limb, conducted by the parasympathetic fibers of the oculomotor nerve (CN III). When light is shone in one eye, there should be direct pupillary constriction of the ipsilateral pupil and consensual constriction of the contralateral pupil because of the following pathway:
   1. Light shone in the right eye activates the photosensitive retinal ganglion cells of the right eye, which convey this information to the right optic nerve.
   2. The right optic nerve sends fibers with input from the nasal retina to the left pretectal nucleus of the upper midbrain (it also sends input from the temporal retina to the right pretectal nucleus, but that is not the focus here).
   3. Axons connect from the left pretectal nucleus of the upper midbrain to neurons in the left and right Edinger-Westphal nuclei.
   4. Each Edinger-Westphal nucleus has axons that run along both the right and left oculomotor nerves.
   5. The right and left oculomotor nerves synapse on the ciliary ganglion neurons of each respective eye, which innervate the constrictor muscles of the irises, thus stimulating bilateral pupillary constriction.
      Note: When light is shone in the left eye, retinal ganglion cells are activated on the left side, and the information continues on the visual pathway, thus also resulting in bilateral constriction of both pupils (Fig. 18.4).

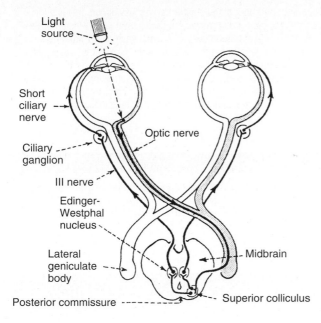

Figure. 18.4. Pathway of pupillary response in the left optic nerve. *(From Lindsay KW, Bone I, Callander R. Neurology and Neurosurgery Illustrated. 3rd ed. Edinburgh: Churchill Livingstone; 2002.)*

Labels in figure: Light source; Short ciliary nerve; Optic nerve; Ciliary ganglion; III nerve; Edinger-Westphal nucleus; Lateral geniculate body; Posterior commissure; Midbrain; Superior colliculus

6. If there is a lesion in the left optic nerve, what would be the pupillary response if a light is shone into the right eye versus the left eye?
   1. Right eye
      Damage to the left optic nerve impairs only the left afferent limb of the reflex, while both the right and the left efferent limbs will be intact because these are conducted by the parasympathetic fibers of the respective left and right oculomotor nerves. Thus, if light is shone into the right eye, there will be bilateral pupillary constriction.
   2. Left eye
      Although the efferent limbs of both eyes are intact, no signal will be transmitted to activate the reflex arc because the afferent limb of the left eye is impaired. Thus, there will be no pupillary constriction in either eye (see Fig. 18.4).

Clinical Pearl

Damage to the optic nerve can be evaluated on physical exam with the swinging-flashlight test. During this test, a light is swung from one eye to the other. The unaffected eye will constrict in response to light, but when the light is swung toward the affected eye, the reflex arc will not be activated and bilateral pupillary constriction will be lost. This is referred to as *Marcus Gunn pupil* (afferent pupillary defect) and is commonly seen in patients with optic neuritis or retinal detachment.

---

7. What will the pupillary response be to shining a light in either eye if there is a lesion in the left oculomotor nerve?
   The key to this question is to recognize that the afferent limb of the reflex arc in both eyes is intact, but the left efferent response is damaged. Thus, if light is shown into either eye, only the right pupil will constrict.

8. What is an Argyll Robertson pupil?
   An Argyll Robertson pupil demonstrates normal pupillary constriction during accommodation, but there is no pupillary constriction in response to light. Accommodation is the physiologic response of the eyes that occurs when focusing on close-up objects through adjustment of the lens shape and pupillary constriction. This is seen in patients with neurosyphilis, systemic lupus erythematosus, diabetes mellitus, Parinaud syndrome, Wernicke encephalopathy, or other lesions of the Edinger-Westphal nucleus.
      Note: Parinaud syndrome is uncommon but important to know for Step 1 because it is most commonly caused by a pinealoma. The syndrome is manifested by Argyll Robertson pupils and vertical gaze palsy.

9. If the oculomotor nerve is paralyzed on one side, why is the eyeball on that side rotated laterally and inferiorly ("down and out")?
   The oculomotor nerve innervates all the extraocular muscles other than the lateral rectus and superior oblique, which are innervated by the abducens nerve (CN VI) and the trochlear nerve (CN IV), respectively (remember the mnemonic LR_6SO_4). The lateral rectus moves the eyeball laterally (abduction), and the superior oblique rotates it inferiorly, giving the "down and out" position in oculomotor nerve palsy. An important neurologic distinction to make when discussing

oculomotor nerve palsy is whether the pupil is involved. A pupil-sparing oculomotor nerve palsy occurs in vascular disorders, such as diabetes, because the motor fibers responsible for eye movement are located on the inside of the nerve, where they are most susceptible to vascular insult by lack of blood flow to the distal vasa nervorum. The parasympathetic fibers responsible for pupillary constriction are located on the outside of the oculomotor nerve, so they are spared in the setting of vascular disorders. The outer location of the parasympathetic fibers also means that they are the first fibers affected by compressive forces, such as increased intracranial pressure, aneurysms, and uncal herniation. Being able to distinguish between a compressive nerve palsy and a diabetic oculomotor nerve palsy is a commonly tested and important distinction, because a compressive oculomotor nerve palsy could indicate a neurosurgical emergency.

STEP 1 SECRET

The pupillary light reflex and functions of the eye muscles are routinely tested on boards. You should know what happens with lesions of specific cranial nerves. As is true for Chapter 17 (Neurology), your most important task is being able to localize the lesion from a set of signs and symptoms. The functions of the extraocular muscles are listed in Table 18.1.

Table 18.1. Functions of Extraocular Muscles

EXTRAOCULAR MUSCLE	INNERVATION	FUNCTION(S)
Inferior rectus	CN III	Depression Extorsion
Superior rectus	CN III	Elevation Intorsion
Lateral rectus	CN VI	Abduction
Medial rectus	CN III	Adduction
Superior oblique	CN IV	Intorsion Depression
Inferior oblique	CN III	Extorsion Elevation
Levator palpebrae superioris	CN III	Elevates eyelid

10. Describe the function of the medial longitudinal fasciculus.

The medial longitudinal fasciculus (MLF) allows both eyes to move in the same direction in an attempt to track an object when one eye is stimulated. For example, when one looks to the left, the following steps occur:

1. The paramedian pontine reticular formation, which is the horizontal gaze center, activates the left abducens nerve (CN VI), which innervates the lateral rectus muscle.
2. Activation of the left abducens nerve simultaneously stimulates the contralateral oculomotor nerve (CN III) nucleus via the MLF.
3. Activation of the contralateral oculomotor nerve, which innervates the medial rectus muscle, causes adduction of the right eye and conjugate eye movements.

Lesions of the MLF are important to recognize because they cause internuclear ophthalmoplegia, which presents on physical exam as nystagmus of the abducting eye and complete lack of movement in the adducting eye. The eye that is unable to adduct indicates the side of the MLF affected. Internuclear ophthalmoplegia is associated with multiple sclerosis, which is discussed further in Chapter 17 (Neurology).

Note: The MLF does not affect convergence, which is the simultaneous inward movement of both eyes toward one another (adduction) and is a disconjugate movement. Convergence is part of a triad that allows us to see nearby objects. The other two components of this triad are accommodation and pupillary constriction (Fig. 18.5).

11. What is pathologic nystagmus?

Pathologic nystagmus refers to an involuntary smooth pursuit movement of the eye in one direction followed by a saccadic movement in the opposing direction. It can occur with damage to the vestibular system, including the semicircular canals, and the vestibulocerebellum. Nystagmus is also common in brainstem and cerebellar strokes and is a side effect of many medications, including phenytoin. Torsional/rotatory or vertical nystagmus can also be seen with intoxication with *N*-methyl-D-aspartate antagonists, such as ketamine, phencyclidine, and dextromethorphan.

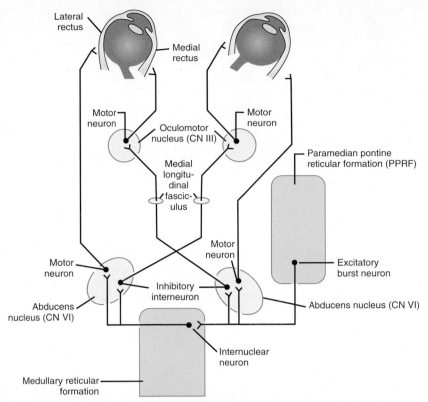

Figure. 18.5. Neural circuit by which the horizontal gaze center elicits conjugate eye movements. Excitation of burst neurons of the right horizontal gaze center causes activation of abducens motor neurons on the right and medial rectus motor neurons on the left. The ascending pathway to the oculomotor nucleus is through the medial longitudinal fasciculus. The left horizontal gaze center is simultaneously inhibited by way of the reticular formation. *(From Berne RM, Levy MN, Koeppen BM, Stanton BA.* Physiology. *5th ed. Philadelphia: Mosby; 2003.)*

CASE 18.1

A 70-year-old hyperopic ("farsighted") man presents with acutely decreased vision, redness, and pain in one eye. Fundoscopic examination reveals cupping of the optic nerve, and a tonometer measurement indicates a significant elevation of the intraocular pressure.

1. What is the most likely diagnosis?
   The most likely diagnosis is glaucoma, which describes a group of diseases associated with elevated intraocular pressure.

2. What is the difference between open-angle glaucoma and closed-angle glaucoma?
   The "angle" refers to the junction of cornea and iris, where the aqueous humor drains through the trabecular meshwork into the canal of Schlemm. In open-angle glaucoma, the angle is clinically open, but drainage is still chronically compromised (Fig. 18.6A). This leads to chronic, painless elevation of pressure and gradual damage to the optic nerve, resulting in peripheral and then central vision loss. In closed-angle glaucoma, the lens moves forward against the posterior surface of the iris, pushing the iris forward against the cornea (Fig. 18.6B). This results in blockage of the trabecular meshwork. An acute obstruction of outflow causes a severe elevation of intraocular pressure, leading to pain, sudden vision loss, rock-hard eye, and halos around lights. This is a true ophthalmic emergency, and if not treated immediately, closed-angle glaucoma can lead to severe optic nerve damage and loss of vision.

3. What is the mechanism by which beta-blockers reduce intraocular pressure in glaucoma?
   Beta-blockers inhibit the production of aqueous humor, thereby lowering the intraocular pressure. Because of some systemic absorption, nonselective beta-blockers should be avoided in individuals with severe asthma (because of their β_2-antagonistic effect on the lungs, which enhances bronchoconstriction).

4. What is the mechanism of action by which topical and oral carbonic anhydrase agents (e.g., acetazolamide) could be used to treat this man's glaucoma?
   Like beta-blockers, carbonic anhydrase inhibitors also inhibit the production of aqueous humor, thereby lowering intraocular pressure.

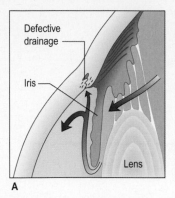

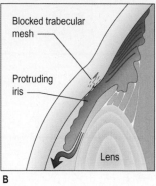

Figure. 18.6. Open-angle glaucoma (A) and closed-angle glaucoma (B). *(From Vaz F, Nishchay M, Hamilton RD. Kumar and Clark's Clinical Medicine. 9th ed. Philadelphia: Elsevier; 2017: 1311–1336, Fig. 30.39.)*

RELATED QUESTIONS

5. Why are cholinomimetics such as pilocarpine and carbachol useful for closed-angle glaucoma?
   One of the mechanisms causing angle closure is iris dilation by the peripheral iris tissue (e.g., triggered by darkness). Angle closure caused by peripheral iris dilation can be relieved by parasympathetic cholinergic nerves stimulating constriction of sphincter pupillae via the M3 receptors. Cholinomimetics such as pilocarpine will constrict the pupil, pulling the iris from the angle and allowing it to open and improve drainage.

6. Why should epinephrine be avoided in closed-angle glaucoma?
   Although epinephrine is useful in open-angle glaucoma by preventing aqueous humor synthesis, it also causes mydriasis by stimulating the pupillary dilator muscle. Mydriasis will increase the obstruction between iris and lens in closed-angle glaucoma.

STEP 1 SECRET

The drugs used to treat glaucoma and their mechanisms of action are far more high yield for boards than the anatomy or pathophysiology of the disease.

SUMMARY BOX: GLAUCOMA

- Presentation
  - Open-angle glaucoma: Typically asymptomatic, but over time can lead to peripheral vision loss
  - Closed-angle glaucoma: Acute onset of visual loss and eye pain
- Pathophysiology: Obstruction of the flow of aqueous humor out of the angle between the cornea and the iris
  - Open-angle glaucoma: Angle is still open, but drainage is chronically compromised
  - Closed-angle glaucoma: Lens moves forward against the posterior surface of the iris with pupillary dilation, causing an acute blockage that leads to a severe elevation of intraocular pressure and damage to the optic nerve
- Complications: Vision loss
- Treatment: Beta-blockers, carbonic anhydrase inhibitors, cholinomimetics for treatment of closed-angle glaucoma
- Prognosis
  - Open-angle glaucoma: Progressive peripheral visual field loss without treatment
  - Closed-angle glaucoma: An ophthalmologic emergency; without timely treatment, permanent vision loss can occur

CASE 18.2

A 70-year-old man who smokes one pack of cigarettes per day presents with central vision loss, describing that straight lines appear wavy. Funduscopic examination reveals abnormal blood vessel growth and bleeding in the macula.

1. What is the most likely diagnosis?
   AMD with choroidal neovascularization ("wet" AMD) is most likely.

2. What is the difference between "dry" and "wet" AMD?
   "Dry" (nonexudative) AMD is the most common form of AMD and occurs because of a breakdown of the photoreceptor cells. Drusen, which are yellow-white deposits of extracellular material, form under the macula and are associated with vision loss. "Wet" (exudative) AMD is less common and attributed to abnormal growth of blood vessels in the choroid. Rupturing of these blood vessels can cause blood to leak into the retina and damage the macula. Note that dry AMD can progress to wet AMD.

3. Where is the macula, and what is its function?

The macula is a yellow spot near the central part of the retina. The fovea is located in the macula. The fovea has the highest concentration of cone photoreceptor cells, allowing us to see at the highest visual acuity.

4. What is the mechanism of action for the intravitreal injection of ranibizumab that will be used to treat this man's AMD?

Ranibizumab is an antibody fragment that can bind to and inactivate vascular endothelial growth factor A, a potent angiogenic factor. Inhibition of vascular endothelial growth factor A can prevent the growth of new vessels, potentially improving vision in wet AMD.

5. What simple diagnostic test can be conducted to detect AMD?

In patients with AMD, straight lines may start appearing wavy. An Amsler grid, which is a grid made up of vertical and horizontal lines, can be used to quickly assess a patient's vision.

6. What treatments are available for dry AMD?

Currently, the only treatments shown to help prevent progression are multivitamin and antioxidant supplements, specifically vitamin C and E, β-carotene, zinc, copper, lutein, and omega-3 fatty acids.

SUMMARY BOX: AGE-RELATED MACULAR DEGENERATION

- Presentation: Central vision loss and reports that "straight lines are appearing wavy"
- Pathophysiology
  - Dry age-related macular degeneration (AMD): Characterized by blurring of central vision, drusen deposits under the macula
  - Wet AMD: Characterized by abnormal blood vessel growth and "leakage of blood," leading to severe vision loss
- Diagnosis: Amsler grid
- Treatment: Multivitamins and antioxidants for dry AMD; ranibizumab (vascular endothelial growth factor A inhibitor) for wet AMD

CASE 18.3

A 60-year-old man with a history of cataract surgery presents with a sudden onset of flashing light in the periphery of his visual fields, floaters, and the feeling that a curtain has been drawn over his field of vision.

1. What is the most likely diagnosis?

Retinal detachment is the most likely diagnosis. Retinal detachment occurs when the retina separates from the underlying retinal pigment epithelium and choroid. This results in rapid ischemia and photoreceptor degeneration. It commonly presents with a sudden onset of floaters and decrease in vision.

2. What are some common risk factors for retinal detachment?

Myopia, cataract surgery, ocular trauma, and ocular inflammation are all risk factors.

3. How is retinal detachment treated?

Retinal detachment is treated with surgical reattachment of the retina. Retinal detachment is especially important to know for Step 1 because permanent vision loss will result if it is not rapidly repaired.

SUMMARY BOX: RETINAL DETACHMENT

- Presentation: Sudden onset of floaters, decrease in vision
- Risk factors: Myopia, cataract surgery, ocular trauma, and ocular inflammation
- Pathophysiology: Separation of retina from underlying blood supply
- Complications: Vision loss
- Treatment: Surgery

BASIC CONCEPTS

1. What is a "diarthrodial" joint?
   A diarthrodial joint is a joint in which bones meet in cartilage-covered surfaces (e.g., shoulder, hip, interphalangeal joints). They are primarily designed for mobility. The diarthrodial joint is the most common type of joint found in the body. These joints are composed of articulating bones covered by cartilage (usually hyaline cartilage). A fibrous capsule surrounds and protects the joint. The diarthrodial joint cavity is lined with a synovial membrane, which produces synovial fluid to lubricate the joint space. Ligamentous connections provide support and typically allow for a large amount of movement (Fig. 19.1).

   Note: In contrast with diarthrodial joints, synarthrodial joints exist where bones meet by fibrous connections without a joint space. These joints prevent motion between bones. The suture lines in the skull are an example of synarthroses. Amphiarthrodial joints consist of bones bound by fibrocartilage, which allows some limited degree of movement. The joints between vertebrae and the pubic symphysis are examples of amphiarthroses.

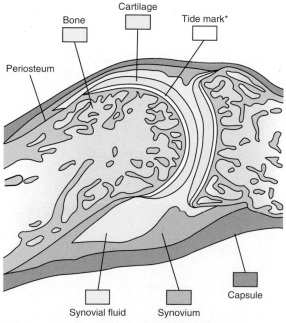

*Interface between calcified and noncalcified cartilage matrix.

Figure 19.1. Normal interphalangeal joint, in sagittal section, as an example of a synovial, or diarthrodial, joint. *Interface between calcified and noncalcified cartilage matrix. *(From Sokoloff L, Bland JH. The Musculoskeletal System. Baltimore: Williams & Wilkins; 1975.)*

2. Which sites within a diarthrodial joint are vulnerable to disease?
   Each of the components of the joint may be involved in disease processes (see Fig. 19.1).

CASE 19.1

A 55-year-old obese woman presents with several months of bilateral knee pain. The pain is worst at the end of the day and is exacerbated by activity but improves with rest. She experiences approximately 10 to 15 minutes of morning stiffness each day but otherwise denies constitutional concerns, such as fever, anorexia, weight loss, or fatigue.

1. What is the differential diagnosis?
   The differential diagnosis for symmetric joint pain is broad and includes rheumatoid arthritis (RA), osteoarthritis (OA), spondyloarthropathies such as ankylosing spondylitis or psoriatic arthritis, crystal arthropathy such as gout or pseudogout, and septic arthritis. In a middle-aged obese woman with involvement of weight-bearing joints and no systemic symptoms, OA seems most likely. A chronic course with asymptomatic periods is not consistent with septic arthritis.

CASE 19.1 CONTINUED:

The patient is moderately obese. None of her joints are warm, swollen, or tender. Aside from some crepitus with passive movement, examination of her knees is normal. The proximal and distal interphalangeal joints in both hands are enlarged but nontender. Plain film of the right knee is shown in Fig. 19.2.

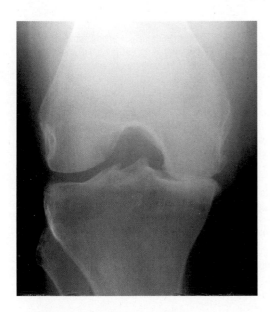

Figure 19.2. Plain film of the knee for patient in Case 19.1. *(From Harris ED, Budd RC, Genovese MC, et al. Kelley's Textbook of Rheumatology. 7th ed. Philadelphia: WB Saunders; 2005.)*

2. What is the likely diagnosis?
   Given the patient's history and x-ray findings (narrowing of the medial compartment joint space), OA (also known as *osteoarthrosis*, *degenerative joint disease*, or *hypertrophic arthritis*) is most likely. OA is the most common joint disease worldwide. It is characterized by loss of articular cartilage, which results in damage to the underlying bone. This process results primarily in pain (especially in weight-bearing joints), as well as stiffness and loss of joint mobility. The process is noninflammatory, so there is no ankylosis (fusion) of the joint. Loss of the smooth articulating surface accounts for the finding of crepitus (crunching sound) when the joint is moved. Pain is typically worse with use of the joint and decreases with rest. Reactive bone formation resulting in osteophytes (bone spurs) also occurs at the joint margins and may cause pain. Joints typically affected include the knees, hips, and proximal and distal interphalangeal (DIP) joints (Bouchard and Heberden nodes, respectively). Fig. 19.3 shows both Bouchard and Heberden nodes.
   Note: Recall that OA typically does *not* affect the metacarpophalangeal joints, while RA typically does *not* affect the DIP joint.

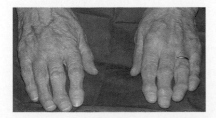

Figure 19.3. Typical hand deformities in osteoarthritis. Heberden nodes are seen on the distal interphalangeal joints, and Bouchard nodes are seen at the proximal interphalangeal joints. *(From Forbes CD, Jackson WF. Color Atlas and Text of Clinical Medicine. 3rd ed. London: Mosby; 2003.)*

3. **Is the pathogenesis of this condition primarily related to degeneration of bone, cartilage, or synovial membrane?**

OA is characterized by degeneration of articular cartilage and is often associated with overuse or trauma to the joint. Chondrocytes produce the type II cartilage that makes up the articular cartilage, and altered chondrocyte function has been demonstrated to occur in OA. When articular cartilage is not maintained properly, the bones in the diarthrodial joint may come into direct contact with one another. This wear and tear leads to abnormal bone proliferation with the formation of osteophytes (bone spurs).

RA differs from OA in that the primary site of damage is the synovium. Unlike OA, RA is characterized by systemic inflammation that is immune mediated. Rheumatoid joints often appear red and swollen (synovitis), whereas joints affected by OA typically do not.

4. **What is the anatomic source of the joint pain in OA?**

Although cartilage is the primary site of injury in this disease, there is no neural input to cartilage and therefore no pain transmission from it. The pain of OA actually comes from the periosteum (dense fibrous tissue) surrounding the bone. The periosteum is highly innervated and is damaged when the cartilage has worn away to the point that bone is rubbing on bone.

Note: Joint cartilage is also completely avascular, which explains why injured cartilage will not heal.

5. **What are some risk factors associated with development of OA?**

Risk factors for OA include anything that increases the mechanical forces to which the joint cartilage is exposed, for example, obesity, occupation (repetitive motions), intense physical activity, joint trauma, and muscle weakness (likely from joint instability). Gender, hormones, and genetics are involved as well. Women are more likely to have OA than men, and elderly populations are affected by this disease much more often than young people. There are certain forms of OA that appear to be heritable.

Note: OA can be classified as primary (idiopathic), the most common, or secondary, with an underlying cause (e.g., trauma, obesity, Paget disease, metabolic disorders). Diseases that involve the systemic deposition of certain compounds, such as hemochromatosis (iron), Wilson disease (copper), and the crystal arthropathies, may be causes of secondary OA.

6. **Would you expect the erythrocyte sedimentation rate or C-reactive protein to be elevated in this patient?**

No. An elevated erythrocyte sedimentation rate (ESR) or C-reactive protein (CRP) is a nonspecific indicator of a systemic inflammatory process. Because OA is a local degenerative disease, these markers would probably not be elevated in this patient. (Note that unlike RA, OA does not result in systemic symptoms.) In addition, although severe joint degeneration caused by OA may lead to inflammation, this inflammatory response is confined to the joint space.

Note: Although OA is classically considered a noninflammatory disease, it is interesting to note that pharmacologic treatment frequently involves the use of nonsteroidal antiinflammatory drugs (NSAIDs), which act by reducing pain and inflammation within the joint space. The efficacy of intra-articular steroid injections for OA have recently come into question based on randomized data failing to show benefit over placebo injection.

7. **How do the findings on x-ray studies generally differ between OA and RA?**

The characteristic radiologic finding in OA is joint space narrowing (see Fig. 19.2) due to the loss of cartilage between the bones. There may also be evidence of bony proliferation, such as increased density of the bones abutting the joint (subchondral sclerosis or eburnation) and presence of osteophytes. Chondrocalcinosis (calcium in the articular cartilage) and subchondral cysts may also be evident.

In RA, in contrast, there are often marginal erosions of bone and osteoporotic changes (demineralization), and the joint space is typically normal. However, if the RA is severe enough, the inflammatory process may eventually destroy articular cartilage and also narrow the joint space.

Fig. 19.4A demonstrates nearly complete loss of the lateral and medial joint spaces in RA, whereas Fig. 19.4B demonstrates loss of only the medial joint space with subchondral sclerosis (increased density) of the underlying bone in OA.

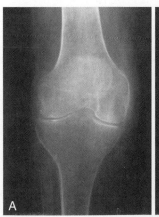
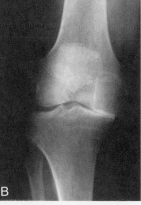

Figure 19.4. Radiographs of the knees in the two most common forms of arthritis: rheumatoid arthritis and osteoarthritis. A, Severe involvement in rheumatoid arthritis, with almost complete symmetric loss of joint space in both the medial and lateral compartments, with little subchondral sclerosis or osteophyte formation. B, Typical osteoarthritis, with severe, near-total loss of joint space of one compartment and a normal or actually increased joint space of the other compartment. *(From Goldman L, Ausiello D. Cecil Textbook of Medicine. 22nd ed. Philadelphia: WB Saunders; 2004.)*

8. NSAIDs and cyclooxygenase-2 inhibitors are both possible treatments for OA. What is similar about their mechanisms of action, and what is different?

Both classes of drug inhibit prostaglandin synthesis by inhibiting cyclooxygenase (COX), an enzyme that converts arachidonic acid to prostanoids (prostaglandins, prostacyclins, and thromboxanes), and by doing so cause relief of pain. All NSAIDs reversibly inhibit COX-1 and COX-2, except aspirin, which irreversibly inhibits them. The selective COX-2 inhibitor inhibits a form of COX induced in inflammatory cells, but not the constitutively expressed COX-1 that is produced for various normal body functions. Thus selective COX-2 inhibitors spare the gastrointestinal (GI) side effects associated with nonselective COX inhibition.

9. What is the principal therapeutic advantage of the COX-2 inhibitors? What can be given to this patient with an NSAID to prevent their principal side effect?

COX-1 is responsible for GI prostaglandin synthesis, which protects and maintains the GI mucosa. NSAIDs disrupt GI prostaglandin synthesis and can result in gastric ulceration, a common side effect of NSAID use. By not inhibiting GI prostaglandin synthesis, COX-2 inhibitors cause less gastric ulceration. Other options for preventing GI ulceration with NSAID use include drugs such as proton pump inhibitors (PPIs), such as omeprazole, although prolonged PPI usage has side effects as well.

Note: NSAID use can also precipitate renal failure in patients with borderline renal function because of reduced synthesis of vasodilatory prostaglandins that help maintain renal perfusion via dilation of the afferent arteriole.

10. Why are COX-2 inhibitors considered dangerous in some patients?

COX-2 inhibitors *do not* inhibit COX-1 found in platelets responsible for synthesis of thromboxane A2, a mediator that promotes platelet aggregation. They therefore leave platelets capable of aggregating and forming thrombi. In addition, COX-2 inhibitors *do* inhibit the production of prostaglandins in endothelial cells, potentially creating a prothrombotic state and promoting vasoconstriction. It is therefore believed that COX-2 inhibitors may pose a cardiovascular threat to certain patients who are at risk for stroke or myocardial infarction, which is why rofecoxib was withdrawn from the market in 2004.

11. Is acetaminophen a reasonable option for treating joint pain in this patient?

Yes. Actually, acetaminophen should be the first-line therapy. Acetaminophen primarily works in the central nervous system (CNS) by raising the pain threshold, and thus acts as an analgesic. Because acetaminophen is not an NSAID and does not inhibit peripheral prostaglandin synthesis to a significant extent, it does not have the potential GI or renal negative side effects of NSAIDs.

12. What sort of analgesic would you prescribe for a patient with preexisting renal disease? Or liver disease? Or pregnancy?

NSAIDs are renally excreted, and they decrease perfusion to the kidneys. They would therefore be relatively contraindicated in a patient with kidney disease, and acetaminophen is a better choice for this patient. Acetaminophen, however, is metabolized primarily by the liver (remember that patients who overdose on acetaminophen develop liver failure). A patient with cirrhosis or other liver disease would be better served by an NSAID than by large doses of acetaminophen. In a pregnant patient, NSAIDs should be avoided, particularly in the third trimester. Acetaminophen is the drug of choice for these patients. Remember, the fetal ductus arteriosus is kept open by prostaglandins, and NSAIDs cause it to close prematurely in utero. However, in the case of a patent ductus arteriosus that persists after birth, indomethacin, which inhibits prostaglandin synthesis, can be given to promote closure.

13. Quick review: Looking only at the left column in Table 19.1, try to list the class of drug, mechanism of action, and major side effects for each drug listed.

Table 19.1. Types of Analgesic			
DRUG	**CLASS OF DRUG**	**MECHANISM OF ACTION**	**SIDE EFFECT(S)**
Celecoxib (Celebrex)	COX-2 inhibitor	Inhibition of prostaglandin synthesis by inflammatory cells	Renal toxicity, increased cardiovascular disease risk
Indomethacin, naproxen, ibuprofen, etodolac, ketorolac (Toradol)	NSAID	Reversible COX-1/COX-2 inhibition	GI ulcers and bleeding, renal damage
Aspirin	NSAID	Irreversible COX-1/COX-2 inhibition	GI ulcers and bleeding, renal damage
Acetaminophen	No class	"Raises pain threshold"	Hepatotoxicity

COX, Cyclooxygenase; *GI,* gastrointestinal; *NSAID,* nonsteroidal antiinflammatory drug.

SUMMARY BOX: OSTEOARTHRITIS

- Epidemiology: Most common joint disease worldwide.
- Presentation: Joint pain is typically worse with activity. Obesity, gender, age, and trauma all contribute to development.
- Pathophysiology: Degradation of hyaline cartilage at articulating bones, noninflammatory condition without systemic (constitutional) symptoms.
- Diagnosis: Radiographs show joint space narrowing, subchondral sclerosis, and osteophytes.
- Treatment: Acetaminophen, cyclooxygenase-2 inhibitors, and nonsteroidal antiinflammatory drugs are the mainstay of pharmacotherapy. Intra-articular glucocorticoid injections may also be an option.
- Prognosis and/or complications: Total joint replacement, most commonly of the knees, hips, and shoulders, may be needed in severe cases.

CASE 19.2

A 52-year-old woman presents with a chief concern of polyarticular joint pain for several months. Her pain is worst in the morning and lessens with activity over the course of the day. She typically experiences 1 hour of stiffness after she wakes up. She also reports malaise, anorexia, night sweats, and a persistent low-grade fever. Her symptoms seem to come and go at will.

1. What is the differential diagnosis?

   The differential diagnosis for polyarticular arthritis includes OA, RA, septic arthritis (e.g., disseminated gonococcal infection), reactive arthritis (e.g., in response to GI or respiratory infections, previously known as Reiter syndrome), systemic lupus erythematosus (SLE), hepatitis, and paraneoplastic syndromes. Although the differential here is broad, her morning stiffness and constitutional concerns are suggestive of an inflammatory arthropathy, such as RA.

CASE 19.2 CONTINUED:

On examination, she has symmetric involvement of the metacarpophalangeal and proximal interphalangeal joints, with sparing of the distal interphalangeal joints (Fig. 19.5). Involved joints in her hands are swollen, warm, and tender to palpation. She has moderate-size bilateral knee effusions. Laboratory tests show elevated erythrocyte sedimentation rate and C-reactive protein concentrations and positive rheumatoid factor. She is prescribed methotrexate, a nonsteroidal antiinflammatory drug, and prednisone.

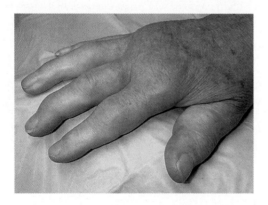

Figure 19.5. Appearance of the proximal interphalangeal and metacarpophalangeal joints of the patient in Case 19.2. *(From Goldman L, Ausiello D. Cecil Textbook of Medicine. 22nd ed. Philadelphia: WB Saunders; 2004.)*

2. What is the diagnosis?

   This patient presents with classic signs of RA, which is an immune-mediated disease of synovial joints. The principal pathologic process in RA is synovitis, inflammation of the synovial membrane, which leads to progressive destruction of the joint. Because RA is a systemic inflammatory condition, patients often present with constitutional symptoms, such as fever, weight loss, and fatigue, in addition to the joint pain. Note that joint involvement in RA is usually symmetric and typically spares the DIP joints.

3. What are the criteria for the diagnosis of RA?

   The following support a diagnosis of RA based on criteria developed in 2010 where a patient has synovitis in a joint, no alternative diagnosis, and a score of at least six based on the following criteria (simplified, as USMLE Step 1 is not going to test specific scores):
   Number of involved joints: more joints and small joint involvement = higher score (maximum 5)
   Serologic abnormality of rheumatoid factor (RF) or anti–citrullinated cyclic peptide: more positive = higher score (maximum 3)
   Elevated ESR or CRP: 1 point
   Symptom duration over 6 weeks: 1 point

This patient has morning stiffness, symmetric arthritis of more than three joints including the hand, elevated inflammatory markers, and positive RF symptoms for longer than 6 weeks. She therefore meets the criteria for the definitive diagnosis of RA.

4. **What sort of damage occurs in the joints of patients with RA?**
   The initial site of damage is the synovium lining the joint space, which becomes the center of an inflammatory process that will involve the entire joint. Lymphocytes, macrophages, osteoclasts, and fibroblasts are all involved and ultimately lead to destruction of the cartilage and bone of the joint. Pannus formation occurs as synovial tissue is aberrantly stimulated to proliferate, and bony erosions develop as the inflammatory process continues. Joints will be painful, show signs of inflammation, and eventually lose normal architecture and mobility.

5. **What is the significance of RF in this disease?**
   RF is a predominantly immunoglobulin M (IgM) autoantibody directed against the Fc region of IgG. This autoantibody forms immune complexes, which deposit throughout the body and are implicated in the extra-articular manifestations of RA. RF is present in roughly 80% of patients with RA, but it is not highly specific for the condition. RF can also appear in lupus, tuberculosis, Sjögren syndrome, and other disorders. It is therefore not necessary for the diagnosis of RA, but it is useful for determining prognosis. Virtually 100% of patients with extra-articular manifestations have a positive RF.
   Note: The current best serologic test for the diagnosis of RA is the anti–citrullinated cyclic peptide antibody. Its sensitivity is the same as that for RF, but it is more specific for RA and is a better predictor of disease progression.

6. **What is the epidemiology of RA?**
   As is the case with most immune-mediated conditions, RA affects women more often than men, and its prevalence increases with age. Genetic susceptibility has been demonstrated, as the disease is associated with certain major histocompatibility complex class II proteins expressed by antigen-presenting cells. The *HLA-DR4* haplotype confers risk for RA, and a specific *HLA-DR* epitope is shared by many people with RA. However, these *HLA* genes do not tell the whole story, and many genes are likely to be responsible for the development of the disease.

7. **What is the typical treatment for RA?**
   Three classes of medications are used to manage RA: analgesics to treat pain, corticosteroids to suppress inflammation, and disease-modifying antirheumatic drugs (DMARDs) to limit progression of the disease. NSAIDs are commonly used as analgesics and have the added benefit of dampening inflammation. Corticosteroids can be injected directly into affected joints and may be used to manage acute flares of RA. DMARDs include a variety of drugs, such as methotrexate, sulfasalazine, and tumor necrosis factor inhibitors (e.g., infliximab). Early use of DMARDs is desirable because these drugs halt progression of irreversible joint damage.

8. **What would be learned from aspiration of this patient's knee?**
   Aspiration would likely not reveal much. The synovial fluid will likely have an inflammatory composition with 2000 to 50,000 white blood cells (WBCs)/mm^3, with the cells being predominantly polymorphonuclear neutrophils (PMNs). If crystals or bacteria are present, or the WBC count is not in this range, another diagnosis should be considered.

CASE 19.2 CONTINUED:

Your patient with RA is lost to follow-up but then returns to your office years later. She describes diffuse arthralgias, weight loss, and shortness of breath. Her hands appear as shown in Fig. 19.6, and subcutaneous nodules are present at the olecranon bilaterally. She has decreased breath sounds at the lung bases, and chest x-ray film shows bilateral pleural effusions and several pulmonary nodules.

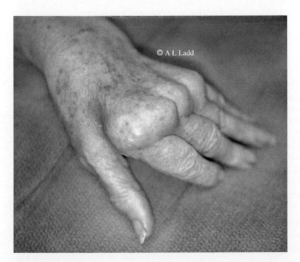

Figure 19.6. Left hand of the patient in Case 19.2. *(Copyright A.L. Ladd.)*

9. What are the characteristic deformities in the hands in advanced RA?

Destruction of the metacarpophalangeal joints leads to ulnar deviation (see Fig. 19.6) as the distal portions of the digits shift toward the ulna. Boutonnière and swan-neck deformities consist of contractions of the fingers at the proximal interphalangeal (PIP) and DIP joints. Remember that the DIP joints are not typically involved with RA, although they may be forced into flexion/extension as a result of involvement of the PIP joints and the tendons of the hand.

STEP 1 SECRET

Symmetric joint involvement, sparing of the distal interphalangeal joints, and morning stiffness longer than 1 hour that resolves with joint use are unique characteristics of rheumatoid arthritis (RA). Be on the lookout for mention of these clues if you suspect a diagnosis of RA.

---

10. What are the extra-articular manifestations of RA?

Because RA is a systemic inflammatory disease, it is not limited to the joints; immune complexes deposit in the vasculature and may affect nearly any organ system. Rheumatoid nodules typically form in the subcutaneous tissue or along tendon sheaths. Pericarditis, pulmonary nodules, interstitial fibrosis, episcleritis, and effusions in the pleural and pericardial space may all be seen in rheumatoid patients. Carpal tunnel syndrome can result from median nerve compression. A normocytic normochromic anemia (anemia of chronic disease) is also common.

Note: Felty syndrome is the combination of seropositive (RF+) RA, granulocytopenia, and splenomegaly.

SUMMARY BOX: RHEUMATOID ARTHRITIS

- Presentation: Pain is worst in the morning, classically lasting more than 1 hour, and improves with use. Bilateral hand involvement is frequent but with sparing of the distal interphalangeal joints. Joints are typically warm, erythematous, swollen, and tender (synovitis). Gender, age, and human leukocyte antigens have been associated.
- Pathophysiology: Systemic inflammatory disease caused in part by immune complex deposition in the joints and potentially various other tissues. The disease process is centered in the synovium of the joint.
- Diagnosis: Can be made clinically with the following supportive features: symmetric arthritis, arthritis of three or more joints, morning stiffness for at least 1 hour, bilateral involvement of the hands (subcutaneous nodules). The presence of a positive rheumatoid factor supports the diagnosis, but remember that the most specific serologic test for rheumatoid arthritis is the anti–citrullinated cyclic peptide antibody. Inflammatory markers such as erythrocyte sedimentation factor and C-reactive protein are commonly elevated.
- Treatment: Nonsteroidal antiinflammatory drugs, glucocorticoids, and disease-modifying antirheumatic drugs (DMARDs). In recent years there has been a strong push to start DMARDs at the time of initial diagnosis to prevent irreversible damage.
- Complications: Extra-articular manifestations include rheumatoid nodules, pericarditis, pleural effusions, pulmonary nodules, pulmonary fibrosis, carpal tunnel syndrome, ocular manifestations, and anemia of chronic disease.

CASE 19.3

A 47-year-old man presents with a 24-hour history of excruciating pain in the right knee. He had been to a banquet the night before and woke up with a red, swollen knee. He tried taking aspirin, but his pain only worsened. He has a history of hypertension treated with hydrochlorothiazide, and his body mass index is 32.

---

1. What is your differential diagnosis?

The differential diagnosis for an acutely inflamed joint includes septic arthritis, cellulitis, gout, pseudogout, and osteomyelitis. However, in a middle-aged man taking hydrochlorothiazide (which reduces uric acid renal excretion) with the acute onset of an excruciatingly painful joint in the setting of suspected excess dietary intake (given the prior night's festivities), acute gout should be suspected.

2. How can crystal and septic arthritis be differentiated?

Examination of joint fluid is of paramount importance. Both conditions will cause a high WBC and PMN percentage in the fluid, but Gram stain and culture must be done to look for infectious causes. Septic arthritis may cause more systemic illness, with symptoms such as fever, malaise, lymphadenopathy, and skin lesions. Organisms responsible for septic arthritis include *Staphylococcus aureus*, *Streptococcus* species, and *Neisseria gonorrhoeae*. Rapid diagnosis and treatment are crucial in septic arthritis.

Note: With septic arthritis, think *N. gonorrhoeae* in a young, otherwise healthy, sexually active patient. Treat septic joint with ceftriaxone and additional azithromycin or doxycycline for possible *Chlamydia* coinfection. For *S. aureus*–mediated septic arthritis, treat with vancomycin until sensitivity results, as empiric methicillin-resistant *S. aureus* coverage should be initiated.

CASE 19.3 CONTINUED:

On examination, the right knee is warm, erythematous, swollen, and tender to touch. The patient is afebrile, and the remainder of his examination is unremarkable. You aspirate cloudy yellow fluid from the joint and find 24,000 white blood cells, 70% polymorphonuclear neutrophils, and needle-shaped crystals that are strongly negatively birefringent under polarized light (Fig. 19.7).

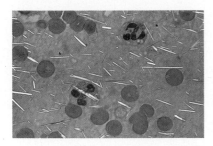

Figure 19.7. Microscopic appearance of synovial fluid under polarized light aspirated from patient in Case 19.3. *(From McPherson RA, Pincus MR.* Henry's Clinical Diagnosis and Management by Laboratory Methods. *21st ed. Philadelphia: WB Saunders; 2006.)*

3. What is the likely diagnosis?

   Gout is an inflammatory arthritis caused by the intra-articular deposition of urate crystals. Although this patient's presentation is consistent with the other diseases listed for the differential diagnosis, the crystals seen here are pathognomonic for gout. Although clinically gout and septic arthritis can coexist (a patient with gout is not immune to septic arthritis), on an examination the patient would have one or the other.

   The term to associate with gout is *negative birefringence*, which means that when the crystals are examined under polarized light, they appear yellow when oriented parallel (yeLLow is paraLLel) to the direction of slow light vibration, and blue when oriented perpendicularly.

4. What is the pathophysiology of this condition?

   Uric acid is the end product of purine nucleotide metabolism and is excreted from the body by the kidneys. High levels of serum uric acid may occur with either overproduction or underexcretion of uric acid. Most of the time ($>$90% of cases), gout is caused by underexcretion. In either situation, uric acid is deposited in synovial fluid in the form of urate crystals, which are phagocytosed and induce a local inflammatory response. Free uric acid crystals also activate synovial cells, leukocytes, and complement proteins, including C5a, which recruits large numbers of PMNs into the joint space.

5. Do most people with hyperuricemia experience gout?

   No. Most people with hyperuricemia do not have gout, and many gout patients do not have high serum levels of urate. The risk for development of gout becomes substantial only with quite high levels of uric acid ($>$9 mg/dL vs. normal level of ≈5 mg/dL). Other risk factors for gout are a purine-rich diet (e.g., seafood, red meat), male gender, age (fifth decade), obesity, hypertension, alcohol intake, renal disease, family history of gout, use of certain drugs including thiazide diuretics, and certain genetic conditions.

6. What is Lesch-Nyhan syndrome, and why might it predispose to gout?

   Lesch-Nyhan syndrome consists of intellectual impairment, spasticity, choreoathetosis, aggressive behavior, self-mutilation, and gouty arthritis. It is due to an X-linked defect in hypoxanthine phosphoribosyltransferase, an enzyme involved in the purine salvage pathway. Absence of hypoxanthine phosphoribosyltransferase and the salvage pathway leads to overproduction of uric acid during purine nucleotide breakdown, resulting in hyperuricemia (see Case 11.4 in Chapter 11, Genetic and Metabolic Disease, for further details).

7. Are there any complications of gout besides the monoarticular inflammatory arthritis?

   The classic location for gouty arthritis is in the metatarsophalangeal joint of the great toe, which is known as *podagra*. In patients with chronic gout, urate crystals can also deposit in subcutaneous tissues, forming nodules called *tophi*. Tophi are often found in the helix of the ear and over the elbow. Fig. 19.8 shows olecranon bursitis in chronic tophaceous gout. Uric acid calculi may form in the renal pelvis or ureters, leading to obstruction of the urinary tract. Crystals may also cause damage to the renal interstitial tissue, a condition termed *gouty interstitial nephropathy*.

8. Are there any medications that can precipitate attacks of gout?

   Drugs that decrease the renal excretion of uric acid may contribute to gout. Such offenders include low-dose salicylates, thiazide diuretics, and furosemide. Our patient may have been predisposed to development of gout because of his hydrochlorothiazide use. Use of aspirin may have exacerbated symptoms by further decreasing uric acid excretion because acid secretion at the proximal nephron is a saturable process. Other precipitants include alcoholic beverages and purine-rich foods (red meat and seafood).

CASE 19.3 CONTINUED:

He is given colchicine and experiences rapid improvement.

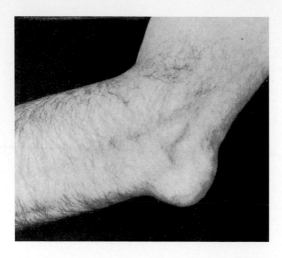

Figure 19.8. Olecranon bursitis in a patient with tophaceous gout. *(From Polley HF, Hunder GG.* Rheumatologic Interviewing and Physical Examination of the Joints. *2nd ed. Philadelphia: WB Saunders; 1978.)*

9. **What other treatment options exist for an acute gout attack?**
Acute attacks can be managed with NSAIDs (typically indomethacin), glucocorticoids, and colchicine, all of which dampen the inflammatory response and inhibit the continued phagocytosis of urate crystals.
   Note: Colchicine works by binding to the molecule tubulin and inhibiting the polymerization of microtubules, thereby preventing mitosis in inflammatory cells. By inhibiting microtubule function, it also serves to limit the mobility of inflammatory cells. A worrisome adverse effect of colchicine is bone marrow suppression. Common negative side effects include intestinal upset and diarrhea.

10. **Who needs chronic treatment for gout, and what does this treatment consist of?**
Patients with recurrent bouts of gouty arthritis, radiographic evidence of joint damage, and extra-articular manifestations such as tophi and urate kidney stones merit chronic treatment. Note that asymptomatic hyperuricemia is *not* a reason for treatment (treat the patient not the lab tests!). Allopurinol, an inhibitor of the uric acid–synthesizing enzyme xanthine oxidase, can be used to treat chronic gout and is now considered a first-line treatment for the management of gout. Probenecid is used for some patients with chronic gout (underexcretors) because it serves to increase renal excretion of uric acid by interfering with the organic anion transporter in the kidney. For boards, patients are designated underexcretors or overproducers using a 24-hour urinary uric acid excretion test, although in clinical practice this is rarely done.
   Note: Patients undergoing treatment for hematologic malignancies are at risk for tumor lysis syndrome. As malignant cells are killed, their DNA is degraded into purine and pyrimidine nucleotides. Allopurinol is often given before radiation therapy or chemotherapy to prevent the production of uric acid through purine catabolism.
   Note: Febuxostat is an alternative to allopurinol and also acts as a xanthine oxidase inhibitor. Although febuxostat has been shown to be more effective than allopurinol at lowering serum urate concentration, it has not been shown to be more clinically efficacious at preventing gouty flares.

11. **What is pseudogout?**
Pseudogout is a crystal arthropathy caused by calcium pyrophosphate dihydrate (CPPD) deposition. Joint symptoms are similar to those seen with gout, but they tend to be less severe. Synovial fluid shows rhomboid, weakly positively birefringent crystals that are blue when parallel to light and yellow when perpendicular (vs. the needle-shaped, strongly negatively birefringent crystals of gout). This condition usually affects larger joints, such as the knees, and occurs in women more often than in men. Radiographs might show chondrocalcinosis, reflecting calcium pyrophosphate dihydrate deposition within cartilage. Hemochromatosis and hyperparathyroidism are two metabolic disorders that predispose to pseudogout.

STEP 1 SECRET

Be sure that you understand the concepts of positive and negative birefringence and their associations with pseudogout and gout, respectively.

ONE LAST CRYSTAL...

A 78-year-old woman with a history of OA presents with increasing left shoulder pain during the past few months. On examination, her shoulder is warm and an effusion is present. Her range of motion is severely limited by pain, and you note obvious crepitus. Aspiration reveals blood but no crystals in the synovial fluid. You order an x-ray study, compare it with one from 3 months ago, and find that the head of her humerus has been severely eroded during this short time.

12. **What is going on here?**
This condition, termed *Milwaukee shoulder syndrome*, is caused by deposition of hydroxyapatite crystals. It typically affects elderly women and causes rapid destruction of the shoulder. These crystals are visible only with electron microscopy.

SUMMARY BOX: GOUT

- Presentation: Sudden onset of extremely painful joint, frequently the great toe (podagra). The joint will be warm, erythematous, swollen, and extremely tender. A history of increased red meat, alcohol, or seafood intake in recent days (all purine rich) may be elicited. Risk factors include a purine-rich diet, male gender, age (fifth decade), obesity, hypertension, alcohol intake, diuretic use, renal disease, and family history.
- Pathophysiology: Intra-articular deposition of urate crystals that triggers a damaging inflammatory cascade. Uric acid is a product of purine nucleotide catabolism. Hyperuricemia is neither necessary nor sufficient for the development of gout.
- Diagnosis: Normally clinically obvious on exam and history, but if need for confirmation, joint aspiration will show needle-shaped crystals that demonstrate strongly negative birefringence under polarized light.
- Diagnosis
  - Acute: nonsteroidal antiinflammatory drugs (NSAIDs), glucocorticoids, and colchicine
  - Chronic: Allopurinol and probenecid; lifestyle modifications
  - Complications: Subcutaneous tophi, renal calculi, and interstitial nephropathy

CASE 19.4

A 42-year-old woman presents with the symptom of "feeling sore all over" with constant aching pain. She describes persistent fatigue as well. She has felt this way for years and has been to see several physicians without receiving a definitive diagnosis.

1. **What is your differential diagnosis for diffuse musculoskeletal pain and fatigue?**
   This is a truly broad differential diagnosis. Hypothyroidism, Lyme disease, sleep apnea, anemia, and many rheumatologic conditions can cause pain and fatigue. Certain medications may cause musculoskeletal pain, particularly statins. Any number of malignancies could be responsible for this presentation as well.

CASE 19.4 CONTINUED:

Your patient states that along with the pain and fatigue, she has alternating episodes of constipation and diarrhea. She has a history of migraine headaches and takes fluoxetine for depression. Physical examination is remarkable only for tenderness to palpation at many points across her body. Laboratory tests show a normal complete blood cell count, erythrocyte sedimentation rate, C-reactive protein concentration, and creatine phosphokinase concentration. Muscle biopsy and electromyography findings are normal.

2. **What is the likely diagnosis?**
   Fibromyalgia, a condition characterized by diffuse musculoskeletal pain, is likely. A diagnosis of fibromyalgia requires the presence of significant widespread pain for at least 3 months. Prior criteria required counting of anatomically specific tender points (Fig. 19.9), but this is no longer part of the diagnosis.

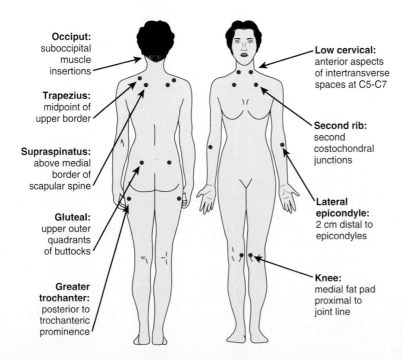

Occiput: suboccipital muscle insertions

Trapezius: midpoint of upper border

Supraspinatus: above medial border of scapular spine

Gluteal: upper outer quadrants of buttocks

Greater trochanter: posterior to trochanteric prominence

Low cervical: anterior aspects of intertransverse spaces at C5-C7

Second rib: second costochondral junctions

Lateral epicondyle: 2 cm distal to epicondyles

Knee: medial fat pad proximal to joint line

Figure 19.9. Location of specific tender points in fibromyalgia. *(From Fibromyalgia syndrome. In: Primer on Rheumatic Diseases. Atlanta: Arthritis Foundation; 1993.)*

3. **What causes fibromyalgia?**
The pathophysiology of this syndrome is poorly understood. Most believe that it is due to abnormalities in the CNS, leading to a heightened sensitivity to painful stimuli (visceral hypersensitivity). Patients with fibromyalgia have been shown to have lower-than-normal levels of serotonin and elevated levels of substance P (a neuropeptide that mediates the transmission of pain signals from the peripheral nervous system to the CNS).

4. **Are steroids indicated?**
No. This is not a primary inflammatory disorder, as evidenced by the lack of laboratory abnormalities, such as ESR and CRP. Steroids should not be used in this situation. Sleep medications, NSAIDs, antidepressants, and muscle relaxants may be of some help. Physical therapy, cognitive-behavioral therapy, and aerobic exercise may be useful as well.

5. **Who is prone to development of fibromyalgia?**
This disorder is seen predominantly in women (affected four to seven times more often than men). Fibromyalgia is often seen alongside mood disorders such as depression and anxiety, sleep disorders, and other disorders involving visceral hypersensitivity, such as migraines, endometriosis, and irritable bowel syndrome.

6. **What laboratory value helps rule out myositis from statin use?**
Polymyalgia rheumatica (PMR) presents similarly to fibromyalgia but oftentimes has abnormal lab values, such as an elevated ESR concentration. In contrast, myositis from statin use traditionally shows increased plasma concentration of creatine phosphokinase.

SUMMARY BOX: FIBROMYALGIA

- Epidemiology: Predominantly affects woman and often coexists with mood disorders, sleep disorders, headaches, and irritable bowel syndrome.
- Presentation: Diffuse musculoskeletal pain of unclear etiology with multiple tender points on exam, along with fatigue and sleep disturbance.
- Pathophysiology: Poorly understood; a possible depletion of serotonin with concomitant increase in substance P, which lowers the pain threshold.
- Diagnosis: Widespread significant pain for at least 3 months.
- Treatment: Exercise is first-line therapy. Other options include sleep medications, nonsteroidal antiinflammatory drugs, antidepressants, and muscle relaxants. Physical therapy and cognitive-behavioral therapy may also be helpful.

CASE 19.5

The next patient is a 57-year-old woman who presents for evaluation of a 4-week history of diffuse aching pain of abrupt onset in her shoulders, hips, and low back. She has lost 8 lb and reports occasional low-grade fever. On examination, she is tender to palpation in the proximal muscles and large joints but shows no signs of muscle atrophy, muscle weakness, or sensory losses. Laboratory tests show an erythrocyte sedimentation rate of 84 mm/h, hematocrit of 35%, mean corpuscular volume of 93 fL, and an elevated ferritin level. Serum creatine phosphokinase is not elevated, and electromyography and muscle biopsy findings are normal as well.

---

1. **What is the diagnosis in this patient?**
This woman has PMR, another immune-mediated rheumatologic condition that presents primarily with diffuse myalgias. Unlike fibromyalgia, PMR is a systemic inflammatory disorder. Proximal muscles of the neck, shoulders, back, and thighs are typically involved. Fever, weight loss, and fatigue may be noted in the history, and a normochromic, normocytic anemia (anemia of chronic disease) occurs in 50% of cases. PMR usually has an abrupt onset.
   Note: PMR and polymyositis both present with fatigue and muscle tenderness. An important distinction is that, unlike in polymyositis, muscle strength is preserved in PMR, and the creatine phosphokinase level is normal.
   Note: Ferritin is one of the acute-phase reactants: a group of proteins synthesized by the liver in response to inflammation. To attribute the high ferritin level to an acute response (vs. iron overload, as in hemochromatosis), one should look for other signs of inflammation, such as an elevated ESR or CRP level.

2. **How is this condition treated?**
PMR is highly sensitive to corticosteroid administration, which is the mainstay of therapy for this disease. It typically responds within days to relatively low-dose prednisone (10–20 mg/day). If symptoms do not rapidly improve, other conditions should be considered.

3. **What else should be looked for in patients with suspected PMR?**
PMR is often associated with giant cell (temporal) arteritis, one of the vasculitides, and patients with PRM should be evaluated for giant cell arteritis. Signs of giant cell arteritis include claudication involving the arms and legs, arterial bruits, and asymmetric blood pressures in the extremities. Involvement of the temporal artery may cause jaw pain and unilateral headaches and, if left untreated, may lead to blindness.

SUMMARY BOX: POLYMYALGIA RHEUMATICA

- Presentation: Proximal muscles of the neck, shoulders, back, and hips are typically involved. Fever, weight loss, and fatigue may be noted in the history, and anemia of chronic disease occurs in 50% of cases. Polymyalgia rheumatica usually has an abrupt onset.
- Pathophysiology: Poorly understood systemic immune-mediated rheumatologic condition causing proximal greater than distal myalgia and weakness.
- Diagnosis: Age > 50 years; proximal and bilateral myalgias of neck, shoulders, torso, or hips for at least 2 weeks; elevated erythrocyte sedimentation rate; and rapid improvement in response to low-dose steroids.
- Treatment: Low-dose corticosteroids.
- Complications: Often associated with giant cell (temporal) arteritis, which, if left untreated, can lead to blindness.

CASE 19.6

A 37-year-old man presents with a several-month history of burning pain in his hands. His wife notices that he often wakes from sleep because of this pain and paces around their bedroom, shaking his hands to relieve the pain. He works for a moving company and spends much of his time lifting furniture. He finds that the pain sometimes shoots up from his wrists into his forearms, and he is beginning to notice hand weakness and difficulty with grasping objects.

1. What is your differential diagnosis?
   This presentation is consistent with a tendonitis, enthesopathy, or neuropathy.
   Note: Pathology at the site of insertion of tendons, ligaments, muscle, and joint capsule into bone is referred to as an *enthesopathy*.

CASE 19.6 CONTINUED:

On examination, you note bilateral thenar atrophy and evoke positive Phalen and Tinel signs.

2. What is the Phalen sign? What is the Tinel sign?
   The Phalen test (Fig. 19.10) consists of having patients flex their wrists and hold their hands together for 60 seconds, which will cause numbness and tingling in the distribution of the median nerve if carpal tunnel syndrome is present. The Tinel sign is positive if similar paresthesias are evoked by simply tapping the wrist over the transverse carpal ligament in the area of the median nerve.
   Note: A 2002 study evaluating these tests in carpal tunnel syndrome confirmed patients and healthy control subjects showed a sensitivity and specificity of 85% and 89%, respectively, for the Phalen test and 66% and 67%, respectively, for the percussion test (Tinel sign).

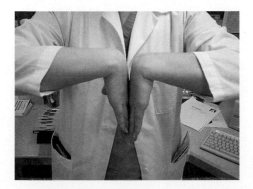

Figure 19.10. Phalen test. *(From Marx JA, Hochberger RS, Walls RM, Adams JG. Rosen's Emergency Medicine: Concepts and Clinical Practice. 6th ed. Philadelphia: Mosby; 2006.)*

3. What is your diagnosis?
   This man has carpal tunnel syndrome, which is a compressive or entrapment neuropathy of the median nerve at the wrist.

4. What causes carpal tunnel syndrome?
   The median nerve passes into the hand via the carpal tunnel. This space is bounded by carpal bones and the transverse carpal ligament (flexor retinaculum). Compression of the nerve in this location leads to carpal tunnel syndrome, which is

characterized by neuropathic pain in the distribution of the median nerve. Repetitive wrist flexion may lead to irritation and inflammation within the carpal tunnel, making carpal tunnel syndrome a common work-related injury. Several medical conditions may also be responsible, including pregnancy, obesity, hypothyroidism, and amyloidosis.

5. **What structures pass through the carpal tunnel?**
Ten anatomic structures reside within this space: four tendons of the flexor digitorum profundus, four tendons of the flexor digitorum superficialis, the tendon of the flexor pollicis longus, and the median nerve.

6. **What does the median nerve innervate in the hand?**
The median nerve originates in spinal roots C6-T1 and supplies the muscles of the anterior forearm. In the hand, it provides sensory innervation to the palmar surface of the first three and a half digits, as well as the distal dorsal portion of these fingers. The median nerve also supplies motor innervation to the thenar (thumb) muscles and the first two lumbrical muscles (Fig. 19.11).

CARPAL TUNNEL SYNDROME

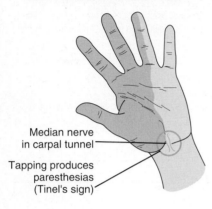

Median nerve in carpal tunnel

Tapping produces paresthesias (Tinel's sign)

Figure 19.11. Distribution of pain and paresthesias (*dark shaded area*) when the median nerve is compressed by swelling in the wrist (carpal tunnel). *(From Arnett FC. Rheumatoid arthritis. In: Andreoli TE, ed. Cecil Essentials of Medicine. 4th ed. Philadelphia: WB Saunders; 1997.)*

7. **What are the treatment options for carpal tunnel syndrome?**
Conservative measures are often tried initially and include splinting and limiting aggravating factors. Steroid injections may be helpful and can also be used in pregnancy. Surgical treatment involves releasing the transverse carpal ligament to reduce pressure in the canal. Although this has traditionally been an open surgery, it is now routinely performed laparoscopically.

SUMMARY BOX: CARPAL TUNNEL SYNDROME

- Presentation: Pain and paresthesias in the distribution of the median nerve (cutaneous innervation to the first three and a half fingers and motor supply to the thumb).
- Pathophysiology: Compressive (entrapment) neuropathy of the median nerve as it travels through the carpal tunnel at the wrist.
- Diagnosis: Wasting of the thenar eminence, + Phalen/Tinel signs (recall the higher sensitivity/specificity of the Phalen sign), and electromyogram showing nerve conduction delay along the median nerve.
- Treatment: Orthotic wrist splints to improve ergonomics, steroid injections, and surgery.
- Prognosis: Excellent with appropriate therapy (often surgery).

CASE 19.7

A 26-year-old man presents with a 9-month history of low-back pain and stiffness that is worse in the morning and generally subsides after a few hours of activity. On examination, you find tenderness to palpation of the sacroiliac joints, reduced flexibility of the lumbar spine, and limited expansion of the chest. Ten years later, x-ray films of the lumbar spine are obtained and are shown in Fig. 19.12.

1. **What is the diagnosis?**
This man has ankylosing spondylitis, one of the seronegative spondyloarthropathies. This disease generally occurs in young men and involves the axial skeleton. The x-ray films show the classic "bamboo spine" (see Fig. 19.12B), which is caused in part by syndesmophytes (see white arrowheads in Fig. 19.12A), curvilinear calcifications linking one vertebral body to another.

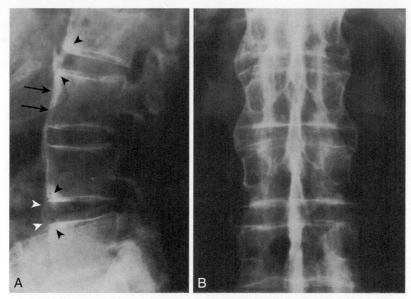

Figure 19.12. A, Early manifestations of ankylosing spondylitis in the lumbar spine include the development of an osteitis (*black arrowheads*) at the corners of vertebral body end plates that results in sclerosis and bone resorption. Early syndesmophytes (*white arrowheads*) are gracile, curvilinear calcifications extending from corner to corner. Mineralization of the anterior longitudinal ligament (*black arrows*) may contribute to the squared appearance of a vertebral body. B, Gracile syndesmophytes at all levels create the "bamboo spine" appearance. *(From Grainger RG, Allison D, Adam A, et al.* Grainger & Allison's Diagnostic Radiology: A Textbook of Medical Imaging. *4th ed. Philadelphia: Churchill Livingstone; 2001.)*

Note: The seronegative spondyloarthropathies are "seronegative" in that patients are typically negative for RF. These diseases all occur most frequently in people who share a certain major histocompatibility complex class I antigen, the *HLA-B27* allele. Not all people with this allele will develop one of the spondyloarthropathies, but most patients with these diseases do have the *HLA-B27* allele. This relationship is not fully understood, but the spondyloarthropathies obviously share a strong genetic component. They tend to affect the axial skeleton, along with the eyes, skin, genitalia, and GI tract.

2. What is the bamboo spine?

As the inflammatory process unfolds in the spine, fibrous and cartilaginous structures are replaced with bone. This leads to diminished flexibility and eventual fusion of the vertebrae, giving the spine the appearance of bamboo on plain x-ray films.

CASE 19.8

A 32-year-old man presents with a 2-week history of pain in multiple joints, painful red eyes, and burning with urination. He has had several sexual partners in the past few months. Polymerase chain reaction assay is positive for *Chlamydia trachomatis* and negative for *Neisseria gonorrhoeae*. You note a few ulcerated lesions of the oral mucosa on examination.

1. What is the likely diagnosis?

This is reactive arthritis, formerly referred to as *Reiter syndrome*. The classic triad of arthritis, conjunctivitis/uveitis, and urethritis makes up the clinical presentation in many cases of this seronegative arthropathy. Symptoms can be remembered by the rhyme "Can't see, pee, or climb a tree."

2. What triggers this condition?

Reactive arthritis occurs in response to an infection in patients with the *HLA-B27* allele. Common agents include *Shigella*, *Yersinia*, *Chlamydia*, and *Salmonella*. Respiratory pathogens also have been implicated. Reactive arthritis is a systemic inflammatory response to these bacterial antigens; it is *not* a septic arthritis, and these bacteria will not be found in any affected joint. This differs from gonococcal arthritis, which typically involves bacterial seeding of affected joints.

CASE 19.9

A 40-year-old man presents with a 3-month history of pain and stiffness in his back, neck, and hands. You note large erythematous scaly plaques over the extensor surfaces of his elbows and knees, which he states he has had for years. There is tenderness to palpation of the left sacroiliac joint, and the distal interphalangeal joints are warm and swollen. You note that the first finger on his left hand is extensively red and swollen all along its length. You examine his feet and find that the toenails have extensive pitting.

1. What is the diagnosis here?

This man has psoriatic arthritis, another member of the group of seronegative spondyloarthropathies. This entity is associated with the dermatologic condition psoriasis, which is characterized by large red plaques covered with silvery white scales over extensor surfaces (Fig. 19.13).

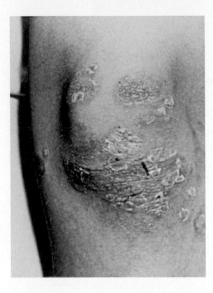

Figure 19.13. Chronic psoriatic plaques on the knee. *(From Behrman RE.* Nelson Textbook of Pediatrics. *16th ed. Philadelphia: WB Saunders; 2000.)*

STEP 1 SECRET

The USMLE loves to include pictures of common dermatologic lesions on the exam. Psoriasis is a particular favorite, but you should make a point of looking at as many images of skin lesions as possible as you encounter them throughout your studies.

2. What joints are affected by psoriatic arthritis?

Commonly the joints of the hands and feet (including the DIP joints) are involved, but the axial skeleton can also be affected. The nails can show characteristic deformities in psoriatic arthritis, including pits, horizontal ridges, and discoloration. Dactylitis, or inflammation of the soft tissue of an entire digit, is seen as well; this is known colloquially as a "sausage digit" (Fig. 19.14).

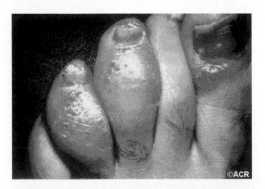

Figure 19.14. Sausage toes, or dactylitis, in a patient with psoriasis. *(From American College of Rheumatology.* Clinical Slide Collection on the Rheumatic Diseases. *Atlanta: American College of Rheumatology; 1998.)*

SUMMARY BOX: SERONEGATIVE SPONDYLOARTHROPATHIES

- The seronegative spondyloarthropathies are associated with the *HLA-B27* allele.
- These conditions are inflammatory arthritides not associated with rheumatoid factor.
- Involvement of the axial skeleton and extra-articular manifestations are common.
- Ankylosing spondylitis affects the spine and leads to fusion of vertebrae.
- Reactive arthritis that occurs in response to an infection (usually gastrointestinal, respiratory, or urogenital).
- Psoriatic arthritis is associated with the dermatologic condition psoriasis.

CASE 19.10

A 33-year-old woman presents with a troublesome concern. She states that when she goes outside in the cold, her fingertips turn white, then blue, then red. The condition is painful and has been occurring for several months. She also describes swelling and puffiness of her fingers, hands, and forearms, which have been persistent for the last few weeks.

1. **What do you think is going on here?**
   This condition of painful fingers that change color in cold is known as *Raynaud phenomenon* (Fig. 19.15). It is caused by vasospasm of small vessels and can affect the hands, feet, nose, and ears. Cold, vibration, and emotional stress may provoke this condition. It is termed *Raynaud disease* when it occurs idiopathically and *Raynaud phenomenon* or *syndrome* when there is an underlying cause such as a rheumatologic disorder.

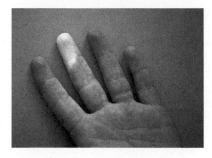

Figure 19.15. Raynaud phenomenon in the acute phase, with severe blanching of the tip of one finger. *(From Forbes CD, Jackson WF. Color Atlas and Text of Clinical Medicine. 3rd ed. London: Mosby 2003.)*

CASE 19.10 CONTINUED:

You educate your patient about Raynaud disease and advise her on ways to avoid the painful episodes. For the puffiness in her hands and feet, you come up with a differential diagnosis that includes thyroid disorders, nephrotic syndrome, venous thrombi, heart failure, and vena cava syndrome. You find no protein in her urine, and her thyroid-stimulating hormone is normal. You realize that the other conditions on your differential diagnosis are highly unlikely in a healthy 33-year-old woman, so you decide to see her back in a few weeks.

Your patient returns several months, rather than weeks, later. Her puffiness is gone, but she feels that the skin over her hands and feet has become thickened. She is now having frequent symptoms of gastroesophageal reflux, including burning in her chest after meals and when she lies down. She reports diffuse arthralgias and also of dry mouth. You are beginning to think you may know what is going on here, so you order a few antibody tests. The results are as follows:

Antinuclear antibody: positive
Anticentromere: negative
Anti-topoisomerase (Scl-70): positive

2. **What is your diagnosis?**
   This woman has systemic sclerosis, also known as *scleroderma*, which is a rheumatologic disease characterized by abnormal proliferation of connective tissue. Scleroderma manifests in several varieties: limited cutaneous, diffuse cutaneous, and localized.

3. **What is the pathogenesis of scleroderma?**
   In this immune-mediated disease, fibroblasts are pathologically stimulated to deposit collagen and other extracellular matrix proteins. The cause of this disease is unknown. As with other immune-mediated diseases, theories posit that infectious agents, environmental factors, and genetics all play a role.

4. **Which sort of scleroderma does this patient have?**
   Your patient has skin and GI involvement, which may occur with either limited or diffuse systemic sclerosis. The antibody findings, however, point to a diagnosis of diffuse scleroderma. The anticentromere antibody is relatively specific for limited disease, but the anti-topoisomerase antibody is associated with diffuse disease. Diffuse systemic scleroderma is associated with a higher mortality rate and more rapid progression than the other forms.

5. **What is the reason for the reflux?**
   With systemic disease, the esophagus may become infiltrated with collagen, and motility is impaired. Reflux occurs as the lower esophageal sphincter loses tone. Gastroparesis may also occur with involvement of the stomach. Any portion of the GI tract may be affected by systemic sclerosis.

CASE 19.10 CONTINUED:

You see your patient again several years later. She now has extensive thickening and tightening of the skin of her extremities and face. The skin on her hands appears thickened and shiny, with several of the fingers contracted (Fig. 19.16). She reports frequent dyspnea. Her blood pressure is 165/98 mm Hg, and her weight is down 12 lb from last year. You note bilateral basilar rales on pulmonary examination. CBC shows a normocytic anemia consistent with chronic inflammatory disease, and her creatinine concentration is 1.6 mg/dL. You order pulmonary function tests, which show a restrictive pattern of lung disease.

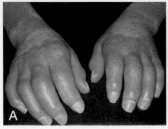
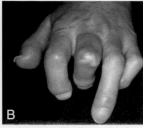

Figure 19.16. Scleroderma involving the hands. A, Edematous phase with diffuse swelling of the fingers. B, Atrophic phase with contracture and thickening sclerodactyly (thick skin over the fingers). *(From Goldman L, Ausiello D.* Cecil Textbook of Medicine. *22nd ed. Philadelphia: WB Saunders; 2004.)*

6. **What are the renal manifestations of diffuse scleroderma?**
   The renal vasculature may be compromised by collagen deposition, limiting blood flow to the kidneys. This leads to activation of the renin-angiotensin-aldosterone system, with a resultant increase in blood pressure. Patients with scleroderma may have malignant hypertension and ultimately renal failure. Before the advent of angiotensin-converting enzyme inhibitors, renal failure was the leading cause of death in patients with scleroderma.

7. **What is the current leading cause of death for these patients?**
   Pulmonary involvement now poses the biggest threat. The lung parenchyma and the pulmonary vasculature can be infiltrated with fibrotic material, leading to both interstitial fibrosis and pulmonary hypertension. Interstitial fibrosis reduces the compliance of the lungs and also limits the diffusing capacity. The increase in pressure in the pulmonary arteries places an afterload burden on the right ventricle, which can lead to heart failure.

8. **What is the CREST syndrome?**
   CREST syndrome is another name for *limited* diffuse scleroderma, and stands for the following:
   C: Calcinosis cutis
   R: Raynaud syndrome
   E: Esophageal dysmotility
   S: Sclerodactyly
   T: Telangiectasias
   Calcium deposits may occur in subcutaneous tissue, tendons, or ligaments. Raynaud syndrome is seen in nearly 100% of patients with scleroderma. Esophageal dysmotility leads to dysphagia and reflux, as mentioned previously. Sclerodactyly is the condition of contracted, hardened skin and soft tissues of the hands. Patients with CREST syndrome tend to have skin involvement only of the distal extremities, with sparing of the trunk. Telangiectasias are groups of dilated superficial blood vessels visible on the skin.

9. **What is localized scleroderma?**
   This form of scleroderma affects only the skin and subcutaneous tissue, not the internal organs. It is sometimes referred to as *morphea* and includes several specific subtypes. Fig. 19.17 shows an example of *en coup de sabre* ("stroke of a sword"), which is a form of localized scleroderma that affects the face and scalp.

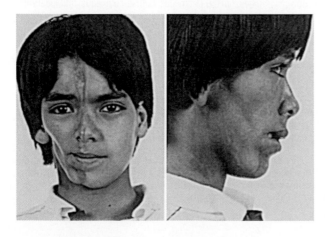

Figure 19.17. Linear scleroderma of the face (*en coup de sabre*) in a 13-year-old boy who had the disease for 8 years. *(From Harris ED, Budd RC, Genovese MC, et al.* Kelley's Textbook of Rheumatology. *7th ed. Philadelphia: WB Saunders; 2005.)*

10. **How is scleroderma treated?**
    Unlike most other rheumatologic diseases, systemic sclerosis does not respond well to immunosuppressant agents, such as steroids. However, a majority of patients do respond to therapy with d-penicillamine. Although its precise mechanism of action remains unclear, d-penicillamine appears to inhibit cytokines such as interleukin-1, which

stimulates fibroblast proliferation and collagen deposition, and retards the maturation of newly synthesized collagen. Other drugs used in the treatment of scleroderma include angiotensin-converting enzyme inhibitors to prevent the progression of renal disease, calcium channel blockers to alleviate the symptoms of Raynaud phenomenon, and H_2 blockers or PPIs to prevent gastric reflux. As mentioned earlier, pulmonary disease is the least treatable complication of scleroderma at this point. Cyclophosphamide is currently being evaluated for treatment of interstitial fibrosis, and prostacyclins and nitric oxide may be helpful in treating pulmonary hypertension.

11. Quick review: Cover the three columns on the right in Table 19.2 and describe the various characteristics of diffuse, limited, and localized scleroderma.

Table 19.2. Types of Scleroderma

	DIFFUSE CUTANEOUS SCLERODERMA	LIMITED CUTANEOUS SCLERODERMA (CREST)	LOCALIZED SCLERODERMA (MORPHEA)
Organ involvement	Extensive and diffuse skin involvement; significant visceral involvement (pulmonary, renal, gastrointestinal, cardiac, other)	Skin involvement, primarily of extremities; little visceral involvement; may evolve to diffuse scleroderma	Limited skin involvement with *no* visceral involvement
Antibodies	+ Anti-topoisomerase (Scl-70)	+ Anticentromere	None/variable
Prognosis	Poor	Better	Good

*CREST, c*alcinosis, *R*aynaud syndrome, *e*sophageal dysmotility, *s*clerodactyly, *t*elangiectasias.

SUMMARY BOX: SCLERODERMA

- Presentation: Raynaud syndrome, thickened skin of the hands and/or feet, heartburn, arthralgias, and dry mouth are common symptoms.
- Pathophysiology: Fibroblasts are pathologically stimulated to deposit collagen and other extracellular matrix proteins to varying extents around the skin and internal organs.
- Diagnosis: Limited scleroderma (CREST syndrome) in which the scleroderma is largely restricted to the skin to the more severe diffuse scleroderma, which involves the lungs and kidneys.
- Treatment
  - D-Penicillamine, which, by inhibiting interleukin-1, slows fibroblast proliferation, collagen synthesis, and collagen deposition.
  - Angiotensin-converting enzyme inhibitors to prevent the progression of renal disease.
  - Calcium channel blockers for Raynaud syndrome.
  - H_2 blockers or proton pump inhibitors for gastroesophageal reflux disease.
- Prognosis
  - Diffuse systemic scleroderma: Poor prognosis. Pulmonology complications are the current leading cause of death in systemic disease.
  - Limited sclerosis (CREST syndrome): Scleroderma largely affects the skin, so there is a much better prognosis than with diffuse systemic sclerosis.

CASE 19.11

A 22-year-old woman presents for evaluation of a painless facial rash that has been present for the past 3 weeks. She otherwise feels well and is taking no medications. She can think of no precipitating factors other than sun exposure during her recent vacation. On examination, the rash involves both cheeks and the bridge of the nose but spares the nasolabial folds. The lesions appear as erythematous patches with scaling and a crusty appearance, similar in appearance to the facial rash shown in Fig. 19.18.

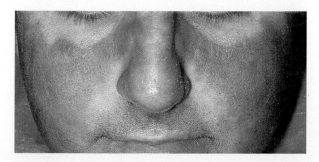

Figure 19.18. Classic appearance of a malar (butterfly) rash. *(From Habif TP. Clinical Dermatology. 4th ed. Philadelphia: Mosby; 2004.)*

1. **What is the likely diagnosis in this patient?**
   In the absence of other symptoms, the differential diagnosis for a malar rash includes rosacea, pellagra, psoriasis, dermatomyositis, and discoid lupus, a poorly understood immune-mediated disease. If symptoms such as arthralgia were present, we would suspect SLE.

2. **How can a diagnosis of discoid lupus be confirmed?**
   Skin biopsy is the method of definitive diagnosis.

3. **What treatment options exist for discoid lupus?**
   Topical corticosteroids and antimalarial agents such as hydroxychloroquine can be used. Patients should be advised of the importance of sun protection as well.

CASE 19.11 CONTINUED:

Your patient's skin improves with the topical steroids, and she remains well for 10 years. She then returns to you with worsening facial rash, as well as diffuse arthralgias and fatigue. She reports constant dryness of her mouth and eyes. Further history reveals that she has had several early miscarriages, and she was diagnosed with syphilis 3 years ago in the absence of clear symptoms or risk factors.

On physical examination, you find an erythematous facial rash in the malar distribution. Her metacarpophalangeal and PIP joints are tender, swollen, and erythematous bilaterally. Her mucous membranes appear dry, and you note the presence of aphthous ulcers (canker sores) and fissures in her lips. You draw several laboratory tests and find a mild anemia, protein in the urine, and the following serum autoantibodies:

Antinuclear antibody: positive
Anti-Smith: positive
Antihistone: negative

---

4. **What is the likely diagnosis?**
   This patient has SLE (lupus), an immune-mediated disease that damages multiple organ systems primarily via pathologic immune complex deposition.

5. **What is the pathogenesis of SLE?**
   The primary immune phenomenon in lupus is the generation of autoantibodies directed against cellular components, a process that forms immune complexes. Note that SLE is a type III hypersensitivity reaction. Although the exact mechanism is not fully understood, there is evidence that immune cells become hyperreactive, leading to a sustained pathologic immune response. It is important to realize that SLE is truly a systemic disease and may manifest in the dermatologic, renal, cardiac, pulmonary, musculoskeletal, hematologic, GI, vascular, and nervous systems.

6. **What causes SLE?**
   As with most immune-mediated diseases, a combination of genetic and environmental factors is thought to be responsible. Lupus tends to occur most frequently in women aged 15 to 40 years, and African Americans are at highest risk. However, SLE may develop in men and women of any age or race.

7. **What are the criteria for diagnosing SLE?**
   SLE is diagnosed on the basis of a combination of clinical and laboratory findings. If four or more of the following criteria are present at *any time* in the patient's history, the diagnosis can be made with 95% specificity.
   1. Malar rash
   2. Discoid rash
   3. Photosensitivity
   4. Oral ulcers
   5. Arthritis
   6. Serositis (pleurisy, pericarditis)
   7. Renal dysfunction ± proteinuria/cellular casts
   8. Neurologic disorder (unexplained seizures or psychosis)
   9. Hematologic disorder (hemolytic anemia, leukopenia, lymphopenia, thrombocytopenia)
   10. Anti–double-stranded DNA (dsDNA), anti-Smith, or antiphospholipid antibodies
   11. Antinuclear antibodies

8. **What are "antinuclear antibodies," and are they sensitive or specific for SLE?**
   The antinuclear antibodies are a diverse group of autoantibodies, all of which bind antigenic targets within the cellular nucleus. Because they are sensitive for SLE (>95% of patients with SLE have them), they are a good screening test for the disease. However, they are not specific because they are present in many other immune-mediated diseases and are often present in healthy elderly adults. Anti-dsDNA and anti-Smith antibodies are very specific for SLE and are useful for confirming the diagnosis. Anti-dsDNA antibodies, in particular, are associated with SLE-induced renal disease and indicate poorer prognosis. Antihistone antibodies are found in drug-induced lupus.

   Note: Understanding which antibodies are sensitive and specific for which condition is very high yield for the STEP 1 exam.

9. What is causing this patient's dry mouth and dry eyes?

The concern of dry mouth (xerostomia) and dry eyes (xerophthalmia) together constitutes sicca complex, also known as *Sjögren syndrome*. This is an immune-mediated disorder of the exocrine glands that can occur either on its own (primary Sjögren) or alongside another immune-mediated disease (secondary), such as lupus, scleroderma, or RA. The anti-Ro (SS-A) and anti-La (SS-B) antibodies are often found in Sjögren syndrome. Anti-Ro is capable of crossing the placenta and can cause third-degree heart block in neonates born to mothers positive for this antibody. Thus babies born to mothers with Sjögren syndrome require immediate cardiac monitoring and, if needed, placement of a permanent pacemaker.

10. What is the reason for the proteinuria?

Immune complexes are deposited in the renal glomeruli, leading to a type III hypersensitivity reaction. This entity is termed *lupus nephritis* and may progress to varying degrees in different patients with SLE. Renal biopsy is often needed to accurately determine prognosis and therapy. Other type III reactions seen in lupus include pericarditis, pleuritis, endocarditis, and the malar rash.

Note: Libman-Sacks endocarditis is a nonbacterial form of endocarditis seen in SLE. Fibrinous vegetations are formed on valve leaflets in response to immune complex deposition. The mitral valve is most commonly involved.

11. What is the reason for this woman's anemia?

Lupus is a chronic inflammatory disorder, and as such, it is capable of causing anemia of chronic disease. This sort of anemia is typically normochromic and normocytic, but it may be hypochromic and microcytic in some cases. Although anemia of chronic disease is the most frequent hematologic manifestation of lupus, other potential complications include immune-mediated hemolytic anemia, leukopenia, lymphopenia, and thrombocytopenia. Lab values for anemia of chronic disease are low serum iron and transferrin, but high ferritin.

12. Why was this patient diagnosed with syphilis without symptoms or risk factors?

Some patients with lupus produce the inaptly named "lupus anticoagulant," which is an antibody directed against certain phospholipid molecules. Although this antibody delays in vitro coagulation assays, it actually predisposes to thrombus formation in vivo. This accounts for the increased incidence of venous and arterial thrombi, fetal loss (first trimester), and thrombocytopenia in patients with lupus. The lupus anticoagulant happens to bind the phospholipid used in the Venereal Disease Research Laboratory assay, which is the reason for the false-positive result when testing for syphilis.

STEP 1 SECRET

The correlation between systemic lupus erythematosus and positive Venereal Disease Research Laboratory test results is a high-yield fact to know for boards.

13. What are the treatment options for SLE?

The mainstay of treatment is the antimalarial medications chloroquine or hydroxychloroquine. Patients with active flares or more severe disease also require systemic glucocorticoids. High doses are used for short periods of active disease, and low doses can be used to prevent flares. The side effects of glucocorticoids are frequently encountered in patients with lupus, who may take these medications for years. The cytotoxic drug cyclophosphamide is also useful in the treatment of lupus nephritis. Many other immunomodulatory medications, such as interferon blocker anifrolumab, are currently under investigation.

Note: Negative side effects of glucocorticoids include hypertension, hyperglycemia, osteoporosis, central obesity, and increased rates of infection.

14. What medications are responsible for drug-induced lupus?

Procainamide, quinidine, hydralazine, isoniazid, sulfonamides, methyldopa, and chlorpromazine have all been shown to cause a disease syndrome that mimics SLE. Drug-induced lupus typically resolves once the offending agent is withdrawn. Remember that with drug-induced lupus, anti-histone antibodies will be present.

15. Quick review: Cover the right column in Table 19.3 and name the primary disease(s) associated with the autoantibodies listed in the left column.

Table 19.3. Autoantibody Summary

AUTOANTIBODY	PRIMARY DISEASE
Antiacetylcholine receptor	Myasthenia gravis
Anticentromere	Limited cutaneous scleroderma (CREST syndrome)
Anti-dsDNA	SLE (specific)

Continued

Table 19.3. Autoantibody Summary—cont'd

AUTOANTIBODY	PRIMARY DISEASE
Anti–glomerular basement membrane	Goodpasture syndrome
Antihistone	Drug-induced SLE
Anti-IgG (RF)	Rheumatoid arthritis
Anti–islet cell	Type 1 diabetes mellitus
Anti-La (SS-B)	Sjögren syndrome
Antimicrosomal	Hashimoto thyroiditis
Antimitochondrial	Primary biliary cirrhosis
Antineutrophil (c-ANCA)	Granulomatosis with polyangiitis (Wegener's)
Antineutrophil (p-ANCA)	Microscopic polyangiitis
Antinuclear	SLE, scleroderma, dermatomyositis
Antiphospholipid	SLE
Anti-Ro (SS-A)	Sjögren syndrome
Anti-Smith	SLE (specific)
Anti–smooth muscle	Chronic autoimmune hepatitis
Anti–tissue transglutaminase	Celiac
Anti-topoisomerase (Scl-70)	Diffuse cutaneous scleroderma

c-ANCA, Cytoplasmic antineutrophil cytoplasmic antibody; *CREST, c*alcinosis, *R*aynaud phenomenon, *e*sophageal dysmotility, *s*clerodactyly, *t*elangiectasia; *dsDNA,* double-stranded DNA; *IgG,* immunoglobulin G; *p-ANCA,* perinuclear antineutrophil cytoplasmic antibody; *RF,* rheumatoid factor; *SLE,* systemic lupus erythematosus.

SUMMARY BOX: SYSTEMIC LUPUS ERYTHEMATOSUS

- Epidemiology: Common immune-mediated disease that primarily occurs in young women.
- Presentation: Classically a young woman with a rash, constitutional concerns, diffuse arthralgias, and an examination showing synovitis of the metacarpophalangeal and proximal interphalangeal joints of the hands. A history of photosensitivity, miscarriages, hematologic disorder, renal dysfunction, and neurologic disorder makes the diagnosis that much more likely.
- Pathophysiology: Caused by autoantibodies directed against nuclear antigens resulting in pathologic immune complex deposition and tissue damage (type III hypersensitivity reaction).
- Diagnosis: Based on a combination of clinical and laboratory findings. Recall that antinuclear antibodies are highly sensitive, but not specific, for systemic lupus erythematosus (SLE), whereas anti-Smith and anti-dsDNA antibodies are highly specific, but not sensitive, for SLE.
- Treatment
  - SLE: Steroids and immunomodulators such as chloroquine
  - Lupus nephritis: Commonly cyclophosphamide
- Complications
  - The lupus anticoagulant is an autoantibody that causes thrombosis, early miscarriages, thrombocytopenia, and false-positive results on Venereal Disease Research Laboratory assays.
  - Drug-induced lupus: Potentially caused by procainamide, quinidine, hydralazine, isoniazid, methyldopa, and chlorpromazine.
  - Lupus nephritis is a type III hypersensitivity reaction associated with high morbidity and mortality rates.

CASE 19.12

A 58-year-old woman presents to your office for evaluation of a several-month history of progressively worsening muscle weakness. She has had difficulty getting into and out of chairs, climbing the stairs, and lifting things over her head. She also reports recently developing a violet-colored rash around her eyes (Fig. 19.19). Review of systems is positive for fatigue, joint stiffness, and an unintentional 10-lb weight loss over the past 6 months. She takes no medications.

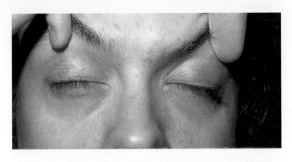

Figure 19.19. Periorbital rash from the patient in Case 19.12. *(From Habif TP. Clinical Dermatology. 4th ed. Philadelphia: Mosby; 2004.)*

1. What is your differential diagnosis?

   This patient has several symptoms of systemic disease (weakness, fatigue, weight loss), as well as a rash and joint pain. One could entertain diagnoses of a thyroid disorder, rheumatic arthritis, myasthenia gravis, PMR, Cushing syndrome, paraneoplastic syndrome or other malignancy, or various myopathies (e.g., muscular dystrophy, dermatomyositis, polymyositis).

CASE 19.12 CONTINUED:

You order several laboratory tests and find elevated levels of creatine kinase (CK), aldolase, and aspartate transaminase. Electromyographic studies are suggestive of myopathy, and a muscle biopsy shows an infiltration of lymphocytes and muscle atrophy.

2. What is the diagnosis?

   This patient has dermatomyositis, one of the idiopathic inflammatory myopathies. This immune-mediated disease causes inflammatory damage to muscle fibers, with resultant proximal muscle weakness and elevated muscle enzymes (CK).

3. What causes this disease?

   Although the exact cause is unknown, a substantial fraction of patients with dermatomyositis have an underlying malignancy. It is therefore important to consider the presence of a neoplastic process in a patient who presents with dermatomyositis.

4. What is the treatment?

   Because this is an inflammatory disorder, immunosuppressant drugs are the mainstay. Prednisone is first-line therapy, and methotrexate can be used if corticosteroids are unsuccessful.

5. What are the other "idiopathic inflammatory myopathies"?

   Dermatomyositis and polymyositis are both inflammatory myopathies characterized by symmetric proximal muscle weakness, elevated serum muscle enzymes, and evidence of myopathy on electromyography. Dermatomyositis often presents with skin findings, such as the heliotrope rash, Gottron papules (Fig. 19.20), and shawl sign; polymyositis does not have these dermatologic manifestations. Dermatomyositis and polymyositis appear distinct on muscle biopsy, with dermatomyositis showing immune complex deposition and polymyositis revealing predominantly T-cell invasion of muscle fibers. Inclusion body myositis is another inflammatory myopathy, which presents with both proximal and distal muscle weakness and normal or mildly elevated muscle enzymes and is associated with distinctive changes on electromyogram and biopsy. Fig. 19.20 shows Gottron papules on the hands in dermatomyositis.

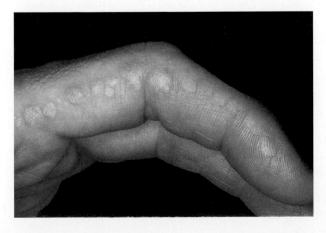

Figure 19.20. Gottron papules, a pathognomonic sign of dermatomyositis, are round, smooth, flat-topped papules that occur over the knuckles and along the sides of the fingers. *(From Habif TP. Clinical Dermatology. 4th ed. Philadelphia: Mosby; 2004.)*

6. What disease that is transmitted by pork can cause similar muscular symptoms?

Trichinosis is caused by eating raw or undercooked meats that contain the viable larvae of the roundworm *Trichinella spiralis.* Although most infections are subclinical, exposure to a heavy inoculum of larvae can result in trichinosis, which may present clinically with diarrhea, myositis, fever, and periorbital edema. Laboratory evaluation will typically reveal hypereosinophilia as well.

SUMMARY BOX: INFLAMMATORY MYOPATHIES

- Dermatomyositis, polymyositis, and inclusion body myositis are idiopathic inflammatory myopathies.
- Dermatomyositis is characterized by proximal muscle weakness, elevated serum muscle enzymes, electromyogram abnormalities, dermatologic manifestations, and characteristic muscle pathologic changes. It is often associated with an underlying malignancy.
- Polymyositis is a similar myopathic process with distinct muscle disease but without skin involvement.
- Inclusion body myositis causes both proximal and distal muscle weakness without markedly raised serum muscle enzymes.
- The inflammatory myopathies are treated with steroids.
- Trichinosis is a parasitic disease that may cause myopathy.

CASE 19.13

The parents of a 3-year-old boy are concerned that he is not walking as well as other boys his age. Both parents are healthy, and there is no family history of neuromuscular disease. He has three older brothers who are healthy. On physical examination, he has large calf muscles and lower extremity proximal muscle weakness, as demonstrated by the need to use his arms and hands to assist in standing from a seated position. Examination is otherwise unremarkable.

1. What is your differential diagnosis?

his child with muscle weakness may have a myopathy such as juvenile dermatomyositis, an inflammatory disease such as juvenile RA, an inherited muscular dystrophy, a neurologic disorder such as Guillain-Barré syndrome, or an infection such as Lyme disease or trichinosis.

CASE 19.13 CONTINUED:

Laboratory tests are significant only for a markedly elevated CK level. A skeletal muscle biopsy reveals complete absence of dystrophin staining.

2. What is the most likely diagnosis?

Duchenne muscular dystrophy is most likely.

3. Is this condition more commonly acquired or inherited?

About two-thirds of cases of Duchenne muscular dystrophy are inherited in an X-linked recessive manner. However, approximately one-third of the cases are secondary to spontaneous mutations within the dystrophin gene. The dystrophin gene is subject to a high rate of spontaneous mutations because of its enormous size ($>2 \times 10^6$ bases). Because his parents were unaffected and he has three healthy older brothers, this condition was likely acquired in this boy following a spontaneous mutation in the dystrophin gene.

STEP 1 SECRET

Boards will often relate genetics questions to pedigrees, which means that you should know the inheritance patterns of the genetic diseases that you study. X-linked recessive diseases are a particular USMLE favorite. These include **G***6PD (glucose-6-phosphate dehydrogenase) deficiency,* **O***cular albinism,* **L***esch-Nyhan syndrome,* **D***uchenne muscular dystrophy,* **W***iskott-Aldrich syndrome,* **B***ruton agammaglobulinemia,* **C***hronic granulomatous disease,* **H***unter syndrome,* **F***abry disease, and* **H***emophilia (A and B).*
You can use this mnemonic to remember the X-linked recessive diseases: **"Good OLD WBCs Hunt and Fight Heroically."**

4. What is the function of dystrophin?

Dystrophin is a cytoskeletal membrane protein that plays an important structural role in skeletal muscle cells. It is absent in Duchenne muscular dystrophy.

5. How do the manifestations of Becker muscular dystrophy differ?

This disease is also due to mutations in the dystrophin gene, but there is some level of protein present rather than a complete absence, so the clinical manifestations are not as severe as in Duchenne muscular dystrophy.

6. Why does this boy have such large calf muscles on examination? What term is used to describe this finding in patients with Duchenne muscular dystrophy?

Patients with Duchenne muscular dystrophy ironically have the appearance of enlarged calf muscles, referred to as *pseudo-hypertrophy of the calf muscles* (Fig. 19.21). This hypertrophy occurs initially in response to hypertrophy of muscle fibers but secondarily in response to fatty infiltration of the muscle and abnormal proliferation of connective tissue within the muscle.

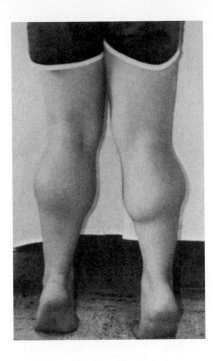

Figure 19.21. Enlarged calf muscles in a patient with Duchenne muscular dystrophy. *(From Fenichel GM.* Clinical Pediatric Neurology. *Philadelphia: WB Saunders; 1997.)*

7. **How is a Gower sign elicited on examination, and what does it indicate?**
   A Gower sign can be elicited by asking the child to stand from a sitting position. Children with muscular dystrophy and other disorders involving muscle wasting will not have the muscle strength to simply stand. They may instead first roll over into a prone position, push themselves onto all fours, and then "walk" their hands up their thighs to a standing position (i.e., positive Gower sign). The presence of a Gower sign indicates marked proximal muscle weakness (Fig. 19.22).

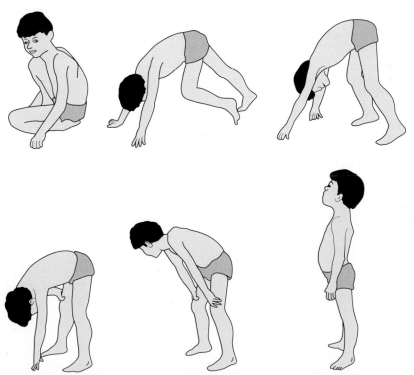

Figure 19.22. Gower sign. *(Redrawn from Siegel IM.* Clinical management of muscle disease. *In: Canale STS.* Campbell's Operative Orthopedics. *5th ed. London: William Heinemann; 1977.)*

A FEW MORE MUSCULAR DYSTROPHIES . . .

CASE 19.14

A patient reports a long history of generalized muscle weakness. On examination, his facial muscles show marked atrophy, and when you ask him to shake your hand, he appears unable to relax his grip for an extended period.

1. What diagnosis might you suspect?

   You might suspect myotonic dystrophy, which is the most common adult dystrophy. The term *myotonia* refers to a sustained involuntary contraction of muscles, which this man is exhibiting by not being able to release his grip.

   Other symptoms of myotonic dystrophy include facial muscle weakness, frontal balding, testicular atrophy, cataracts, cardiac conduction defects, and glucose intolerance.

2. What is the mechanism of inheritance of myotonic dystrophy?

   Myotonic dystrophy results from impaired expression of the myotonin protein kinase gene. The mechanism causing impaired expression involves expansion of a trinucleotide repeat sequence located in the 3′ untranslated region of the myotonin protein kinase gene. This disorder is inherited as an autosomal dominant disease, and because this mechanism involves expansion of trinucleotide repeat sequences (CTG), the phenomenon of anticipation is seen (i.e., family members get the disease at earlier and earlier ages throughout the generations).

   Note: Other trinucleotide repeat disorders include Huntington disease (CAG), fragile X syndrome (CGG), and Friedreich ataxia (GAA).

CASE 19.15

An adult patient with a long history of muscle weakness has maintained a slow, steady course of declining function and is now wheelchair bound. His weakness is most prominent in proximal muscles, with complete sparing of facial and extraocular musculature. A muscle biopsy shows normal dystrophin expression. The patient's father and grandfather had similar courses.

1. What is the diagnosis?

   This is limb-girdle muscular dystrophy, which is actually a group of myopathies that affect the shoulder and pelvic girdles. Limb-girdle dystrophies can be inherited in both autosomal dominant and recessive fashion and may display a heterogeneous phenotype. The recessive form of the disease tends to have an earlier onset and progresses more quickly, whereas the dominant form follows a slower and more variable course. Several different genes have been implicated in this disease.

SUMMARY BOX: THE MUSCULAR DYSTROPHIES

- Duchenne muscular dystrophy is a usually inherited loss of the dystrophin protein, which is a structural component of skeletal muscle cells.
- Duchenne muscular dystrophy is inherited in a recessive X-linked fashion, or it may be an acquired spontaneous mutation.
- Becker muscular dystrophy is an inherited defect in dystrophin that results in partial loss of the dystrophin protein.
- Myotonic muscular dystrophy is a trinucleotide repeat disorder.
- Limb-girdle muscular dystrophy is a heterogeneous group of heritable defects in proteins that result in proximal muscle weakness and atrophy.
- Gower sign indicates proximal muscle weakness.

CASE 19.16

Dr. Rheumatoid is a specialist widely known for his interest and skill in treating rare disorders of the musculoskeletal system. His particular expertise is in diagnosing and treating metabolic and developmental disorders of bone. A third-year medical student working with him one afternoon is delighted to encounter one "zebra" after another in clinic.

CASE 19.17

The first patient was referred to Dr. Rheumatoid with bone pain and a diagnosis by a hematologist of myelophthisic anemia. A bone scan reveals abnormally thick and dense bones with an "Erlenmeyer flask" deformity (Fig. 19.23).

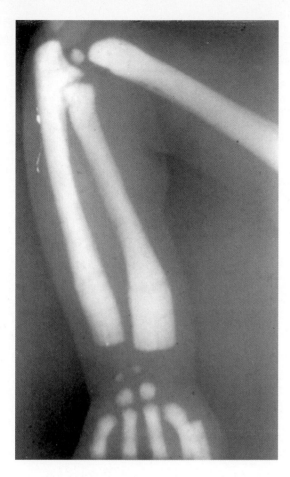

Figure 19.23. Radiograph of the upper extremity in a patient with osteopetrosis. *(From Kumar V, Abbas AK, Fausto N.* Robbins and Cotran Pathologic Basis of Disease. *7th ed. Philadelphia: WB Saunders; 2005.)*

1. **What is your diagnosis?**
   Osteopetrosis (also known as *marble bone disease*) is the diagnosis.

2. **What causes the bones to be dense and thick in this patient?**
   In osteopetrosis, osteoclasts are less active than normal (or inactive entirely) and therefore do not resorb bone effectively during bone remodeling. This generally is the result of failure of the osteoclasts to acidify the resorption pit (as a result of carbonic anhydrase or chloride channel gene mutations). In addition, the process whereby woven (immature) bone is converted to compact (mature) bone is disrupted in osteopetrosis. This combination of reduced remodeling of bone and inadequate bone "maturation" results in thick and brittle bones.

3. **Why might you see anemia in osteopetrosis, and why is it referred to as a** *myelophthisic anemia*?
   The term *myelophthisis* describes the replacement of hematopoietic tissue in the bone marrow with abnormal tissue. Myelophthisic anemia is therefore caused by the replacement of bone marrow by abnormal tissue. In the case of osteopetrosis, the failure of osteoclasts to remodel existing bone allows newly formed bone to encroach on the space of the bone marrow, making hematopoiesis less effective and resulting in pancytopenia (anemia, thrombocytopenia, and leukopenia).

4. **Should you observe any laboratory value abnormalities in a patient who has osteopetrosis?**
   No. Serum calcium, phosphate, alkaline phosphatase, and parathyroid hormone levels are normal in osteopetrosis.
   Note: You do not need to know exact laboratory value ranges, but you should be able to compare them with normal values using relative terms (increased, decreased, normal).

STEP 1 SECRET

Laboratory value abnormalities associated with various bone disorders are high yield for Step 1. When studying this topic, you should classify these disorders according to their unique clinical and radiographic features, as well as their expected laboratory values (e.g., calcium, phosphate, alkaline phosphatase, parathyroid hormone).

CASE 19.18

A 13-year-old boy with sickle cell anemia is referred for persistent right hip pain and intermittent fevers, although he cannot recall any specific trauma to the hip. An x-ray of the hips suggests avascular necrosis of the femoral heads.

1. **Infection with what organisms should be suspected?**

   Although *S. aureus* is the most common organism responsible for osteomyelitis, patients with sickle cell anemia are uniquely susceptible to *Salmonella* bacteremia and osteomyelitis. This susceptibility stems from the impaired splenic and mononuclear cell function associated with sickle cell anemia because *Salmonella* is an encapsulated organism.

CASE 19.19

A 42-year-old woman with end-stage renal failure is referred to Dr. Rheumatoid because recent bone scans revealed marked osteopenia throughout her body.

1. **What most likely explains this?**

   The most likely explanation is osteomalacia caused by vitamin D deficiency secondary to renal failure. Recall that an important endocrine function of the kidneys is the production of 1,25-dihydroxycholecalciferol, the active form of vitamin D. Because vitamin D is necessary for bone mineralization and because bone is constantly being remodeled, impaired mineralization results in an imbalance between mineralization and degradation, causing marked osteopenia (Fig. 19.24).

   Note: Additional causes of renal osteodystrophy include bone buffering of excess acid and hypocalcemia from calcium phosphate precipitation in hyperphosphatemia.

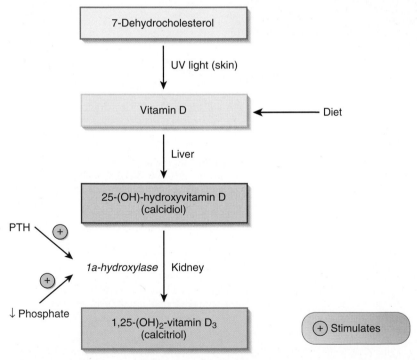

Figure 19.24. Vitamin D synthesis. PTH, parathyroid hormone; UV, ultraviolet. *(From Brown T. Rapid Review Physiology. 2nd ed. Philadelphia: Mosby; 2011.)*

CASE 19.20

A 6-year-old boy is brought to the clinic by his mother because he has had multiple bone fractures throughout his short life. These fractures were all unexpected because they invariably occurred in response to very minor accidents. In addition, the boy has been doing poorly in school recently because he is having trouble hearing the teacher. The examination is remarkable only for slightly blue sclerae. X-ray of the lower extremity shows marked bowing of the bones (Fig. 19.25).

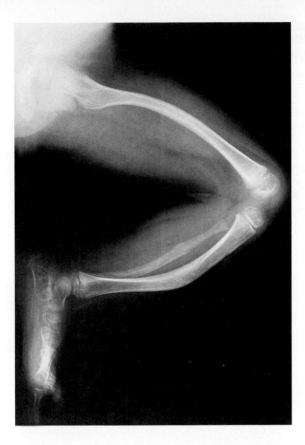

Figure 19.25. Lateral view of the lower extremities shows marked bowing of the bones caused by softening and multiple fractures that occur as a result of this congenital bone dysplasia. *(From Mettler FA.* Essentials of Radiology. *2nd ed. Philadelphia: WB Saunders; 2005.)*

1. What is your diagnosis, and what is the etiology of this condition?

   Osteogenesis imperfecta is due to genetic defects that result in structural or quantitative abnormalities of type I collagen, which is the primary component of the extracellular matrix of bones, including the middle ear bone (explaining the hearing loss seen in this child). Type I collagen is also found in corneal tissues. A defect in type I collagen results in translucency of the connective tissue over the vascular choroid layer of the eye such that the veins impart a blue appearance to the sclerae.

   Note: A wide spectrum of genotypes and phenotypes is associated with osteogenesis imperfecta, ranging from fairly minor to very severe.

2. Quick review: Cover the right column in Table 19.4 and list the pathophysiologic abnormality associated with each of the rheumatologic disorders listed in the left column.

Table 19.4. Rheumatologic Disorders

DISORDER	PATHOPHYSIOLOGY
Achondroplasia	Mutation in fibroblast growth factor receptor prevents endochondral ossification and limits long bone growth
Gout	Increased uric acid production or decreased uric acid excretion
Osteoarthritis	Degeneration of joint cartilage
Osteogenesis imperfecta	Genetic defects in type I collagen weaken bone
Osteomalacia	Impaired bone mineralization in adults
Osteopetrosis (marble bone disease)	Decreased osteoclast activity, bony invasion of bone marrow leading to myelophthisic anemia
Paget disease	Increased rate of osteoclast activity (perhaps secondary to viral infection of osteoclasts), resulting in increased rates of bone resorption, formation, and mineralization, with consequent deposition of woven rather than lamellar bone

Continued

Table 19.4. Rheumatologic Disorders—cont'd

DISORDER	PATHOPHYSIOLOGY
Pseudogout (chondrocalcinosis)	Calcium pyrophosphate deposition
Rheumatoid arthritis	Inflammation of synovial membrane
Rickets	Impaired bone and cartilage mineralization in children

SUMMARY BOX: OSTEOPETROSIS, SICKLE CELL AVASCULAR NECROSIS, AND OSTEOGENESIS IMPERFECTA

- Osteopetrosis is a disorder of osteoclasts that results in thick, brittle bones and myelophthisic anemia.
- Patients with sickle cell disease are prone to osteomyelitis caused by *Salmonella* species.
- End-stage renal failure results in vitamin D deficiency and osteomalacia, also known as *renal osteodystrophy*.
- Osteogenesis imperfecta is a highly variable disease caused by a defect in type I collagen.

VASCULITIDES

BASIC CONCEPTS

1. What are the vasculitides, and how do they typically present clinically?

   The best way to think of the vasculitides is as a group of poorly understood autoimmune disorders involving the blood vessels. They are defined by the presence of leukocytes in the vessel walls, and as inflammatory diseases, they typically present with vague constitutional signs, such as fever, malaise, and arthralgias or myalgias. There is often associated ischemia and damage to the organs supplied by the affected vessels. A biopsy of affected blood vessels can be very helpful in making a definitive diagnosis, although obtaining a segment of affected vasculature can be difficult. Although it appears that most vasculitides are caused by an immune-mediated mechanism, other possible etiologies include drug hypersensitivity reactions and viral infections resulting in immune complex deposition within the vasculature.

2. Along with constitutional concerns, what clinical signs and patterns of organ involvement suggest a vasculitic syndrome?

   Palpable nonblanching purpura may indicate vasculitides, such as hypersensitivity vasculitis (also known as leukocytoclastic vasculitis or cutaneous small vessel vasculitis), Henoch-Schönlein purpura, and microscopic polyangiitis (MPA).

   Mononeuritis multiplex, a clinical picture that arises from simultaneous disease to multiple individual nerves, typically affects sensory and motor function. In the United States, diabetes is the most common cause of this neuropathy, but in the nondiabetic person, it is very suggestive of vasculitis, particularly polyarteritis nodosa (PAN). Pulmonary-renal involvement, such as hemoptysis and hematuria, are suggestive of a pulmonary-renal syndrome, such as granulomatosis with polyangiitis (GPA; formerly known as Wegener granulomatosis).

3. How are the vasculitides classified?

   The vasculitides are generally classified by the size and types of blood vessel that are typically affected in patients with each disorder.

   Large vessel vasculitis:
   - Takayasu arteritis affects the aorta and its major branches.
   - Temporal arteritis, also known as giant cell arteritis (GCA), most commonly affects the branches of the external carotid artery, characteristically including the temporal artery. It can also involve the aorta and its major branches.

   Medium vessel vasculitis:
   - PAN affects medium-size muscular arteries.
   - Kawasaki disease actually affects large, medium, and small arteries, but the most important association is that, if untreated, it can affect the coronary arteries causing aneurysms.
   - Thromboangiitis obliterans, also known as *Buerger disease*, affects small- to medium-size arteries and, as such, is typically classified as a medium vessel vasculitis.

   Small vessel vasculitis:
   - Eosinophilic GPA (Churg-Strauss syndrome) affects the arteries of the lungs and of the skin.
   - GPA (Wegener granulomatosis) and MPA affect medium- and small-size vessels, particularly in the respiratory tract and kidneys.

- Cryoglobulinemic vasculitis affects capillaries, arterioles, and venules.
- Henoch-Schönlein purpura (IgA vasculitis) primarily affects small-size vessels.
- Vasculitis secondary to hypersensitivity reaction, viral infection, or connective tissue disorder typically affects small vessels.

4. Cover the right column in Table 20.1 and attempt to describe the "classic presentation" for each of the listed vasculitides.

Table 20.1. Classic Presentation of the Vasculitides

VASCULITIS	TYPICAL PATIENT	CLASSIC PRESENTATION	CHARACTERISTIC LABS
Temporal (giant cell) arteritis	Caucasian female > 50 years old	Fever, unilateral headache, jaw claudication, vision loss	Markedly elevated ESR
Granulomatosis with polyangiitis (Wegener)	Older Caucasian	Constitutional symptoms, hemoptysis, hematuria, ENT symptoms (saddle nose, sinusitis, epistaxis, nasopharyngeal ulcers, nasal septal perforation)	c-ANCA (directed against proteinase 3) Elevated ESR Granulomatous changes
Microscopic polyangiitis	Older Caucasian	Constitutional symptoms, hemoptysis, hematuria. Spares the upper respiratory tract (e.g., nasopharynx)	p-ANCA (directed against myeloperoxidase) Elevated ESR No granulomatous changes
Kawasaki syndrome	Asian child < 5 years old	Unexplained fever, polymorphous rash, bilateral nonexudative conjunctivitis, cervical lymphadenopathy, extremity changes (hands/feet), and mucosal changes (e.g., strawberry tongue)	Elevated ESR, CRP
Polyarteritis nodosa	Middle-aged or older patient with HBV	Generally affects vessels of the kidney, heart, liver, and GI system Pulmonary vasculature spared Hepatitis B antigen positivity is common; arterial biopsy reveals transmural inflammation and fibrinoid necrosis in varying stages	No ANCA association Aneurysms in mesenteric or renal arteries on angiography/imaging ("string of pearls" appearance)
Eosinophilic granulomatosis with polyangiitis (Churg-Strauss syndrome)	Middle-aged patient, rare in children and elderly	History of asthma, sinusitis, peripheral neuropathy, skin lesions; can have cardiac involvement	Eosinophilia (>10% on WBC differential) p-ANCA (directed against myeloperoxidase)
Takayasu arteritis ("pulseless disease")	Asian women < 40 years old	Fever, night sweats, arthritis, myalgia, vision problems, differential blood pressures in the upper extremities	Elevated ESR and CRP support clinical findings MRI or CTA to confirm
Henoch-Schönlein purpura (IgA vasculitis)	Child from age 3–15 years	Abdominal pain, arthritis, arthralgia, hematuria with RBC casts (IgA nephropathy), maculopapular rash on lower extremities (palpable purpura) Associated with IgA nephropathy after upper respiratory infection; increased risk for intussusception	No specific testing Elevated IgA in 50–70% of cases
Mixed essential cryoglobulinemia	Patient in 50s–60s with HCV	Arthralgias, hepatosplenomegaly, hypocomplementemia, palpable purpura, proteinuria, and hematuria; confirmed by presence of circulating cryoglobulins; strongly associated with HCV infection	Elevated cryoglobulins Hypocomplementemia
Thromboangiitis obliterans (Buerger disease)	Male smoker aged 40–45 years	Young male smoker with distal extremity cold intolerance, may lead to gangrene and autoamputation of digits; strongly associated with heavy smoking	Normal ESR/CRP, complement levels

c-ANCA, Cytoplasmic antineutrophil cytoplasmic antibodies; *CRP,* C-reactive protein; *CT,* computed tomography angiography; *ENT,* ear, nose, throat; *ESR,* erythrocyte sedimentation rate; *GI,* gastrointestinal; *HBV,* hepatitis B virus; *HCV,* hepatitis C virus; *IgA,* immunoglobulin A; *MRI,* magnetic resonance imaging; *p-ANCA,* perinuclear antineutrophil cytoplasmic antibodies; *RBC,* red blood cell; *WBC,* white blood cell.

CASE 20.1

A 75-year-old Caucasian woman is evaluated for a 1-week history of anorexia, fatigue, and unilateral severe headache. She denies any recent visual problems or photophobia.

1. **What are the main considerations in your differential diagnosis?**
   Constitutional concerns such as anorexia and fatigue are suggestive of malignancy, depression, infection, and vasculitis. The headache could be caused by a migraine, meningitis, brain mass, intracranial hemorrhage, or vasculitis. However, for the boards, unilateral headache in an adult older than 50 years in the absence of fever or head trauma is temporal arteritis until proven otherwise.

CASE 20.1 CONTINUED:

Physical examination is significant for right-sided scalp tenderness. Laboratory tests reveal a markedly elevated erythrocyte sedimentation rate.

2. **What is the likely diagnosis?**
   Temporal arteritis or GCA is the likely diagnosis. Temporal arteritis occurs almost exclusively in patients older than 50 years. Women are more likely than men to be affected, and rates are highest in Caucasians. Unilateral headache and scalp tenderness are classic for temporal arteritis, as is the elevated erythrocyte sedimentation rate (ESR). Temporal arteritis also commonly presents with jaw claudication (jaw pain brought on by mastication and relieved by stopping). Vision impairment (*amaurosis fugax*) or blindness may result in the most serious cases.
   The name *temporal arteritis* is derived from the fact that the disease preferentially targets the extracranial branches of the carotid arteries, frequently affecting the superficial temporal artery. The ophthalmic, vertebral, and carotid arteries may also be affected. Involvement of intracranial/intradural arteries is rare, possibly because of fewer elastic fibers in the media and adventitia and absence of vasa vasorum in these arteries (see subsequent discussion regarding events that lead to inflammation).

3. **What does the elevated ESR suggest?**
   The ESR and C-reactive protein (CRP) are the most widely used indicators of the acute-phase protein response. Although these measurements lack specificity (commonly elevated in other vasculitides, infections such as endocarditis, and malignancies), they are useful because the acute-phase protein response may reflect the presence and intensity of an inflammatory process.
   Specifically, the ESR represents the rate at which erythrocytes fall (sediment) through plasma, which depends largely on the plasma concentration of fibrinogen, a protein seen in higher concentrations during an inflammatory process.

4. **In temporal arteritis, what events lead to inflammation of the artery?**
   It is likely that T cells and macrophages enter the artery wall via the vasa vasorum. How they become activated and targeted is unknown. CD4$^+$ T cells release interferon gamma (IFN-γ), and macrophages release interleukins (IL-1, IL-6) and platelet-derived growth factor. IFN-γ mediates the inflammatory response in the vessel wall, IL-6 is largely responsible for systemic signs of inflammation and destruction of vessel wall structures (e.g., internal elastic lamina), and platelet-derived growth factor promotes proliferation of smooth muscle cells and intimal hyperplasia. This intimal hyperplasia leads to occlusion of the arterial lumen and ultimately symptoms of ischemia.

CASE 20.1 CONTINUED:

The patient is started on high-dose steroids; the following day, a biopsy of a 3-cm section of the right side of the temporal artery returns negative for signs of inflammation.

5. **Why might it still make sense to treat this patient?**
   Temporal arteritis affects the temporal artery in a segmental fashion, and this could explain a negative biopsy result even in the presence of the disease. Furthermore, in some cases, GCA may affect other extracranial branches of the carotid artery and spare the superficial temporal artery. Therefore, if the clinician has a high index of suspicion for temporal arteritis, the patient should be treated regardless of biopsy results (making biopsy of questionable clinical value).

6. **What severe complication of this disorder may be avoided by initiating immunosuppressive therapy as soon as possible?**
   Partial or total blindness can occur suddenly and without warning. This is caused by occlusion of the ophthalmic artery, leading to ischemia of the optic nerve. Blindness may be preceded by amaurosis fugax, which is transient visual loss, often with heat or exercise. Blindness is usually permanent but can be prevented by adequate treatment with corticosteroids, making timely diagnosis and treatment of GCA crucial. Studies have also shown further loss of vision in the unaffected eye in a considerable fraction (25%–50%) of untreated patients. As demonstrated in this case, patients with GCA are treated with high-dose steroids to prevent blindness.

7. **What other symptomatic manifestations may be expected as a result of arterial inflammation in patients with GCA?**

Decreased blood flow in the extracranial branches of the carotid arteries caused by inflammation of those vessels can lead to symptoms such as jaw claudication, especially when prolonged talking or chewing causes an increase in oxygen demand. Occasionally, respiratory symptoms such as nonproductive coughing can be seen with GCA and are believed to be a result of inflammatory involvement of branches of the pulmonary artery involved in the cough reflex pathway.

In a subset of patients, the predominant symptoms of GCA may be constitutional signs of systemic inflammation, such as fever, fatigue, and anorexia. Fatigue is often also noted in patients with more typical presentations, such as headache or scalp tenderness. This is evidence that immune activation is not necessarily limited to vascular lesions. Patients with GCA have elevated levels of circulating monocytes, which produce IL-1 and IL-6, and the latter is a potent inducer of the acute-phase response. Release of IL-6 therefore not only leads to the elevation of ESR in these patients but also helps explain the nonspecific systemic symptoms.

8. **How can response to corticosteroids be monitored?**

Remember the ESR? The drop in ESR or CRP, along with the clinical response, can be used to gauge effectiveness of corticosteroid therapy.

9. **With what other disease is GCA associated?**

Polymyalgia rheumatica (PMR), which is an inflammatory disorder characterized by bilateral pain in the muscles of the neck, shoulder, and pelvic girdle, along with morning stiffness and elevated ESR. PMR is often considered to be a form of GCA that lacks the fully developed vasculitis. Both GCA and PMR respond to steroid therapy. Whereas high-dose steroids are used to treat GCA, low-dose steroids are used to treat PMR.

STEP 1 SECRET

Temporal arteritis is a favorite on the USMLE. Be on the lookout for symptoms of unilateral headache, jaw claudication, vision problems, and musculoskeletal pain (PMR association).

SUMMARY BOX: TEMPORAL ARTERITIS

- Presentation: Unilateral headache, scalp tenderness, jaw claudication, and constitutional signs (fever, fatigue, and weight loss)
- Epidemiology: Adults > 50 years old, usually Caucasian women
- Pathogenesis: Inflammation of the walls of extracranial branches of carotid arteries
- Diagnosis: Elevated erythrocyte sedimentation rate and C-reactive protein
  - Biopsy of the superficial temporal artery, showing granulomatous infiltration of the arterial wall, may be helpful but is associated with a high false-negative rate because of skip lesions
- Complications: Partial/complete blindness
- Treatment: High-dose corticosteroids

CASE 20.2

A 4-year-old girl is evaluated for a 5-day history of high fever and desquamating rash of her palms and soles with swelling of her hands and feet (Fig. 20.1). Examination is significant for cervical lymphadenopathy, injected conjunctiva, and "cherry-red" lips with fissuring and crusting. Laboratory evaluation reveals an elevated ESR and platelet count.

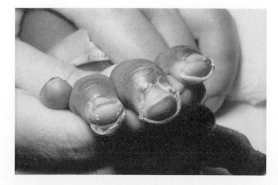

Figure 20.1. Kawasaki disease. *(From Shah BR, Laude TA.* Atlas of Pediatric Clinical Diagnosis. *Philadelphia: WB Saunders; 2000.)*

1. **What are the considerations in your differential diagnosis?**

   The desquamating rash is concerning for staphylococcal scalded skin syndrome (SSSS), in which epidermolytic toxins are produced by *Staphylococcus aureus* infection. Children are thought to be at increased risk for SSSS because they have not previously been exposed to the epidermolytic toxins and thereby lack protective antibodies to the toxins. The presentation is also concerning for toxic shock syndrome, in which superantigen toxins from streptococcal or staphylococcal infections (often following use of tampons, contraceptive devices, or nasal packing) are produced. These toxins overstimulate the immune system, resulting in fever, a rash that may desquamate, and a myriad of other signs and symptoms. Remember that superantigens nonspecifically activate many T cells at once, resulting in release of large quantities of cytokines (IL-1, IL-2, tumor necrosis factor α and β, IFN-γ) that trigger a massive inflammatory response.

   Scarlet fever is another concern in this child. Scarlet fever is an exotoxin-mediated disease associated with streptococcal pharyngitis, impetigo, or other streptococcal infections. It is characterized by fever, rash, and a "strawberry tongue."

   Finally, we need to consider Kawasaki disease (also called *mucocutaneous lymph node syndrome*), an acute febrile systemic illness of childhood affecting medium-size vessels. It is more common in Asian children and can also present with many of the previously mentioned symptoms.

CASE 20.2 CONTINUED:

The attending physician is not interested in an impressive differential diagnosis but rather wants a specific diagnosis for the child.

2. **What is your diagnosis?**

   Kawasaki disease could explain all of this girl's symptoms. The diagnosis of Kawasaki disease requires unexplained fever for at least 5 days, accompanied by at least four of the five following criteria:
   1. Bilateral nonexudative conjunctivitis
   2. Oral mucous membrane changes, such as cracked lips, throat redness, or "strawberry tongue"
   3. Peripheral extremity changes, such as palmar erythema or edema of the hands and feet
   4. Polymorphous rash (different appearance depending on the patient with temporal variation, but generally maculopapular [small, flat discolored areas with small, raised bumps] and involving the trunk)
   5. Cervical lymphadenopathy

   A popular mnemonic that is used to remember these criteria is "CRASH and burn" ("CRASH" stands for **C**onjunctivitis, **R**ash, **A**denopathy, **S**trawberry tongue, **H**and and feet swelling, erythema, and peeling, and "burn" refers to 5 days of fever). If these conditions are not strictly met, the patient may have an "incomplete Kawasaki disease," which can potentially lead to the same cardiac sequelae as typical disease. Of the criteria found in typical disease, mucous membrane changes are most common. Incomplete Kawasaki disease (previously called atypical) is diagnosed if two to three clinical criteria are met and there is a suspicion of Kawasaki disease and laboratory findings are consistent with the disease. First, an ESR and/or CRP must be elevated, and then various lab parameters are checked. If at least three supplemental laboratory criteria are positive, incomplete Kawasaki disease is diagnosed and the treatment is identical to that of Kawasaki disease. The term *incomplete* is preferred to *atypical* because the patients have typical courses and have high risk for cardiovascular sequelae.

   It may be helpful to remember the other term for Kawasaki disease: *mucocutaneous lymph node syndrome*. This name is derived from the typical signs and symptoms, which include *mucosal* inflammation, *cutaneous* maculopapular rash, and *lymph node* enlargement, all with an unexplained high fever.

3. **What is the major concern in patients with this disease who do not receive adequate therapy?**

   Coronary artery aneurysms are the major cause of morbidity and mortality in Kawasaki disease, occurring in 20% to 25% of untreated children. A much smaller percentage ($\approx$4%) of those adequately treated (see later discussion for treatment) will develop coronary artery aneurysms. Coronary artery inflammation can lead to myocardial inflammation, arrhythmias, or death. In fact, roughly 1% of all children who develop Kawasaki disease will die of rupture of a coronary artery aneurysm or coronary artery thrombosis and infarction. Pericardial effusions are seen in approximately 20% of cases, and myocarditis can lead to tachycardia. Otherwise, the course of this disease is self-limiting, with fever and acute manifestations lasting an average of 12 days without therapy.

4. **What is the pathogenesis of Kawasaki disease?**

   The exact pathogenesis of Kawasaki disease is unknown, but it is speculated that an infectious agent may trigger vasculitis in genetically susceptible individuals. Overactivation of immune-competent cells and an overproduction of cytokines cause endothelial cell injury and blood vessel wall damage. Inflammation in blood vessels is primarily mediated by activated T cells, monocytes, and macrophages. Coronary arteries are preferentially affected, which can lead to myocardial infarction.

5. **How is this disease treated?**

   Intravenous immunoglobulin (IVIG) and aspirin are given to prevent coronary aneurysms. IVIG has anti-inflammatory properties, while aspirin has both anti-inflammatory and antiplatelet properties.

   Note: Aspirin is generally contraindicated in children with a febrile illness because of the risk of developing Reye syndrome (encephalopathy and hepatic dysfunction), especially in children with varicella or influenza. However, the benefits are thought to outweigh the risks in Kawasaki disease. Aspirin should be discontinued (with continuation of IVIG) if exposure to varicella or influenza occurs during treatment.

6. Describe the epidemiology of this disease.

This is a disease of unknown cause that is seen in children and is most common in Asian populations. Eighty percent of cases occur in children younger than 5 years, with the peak incidence at 2 years of age. The disease is more common in boys than in girls. Interestingly, there is a twofold increased risk in a child who has at least one parent who was affected as a child, suggesting a possible genetic component to the disease. Seasonal variation in incidence, with increased incidence in late winter and early spring, and the "epidemic" nature of the disease suggest some environmental component.

SUMMARY BOX: KAWASAKI DISEASE

- Presentation: Fever for ≥5 days, erythema of lips and oral mucosa, rash, bilateral nonexudative conjunctivitis
- Epidemiology: 80% of cases occur in children younger than 5 years; more common in males and Asians
- Pathogenesis: Immune overactivation and excessive cytokine production result in endothelial cell and vascular wall damage
  - Speculated to be triggered by an infectious agent
- Diagnosis: Unexplained fever for ≥5 days, accompanied by at least four of the five following criteria:
  1. Bilateral nonexudative conjunctivitis
  2. Oral mucous membrane changes, such as cracked lips, throat redness, or strawberry tongue
  3. Peripheral extremity changes, such as palmar erythema or edema of the hands and feet
  4. Polymorphous rash
  5. Cervical lymphadenopathy
- Complications: Coronary artery aneurysms, leading to myocardial infarction or fatal arrhythmias
- Treatment: Intravenous immunoglobulin and aspirin

CASE 20.3

A 40-year-old man is evaluated for a 1-year history of recurrent ear and sinus infections and headache. He has a history of pollen allergy and assumed that the sinus congestion resulted from increased allergies this season. Recently, however, he began to notice blood-tinged sputum and a slight cough.

---

1. What is your differential diagnosis?

Upper airway involvement and constitutional concerns (anorexia, fatigue, weakness) are suggestive of a variety of conditions. Recurrent sinusitis with hemoptysis due to acute bronchitis—the most common cause of hemoptysis—is one possibility, but this seems unlikely. Other diagnoses to consider include Churg-Strauss syndrome (eosinophilic GPA), GPA, MPA, Goodpasture syndrome, and bronchogenic carcinoma.

Churg-Strauss syndrome is a systemic vasculitis that occurs in the setting of allergic rhinitis, asthma, and eosinophilia. Pulmonary infiltrates may occur. Asthma typically precedes this disease by many years, and the allergic nasal and sinus disease are generally not destructive.

Another vasculitic syndrome to consider is GPA. Patients with GPA often present with sinus, tracheal, or ear concerns. MPA presents very similarly to GPA but does not have any nasopharyngeal involvement and is less likely. Goodpasture syndrome (also known as *anti–glomerular basement membrane disease*) is a pulmonary-renal syndrome that can also present with cough and hemoptysis.

Finally, pulmonary vascular disorders, such as pulmonary embolism or elevated pressure in the pulmonary vasculature, can lead to hemoptysis, although nothing in this patient's history so far would indicate pulmonary embolism or pulmonary hypertension.

CASE 20.3 CONTINUED:

A chest x-ray study reveals bilateral nodular and cavitary infiltrates. Laboratory workup is significant for an elevated ESR and the presence of cytoplasmic antineutrophil antibodies directed against proteinase 3.

---

2. What is the likely diagnosis?

The presentation of upper and lower respiratory airway symptoms with a workup significant for cavitary infiltrates and elevated inflammatory biomarkers with positive cytoplasmic antineutrophil antibodies is classic for GPA. This disease can occur at any age and affects mostly Caucasian individuals.

3. What is the pathogenesis of this disease?

Antibodies to neutrophil cytoplasmic antigens lead to aseptic inflammation and granuloma formation. Inflammation causing vascular injury leads to damage in the respiratory tract and kidneys, specifically causing glomerulonephritis. Granuloma formation occurs both within arterial walls, causing further vasculitic damage, and outside vascular structures, causing lesions that may cavitate and damage pulmonary tissue.

4. **What is the usual progression of symptoms in this disease? What other organ systems will likely become involved?**

Approximately 85% of patients with GPA will eventually develop sinopulmonary disease. Ear, nose, and throat manifestations include refractory rhinosinusitis, epistaxis, nasopharyngeal ulcerations, and nasal septal perforation. Saddle nose deformity may be a complication of untreated disease. Lower respiratory tract involvement is more life-threatening and may include symptoms such as cough, hemoptysis, and dyspnea. About 75% of patients will develop glomerulonephritis, which will almost always be asymptomatic until the development of advanced uremia.

A diagnosis of GPA before the 1970s meant that the patient had a 50% 5-month survival rate, and 82% of patients died within a year of diagnosis, most commonly from infection and renal failure. Besides pulmonary involvement and glomerulonephritis, musculoskeletal symptoms can occur, usually consisting of severe pain that is disproportionate to the signs of inflammation. Peripheral nerves can also be affected in some cases.

5. **How is GPA treated?**

The recommended therapy for GPA and other severe vasculitides (e.g., MPA) consists of corticosteroids combined with cyclophosphamide. Doses are increased until symptoms are reduced and the leukocyte count returns to normal values. Steroids are then tapered gradually. Maintenance of remission with cyclophosphamide is continued, often for a year after symptomatic improvement. Keep in mind that long-term daily cyclophosphamide therapy is associated with bladder cancer and myelodysplasia. Long-term immunosuppressive therapy also makes patients susceptible to opportunistic disease.

SUMMARY BOX: GRANULOMATOSIS WITH POLYANGIITIS (WEGENER GRANULOMATOSIS)

- Presentation: Sinus congestion, headache, hemoptysis, nasopharyngeal ulcerations, nasal septal perforation
- Epidemiology: Any age, more common in Caucasians
- Pathogenesis: Antibodies to neutrophil cytoplasmic antigens lead to aseptic inflammation and granuloma formation, causing damage to the vasculature
- Diagnosis: Positive cytoplasmic antineutrophil cytoplasmic antibodies directed against proteinase 3, cavitary nodules on chest x-ray, microscopic hematuria with red blood cell casts on urinalysis; confirm diagnosis with biopsy of affected tissue, which will show granulomatous vasculitis
- Complications: Necrotizing pulmonary granuloma formation (resulting in hemoptysis) and kidneys (resulting in glomerulonephritis)
- Treatment: Corticosteroids with cyclophosphamide

CASE 20.4

A 61-year-old man is evaluated for a 5- to 6-week history of fever, myalgias, fatigue, anorexia, and postprandial abdominal pain. He also describes painful paresthesias of the hands and has noticed a netlike rash on his legs. His girlfriend has noticed him dragging his right foot lately. He denies a history of tick bites or unprotected sexual intercourse. Workup reveals that he is positive for hepatitis B surface antigen, although to his knowledge, he has never been diagnosed with hepatitis. An arterial biopsy shows inflammation of the tunica intima, media, and adventitia.

---

1. **What is the diagnosis?**

Polyarteritis nodosa (PAN), a necrotizing vasculitis affecting small- to medium-size arteries with a predilection for the arteries supplying peripheral nerves, skin, gastrointestinal tract, and kidneys. Greater than 80% of people with PAN develop neuropathy, often in the pattern of mononeuritis multiplex (see later discussion). This neuropathy explains the tingling in this patient's hand and the foot drop. The postprandial abdominal pain or "intestinal angina" is also classic for PAN.

2. **What is the significance of the positive hepatitis B surface antigen in this patient?**

About 20% of cases of PAN are associated with hepatitis B viral infection. Other microbial pathogens, such as hepatitis C, may also be a factor, but there are fewer reported cases in the literature.

It is believed that immune complex depositions with antigens may be a cause of the disease. Inflammatory cells, predominantly neutrophils, form an infiltrate in arterial walls, which eventually leads to fibrinoid necrosis and varying degrees of transmural proliferation. Subsequent luminal narrowing and thrombosis of affected arteries result in tissue ischemia and the symptoms and complications described here.

The lesions of PAN are segmental and favor the branch points of the smaller arteries. A key pathologic feature is the *absence* of granulomas or granulomatous infiltration.

STEP 1 SECRET

Hepatitis B association with polyarteritis nodosa is a commonly tested fact on Step 1.

CASE 20.4 CONTINUED:

The patient returns to the clinic several weeks later for evaluation of severe hand pain. Examination of his hands reveals severe digital cyanosis and edema, as shown in Fig. 20.2.

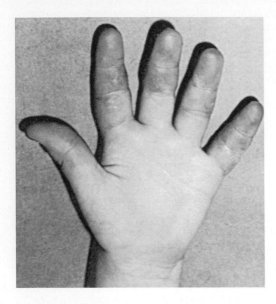

Figure 20.2. Marked digital cyanosis and swelling. *(From Harris ED, Budd RC, Genovese MC, et al.* Kelley's Textbook of Rheumatology. *7th ed. Philadelphia: WB Saunders; 2005.)*

3. What are the clinical manifestations of PAN?

   The rash on this patient's legs is livedo reticularis, a mottled blue-red discoloration that may affect large areas of the legs, arms, or abdomen. Painful nodules, purpura, and splinter hemorrhages may also be seen. Later in the course of this disease, patients may develop gangrene of the digits after occlusion of the arteries in the hands or feet. Gastrointestinal tract involvement is typically evidenced by postprandial periumbilical pain. Potential life-threatening consequences include rupture of mesenteric aneurysms and perforation of ischemic bowel. Finally, renal involvement, which is almost always seen on autopsy, presents as renin-mediated hypertension caused by occlusion of interlobar renal vessels. Curiously, the disease spares the pulmonary vasculature.

4. How can the diagnosis of PAN be confirmed?

   Diagnosis is based mainly on clinical suspicion. Angiography of the mesenteric or renal arteries may show aneurysms, as is suggested by the name polyarteritis "nodosa." Diagnosis should be confirmed with arterial biopsy, which will classically reveal varying stages of transmural inflammation, fibrinoid necrosis, and inflammatory infiltrate without granulomas.

CASE 20.4 CONTINUED:

The patient is placed on high doses of corticosteroids for his polyarteritis nodosa (PAN). Without immunosuppressive therapy, the prognosis for PAN is poor because of complications from renal failure and mesenteric, cardiac, or cerebral infarction.

5. Given the high-dose steroids, what prophylaxis needs to be considered?

   Prophylaxis against *Pneumocystis jiroveci* with trimethoprim-sulfamethoxazole should be considered.

SUMMARY BOX: POLYARTERITIS NODOSA

- Presentation: Hypertension from stenosis of renal arteries. Skin involvement manifesting as mottled blue-red rash (livedo reticularis) on arms, legs, and abdomen; painful skin nodules; purpura; and splinter hemorrhages. Gastrointestinal involvement manifesting as postprandial periumbilical pain ("intestinal angina")
- Epidemiology: Middle-aged or older adult. Associated with hepatitis B virus!
- Pathophysiology: Immune-complex deposition in arterial walls accompanied by neutrophilic inflammatory infiltrates, leading to fibrinoid necrosis and transmural inflammation that results in artery occlusion and thrombosis
- Diagnosis: Clinical suspicion and arterial biopsy showing neutrophilic infiltration of the arterial walls
- Complications: Rupture of mesenteric aneurysms, ischemic bowel perforation, gangrene, renin-mediated hypertension
- Treatment: Corticosteroids
- Prognosis: Poor without treatment from complications related to renal failure, stroke, mesenteric infarction, and cardiac infarction

CASE 20.5

A 51-year-old Caucasian woman is evaluated for a 2-week history of fatigue, diffuse myalgias, anorexia, and unintentional weight loss. She was found to be very mildly anemic, and iron supplementation therapy was begun. She is presenting to the emergency department today with a new concern. She states that since beginning to feel fatigued weeks ago, she became more interested in her personal health, attempting to exercise every day and taking her own blood pressure (BP) before and after her morning walks. Yesterday, she was unable to get a BP reading in her left arm before exercising. Her BP in her right arm was 110/60 mm Hg, per her report. She had assumed that there had been some problem with the BP cuff, but the same thing happened again this morning. She could not obtain a BP from her left arm, and her right arm read 100/60 mm Hg. She also states, somewhat fearfully, that her left arm feels cool today, and that in retrospect, her left arm has frequently been "tingly" over the past week.

1. What is the likely diagnosis in this patient?

   Given the difficulty obtaining a BP in this patient's left arm and the coolness in the left upper extremity, consider involvement of the aortic arch and its major branches or occlusion of the arteries of the upper extremity. This vascular compromise would also explain the tingling in the arm. Other, nonvascular explanations of paresthesias, such as brachial plexus damage, would not explain the difficulty in obtaining the BP. The patient does not present with severe back pain, which would raise concern for a ruptured aortic aneurysm. The onset later in life makes congenital coarctation of the aorta unlikely. Given the very specific presentation, Takayasu arteritis should be considered.

2. What is Takayasu arteritis?

   This is a vasculitis of the large elastic arteries, including the aorta and its main branches. It can also affect the coronary and pulmonary arteries. Inflammatory injury to the arterial wall leads to aneurysm formation or occlusion of the arteries, leading to the symptoms of decreased blood flow to the upper extremity in this patient. Takayasu arteritis is also known as *pulseless disease*, because of the possibility of losing the pulse in one or both upper extremities.

   The cause of this disease is unknown. Granulomas and giant cells are characteristically found in the media of the large elastic arteries, and the adventitia is usually profoundly thickened. Destruction of the media by granulomatous inflammation leads to replacement with fibrotic tissue and subsequent aneurysm formation. Thickening of the adventitia, in contrast, leads to occlusion of the vascular lumen.

3. What makes this patient different from the typical presentation of Takayasu arteritis?

   Although different BPs in the upper extremities is a classic presentation for Takayasu arteritis, this patient does not demonstrate the typical epidemiologic features of this disease. This disease is most common among Asian women (specifically those of Japanese, Chinese, or Korean descent; incidence is also relatively high among Indian women). Furthermore, it is a disease of adolescent girls and young women. Some diagnostic criteria for the disease require that the patient be younger than 40 years at onset. Our patient, as a 51-year-old Caucasian woman, is therefore atypical.

4. Ischemic complications as a result of vascular involvement of the aortic arch and its major branches led to this patient's symptoms. What other symptoms can be expected from persistent ischemia in a patient with Takayasu arteritis?

   The carotid and vertebral arteries can also be involved, leading to symptoms including headache, syncope, or visual disturbance. Stroke can sometimes occur. The following may also be seen:

   - Involvement of the coronary arteries can produce symptoms of myocardial ischemia.
   - Involvement of the renal arteries can cause renin-induced hypertension, which is classically the presenting symptom in some specific ethnic groups, such as Indians.
   - Involvement of the mesenteric arteries is less common but may include symptoms such as postprandial abdominal pain, nausea, and vomiting.
   - Progressively enlarging aneurysms can occur, typically along the aorta. However, these are frequently asymptomatic.

5. How is the diagnosis made?

   In this patient, physical examination would include listening for a bruit over the subclavian arteries or abdominal aorta and documenting a lower BP in the left arm compared with the right arm, as well as observing for extremity claudication with activity. Noninvasive magnetic resonance angiography or computed tomography angiography is indicated to confirm the diagnosis and to document the extent of arterial wall inflammation. The effects of therapy are usually monitored by documenting change in arterial wall inflammation on angiography and monitoring the diameter of the aortic root.

6. How is this disease treated?

   Corticosteroids are used for the treatment of Takayasu arteritis. Methotrexate may be used to enable a lower dose of steroids to be given.

SUMMARY BOX: TAKAYASU ARTERITIS

- Presentation: Nonspecific symptoms including fatigue, myalgias, and weight loss, followed by signs of extremity involvement, including coolness, pain with use (claudication), and tingling
- Epidemiology: Characteristically seen in young Asian women but can be seen in other races as well
- Pathophysiology: Mechanism is poorly understood but thought to result from cell-mediated inflammatory injury to the arterial wall that causes fibrosis and adventitial thickening, leading to aneurysm formation and vascular occlusion
- Diagnosis: Physical examination findings include decreased brachial pulses, BP difference between the arms, and bruit over subclavian arteries or abdominal aorta. Clinical suspicion is confirmed by noninvasive magnetic resonance angiography or computed tomography angiography (CTA)
- Complications: Angina or myocardial infarction from involvement of coronary arteries, renin-induced hypertension from involvement of renal arteries, bowel ischemia from involvement of mesenteric arteries, stroke or transient ischemic attack from intracerebral artery involvement, and aortic aneurysms
- Treatment: Corticosteroids

BACTERIAL DISEASES

BASIC CONCEPTS PART I: BACTERIAL MORPHOLOGY AND VIRULENCE FACTORS

1. What makes an organism gram-positive or gram-negative?

   Both gram-positive and gram-negative organisms have an internal cell membrane and cell wall made of *peptidoglycan*. The cell wall of gram-positive organisms tends to be thicker than their gram-negative counterparts and contain *teichoic acid*. The thicker, meshlike cell wall in gram-positive bacteria retains *crystal violet dye* and stains *purple*. In contrast, gram-negative bacteria have a very thin cell wall and cannot retain crystal violet dye. They are counterstained with *safranin* or *fuchsine*, giving them a *pink* coloring instead. However, gram-negative bacteria do have an extra outer membrane outside the cell wall that is largely composed of *lipopolysaccharide* (LPS), an endotoxin (Fig. 21.1).

Gram-negative (–) cell wall

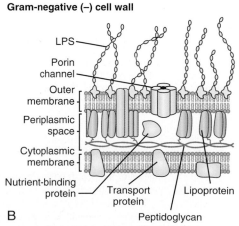

Gram-positive (+) cell wall

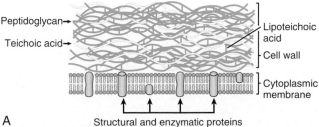

A

B

Figure 21.1. Structure of the cell wall in gram-positive and gram-negative bacteria. A, Gram-positive bacteria have a thick peptidoglycan layer that contains teichoic and lipoteichoic acids. B, Gram-negative bacteria have a thin peptidoglycan layer that is connected by lipoproteins to an outer membrane. *LPS,* Lipopolysaccharide. *(From Rosenthal K.* Rapid Review Microbiology and Immunology. *3rd ed. Philadelphia: Elsevier; 2010.)*

2. Why are gram-negative organisms more likely to cause bacterial sepsis?
Gram-negative organisms are more likely to cause sepsis because of *lipid A*, an *endo*toxin that is part of the LPS component of the outer membrane of gram-negative bacteria. Lipid A is released on bacterial death and has potent proinflammatory effects.

Lipid A binds to the *Toll-like receptor* 4/CD14/MD2 receptor complex on the surface of many different types of immune cell (e.g., macrophages). This stimulates the immune cell to secrete a host of inflammatory cytokines, including *interleukin-1* (IL-1) and *tumor necrosis factor alpha* (TNF-α), otherwise known as *acute-phase cytokines*. IL-1 stimulates the fever response, while TNF-α triggers tissue necrosis and shock. Lipid A also stimulates the release of nitric oxide from endothelial cells, causing vasodilation that may lead to intravascular coagulation and shock.

3. What are exotoxins?
*Exo*toxins are proteins *released* by both gram-positive and gram-negative bacteria during their normal life cycle. This is in contrast with *endo*toxins, which are present *within* the cell membrane of gram-negative organisms and are released only after bacterial cells are lysed. Exotoxins released into food can cause food poisoning (e.g., *Bacillus cereus* and *Staphylococcus aureus*). Pyrogenic exotoxins released by *S. aureus* and *Streptococcus pyogenes* can cause rash, fever, and toxic shock syndrome. Exotoxins act on various organ systems throughout the body, such as the gastrointestinal (GI) system (enterotoxins) or nervous system (neurotoxins). For example, infectious diarrhea is caused by enterotoxins produced by *Vibrio cholerae*, *Escherichia coli*, *Campylobacter jejuni*, and *Shigella dysenteriae*.

STEP 1 SECRET

Use the mnemonics below to help you keep the definitions and origins of endotoxins versus exotoxins straight in your mind on test day.
  ENDOtoxin = from **ENDO**genous source (i.e., made from bacterial chromosome), **EN**tegral to outer membrane of most gram-negative bacteria (and *Listeria* spp.), released when the cell's life **END**s (i.e., the cell is lysed).
  EXotoxin = from **EX**ogenous source (i.e., plasmid or bacteriophage) and released by **EX**cretion from living bacteria.

4. What is a capsule, and what purpose does it serve?
Certain species of bacteria produce a slippery outermost covering called a *capsule*. This covering consists of high-molecular-weight polysaccharides that help the bacteria evade phagocytosis by neutrophils and macrophages. Note that *Bacillus anthracis* has a proteinaceous capsule made of D-*glutamic acid*. The capsule is not essential for growth and serves an exclusively protective role. The most common medically relevant encapsulated organisms are **S**treptococcus *pneumoniae*, **K**lebsiella *pneumoniae*, **H**aemophilus *influenzae* type b, **P**seudomonas *aeruginosa*, **N**eisseria *meningitidis*, and **C**ryptococcus *neoformans* (a fungus).

Remember that **S**ome **K**illers **H**ave **P**erfectly **N**asty **C**apsules. This mnemonic will help you recall the encapsulated organisms that are important to know for board exams. A mnemonic to help remember the unique proteinaceous capsule of *Bacillus anthracis* is **BAD**: **B**acillus **a**nthracis's capsule contains D-glutamate.

Note: To test for the presence of encapsulated bacteria, the *Quellung reaction* is used in which bacteria with a capsule will swell when exposed to specific antibodies. The *latex agglutination assay* and *India ink stain* are two additional methods for detecting capsular presence.

STEP 1 SECRET

*Although the Quellung reaction and several other techniques in this book may be clinically outdated, many authors of the USMLE Step 1 exam expect you to know the names and basic science principles illustrated by these tests. You should focus only on learning the techniques listed in this book and in First Aid, because students are **not** expected to know controversial or cutting-edge technologies for their USMLE exams.*

5. What characteristics make an individual more susceptible to infection by encapsulated bacteria?
Asplenic patients or those with opsonization/complement protein defects are increasingly susceptible to infection by encapsulated bacteria because the spleen normally sequesters these microorganisms. Patients who have undergone splenectomy (e.g., patients with sickle cell disease or hemolytic anemias) are at a greater risk for incurring infection by encapsulated bacteria. Patients with opsonization defects and complement protein deficiencies are also vulnerable to infection by encapsulated bacteria (see Chapter 15, Immunology, Table 15.3). *C5-C9 complement deficiency* and subsequent predisposition to *Neisseria meningitides* is a classic vignette you may encounter in practice questions or on the USMLE Step 1 exam.

6. Identify the Gram stain and the morphology of the organisms in Table 21.1.

Table 21.1. Noteworthy Bacterial Histologic Images

IMAGE	GRAM STAIN AND MORPHOLOGY
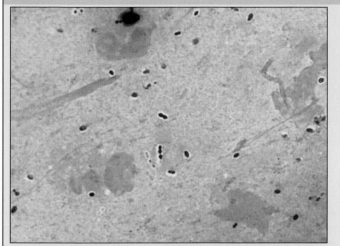 Gram stain of a sputum sample infected with *Streptococcus pneumoniae*	Gram-positive cocci in pairs: *S. pneumoniae*
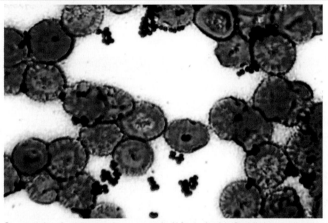 Gram stain of a blood culture sample infected with Staphylococcus aureus	Gram-positive cocci in clusters: *Staphylococcus aureus*
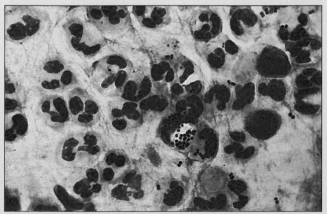 Sputum smear with Gram stain, shows many neutrophils and intracellular gram-negative diplococci suggestive of *Neisseria meningitidis* infection (oil immersion)	Gram-negative cocci in pairs: *Neisseria* spp.

Continued

Table 21.1. Noteworthy Bacterial Histologic Images—cont'd

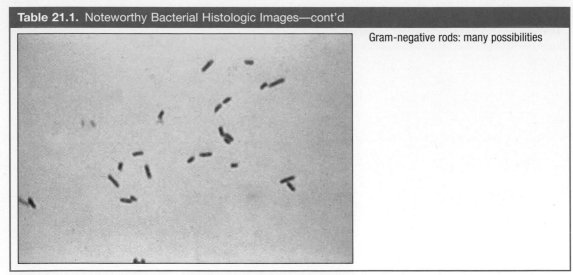

Gram-negative rods: many possibilities

Staphylococcus aureus image from Murray PR, Rosenthal KS, Pfaller MA. *Medical Microbiology.* 8th ed. Philadelphia: Elsevier; 2016. Images of *Streptococcus pneumoniae, Neisseria meningitidis,* and gram-negative rods are from McPherson RA, Pincus MR. *Henry's Clinical Diagnosis and Management by Laboratory Methods.* 22nd ed. Philadelphia: Saunders; 2011.

7. Review Tables 21.2 through 21.9 to test your knowledge of these high-yield bacteria.

Table 21.2. Commonly Tested Gram-Positive Cocci

ORGANISM	ASSOCIATED DISEASE(S)	TOXIN	LABORATORY INFO	PEARLS TO REMEMBER
Staphylococcus aureus	Cellulitis Acute endocarditis (in previously healthy valve) Septic arthritis Osteomyelitis Pneumonia Carbuncles/furuncles Stye	Protein A (binds Fc portion of IgG) Toxic shock syndrome toxin-1	Catalase positive Coagulase positive Ferments mannitol	Toxin-mediated diseases: Staphylococcal toxic shock syndrome Scalded skin syndrome Staphylococcal gastroenteritis MRSA: resistant to methicillin because of alteration in PBP; treat with vancomycin, linezolid, or daptomycin
Staphylococcus epidermidis	Prosthetic valve endo-carditis Prosthetic joint infec-tions Bacteremia from indwelling catheters	—	Novobiocin sensitive Urease positive	Normal skin flora Produces adherent biofilm
Staphylococcus saprophyticus	Cystitis in young women Second most common cause of UTI in sexu-ally active women (behind *Escherichia coli*)	—	Novobiocin resistant Urease positive	Normal flora of female genital tract
Streptococcus pneumoniae	Most common cause of: Meningitis Otitis media Pneumonia Sinusitis ("MOPS")	IgA protease	α-Hemolysis Bile soluble Optochin sensitive	Encapsulated, lancet-shaped Rust-colored sputum Sepsis in asplenic patients

Table 21.2. Commonly Tested Gram-Positive Cocci—cont'd

ORGANISM	ASSOCIATED DISEASE(S)	TOXIN	LABORATORY INFO	PEARLS TO REMEMBER
Viridans streptococci	Dental caries (*Streptococcus mutans*) Subacute bacterial endocarditis (*Streptococcus sanguinis*)	—	α-Hemolysis Optochin resistant	Normal oral flora
Streptococcus agalactiae (group B streptococci)	Neonatal pneumonia, meningitis, and sepsis Chorioamnionitis	—	β-Hemolysis Bacitracin resistant Hippurate positive	Normal vaginal flora Screen pregnant women at 35–37 weeks of gestation
Streptococcus bovis	Subacute endocarditis	—	—	Strong association with colon cancer
Enterococcus spp.	UTI Bacteremia/sepsis Endocarditis Abdominal abscess		α- or γ-Hemolysis PYR positive Grow in 6.5% NaCl and bile	Part of normal bowel flora that causes disease when host is immunocompromised or gastrointestinal tract has been breached

MRSA, Methicillin-resistant *Staphylococcus aureus; PBP,* penicillin-binding protein; *PYR,* pyrrolidonyl aminopeptidase; *UTI,* urinary tract infection.

Table 21.3. Commonly Tested Gram-Positive Bacilli

ORGANISM	ASSOCIATED DISEASE(S)	TOXIN	LABORATORY INFO	PEARLS TO REMEMBER
Bacillus anthracis	Cutaneous anthrax (most common form) Pulmonary anthrax	Lethal factor Edema factor (increases cAMP)	Spore-forming	Painless black eschars with cutaneous anthrax Pulmonary anthrax (Wool-sorter's disease) D-Glutamate polypeptide capsule
Corynebacterium spp.	Diphtheria Granulomatous lymphadenitis Pneumonitis Pharyngitis Skin infections Endocarditis	Diphtheria toxin (RNA translational inhibitor that inactivates EF-2 via ADP ribosylation)	Grows on tellurite agar	Normal skin flora Pseudomembrane (gray-white) or esophageal web Metachromatic granules
Listeria monocytogenes	Listeriosis	Listeriolysin O	Exhibits characteristic tumbling motility Grows well at 4°–10°C	Perinatal/neonatal infections Immunocompromised persons at risk Associated with raw milk, cold deli meat, and dairy products

ADP, Adenosine diphosphate; *cAMP,* cyclic adenosine monophosphate; *EF-2,* elongation factor 2; *RNA,* ribonucleic acid.

Table 21.4. Commonly Tested Gram-Negative Cocci

ORGANISM	ASSOCIATED DISEASE(S)	TOXIN	LABORATORY INFO	PEARLS TO REMEMBER
Neisseria meningitidis (meningococcus)	Meningitis Septicemia Waterhouse-Friderichsen syndrome	IgA protease	Maltose fermentation	Encapsulated Purpuric, nonblanching rash Vaccine available
Neisseria gonorrhoeae (gonococcus)	Infects superficial mucosal surfaces lined with columnar epithelium: Urethra: urethritis (gonorrhea) Vagina: vulvovaginitis in young girls Rectum: proctitis Conjunctiva: ophthalmia neonatorum	IgA protease	No maltose fermentation	No capsule No vaccine (unlike *N. meningitidis*, *N. gonorrhoeae*'s pilus protein undergoes antigenic variation) Main cause of infectious arthritis in sexually active persons

Table 21.5. Commonly Tested Enteric Gram-Negative Rods

ORGANISM	ASSOCIATED DISEASE(S)	TOXIN	LABORATORY INFO	PEARLS TO REMEMBER
Campylobacter jejuni	Enteritis	—	Grows at 42°C Oxidase positive Comma-shaped	Present in animal feces Associated with Guillain-Barré syndrome and reactive arthritis
Escherichia coli	Enteritis UTI Meningitis Peritonitis Mastitis Septicemia Gram-negative pneumonia HUS	K Capsule (can cause pneumonia) Labile toxin (increases cAMP) Stable toxin (increases cGMP)	—	Normal gut flora EHEC 0157:H7—a particularly virulent pathologic strain associated with HUS
Salmonella spp.	Food-borne illness Typhoid fever (*Salmonella typhi*)	—	Produces H_2S	Osteomyelitis in patients with sickle cell anemia
Shigella spp.	Shigellosis (bacterial dysentery)	Shiga toxin (inhibits protein synthesis in target cells)	Does not produce H_2S	Bloody diarrhea Fecal-oral route of transmission Low inoculum required (toxin mediated)
Vibrio cholerae	Diarrhea	Cholera toxin (permanently activates G_s)	Grows in alkaline media Oxidase positive Comma-shaped	"Rice-water" diarrhea Transmitted through contaminated water or seafood Prompt oral rehydration necessary
Helicobacter pylori	Peptic ulcer disease Gastritis Duodenitis Gastric cancer MALT lymphoma	—	Positive urea breath test as a result of presence of urease enzyme Catalase positive Oxidase positive	Lives in stomach but common in duodenal ulcers Triple therapy: amoxicillin, clarithromycin, and PPI

cAMP, Cyclic adenosine monophosphate; *cGMP,* cyclic guanosine monophosphate; *EHEC,* enterohemorrhagic *Escherichia coli; HUS,* hemolytic uremic syndrome; H_2S, hydrogen sulfide; *MALT,* mucosa-associated lymphoid tissue; *PPI,* proton pump inhibitor; *UTI,* urinary tract infection.

Table 21.6. Other Commonly Tested Gram-Negative Rods

ORGANISM	ASSOCIATED DISEASE(S)	TOXIN	LABORATORY INFO	PEARLS TO REMEMBER
Bordetella pertussis	Pertussis (whooping cough)	Pertussis toxin (inactivates G_i, leading to high amounts of cAMP)	Grown on Bordet-Gengou agar	Highly contagious; spread by coughing and nasal drops Three stages: 1. Catarrhal: low-grade fevers and sinusitis 2. Paroxysmal: paroxysms of intense cough followed by inspiratory "whoop"; coughing can lead to vomiting 3. Convalescent: months-long recovery phase with milder cough
Brucella spp.	Brucellosis ("undulant fever")	—	—	Transmitted via contaminated or unpasteurized milk
Francisella tularensis	Tularemia ("rabbit fever")	—	—	Reservoir in rabbits; transmitted by tick Symptoms/signs similar to those of plague Culture, drainage contraindicated because of high virulence
Haemophilus influenzae	Meningitis (type b) Bacteremia Cellulitis Pneumonia Sinusitis Epiglottitis ("cherry red")	IgA protease	Grown on chocolate Agar supplemented with Factors V (NAD+) and X (hematin)	Type b: encapsulated and more virulent Vaccine available for type b strain
Pseudomonas aeruginosa	Pneumonia in patients with cardiac failure Otitis externa Osteomyelitis in diabetics Endocarditis UTI Hot tub folliculitis Sepsis	Exotoxin A (inactivates EF-2, similar to diphtheria toxin)	Produces the blue-green pigment pyocyanin Oxidase positive	Think *Pseudomonas* infection in burn patients and intravenous drug users Can cause black skin lesions Resistant to many antibiotics
Legionella pneumophila	Legionnaires disease Pontiac fever	—	Readily visualized with silver stain Grown on charcoal yeast extract with iron and cysteine Detected with urine test	Legionnaires disease: acute pneumonia with multisystem involvement; from water source, so no person-to-person spread Pontiac fever: similar to flu Hyponatremia is a common laboratory finding
Yersinia pestis	Bubonic plague	—	—	Transmitted by fleas from rodents to humans Black buboes
Yersinia enterocolitica	Enterocolitis	—	—	Pseudoappendicitis (can mimic Crohn disease as well) Seen in nursery schools Transmitted from pet feces and pork chitterlings

cAMP, Cyclic adenosine monophosphate; *EF-2,* elongation factor 2; *NAD,* nicotinamide adenine dinucleotide; *UTI,* urinary tract infection.

Table 21.7. Commonly Tested Anaerobes

ORGANISM	ASSOCIATED DISEASE(S)	TOXIN	LABORATORY INFO	PEARLS TO REMEMBER
Clostridium perfringens	Anaerobic cellulitis Gas gangrene (myonecrosis) Food poisoning	Alpha toxin (lecithinase)	Spore-forming	Crepitus is associated with gas gangrene
Clostridium tetani	Tetanus Trismus ("lockjaw") Risus Sardonicus (grinning and raised eyebrows)	Exotoxin causes spastic paralysis by blocking inhibitory glycine and GABA release from Renshaw cells in spinal cord	Spore-forming	Vaccine is available Treat with antitoxin
Clostridium botulinum	Botulism Floppy baby syndrome (ingestion of spores in honey)	Food poisoning that causes flaccid paralysis Preformed toxin prevents release of acetylcholine at presynaptic terminals	Spore-forming	Classic scenario from consumption of dented home-canned goods or honey Local Botox injections use this toxin
Clostridioides difficile	Pseudomembranous colitis	Toxin A (acts on brush border of gut) Toxin B (causes pseudomembranes)	Spore-forming	Often preceded by antibiotic use, especially clindamycin or ampicillin Treat with oral vancomycin or rifaximin

Table 21.8. Commonly Tested Spirochetes

ORGANISM	ASSOCIATED DISEASE(S)	LABORATORY INFO	PEARLS TO REMEMBER
Borrelia burgdorferi	Lyme disease	Best visualized with Wright or Giemsa stain	Bull's-eye rash Late stage of infection is associated with arthritis and neurologic symptoms
Borrelia recurrentis	Relapsing fever	—	Organism switches surface proteins to evade immune response, leading to intermittent fevers
Treponema pallidum	Syphilis	Visualized via dark-field microscopy	Spread through sexual contact or through vertical transmission Palms-and-soles rash Neurosyphilis results in tabes dorsalis causing an ataxic gait Argyll Robertson pupil
Leptospira interrogans	Leptospirosis Weil disease	—	Transmitted by water that is contaminated by animal urine through cracks in the skin, eyes, or mucous membranes

Table 21.9. Commonly Tested Intracellular Organisms

ORGANISM	ASSOCIATED DISEASE(S)	LABORATORY INFO	PEARLS TO REMEMBER
Mycoplasma pneumoniae	Atypical ("walking") pneumonia	Best grown on Eaton agar Blood shows IgM "cold agglutinins"	No cell wall Treat with macrolides Chest radiograph demonstrates diffuse interstitial infiltrates; radiographic changes often more extensive than expected from patient's symptoms
Chlamydia trachomatis	Urethritis Pelvic inflammatory disease Blindness Lymphogranuloma venereum Neonatal conjunctivitis	Visualized with Giemsa stain Cell wall lacks muramic acid	Treat neonates with erythromycin eye drops for conjunctivitis prophylaxis Also frequently associated with reactive arthritis
Chlamydia psittaci	Psittacosis (flulike syndrome)	—	Transmitted from bird droppings via aerosol
Chlamydia pneumoniae	Atypical pneumonia	—	Transmitted via aerosols
Mycobacterium tuberculosis	Tuberculosis	Ziehl-Neelsen stain for acid-fast bacilli Grows on Lowenstein-Jensen agar	Associated with granulomas and caseous necrosis Ghon complex indicates active primary infection or resolved infection
Mycobacterium leprae	Leprosy (Hansen disease)	—	Tuberculoid form: milder with few organisms in lesions Lepromatous form: severe with many organisms in lesions Grows in cool temperatures, so affects distal sites Treat with dapsone and rifampin
Rickettsia rickettsii	Rocky Mountain spotted fever	Weil-Felix test will be positive for rickettsial diseases	Rash that starts on palms and soles and migrates centrally (centripetal migration) Treat with doxycycline

BASIC CONCEPTS PART II: ANTIBACTERIAL PHARMACOLOGY

1. Describe the difference between *bacteriostatic* and *bactericidal* antibiotics.

   Bacteriostatic antibiotics work by inhibiting the growth or reproduction of infectious bacteria; they do *not* kill the organism. These include most ribosomal-acting antibiotics (e.g., tetracyclines and macrolides), which block bacterial protein translation by inhibiting ribosomal subunits.

   In contrast, *bactericidal* agents kill the bacteria. These antibiotics include agents that disrupt the cell wall, such as β-lactam antibiotics (e.g., penicillins, cephalosporins, carbapenems), and other antibiotics with different mechanisms, such as aminoglycosides, fluoroquinolones, and metronidazole.

2. Describe the most common mechanisms by which antibiotic agents work.

   Antibiotics generally work via one of four mechanisms:
   1. Disruption of cell wall synthesis (β-lactam antibiotics)
   2. [Direct] inhibition of bacterial DNA replication (fluoroquinolones)
   3. [Indirect] inhibition of bacterial DNA synthesis (trimethoprim, sulfamethoxazole)
   4. Impairing the function of bacterial ribosomes (macrolides, tetracyclines, aminoglycosides, chloramphenicol, clindamycin, linezolid)

3. **What are the β-lactam antibiotics, and what is their mechanism of action?**
The β-lactam antibiotics include the penicillins, cephalosporins, and carbapenems (e.g., imipenem, meropenem). By virtue of their β-lactam chemical moiety, they act by blocking bacterial cell wall synthesis through the inhibition of bacterial *transpeptidase*, also known as *penicillin-binding protein*. Resistance to these antibiotics is mediated by bacterially synthesized β-lactamase enzymes that destroy the β-lactam ring.

4. **Why are clavulanic acid, sulbactam, and tazobactam added to some penicillins?**
These agents *inhibit β-lactamase*, thereby reducing resistance of bacterial species to penicillins. Typical combinations include amoxicillin-clavulanic acid, ampicillin-sulbactam, and piperacillin-tazobactam.

STEP 1 SECRET

Antibiotics that inhibit the bacterial ribosome can be recalled with the mnemonic "These Malicious Antibiotics Cripple Little Critters" (Tetracyclines, Macrolides, Aminoglycosides, Chloramphenicol, Linezolid, Clindamycin). It is also crucial to know which subunit of the ribosome is inhibited by a particular antibiotic. The 50S subunit is targeted by chloramphenicol, clindamycin, linezolid, and the macrolides, while the 30S subunit is targeted by aminoglycosides and tetracyclines.

---

5. **What percentage of patients allergic to penicillin are also allergic to cephalosporins?**
Only a small percentage of individuals with a penicillin allergy will also have a hypersensitivity reaction to cephalosporins, which presents with pruritus, urticaria, bronchospasm, laryngeal edema, and hypotension. There is no cross-reactivity between penicillins and aztreonam.

6. **What is the antibacterial spectrum of the various subclasses of penicillins and cephalosporins?**
The spectrum of action of antibiotics is complicated, but thankfully the USMLE does not expect you to have a specialist's understanding. Instead, you should focus on overall themes. Note that new antibiotic classes were created in response to increased resistance to the "older" versions. Thus, each new antibiotic class typically demonstrates broader or improved coverage.
Natural penicillins have largely gram-positive coverage, while extended-spectrum penicillins (e.g., ampicillin and amoxicillin) were developed to include better gram-negative coverage; importantly, they also cover *enterococcus* species. To combat the growing issue of penicillinase-producing bacteria, penicillinase-resistant penicillins were developed (e.g., methicillin, oxacillin, nafcillin, and dicloxacillin). These antibiotics are used largely for treatment of methicillin-sensitive *Staphylococcus aureus*. Finally, antipseudomonal penicillins (e.g., ticarcillin and piperacillin) were developed.
Cephalosporins can be thought of as "stronger" penicillins because they have a similar mechanism of action but are less susceptible to the effects of β-lactamases. There are a multitude of drugs in this class, and you are not expected to know all of their names, but important cephalosporins are highlighted in Table 21.10. First-generation and second-generation cephalosporins largely have gram-positive coverage, while third-generation cephalosporins also have robust gram-negative coverage. Fourth-generation cephalosporins (e.g., cefepime) have a similar coverage spectrum as third-generation cephalosporins, but they also cover *Pseudomonas aeruginosa*.

7. **What is the antibacterial spectrum and mechanism of action of vancomycin?**
Vancomycin is effective against gram-positive bacteria and often is used for drug-resistant organisms, such as methicillin-resistant *Staphylococcus aureus* (MRSA). It is also commonly used for *Clostridioides difficile* infections, because it is poorly absorbed from the intestinal tract. Therefore, it is primarily administered orally for infections of the colon, such as *C. difficile* colitis; otherwise, vancomycin is given intravenously.
Vancomycin acts by binding to the *D-Ala-D-Ala* site of gram-positive bacteria, inhibiting cell wall synthesis. However, some bacteria have developed resistance to vancomycin by altering their binding site to D-Ala-D-Lac, thereby reducing the antibiotic's effectiveness.
Intravenous (IV) vancomycin is commonly used in the hospital for treatment of MRSA. Other less common but effective antibiotics used to cover MRSA include linezolid and daptomycin.

8. **What is the antibacterial spectrum of the fluoroquinolones, and what is their mechanism of action?**
This class has a broad spectrum of activity, including both gram-positive and gram-negative organisms. They also cover *Pseudomonas*, making them similar in spectrum to the antipseudomonal penicillins. Fluoroquinolones work by inhibiting bacterial DNA synthesis through inhibition of the bacterial *topoisomerase* (DNA gyrase) protein. You can recognize them by their suffix "-floxacin" (e.g., levofloxacin, ciprofloxacin, and moxifloxacin). They are frequently used to treat respiratory infections (e.g., pneumonia) and urinary tract infections.

Table 21.10. Antibacterial Pharmacology

DRUG CLASS *EXAMPLES*	COVERAGE	MECHANISM OF ACTION	MECHANISM OF RESISTANCE	ADVERSE DRUG EFFECTS	NOTES
Penicillin-Based Antibiotics					
Natural penicillin *Penicillin*	Mostly gram-positive organisms	Inhibits transpeptidase and stimulation of autolysis	Formation of β-lactamases that break the β-lactam ring		Increasing resistance limits use, antibiotic of choice for syphilis (intramuscular or intravenous penicillin G)
Extended-spectrum penicillins *Ampicillin* *Amoxicillin*	Gram positive with improved gram-negative coverage, includes enterococcus				
Antistaphylococcal (penicillinase-resistant) penicillins *Dicloxacillin* *Cloxacillin* *Methicillin* *Oxacillin*	MSSA				Better resistance to β-lactamases as a result of bulk side chain
Antipseudomonal penicillins *Ticarcillin* *Piperacillin*	Increasing gram-negative coverage includes *Pseudomonas*				
Penicillin plus β-lactamase inhibitor *Ampicillin-sulbactam* *Amoxicillin-clavulanic acid* *Piperacillin-tazobactam*	β-Lactam-resistant bacteria. Piperacillin-tazobactam covers *Pseudomonas*				
First-generation cephalosporins *Cephalexin* *Cefotetan* *Cefazolin*	Mostly gram positive				Ten percent cross-reactivity with penicillin allergy (all generations)
Second-generation cephalosporins *Cefuroxime* *Cefaclor* *Cefoxitin*	Mostly gram positive				

Continued

Table 21.10. Antibacterial Pharmacology—cont'd

DRUG CLASS *EXAMPLES*	COVERAGE	MECHANISM OF ACTION	MECHANISM OF RESISTANCE	ADVERSE DRUG EFFECTS	NOTES
Third-generation cephalosporins *Ceftazidime* *Ceftriaxone* *Cefotaxime*	Mostly gram-negative coverage, including invasive infections such as meningitis and pneumococcal pneumonia, as well as gonorrhea. Ceftazidime covers *Pseudomonas*				
Fourth-generation cephalosporins *Cefepime*					
Monobactam					No penicillin cross-reactivity
Carbapenems					Imipenem is administered with cilastatin to inhibit metabolism by renal dehydropeptidase I
Ribosomal Antibiotics Aminoglycosides *Gentamicin* *Tobramycin* *Streptomycin* *Neomycin* *Amikacin*	Gram negative	Impairs proper assembly of the ribosome, causing the 30S subunit to misread the genetic code	Acetylation, adenylation, phosphorylation	Nephrotoxicity and ototoxicity	Only bactericidal ribosomal antibiotic
Tetracyclines *Doxycycline* *Tetracycline* *Demeclocycline*	Lyme, *Rickettsia, Chlamydia*	Bind to the 30S subunit of the bacterial ribosome, inhibiting protein synthesis	Decreased transport into the cell and increased transport out of the cell	GI upset, toxicity in renal impairment, photosensitivity; alters bone growth and discolors teeth in children	Demeclocycline more commonly used to treat SIADH. Tetracyclines block tRNA from binding A-site and discolors teeth
Clindamycin	Gram positive, anaerobes	Binds 50S subunit to prevent peptide bond formation		Common cause of antibiotic-associated *Clostridioides difficile*	

Drug	Coverage	Mechanism	Resistance	Side Effects	Notes
Chloramphenicol	Gram positive, gram negative, anaerobes	Reversibly inhibits protein synthesis by binding to the 50S subunit	Acetylation	Aplastic anemia, gray baby syndrome	Cytochrome P-450 inhibitor; not used in the United States because of gray baby syndrome; can cause aplastic anemia
Macrolides *Azithromycin Erythromycin*	Gram-positive, atypicals (*Mycoplasma, Legionella, Chlamydia*), neonatal conjunctivitis prophylaxis (topical erythromycin), MAC prophylaxis in HIV	Binds to 50S subunit of ribosome, inhibiting translocation	Methylation	GI upset, acute cholestatic hepatitis, prolonged QT	Cytochrome P-450 inhibitor; bacteriostatic alone; erythromycin also used for GI motility
Unique Antibiotics					
Vancomycin	Gram-positive coverage only; MRSA (IV), *C. difficile* (oral)	Inhibits cell wall synthesis by binding D-alanine	D-Alanine replaced with D-lactate	Nephrotoxicity, ototoxicity, thrombophlebitis, red man syndrome	Administer antihistamine and slow infusion rate to treat red man syndrome
Metronidazole	Giardia, *Entamoeba, Trichomonas, Gardnerella,* anaerobes, *C. difficile*	Converts to a toxic metabolite that prevents cell wall synthesis		Disulfiram-like reaction, metallic taste	
Fluoroquinolones *Ciprofloxacin Levofloxacin Moxifloxacin*	Gram-negative rods, UTIs, respiratory infections	Inhibits DNA gyrase, preventing DNA replication	Efflux pump and mutated DNA gyrase	Cartilage damage in children, tendon rupture in adults	Cytochrome P-450 inhibitor
TMP-SMX	UTIs, MRSA, PCP and toxoplasmosis, and PCP prophylaxis in HIV	Inhibits folic acid synthesis		Megaloblastic anemia, leukopenia, granulocytopenia; sulfonamides component can cause allergic reaction, hemolysis in G6PD deficiency, photosensitivity	Treat bone marrow suppression with leucovorin rescue

Continued

Table 21.10. Antibacterial Pharmacology—cont'd

DRUG CLASS *EXAMPLES*	COVERAGE	MECHANISM OF ACTION	MECHANISM OF RESISTANCE	ADVERSE DRUG EFFECTS	NOTES
Linezolid	MRSA	Binds to 50S subunit to prevent protein synthesis			Can cause serotonin syndrome
Daptomycin	MRSA, VRE	Disrupts bacterial plasma membrane by altering electrical charge		Myopathy, elevated CPK	
Mycobacterial Drugs					
Isoniazid	*Mycobacterium tuberculosis*	Activated by mycobacterial KatG, product inhibits mycolic acid synthesis		Hepatotoxicity, peripheral neuropathy, drug-induced lupus	Cytochrome P-450 inhibitor Administer with B6 to prevent peripheral neuropathy
Ethambutol		Obstructs formation of mycobacterial cell wall by inhibiting arabinosyl transferase		Red-green color blindness, hepatotoxicity	
Pyrazinamide		Mechanism unknown		Hepatotoxicity	
Rifampin		Inhibitor of bacterial DNA-dependent RNA polymerase		Hepatotoxicity, turns body fluids orange	Cytochrome P-450 inducer
Streptomycin		Blocks 30S subunit of bacterial ribosome	Acetylation, adenylation, or phosphorylation	Nephrotoxicity and ototoxicity	See also aminoglycosides

CPK, Creatine phosphokinase; *G6PD*, glucose-6-phosphate dehydrogenase; *GI*, gastrointestinal; *HIV*, human immunodeficiency virus; *IV*, intravenous; *KatG*, catalase-peroxidase enzyme; *MAC*, *Mycobacterium avium* complex; *MRSA*, methicillin-resistant *Staphylococcus aureus*; *MSSA*, methicillin-sensitive *Staphylococcus aureus*; *PCP*, *Pneumocystis* pneumonia; *SIADH*, syndrome of inappropriate secretion of antidiuretic hormone; *TMP-SMX*, trimethoprim-sulfamethoxazole; *tRNA*, transfer RNA; *UTI*, urinary tract infection; *VRE*, vancomycin-resistant enterococci.

9. **What are the antimicrobial spectrum and mechanism of action of the macrolides?**
Macrolides have good gram-positive coverage and also cover *Mycoplasma*, *Legionella*, and *Chlamydia* (recall that this is one of "our favorite drugs for intracellular bugs"). Macrolides are also used prophylactically against *Mycobacterium avium complex* (MAC) species in patients with human immunodeficiency virus (HIV) with CD4 counts less than 50 cells/mm³. They work by inhibiting bacterial protein synthesis via the 50S ribosomal subunit. Examples include azithromycin, clarithromycin, and erythromycin. An important negative side effect of macrolides to remember is that they can prolong the QT interval and may cause torsades de pointes arrythmia.

10. **What is the mechanism of action, side effects, and spectrum of activity of tetracyclines?**
Tetracyclines work by binding to the 30S ribosomal subunit and inhibiting bacterial protein synthesis. These agents are bacteriostatic. Important side effects of tetracyclines include the discoloration of teeth in children, photosensitivity, and renal impairment. These drugs are the most important agents for the treatment of infection with intracellular organisms, such as *Chlamydia* and rickettsia species.
Note: Tetracyclines prevent transfer RNA from binding at the A-site, and also may discolor teeth.

11. **What is the mechanism of action and spectrum of the aminoglycosides?**
Aminoglycosides are irreversible inhibitors of protein synthesis (via the 30S ribosomal subunit) that are generally effective only against gram-negative rods. However, they may be used in combination with penicillins for enterococcal endocarditis (a gram-positive organism). Aminoglycosides are frequently combined with ampicillin for broad-spectrum gram-positive and gram-negative coverage. They are also the only bactericidal ribosomal antibiotics. Important negative side effects to know for this class are ototoxicity and nephrotoxicity. Aminoglycosides can be recognized by the suffix "-mycin" (e.g., streptomycin, tobramycin, neomycin) or "-micin" (e.g., gentamicin).

STEP 1 SECRET

*Aminoglycosides are the only bactericidal ribosomal agents and they bind to the 30S subunit (like tetracyclines). Remember this by recalling that the month of April (**A** for **A**minoglycoside) has **30** days.*
*You can think of a mean kid shouting in your ear to remember that a-**MEAN**-oglycosides are toxic to the **KID**ney and the **EAR**.*

12. **How does chloramphenicol work, and why is it rarely used?**
Chloramphenicol inhibits protein synthesis via the 50S ribosomal subunit. It is associated with aplastic anemia, a life-threatening side effect that limits its use in industrialized nations. Another commonly tested side effect of chloramphenicol is "gray baby syndrome," which is also potentially fatal. It occurs in premature infants and neonates who are unable to fully metabolize the drug, leading to shock and cyanosis (hence the name "gray baby syndrome").

13. **How does trimethoprim work? Why is it commonly given in combination with sulfamethoxazole as TMP-SMX?**
Both trimethoprim and sulfamethoxazole ultimately inhibit the formation of *tetrahydrofolic acid*, an essential precursor of *thymidine*. This lack of thymidine brings the synthesis of bacterial DNA to a halt. Because these agents inhibit tetrahydrofolic acid synthesis at different steps, their combination is synergistic. Trimethoprim inhibits the enzyme *dihydrofolate reductase*, while sulfamethoxazole inhibits *dihydropteroate synthetase* (Fig. 21.2).

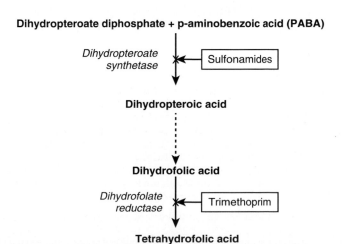

Figure 21.2. Mechanism of trimethoprim and sulfamethoxazole to inhibit folate synthesis. *(From Wikipedia, available at: http://en.wikipedia. org/wiki/Trimethoprim/sulfamethoxazole, accessed January 19, 2021.)*

14. Test yourself on the coverage, mechanism of action, resistance, and common side effects for the antibiotic classes using Table 21.10.

STEP 1 SECRET

The list of antibiotics to know for the USMLE Step 1 is quite extensive, leaving students to wonder how in-depth their knowledge must be to excel on board exams. Our recommendation is that you should expect anywhere from three to five questions on antibiotics. First Aid has a detailed review of this topic, with valuable explanations and additional information included in these pages. If you find yourself short on time while studying, go for the highest-yield points. For each antibiotic, we recommend learning the information systematically in the following order:

- Mechanism of action and mode of resistance
- Unique side effects and toxicity symptoms: Note that we said you should learn the *unique* side effects of each drug. Board exams will not test you on the fact that certain antibiotics can cause occasional gastrointestinal (GI) upset or headache. These symptoms are too commonplace and not specific enough to make for good test questions. Focus on the toxicities listed in Table 21.10.
- Clinical uses: Note that you should know the general uses for each drug (e.g., vancomycin is used for gram-positive organisms, aminoglycosides for serious gram-negative infections, aztreonam for gram-negative rods, metronidazole and clindamycin for anaerobes, etc.), but you do not need to learn the individual organisms affected by each antibiotic. We are not insinuating that this material is not important for your clinical years or fair game for board exams, but it is less likely to be tested than the previous two points. However, you should know which drugs can be used for select high-yield bacterial species—namely, *Pseudomonas* (i.e., piperacillin-tazobactam, ciprofloxacin, cefepime, imipenem), methicillin-resistant *Staphylococcus aureus* (MRSA) (i.e., vancomycin, linezolid, daptomycin), and *Enterococcus* (i.e., ampicillin, vancomycin).

CASE 21.1

A 64-year-old man is evaluated for a 3-day history of sudden-onset productive cough, fever, and chills. He describes his phlegm as "rust colored" and notes that his ribs hurt when he takes a deep breath. On exam, the patient is febrile with a temperature of 101.5°F and an O_2 saturation of 89%. Crackles are heard in the right lower posterior lung field. Laboratory workup reveals a significant leukocytosis. Chest x-ray study and sputum culture are pending.

1. What is the most likely diagnosis?
   The combination of fever, chills, pleuritic chest pain, hypoxemia, and productive cough is suggestive of pneumonia. Furthermore, the rust-colored sputum is indicative of streptococcal pneumonia.

STEP 1 SECRET

Gram-positive cocci in pairs, *and* rust-colored sputum *are common buzzwords for* Streptococcus pneumoniae. *You should know the buzzwords associated with various microorganisms, because they are likely to be useful hints on your exam.* Currant-jelly sputum *suggests* Klebsiella *infection, while* frank blood *or* hemoptysis *suggests tuberculosis. We will continue to draw attention to these buzzwords throughout the microbiology chapters.*

2. What defense mechanisms prevent pneumonia in a healthy individual?
   The respiratory tract has many defenses in place to prevent pathogens from gaining access to the lungs. The nasal hairs, mucosa, and dynamics of airflow all act to prevent inhalation of microorganisms. The epiglottis and cough reflex both act to prevent particulate matter from traveling into the deeper airways. The respiratory tract is lined with mucus all the way to the terminal bronchioles. Mucus is propelled upward by ciliated epithelium, eliminating foreign material as expectorant. The last line of defense is composed of alveolar macrophages, infiltrating leukocytes (e.g., lymphocytes, neutrophils), immunoglobulin, and complement. These components will become hyperactive during an infection.
   Note: Any state that alters a patient's level of consciousness (e.g., anesthesia, seizure, intoxication, sedation, or neurologic disorders such as coma) predisposes to aspiration pneumonia because of suppression of the cough reflex. The organisms causing this type of infection are usually anaerobes from the mouth or refluxed gastric contents (e.g., *Bacteroides* species).

3. Why might a patient in the intensive care unit who is intubated be at increased risk for development of pneumonia?
   Mechanical ventilation bypasses the normal host defenses (e.g., mucociliary clearance) that would otherwise prevent contamination of the sterile lower respiratory segments. For each day on mechanical ventilation, it is estimated that the

patient has a 1% increased chance of developing nosocomial (i.e., hospital-acquired) pneumonia. The expected duration of intubation must be carefully considered when deciding whether to place a patient on mechanical ventilation.

4. Why is it important to distinguish between community-acquired and nosocomial pneumonia?
There is a different spectrum of organisms that cause these two types of pneumonia, leading to differences in empiric antibiotic selection. The most common pathogens causing community-acquired pneumonia include *S. pneumoniae*, *H. influenzae*, *Legionella pneumophila*, and *Mycoplasma pneumoniae*. The most common pathogen causing nosocomial pneumonia is *S. aureus*, but *P. aeruginosa* should always be considered as well.

5. What is atypical ("walking") pneumonia, and is the patient in this case more likely to have typical or atypical pneumonia?
Atypical or "walking" pneumonia has a more insidious onset than the sudden onset described in this case. On USMLE exams, it classically occurs in younger individuals who live in close quarters (e.g., college dormitory or military barracks). Atypical pneumonia is characterized by headache, nonproductive cough, low-grade fever, and a nonspecific *diffuse* interstitial infiltrate on chest x-ray that typically looks worse than might be expected from the patient's appearance. Atypical pneumonia is generally caused by viruses, intracellular bacteria (e.g., *Legionella* and *Mycoplasma* species), and species of *Chlamydia* (e.g., *Chlamydia psittaci*). *Mycoplasma pneumoniae* is the classic causative organism and can be distinguished from other causes based on a high titer of *cold agglutinins* (immunoglobulin M [IgM]). Most of the bacterial causes of atypical pneumonia can be treated with a macrolide (e.g., azithromycin) or tetracycline. Remember that macrolides are "our favorite drugs for intracellular bugs"!

This patient most likely has a typical case of pneumonia based on the rapidity of onset and productive cough.

STEP 1 SECRET

Note: The term cold agglutinins *refers to the fact that immunoglobulin M antibodies bind optimally to red blood cells at low temperatures and cause them to agglutinate, or stick together. This can be demonstrated at the bedside when a blood sample becomes clumpy when placed in ice and returns to its fluid state when rewarmed. Board exams commonly test students on the association between cold agglutinins and* Mycoplasma pneumoniae.

CASE 21.1 CONTINUED:

The chest x-ray film of this patient is shown in Fig. 21.3A. Sputum Gram stain reveals large numbers of slightly elongated, gram-positive cocci in pairs and chains (Fig. 21.3B).

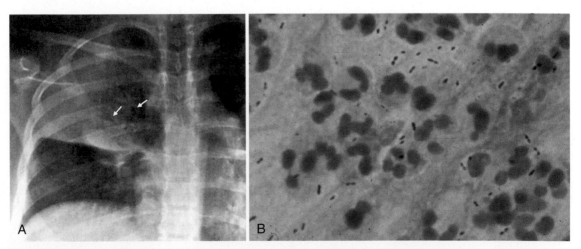

Figure 21.3. A, Chest x-ray film showing classic pneumococcal pneumonia (*arrows*). B, Gram-stained sputum from the patient in Case 21.1 at 1000× magnification. *(A, From Brown TA, Brown D. USMLE Step 1 Secrets. Philadelphia: Hanley & Belfus; 2004; B, from Goldman L, Schaffer A. Goldman-Cecil Medicine. 25th ed. Philadelphia: Elsevier; 2016.)*

6. What is the diagnosis?
Gram-positive cocci in pairs are suggestive of streptococcal infection. For the sake of completeness, the chest x-ray shows opacification (consolidation) of the right upper lobe, consistent with a *lobar* pneumonia. In contrast, atypical pneumonia would show diffuse *interstitial* infiltrates without evidence of lobar consolidation (Fig. 21.4).

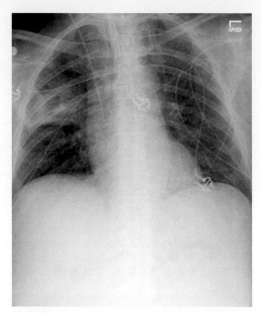

Figure 21.4. Lobar pneumonia and bronchopneumonia. Chest x-ray film showing right upper lobe pneumonia. *(From Husain AN.* High-Yield Thoracic Pathology. *Philadelphia: Elsevier; 2012.)*

7. How should this patient be treated pharmacologically?

   Although penicillin G has previously been considered first-line therapy for community-acquired pneumonia, a rising incidence of penicillin resistance among strains of *Streptococcus pneumoniae* often requires the use of an alternative agent (e.g., the third-generation cephalosporin ceftriaxone). Notice that as a third-generation cephalosporin, ceftriaxone can cover the more common gram-positive *and* gram-negative organisms that lead to community-acquired pneumonia (e.g., pneumococci and *H. influenzae*, respectively). Ceftriaxone is only intravenous, so if the patient could be discharged on oral therapy, a combination of either amoxicillin (if no medical problems) or amoxicillin-clavulanate and a macrolide such as azithromycin (if any risk factors for more severe disease) would be reasonable.

8. Use Table 21.11 to quiz yourself on the most common causes of pneumonia in different age groups.

Table 21.11. Most Common Causes of Pneumonia by Age

NEONATES (0–6 WEEKS)	CHILDREN (6 WEEKS TO 18 YEARS)	ADULTS (18–40 YEARS)	ADULTS (40–65 YEARS)	ELDERLY ADULTS (>65 YEARS)
Group B streptococci *Escherichia coli*	Viruses *Mycoplasma* *Chlamydia pneumoniae* *Streptococcus pneumoniae*	*Mycoplasma* *C. pneumoniae* *Streptococcus pneumoniae*	*S. pneumoniae* *Haemophilus influenzae* Anaerobes Viruses *Mycoplasma*	*S. pneumoniae* Viruses Anaerobes *H. influenzae* Gram-positive rods

9. Use Table 21.12 to quiz yourself on the important distinguishing characteristics of the microorganisms known to cause pneumonia.

Table 21.12. Characteristics of Organisms That Cause Pneumonia

Streptococcus pneumoniae

Seen in:	Community-acquired pneumonia
Stain	Gram-positive
Morphology	Cocci in pairs
Catalase	Negative
Hemolysis	Alpha
Optochin	Sensitive
Quellung reaction	Positive
Bile solubility	Soluble
Sputum	Rust colored

Staphylococcus aureus

Seen in:	Nosocomial pneumonia
Stain	Gram-positive
Morphology	Cocci in clusters
Catalase	Positive
Coagulase	Positive
Hemolysis	Beta

Klebsiella spp.

Seen in:	Alcoholics
	Diabetics
	Aspiration
Stain	Gram-negative
Morphology	Rods
Lactose fermentation	Positive
Sputum	Red currant jelly

Pseudomonas aeruginosa

Seen in:	Cystic fibrosis, nosocomial infection
Stain	Gram-negative
Morphology	Rod
Lactose fermentation	Negative
Oxidase	Positive

Group B Streptococci

Seen in:	Neonates
Stain	Gram-positive
Morphology	Cocci in chains
Catalase	Negative
Hemolysis	Beta
Bacitracin	Resistant

Mycoplasma spp.

Seen in:	Atypical pneumonia
Stain	None
Growth medium	Eaton agar
Blood test	Cold agglutinins (immunoglobulin M)

Escherichia coli

Seen in:	Neonates
Stain	Gram-negative
Morphology	Rod
Lactose fermentation	Positive

Chlamydia pneumoniae

Seen in:	Atypical pneumonia
Stain	Giemsa

SUMMARY BOX: PNEUMONIA

- Presentation
  - Lobar pneumonia: Sudden onset of productive cough, fever, chills, pleuritic chest pain
  - Rust-colored sputum often accompanies streptococcal pneumonia
  - Atypical pneumonia: More insidious onset with a classic clinical presentation of headache, nonproductive cough, low-grade fever
- Epidemiology
  - Lobar pneumonia typically affects older patients and immunocompromised individuals
  - Atypical pneumonia classically affects young, healthy patients (e.g., adolescents living in dormitory or barracks settings)
- Pathophysiology
  - Lobar pneumonia is commonly caused by *Streptococcus pneumoniae*
  - Most common causes of nosocomial pneumonia are *Staphylococcus aureus* and *Pseudomonas aeruginosa*
  - Atypical pneumonia is commonly caused by *Mycoplasma pneumoniae*
- Diagnosis
  - Crackles on lung auscultation, leukocytosis, chest x-ray (lobar opacification [lobar pneumonia] or diffuse patchy infiltrates [atypical pneumonia]), decreased O_2 saturation, sputum culture
- Treatment: Antibiotics appropriate for the causative organism

CASE 21.2

A 26-year-old woman presents to your office with nausea, vomiting, and severe diarrhea for the past day. She informs you that her bowel movements are watery, but she denies the presence of blood in her stool. She just returned from a week-long trip to Mexico, where she drank only bottled water supplemented with ice from her hotel room. She has no other reports or problems. Examination is remarkable for tachycardia and dry mucous membranes.

1. What is the most likely diagnosis?

   The most likely diagnosis is *traveler's diarrhea*, which is typically caused by enterotoxigenic *E. coli* (ETEC). Despite her best efforts to drink only bottled water, she has made a common mistake among travelers: she used ice made with local water.

2. What other types of diarrhea can be caused by *E. coli*?

   Enterohemorrhagic *E. coli* and enteroinvasive *E. coli* both cause a dysentery-like syndrome with fever and *bloody* stools, which distinguishes them from the *watery* stools of ETEC. Enteropathogenic *E. coli* is a common cause of diarrhea in infants, and enteroadherent *E. coli* is another cause of traveler's diarrhea. Use Table 21.13 to review the types of *E. coli* and the pathologic syndromes they cause.

Table 21.13. *Escherichia coli* Strains

STRAIN	SYNDROME
Enterotoxigenic (ETEC)	Traveler's diarrhea
Enteroadherent	Traveler's diarrhea
Enteropathogenic (EPEC)	Infantile diarrhea
Enterohemorrhagic (EHEC)	Bloody diarrhea; hemorrhagic colitis, and hemolytic uremic syndrome (0157:H7)
Enteroinvasive (EIEC)	Bloody diarrhea (dysentery)
Enteroaggressive	Persistent diarrhea in children and HIV-infected patients

HIV, Human immunodeficiency virus.

STEP 1 SECRET

It is important to remember that the enterohemorrhagic E. coli *serotype 0157:H7 is strongly associated with hemolytic uremic syndrome. Hemolytic uremic syndrome is a condition that causes anemia, thrombocytopenia, and renal failure (most often in children) because of damage to the blood vessels in the kidney.*

3. **What is the difference between** *osmotic* **and** *secretory* **diarrhea? Name a cause for each type.**
   Secretory diarrhea is caused by *active secretion* of fluids by the intestines. Examples of pathogens that cause this type of diarrhea include *Vibrio cholerae* (Fig. 21.5) and ETEC. However, these two organisms have different mechanisms of action. *Vibrio cholerae* has an exotoxin that permanently *activates* G_S receptors, leading to *chloride ion efflux* and subsequent secretion of water and other ions into the intestinal lumen. ETEC has a *heat-labile toxin* (**LT**) that stimulates *cyclic adenosine monophosphate* (c**A**MP) (remember "**L**abile like the **A**ir") and a *heat-stable toxin* (**ST**) that stimulates *cyclic guanosine monophosphate* (c**G**MP) (remember "**S**table like the **G**round"). Both toxins promote excess fluid secretion by intestinal epithelial cells into the intestinal lumen (Table 21.14).

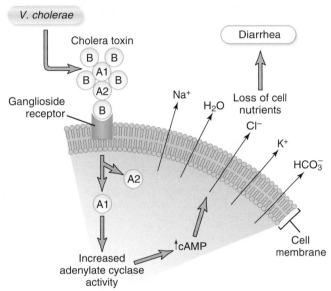

Figure 21.5. Mechanism of cholera toxin, an A-B type toxin. *cAMP*, Cyclic adenosine monophosphate. *(From Rosenthal K. Rapid Review Microbiology and Immunology. 3rd ed. Philadelphia: Elsevier; 2010.)*

Table 21.14. Commonly Tested Causes of Watery Diarrhea

INFECTIOUS AGENT	COMMENTS	TREATMENT
ETEC	Causes traveler's diarrhea and is an important cause of diarrhea in children <2 years of age in the developing world; heat-labile toxin acts on adenylate cyclase; heat-stable toxin acts on guanylate cyclase	Fluid and electrolyte replacement
Vibrio cholerae	Activates G_S protein to stimulate adenylate cyclase, leading to increased Cl^- release into lumen of gut; possible "rice water" diarrhea	Fluid and electrolyte replacement
Giardia (protozoan)	Transmitted by cysts in water and diagnosed by trophozoites in stool; steatorrhea; hiking	Metronidazole
Norwalk virus	Calicivirus	Fluid and electrolyte replacement
Rotavirus	Cause of fatal diarrhea in children and often found in day care centers	Fluid and electrolyte replacement
Cryptosporidium (protozoan)	Can be severe in AIDS	Fluid and electrolyte replacement and treatment of underlying HIV/AIDS. Occasionally may antimicrobial therapy with nitazoxanide.

AIDS, Acquired immunodeficiency syndrome; *ETEC*, enterotoxigenic *Escherichia coli*.

Osmotic diarrhea is caused by osmotically active agents within the gut lumen that *draw water into* the intestinal lumen along osmotic gradients. An example of osmotic diarrhea occurs in nutritional malabsorption (e.g., celiac sprue or pancreatic insufficiency), where osmotically active nutrients pull water into the intestines.

4. What predisposes patients to *C. difficile* colitis, and what sort of diarrhea does this cause?

The use of antibiotics (especially ampicillin and clindamycin) must be carefully monitored to avoid inducing *C. difficile* colitis, also known as *pseudomembranous colitis*. Pseudomembranous colitis occurs when a member of the normal intestinal flora (*C. difficile*) proliferates in excess after elimination of competitor species following broad-spectrum antibiotic use, resulting in superinfection. *C. difficile* is associated with two exotoxins (*toxins A and B*) that result in secretory diarrhea and damage the gut mucosa. Toxin A is an *enterotoxin* that causes diarrhea, while toxin B is a *cytotoxin* that acts on colonic cells. Colonoscopy generally reveals inflamed mucosal surfaces and the presence of pseudomembranes (i.e., layers of exudate resembling membranes) after *C. difficile* infection. Detection of toxin B in the stool can be used to confirm *C. difficile* infection. Treatment consists of oral vancomycin or rifaximin. In the past, metronidazole used to be the standard treatment, but that is no longer the case due to higher rates of treatment failure.

5. How is diarrhea treated?

Generally, supportive therapy to replace lost fluids and electrolytes is all that is needed. For the more serious microorganisms, such as those that cause bloody diarrhea, broad-spectrum antibiotics may be helpful. However, you must remain vigilant of the fact that this increases the risk for inducing *C. difficile* infection (Tables 21.14 and 21.15).

Table 21.15. Commonly Tested Causes of Bloody Diarrhea

INFECTIOUS AGENT	COMMENTS	TREATMENT
Shigella	Low inoculum (10^1); nonmotile; transmitted by 4 Fs (fingers, food, feces, flies); does not invade beyond gut mucosa	TMP-SMX
Salmonella	Higher inoculum (10^5); motile; transmitted from animal products, especially poultry and eggs; can become disseminated	TMP-SMX
EHEC	Shiga-like toxin that can cause HUS, especially O157:H7	Fluid and electrolyte replacement (with glucose)
EIEC	Signs/symptoms similar to those of shigellosis; begins as watery and can proceed to bloody diarrhea	Fluid and electrolyte replacement; antibiotics for severe infections
Campylobacter	"Thermophilic" (optimal growth temperature is 42°C); characteristic comma or S shape; oxidase and catalase positive	Usually self-limiting; give fluid and electrolyte replacement
Clostridioides difficile	Causes pseudomembranous colitis; may be seen after the administration of clindamycin or ampicillin	Oral vancomycin or rifaximin
Yersinia enterocolitica	Transmitted via pet feces, milk, or pork; causes day care outbreaks with symptoms/signs similar to those of appendicitis, called *pseudoappendicitis*	Fluid and electrolyte replacement (although antibiotics are indicated if infection is invasive)
Entamoeba histolytica (protozoan)	Transmitted by cysts in water	Metronidazole

EHEC, Enterohemorrhagic *Escherichia coli; EIEC,* enteroinvasive *E. coli; HUS,* hemolytic uremic syndrome; *TMP-SMX,* trimethoprim-sulfamethoxazole.

SUMMARY BOX: TRAVELER'S DIARRHEA

- Presentation: Abrupt onset of nausea, vomiting, and watery diarrhea in a patient with recent travel history
- Risk factors: Consumption of contaminated water (including ice) in endemic areas
- Pathophysiology: Mediated by the enterotoxigenic (ETEC) or enteroadherent strains of *Escherichia coli*
  - ETEC-associated heat-labile toxin (LT) and heat-stable toxin (ST) promote excess fluid secretion by intestinal epithelial cells into the intestinal lumen
- Diagnosis: History, physical exam (i.e., dry mucous membranes, tachycardia), stool culture
- Treatment: Supportive (replacement of lost fluids and electrolytes)
- Prognosis: Good prognosis with appropriate fluid and electrolyte replacement

CASE 21.3

A 65-year-old Polish woman with a history of hypertension and rheumatic fever as a child is evaluated for a 2- to 3-week history of night sweats, fever, malaise, and myalgias. Cardiac auscultation reveals a previously undetected faint diastolic murmur. Findings on inspection of the fingers and funduscopic examination are as shown in Figs. 21.6 and 21.7. Echocardiogram and blood culture results are pending.

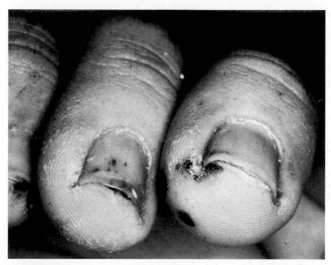

Figure 21.6. Finger inspection of the patient in Case 21.3. *(From Korzeniowski OM, Kaye D. Infective endocarditis. In Braunwald E, ed.* Heart Disease. *4th ed. Philadelphia: WB Saunders; 1992.)*

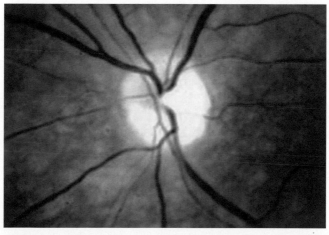

Figure 21.7. Funduscopic examination of the patient in Case 21.3. *(From Newman NJ.* Neuro-Ophthalmology. *Philadelphia: Elsevier; 2008.)*

1. **What is the most likely diagnosis?**
   This case describes the presentation of acute bacterial endocarditis, an infection of the endothelial lining of the heart (Fig. 21.8).

STEP 1 SECRET

Bacterial endocarditis is a high-yield topic for the USMLE Step 1 exam. Students may see images similar to those in Fig. 21.8 on their examinations.

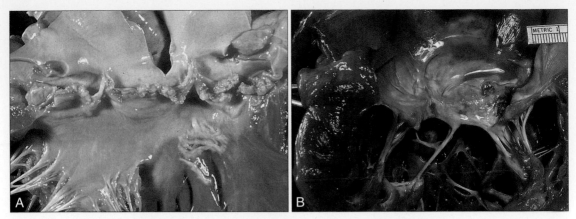

Figure 21.8. A, Acute rheumatic endocarditis. Gross photograph of an aortic valve with small vegetations (verrucae) along the lines of valve closure. B, Chronic rheumatic endocarditis. Gross photograph of a mitral valve with massive fibrosis and distortion of the leaflets and fusion of the chordae tendineae. *(From King T. Elsevier's Integrated Pathology. Philadelphia: Mosby; 2007.)*

2. **What are the major risk factors for development of bacterial endocarditis?**
   The major risk factor for the development of bacterial endocarditis is a structurally abnormal heart valve causing aberrant blood flow. Common structural abnormalities are *prosthetic valves* or *native valve lesions*, *calcifications*, *rheumatic heart disease*, and *congenital abnormalities*. Most infections occur in the left side of the heart (the *mitral valve* is the most frequently affected valve in bacterial endocarditis, but the *aortic valve* may also be involved), but with *IV drug use*, right-sided *tricuspid valve* lesions may occur as a result of direct inoculation of pathogens into the venous system. Bacterial species associated with IV drug use include *S. aureus* and *P. aeruginosa*, and fungal cases with *Candida albicans* have also been reported.

3. **What are the clinical signs of bacterial endocarditis?**
   Bacterial endocarditis commonly presents with low- to high-grade fever, new-onset heart murmur, chills, night sweats, weight loss, fatigue, and mild anemia of chronic disease. The timeline of this presentation depends on whether the endocarditis is acute or subacute. Bacterial endocarditis also presents with *Roth spots* (white dots on the retina surrounded by areas of hemorrhage; see Fig. 21.7), *Osler nodes* (painful, elevated lesions on the pads of the fingers and toes), *Janeway lesions* (painless, flat discolorations on the palms and soles), and *splinter hemorrhages* (see Fig. 21.6). The aforementioned symptoms are manifestations of small bacterial emboli (Table 21.16) and can aid in the diagnosis of bacterial endocarditis. Echocardiography and blood cultures are useful diagnostic tools for this condition.

Table 21.16. Symptoms and Signs of Bacterial Endocarditis

SYMPTOMS/SIGNS	DESCRIPTION
Fever	Can be spiking
Roth spots	Retinal hemorrhages with pale white centers composed of fibrin
Osler nodes	Tender, raised lesions of finger or toe pads
Cardiac murmur	New or changing as a result of valvular damage
Janeway lesions	Nontender, erythematous macules on palms or soles
Anemia	Anemia of chronic disease
Nail bed hemorrhages	Often called *splinter hemorrhages* and can be seen under the nail bed; caused by microemboli blocking smaller vessels
Emboli	Can lead to stroke or gangrene of distal extremities

4. **What are the clinical signs of rheumatic fever?**
   Rheumatic fever is an inflammatory sequela of *Streptococcus pyogenes* (group A, β-hemolytic) pharyngitis that is thought to result from cross-reactivity of streptococcal-specific antibodies against the myocardium and joints (type II hypersensitivity reaction; see Chapter 15, Immunology, Table 15.7). Rheumatic heart disease is a risk factor for subsequent bacterial endocarditis because of damage inflicted on the heart valves. Acute rheumatic fever most

commonly occurs in children but has also occasionally been seen in adults. The symptoms of acute rheumatic fever usually occur 2 to 3 weeks after pharyngitis and can be prevented with prompt administration of penicillin.

Rheumatic fever is diagnosed using the *Jones criteria* (Table 21.17). The diagnosis of rheumatic fever is made when at least two major criteria or one major criterion plus two minor criteria are met. The five major criteria can be easily remembered using the acronym **JONES**, which stands for **J**oints (*migratory arthritis*), carditis (**O** is circular like a heart), *subcutaneous **N**odules*, **E**rythema marginatum, and **S**ydenham chorea.

Note: *Aschoff bodies* are the pathognomonic histologic finding in rheumatic heart disease. They are found in the myocardium and consist of regions of fibrinoid necrosis with mononuclear and multinucleated giant cell infiltrates (Fig. 21.9). Also, the *antistreptolysin O* titer is used to detect a recent *Streptococcus pyogenes* infection and will be elevated in cases of acute rheumatic fever as a result of recent streptococcal infection.

Table 21.17. Criteria to Diagnose Acute Rheumatic Fever

SYMPTOM/SIGN	DESCRIPTION
Major Jones Criteria	
Migratory arthritis	Multiple joint involvement, but each persists for only a short period; arthritis is usually the initial manifestation
Carditis	New or changing murmurs may appear; pericardium, epicardium, myocardium, and endocardium are all affected; may see cardiomegaly on radiologic studies
Subcutaneous nodules	Most commonly seen over bony prominences; nonpainful and noninflammatory
Erythema marginatum	A rash similar to that of Lyme disease, in which the erythematous region extends outward as the center becomes pale, forming a ring; most often seen on trunk and not the face; occurs early in the disease and persists throughout its course
Sydenham chorea	"St. Vitus dance"—sudden, nonrhythmic, purposeless movement; may be associated with muscle weakness and behavioral changes
Minor Jones Criteria	
Fever	
Arthralgias	
Previous episode of rheumatic fever	
Elevated inflammatory markers (ESR/CRP)	
Prolonged PR interval on ECG	
Leukocytosis	

CRP, C-reactive protein; *ECG*, electrocardiogram; *ESR*, erythrocyte sedimentation rate.

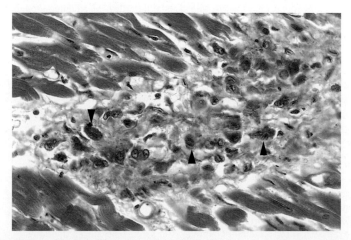

Figure 21.9. Microscopic appearance of an Aschoff body in a patient with acute rheumatic carditis; there is central necrosis with a circumscribed collection of mononuclear inflammatory cells, some of which are activated macrophages (Anitschkow cells) with prominent nucleoli (*arrowheads*). *(From Kumar V, Cotran R, Robbins S. Robbins Basic Pathology. 8th ed. Philadelphia: WB Saunders; 2008.)*

5. **Which bacteria are most commonly associated with bacterial endocarditis?**

   Bacterial endocarditis can be classified into acute or subacute types depending on the time course. Acute infections occur within days or weeks, and patients are extremely sick during this time. *Streptococcus* and *Staphylococcus* are the common pathogens involved in acute infection. Subacute infections present with milder symptoms and are characterized by a consistently low-grade illness for 3 to 4 weeks. They are frequently caused by viridans group streptococci and group D streptococci (e.g., *Streptococcus bovis*) (Table 21.18).

   Note: Bacterial endocarditis that occurs shortly after *prosthetic valvular surgery* is commonly due to *Staphylococcus epidermidis* infection after intraoperative contamination.

Table 21.18. Acute Versus Subacute Endocarditis

CHARACTERISTIC	ACUTE	SUBACUTE
Organisms	*Staphylococcus aureus*	Viridans group streptococci (*S. sanguinis*) after dental procedures
Onset	Rapid (days to weeks)	Insidious (3–4 weeks)
Clinical manifestations	Severe sickness	Mild sickness
Vegetation size	Large	Smaller
Types of valve affected	Previously normal valves	Damaged or congenitally abnormal valves

6. **What drugs could be used to treat this patient?**

   Because acute endocarditis can be caused by *Streptococcus* species and *S. aureus*, the drug chosen will need to cover both organisms. If there is no suspicion of MRSA, then either oral dicloxacillin or IV nafcillin would be effective, but if MRSA is suspected, then IV vancomycin would be the drug of choice. In some cases, surgical intervention may also be necessary.

7. **How does bacterial endocarditis differ from Libman-Sacks endocarditis?**

   Libman-Sacks (LS) endocarditis, which is seen in *systemic lupus erythematosus*, is an *aseptic* inflammation of the heart valves. The vegetations in LS endocarditis involve *both* sides of the valve, which differs from bacterial endocarditis in which the vegetations are due to bacterial deposition and occur primarily on the "downstream" side of the affected cardiac valve. It is also worth noting that the vegetations in LS endocarditis will *not* embolize.

SUMMARY BOX: ENDOCARDITIS

- Presentation: Fever, chills, night sweats, weight loss, and fatigue
- Risk factors: Structurally abnormal heart valves or history of rheumatic fever (classically affecting the left-sided mitral or aortic valves) and intravenous drug use (classically affecting the right-sided tricuspid valve)
- Pathophysiology
  - Causes:
  Staphylococcus aureus is the most common cause of acute bacterial endocarditis.
  Viridans group streptococci are an important cause of subacute endocarditis that should be considered in a patient who has undergone a recent dental procedure
- Complications: Significant structural heart damage, anemia of chronic disease
- Diagnosis: Physical exam (e.g., new-onset heart murmur, Roth spots, Osler nodes, Janeway lesions, splinter hemorrhages), positive blood cultures, echocardiography
- Treatment: Antibiotic therapy and potential surgery

CASE 21.4

A 20-year-old man is evaluated for a new genital lesion. The patient returned from spring break last month and recently noticed a painless ulcer on his penis. He is quite concerned and admits to several instances of unprotected intercourse. On physical examination, there is a well-demarcated, 2-cm painless lesion with a raised border on the shaft of the penis (Fig. 21.10). The remainder of the examination is unremarkable.

1. What is the likely diagnosis?

   This patient most likely has syphilis resulting from *Treponema pallidum* infection. This *spirochete* enters the body through broken epithelium or direct mucosal contact. The classic syphilitic chancre is *painless* and has a clean, nonpurulent base with a sharply defined border (see Fig. 21.10).

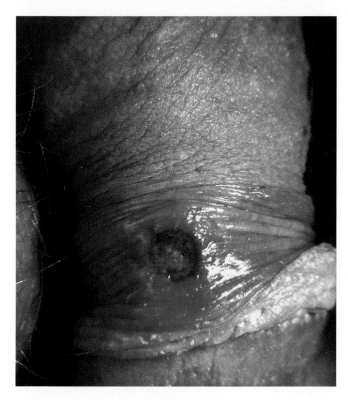

Figure 21.10. Physical examination of the genitalia of the patient in Case 21.4. *(From Habif TP. Clinical Dermatology. 6th ed. Philadelphia: Elsevier; 2016, Fig. 10-9.)*

2. Based on this patient's presentation, in which "stage" of syphilitic infection is he most likely to be?

   Syphilis progresses through three stages: primary, secondary, and tertiary. This patient displays the classic painless genital chancre of *primary* syphilis, which appears 3 to 6 weeks after initial infection. This lesion is highly infectious and continuously sheds motile spirochetes. The primary stage will last 4 to 6 weeks and then resolve, often fooling patients into thinking that they were spontaneously cured.

3. What stage of syphilis would you suspect in a patient with a diffuse maculopapular rash?

   This presentation is classic for *secondary* syphilis. The secondary stage of syphilis will begin approximately 6 weeks after the primary chancre has healed. This phase is characterized by a generalized maculopapular rash, often *involving the palms of the hands and soles of the feet*, with or without the fleshy, painless genital warts termed *condyloma lata*. The secondary stage of syphilis resolves in 6 weeks and enters the *latent* phase. If the infection is not treated, it will progress from the latent phase to tertiary syphilis in approximately one-third of patients.

STEP 1 SECRET

You should know which bacteria and viruses cause genital lesions and whether these lesions are painful or painless. Remember that the two bugs associated with painful genital lesions are herpes simplex virus 2 (HSV-2) (genital herpes) and Haemophilus ducreyi. An easy way to keep this in mind is to remember that "those with genital herpes do cry (ducreyi) in pain." By contrast, genital lesions associated with syphilis, lymphogranuloma venereum (LGV), and human papillomavirus (HPV) will be described as painless on the USMLE Step 1 exam.

STEP 1 SECRET

When distinguishing the likely cause of a rash, involvement of the palms and soles *is an important clue, because very few rashes involve these areas. Syphilis* (Treponema pallidum), *Rocky Mountain spotted fever* (Rickettsia rickettsii), *hand-foot-and-mouth disease* (coxsackievirus A), *and the noninfectious Kawasaki disease are the four palms-and-soles rash pathologies most commonly tested on the USMLE Step 1. The mnemonic **CARS** is helpful to remember the infectious causes (Coxsackie **A**, **R**ickettsia, and **S**yphilis) of this unique rash because you use your hands (palms) and feet (soles) to maneuver your vehicle while driving.*

CASE 21.4 CONTINUED:

This patient does not seek treatment and presents to your office 10 years later with an ataxic gait and regurgitant cardiac murmur heard best over the right second intercostal space.

4. What is the likely diagnosis?

   This patient is presenting with symptoms of *tertiary* syphilis, which can develop anywhere from 5 to 35 years after the initial syphilitic infection. Tertiary syphilis is a systemic disease with three major components: granulomatous cutaneous lesions (*gummas*), *cardiovascular* syphilis, and *neurosyphilis*. Inflammatory destruction is the pathophysiologic mechanism that underlies all three components. It is important to know that cardiovascular syphilis may result in *aortic valve insufficiency* and *thoracic aortic aneurysm* (caused by involvement of the *vasa vasorum*). Neurosyphilis can cause *tabes dorsalis*, a condition that affects the *dorsal column* of the spinal cord and subsequently presents with *ataxia*. Another common association is *Argyll Robertson pupils*, which react (i.e., constrict) during accommodation maneuvers but do not react when exposed to light.

5. Use Table 21.19 to quiz yourself on the three stages of syphilitic infection.

Table 21.19. Stages of Syphilis

PARAMETER	PRIMARY	SECONDARY	TERTIARY	CONGENITAL
Timing	Three weeks of incubation followed by emergence of papule	Weeks to months after emergence of papule	1–30 years after primary infection (because of latent period between secondary and tertiary)	Transmitted to fetus
Characteristic symptoms/signs	Painless papule on genitals	Disseminated disease with constitutional symptoms; possible rash that can involve palms and soles; condyloma lata are white lesions on genitals; most infectious stage	Gummas (granulomas), aortitis, tabes dorsalis (neurosyphilis of dorsal columns), Argyll Robertson pupil (constriction to accommodation but not to light)	Stillbirth, "saber shins," saddle-nose deformity, Hutchinson teeth, deafness
Treatment	Penicillin G	Penicillin G	None	Symptom dependent

6. What diagnostic tests could be done to definitively diagnose syphilis across each stage of the disease?

   Direct visualization by *dark-field microscopy* can be done during the active phases of primary and early secondary syphilis. This is conducted by obtaining a sample from the lesion and observing the motile spirochetes. Serologic tests were also developed to satisfy the need for a syphilis screen. The Venereal Disease Research Laboratory (VDRL) and the rapid plasma reagin (RPR) tests were developed to detect antibodies present against certain components released after cell death. These tests are nonspecific and highly sensitive and, if positive, require confirmation with the fluorescent treponemal antibody absorption (FTA-ABS) test. The key point is that the VDRL and the RPR tests are effective for screening high-risk patients. The VDRL test is easier and less expensive, so it is usually done first. However, it can have false-positive results because it cross-reacts in the presence of various **V**iruses, **D**rugs, **R**heumatologic diseases, and

Lupus or **L**eprosy. These can be easily remembered because they start with the letters **V**, **D**, **R**, and **L**. The VDRL test will become positive in late primary syphilis, but it will become negative again in late secondary syphilis. In addition to being more specific, the FTA-ABS test also becomes positive earlier and stays positive for a longer period. Therefore the FTA-ABS test can be used to diagnose tertiary syphilis and to confirm a positive VDRL test result (Table 21.20). **Remember:** The VDRL test is *sensitive* and is used for screening, while the FTA-ABS test is *specific* and is used for confirmation of the diagnosis (recall the **Sp**in and **Sn**out mnemonics from Chapter 25, Biostatistics).

Table 21.20. Syphilis Tests

TEST	USE
Dark-field microscopy	Test of choice when a chancre is present and a biopsy of the lesion can be taken for direct observation
VDRL	First test used when secondary syphilis is suspected; must be confirmed by FTA-ABS testing because of high number of false-positive results
FTA-ABS	Test of choice for tertiary syphilis; used to confirm a positive result on VDRL test

FTA-ABS, Fluorescent treponemal antibody absorption; *VDRL,* Venereal Disease Research Laboratory.

7. How would you treat this patient?

Fortunately, syphilis is one of the easiest diseases to treat. *Penicillin G* is the first-line treatment, followed by *tetracycline* or *doxycycline* if the patient is allergic to penicillin. It is important to remember that only primary and secondary syphilis can be cured with these medications, because antibiotics will not restore the neurodegenerative changes that define tertiary syphilis.

8. Later that night, the patient calls you at home with serious concerns about a reaction to penicillin. He states that several hours after taking the first dose of penicillin G he developed a new rash, along with fever, headache, and muscle aches. What are you concerned about in this patient?

Resist the urge to call this an allergic reaction! This patient has likely suffered from a common reaction to the penicillin treatment of syphilis known as the *Jarisch-Herxheimer reaction.* This side effect of treatment is due to the immune system's robust reaction after the lysis of treponemes. When exposed to the tremendous load of foreign treponemal antigens, the body releases high volumes of IL-1 and TNF-α, causing fever and possibly shock. The Jarisch-Herxheimer reaction should not be confused with an allergy to penicillin and requires only supportive care and close monitoring because most patients recover quickly and spontaneously.

SUMMARY BOX: SYPHILIS

- Presentation
  - Primary: Painless genital chancre in an individual with a history of unprotected sexual intercourse
  - Secondary: Diffuse maculopapular rash (involving the palms and soles), condyloma lata
- Pathophysiology: Results from *Treponema pallidum* spirochete infection through direct mucosal contact
- Diagnosis: The Venereal Disease Research Laboratory (VDRL) assay followed by confirmatory fluorescent treponemal antibody absorption (FTA-ABS) test; direct visualization by dark-field microscopy
- Complications: Progression to tertiary syphilis if untreated (gummas, aortic valve insufficiency, thoracic aortic aneurysm, tabes dorsalis, Argyll Robertson pupils)
- Treatment: Intravenous penicillin G, followed by tetracycline or doxycycline if the patient has an allergy to penicillin
  - The Jarisch-Herxheimer reaction may occur after initial penicillin treatment because of widespread treponemal lysis and the ensuing antigen release
- Prognosis: Primary and secondary syphilis are easily curable with the appropriate antibiotics; the neurodegenerative changes of tertiary syphilis will *not* respond to antibiotics

CASE 21.5

A frantic mother has brought her 8-year-old son in for an emergent visit. She is concerned about an enlarging rash located on the child's back, where she had found an attached tick. She adds that he has been complaining of a flulike illness since the family's return from a hiking trip in New England 3 weeks ago. On examination, you note a large, well-demarcated, 20-cm erythematous rash with central clearing (Fig. 21.11) and some regional adenopathy.

1. **What is the most likely diagnosis?**

   Lyme disease, caused by the spirochete *Borrelia burgdorferi*, is the most likely diagnosis. This bug is transmitted from the bite of an *Ixodes* tick, endemic to the woodlands of New England and the northeastern United States. The image in Fig. 21.11 shows an expanding erythematous lesion known as *erythema chronicum migrans* ("bull's-eye" rash) that is also common in the early stages of Lyme disease.

   Note: The *Ixodes* tick is the vector for *Borrelia burgdorferi* (Lyme disease), *Babesia* (babesiosis), and *Anaplasma phagocytophilum* (granulocytic ehrlichiosis), making coinfection possible. Other arthropod vectors include the dog tick (*Dermacentor variabilis*) and Rocky Mountain wood tick (*Dermacentor andersoni*), which carry Rocky Mountain spotted fever, as well as the lone star tick (*Amblyomma americanum*), which carries *Ehrlichia chaffeensis* (human monocytic ehrlichiosis).

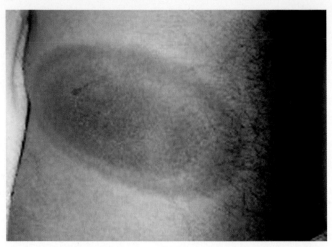

Figure 21.11. Cutaneous lesion from the patient in Case 21.5. Note the variation in color and target-like appearance of the lesion. The bite site is visible in the center.

STEP 1 SECRET

The USMLE Step 1 exam commonly asks students about vectors for various bacterial and parasitic infections. Coinfection with Lyme disease and a parasitic infection such as babesiosis or anaplasmosis are regularly tested because both pathogens share the same vector, the Ixodes *tick.*

2. **What stage of Lyme disease would you suspect in this child?**

   Our patient has manifestations consistent with *stage 1* or "early localized" Lyme disease. Lyme disease is similar to syphilis in that both illnesses are caused by the dissemination of an infectious spirochete and progress through three stages: an *early localized* stage, an *early disseminated* stage, and a *late* stage (stages 1, 2, and 3, respectively). This patient is in stage 1, which consists of the expanding erythematous lesion known as *erythema chronicum migrans*. A *flulike syndrome* and *regional lymphadenopathy* often accompany the characteristic rash of stage 1 Lyme disease. A formal diagnosis is typically made by enzyme-linked immunosorbent assay (ELISA), which can detect antibodies against *B. burgdorferi*. Western blot is used to confirm the diagnosis if the ELISA test is positive.

3. **How would your diagnosis change if this patient presented with a similar history but had reports of various painful swollen joints and a diffuse macular rash all over his body?**

   He would then mostly likely have stage 2 (i.e., early disseminated) Lyme disease. This stage is characterized by the spread of *B. burgdorferi* to four main areas of the body: joints, heart, nervous tissue, and skin. Migratory musculoskeletal pains and swelling occur, usually affecting large joints, such as the knee. Cardiac complications can vary, ranging from atrioventricular conduction block to myocarditis, and neural issues range from viral meningitis to nerve palsies (classically a *bilateral Bell palsy*). The skin lesions of stage 2 Lyme disease are similar to stage 1 rashes but are smaller and more widely distributed over the body surface. A summary of the symptoms of stage 2 Lyme disease can be remembered by the acronym **CANE** (**C**ardiac block, **A**rthritis, **N**eural issues, **E**rythema migrans).

4. **If this patient does not receive appropriate treatment, what is the likelihood that the infection will progress to stage 3 Lyme disease?**

   The late stage of Lyme disease (stage 3) occurs in only 10% of untreated patients and is characterized by the development of a chronic arthritis involving multiple large joints and a progressive central nervous system (CNS) disease (Table 21.21).

Table 21.21. Stages of Lyme Disease

STAGE	CHARACTERISTIC SYMPTOMS
Early local (stage 1)	Erythema chronicum migrans; flulike symptoms; occurs within 1 month of tick bite
Early systemic (stage 2)	Monoarticular or oligoarticular arthritis, Bell palsy or other cranial nerve palsy, and atrioventricular conduction blocks; can occur days to months after tick bite
Late (stage 3)	Migratory polyarthritis and neurologic symptoms; occurs months to years after initial infection

5. What is the treatment for Lyme disease? Name a preventive measure that can be taken to protect against development of Lyme disease.

Early Lyme disease in adults is effectively treated with *doxycycline*, while later stages should be treated with ceftriaxone. Note that children aged 8 years and younger are treated with *amoxicillin* because of the potential side effect profile of doxycycline. Recently, an effective vaccine has been developed and is routinely administered to pets in Lyme-endemic areas. The vaccine for humans is no longer available.

Note: Lyme disease is commonly transmitted during the summer, making the spring the ideal time for pet vaccination.

6. Describe the *Ixodes* life cycle.

Remember, the *Ixodes* tick is only the *vector* for the infectious spirochete *B. burgdorferi*. The *Ixodes* life cycle extends over 2 years and is outlined in Fig. 21.12. Eggs are laid in the spring and will develop into larvae that feed in the summer, typically on mice. The mice act as the *reservoir* for *B. burgdorferi* and the source of the spirochete for the *Ixodes* tick to then transmit. *Ixodes* is dormant in the fall and winter, but will become a nymph in the following spring. It feeds on both mice and humans (but note that a human is *not* necessary for the life cycle of the tick). After feeding, the tick becomes an adult and will mate, often on a deer. Note that ticks typically require a minimum 48-hour attachment period to transmit Lyme disease, although other diseases may be transmitted more quickly.

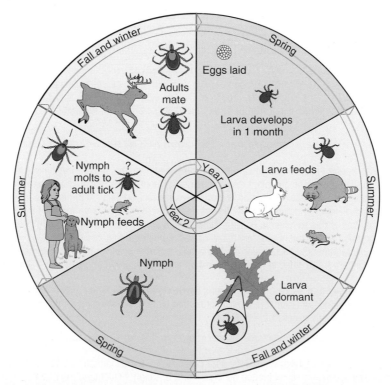

Figure 21.12. Life cycle of *Ixodes scapularis* (also known as *Ixodes dammini*). *(Adapted from an illustration by Nancy Lou Makris in Rahn DW, Malawista SE. Lyme disease. West J Med. 1991;154(6):708.)*

SUMMARY BOX: LYME DISEASE

- Presentation: Appearance of a bull's-eye rash and development of flu-like symptoms that occur within a few days after a tick bite
- Risk factors: Increased prevalence in hikers, particularly those located in New England and the northeastern United States
- Pathophysiology: Caused by *Borrelia burgdorferi*, a spirochete transmitted by the *Ixodes* tick
- Diagnosis: History and physical examination (rash, regional lymphadenopathy), enzyme-linked immunosorbent assay (ELISA), and confirmatory Western blot
- Complications: Progression to stage 2 or stage 3 Lyme disease, coinfection with other microorganisms also known to infect the *Ixodes* tick (i.e., *Babesia* and *Anaplasma* species)
  - Stage 2 Lyme disease: **CANE** symptoms (**c**ardiac block, **a**rticular disease, **n**eural issues [Bell palsy], **e**rythema migrans)
  - Stage 3 Lyme disease: Migratory arthritis and neurologic symptoms
- Treatment: Doxycycline in early stages and ceftriaxone in later stages. If the patient is 8 years or younger, give amoxicillin or ceftriaxone for any stage to prevent the side effects associated with doxycycline.

CASE 21.6

While you are in Pakistan on a medical mission, a patient presents with an 8-week history of fever, night sweats, and a productive cough, at times tinged with blood. He has lost 20 lb during this time and has been generally fatigued and weak. A chest x-ray reveals a pulmonary infiltrate, and a purified protein derivative (PPD) skin test is positive. The patient reports that the same test was negative a year ago. A sputum stain for acid-fast bacilli is positive.

1. What is the presumptive diagnosis?

   Based on this patient's clinical symptoms and laboratory results, tuberculosis (TB) is the presumptive diagnosis, caused by infection with *Mycobacterium tuberculosis*. Note that this is a presumptive rather than definitive diagnosis, which must be confirmed with DNA testing. Several pathogenic mycobacteria, such as *Mycobacterium avium-intracellulare* (MAC), can produce a similar clinical presentation and positive acid-fast stain result. Epidemiologic clues may help you, because TB often occurs in immigrants from developing nations or in persons who have spent significant time in prisons or homeless shelters. MAC commonly occurs in elderly women who are otherwise healthy and in patients with HIV who are severely immunocompromised.

2. How is this disease primarily transmitted?

   TB is primarily transmitted through aerosolization of contaminated respiratory secretions (e.g., coughing).

3. Why is the acid-fast stain required to visualize this bacterium?

   Mycobacterium species, such as TB and MAC, do not stain well with the Gram stain because they contain *mycolic acids* in their cell wall instead of peptidoglycan. However, they do stain well with the acid-fast (Ziehl-Neelsen) stain, which is why mycobacterium is referred to as an *acid-fast bacterium*. *M. tuberculosis* is grown on *Lowenstein-Jensen agar*.

4. Does this patient most likely have primary TB, latent TB, or recrudescent (i.e., reactivated or secondary) TB?

   Because his previous purified protein derivative (PPD) test was negative, this patient most likely has *primary* TB, which results from initial infection with the organism. More specifically, he probably has a "progressive" primary infection, in which symptoms manifest. This latter distinction is made because most patients who become infected with the mycobacterium do not develop symptoms. *Latent* TB develops after symptoms have resolved from primary TB (if there were any symptoms) and is due to tubercle bacilli *residing in macrophages. Recrudescent* TB develops after immunologic compromise allows latent tubercle bacilli to begin proliferating again (Fig. 21.13).

   Note: About 10% of patients infected with TB in the United States will eventually develop secondary TB. *Miliary* TB occurs when the bacilli are transmitted and cause foci of infection *throughout the body*, usually in the lungs, liver, and bone marrow.

   A *Ghon complex* refers to a region of the lung (and associated *perihilar lymph nodes*) that have been exposed to TB and become granulomatous. A Ghon complex indicates that either the patient currently has an active primary infection or has been previously exposed to TB and fully recovered.

5. What are the first-line medications for treating active TB, and why are they always used in combination?

   These agents include **R**ifampin, **I**soniazid (also used for prophylaxis), **P**yrazinamide, and **E**thambutol (remember the mnemonic **RIPE**). They are used in combination because there is a high incidence of resistance; in fact, in the United States, about 10% to 15% of mycobacterium isolates have resistance to one of these drugs before treatment. Latent TB can be treated with isoniazid and pyridoxine for 9 months.

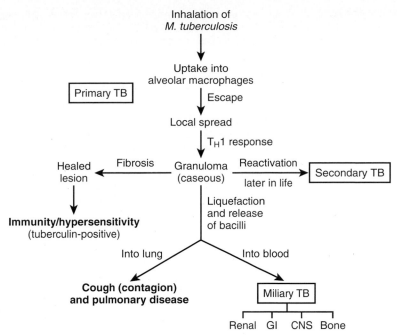

Figure 21.13. Pathogenesis and clinical course of tuberculosis (TB) caused by *Mycobacterium tuberculosis. CNS,* Central nervous system; *GI,* gastrointestinal; T$_H$1, T helper 1. *(From Rosenthal K, Tan J. Rapid Review Microbiology and Immunology. 2nd ed. Philadelphia: Mosby; 2007.)*

6. If this patient is treated with isoniazid as part of his regimen, why should he also receive supplemental pyridoxine (vitamin B₆)?

   One of the main side effects of isoniazid treatment is *peripheral neuropathy*. Isoniazid stimulates pyridoxine excretion, creating a relative pyridoxine deficiency. One of the features of pyridoxine deficiency is peripheral neuropathy.

   Note: Isoniazid is well known for its hepatotoxicity and can even cause hepatitis with nausea, vomiting, jaundice, and right upper quadrant pain. Isoniazid is also known to cause a lupus-like syndrome and can lead to hemolysis in patients with glucose-6-phosphate dehydrogenase deficiency. In addition, it is an *inhibitor* of the cytochrome P-450 system.

7. If this patient is treated with rifampin as part of his regimen, why may he need larger doses of opioid analgesics for pain control in other illnesses/injuries?

   Rifampin *induces* hepatic cytochrome P-450 enzymes, including those that metabolize opioids. Induction of the cytochrome P-450 system reduces the effectiveness of these medications.

8. Three weeks after starting a therapeutic regimen with the RIPE protocol, the patient reports orange urine. What is probably causing this?

   This is a common side effect of *rifampin*. Rifampin also causes an orange discoloration of sweat, tears, and contact lenses.

9. If this patient begins describing vision problems, what would you suspect is the cause?

   Ethambutol is known to cause optic neuropathy (i.e., decreased visual acuity and red-green color blindness).

10. Why is the standard duration of treatment for TB so prolonged?

    Several characteristics of the tubercle bacillus make it difficult to control quickly. One problem is its intracellular location, making it difficult for therapeutic agents to access the offending microorganisms. In addition, the bacillus is often found in large cavities with avascular centers, another region that is difficult for medication therapy to access. Finally, the tubercle bacillus has a slow generation time between 12 and 16 hours.

RELATED QUESTIONS

11. Is cell-mediated or humoral immunity more important for fighting TB? Why?

    Because the tubercle bacillus resides intracellularly in macrophages, *cell-mediated immunity* is more important for fighting TB because it can better target intracellular pathogens.

12. How does the PPD skin test work?

    PPD is made from the bacterial cell wall of *M. tuberculosis*. When injected into an individual whose immune system has already been exposed to the tubercle bacilli (i.e., current or previous infection), the PPD elicits a *type IV hypersensitivity* response, which manifests as an indurated area at the site of injection within roughly 48 hours.

Patients with a compromised immune system (e.g., HIV-infected patients) may not mount the appropriate immune response and may have a false-negative PPD result. In contrast, patients who have been previously infected with TB or who have previously received the Bacillus Calmette–Guérin vaccine (used abroad in many nations) will always have a positive result despite lack of current infection.

13. **Why is reactivated TB more likely to occur in the apical lungs rather than in the lower lobes?**
Because mycobacteria are obligate aerobes, the higher oxygen tension in the apex of the lung facilitates their growth. However, primary infections are more likely to occur in the lower segments where the bacteria are initially deposited.

14. **What type of necrosis is associated with granulomatous cell death in TB?**
Caseous necrosis, which has a cheesy white appearance. For board exams, other types of necrosis include *liquefactive* (e.g., stroke), *coagulative* (e.g., myocardial infarction), *fat* (e.g., pancreatitis), and *gangrenous* (e.g., bacterial infection) necrosis.
   Note: TB is the only granulomatous disease associated with caseous necrosis. Other granulomatous diseases (e.g., syphilis, cat scratch fever, leprosy, Crohn disease, chronic granulomatous disease, granulomatosis with polyangiitis, berylliosis, sarcoidosis, systemic fungal infections, *Listeria* infection, and foreign bodies) are *noncaseating*.

15. **What type of secondary infection may occur in the residual pulmonary cavitations that remain after infection with TB?**
Aspergillus, which can colonize in previously formed lung cavities, is a commonly tested secondary infection. These colonies are often called *aspergillomas*, *aspergillus balls*, or *fungus balls*.

16. **How can TB cause a urinalysis to show microscopic pyuria and hematuria (with red blood cell casts) in the face of a "sterile" culture ("sterile pyuria")?**
Hematogenous spread of TB to the kidneys can cause pyelonephritis. TB is notoriously difficult to culture, and urine is not cultured routinely unless specifically requested.

17. **Why might *Pott disease* be suspected in a patient with TB who has new-onset back pain and denies any trauma that might otherwise explain the pain?**
Hematogenous spread of TB to the spine can lead to vertebral osteomyelitis, referred to as *Pott disease*. The lower thoracic and upper lumbar vertebrae are the most common sites of spread.

SUMMARY BOX: TUBERCULOSIS

- Presentation: Fever, weight loss, night sweats, hemoptysis
- Epidemiology: Often occurs in immigrants from developing nations, individuals who have traveled to endemic areas, or individuals who have spent significant time in prisons or homeless shelters
- Pathophysiology:
  - *Mycobacterium tuberculosis* is inhaled and resides inside alveolar macrophages (primary infection), stimulating granuloma formation
- If the infection is reactivated later in life secondary to immunologic compromise, caseous necrosis, pulmonary symptoms, and signs of disseminated infection may develop
- Diagnosis: Positive purified protein derivative (PPD) or acid-fast stain, chest x-ray findings (Ghon complex), diagnosis confirmed via DNA testing
- Complications
  - Reactivation of TB leads to apical lung disease
  - Hematogenous spread can cause Pott disease and pyelonephritis
  - *Aspergillus* can infect old lung cavitations, leading to aspergillomas
- Treatment: Drug combination (**R**ifampin, **I**soniazid, **P**yrazinamide, **E**thambutol [RIPE]) to prevent antibiotic resistance; latent TB can be treated with isoniazid and pyridoxine for 9 months

---

CASE 21.7

A 21-year-old woman presents to your clinic because of abdominal discomfort that she describes as progressing in severity over the past week. She has also noticed yellow, malodorous vaginal discharge, as well as occasional vaginal bleeding following sexual intercourse. It is becoming more uncomfortable for her to urinate, but there has been no change in urinary urgency or frequency. She has had three sexual partners over the last 3 months and changed her intrauterine device (IUD) 2 weeks ago. On physical examination, she has purulent drainage from the cervical os and significant cervical motion tenderness.

1. **What is the most likely diagnosis?**
Pelvic inflammatory disease (PID), which is most often caused by *Chlamydia trachomatis* or *Neisseria gonorrhoeae*.

2. **How are *Chlamydia trachomatis* and *Neisseria gonorrhoeae* transmitted?**
By contact with infected genitals, most commonly via sexual contact or during childbirth.

3. How does PID develop, and why can it lead to pelvic discomfort, vaginal discharge, and vaginal bleeding?

PID is the result of a cervical or vaginal infection that ascends the female reproductive tract to cause endometritis and/or salpingitis. Inflammation of the uterine lining or fallopian tubes leads to pelvic discomfort. The original infection of the lower reproductive tract and the resulting inflammatory response can result in vaginal or cervical discharge. The infected epithelium is more likely to bleed even with mild contact.

CASE 21.7 CONTINUED:

The histology results report the presence of cytoplasmic inclusions but no gram-negative diplococci.

4. Based on these results, what is the definitive diagnosis?

Chlamydia trachomatis infection. A Gram stain is helpful to distinguish between *Chlamydia trachomatis* and *Neisseria gonorrhea* because the former is an obligate intracellular organism, whereas *Neisseria gonorrhoeae* is a gram-negative diplococcus (Fig. 21.14).

Chlamydia trachomatis are obligate intracellular organisms because they cannot make their own adenosine triphosphate. Therefore, when stained with Giemsa, they will be seen in the cytoplasm of the infected cell. *Rickettsia* is another example of an obligate intracellular organism.

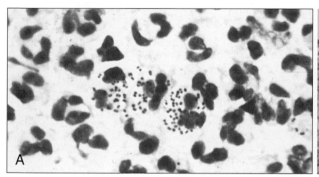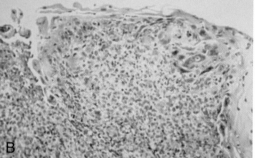

Figure 21.14. A, *Neisseria gonorrhoeae.* Gram stain of urethral exudate in gonorrhea, showing intracellular gram-negative reniform diplococci. *(From Hochberg M, Silman, A, Smolen J, et al.* Rheumatology. *6th ed. Philadelphia: Hochberg; 2015). B, Gram stain of* Chlamydia trachomatis. *(Courtesy Centers for Disease Control and Prevention; from Bailey HR.* Colorectal Surgery. *Philadelphia: Elsevier; 2012.)*

5. What should be prescribed as a treatment for this patient?

Chlamydial infections respond best to antibiotics that target the 30S ribosomal subunit and work best against intracellular organisms (e.g., macrolides and tetracyclines). *Azithromycin* is commonly used to treat *Chlamydia trachomatis* infections. Note that the chlamydial peptidoglycan *lacks muramic acid*, rendering β-lactam antibiotics useless. Because patients with chlamydial infection are at risk for coinfection with gonorrhea, you should *also treat them with ceftriaxone.*

Mounting evidence also shows that empiric anaerobic bacteria coverage with metronidazole may improve outcomes but would not be standardly tested.

6. If the patient's current and past sexual partners do not have any symptoms, should they also receive treatment?

Yes. Anyone who has had sexual contact with the patient in the 60 days leading up to her symptoms should also be treated for presumed infection. *Chlamydia trachomatis* genital infections are often asymptomatic and are an important reservoir for the infectious cycle. Even though they can be asymptomatic, chlamydial infections can lead to sterility in women because of the inflammatory effects and resulting scar tissue on the fallopian tubes and uterine lining.

7. Why is the fact that the patient was using an IUD significant in this case?

An IUD may help the infection ascend from the lower reproductive tract into the endometrium of the uterus during IUD insertion. This was a common problem with older models of IUDs, as a braided string allowed for easy ascension of bacteria into the upper reproductive tract. Current IUDs have a straight string to reduce the risk for this complication.

8. What are other risk factors for the development of PID?

Any act that may help the passage of an infection from the lower genital tract into the upper genital tract (e.g., douching, aborting a pregnancy, and parturition) is a potential risk factor for PID.

9. If this patient was not using any birth control and had been trying to become pregnant, what other concerns would you need to take into account?

PID increases the risk of *ectopic pregnancy* and can also lead to infertility because of scarring of the fallopian tubes (a sequela of the inflammatory response).

10. What is reactive arthritis (previously called Reiter syndrome)?

This autoimmune disease develops when the antibodies formed against *Chlamydia trachomatis* react against antigens on the urethra, joints, and uveal tract. This results in the classic triad of uveitis, urethritis, and arthritis ("Can't see, can't pee, can't climb a tree"). Remember that although reactive arthritis is commonly associated with chlamydial infection, it can occur with other bacterial infections (e.g., *Salmonella*, *Shigella*, *Campylobacter*, and *N. gonorrhoeae*) and is also an HLA-B27-linked condition.

11. Describe the unique life cycle of a chlamydial infection.

Infection begins when an *elementary body* attaches to and enters an epithelial cell. The elementary body will then transform into a *reticulate body*, which will divide multiple times through binary fission. The reticulate bodies will then be organized into elementary bodies and become visible microscopically as *cytoplasmic inclusion bodies*. The elementary bodies will be released from the cell, and each is then capable of infecting another epithelial cell (Fig. 21.15).

12. What are the serotypes of *Chlamydia trachomatis* that can cause PID?

PID is caused by *Chlamydia trachomatis* serotypes D through K. See Table 21.22 for diseases caused by other *Chlamydia trachomatis* serotypes.

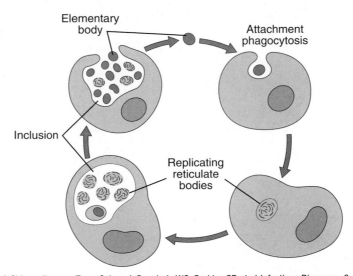

Figure 21.15. Life cycle of *Chlamydia* spp. *(From Cohen J, Powderly WG, Berkley SF, et al. Infectious Diseases. 3rd ed. Philadelphia: Saunders; 2010.)*

Table 21.22. Serotypes of *Chlamydia trachomatis*

SEROTYPES	DISEASE
A–C	Blindness in Africa as a result of chronic infections
D–K	Pelvic inflammatory disease, neonatal pneumonia, neonatal conjunctivitis
L1–L3	Lymphogranuloma venereum

13. What are the other species of *Chlamydia*, and what diseases do they cause?

Table 21.23 outlines the diseases, modes of transmission, and recommended treatments for other *Chlamydia* species that you may see on the USMLE Step 1 exam.

Table 21.23. Chlamydial Species and Associated Diseases

SPECIES	DISEASE	TRANSMISSION	TREATMENT
Chlamydia trachomatis	Reactive arthritis, nongonococcal urethritis, conjunctivitis, blindness, lymphogranuloma venereum	Sexual intercourse or passage through birth canal	Tetracycline Azithromycin Erythromycin eye drops for neonatal conjunctivitis prophylaxis
Chlamydia pneumoniae	Atypical pneumonia	Aerosol	Tetracycline or erythromycin
Chlamydia psittaci	Atypical pneumonia with avian reservoir	Aerosol	Tetracycline or erythromycin

SUMMARY BOX: *CHLAMYDIA TRACHOMATIS* INFECTION

- Presentation: Abdominal discomfort, malodorous cervical discharge, vaginal bleeding, dysuria
- Epidemiology: Sexually active patients who do not use barrier protection
- Diagnosis: History, physical exam (i.e., cervical motion tenderness, drainage from cervical os), Gram stain to rule out gonorrhea, Giemsa stain
- Pathophysiology
  - Obligate intracellular microorganism
  - Two phases of the chlamydial life cycle:
    1. *Elementary bodies* infect new cells
    2. *Reticulate bodies* divide within cells
  - Serotypes A to C cause blindness (i.e., trachoma), serotypes D to K cause pelvic inflammatory disease (PID), and serotypes L1 to L3 cause lymphogranuloma venereum (LGV)
- Complications: PID, infertility, ectopic pregnancy, Reiter syndrome
- Treatment: Azithromycin and ceftriaxone (for potential gonorrheal coinfection)
  - All sexual contacts within past 60 days should be treated as well

CASE 21.8

A 20-year-old university music major is brought to your clinic by one of his roommates, who reports that the patient was complaining of a headache last night and was confused when he was awakened this morning. On questioning, the patient knew his name but thought that he was in a different city and that the year was 2008. He reports having a severe headache and asks for the lights to be turned down in the office. His roommate says that he has no history of migraines and that they have known each other for the past 3 years. His temperature is taken and shown to be elevated at 38.7°C. On examination, he has positive Brudzinski and Kernig signs.

1. What is the most likely diagnosis?
   Meningitis is the most likely diagnosis.

2. What is the classic triad of symptoms associated with meningitis?
   Fever, nuchal rigidity, and altered mental status (confusion). However, only about one-third of patients with meningitis will present with all three of these symptoms. Photophobia and headache are also commonly seen in meningitis, but they are not considered to be part of the classic triad.

3. What are the most common causes of meningitis by age group? Use Table 21.24 to quiz yourself.

CASE 21.8 CONTINUED:

Lumbar puncture is performed on the patient to obtain cerebrospinal fluid (CSF; see Chapter 26, Clinical Anatomy, Case 26.4, Part A, for more details). A Gram stain of the CSF is provided in Fig. 21.16.

4. What is the most likely cause of this patient's meningitis?
   Neisseria meningitidis is the most likely causative agent based on this patient's Gram stain results (gram-negative cocci in pairs) and the patient's age.

Table 21.24. Most Common Causes of Meningitis by Age

0–2 YEARS	2–18 YEARS	18–60 YEARS	60+ YEARS
Escherichia coli	Neisseria meningitidis	N. meningitidis	S. pneumoniae
Group B streptococci	Streptococcus pneumoniae	S. pneumoniae	L. monocytogenes
Listeria monocytogenes	Haemophilus influenzae	H. influenzae	N. meningitidis
		L. monocytogenes	Group B streptococci
			H. influenzae

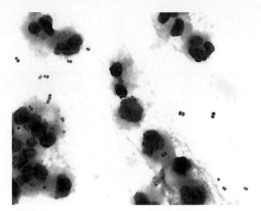

Figure 21.16. Gram stain of the cerebrospinal fluid (CSF) sample from the patient in Case 21.8. *(From Murray P, Rosenthal K, Pfaller M. Medical Microbiology. 8th ed. Philadelphia: Elsevier; 2016.)*

5. **What other potential complications should we be aware of in this patient?**
   In patients with meningococcal infection, it is important to look out for *Waterhouse-Friderichsen syndrome*, which results from hemorrhage into the adrenal glands and subsequently results in adrenal failure.

6. **When would be an appropriate time to initiate antibiotic therapy in this patient, and what antimicrobial agent could be used?**
   Antibiotic therapy must be initiated *immediately* when bacterial meningitis is suspected because of its severity. Based on the age of the patient and the morphology on the Gram stain, an appropriate antimicrobial agent can be chosen. Often a combination of IV *vancomycin and ceftriaxone* is used because of their CNS penetration and broad coverage. Ampicillin can be added if you are concerned that *Listeria* may be the cause of the meningitis (more common in newborns and the elderly).
   Note: Close contacts of a patient with bacterial meningitis (e.g., this patient's roommate) should be treated prophylactically with *rifampin.*

7. **In a patient with HIV, what infective microorganisms may be more likely to cause meningitis than in a patient who has a fully competent immune system?**
   In a patient with HIV, opportunistic infections, such as toxoplasmosis, *Cryptococcus neoformans*, and JC virus, must be considered in the differential diagnosis. If these organisms are discovered to be the causative pathogens in otherwise healthy individuals, those patients should be worked up for possible underlying immunodeficiencies.

SUMMARY BOX: MENINGITIS

- Presentation: Fever, nuchal rigidity, altered mental status, headache, and photophobia
- Pathophysiology: The most common causes of meningitis vary based on age (see Table 21.24)
- Diagnosis: Positive Brudzinski and Kernig signs, lumbar puncture
- Complications: Waterhouse-Friderichsen syndrome (i.e., adrenal insufficiency)
- Treatment: The combination of vancomycin and ceftriaxone is often used to treat bacterial meningitis because of good central nervous system penetration; ampicillin should be added if *Listeria* is a concern (i.e., newborn or elderly patients)

CHAPTER 22

VIRAL, PARASITIC, AND FUNGAL DISEASES

Insider's Guide to Viral, Parasitic, and Fungal Diseases for the USMLE Step 1

Preparing for microbiology does not end after you master the bacterial diseases that were discussed in the previous chapter. These remaining critters are important, too. Fungi are becoming particularly high yield on the USMLE Step 1 exam. In fact, some students report having as many questions on fungi as on bacteria, so make sure you have this section down. Viruses and protists also show up rather frequently on board exams, although perhaps not as often as bacteria and fungi. We recommend that you study for this section in the same way that you learned the bacteria in Chapter 21 (Bacterial Diseases). A resource many students find particularly useful is *Clinical Microbiology Made Ridiculously Simple* and *Sketchy Micro*. Our strongest suggestion is to try to study this material early and often—there are many specific details that need to be remembered for test day, and the more often you review them, the more likely you will remember them when the exam clock is ticking.

BASIC CONCEPTS—VIROLOGY

1. What characteristics are used to categorize viruses?
   Viruses can be categorized as follows (Fig. 22.1):
   - Genetic material
     - Ribonucleic acid (RNA) or deoxyribonucleic acid (DNA)
     - Single-stranded or double-stranded
     - Linear or circular
     - Segmented or nonsegmented
   - Capsid symmetry (icosahedral vs. helical)
   - Presence or absence of an envelope (nonenveloped viruses are called *naked* viruses)

STEP 1 SECRET

Although it is of little clinical relevance, you are expected to know how to classify viruses according to their genomes (DNA vs. RNA, single- vs. double-stranded, linear vs. circular), capsids (helical or icosahedral), and presence or absence of an envelope. For instance, you may be given a clinical vignette with a question that asks you to complete the following sentence: "The causative agent of this patient's disease is _____." Instead of naming viruses, you might see answer choices that reflect the composition of the virus (e.g., "a dsDNA virus with a circular genome"). Remember, the USMLE test makers love to ask second- and third-order questions!

Unfortunately, the only way to learn this information is to simply memorize it. At first it may seem difficult to keep track of all the small details that distinguish one virus from another. First try to recognize the general rules, then learn the few exceptions to each rule. Tricks and mnemonics are of great use here.

RNA viruses are most easily categorized by their capsid symmetry and nucleic acid polarity. The nucleic acid polarity is either positive (+) or negative (−) sense. Viruses with + sense polarity have RNA strands that function directly as messenger RNA (mRNA) and do not need any further modification before they can be translated into viral protein. All + sense RNA viruses have icosahedral capsids except the coronavirus, which has a helical capsid. In contrast, RNA viruses that contain − sense genomes rely on RNA-dependent RNA polymerases to make a + sense template before they can be used to create viral protein. All − sense RNA viruses have helical capsids except the delta virus responsible for hepatitis D, whose capsid symmetry is unknown. All RNA viruses contain single-stranded RNA (ssRNA) except rotavirus, which is a member of the reovirus family and contains a double-stranded RNA (dsRNA) genome. There are four naked RNA virus families: the reoviruses (rotavirus), picornaviruses (polio, rhinovirus, coxsackie A and B, hepatitis A, and echovirus), caliciviruses (norovirus), and hepeviruses (hepatitis E). All other RNA viruses are enveloped.

All DNA viruses contain dsDNA except the parvovirus family, which contains ssDNA (remember this by remembering that the root word parvo *is derived from the Latin word meaning "small"). All DNA viruses are enveloped except parvovirus, adenovirus, and the papovaviruses (papillomavirus and polyomavirus). All DNA viruses have linear genomes except those with a virus core name ending with the letter a (papilloma, polyoma, hepadna), which each having circular genomes. Nearly all DNA viruses replicate in the nucleus because they rely on host machinery for transcription. The only exception is poxvirus, which replicates in the cytoplasm because it is large enough to carry its own DNA-dependent RNA polymerase.*

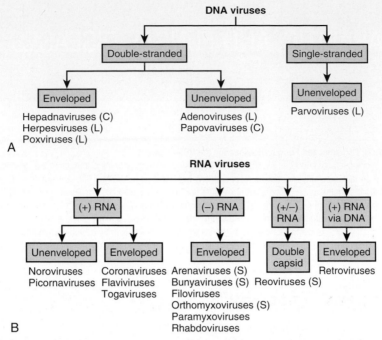

Figure 22.1. Classification of major viral families based on genome structure and virion morphology. A, DNA viruses. B, RNA viruses. + or − refers to nucleic acid polarity (see text). C, circular genome; L, linear genome; S, segmented genome. *(From Rosenthal K, Tan J.* Rapid Review Microbiology and Immunology. *Philadelphia: Mosby; 2007.)*

2. What is the difference between genetic shift and genetic drift?

   Also called *antigenic shift* and *antigenic drift*, these describe two mechanisms by which viral genomes undergo change over time. Genetic **s**hift involves the **s**udden rea**ss**ortment of **s**egmented genomes from two **s**eparate viruses or separate strains of the same virus—to remember this on test day, note the association with the letter *s*. Genetic **d**rift is a gra**d**ual change resulting from ran**d**om mutations within one **d**istinct virus (most commonly in influenza within the genes that code for hemagglutinin [HA] and neuramini**d**ase [NA])—note the association with the letter *d*.

3. Name the disease associated with each DNA virus listed in Table 22.1.

Table 22.1. DNA Viruses

FAMILY	MEMBER VIRUS(ES)	DISEASE(S)
Parvovirus	Parvovirus B19	Fifth disease (also called erythema infectiosum or slapped-cheek disease), aplastic anemia (in sickle cell patients), arthritis (in adults), hydrops fetalis (in utero)
Herpesviruses	Herpes simplex virus types 1 and 2 (HSV-1 and HSV-2)	Oral and genital lesions, keratoconjunctivitis, herpetic whitlow, erythema multiforme Temporal lobe encephalitis
	Varicella-zoster virus (VZV)	Chickenpox, shingles (followed by postherpetic neuralgia), herpes zoster ophthalmicus
	Epstein-Barr virus (EBV)	Infectious mononucleosis, Burkitt lymphoma, Hodgkin lymphoma, nasopharyngeal carcinoma (in adult Asian men), primary central nervous system lymphoma (immunocompromised patients)
	Cytomegalovirus (CMV)	Immunocompromised or transplant patients: CMV retinitis, esophagitis, pneumonia In utero: hydrops fetalis, congenital deafness with hepatosplenomegaly and periventricular calcifications
	Human herpesvirus types 6 and 7 (HHV-6 and HHV-7)	Roseola infantum (exanthema subitum)
	HHV-8	Kaposi sarcoma (immunocompromised patients)

Table 22.1. DNA Viruses—cont'd

FAMILY	MEMBER VIRUS(ES)	DISEASE(S)
Poxviruses	Variola	Smallpox
	Molluscum contagiosum virus	Fleshy, centrally umbilicated papules
Hepadnavirus	Hepatitis B	Hepatitis, hepatocellular carcinoma
Adenovirus	Adenovirus	Conjunctivitis, acute hemorrhagic cystitis, pneumonia, gastroenteritis, pharyngitis
Papovaviruses	Human papillomavirus (HPV)	High-risk serotypes (16, 18, 31, 33): cervical dysplasia and cancer Low-risk serotypes (6, 11): condyloma acuminata (genital warts), laryngeal papillomatosis
	Polyomavirus	John Cunningham (JC) virus: progressive multifocal leukoencephalopathy (PML) BK virus: renal dysfunction ***Note:*** *You are most likely to encounter these viruses on test questions about immunocompromised or transplant patients.*

STEP 1 SECRET

Herpes simplex virus 1 (HSV-1) can cause genital lesions, but more commonly causes oral lesions. Compare this with HSV-2, which is the more common cause of genital herpes. Just remember: "Head to groin—1, 2."

4. Cover the right-hand column in Table 22.2 and determine the most likely viral infection from the clinical description provided.

Table 22.2. Classic Clinical Manifestations of Commonly Tested Viral Infections

DESCRIPTION	VIRUS(ES)
Child with rash and "slapped cheek" appearance	Parvovirus B19
Descending maculopapular rash with cough, coryza, and Koplik spots; possibility of subacute sclerosing panencephalitis (SSPE) 10–20 years later	Measles (rubeola) virus
Typically causes gastroenteritis but may cause asymmetric lower extremity paralysis because of destruction of anterior horn cells; prevented with Salk (killed) or Sabin (live attenuated) vaccines	Poliovirus
Cervical cancer in sexually active smoker	HPV (serotypes 16, 18, 31, or 33)
Parotitis, orchitis, and decreased fertility in males	Mumps virus
Neonatal cataracts with heart murmur (PDA) and sensorineural hearing loss	Rubella virus
Painful vesicular lesions in dermatomal pattern; virus remains dormant in dorsal root ganglion	VZV
Acute retinitis (cotton wool spots) in patient with AIDS or recent transplant recipient	CMV
Genital warts (condyloma acuminata)	HPV (serotypes 6, 11)
Painful genital vesicular lesions on an erythematous base	HSV-2 (occasionally HSV-1)
Hepatitis in pregnant women, with high mortality rate	Hepatitis E virus
Fatigue, splenomegaly, and lymphadenopathy in a teenager; positive heterophile antibody (monospot) test result	EBV
Gastroenteritis on cruise ship	Norovirus
Common cause of gastroenteritis in children	Rotavirus

Continued

Table 22.2. Classic Clinical Manifestations of Commonly Tested Viral Infections—cont'd

DESCRIPTION	VIRUS(ES)
Common cold viruses	Coronavirus, rhinovirus
Most common cause of bronchiolitis in children	RSV
8-segment genome can undergo reassortment, causing pandemic shift pneumonia as a result of hemagglutinin and neuraminidase antigens; intramuscular (killed) and intranasal (live attenuated) vaccines available	Influenza A virus
Severe encephalitis and hydrophobia after an animal bite; intracytoplasmic Negri bodies in neurons; binds to ACh receptors and uses dynein motors to travel retrograde along nerve axons to the CNS	Rabies virus
Neonatal encephalitis	HSV or CMV
"Barking" cough with inspiratory stridor in children; steeple sign on x-ray	Parainfluenza virus

ACh, Acetylcholine; *AIDS,* acquired immunodeficiency syndrome; *CMV,* cytomegalovirus; *CNS,* central nervous system; *EBV,* Epstein-Barr virus; *HPV,* human papillomavirus; *HSV,* herpes simplex virus; *PDA,* patent ductus arteriosus; *RSV,* respiratory syncytial virus; *VZV,* varicella-zoster virus.

BASIC CONCEPTS—PARASITOLOGY

1. What are protozoa?
   Protozoa are single-celled eukaryotic parasites. The medically relevant and most commonly tested protozoa are listed in Table 22.3 alongside their associated diseases.

Table 22.3. Clinical Manifestations of Commonly Tested Protozoa Infections

PROTOZOAN	DESCRIPTION
Entamoeba histolytica	Bloody diarrhea; "flask-shaped" liver abscess with "anchovy paste" exudate
Giardia lamblia	Bloating with foul-smelling steatorrhea; often in hikers drinking contaminated water
Cryptosporidium spp.	Severe watery diarrhea in an immunocompromised patient
Trichomonas vaginalis	Vaginitis with frothy green discharge; burning sensation; "strawberry" cervix; motile organisms seen on wet mount
Plasmodium falciparum, Plasmodium vivax, Plasmodium ovale, Plasmodium malariae	Malaria (fever, anemia, malaise, splenomegaly); spread by Anopheles mosquito; trophozoite ring within RBCs on blood smear Only *P. vivax* and *P. ovale* cause recurrent infection due to dormant liver hypnozoite stage Fever cycles: tertian—every 48 hours (*P. vivax, P. ovale*); quartan—every 72 hours (*P. malariae*); constant (*P. falciparum*). Treatment with primaquine may cause adverse reaction (hemolytic anemia) in patients with G6PD deficiency
Babesia	Babesiosis presents similarly to malaria. Key differences: spread by Ixodes tick (not Anopheles mosquito); "Maltese cross" on blood smear
Toxoplasma gondii	Toxoplasmosis (from cat feces or contaminated meat) Can cause multiple ring-enhancing cystic brain lesions in HIV-infected individuals Congenital infection: hydrocephalus, chorioretinitis, and intracranial calcifications
Leishmania spp.	Cutaneous and/or visceral lesions with hepatosplenomegaly and pancytopenia Transmitted by sandfly
Trypanosoma brucei	African sleeping sickness (African trypanosomiasis) Transmitted by tsetse fly
Trypanosoma cruzi	Chagas disease (American trypanosomiasis) transmitted by reduviid kissing bug Sequelae include dilated cardiomyopathy, dementia, and megacolon

G6PD, Glucose-6-phosphate dehydrogenase; *HIV,* human immunodeficiency virus; *RBC,* red blood cell.

Table 22.4. Clinical Manifestations of Commonly Tested Helminth Infections

HELMINTH	DESCRIPTION/MECHANISM(S) OF INFECTION
Cestodes (Flatworms)	
Taenia solium (pork tapeworm)	Ingestion of larvae in undercooked pork leads to intestinal worm; ingestion of eggs causes cysts to encrust in brain (neurocysticercosis)
Taenia saginata (beef tapeworm)	Transmitted by undercooked beef (mostly asymptomatic)
Diphyllobothrium latum (fish tapeworm)	Extremely long intestinal tapeworm that causes vitamin B_{12} deficiency and megaloblastic anemia; can be acquired by eating raw fish
Echinococcus granulosus	Ingestion of eggs from dog feces; hydatid cysts with "eggshell calcifications" in liver, lungs, and brain Rupture of cysts may cause anaphylaxis
Nematodes (Roundworms)	
Enterobius vermicularis (pinworm)	Anal itching at night/on waking; fecal-oral transmission; positive Scotch tape test
Ascaris lumbricoides (giant roundworm)	Intestinal infection may cause ileocecal obstruction; worms migrate from intestine to lungs Marked eosinophilia Eggs have rough, bumpy surface
Ancylostoma duodenale or *Necator americanus* (hookworms)	Larvae directly penetrate the skin (often after walking in sand) and attach to intestinal mucosa, causing chronic blood loss and anemia
Trematodes (flukes)	
Schistosoma haematobium	Hematuria after swimming in the Nile Egg has small terminal spine Increased risk for bladder squamous cell cancer
Schistosoma mansoni or *Schistosoma japonicum*	Free-swimming cercariae released from snails infect the human host Eggs have small lateral spine and are antigenic, may induce granuloma formation Pipestem fibrosis of liver may cause portal hypertension, cirrhosis, or jaundice
Clonorchis sinensis	Pigmented gallstones causing biliary obstruction; associated with cholangiocarcinoma
Paragonimus westermani	Transmitted by eating raw crab meat, resulting in gastrointestinal and pulmonary disease

2. What is the difference between cestodes, nematodes, and trematodes?
   Cestodes, nematodes, and trematodes are all helminths (worms) but differ in worm morphology. Cestodes are flatworms (tapeworms), nematodes are roundworms, and trematodes are flukes.

3. Cover the left-hand column in Table 22.4 and determine the most likely helminth infection from the clinical description provided.

BASIC CONCEPTS—MYCOLOGY

1. What are the two morphologic types of pathogenic fungus?
   Filamentous mold and unicellular yeast are the two morphologic types of pathogenic fungus. An example of a filamentous mold is *Aspergillus*. Inhalation of spores, often found in hay and dead organic matter, is responsible for allergic bronchopulmonary aspergillosis, angioinvasive aspergillosis, and pneumonia with apical "fungus balls" visible on chest x-ray. The pathognomonic microscopic appearance of *Aspergillus* is septate hyphae with a 45-degree branching pattern (Fig. 22.2). Other pathogenic filamentous molds include *Mucor* and *Rhizopus*, which branch at wide angles. Remember the alliteration "**A**spergillus has **a**cute angles, the **o**thers are **o**btuse" to keep the hyphae branching patterns of *Aspergillus*, *Mucor*, and *Rhizopus* straight in your mind. For test purposes, remember that *Aspergillus* infections are also associated with eosinophilia, and *Mucor* and *Rhizopus* infections are associated with diabetic ketoacidosis and a necrotic eschar on the patient's face.
   Cryptococcus neoformans is a unicellular (yeast) encapsulated fungus that can cause cryptococcal meningitis in immunocompromised patients. The capsule is antiphagocytic, responsible for conferring virulence, and characteristically excludes India ink.

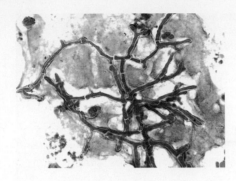

Figure 22.2. *Aspergillus* in tissue showing acute-angle branching. *(From Murray P, Rosenthal K, Pfaller M. Medical Microbiology. 8th ed. Philadelphia: Elsevier; 2016, Fig. 60-3.)*

STEP 1 SECRET

You should know the histologic appearances of all the medically relevant fungi. It is common for the USMLE test makers to ask students to identify fungi based on images.

2. **What is meant by the term** *dimorphic* **fungi?**
   Dimorphic fungi can exist in either the filamentous mold form or the unicellular yeast form, depending on the temperature of their surrounding conditions. In the environment (roughly 20°C), they exist as mold. In the host (37°C), they live as yeast. As a general rule of thumb, all dimorphic fungi are responsible for systemic infections that mimic tuberculosis (i.e., they often lead to granuloma formation). The most notable exception to this rule is *Candida albicans*, which does not cause granuloma formation.
      Histoplasma capsulatum, *Blastomyces*, and *Candida* are dimorphic fungi that can cause pathogenic infections. *Histoplasma* causes an atypical pneumonia (occasionally with cavitations) endemic to the Ohio and Mississippi river valleys. *Blastomyces* is endemic to the northern Midwest United States (also called the Great Lakes region) and may present with skin and bone lesions in addition to respiratory symptoms. *Candida* causes a variety of mucocutaneous and systemic infections (thrush, intertrigo, diaper rash, paronychia, vaginitis, urinary tract infections, endocarditis in intravenous [IV] drug users, and pneumonia) and is not associated with any particular geographic region.
      Note: Certain systemic fungal infections typically occur only in patients with severely compromised immune systems, especially with defects in cell-mediated immunity. These fungi include *Candida*, *Cryptococcus*, and *Aspergillus fumigatus*.

STEP 1 SECRET

It is critical that you know the geographic regions where each fungus is found (Fig. 22.3). You will often receive this information in the question stem, and it may be the only clue to the causative organism in an otherwise vague vignette.

3. **How do the antifungal "-azole" agents work?**
   These agents all inhibit the synthesis of ergosterol, a key component of fungal cell membranes. Examples of this class of drug are fluconazole, ketoconazole, and itraconazole.
      Note: Ketoconazole use in men is also associated with reversible gynecomastia. This side effect is suspected to be due to inhibition of hepatic enzymes, as well as adrenal and gonadal steroid synthesis.

4. **What is the mechanism of action for amphotericin B and nystatin?**
   Both of these agents bind to ergosterol in the fungal membrane, creating pores that affect membrane permeability and stability. Remember that "ampho**ter**icin will **tear** a pore in the membrane."
      Note: Amphotericin B is very nephrotoxic and can cause distal (type 1) renal tubular acidosis.

5. **Cover the right-hand column in Table 22.5 and determine the most likely fungal infection based on the clinical description provided.**

CASE 22.1

A 45-year-old woman presents to the clinic with a flulike illness. The patient is currently employed as a nurse and has recently taken several days off for sick leave. She states that approximately 1 month ago she started feeling fatigued and feverish, followed by achy abdominal pain in the right upper quadrant (RUQ) with occasional nausea and a decrease in appetite. Last week she noticed that her urine was darker than usual.

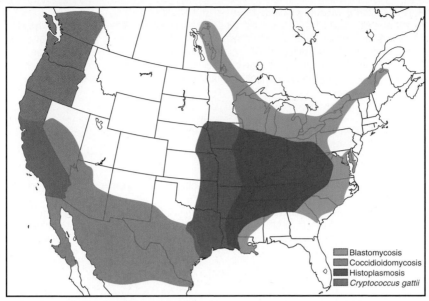

Figure 22.3. Map of systemic fungal infections with geographic associations.

Table 22.5. Clinical Manifestations of Commonly Tested Fungal Infections

DESCRIPTION	FUNGAL PATHOGEN(S)
Diffuse bilateral interstitial markings on chest radiograph in patients with HIV who presents with shortness of breath Positive silver staining Prophylax with TMP-SMX or dapsone if CD4$^+$ count <200 cells/mm^3	*Pneumocystis jiroveci* **Note:** Most common opportunistic infection in HIV-infected individuals
Thrush in patient with cancer receiving high-dose chemotherapy; endocarditis in an IV drug user; vulvovaginitis in a female patient with diabetes	*Candida albicans*
Signs and symptoms of meningitis in an HIV-infected patient Positive India ink staining of CSF obtained by lumbar puncture	*Cryptococcus neoformans*
Lung granulomas in former or current resident of Ohio River Valley; associated with caves and bat feces Intracellular yeast	*Histoplasma capsulatum*
Tinea cruris, corporis, and pedis Hyphae on KOH preparation	*Trichophyton, Epidermophyton*, or *Microsporum*
Pityriasis versicolor; melanocyte destruction; "spaghetti and meatball" appearance on KOH preparation	*Malassezia* spp.
Lung granulomas, erythema nodosum, and/or arthralgias caused by dissemination to skin/bone; southwestern United States and Mexico Spherule with endospores	*Coccidioides* spp.
Fungus ball in cavitary lung lesion; **a**cute **a**ngle branching of septate hyphae; eosinophilia; may produce **a**flatoxin (associated with hepatocellular carcinoma) Can be angioinvasive	**A**spergillus
Systemic mycoses involving lungs with bone and skin lesions; granuloma formation **B**road-**b**ased, **b**udding yeast	**B**lastomyces
Ascending lymphangitis after puncture by a thorn; "cigar-shaped" budding yeast	*Sporothrix schenckii*
Severe rhinocerebral infection in diabetic ketoacidosis; penetration of cribriform plate; black eschar formation	Mucormycosis (typically *Mucor* or *Rhizopus*)
Nonseptate hyphae with wide branching pattern	Angioinvasive fungi (typically *Mucor* or *Rhizopus*)

CSF, Cerebrospinal fluid; *HIV,* human immunodeficiency virus; *KOH,* potassium hydroxide; *TMP-SMX,* trimethoprim-sulfamethoxazole.

1. With this initial history, what is your differential diagnosis?

   There are several causes of acute right upper quadrant (RUQ) pain—biliary disease (colic, cholecystitis, choledocholithiasis, ascending cholangitis), acute pancreatitis, peptic ulcer disease, dyspepsia, lower lobe pneumonia, or an atypical presentation of myocardial infarction. In a 45-year-old woman, a gallstone should be high on your differential list. Her report of darkened urine suggests conjugated bilirubinuria and further supports a potential obstruction. It is also possible that this clinical picture could be caused by an intrahepatic process.

CASE 22.1 CONTINUED:

On further questioning, you learn that she is quite concerned about possible infection with human immunodeficiency virus (HIV) due to a needlestick exposure a few months earlier. On examination, the patient's skin and sclera appear jaundiced.

2. How does the preceding information alter the differential diagnosis, and what information could help confirm the diagnosis?

   Given the needlestick exposure, you should now be considering an infection such as HIV or, even more likely, hepatitis B. At this point, you should check liver enzymes and order serologic markers for evidence of viral hepatitis and HIV. These tests may also help clarify whether her pain is related to gallbladder disease and whether an abdominal ultrasound is necessary.

CASE 22.1 CONTINUED:

Laboratory results show that this patient's alanine aminotransferase (ALT) and aspartate aminotransferase (AST) levels are each over 1000, and her alkaline phosphatase and γ-glutamyltransferase (GGT) are both within normal limits. The hepatitis serologic assays return positive for hepatitis B core immunoglobulin M antibody (HBcAb IgM) and hepatitis B surface antigen (HBsAg).

3. What is the diagnosis?

   Based on the laboratory testing and serologic results, this patient is diagnosed with an acute hepatitis B infection. Hepatitis B can be acute or chronic (>6 months). Acute hepatitis B often manifests weeks to months after infection with constitutional symptoms, RUQ abdominal pain, and jaundice. Because hepatitis B can be transmitted parenterally, this patient was likely infected by her reported needlestick injury.

4. Why are the aspartate aminotransferase and alanine aminotransferase values elevated in this patient, and what is the significance of this patient's normal levels of alkaline phosphatase and γ-glutamyltransferase?

   Hepatitis is an inflammatory disease of the liver. The viral particles infect hepatocytes, and in an effort to clear the infection, the host immune system destroys any infected cells. This hepatocyte destruction causes a massive leakage of hepatic enzymes. The elevated aspartate aminotransferase (AST) and alanine aminotransferase (ALT) levels are therefore markers of hepatocyte death, *not liver function* (the term *transaminitis* indicates an increased AST and ALT). In comparison, a "cholestatic" pattern suggests an obstructive process (intrahepatic or extrahepatic) and typically includes elevated alkaline phosphatase and γ-glutamyltransferase (GGT). The fact that this patient's alkaline phosphatase and GGT were within normal limits suggests that the illness is due to intrinsic hepatocyte dysfunction and not an obstruction farther along the biliary tract.

5. What are the three different antigens of hepatitis B, and which antibody can be measured first in an acute infection?

   The three different antigens of hepatitis B are **s**urface antigen (HB**s**Ag), **c**ore antigen (HB**c**Ag), and **e** antigen (HB**e**Ag), each with their own clinical significance (Table 22.6). It may seem confusing at first when trying to learn the many different hepatitis B antigen–antibody combination possibilities, but remember these three cardinal rules to guide your analysis:

   - The presence of HBsAg means *current* infection—it may be acute or it may be chronic (depending on which other serologic markers are present), but the infection has *not* resolved yet.
   - If the only positive serology result is immunoglobulin G (IgG) surface antibody (HBsAb IgG), this patient was never actually infected with hepatitis B—they received the hepatitis B vaccine.
   - The presence of any IgM antibody represents an acute immune response, while an IgG antibody represents a chronic immune response.

   Hepatitis B core IgM antibody (HBcAb IgM) is the first to be made. The presence of IgM HBcAb plus the HBsAg indicates acute infection. Compare this with the presence of IgM HBcAb and absence of HBsAg, which indicates a recent but resolved acute infection.

6. What other viruses cause hepatitis, and what is their usual course of infection?

   Hepatitis A, C, D, and E viruses are all RNA viruses that cause hepatitis—hepatitis B virus is the only hepatitis-related DNA virus (Table 22.7). Hepatitis A and E cause acute infections only and are transmitted by the fecal-oral route, typically through contaminated water or food. Hepatitis **A** and **E** are also the two naked hepatitis viruses—note that the letters *a* and *e* are conveniently also the two vowels included in the word *naked*.

Table 22.6. Serologic Markers in Hepatitis B Infection

MARKER	ABBREVIATION	SIGNIFICANCE
Hepatitis B surface antigen	HBsAg	Indicates active infection (acute or chronic)
Hepatitis B surface antibody	HBsAb	Indicates successful eradication of infection or immunized status
Hepatitis B core antibody immunoglobulin M	HBcAb IgM	First antibody produced in acute hepatitis B infection
Hepatitis B e antigen	HBeAg	Indicates high level of viral infectivity

Table 22.7. Hepatitis Viruses

VIRUS	MODE OF TRANSMISSION	TIME COURSE	TREATMENT
Hepatitis A virus	Fecal-oral	Acute	Pooled intravenous immunoglobulin (IVIG); vaccine for travelers to endemic areas
Hepatitis B virus	Usually sexual contact, but also parenteral and vertical	Chronic	Vaccine for persons at high risk Interferon-α and lamivudine
Hepatitis C virus	Usually parenteral, but also sexual contact and vertical	Chronic	Ledipasvir/sofosbuvir Interferon-α and ribavirin
Hepatitis D virus	Sexual contact, parenteral, and vertical	Chronic	Prevention of hepatitis B infection through vaccination
Hepatitis E virus	Fecal-oral	Acute	Symptomatic relief

Hepatitis B, C, and D can cause acute or chronic infections and are transmitted sexually, parenterally (IV drug use, transfusion, or needlestick), and vertically (mother to baby). Remember that these "chronic" viruses are so labeled because they often persist beyond 6 months. Hepatitis D is a uniquely defective virus: It requires coinfection with hepatitis B before it can cause disease. Thus ordering a serum test for anti–hepatitis D Ab is indicated only if the HBsAg is positive.

7. **Which hepatitis viruses have U.S. Food and Drug Administration–approved vaccines available?**
Vaccines are available for hepatitis A, B, and D. The hepatitis A vaccine is typically offered to travelers planning to visit countries outside the United States. The hepatitis B vaccine is now routinely administered to infants, children, and high-risk individuals such as health care workers. There is currently no vaccine available for hepatitis C or E. Although a vaccine does exist for hepatitis D, the best method to prevent infection with hepatitis D is to prevent hepatitis B infection.

8. **Describe the association between viral hepatitis and hepatocellular carcinoma.**
Both hepatitis B and hepatitis C are strongly associated with hepatocellular carcinoma (HCC), because hepatitis B and C are both capable of becoming chronic infections. In fact, hepatitis C is estimated to be the causative agent behind approximately one-third of HCC cases.

SUMMARY BOX: HEPATITIS

- Epidemiology
  - Fecal-oral transmission (hepatitis A and E)
  - Sexual, parenteral, or vertical transmission (hepatitis B, C, and D)
  - Hepatitis D requires coinfection with hepatitis B
- Symptoms: constitutional symptoms, nausea and/or vomiting, jaundice, and right upper quadrant (RUQ) abdominal pain
- Pathophysiology: Immune-mediated destruction of virally infected hepatocytes
- Diagnosis: Significantly elevated aspartate aminotransferase (AST) and alanine aminotransferase (ALT) levels (typically >1000) in a patient with symptoms of viral hepatitis and confirmatory viral titers (see Table 22.6)
- Treatment: See Table 22.7
- Vaccines are available for hepatitis A, B, and D only
- See Chapter 7 (Hepatology) for a more detailed analysis of hepatitis B

CASE 22.2

A 51-year-old Mexican-American man presents to the emergency department in a moderately stuporous condition with new-onset seizure and headache. He is confused and unable to answer questions. His wife describes an approximate 1-month history of worsening headache that has not been relieved with ibuprofen. Three days ago, he awoke in the middle of the night feeling nauseated and collapsed on the way to the bathroom. He was found unconscious on the bedroom floor and regained consciousness minutes later. Today, the patient is reporting an acrid, burning smell at breakfast, and his right arm began to twitch uncontrollably. He then slumped in his chair and seized violently.

1. **What is the differential diagnosis for new-onset seizure in adults?**
   New-onset seizure in an adult is an ominous sign. It can be associated with a space-occupying lesion, head trauma, medications, alcohol withdrawal, illicit drug use, or intracranial infection.

CASE 22.2 CONTINUED:

On admission, the patient is obtunded and oriented to person only. His speech is disorganized and incoherent. He is afebrile with no lymphadenopathy or nuchal rigidity. Further history is elicited from his wife, who reports that their daughter was recently treated for a *Taenia solium* infection.

2. **What is the significance of a close contact with previous taeniasis?**
   Humans can serve as the intermediate or definitive host of *T. solium*, depending on which stage of the parasite is ingested. Taeniasis is caused by consumption of cysticerci (larvae) in undercooked pork, with subsequent growth of the adult tapeworm in the intestine. Ova (eggs) are shed in the feces of a human carrier and, if ingested, may disseminate to the skin, striated muscle, and brain, causing neurocysticercosis.

3. **How is the diagnosis of neurocysticercosis made?**
   Diagnosis is typically based on radiographic findings, symptomatology, and exposure history. Computed tomography can show a single lesion that is often calcified, serving as a substrate for seizures, or hundreds of lesions distributed diffusely through the cerebral cortex. Examination of the stool for parasite eggs may detect concurrent taeniasis, but a positive finding in the stool is not diagnostic of neurocysticercosis.

CASE 22.2 CONTINUED:

The patient is given intravenous lorazepam to terminate his seizure. Blood work and chest x-ray film are unrevealing. A computed tomography scan of the head shows viable cysts as diffuse radiolucent defects (*small arrow* in Fig. 22.4) and as calcified (nonviable) cysts (*large arrow* in Fig. 22.4).

   Based on this radiographic evidence, history of likely exposure in an endemic area, and clinical symptoms including new-onset seizures, the diagnosis of neurocysticercosis is made. The stool sample for *Taenia solium* ova is positive, indicating active concurrent gastrointestinal infection.

4. **How is neurocysticercosis managed?**
   Asymptomatic disease is not treated. Symptomatic neurocysticercosis with few parenchymal lesions is managed only with anticonvulsant therapy. Cysticidal agents such as albendazole, paired with prophylactic IV corticosteroids, are reserved for symptomatic disease with a high burden of cysts.

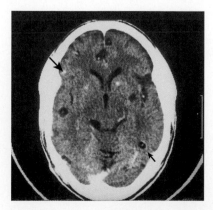

Figure 22.4. Computed tomography head scan demonstrating cysts in patient from Case 22.2. *(From Cohen J, Powderly WG, Berkley SF, et al.* Infectious Diseases. *2nd ed. Edinburgh: Mosby; 2004.)*

CASE 22.2 CONTINUED:

An infectious disease consult suggests that the patient should be started on intravenous dexamethasone to limit the anticipated inflammatory response to anthelminthic therapy. Within 12 hours, the patient's mental status improves. A 15-day course of albendazole is initiated.

5. What does neurocysticercosis look like pathologically?

The brain parenchyma is infiltrated with fluid-filled cysts surrounded by a dense fibrotic capsule. Inflammation is scant and mainly lymphocytic.

6. What is the epidemiology of neurocysticercosis?

Neurocysticercosis is the most common parasitic disease of the central nervous system (CNS). It is caused by the cestode *Taenia solium*, a parasite endemic to Central and South America, sub-Saharan Africa, and parts of Asia. It is the leading cause of late-onset seizure in these regions. Infections in the United States have also been reported, primarily in large urban centers among immigrants and travelers.

SUMMARY BOX: NEUROCYSTICERCOSIS

- Epidemiology: Most common parasitic disease of the central nervous system (CNS)
- Symptoms: Headache, late-onset seizure
- Pathophysiology: *Taenia solium* infection
  - Ingestion of ova (eggs) shed in the feces of a human carrier leads to cysticercosis with hematogenous dissemination of the organism
- Diagnosis: Cortical cysts on computed tomography scan with expected symptomatology and exposure history
- Treatment
  - Anticonvulsant therapy for seizures
  - Cysticidal agent (albendazole) paired with prophylactic intravenous (IV) corticosteroids for symptomatic disease with high cyst burden

---

CASE 22.3

A 35-year-old man with acquired immunodeficiency syndrome presents to the emergency department reporting fever, stiff neck, and a mild but persistent headache. One month ago, he experienced an upper respiratory tract infection that resolved on its own. A chest x-ray film at that time was normal. Over the last 48 hours he has vomited twice, and he now reports that it hurts his eyes to go outside because "it is too bright." He denies night sweats or recent weight loss. Examination is significant for nuchal rigidity and positive Kernig and Brudzinski signs. Laboratory tests from his last visit show a CD4$^+$ count of 105 cells/mm^3 (normal: 500–1500 cells/mm^3).

1. What diagnosis do you suspect?

Fever, nuchal rigidity, and photophobia are classic for meningitis. The causes of meningitis vary considerably based on age and immune status, and it is important to know likely pathogens in the different age groups (Table 22.8).

In immunocompromised patients, the differential diagnosis for meningitis is fairly broad. CNS symptoms can be caused by cytomegalovirus (CMV) encephalitis, toxoplasmosis, cryptococcosis, primary CNS lymphoma, and progressive multifocal leukoencephalopathy (PML). CMV typically occurs in patients with HIV with a CD4$^+$ count below 50 cells/mm^3. PML is a rare, rapidly fatal development in immunocompromised patients after recrudescence of John Cunningham (JC) virus (a polyomavirus) and typically presents with signs of increased intracranial pressure and focal neurologic deficits rather than the true meningismus described by this patient. Primary CNS lymphoma is almost always accompanied by night sweats and weight loss and is typically associated with EBV infection. In this patient, the clinical picture suggests either toxoplasma encephalitis or cryptococcal meningitis as the leading differential diagnoses.

Table 22.8. Causes of Meningitis in Different Age Groups

NEWBORNS (0–6 MONTHS)	CHILDREN	ADULTS	ELDERLY (65+ YEARS)
Group B streptococci (*Streptococcus agalactiae*) *Escherichia coli* *Listeria*	*Streptococcus pneumoniae* *Neisseria meningitidis* *Haemophilus influenzae* type b Enterovirus (echovirus, coxsackievirus B)	*S. pneumoniae* *N. meningitidis* Enterovirus (echovirus, coxsackievirus B)	*S. pneumoniae* *E. coli* *Listeria*

CASE 22.3 CONTINUED:

A head computed tomographic scan is performed, and no contraindications to lumbar puncture are identified. An elevated opening pressure is noted.

2. **How do the cerebrospinal fluid findings differ among viral, fungal, and bacterial meningitis?**
   First, look at the glucose level to distinguish viral from fungal and bacterial meningitis. Glucose is consumed by living organisms and will therefore be low in cases of bacterial and fungal meningitis but normal in cases of viral meningitis. To distinguish fungal from bacterial meningitis, look at the white blood cell differential. Fungal meningitis will demonstrate increased lymphocytes, while bacterial meningitis will demonstrate increased neutrophils. See Table 22.9 for a comparison of these findings.

CASE 22.3 CONTINUED:

Cerebrospinal fluid (CSF) analysis reveals a lymphocytosis, mildly decreased glucose, increased opening pressure, and slightly elevated CSF protein. Gram stain is unremarkable. Serum is negative for toxoplasma antibodies. An India ink preparation of the CSF is as shown in Fig. 22.5.

3. **What is the diagnosis?**
   Based on the clinical presentation, CSF results, and India ink preparation, cryptococcal meningitis is diagnosed. The India ink stain (see Fig. 22.5) shows encapsulated cryptococci with classic "halo" sign; note the large capsules surrounding the smaller organisms. More commonly, a latex agglutination assay for the polysaccharide cryptococcal capsular antigen is done. *Cryptococcus* can also be cultured on Sabouraud agar or stained red with mucicarmine.

4. **What is aseptic meningitis?**
   Aseptic meningitis is inflammation of the meninges caused by nonbacterial pathogens. More than 80% of aseptic meningitis diagnoses are due to viral infections (commonly by enteroviruses such as echovirus and coxsackievirus B), but other causes include mycobacteria, fungi, rickettsiae, spirochetes, malignancy, and medications (e.g., IV immunoglobulin and trimethoprim-sulfamethoxazole).

5. **Why is the distinction between aseptic meningitis and bacterial meningitis important?**
   The prognosis and treatment of meningitis varies tremendously depending on whether the cause is viral, fungal, or bacterial. Acute bacterial meningitis can be life-threatening and often responds well to antibiotics. Fungal meningitis likewise requires emergent therapy. In contrast, aseptic viral meningitis is usually self-limited. After 48 hours of negative CSF cultures, patients will be taken off empiric antibiotics and monitored for any change in course. Viral encephalitis, in which both the meninges and the brain parenchyma itself become inflamed, frequently has devastating outcomes.

Table 22.9. Cerebrospinal Fluid Findings in Meningitis

INFECTION	COLOR	WBC DIFFERENTIAL	GLUCOSE	PROTEIN	OPENING PRESSURE
Viral (aseptic)	Clear	Increased lymphocytes	Normal	Normal	Normal or mildly increased
Fungal/TB	Clear	Increased lymphocytes	Low	Normal to elevated	Elevated
Bacterial	Cloudy	Predominantly neutrophils	Low	High (>40 mg/dL)	Elevated

TB, Tuberculosis; *WBC,* white blood cell.

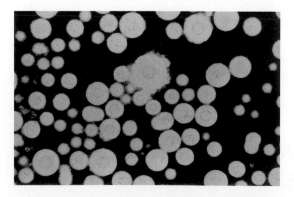

Figure 22.5. India ink preparation of cerebrospinal fluid revealing "halo" of encapsulated cryptococci. *(From Andreoli TE. Cecil Essentials of Medicine. 4th ed. Philadelphia: WB Saunders; 1997.)*

6. **What is the treatment of cryptococcal meningitis?**
Amphotericin B plus 5-flucytosine for induction therapy is the treatment of choice for cryptococcal meningitis. Maintenance therapy requires the addition of fluconazole; depending on the severity of infection, fluconazole may also be continued for life if well tolerated.

SUMMARY BOX: MENINGITIS

- Epidemiology: Causal organisms vary by age group (see Table 22.8)
  - Symptoms: Fever, nuchal rigidity, photophobia
- Diagnosis: Cerebrospinal fluid (CSF) analysis (see Table 22.9), positive Kernig and Brudzinski signs
  - Diagnosis of cryptococcal meningitis requires India ink stain or latex agglutination assay
- Treatment: Dependent on cause of infection
- Bacterial meningitis: Antibiotics
- Cryptococcal meningitis: Amphotericin B plus 5-flucytosine
- Viral meningitis: Self-limited

CASE 22.4

A 6-year-old boy is evaluated for a 2-day history of headache, runny nose, and nausea. He also reports diffuse muscle aches but denies neck stiffness or photophobia. He does not know of any sick contacts but was recently transferred to a new elementary school. Physical examination is significant for fever and pink, edematous ("boggy") nasal turbinates but is otherwise unrevealing.

---

1. **Given this patient's history and examination findings, what are your first impressions?**
This is a common story for young children. The cause of new-onset fever accompanied by headache and nausea is very broad. This clinical picture could be caused by something as commonplace as a viral infection (e.g., common cold, influenza, gastroenteritis) or an ear infection, as well as something more serious like a developing meningitis. Influenza should be eliminated from the differential with a rapid flu test if there is a high index of suspicion, and ear infections and meningitis should be eliminated by clinical examination. Most commonly, reassurance and clinical follow-up are all that is necessary, particularly once life-threatening illnesses have been ruled out.

2. **What is the most common presentation of influenza in children? In adults?**
In both adults and children, influenza virus infection classically presents with acute-onset, high-grade fever ($>102.2°F$) with myalgia, malaise, and headache. Other common symptoms include nonproductive cough and rhinitis. In a child without comorbidities, infection with influenza virus is typically self-limited. The same is true in adults, and most will recover within a week or two without significant sequelae.

   An important complication of influenza to keep in mind for the USMLE Step 1 exam is bacterial coinfection on top of an existing influenza infection that causes secondary bacterial pneumonia. Secondary bacterial pneumonia most commonly affects older adults (ages 65+ years) and presents with worsening respiratory symptoms and recurrent fever after initial improvement. *Streptococcus pneumoniae* is responsible for the majority of these cases, although *Staphylococcus aureus* accounts for an increasing proportion of cases.

3. **What is the significance of H and N typing? How do these proteins help influenza virus infect host cells?**
H and N (HA and NA) refer to the major antigenic determinants found on the surface of influenza viruses, which provide a means of categorizing virus subtypes. The specific type of HA also determines where in the respiratory tract the virus will bind, with certain subtypes having tropism for sites in more proximal or distal airways.

   After virus aerosols or droplets are inhaled, HA binds to sialic acid on the surface of epithelial cells in the bronchioles, bronchi, and trachea. This facilitates endocytosis of the virus, allowing viral RNA to be released into the cytoplasm. From there, the viral material is transported into the nucleus for replication and transcription. Once complete, buds containing new virus are released from the host cell membrane in a process enabled by NA. NA catalyzes the hydrolysis of sialic acid from the virions and host cell receptors, thus allowing viruses to leave and infect other cells. Oseltamivir (Tamiflu) and zanamivir (Relenza) competitively inhibit viral NA, which prevents viral budding.

CASE 22.4 CONTINUED:

A rapid flu test is negative. Several days later, an erythematous macular rash develops in the malar distribution. The patient's abdomen and extremities are also covered diffusely by a reticular pattern. No desquamation is noted. Antistreptolysin O (ASO) titer is negative.

4. Based on this information, what is the most likely diagnosis?

Erythema infectiosum is the most likely diagnosis. Given the description of the diffuse rash, it is important to rule out exotoxin-mediated scarlet fever with an antistreptolysin O (ASO) titer, as well as rarer vasculitides, such as Kawasaki disease, via clinical examination and history (e.g., absence of desquamation, conjunctivitis, and cervical lymphadenopathy).

Clinical Pearl

In practice, the sensitivity of the rapid flu test ranges from 30% to 70%. Whereas a positive result can be very helpful in ruling in disease because of the test's high specificity ($\approx$98%), a negative test should not be used to rule out influenza infection if clinical suspicion is high. For the purposes of your USMLE Step 1 exam, however, you can consider a reported test result to be a true positive or true negative.

---

5. What is erythema infectiosum?

Erythema infectiosum (also known as *fifth disease* or *slapped cheek disease*) is a self-limited illness most often affecting school-age children. It is a viral exanthem caused by parvovirus B19. The virus infects erythroid progenitor cells in the bone marrow and peripheral blood, resulting in defective erythropoiesis.

Often it presents as a biphasic illness, with a viremic period marked by fever, headache, and myalgia. Up to a week later, the characteristic slapped–cheek rash can appear and evolve to include the whole body. The illness may persist for several weeks to months and is exacerbated by stress, increased physical activity, and exposure to sun.

6. What are the other viral exanthems?

See Table 22.10.

7. What are other clinical manifestations of infection with parvovirus B19?

Remember the other presentations of B19 as the three As—**a**nemia, **a**rthritis, and **a**bortion.

- Aplastic *anemia* (transient anemic crisis) usually causes pure red blood cell aplasia but can also affect other hematopoietic cell lines. Severe anemia most often occurs in patients with extant hematologic abnormalities such as sickle cell disease, thalassemia, and hereditary spherocytosis. Severity varies, and transfusions are occasionally necessary.
- *Arthritis* is typically monoarticular or pauciarticular in nature. Symptoms are usually symmetric and involve the small joints of the hands, knees, and feet. The arthritis is nondestructive.
- *Abortion:* In pregnant women, parvovirus can cause miscarriage, intrauterine fetal death, and nonimmune hydrops fetalis. When infection occurs before 20 weeks of gestation, outcomes are worse.

8. Describe the structure of the B19 virion. How is it transmitted?

Parvovirus B19 is a nonenveloped ssDNA virus. It is transmitted primarily by respiratory aerosols but can also pass hematogenously and transplacentally. Approximately 50% to 70% of Americans older than 18 years are seropositive.

9. How is parvovirus B19 infection diagnosed?

Serologic testing for B19-specific IgM is used to detect acute infection. Detectable levels can be found within 7 to 10 days of exposure and remain elevated for several months. Another method to diagnose acute infection is detection of B19 DNA by polymerase chain reaction (PCR). This test, however, has the drawback of remaining positive for several years and does not reliably indicate acute infection.

10. What is the treatment for parvovirus infection?

There is no specific treatment for B19 infection. Passive immunity via immunoglobulin transfer may be beneficial to compromised hosts with chronic infection but plays no role in acute disease. Currently, no vaccine is available. Prevention of disease by good infection-control practices is the best method to decrease transmission.

SUMMARY BOX: PARVOVIRUS B19

- Epidemiology: Most commonly affects school-age children
- Symptoms: Fever, nausea, and myalgia, with subsequent development of the slapped-cheek rash characteristic of erythema infectiosum (fifth disease)
  - Other clinical manifestations include aplastic anemia, arthritis, and spontaneous abortion
- Pathophysiology: Caused by single-stranded DNA virus that infects early-stage red blood cells (RBCs)
- Diagnosis: Serum immunoglobulin (IgM) levels or polymerase chain reaction (PCR)
- Treatment: Self-limited. No specific treatment or vaccine is available

---

CASE 22.5

A 28-year-old man presents to the emergency department with a 3-day history of high fever, headache, fatigue, and muscle aches. Over the last 24 hours, he has developed vomiting and diarrhea and "hasn't been able to keep anything down." His eyes appear reddened.

Table 22.10. Childhood Exanthems

DISEASE	ETIOLOGY	AGE RANGE	RASH	ASSOCIATED SYMPTOMS	COMPLICATIONS
Measles (first disease)	Rubeola (paramyxovirus; enveloped – ssRNA virus)	3–5 years	Maculopapular erythematous rash that spreads from face to trunk and extremities over ≈3 days. Typically becomes confluent, unlike rubella	Cough, coryza, conjunctivitis, Koplik spots (white spots on oral mucosa). Often associated with fever and toxic appearance	Otitis media, encephalitis, PNA; rarely SSPE 10–20 years after infection Vitamin A supplementation may reduce morbidity and mortality
Chickenpox (second disease)	Varicella-zoster virus (enveloped herpesvirus dsDNA, also known as *HHV-3*)	Usually before age 10 years	"Dew drops on rose petal" appearance—papular/vesicular rash on an erythematous base Starts as localized groups of erythematous macules, progresses to papules that eventually become vesicular and rupture with associated crusting Often intensely pruritic with lesions in various stages of healing across entire body. Palms and soles are usually spared. Usually occurs 24 h or less after mild prodrome	Malaise, intense pruritis, decreased appetite, low-grade fever	Herpes zoster ophthalmicus (latent in trigeminal ganglia) Shingles from reactivation of dormant virus in dorsal root ganglia. Causes dermatomal rash, often followed by postherpetic neuralgia Effective vaccine since 1995 has reduced rates of infection and complications
German measles (third disease)	Rubella (togavirus; enveloped + ssRNA)	School age to young adult	Rapidly progressive rash (vs. measles) Starts on face and progresses to trunk and extremities. Pruritic/maculopapular, but fainter than measles	Low-grade fever, generally not toxic appearing. Tender suboccipital and posterior auricular lymphadenopathy are unique features Older patients may have arthralgias as predominant symptom	In pregnancy, can cause congenital rubella syndrome (MR, cataracts, PDA) or miscarriage. Also a notable cause of encephalitis and/or TTP in neonates.
Scarlet fever (fourth disease)	*Streptococcus pyogenes*	School age to young adult	Perioral pallor with flushed face, fine red sandpaper rash on abdomen and trunk. Lasts about a week followed by peeling skin (desquamation)	Abrupt-onset high fever, headache, and severe sore throat	Rheumatic fever, glomerulonephritis, peritonsillar abscess
Erythema infectiosum (fifth disease)	Parvovirus B19 (naked ssDNA virus)	4–10 years, pregnant patients	Bright red "slapped-cheek" pruritic facial rash. When facial rash fades, can progress to trunk and extremities as an erythematous reticular rash	50% of affected individuals will have no symptoms Malaise, low-grade fever, sore throat. Joint pain more common in young women and adults	Hydrops fetalis, fetal demise. Aplastic crisis in sickle cell patients
Roseola infantum (sixth disease)	HHV-6 and HHV-7 (enveloped herpesvirus dsDNA)	6–36 months	High-spiking fever followed by rash that begins after the fever has resolved. Pink macules and papules with white halos appearing on trunk and spreading to neck, face, and proximal extremities. Rash often improves or disappears entirely within 24 h	Abrupt-onset high-grade fever but generally not toxic appearing Just as abrupt defervescence, with no new symptoms for a few days. Rash follows as fever resolves	Rapidly developing high-grade fever (>104°F) can lead to febrile seizures Key to recognizing this disease is the timing: the onset of the rash occurs *after* the fever has resolved

ds, Double-stranded; HHV, human herpesvirus; MR, mental retardation; PDA, patent ductus arteriosus; PNA, pneumonia; ss, single-stranded; SSPE, subacute sclerosing panencephalitis; TTP, thrombocytopenic purpura.

1. With this initial history, what is your differential diagnosis?

   This patient's presentation suggests an infectious etiology. Influenza, typhoid, malaria, and Ebola are all infections to be considered in this patient. Because some of these are extremely serious infections, recent travel history should be obtained.

CASE 22.5 CONTINUED:

On further questioning, the patient reports travel to Liberia 2 weeks ago.

2. Based on this additional information, what is your leading diagnosis?

   Considering the patient's history of recent travel to West Africa, Ebola infection is a strong possibility. Ebola virus is a nonsegmented, ssRNA virus that belongs to the *Filoviridae* family.

   Note: The 2014 Ebola outbreak in West Africa was the largest Ebola outbreak in history. The highest number of cases was recorded in Liberia.

3. How is Ebola virus transmitted?

   The Ebola virus is transmitted through direct contact with body fluids from an infected individual. Patients with Ebola typically develop acute onset of symptoms within 2 to 21 days after initial exposure.

4. What are the typical symptoms of Ebola infection?

   Typical symptoms include fever, myalgias, weakness, vomiting, diarrhea, and rash. Some patients experience unexplained bleeding (i.e., ecchymosis, blood in the stool); major bleeding is a manifestation of the terminal phase of the infection. Bleeding results from massive, virally triggered cytokine release (a phenomenon known as *cytokine storm*), which increases the permeability of blood vessels.

CASE 22.5 CONTINUED:

The patient is quickly isolated, and the local health department is notified of the possible Ebola case. Rapid blood testing for Ebola virus by reverse transcription polymerase chain reaction (RT-PCR) is positive.

5. How is Ebola infection managed?

   Ebola is managed with supportive care, as there is no known cure. Important measures include repletion of fluids lost through vomiting, bleeding, and diarrhea; correction of electrolyte abnormalities; and prevention of shock.

SUMMARY BOX: EBOLA INFECTION

- Epidemiology: The most widespread Ebola epidemic in history (2014) was based in West Africa, with the highest number of cases reported in Liberia
  - Transmission occurs through direct contact with bodily fluids of infected individuals
- Symptoms: Flulike symptoms with vomiting, diarrhea, and bleeding
- Diagnosis: Exposure history, reverse transcription polymerase chain reaction (RT-PCR)
- Treatment: Supportive care (i.e., fluid and electrolyte repletion)

PHARMACOLOGY AND TOXICOLOGY

BASIC CONCEPTS

1. Describe the relationship between absorption, metabolism, excretion, distribution, and the current concentration of a drug within the bloodstream.

   The law of conservation of mass states that matter cannot be created or destroyed. Therefore a drug's current concentration within a person's bloodstream must be equal to any amount of drug that has entered the bloodstream (i.e., through absorption) minus the amount of drug that has been removed from the bloodstream through transforming it into another product (metabolism), transferred into an inactive compartment such as fatty tissue (distribution), and cleared from the bloodstream through the renal system (excretion).

$$\text{Absorption} - \text{excretion} - \text{metabolism} - \text{distribution} = \text{current concentration (in plasma)}$$

2. How does the route by which a drug is administered affect its metabolism?

   Most drugs that are taken orally enter the bloodstream at the level of the portal circulation and encounter the liver almost immediately. There, they undergo first-pass metabolism, which renders them less efficacious than if they had reached their target organs first. As such, the rate of portal blood flow is a major determinant of first-pass metabolism. First-pass metabolism can be circumvented by administering the medication parenterally (e.g., intravenously, intramuscularly, or subcutaneously). Because the drug can reach its target faster and relatively unaltered, its onset of action is more rapid. In comparison with the oral route, the advantage of parenteral administration is that the clinician is able to observe the effects of the drug almost instantaneously and manage dosing appropriately. Disadvantages include more rapid induction of drug side effects, complications associated with venipuncture (e.g., hematoma, phlebitis, extravascular injection), and the need for frequent dosing in cases where a sustained effect is desired.

   Other routes of delivery include inhalation (rapid effect, targeted delivery), intrathecal (into the cerebrospinal fluid), sublingual (rapid onset, avoids first-pass metabolism), rectal (note that some of the delivered drug will undergo first-pass metabolism because the superior rectal vein drains into the *portal* circulation, but the middle and inferior rectal veins drain to the *systemic* circulation), topical (for local effect), and transdermal (sustained delivery).

The concentration of a drug in the body is dependent on the route of administration because this influences the bioavailability (F) of the drug. A drug administered intravenously has 100% bioavailability ($F = 1$), but drugs administered orally have a bioavailability of less than 1 ($F < 1$). You should know how to calculate the concentration of a drug based on dose administered, bioavailability, and volume of distribution (V_D), which is essentially the ability of a drug to penetrate the tissues of the body.

$$V_D = \text{amount of drug in body}/\text{plasma drug concentration} \qquad [23.1]$$

A drug that remains mostly in the bloodstream has a low V_D, whereas a drug that can be absorbed into the body's adipose tissue has a high V_D. Thus small, nonpolar (lipid-soluble), and unionized drugs can better enter fatty tissue and will have a greater V_D than larger, polar (water-soluble), and ionized drugs, which will mostly stay within the plasma. If a drug can enter more tissue, it should, therefore, be more difficult to excrete compared with a drug that stays mostly in the circulation, where renal excretion is accessible. As such, a drug with a large V_D will have a greater half-life.

$$\text{Plasma concentration} = \text{dose} \times F/V_D \qquad [23.2]$$

3. What is phase I versus phase II drug metabolism?
Phase I drug metabolism is carried out by cytochrome P-450 (CYP-450) enzymes of the liver. Certain drugs can either increase or decrease the activity of the CYP-450 enzymes and can thereby alter the concentrations of other coadministered drugs. CYP-450 inhibitors will increase the concentration (and effects) of drugs that are normally metabolized by CYP-450 enzymes, while the opposite will be true of CYP-450 inducers. This is a very commonly tested concept on Step 1. Therefore it is important to be familiar with drugs that are commonly metabolized by CYP-450 enzymes (warfarin, oral contraceptive pills (OCPs), statins, and antiepileptic drugs are the highest-yield examples). Likewise, you should know some examples of the CYP-450 inhibitors and inducers. *Phase II drug metabolism* occurs after CYP-450 metabolism and is carried out by conjugating enzymes. These enzymes can participate in glucuronidation, acetylation, or sulfation of the drug metabolite to form a highly polar and inactive metabolite that can be excreted through the kidney. Some individuals are genetically "slow acetylators"; this decreases their rate of metabolism for certain drugs and can expose them to drug effects for a longer-than-anticipated period. The classic case of delayed acetylation is an individual who is given isoniazid and contracts drug-induced lupus. Slow acetylation causes metabolites of these drugs to accumulate and react with free radicals generated by the oxidative burst that occurs in white blood cells. These radical–metabolite complexes are recognized as foreign by the body's immune system, which then produces antibodies (especially *antihistone antibodies*) in response. This immune response generates lupus-like symptoms, including rash, joint and muscle pain, fatigue, and soft tissue inflammation. Hydralazine (antihypertensive) and procainamide (antiarrhythmic) are also highly associated with drug-induced lupus. Symptoms resolve when the drug is removed.

4. Describe the Henderson-Hasselbalch equation. How can it be used to calculate whether a weak acid will cross the blood-brain barrier?
A simple rule of pharmacology is that for a drug to move as freely as possible across various membranes in the body, it must be uncharged. Most drugs are either weak acids (i.e., uncharged while they still have their proton) or weak bases (i.e., uncharged in their conjugate acid form). The amount of a medication that ends up being uncharged in solution depends on the drug (specifically, the pK_a of the drug) and the pH of the solution. The following simplification is derived from the Henderson-Hasselbalch equation:
For acids (the acid itself is uncharged):

$$pH = pK_a + \log[\text{conjugate base}]/[\text{acid}] \qquad [23.3]$$

If given a list of drugs that are weak acids and asked which will readily cross the blood-brain barrier, simply subtract the pK_a of the drug from the pH of the solution:

$$pH - pK_a = \log[\text{conjugate base}]/[\text{acid}] \qquad [23.4]$$

The drug with the most negative difference will primarily end up being uncharged at that pH. Why is this the case? Recall that the log of a number less than 1 will be negative. Therefore a higher concentration of acid (uncharged) will produce a number even smaller than 1, and the subsequent log[conjugate base]/[acid] will be more negative.

Although you are not expected to calculate logarithms on your exam, we provide the following example calculation to illustrate the aforementioned principle:

Drug X has a pK_a of 3.5, Drug Y has a pK_a of 7.5, and Drug Z has a pK_a of 9.8.

Which will most readily cross the blood-brain barrier (serum pH is approximately 7.4)?
First, we need to determine which drug will be uncharged in the serum by subtracting the pK_a from the pH, as described previously.

Drug X: $7.4 - 3.5 = 3.9$
Drug Y: $7.4 - 7.5 = -0.1$
Drug Z: $7.4 - 9.8 = -2.4$

Because the difference between pH and pK_a is most negative for Drug Z, it will have the highest concentration of conjugate acid (uncharged particles) in the serum.

For bases (the conjugate acid is uncharged):

$$pH = pK_a + \log[\text{conjugate base}]/[\text{acid}]$$

If given a list of weak bases and asked the same question, again subtract the pK_a from the pH. This time, however, the more positive this number is, the greater the amount of that drug in the uncharged form. Look at these equations and convince yourself of the reason that the preceding simplification holds true.

Overdoses of weakly acidic or basic drugs can sometimes be treated by "trapping" the drug in its ionized form to encourage renal excretion. Exposing weakly acidic drugs, such as aspirin (acetylsalicylic *acid*), to a proton-removing base (e.g., bicarbonate) will produce the anionic form of aspirin. Exposing weakly basic drugs, such as amphet*amines* (remember that *amines* are nitrogen-containing bases), to a proton-donating acid (e.g., ammonium) will likewise generate the cationic form of the drug.

5. What is the difference between zero-order kinetics and first-order kinetics?

After a certain period in the body, most drugs are inactivated in the liver. Enzymes conduct this biotransformation in one of two ways: first-order or zero-order kinetics. If a drug is metabolized according to zero-order kinetics, this means that a constant amount of drug is metabolized in a given period *regardless of the initial dose or half-life of the drug*. In other words, enzymes metabolize the same amount of drug per unit time and do not respond to increased workload by increasing their rate of work. The drugs that you should know that are metabolized by zero-order kinetics are phenytoin, ethanol, and aspirin.

In first-order kinetics, a constant *fraction* of a drug dose is metabolized per unit time. If the concentration of the drug is steadily increased, metabolic enzymes increase the rate at which they work to abide by the rule of metabolizing a certain fraction per unit time. As such, the quantity of drug metabolized is directly proportional to the dose administered. First-order kinetics takes half-life into account (see question 6).

6. What is half-life?

The half-life ($t_{1/2}$) of a drug refers to the amount of time required for half of a drug dose to be metabolized.

After one half-life, 50% of a drug will disappear. After two half-lives, another 50% of the remaining drug dose will disappear (75% of the original dose). After four half-lives, 94% of the original drug dose will have been metabolized. For boards, it is very important to know that steady state is reached after four to five half-lives. Only two things affect a substance's half-life: its affinity for tissues (V_D) and its rate of elimination (i.e., clearance).

$$t_{1/2} = 0.7 \times V_D/\text{clearance} \tag{23.5}$$

There is a direct relationship between V_D and $t_{1/2}$—if a molecule has a high affinity for the tissues of the body, it will have a longer half-life because it will be more difficult to eliminate. If there is a high rate of clearance of the molecule, it will have a short half-life (inverse relationship between $t_{1/2}$ and clearance).

7. What is the difference between loading dose and maintenance dose, and how is this affected by liver and renal disease?

Loading dose refers to the dose of drug that is given at the start of a treatment course. Loading dose is calculated using the formula shown in Eq. 23.6:

$$\text{Loading dose} = \text{target plasma concentration} \times V_D/F \tag{23.6}$$

where V_D is the volume of distribution and F is the bioavailability of the drug.

Maintenance dose refers to the amount of drug required to keep a steady-state concentration within the body after administration of a loading dose. Conceptually, it is the required amount of drug required to replace the amount that is cleared. It is calculated using the formula shown in Eq. 23.7:

$$\text{Maintenance dose} = \text{target plasma concentration} \times Cl/F \tag{23.7}$$

where Cl is the clearance of the drug.

You will notice that loading dose takes V_D into account, while maintenance dose takes clearance into account. Because clearance is altered in renal and liver disease, the maintenance dose must be decreased in these patients, but the loading dose is unaffected.

8. What is therapeutic index?

Therapeutic index is used as a tool to measure the safety and efficacy of a drug. Therapeutic index is calculated using the formula shown in Eq. 23.8:

$$\text{Therapeutic index} = \text{Median lethal dose}/\text{Median effective dose} \tag{23.8}$$

The higher the therapeutic index, the safer is the drug. Beta-blockers, calcium channel blockers (CCBs), and diazepam are examples of drugs with large therapeutic indices, which may account for why they are so widely used (although still very dangerous in large overdose). Drugs with low therapeutic indices include phenobarbital, theophylline, digoxin, and warfarin. These drugs must therefore be monitored closely in patients who receive them.

9. What are the differences between competitive and noncompetitive inhibitors?

Competitive inhibitors bind to the same active site of an enzyme as the substrate of interest. In competitive inhibition, the enzyme is bound to either the substrate or the inhibitor at any given point. This is because the inhibitor closely resembles the substrate. Competitive inhibition can be overcome by overwhelming the system with increasing concentrations of substrate, which compete with the inhibitor for the active site of the catalytic enzyme. In contrast, *noncompetitive inhibitors* bind to alternate sites of the enzyme rather than the active site. They do not resemble the substrate, but binding of the noncompetitive inhibitor to the enzyme of interest distorts the enzyme such that it can no longer bind to the substrate. Noncompetitive inhibition is often irreversible and cannot be overcome by saturating the system with increasing concentrations of substrate.

10. What is a partial agonist?

Partial agonists are a curious phenomenon in pharmacology. As their name implies, they can bind to the active site of an enzyme but do so with less efficacy than a full agonist. As such, they can achieve only a fraction of the enzyme's maximal effect (V_{max}) when compared with the full agonist. Thus partial agonists decrease the enzyme's *efficacy*. If the full agonist is present, partial agonists actually act as a *competitive inhibitor* for the enzyme by preventing the full agonist from binding to the active site. This concept is often tested in the context of opioids and opioid withdrawal with exposure to certain drugs, such as buprenorphine and butorphanol. Buprenorphine and butorphanol are both μ-receptor *partial agonists*. Butorphanol is a powerful analgesic and also a κ-receptor agonist, which gives it less abuse potential. Buprenorphine is often used in combination with naloxone as a treatment for opioid use disorder and opioid withdrawal. Because of their partial agonist properties, if either drug is also taken while a full agonist is still present in their system (such as heroin), it will behave as a competitive inhibitor and can precipitate withdrawal.

SECRETS FOR UNDERSTANDING MAXIMAL EFFECT AND SUBSTRATE CONCENTRATION FOR THE USMLE STEP 1

It is common for inhibition principles to be tested on Step 1 in the context of their effects on the pharmacologic concepts of V_{max} and substrate concentration (K_m). These concepts are somewhat abstract and can sometimes appear daunting. However, the following simplified approach should provide a solid framework to approach such questions.

An enzyme's "velocity" refers to the rate at which the enzyme catalyzes a given reaction. *Maximum velocity*, or V_{max}, refers to the maximum rate achieved by the enzyme at infinite (i.e., saturating) K_m. Assuming that all enzymes are functioning at maximal capacity, V_{max} is directly dependent on the number of active enzymes available to do work.

Let's use the analogy of a sweater factory: If the factory has an unlimited amount of wool and all factory workers are knitting at maximal speed, the factory is operating at V_{max}. The only way to increase the V_{max} of the factory at this point would be to add more employees to the staff. If employee numbers were doubled and each was capable of working at maximal speed, the V_{max} of the factory would also double. As such, increasing the number of available enzymes (i.e., "enzyme concentration") should increase the V_{max}, whereas decreasing the number of available enzymes should have the opposite effect.

As previously mentioned, irreversible enzyme inhibitors (competitive irreversible and noncompetitive inhibitors) will take enzymes out of commission and thus lower the V_{max} of a reaction. Because of their effects as antagonists in the presence of a full agonist, *partial agonists* can also lower an enzyme's V_{max} in certain circumstances. However, Step 1 questions are usually not explicit in their wording. They may, for instance, describe a drug that "increases the gene transcription" of a particular enzyme. This is, in fact, synonymous with saying that the drug increases the enzyme concentration, and thus such a drug will increase the enzyme's V_{max}. It is also important to note that an enzyme's "efficacy" describes the magnitude of its V_{max}.

Another important principle to understand is that of K_m. K_m is the substrate concentration at half of the V_{max}. Let us go back to our sweater factory analogy to make sense of this. If the V_{max} of the factory were 100 sweaters per day, then K_m would be equal to the amount of wool required to make 50 sweaters per day. A high K_m indicates a low affinity of an enzyme for its substrate because a great deal of substrate must be provided to produce a decent amount of product from the enzyme. For example, if the K_m for our sweater factory were high, it would require a great deal of wool to make only 50 sweaters. Conversely, if the K_m were low, it would indicate that the factory can make quick and efficient use of its materials. Thus low K_m indicates *high* affinity between enzyme and substrate. It is important to note that in terms of enzymes and pharmacodynamics, the term *potency* is synonymous with *affinity*.

Increasing or decreasing the number of available enzymes is really the only way to affect V_{max}. What factors affect K_m? Because K_m is a measure of an enzyme's affinity for its substrate, it will be affected by anything that alters the interaction between the enzyme and substrate. K_m is affected by changes in the enzyme's *active site* and therefore would be affected by *reversible* competitive inhibitors, but *not* by noncompetitive inhibitors, because these do not bind to the enzyme's active site. Likewise, K_m is not affected by *irreversible* competitive inhibitors because they take the enzyme completely out of commission (preventing further binding of the enzyme with substrate).

CASE 23.1

A 2-year-old girl is evaluated for a 2-day history of fever, vomiting, and diarrhea. Since being administered over-the-counter medications this morning, she has become increasingly sleepy. Examination is significant for fever, tachycardia, tachypnea, hypotension, somnolence, and decorticate posturing. Urgent workup reveals normal electrolytes, normal head computed tomography scan, stool positive for rotavirus antigen, and markedly elevated liver enzymes.

1. Given the preceding clinical picture, what is the most likely explanation for this patient's presentation?

   This patient appears to have started out with a viral gastroenteritis that was then compounded with an over-the-counter medication, which is now causing confusion, somnolence, and fulminant hepatitis. Given this presentation, the most likely culprit is acetylsalicylic acid (aspirin) exposure, which led to Reye syndrome (fulminant hepatic failure and encephalopathy). In children, aspirin can inhibit mitochondrial enzymes and decrease fatty acid beta oxidation, leading to fatty change of the liver and cerebral edema. Aspirin is a nonsteroidal antiinflammatory drug (NSAID) that is contraindicated in children for this exact reason. To treat this patient, one needs to alkalinize the urine (bicarbonate is commonly used) to facilitate aspirin excretion from the body. Consider the pharmacologic principles by which this process occurs: Ionized species can be trapped in urine and eventually excreted, but neutral substances are reabsorbed into the bloodstream (review Basic Concepts, question 3). Aspirin is a weak acid and is thus ionized in an alkaline environment from $RCOOH \rightleftharpoons RCOO^- + H^+$. This ionized form is then excreted in the urine.

2. What are the pharmacotherapeutic actions of aspirin and other NSAIDs?

   Aspirin and other NSAIDs have antiinflammatory, antipyretic, and analgesic actions. Because of its potency as an antiinflammatory agent, aspirin is the NSAID to which all other NSAIDs are typically compared. These other NSAIDs include ibuprofen, indomethacin (drug of choice for a gout flare or for closing a patent ductus arteriosus), ketorolac, and naproxen.

3. What is the mechanism of action of NSAIDs?

   Injurious stimuli induce involved cells to release arachidonic acid. The two general pathways by which arachidonic acid is broken down in the body are referred to as the *cyclooxygenase (COX) pathway* and the *lipoxygenase (LOX) pathway*. The COX pathway eventually produces prostaglandins (PGs), while the LOX pathway produces leukotrienes (Fig. 23.1). NSAIDs play a role in inhibiting the COX pathway, thus reducing PG production. PGs are a group of hormone-like lipid compounds. They are proinflammatory, heighten sensitivity to painful stimuli, and alter hypothalamic temperature homeostasis, promoting fever. Aspirin is notable for being an *irreversible* COX-1 and COX-2 inhibitor—it covalently acetylates the COX enzyme, which renders it permanently inactive. Most other NSAIDs are reversible.

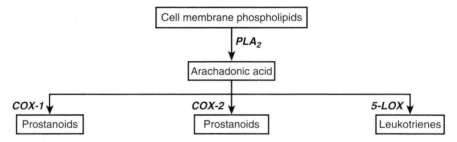

Figure 23.1. Nonsteroidal antiinflammatory drug mechanisms of action. *COX*, Cyclooxygenase; *LOX*, lipoxygenase; *PLA₂*, phospholipase A₂.

4. What are some negative side effects of NSAIDs, and what alternative medications exist that circumvent these side effects?

   The COX pathway is run by one of two isozymes, depending on where in the body the reaction is occurring. COX-1 is the isozyme involved almost anywhere in the body, whereas COX-2 is typically active at the site of inflammation. Ideally, selective inhibition of the latter would achieve the goal of decreasing inflammation. NSAIDs in general are not selective for COX-2 and thus cause effects in other tissues as well. These other sites include platelets (where inhibition of thromboxane A_2 leads to inability of these cells to aggregate into a clot) and gastric mucosa (where reduction of PGs PGE_2, PGF_2, and PGI_2 compromises the protective lining of the stomach and increases acid secretion, thus predisposing to ulcers). Long-term NSAID use can also lead to kidney disease, namely, acute renal failure and interstitial nephritis. Selective COX-2 inhibitors (e.g., celecoxib) do exist that purportedly have less renal and gastric mucosal toxicity. However, by diverting arachidonic acid metabolism solely through COX-1, more thromboxane A_2 is produced, which could potentially lead to increased platelet aggregation/thrombosis and increased risk for stroke and myocardial infarction. (Rofecoxib was a COX-2 inhibitor that was taken off the market as a result of these effects.) Alternatively, acetaminophen may be given to patients with coagulopathy or history of gastric ulcers.

STEP 1 SECRET

Aspirin toxicity is also notable for causing tinnitus and respiratory alkalosis with superimposed metabolic acidosis, which is fairly unique among toxidromes. The mechanism of these processes is high yield for Step 1. The respiratory alkalosis occurs first because salicylates stimulate the respiratory centers of the brain, leading to hyperventilation and decreased partial pressure of carbon dioxide (Pco_2). Aspirin also uncouples oxidative phosphorylation in the mitochondria, eventually causing accumulation of lactic acid and ketoacids, leading to a metabolic acidosis. Be on the lookout for decreased pressure of carbon dioxide, arterial ($Paco_2$) and decreased HCO_3^- with either elevated, decreased, or even normal pH in a patient with aspirin toxicity.

5. **If given the choice of aspirin or acetaminophen, which would you administer to a child with a fever?**
Aspirin given to a child during a viral infection can lead to Reye syndrome, which can be fatal. To avoid this possibility, always pick acetaminophen over aspirin for children. The exception to this rule is Kawasaki disease. Children with this condition should be treated with high-dose aspirin to prevent coronary artery thrombosis. The coronary artery aneurysms in Kawasaki disease predispose to clot formation, so it is critical to prevent platelet aggregation in these patients. On a side note, aspirin does not affect the risk for development of coronary artery aneurysms; only the intravenous immunoglobulin dose plays a role in that aspect.

SUMMARY BOX: NONSTEROIDAL ANTIINFLAMMATORY DRUGS AND REYE SYNDROME

- Indications: Reduces pain, fever, and inflammation
- Mechanism of action: Inhibition of the cyclooxygenase pathway, thus reducing prostaglandin production
- Side effects: Gastric ulceration, bleeding problems, acute renal failure, and interstitial nephritis (long-term use)
- Toxicity: Tinnitus and mixed respiratory alkalosis-metabolic acidosis
- Contraindications: Children (can lead to Reye syndrome)
  - Exceptions: Should be used in children with Kawasaki disease
- Antidote: Sodium bicarbonate to alkalinize the urine

CASE 23.2

A 14-year-old obtunded boy is brought to the emergency department by his friends, who subsequently leave without providing a history. Vital signs reveal a heart rate of 45 beats/min, respiratory rate of 8 breaths/min, and oxygen saturation of 90% on room air. Examination is significant for pinpoint pupils. There is no sign of trauma. He does not smell of alcohol, no needle track marks are evident, and there is no indication of an irritated or perforated nasal septum. The patient has several chewed-up pieces of plastic that resemble pharmacologic dermal patches in his possession.

---

1. **From the preceding information, what is the likely cause of this patient's presentation?**
The patient is intoxicated on a substance that is depressing both his mental status and cardiorespiratory status, as well as inducing pinpoint pupils. The substance was probably introduced into his bloodstream sublingually, considering the chewed-up dermal patches that were recovered. Given this presentation, the culprit is likely to be an opioid that is available in a transdermal form (e.g., fentanyl).

2. **What is the mechanism of action of opioids?**
There are four types of opioid receptors: μ, κ, σ, and δ. The μ receptors, in particular, are concentrated in central and peripheral pain pathways and account for the analgesic effects of opioids. The μ receptor is coupled to a G_i protein, which causes a decrease in cyclic adenosine monophosphate (cAMP) levels and leads to cell hyperpolarization. This, in turn, makes it difficult for the cell to reach its firing threshold. As a result, release of neurotransmitters associated with the perception of pain (e.g., substance P, norepinephrine [NE], acetylcholine, glutamate, and serotonin) is hindered, and the painful stimulus is not conducted through the nervous system.
   In addition to their analgesic effects, opioids also have anxiolytic effects. It is this ability to relieve anxiety and induce a state of euphoria that has led to the illicit use of opioids. Among the family of opioids, heroin ranks toward the top in terms of being able to cross the blood-brain barrier, possibly explaining its use as an illicit agent.

3. **List a few members of the opioid family.**
Morphine, fentanyl (often delivered through a transdermal patch), codeine, loperamide, meperidine, and methadone are some examples of opioids. Unlike other opioids, meperidine has antimuscarinic effects and does not cause miosis or gastrointestinal upset; however, it can cause tachycardia. Dextromethorphan is an opioid found in some cough syrups. The classic case of opioid abuse to be aware of for Step 1 is a teenager binging on cough syrup.

4. **What are some signs/symptoms of opioid intoxication? Is it life-threatening?**
See Table 23.1. Because opioids decrease release of NE, among other neurotransmitters, there is a shift toward a parasympathetic state, which induces pupillary constriction (miosis). Opioids also cause constipation and abdominal discomfort by acting on μ receptors in intestinal smooth muscle and decreasing peristalsis.

Table 23.1. Opioid Intoxication

STRUCTURE/SYSTEM AFFECTED	MANIFESTATIONS
Eyes	Miosis ("pinpoint pupils") caused by stimulation of the parasympathetic outflow to the eye
Central nervous system	Confusion, obtundation, euphoria
Lungs	Central respiratory depression resulting in hypercapnic respiratory failure, which can be life-threatening
Gastrointestinal	Constipation, spasm of sphincter of Oddi

5. How does opioid tolerance occur?

Unlike persistent use of many other drugs, persistent use of opioids does not alter the μ receptor itself. Instead, the frequent stimulation of G_i receptors and decreased cAMP production eventually cause the cell to upregulate other G proteins to increase cAMP. This negates the effects of the drug and produces a tolerant state. Because of this tolerance, greater quantities of the drug are needed to produce the desired effect, which can lead to overdose. *It is enormously high yield to know that tolerance does not affect symptoms of miosis and constipation.* Opioid overdose is the most common cause of overdose death in the United States, and this is also a high-yield fact for Step 1!

6. How can an opioid overdose be reversed?

Because opioid intoxication is life-threatening, cases of overdose need to be rapidly treated. To this end, naloxone is a competitive antagonist that quickly (in seconds to minutes) displaces opioids already bound to receptors. Note that the administration of naloxone may precipitate immediate withdrawal in opiate-dependent patients.

7. What is the difference between naloxone and naltrexone?

Naltrexone has a longer duration of action and is therefore better suited for long-term management of opioid dependence (rather than acute cases of intoxication, for which naloxone would be a better option). Because the euphoria associated with alcohol dependence is also related to stimulation of opioid receptors, naltrexone can be used to manage alcohol dependence as well.

8. What role can methadone play in treating opioid dependence?

Methadone is a long-acting opioid used for detoxification and maintenance therapy for opioid addiction. However, methadone does not cause the euphoric symptoms that drew the patient to opioids initially. The patient is then weaned off methadone slowly. Because the withdrawal symptoms of methadone are not as severe and take longer to develop compared with other opioids, the process is more tolerable.

9. What are signs/symptoms of opioid withdrawal?

Because opioids cause decreased release of NE (among other neurotransmitters), the body compensates by increasing the number of available α- and β-adrenergic receptors. Removal of the drug will cause a sudden increase in NE, which can bind to the excess α and β receptors and induce a massive sympathetic response, including sweating, fever, and nausea. Pupillary dilation is an important symptom of opioid withdrawal (remember that opioid intoxication causes *pinpoint pupils*). Piloerection (e.g., hair standing up on arms), abdominal pain, diarrhea, yawning, and lacrimation can all occur. Note that opioid withdrawal is *not* life-threatening.

SUMMARY BOX: OPIOIDS

- Indications: Pain control
- Mechanism of action: Bind μ receptors on neurons, hyperpolarizing the cell and decreasing pain conduction
- Toxicity: Miosis, constipation, obtundation, euphoria, respiratory depression
  - Miosis and constipation do *not* diminish with tolerance
- Antidote
  - Acute opioid intoxication is reversed with naloxone
  - Opioid dependence can be treated with naltrexone, methadone, or buprenorphine

---

CASE 23.3

A 22-year-old man with no prior medical history is brought to the emergency department after he had a seizure on the floor of his office an hour ago. His coworkers describe him as a very energetic individual who regularly forgoes sleep to excel at his job. He is not taking any medications, and there is no recent history of head trauma. Examination reveals a diaphoretic and confused young man with a heart rate of 140 beats/min, dilated but reactive pupils, and an eroded nasal septum. No focal neurologic deficits or needle-track marks can be appreciated.

---

1. Given this clinical picture, what is the most likely explanation for this patient's presentation?

This young man was brought in because of a recent seizure. His tachycardia, hyperthermia, dilated pupils (mydriasis), and perforated nasal septum suggest cocaine intoxication, likely through the intranasal route.

2. What is the mechanism of action of cocaine?

Cocaine acts both centrally and peripherally to block the reuptake of NE, serotonin, and dopamine. When this occurs centrally, the result is an increase in mental awareness, hallucinations, delusions, and paranoia. At high-enough doses, tremors, convulsions, and even sudden cardiac death can result from these effects. When reuptake of these neurotransmitters is blocked peripherally, sympathomimetic effects (tachycardia, hypertension [HTN], and pupillary dilation) can occur as a result.

3. The net effects of cocaine on the body can mimic those of which other illicit drug?

It should be apparent that cocaine is a stimulant, similar to amphetamines.

4. **What is the explanation for development of tolerance to cocaine use?**
   The euphoric effects of cocaine are due to prolongation of dopaminergic effects. Over the long term, however, dopamine levels become depleted, and the person craves more cocaine to achieve the same degree of euphoria (this phenomenon is called *tolerance*). Put another way, dopamine levels become depleted, but the threshold at which dopamine causes euphoria remains the same. To reach that same threshold, more cocaine is needed to elicit dopamine release.

5. **Aside from tolerance and dependence, what are some other adverse effects of cocaine?**
   Cocaine can cause cardiac arrhythmias and seizures. Tactile hallucinations can be managed with antipsychotics, such as haloperidol. As with use of other stimulants, cocaine use is followed by post-use "crash" in which the person is physically and emotionally depressed. Cocaine can also lead to coronary vasoconstriction and subsequent nonatherosclerotic myocardial infarction. Beware giving beta-blockers on a test question to an individual with cocaine still within their system, because this can theoretically trigger unopposed α-adrenergic stimulation and worsen vasoconstriction (this frequently tested concept of unopposed α stimulation is the same reason to avoid beta blockers in pheochromocytomas until α-blockade has been established). However, mixed alpha-/beta-blockers (e.g., labetalol, carvedilol) may be considered.

AMPHETAMINES

6. **How does the mechanism of action of amphetamines differ from that of cocaine?**
   As mentioned earlier, amphetamines are stimulants, similar to cocaine. Unlike cocaine, which inhibits reuptake of neurotransmitters, amphetamines induce release of catecholamines. Think of the two drugs as being analogous to filling a kitchen sink; the amount of water in the sink (i.e., the amount of the neurotransmitter in the synaptic cleft) can be increased in one of two ways: the drain can be plugged (similar to what cocaine does), or the faucet can be turned on high (what amphetamines do).

   When amphetamines act centrally, the result is a release of dopamine. Dopamine increases mental awareness, while decreasing fatigue, appetite, and the need for sleep. Because of these effects, amphetamines can be used therapeutically to treat depression, an abnormally high appetite, and narcolepsy. Paradoxically, they can also be used to treat attention-deficit/hyperactivity disorder [ADHD] in children. When amphetamines act peripherally, the result is a release of NE that causes tachycardia, HTN, and pupillary dilation.

7. **What are some adverse effects of amphetamines?**
   Through their effects on the central nervous system (CNS), amphetamines can cause insomnia, irritability, tremor, and panic. Long-term use can lead to development of psychosis (i.e., hallucinations, delusions, loose thought process) that resembles schizophrenia.

   Through their peripheral effects, amphetamines can cause cardiac arrhythmias, HTN, headache, diaphoresis, anorexia, and diarrhea.

LYSERGIC ACID DIETHYLAMIDE

8. **What is the mechanism of action of lysergic acid diethylamide and its effects on the body?**
   Lysergic acid diethylamide (LSD) is a serotonin agonist. It stimulates the sympathetic nervous system and causes tachycardia, HTN, pupillary dilation, and other similar effects. It also causes *visual* hallucinations of bright colors (in contrast with opioids, for which *tactile* hallucinations predominate). These hallucinations can be treated with antipsychotics (e.g., haloperidol), while agitation is treated with benzodiazepines.

PHENCYCLIDINE

9. **What is the mechanism of action of phencyclidine and its resultant effects on the body?**
   Phencyclidine (PCP) is an *N*-methyl-D-aspartate (NMDA) antagonist. The result is a feeling of numbness, staggering gait, slurred speech, rigidity, and *hostile* behavior. Due to the proclivity for violent behavior during PCP intoxication, the most common cause of death in a PCP user is *trauma* (a high-yield Step 1 fact). A key sign of PCP use is nystagmus. If a board question mentions nystagmus and illicit drug use is implied, PCP is most likely the causative agent. PCP intoxication is treated with benzodiazepines and antipsychotics.

   PCP derivatives have some clinical value. An example is ketamine, which is used to produce anesthesia without loss of consciousness. A major side effect of ketamine is hallucinations and bad dreams (after all, it is still a PCP derivative).

TETRAHYDROCANNABINOL

10. **What is the mechanism of action of tetrahydrocannabinol and its resultant effects on the body?**
    Tetrahydrocannabinol (THC) is an ingredient in marijuana. Although its exact mechanism of action is unknown, its effects are mediated by binding to cannabinoid receptors in the brain. This causes a feeling of euphoria, drowsiness, xerostomia, visual hallucinations, impaired judgment, and increase in appetite. *Conjunctival injection* is a key buzzword that examiners like to use to describe the red eyes seen with THC intoxication. Because THC is stored in the body's adipose tissue, it can sometimes be detectable in a blood test up to 30 days after use. Urine tests can detect THC about 4 to 10 days after its use.

SUMMARY BOX: COCAINE, AMPHETAMINES, AND OTHER ILLICIT DRUGS

Drugs of Abuse

- Cocaine: Blocks catecholamine reuptake, leading to increased mental awareness, hallucinations, delusions, paranoia, tremors, convulsions, and risk of death (myocardial infarction or cardiac dysrhythmia).
- Amphetamines: Has effects similar to cocaine but induce *release* of catecholamines rather than blocking catecholamine reuptake.
- Phencyclidine (PCP): Causes numbness, ataxia, slurred speech, belligerence, and nystagmus (key sign). Trauma is the most common cause of death after PCP use.
- Tetrahydrocannabinol (THC): Induces euphoria, drowsiness, xerostomia, visual hallucinations, and increased appetite. Conjunctival injection is a distinct feature of THC intoxication.

CASE 23.4

A 26-year-old woman with an unremarkable medical history is evaluated for a several-hour history of confusion, dizziness, blurred vision, dyspnea, and nausea/vomiting. These symptoms started this morning after she drank herbal tea that was prepared using leaves from a foxglove plant. Examination is significant for an irregular heart rate of 52 beats/min, confusion, and normally reactive pupils. An electrocardiogram (ECG) shows what is termed *paroxysmal atrial tachycardia* with a 2:1 atrioventricular (AV) heart block. Blood work shows a moderately elevated potassium (K) level of 5.7 mEq/L.

1. Based on this presentation, what is the likely culprit?

   Digitalis is the likely culprit. This patient became acutely symptomatic after ingesting extracts from a foxglove plant. A reader who is familiar with the pharmaceutical uses of this plant can quickly infer that this is a case of digitalis toxicity. Even if the reader is unfamiliar with this use, physical examination of this patient nonetheless points to cardiac manifestations (bradyarrhythmia, heart block) and hyperkalemia, both of which suggest digitalis toxicity.

   Digitalis belongs to a class of drugs called *cardiac glycosides*. Included in this group are digitoxin and digoxin. In terms of their action, glycosides are considered inotropes, which are drugs that increase cardiac contractility by increasing intracellular calcium.

2. What is the mechanism of action of digitalis?

   Cardiomyocytes have sodium/potassium-adenosine triphosphatase (Na/K-ATPase) pumps embedded in their membranes that transport sodium out of the cell in exchange for K into the cell. Digitalis inhibits this pump by binding to the K-binding site. As a result, the amount of intracellular sodium accumulates, and this indirectly inhibits the sodium-calcium exchanger in the cell membrane that transports sodium into the cell in exchange for calcium out of the cell. The increase in intracellular calcium means that calcium influx during depolarization of the cell no longer has to be very significant to trigger calcium release from the sarcoplasmic reticulum (i.e., calcium-induced calcium release is "easier" to achieve). Because of the phenomenon of excitation-contraction coupling in cardiomyocytes, the hyperexcitable cell is now able to contract more readily and, together with other similar cells, return the ejection fraction of the heart toward normal. With increased output, sympathetic stimulation to the heart and peripheral vasculature begins to taper, heart rate slows, and peripheral resistance decreases.

3. What are the clinical indications for using glycosides?

   Glycosides increase the force of contraction (+ inotropic effect) and are therefore well suited for treatment of heart failure. They also slow conduction velocity through the atrioventricular (AV) node (negative chronotropic effect) by increasing vagal tone and are therefore used to treat supraventricular tachycardias, such as atrial fibrillation, atrial flutter, and atrial tachycardia.

4. What are some adverse effects of glycosides?

   Because glycosides have an affinity for extravascular proteins, they tend to get widely distributed in the body and are thus difficult to dose (especially when coadministered with other medications). For this reason, cases of glycoside toxicity are not uncommon. The typical symptoms of glycoside toxicity are nausea, vomiting, confusion, and visual disturbances with *blurry yellow "halos."* Remember that cardiac glycosides can decrease AV node conduction as a treatment for supraventricular arrhythmias; as such, toxicity can cause AV block, which can lead to "escape beats" with potential for subsequent ventricular fibrillation and death. Because of this AV block, it should make sense that ECGs during cardiac glycoside toxicity can show *prolonged PR intervals*. ECGs can also show "scooped-out" ST segments, which is a sign of digoxin usage, but not necessarily toxicity (it is present at therapeutic ranges as well).

   Recall that digitalis prevents the cell from exporting Na and importing K (i.e., it blocks the Na/K-ATPase pump). The repercussion of having increased intracellular Na has been described earlier, because it directly results in the therapeutic use of this medication.

   The consequence of having elevated serum K is that it can lead to arrhythmias and even complete heart block. Note that hypokalemia is an additional risk factor for cardiac glycoside toxicity because the K-binding site on the Na/K-ATPase has an increased chance of being vacant, allowing glycosides to bind the pump more readily. Many patients with congestive heart failure are typically prescribed thiazide or loop diuretics in addition to digitalis. These drugs can predispose to a hypokalemic state, thus increasing the risk for digitalis toxicity.

5. **What is the treatment for digitalis toxicity?**
Digitalis toxicity is treated with antidigoxin Fab fragments, which bind circulating digitalis molecules and render them inactive. Magnesium is also given to patients with digitalis toxicity to prevent arrhythmias. Finally, as mentioned earlier, it is critical to normalize the elevated serum K level. Drugs used for this purpose include loop diuretics, insulin (recall that insulin increases the activity of the Na/K-ATPase), and ion exchange resins such as sodium zirconium cyclosilicate. Hemodialysis can also be used to normalize serum potassium levels.

SUMMARY BOX: GLYCOSIDES AND DIGITALIS TOXICITY

- Indications: Heart failure, tachyarrhythmias (especially atrial fibrillation)
- Mechanism of action: Increases intracellular calcium indirectly by inhibiting the Na/K-ATPase pump. Increased intracellular calcium leads to increased cardiac contractility.
- Toxicity: Nausea, vomiting, confusion, "blurry yellow vision," hyperkalemia, arrhythmias, heart block
- Antidotes: Antidigoxin Fab fragments to neutralize the drug particles; magnesium to prevent arrhythmias; and loop diuretics, insulin, ion exchange resins, or hemodialysis to normalize elevated serum K levels

CASE 23.5

A 58-year-old man is brought to the emergency department with reports of headache, dizziness, drowsiness, excessive fatigue, and two episodes of fainting. These symptoms started 2 days ago. He denies recent trauma or dehydration. He has no history of neurologic deficits or metabolic anomalies. His medical history is notable for congestive heart failure, which has been well controlled and without issues for the past 3 years. He also has a history of hypertension (HTN), which persists despite being on beta-blockers. He was seen 4 days ago by his primary care physician, who prescribed verapamil in addition to his beta-blocker. He is not taking any other medication. The patient has no allergies. The review of systems is otherwise negative. Physical examination is notable for a heart rate of 44 beats/min and a blood pressure of 110/70 mm Hg.

1. **What is likely causing this patient's symptoms?**
This patient, who has a history of chronic HTN, is being forced to function at a much lower perfusion pressure and evidently is unable to do so. Because beta-blockers alone were not sufficient in controlling his HTN, his regimen was supplemented with verapamil (a CCB), which is the likely cause of his bradycardia, relative hypotension, and other symptoms. A different CCB would have been a better choice in this case (see following questions).

2. **What is the mechanism of action of CCBs?**
The concentration of intracellular calcium is important when considering any excitable cell in the body. In muscle cells specifically, there is a concept of calcium-induced calcium release. CCBs block the voltage-dependent L-type calcium channel (the one in the cell membrane, *not* the one associated with the sarcoplasmic reticulum). By decreasing the initial influx of calcium into the cell, the likelihood of a massive release of calcium from the sarcoplasmic reticulum is also decreased. The net effect of this phenomenon is interference with the excitation-contraction couplet that is typical of myocytes and resultant relaxation of these cells. In the heart, this effect translates into lower cardiac output. Peripherally, calcium channel blockade results in decreased vascular resistance.

Clinical Pearl

An important use of calcium channel blockers (CCBs), specifically nimodipine, is prevention of cerebral vasospasm after subarachnoid hemorrhage. This may be tested on Step 1.

---

3. **What are the different types of CCB?**
CCBs are divided into three different classes based on chemical properties. The names of these classes are less important than the members themselves. The three members that are important to know are verapamil, diltiazem, and nifedipine. Aside from their different classes, a feature that directly influences their eventual clinical application is their site of action.

Verapamil is a nondihydropyridine CCB that predominantly exerts its effects at the level of the heart. The effects of verapamil on the heart include dilation of the coronary arteries and decrease in contractility. It also slows the heart by suppressing conduction through the sinoatrial (SA) and AV nodes. Peripherally, it causes dilation of the arteries, with a resultant decline in BP. Clinically, verapamil is used to treat/prevent angina, arrhythmias, and HTN. Its use should be avoided in those with a history of congestive heart failure because it not only slows the rate of contraction but also decreases contractility, thus exacerbating failure. Moreover, its combined use with beta-blockers should be avoided because this can lead to profound bradycardia and hypotension.

Nifedipine and other dihydropyridines (CCBs ending in "-dipine") are much more influential at the level of peripheral vasculature than at the heart. Nifedipine can decrease BP but causes reflex tachycardia by stimulating the baroreceptor reflex as well. For this reason, it would have been the most ideal CCB for this patient because it would have supplemented the beta-blocker in decreasing BP without suppressing the heart's compensatory response.

Diltiazem is the other nondihydropyridine CCB that does not decrease contractility to the same extent as is typical with verapamil. Peripherally, it decreases BP by inducing vasodilation of the arteries. Its clinical indications are more or less the same as those for verapamil, although its side effect profile is relatively more benign. Think of diltiazem as a "happy medium" between the cardiac-predominant effects of verapamil and the peripheral vasculature-predominant effects of nifedipine and other dihydropyridines.

Table 23.2 reviews the major subtypes of CCB.

Table 23.2. Calcium Channel Blockers

AGENT	SITE OF ACTION	EFFECT	CLINICAL INDICATION(S)
Verapamil	Heart/vasculature	Dilates coronary arteries, decreases cardiac contractility, suppresses SA/AV nodes Causes peripheral vasodilation without reflex tachycardia (because of its negative chronotropic/inotropic effects on the heart)	Vasospastic (Prinzmetal) angina Obstructive (exertional) angina Arrhythmias (especially supraventricular tachyarrhythmias) Hypertension
Diltiazem	Vasculature > heart	Dilates coronary arteries, suppresses SA/AV nodes Causes peripheral vasodilation without reflex tachycardia (because of its suppression of SA/AV nodes)	Vasospastic (Prinzmetal) angina Obstructive (exertional) angina Arrhythmias (especially supraventricular tachyarrhythmias) Hypertension
Nifedipine	Vasculature	Dilates coronary arteries Causes peripheral vasodilation with reflex tachycardia (no chronotropic/inotropic effects on the heart)	Vasospastic (Prinzmetal) angina Not useful in obstructive (exertional) angina because reflex tachycardia increases oxygen demand Ideal for hypertension with bradycardia because it causes a reflex tachycardia

AV, Atrioventricular; *SA,* sinoatrial.

4. **What are some general side effects of CCBs?**
   Although CCBs are fairly selective for cardiomyocytes and vascular smooth muscle, they do have limited activity at gastrointestinal smooth muscle, which usually manifests as constipation. Their vascular effects in the brain can cause headaches. Excessive hypotension may manifest as generalized fatigue or lead to reflex tachycardia. Peripheral edema and flushing, which are caused by peripheral vasodilation, are commonly tested side effects. Gingival hyperplasia and peripheral edema are also important side effects of CCBs.

SUMMARY BOX: CALCIUM CHANNEL BLOCKERS

- Indications: Antihypertensive, heart rate control, antiarrhythmic, prevention of cerebral vasospasm in subarachnoid hemorrhage
- Mechanism of action: Block the L-type calcium channel, thus decreasing the initial influx of calcium into the cell and reducing both cardiac contractility and peripheral vascular resistance
- Side effects: Peripheral edema, flushing, and gingival hyperplasia
- Toxicity: Profound bradycardia and hypotension (especially with verapamil and diltiazem)

CASE 23.6

An otherwise healthy 35-year-old man is brought to the emergency department by his coworker, who found him to be excessively drowsy and slurring his speech when he showed up to work this morning. The friend mentions that the patient's medical history is notable for anxiety and insomnia, for which he was recently prescribed "some medication." There is no history of trauma, neurologic or metabolic anomalies, or alcohol/drug abuse. On physical examination, the patient has a heart rate of 55 beats/min, blood pressure of 120/70 mm Hg, respiratory rate (RR) of 9 breaths/min, and temperature of 37°C. The remainder of the examination is unremarkable.

1. **Given the preceding presentation, which types of item are at the top of the differential diagnosis and would be worth exploring?**
   This patient presents in a generally depressed cognitive state, and his vital signs are similarly somewhat diminished. The process appears to be acute in onset, but there is no history of trauma, and the patient is afebrile. This history immediately moves injuries, infections, and chronic processes down the differential list and shifts other items, such as alcohol intoxication, hypoglycemia, and medication involvement, up the list. History also reveals that he was recently started on pharmacologic therapy for his anxiety and insomnia. Medications typically used for this purpose tend to be general depressants (e.g., alprazolam, zolpidem) that, if misused, could precipitate a presentation similar to this one. This patient should have his blood glucose checked, as well as his serum levels of alcohol and other depressants (e.g., barbiturates and benzodiazepines).

2. **What is the mechanism of action of benzodiazepines?**
   Benzodiazepines bind sites on the cell membrane that are adjacent to but separate from γ-aminobutyric acid (GABA) receptors. Their presence enhances the affinity that GABA A ($GABA_A$) receptors have for their ligand, GABA. (Recall that increased affinity between receptor and substrate leads to a decreased K_m value—benzodiazepines are a commonly used example of this pharmacodynamic principle!) This translates into a higher frequency of GABA–$GABA_A$ receptor interaction and, therefore, *more frequent* opening of chloride channels in the cell membrane. The chloride influx hyperpolarizes the cell, making it "more difficult" to reach the firing threshold. The end effect is that benzodiazepines enhance the actions of a major inhibitory neurotransmitter in the CNS—namely, GABA—and bring about depressive effects overall.

   Notably, benzodiazepines themselves do not cause the chloride channel to open—this can be done only if GABA is already present and bound to the $GABA_A$ receptor. Benzodiazepines facilitate this process, but their effects are limited by the amount of GABA that is released. Because there is a finite supply of GABA in the body, the effects of benzodiazepines usually plateau before life-threatening respiratory depression, coma, or death ensues. This is not to say that respiratory depression does not occur with benzodiazepines, but it is less likely when compared with drugs such as barbiturates or ethanol. As such, benzodiazepines are considered to be "safer" drugs.

   The sedative effects of benzodiazepines are additive with other CNS depressants, so they can have dangerous effects if taken with alcohol, barbiturates, first-generation antihistamines, or other depressants.

STEP 1 SECRET

It is important to note that benzodiazepines increase the affinity of the γ-aminobutyric acid A ($GABA_A$) receptor. Activation of the $GABA_B$ receptor causes opening of a nearby potassium (not chloride) channel, leading to K^+ efflux and cellular hyperpolarization. Baclofen (an antispasmodic) is a notable example of a drug that binds the $GABA_B$ receptor.

3. **What are a few clinical indications for using benzodiazepines?**
   See Table 23.3.

Table 23.3. Benzodiazepines

INDICATION/USE	COMMENTS
Anxiolytic	Alprazolam (Xanax) helps calm patients with intense fear of flying before boarding plane
Sedative-hypnotic	Induces sleep
Anticonvulsant	Diazepam, midazolam, and lorazepam can terminate seizures and are used for treatment of status epilepticus Clonazepam may be used for long-term treatment of epilepsy
Alcohol withdrawal	Chlordiazepoxide, diazepam, and oxazepam can be used in acute withdrawal

One means of categorizing benzodiazepines is based on their duration of action (Table 23.4).

Table 23.4. Categories of Benzodiazepines Based on Duration of Action

Short-acting	Triazolam, oxazepam, midazolam, alprazolam
Intermediate-acting	Clonazepam, alprazolam, temazepam, lorazepam, estazolam
Long-acting	Chlordiazepoxide, diazepam

4. **What are some common adverse effects of benzodiazepines?**
Given that benzodiazepines are generally depressants, it is no surprise that they can produce oversedation, predisposing the patient to falls, fractures, or work injuries; cause cognitive impairment (e.g., memory loss); exacerbate respiratory problems (e.g., emphysema); and lead to dependence. Given the risk for dependence, benzodiazepines should not be prescribed for prolonged durations.

Benzodiazepine intoxication can be reversed with flumazenil (a GABA$_A$ receptor competitive antagonist); however, it is rarely used because of risk for precipitating benzodiazepine withdrawal seizures (in patients with long-term dependence). Withdrawal should be treated symptomatically using long-acting benzodiazepines.

5. **What are the symptoms of benzodiazepine intoxication and withdrawal?**
See Table 23.5.

Table 23.5. Benzodiazepine Intoxication and Withdrawal

Intoxication	Slurred speech, drowsiness, decreased respiratory rate and tidal volume, bradycardia
Withdrawal	Shaking, diaphoresis, anxiety, irritability, insomnia, cardiac palpitations, painful abdominal cramps, seizures (if long-term dependence)

SUMMARY BOX: BENZODIAZEPINES

- Indications: Anxiolytic, antiepileptic, sedative (for insomnia), and treatment of alcohol withdrawal
- Mechanism of action: Enhances the affinity of γ-aminobutyric acid A (GABA$_A$) receptors for GABA, resulting in chloride influx that hyperpolarizes the cell and leads to depressive effects
- Side effects: Oversedation, memory loss, and dependence (especially with short-acting agents)
- Toxicity
  - If taken alone, effects of overdose are minimal (drowsiness).
  - Respiratory depression is more likely if taken in combination with barbiturates or ethanol.
- Antidote: Flumazenil, a GABA$_A$ receptor competitive antagonist

CASE 23.7

A 48-year-old woman is brought to the emergency department (ED) by her son, who found her to be unarousable this morning from last night's sleep. There is no history of trauma or drug abuse. Her medical history is notable for insomnia, for which she was started on secobarbital recently. Her son brought the pill bottle to the ED with him, and all the pills are accounted for. She takes no other medication and has no known allergies. When questioned, the patient's son notes that his mother did have a few beers last night, although she was not overtly intoxicated. Physical examination reveals a somnolent woman with slurred/unintelligible speech, constricted pupils, diminished deep tendon reflexes, a heart rate of 48 beats/min, a blood pressure of 100/60 mm Hg, and a respiratory rate (RR) of 8 breaths/min.

1. **Given this clinical picture, what scenario best explains this patient's presentation?**
This patient has a history of insomnia and was therefore recently started on a barbiturate (secobarbital). To this, she added another depressant (alcohol) and is now presenting with CNS, respiratory, and cardiac depression.

Although alkalinizing her urine using intravenous bicarbonate may help facilitate bodily excretion of secobarbital (barbiturates are weak acids—see Basic Concepts, question 3), there is no specific antidote for barbiturates. In this case, the best approach is to monitor her respiration (and intubate if warranted) and prevent cardiovascular collapse (give intravenous fluids and possibly administer inotropics/vasopressors, such as dopamine or NE).

2. **What is the mechanism of action of barbiturates?**
Although their binding site is different, barbiturates act very similarly to benzodiazepines in that they potentiate the effect of GABA on the chloride channel. The result is a hyperpolarized cell that is less excitable. However, instead of increasing the frequency of chloride channel openings as benzodiazepines do, barbiturates increase the *duration* for which the channel is open. It is critical to remember this distinction!

In addition, barbiturates also diminish activity of the excitatory neurotransmitter, glutamate. Barbiturates do this by blocking a type of glutamate receptor that is found almost exclusively in the CNS. Although its actual name is much longer (and relatively unimportant), this receptor is commonly referred to by the acronym AMPA.

3. **What are some common indications for using barbiturates?**
Although barbiturates have largely been replaced by benzodiazepines because they have a better side effect profile and less potential for abuse, barbiturates continue to have utility in some clinical settings. For example, they are still used in induction of anesthesia and as anticonvulsants to treat seizures.

One means of categorizing barbiturates is based on the duration of action—long-acting, short-acting, or ultrashort-acting. Phenobarbital is a long-acting agent that can be used to treat seizures on a long-term basis; thiopental is ultrashort-acting and used to induce anesthesia. Thiopental is highly lipid soluble and will quickly diffuse out of the bloodstream and into adipose tissue (thus decreasing its plasma concentration).

4. What are some common adverse effects of barbiturates?

Similar to benzodiazepines, barbiturates are generally depressants. At the level of the CNS, this manifests as drowsiness. In cases of overdose, respiratory depression caused by blockade of the body's response to hypoxia/hypercapnia is also a very real risk. Barbiturates are much more likely to cause respiratory depression than the similarly acting benzodiazepines for reasons explained earlier in this chapter (see Case 23.6, question 2). At toxic doses, barbiturates can also cause severe bradycardia to the point of causing a shocklike condition. In contrast with benzodiazepines, there is no pharmacologic treatment for barbiturate overdose. Treatment consists of supportive care and symptom management.

As noted earlier, barbiturates do have hypnotic/anxiolytic effects that can precipitate dependence and abuse. On withdrawal, symptoms such as tremors, anxiety, seizures, delirium, and cardiac arrest can result. This ability to cause death with both intoxication and withdrawal is a feature that sets barbiturates and benzodiazepines apart from other drugs of abuse and is more reason not to combine the two with other general depressants such as alcohol.

A noteworthy complication of barbiturate use is their exacerbation of porphyria in susceptible individuals. This occurs because barbiturates induce the activity of d-ALA (aminolevulinic acid) synthase, which is the rate-limiting enzyme in the heme synthesis pathway. In individuals with porphyria, this causes an increased accumulation of heme precursors and a flare of porphyria symptoms. Many CYP-450 inducers can do this, but barbiturates are by far the most commonly tested of the bunch.

STEP 1 SECRET

Barbiturates and benzodiazepines are commonly encountered drugs on Step 1. You should know their mechanisms of action, clinical uses, adverse effects, and treatment for overdose.

SUMMARY BOX: BARBITURATES

- Indications: Induction of anesthesia, anticonvulsant, anxiolytic, and treatment of alcohol withdrawal
- Mechanism of action: Modulate γ-aminobutyric acid (GABA) receptors to increase the duration of chloride channel opening, which hyperpolarizes the cell and decreases excitability
- Side effects: Drowsiness
- Toxicity: Respiratory depression, severe bradycardia. Contraindicated in porphyria because of their induction of d-ALA synthase in the heme synthesis pathway
- Antidote: None
  - Can provide supportive care and sodium bicarbonate to alkalinize the urine

CASE 23.8

You are on call overnight and are paged about a 54-year-old patient who is reportedly having a generalized tonic-clonic seizure. The patient underwent an uncomplicated emergent appendectomy approximately 72 hours earlier. Over the past 48 hours, the nursing staff reports the patient to have deteriorated from being fairly pleasant soon after his operation to being quite anxious, diaphoretic, tremulous, and unable to sleep. More recently, the patient is said to have been experiencing visual and auditory hallucinations. His medical history is notable for a simple hand fracture sustained during a bar fight; he is not currently on any medications, nor does he have any allergies. He has no history of prior seizures. He lives alone and is unemployed and twice divorced. A comparison of his daily vital signs shows that his heart rate, blood pressure, and temperature have been progressively increasing over the past 48 hours.

1. Given his recent uncomplicated hospital course and his benign medical history, what condition is this patient likely experiencing?

This patient has no history of epilepsy and is not taking any medications that would predispose him to seizures. In contrast, he has several risk factors for depression and substance abuse (e.g., living alone, inability to hold a job or establish close relationships). The most likely cause of his seizure is alcohol withdrawal syndrome, which usually presents 2 to 3 days after a chronic alcohol abuser stops his intake of alcohol. Symptoms of withdrawal can range from insomnia and tremulousness to severe complications, such as seizures and even delirium tremens (visual/tactile/auditory hallucinations, autonomic hyperactivity, disorientation, agitation, nightmares, and uncontrollable tremors).

2. **What are the symptoms of acute alcohol toxicity, and how can these effects be explained at the molecular level?**

Alcohol has a depressive effect on the brain. It impairs motor function, cognition, judgment, speech, and respiration, and it disinhibits behavior.

At the molecular level, think of the brain as being a teeter-totter that is balanced by an inhibitory neurotransmitter (GABA) at one end and an excitatory neurotransmitter (glutamate) at the other end. Alcohol enhances the effects of GABA on the GABA$_A$ receptor and blunts the effects of glutamate on the NMDA receptor (thus weighing the teeter-totter in favor of a net inhibitory effect).

If exposure to alcohol is chronic, then the brain will enact certain compensatory measures to reestablish balance. On the GABA end, the brain will downregulate the number of GABA$_A$ receptors, and on the glutamate end, the brain will upregulate the number of NMDA receptors. Not only is more alcohol needed to attain the same degree of inhibitory effect (i.e., tolerance), but if alcohol exposure is halted suddenly, then there will also be pronounced hyperexcitability because of the increased number of NMDA receptors (i.e., withdrawal).

3. **What are symptoms of chronic alcohol abuse?**

Hepatic manifestations are fairly common with chronic exposure and include fatty liver, hepatitis, cirrhosis, and liver failure. Other findings include pancreatitis, nutritional deficiencies, peripheral neuropathy, and cerebellar degeneration.

4. **What is the relationship between alcohol and benzodiazepines in terms of their effect on the brain?**

They both enhance the effects of GABA on the GABA$_A$ receptor. As described earlier, if the duration of exposure to alcohol is prolonged, then the number of GABA$_A$ receptors will be downregulated to reestablish homeostasis. As a result, just as a chronic abuser of alcohol builds a tolerance to alcohol so that a higher dose is required to achieve the same effect, the same patient will require a higher-than-normal dose of benzodiazepines to achieve sedation in a medical setting (i.e., cross-tolerance).

The notion of cross-reactivity between alcohol and benzodiazepines can be used therapeutically to manage alcohol withdrawal. For example, an intermediate-acting benzodiazepine (e.g., lorazepam) can be used as a substitute for alcohol to ameliorate the hyperexcitable state that is characteristic of alcohol withdrawal. Once the teeter-totter is balanced, the intermediate-acting benzodiazepine can be tapered slowly or replaced with a long-acting benzodiazepine (e.g., chlordiazepoxide) that has less abuse potential. Eventually, the number of GABA$_A$ and NMDA receptors will be recalibrated to levels present before alcohol exposure, and the benzodiazepines can be stopped altogether.

5. **How is alcohol metabolized in the body?**

Most of the metabolism occurs in the liver, where alcohol is oxidized by alcohol dehydrogenase (ADH) to acetaldehyde, which is subsequently oxidized by aldehyde dehydrogenase (aldehyde-DH) to acetate (Fig. 23.2).

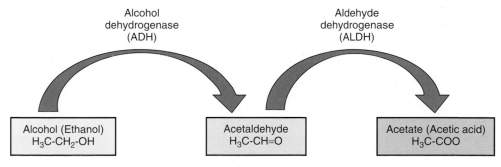

Figure 23.2. Metabolism of alcohol.

Disulfiram is a drug used to manage alcoholism. It inhibits aldehyde-DH, thus causing accumulation of acetaldehyde. Acetaldehyde, in turn, causes nausea, vomiting, severe headaches, and flushing. These negative effects are intended to discourage further alcohol use.

Certain medications can also inadvertently inhibit aldehyde-DH, causing a "disulfiram-like reaction" with the aforementioned side effects. As such, patients are instructed not to consume alcohol while taking such drugs. This is a commonly tested feature of the antibiotic metronidazole. Other medications, such as griseofulvin and first-generation sulfonylureas, also have this effect, although this is less commonly tested. Polymorphisms in acetaldehyde dehydrogenase result in accumulation of acetaldehyde and are particularly common among people of Asian descent.

SUMMARY BOX: ALCOHOL

- Indications: Drug of abuse
- Mechanism of action: Enhances the effects of γ-aminobutyric acid (GABA) on the $GABA_A$ receptor and blunts the effects of glutamate on the N-methyl-D-aspartate (NMDA) receptor, leading to depressive symptoms.
- Withdrawal: Usually 2 to 3 days after a chronic abuser stops intake; symptoms include insomnia, tremulousness, seizures, and delirium tremens.
- Toxicity: Chronic exposure can damage the liver, pancreas, and nervous system and can also lead to nutritional deficits.
- Management
  - Benzodiazepines are used to manage withdrawal.
  - Disulfiram can be used to manage alcoholism by inhibiting aldehyde-DH and causing unpleasant symptoms. Other options include naltrexone and acamprosate.
  - Several drugs (e.g., metronidazole) can have a disulfiram-like effect if alcohol is consumed.

CASE 23.9

A 52-year-old woman is brought to the emergency department by ambulance 3 hours after an apparent suicide attempt by ingestion of medication. Her symptoms include nausea, vomiting, and right upper quadrant pain. Her medical history is positive for depression and chronic alcohol abuse. Her physical examination reveals normal vital signs and some mild tenderness in her right upper quadrant. A serum panel is positive for acetaminophen, but levels are below the toxic threshold.

1. Given this presentation, which other laboratory values would prove informative? Should this patient be treated based on the information provided?

   Acetaminophen is metabolized by the liver, and one of its by-products (N-acetyl-p-benzoquinone imine [NAPQI]) is toxic to hepatocytes. Therefore anytime a toxic level of this drug is ingested, liver necrosis is a real danger. Fortunately, NAPQI can be inactivated by glutathione, which is an antioxidant regenerated in the body by the enzyme glutathione reductase. However, patients whose reserves of glutathione are decreased (e.g., alcoholics, diabetics) or those who ingest massive quantities of acetaminophen that overwhelm the glutathione system are at risk for hepatocyte damage by NAPQI. To assess the degree of damage to the liver, levels of liver function enzymes and coagulation panels are typically acquired. Although this patient's serum level of acetaminophen is below the toxic threshold, given her history of alcohol abuse, it is wise to treat her with N-acetylcysteine to prevent liver failure. Recall that N-acetylcysteine replenishes glutathione supply.

2. What is the mechanism of action of acetaminophen?

   Central (CNS) COX pathway inhibition is the mechanism of action. Cell membranes are composed of fatty acids, and one of these fatty acids is arachidonic acid. When the membrane is damaged, arachidonic acid begins to be broken down along one of two pathways—the COX pathway or the LOX pathway. The COX pathway results in PG production; the LOX pathway produces leukotrienes.

   PGs are among a handful of molecules that mediate inflammation, pain, and fever. If the objective is to decrease inflammation, pain, and fever, then inhibiting the COX pathway is a good start. Acetaminophen reversibly inhibits this pathway. Ibuprofen and aspirin (both NSAIDs) act on the same enzyme, COX, albeit peripherally. Steroids (e.g., hydrocortisone, prednisone) inhibit a different enzyme, phospholipase A_2, which plays a role earlier along this same pathway.

   Although it inhibits COX, acetaminophen is not considered an NSAID. Acetaminophen acts centrally (in the CNS) to inhibit PG synthesis by COX, whereas NSAIDs inhibit the same pathway in peripheral tissues. This difference in location accounts for the analgesic/antipyretic effects of acetaminophen and the antiinflammatory effects of NSAIDs.

SUMMARY BOX: ACETAMINOPHEN

- Indications: Pain and fever reduction
- Mechanism of action: Reversibly inhibits the cyclooxygenase (COX) pathway in the central nervous system (CNS), leading to decreased prostaglandin synthesis
- Toxicity: Liver necrosis
- Antidote: N-acetylcysteine (replenishes glutathione supply)

CASE 23.10

A 74-year-old man with Alzheimer disease is brought to the emergency department by ambulance. His grandson had found him on the bathroom floor, along with a half-empty bottle of his "Alzheimer medication." The patient apparently ingested the medication within the last 3 hours because this was the last time his grandson saw the patient before finding him unconscious. He reports his grandfather to have vomited a few times before being found, and several pills could be seen in the vomitus. The patient's other symptoms include diaphoresis, drooling, and urinary incontinence. Physical examination is notable for a low heart rate and respiratory rate, mydriasis, and fasciculations.

1. Given this patient's presentation, which group of medications is the likely culprit?
   Alzheimer disease is thought to be due in part to a deficiency of acetylcholine (ACh) in the CNS. One way of managing an ACh deficiency is to use a group of medications generally referred to as *cholinergics*. In the case of Alzheimer disease specifically, this means using drugs that can cross the blood-brain barrier and block acetylcholinesterase (AChE), thus decreasing the rate of breakdown of ACh. A few AChE inhibitors used in this way include donepezil, rivastigmine, and tacrine.

   However, if AChE inhibitors are used in excessive amounts, ACh levels can reach toxic proportions. This in turn can cause more global effects because of the interaction of ACh with nicotinic receptors (e.g., fasciculations, muscle weakness), as well as muscarinic receptors (e.g., nausea, vomiting, diarrhea, urinary incontinence, mydriasis, diaphoresis, hypersalivation, bradycardia, hypotension).

   Using an anticholinergic agent such as atropine to reverse these effects is a reasonable therapeutic approach.

2. In general terms, how is the nervous system organized?
   The nervous system can be divided according to function (sensory/motor) or anatomy (central/peripheral). For discussion of anticholinergics, it is best to adopt the former approach and consider only the motor half of the nervous system.

   The motor branch can be further categorized into ANS and SNS, respectively. The SNS and ANS can also be viewed in terms of either anatomy or function. In terms of function, the SNS is the voluntary portion of the nervous system, whereas the ANS is the involuntary portion. In terms of anatomy, the SNS is relatively simple in that a single neuron leaves the CNS and travels directly to the target organ, where it delivers ACh to a nicotinic receptor that is located on striated muscle.

   In terms of anatomy, the ANS is a bit more specialized than the SNS in that instead of relying on a single neuron, it involves two neurons connecting the CNS to target organs. These two neurons are connected to each other via a synapse. The specifics of this synapse are easy to remember because its anatomy is very similar to that of the SNS; that is, it always involves delivery of ACh to a nicotinic receptor.

   The anatomic feature that really sets the ANS apart from the SNS is how the postsynaptic neuron delivers the message from the synapse to the target organ. In fact, the ANS is divided into three groups based on the anatomy of this second neuron:
   1. Parasympathetic division delivers ACh to muscarinic receptors.
   2. Sympathetic division delivers NE to adrenergic receptors.
   3. The third division is actually partially endocrine and delivers epinephrine (Epi; from the adrenal medulla) to an adrenergic receptor. Because this division also involves a catecholamine as its primary neurotransmitter, it is usually considered part of the sympathetic nervous system. The organization of the sensory and motor components of the nervous system is outlined in Table 23.6.

Table 23.6. Organization of the Nervous System		
SENSORY	**MOTOR**	
ANS	SNS	
Involuntary	Voluntary	
2 neurons/1 synapse	1 neuron/no synapse	
Synapse (preganglionic) = ACh → Nct	ACh → Nct (at NMJ)	
PARASYMPATHETIC (POSTGANGLIONIC)	**SYMPATHETIC (POSTGANGLIONIC)**	**ENDOCRINE**
ACh → M	NE → Adr	Epi (from adrenals) → Adr

ACh, Acetylcholine; *Adr*, adrenergic; *ANS*, autonomic nervous system; *Epi*, epinephrine; *M*, muscarinic; *Nct*, nicotinic receptor; *NE*, norepinephrine; *NMJ*, neuromuscular junction; *SNS*, somatic nervous system.

3. Which neurotransmitter can be said to be pivotal to the function of the entire motor nervous system?
   Because it is the lone neurotransmitter in the SNS, and thus the only means of connecting the two neurons in a typical ANS pathway, ACh is pivotal to the function of the motor nervous system. If ACh release is hindered (as occurs in botulinum toxicity), the entire motor nervous system can be blocked, thus producing flaccid paralysis.

4. Is there a way to selectively affect the parasympathetic nervous system?
   Yes, the PNS can be selectively affected by stimulating/inhibiting muscarinic receptors, which are exclusive to this branch of the ANS. The two most common stimulants include bethanechol (used to induce urination in nonobstructive urinary retention) and pilocarpine (used to reduce intraocular pressure in glaucoma).

   The two most common antimuscarinics are atropine and ipratropium. Atropine drips can be used in the eye to induce mydriasis (cholinergic input into the eye causes miosis or pinpointing; if this function is blocked by antimuscarinics, then sympathetic input goes unchecked to induce mydriasis or dilation). At high doses, atropine causes tachycardia by blocking muscarinic receptors at the SA node. Ipratropium is a derivative of atropine and comes in an inhaled form that is used to treat asthma and chronic obstructive pulmonary disease.

Several other drugs have antimuscarinic side effects that mimic the effects of atropine. These drugs include antihistamines, antipsychotics, quinidine, and tricyclic antidepressants (TCAs). TCAs are particularly notable for their antimuscarinic effects and classic "three Cs" triad—coma, cardiotoxicity (torsades de pointes), and convulsions (seizures). Older individuals are particularly susceptible to antimuscarinic effects, and for this reason, these drugs are typically avoided in their care.

STEP 1 SECRET

Antimuscarinic/atropine toxicity is commonly tested on Step 1. Symptoms of atropine toxicity can be remembered with the mnemonic "Hot as a hare, dry as a bone, red as a beet, blind as a bat, mad as a hatter, and full as a flask," which describes increased body temperature (hot), dry skin as a result of decreased sweating (dry), flushed skin (red), cycloplegia or inability to accommodate vision for close-up objects (blind), disorientation secondary to atropine entering the central nervous system (CNS) (mad), and urinary retention (full). The antidote for atropine toxicity is physostigmine, an acetylcholinesterase inhibitor that causes an increased concentration of acetylcholine (ACh) to displace atropine from muscarinic receptors. Physostigmine is the only acetylcholinesterase (AChE) inhibitor capable of crossing the blood-brain barrier and alleviating the CNS side effects of antimuscarinic drugs; other AChE inhibitors, such as neostigmine, are not used as antidotes for antimuscarinic toxicity.

5. What is one way to reduce the side effects of a drug that stimulates both nicotinic and muscarinic receptors?
   By limiting its physical distribution in the body, one can localize the effects of a drug that would otherwise act on a global level. An example of this approach is using carbachol eye drops to reduce intraocular pressure.

6. Are there nicotinic receptor blockers that are selective for the entire motor nervous system?
   Yes. Nicotinic receptor blockers that are selective for receptors located on skeletal muscle (i.e., are SNS selective) are called *neuromuscular blocking agents*. There are two classes of neuromuscular blockers: depolarizing and nondepolarizing (Fig. 23.3). Nondepolarizing neuromuscular blockers compete with ACh (i.e., they are competitive antagonists). The parent compound for nondepolarizing blockers is curare, and as a result, drugs in this class have some variation of this word incorporated into their names (e.g., tubocurarine). These agents are typically used as general anesthetics to achieve skeletal muscle relaxation during surgical procedures. Their effects can be overcome by increasing the concentration of their competitor (ACh). This can be achieved with AChE inhibitors (Table 23.7), particularly neostigmine, because it cannot cross the blood-brain barrier and thus reduces any risk of CNS effects.

   Depolarizing neuromuscular blockers bind the sodium ion channel at the neuromuscular junction (NMJ), thereby prolonging depolarization and preventing the myocyte from repolarizing. The net effect of this inability to repolarize is flaccid paralysis. The only depolarizing blocker you need to know for Step 1 is succinylcholine, which is used in brief procedures (e.g., endotracheal intubations just before surgical procedures). Unlike nondepolarizing neuromuscular

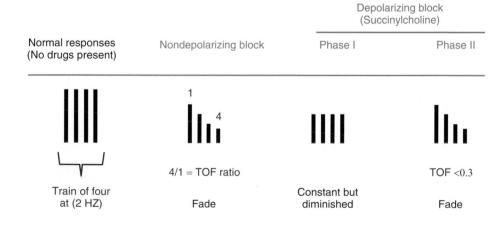

Figure 23.3. Neuromuscular blockade.

Table 23.7. Acetylcholine Agonists and Antagonists

CATEGORY	MUSCARINIC RECEPTORS	NICOTINIC RECEPTORS
Agonist	Bethanechol, pilocarpine, carbachol	Nicotine
Antagonist	Atropine, ipratropium	Succinylcholine (a depolarizing neuromuscular junction blocker), tubocurarine (a nondepolarizing neuromuscular junction blocker)

blockers, a succinylcholine NMJ block occurs in two phases. During phase I, the ACh receptor channel undergoes "prolonged depolarization," and the block cannot be reversed. In fact, giving cholinesterase inhibitors will only cause continued depolarization and will prolong the paralytic effects of succinylcholine. Succinylcholine can be reversed only during phase II, at which point the channel has repolarized but is still blocked by succinylcholine. At this point, AChE inhibitors can be administered, and the block can be reversed. Certain individuals can have an autosomal recessive *pseudocholinesterase deficiency*, meaning that they metabolize succinylcholine at a much slower rate. These individuals can remain paralyzed for hours. (A normal dose of succinylcholine should paralyze a typical individual for only about 5 minutes.) Such patients can remain in phase I for prolonged periods, so it is especially important not to administer AChE inhibitors until it is certain that they have reached phase II. This can be determined by administering nerve stimulation four consecutive times and evaluating the muscle responses ("train of four" responses). In phase I, all four responses should have the same amplitude, which will increase over time. Once in phase II, the muscle responses demonstrate a "fading" pattern (this fading pattern is also always seen with nondepolarizing agents). The phase II pattern indicates it is now safe to administer AChE inhibitors to reverse the NMJ blockade. Giving AChE inhibitors too early can prolong paralysis even further and possibly lead to respiratory failure and death.

7. **How can a cholinergic drug help diagnose myasthenia gravis?**
Myasthenia gravis is a neuromuscular disease marked by autoantibodies that occupy ACh receptors at the NMJ (type II hypersensitivity reaction). The typical patient tends to fatigue unusually quickly with increasing activity. The reason for this is that the autoantibodies that occupy ACh receptors prevent the neurotransmitter from contacting its target, and ACh is degraded by AChE before it has a chance to displace the autoantibody. Ptosis and diplopia are common initial findings. Weakness in proximal muscles and the diaphragm often follows. Patients may also present with dysphagia to solids and liquids.

With use of a fast-acting AChE inhibitor such as edrophonium, the exposure time of the receptor to ACh is increased, and the autoantibodies are therefore displaced. A completely fatigued patient may then momentarily regain his or her strength and energy. This is in contrast with a genuinely fatigued patient, who will not respond because the muscle itself is fatigued. This test, called the *Tensilon test*, is used to diagnose myasthenia gravis. Pyridostigmine is used for long-term treatment of myasthenia gravis.

STEP 1 SECRET

Myasthenia gravis is a popular Step 1 topic. Be on the lookout for patients who experience muscle fatigue with increasing use (in contrast with Lambert-Eaton syndrome). Note that myasthenia gravis is also associated with thymoma, which may be presented to you on a chest x-ray.

SUMMARY BOX: CHOLINERGICS/ANTICHOLINERGICS

- Muscarinic receptors are exclusive to the parasympathetic branch of the autonomic nervous system (ANS).
- Botulinum toxin inhibits release of acetylcholine (ACh), thus causing flaccid paralysis.
- Muscarinic agonists: Bethanechol (induces urination) and pilocarpine (reduces intraocular pressure)
- Muscarinic antagonists: Atropine (induces mydriasis, causes tachycardia at high doses) and ipratropium (bronchodilator)
- Nondepolarizing neuromuscular blockers ("curares"): Competitive ACh antagonists (skeletal muscle relaxation during surgical procedures or intubation), most commonly rocuronium
  - Antidote: Acetylcholinesterase (AChE) inhibitors (e.g., neostigmine or edrophonium) or more recently sugammadex, which binds rocuronium or vecuronium
- Depolarizing neuromuscular blockers: Succinylcholine (flaccid paralysis for brief procedures, i.e., intubation)
  - Antidote: AChE inhibitors only after nerve stimulation demonstrate a "fading" pattern (phase II pattern). Giving AChE inhibitors too early will prolong paralysis.

CASE 23.11

A 22-year-old man is brought to the emergency department by his parents, who report that he recently ingested his father's antihypertensive medication in an apparent suicide attempt. His medical history is notable for depression and asthma. On physical examination, the patient is bradycardic, hypotensive, tachypneic, and in respiratory distress. The patient's mental status is also depressed.

1. **Given this presentation, to which group of antihypertensives does the likely culprit belong?**
Very few antihypertensive medications precipitate respiratory crisis in a patient with a history of asthma. From that standpoint, the drug in question is likely a beta-blocker (more on beta-blockers later). Management of this patient requires intravenous fluid, adrenergic agents, and inotropic/chronotropic drugs that bypass the beta receptors altogether and work to restore heart rate and BP. If this patient's respiratory crisis is unresponsive to beta-agonists, endotracheal intubation may be warranted as well.

2. **In the sympathetic nervous system, what are the two types of neurotransmitter and the two main adrenergic receptors?**
The two main neurotransmitters are NE and Epi. Both are derived from the amino acid tyrosine (Fig. 23.4).
   The two main types of receptor in the sympathetic nervous system are α-adrenergic and β-adrenergic receptors. Dopaminergic receptors also exist but are not the predominant subtype.

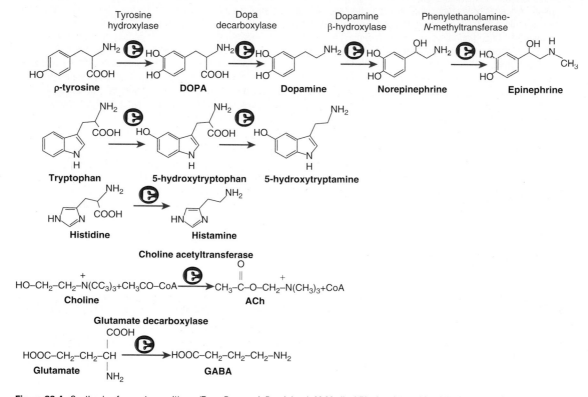

Figure 23.4. Synthesis of neurotransmitters. *(From Baynes J, Dominiczak M. Medical Biochemistry. 4th ed. Philadelphia: Saunders; 2014.)*

3. **Describe α receptors in terms of their distribution in the body and a few of their agonists/ antagonists.**
There are actually two types of α-adrenergic receptor: α_1 and α_2.
   α_1 receptors are located in the radial muscle of the eye (causes mydriasis) and in the smooth muscle of the vasculature (causes vasoconstriction). An example of an α_1-agonist is phenylephrine, which is used to treat nasal congestion by inducing vasoconstriction. An example of an α_1-blocker is prazosin, which is used to treat urinary tract obstruction in benign prostatic hyperplasia (BPH), HTN by causing smooth muscle relaxation, and posttraumatic stress disorder by reducing nightmares.
   α_2 receptors are located centrally, and stimulating them actually inhibits NE release from synaptic vesicles. As a result, these receptors can be regarded as part of the inhibitory arm of the sympathetic nervous system. α_2-agonists include clonidine and α-methyldopa. Clonidine is used to treat severe HTN and opioid withdrawal. α-Methyldopa is used to treat HTN, especially in pregnancy. An example of an α_2-blocker is mirtazapine, which is used in the treatment of depression. By inhibiting the inhibitory arm of the sympathetic nervous system, it increases catecholamine activity (Table 23.8).

Table 23.8. α-Adrenergic Receptors

CATEGORY	α₁ RECEPTORS	α₂ RECEPTORS
Agonists	Phenylephrine, midodrine	Clonidine, guanfacine, α-methyldopa, tizanidine
Antagonists	Prazosin, terazosin, phentolamine (nonselective), phenoxybenzamine (nonselective)	Mirtazapine

4. Describe β receptors in terms of their distribution in the body and a few of their agonists/antagonists.

There are three types of β-adrenergic receptor: β_1, β_2, and β_3.

β_1 receptors are located in the heart, and stimulating them increases cardiac output by increasing conduction velocity and contractility. An agonist selective for this receptor is dobutamine, which is used to increase cardiac output in cardiogenic shock. Blocking these receptors decreases cardiac output and hence BP. A few antagonists selective for this receptor are metoprolol, esmolol, and atenolol.

β_2 receptors are located in the lungs, and stimulating them causes dilation of the bronchi. An example of a selective agonist is albuterol, which is used in the management of asthma. Blocking these receptors can constrict the airways and precipitate an asthma attack in those predisposed to such an event. Because there is little therapeutic advantage to selectively blocking these receptors, there are few such agents available. The drugs that happen to block these receptors do so as a side effect of their nonselective beta-blocking activity. These agents include timolol, nadolol, and propranolol, and they are contraindicated in patients with asthma (Table 23.9). β_2 receptors are also located in the eye (stimulate aqueous humor production), pancreas (stimulates insulin secretion), and uterus (tocolytic).

Table 23.9. β-Adrenergic Receptors

CATEGORY	β₁ RECEPTORS	β₂ RECEPTORS
Agonists	Dobutamine, isoproterenol	Albuterol
Antagonists	Metoprolol, esmolol, atenolol, timolol (nonselective), nadolol (nonselective), propranolol (nonselective)	

β_3 receptors are located in the skeletal muscle and urinary bladder. In the skeletal muscle, stimulation of the receptors promotes thermogenesis, whereas in the bladder, stimulation of the receptors promotes bladder relaxation and prevents urination. In this way, β_3-agonists can be used to treat overactive bladder and urinary incontinence. One such agent is mirabegron.

5. What antidote should be given to this patient?

Glucagon is a must-know antidote for beta-blocker toxicity—it is commonly asked on Step 1. Glucagon increases heart rate, contractility, and AV conduction possibly via a mechanism that bypasses the β receptor.

SUMMARY BOX: SYMPATHOMIMETIC PHARMACEUTICALS

- α_1 receptors: Phenylephrine is an α_1-agonist (used to treat nasal congestion), and prazosin is an α_1-blocker (used to treat hypertension [HTN], benign prostatic hyperplasia [BPH], and posttraumatic stress disorder). Tamsulosin is a newer generation α_1-blocker that is more selective for prostatic receptors and therefore causes fewer side effects than BPH.
- α_2 receptors: Clonidine (used to treat severe HTN and opioid withdrawal) and α-methyldopa (used to treat HTN in pregnancy) are α_2-agonists. Mirtazapine is an α_2-blocker (used in the treatment of depression).
- β_1 receptors: Dobutamine is a β_1-agonist (used to manage congestive heart failure). Metoprolol, esmolol, and atenolol are beta$_1$-blockers (used to treat HTN).
- β_2 receptors: Albuterol is a β_2-agonist (used to manage asthma). Timolol, nadolol, and propranolol are nonselective β-blockers, which are contraindicated in patients with asthma because they can precipitate an asthma attack.
- β_3 receptors: Mirabegron is a β_3-agonist (used to treat overactive bladder).
- Antidote: Glucagon is a must-know antidote for beta-blocker toxicity.

CASE 23.12

A 40-year-old farmer arrives at the emergency department reporting that he cannot breathe. Physical examination reveals pulse of 48 beats/min and blood pressure of 94/58 mm Hg. He also demonstrates excessive lacrimation, salivation, and pinpoint pupils.

1. **What is the likely cause of this man's symptoms?**
   Organophosphate poisoning is the likely cause. Organophosphates are components of insecticides, and toxicity is often suspected in farmers who present with symptoms of excessive cholinergic release.

STEP 1 SECRET

Organophosphate poisoning in a farmer is one of the most commonly encountered clinical vignettes on Step 1.

2. **How does organophosphate poisoning result in this patient's symptoms?**
   Organophosphates are AChE inhibitors. AChE is an enzyme responsible for degradation of ACh. Inhibition of AChE results in accumulation of ACh. Excessive ACh results in the **DUMBBELSS** symptoms:
   - **D**iarrhea
   - **U**rination
   - **M**iosis
   - **B**radycardia
   - **B**ronchospasm
   - **E**xcitation of skeletal muscles (muscle fasciculations, twitches, and trembling)
   - **L**acrimation
   - **S**alivation
   - **S**weating

3. **What is the treatment for organophosphate poisoning?**
   Atropine and pralidoxime are used. Atropine is a cholinergic antagonist, which directly inhibits ACh receptors. Pralidoxime is used to regenerate AChE.
   Note: Atropine toxicity is treated with physostigmine, an indirect agonist of AChE (inhibits AChE).

4. **Atropine administration relieves all DUMBBELSS symptoms except one. Which symptom is not relieved by atropine?**
   Excitation of skeletal muscle is not relieved by atropine. The synapses at the NMJ are nicotinic receptors, and atropine is a muscarinic antagonist. Therefore atropine will not block the nicotinic receptors at the NMJ.

STEP 1 SECRET

Question 4 is a perfect example of the type of tricky question you can expect to see on boards. At first, you may panic if you cannot recall seeing the direct answer in a textbook. However, if you take a deep breath and just think about what the question is asking, you will realize that you can integrate and apply your knowledge to arrive at the correct answer. The purpose of boards, after all, is to see if you can apply the basic science knowledge you have gained in the first and second years of medical school toward clinical problem solving.

SUMMARY BOX: ORGANOPHOSPHATES

- Indications: No medical uses; found in insecticides and herbicides (suspect in farmers!)
- Mechanism of action: Block action of acetylcholinesterase (AChE), leading to increased circulating quantities of acetylcholine (ACh)
- Toxicity: Excessive ACh release results in the DUMBBELSS symptoms
- Antidote: Atropine (blocks ACh receptors) and pralidoxime (regenerates AChE)

CASE 23.13

A 25-year-old woman presents with 3-day history of malaise, headache, low-grade fever, and a rash on her left calf. Her social history reveals that she was hiking in the woods near her Connecticut home about 10 days ago. Vital signs show temperature of 100.3°F, heart rate 100 beats/min, blood pressure 118/82 mm Hg, respiratory rate (RR) 16 breaths/min, and SaO$_2$ 99% on room air. Examination reveals a 3-cm circular red rash on her left posterior calf. You make the presumptive diagnosis of Lyme disease. Anti–*Borrelia burgdorferi* antibodies are found on serology. The patient has a history of tetracycline allergy, so you begin a course of rifampin. On follow-up several weeks later, the patient reveals that her Lyme symptoms resolved, but she still feels "off." She took multiple home pregnancy tests, which were positive. Serum β-human chorionic gonadotropin is 400 mIU/mL. She is sexually active with her boyfriend of 2 years but tells you it is impossible for her to be pregnant because she takes oral contraceptive pills daily as instructed. She asks you how this could have happened.

The purpose of this excessively detailed history is to demonstrate a critical test-taking strategy for Step 1. Always read the question's last sentence before reading the entire vignette! If you had read the vignette from the beginning, you may have found yourself being distracted by certain buzzwords and clues—the patient's Lyme symptoms, the history of hiking in the woods, the erythema chronicum migrans rash, etc. You may have also been scanning your memory for an alternative antibiotic for Lyme disease if doxycycline cannot be prescribed. If so, you were probably disappointed to find that the vignette had done all of the work for you—diagnosed the illness, identified the organism, and prescribed the appropriate treatment. Step 1 questions can contain lots of irrelevant information. Knowing the question before reading the vignette allows you to hone in on the salient points without being distracted by extraneous details.

1. What is the most likely explanation for this patient's pregnancy?
   Rifampin-induced CYP-450 activation and subsequent consumption of OCP metabolites. You must know some common examples of CYP-450 substrates, inhibitors, and inducers (Table 23.10). A CYP-450 substrate is simply consumed by the enzyme but does not alter its activity. Inducers, as the name suggests, will increase the activity of CYP-450 and thereby *decrease* the concentration of the substrate. Inhibitors will have the opposite effect. In the case of this patient, the rifampin she took for Lyme disease acted as a CYP-450 inducer and caused her OCP metabolites to be metabolized at a higher-than-normal rate. As such, the OCPs did not last long enough to have their intended effect, and she became pregnant as a result.

Table 23.10. Cytochrome P-450 Interactions

SUBSTRATES	INHIBITORS	INDUCERS
Warfarin	"Azole" antifungals	Barbiturates
Oral contraceptive pills	Macrolides Fluoroquinolones	Rifampin
Statins	Sulfonamides	Phenytoin
Antiepileptics	Cimetidine	Quinidine
Antidepressants	Ciprofloxacin Grapefruit juice Protease inhibitors ("navirs") Acute alcohol abuse Isoniazid Valproic acid Proton pump inhibitors	Carbamazepine Griseofulvin St. John's wort Chronic alcohol abuse

Warfarin is an often-cited example of a CYP-450 substrate. The classic Step 1 vignette will mention a patient who is being treated for atrial fibrillation (they may not explicitly say that the patient is taking warfarin—this is something they may expect you to infer) and is then put on azithromycin for atypical pneumonia. The vignette will then reveal that the patient's international normalized ratio is too high (the target range for atrial fibrillation is 2–3) and ask you why. You, of course, will know the answer: macrolides (including azithromycin) act as CYP-450 inhibitors that will prevent CYP-450 consumption of warfarin, leading to a greater anticoagulant effect.

SUMMARY BOX: CYTOCHROME P-450 DRUG METABOLISM

- CYP-450 is involved in phase I of drug metabolism.
- Key substrates to know: Oral contraceptive pills (OCPs), warfarin, statins, antiepileptics
- Key inhibitors to know: Macrolides, azole antifungals, sulfonamides, ciprofloxacin
- Key inducers to know: Phenytoin, barbiturates, rifampin, chronic alcohol abuse

CHAPTER 24

BEHAVIORAL SCIENCES

Insider's Guide to Behavioral Sciences for the USMLE Step 1

Behavioral science is often overlooked by medical students taking the USMLE Step 1, but in our opinion, this is a huge mistake. Most students say that they wish they had studied more for this section because it can be a huge score booster for those comfortable with the material. Expect to see multiple questions that will present ethical dilemmas and then ask you what you would do in those situations. The ideal way to prepare for such questions is to practice reading through as many ethical scenarios as possible. Your best resources will be the cases in this chapter and those presented to you in question bank software programs. Be sure to pay special attention to exceptions for any rules that apply to ethical situations. Other high-yield behavioral sciences topics include developmental milestones and the physiology and pathophysiology of sleep. You should also know about informed consent, advance directives, and care for minors.

BASIC CONCEPTS

1. Describe the four principles of biomedical ethics.
   - Autonomy: personal rule of the self that is free from controlling influences; physician must honor each patient's preferences in accepting medical care and create conditions that facilitate individuality, autonomous choice, and informed consent (see question 2).
   - Beneficence: fiduciary duty to act in the patient's best interest regardless of what is best for one's self or for society.
   - Nonmaleficence: responsibility to "do no harm"; must be balanced against beneficence if benefits and risks are both present.
   - Justice: responsibility to treat all patients fairly and equitably.

2. What is informed consent?
   Informed consent is the process of obtaining permission before conducting a health care procedure or initiating a particular treatment. To obtain informed consent, all pertinent information (including risks, benefits, and alternative options) must be disclosed to the patient, and the patient must have the ability to comprehend this information, reason through and make their own decision, and be free of coercion. The patient must also be told that they can revoke consent at any time.

   Notable exceptions to informed consent include patients who lack decision-making capacity (see question 3), patients who waive the right to informed consent, or the very uncommon situation of therapeutic privilege (withholding information if it could cause serious psychological damage to the patient). Implied consent can be granted in the case of an emergency.

3. How is decision-making capacity determined?
   To be psychologically and legally capable of making a health care decision, the patient must be:
   - An adult or an emancipated minor
   - Informed
   - Able to make and communicate a choice
   - Able to make a stable decision that is consistent with their values
   - Free of hallucinations, delusions, delirium, or active mood disorders that may directly influence decision-making capacity

4. What should a physician do if a patient requires a treatment not covered by their insurance?
   It is never appropriate to deny a patient proper care because of limitations in time or money. You must discuss all treatment options with the patient regardless of insurance status.

CASE 24.1

A 37-year-old man presents to a psychiatrist for evaluation of symptoms he believes might indicate depression. He reports difficulty sleeping for the last 6 months and that he does not feel rested after 7 to 8 hours of sleep. He also notices difficulty concentrating at work.

---

1. What is the differential diagnosis?
   Depression, sleep apnea, sleep disorders (dyssomnias), adjustment disorder, hypothyroidism, substance abuse or withdrawal, and anxiety should be considered.

CASE 24.1 CONTINUED:

He has had relationship troubles with his spouse and is recently divorced. He reports that her primary reason for leaving him was that he no longer seemed to care about her, as he never wanted to go out or do the things they used to do. She even went so far as to accuse him of having an affair. They stopped sleeping in the same room 2 years ago because of his excessive snoring, with intermittent bursts of awakening short of breath, which kept her up at night. He says he just does not have energy to do things anymore. He also relates having been recently reprimanded at work for falling asleep. On examination, he is a moderately obese, otherwise healthy-appearing middle-aged man. His mental status examination is unremarkable. He denies any thoughts of suicide, appetite disturbances, or feelings of guilt or hopelessness but feels as though he has had a depressed mood since his wife has left.

2. In addition to a diagnosis of adjustment disorder with depressed mood, what sleep-related disorder likely explains most of his symptoms?
   This patient has sleep apnea and would be appropriately diagnosed with a breathing-related sleep disorder. These patients are often obese (a collar size >17 inches should be a red flag); presumably, the weight of the fat around the neck collapses the airway. Sleep is often interrupted at night because of the occluded airway, leading to excessive daytime sleepiness and fatigue. Chronic poor sleep can lead to irritability, poor concentration, and the need to "nap" during the day.

STEP 1 SECRET

Associate "excessive daytime sleepiness" with narcolepsy and obstructive sleep apnea. Both diseases are favorites on the USMLE Step 1.

3. What treatment can be used to allow this man to sleep at night?
   Continuous positive airway pressure (CPAP), which involves pressurizing the airway to keep it patent, could be used. The patient wears a mask that provides positive airway pressure to keep the airway from being obstructed. CPAP is only one treatment option for those patients who suffer from obstructive sleep apnea. As always, lifestyle modifications are important as well. This patient should be encouraged to lose weight, which should reduce the compressive forces on the airway and thereby decrease the airway obstruction. Uvuloplasty or nasal surgery may also be indicated if there are anatomic contributors.
   Note: Sleep studies will show apneic episodes with increasing breathing effort against an obstructed airway, frequent arousals, and decreased rapid eye movement (REM) sleep.

SUMMARY BOX: SLEEP APNEA

- Presentation: Loud snoring, difficulty concentrating, poor memory, and waking up feeling unrested after sleep
- Epidemiology: Most commonly occurs in obese individuals
- Diagnosis: Sleep studies will show apneic episodes, frequent arousals, and decreased rapid eye movement (REM) sleep
- Treatment: May consist of lifestyle modifications and nasal continuous positive airway pressure (CPAP)

CASE 24.2

A 29-year-old woman presents after an automobile accident in which she fell asleep at the wheel. She notes that she frequently falls asleep during the day and feels rested after these episodes.

1. What is the differential diagnosis?
   Sleep deprivation, primary hypersomnia, narcolepsy, sleep apnea, substance abuse or withdrawal, hypothyroidism, and anemia are considerations.

CASE 24.2 CONTINUED:

The patient states that sometimes she awakens but is utterly "unable to move a muscle." She confirms that she has always been able to fall asleep quickly. She denies any use of drugs or medications. You excuse yourself to answer a page and find her asleep when you return to your office. On awakening she is startled at first but then seems to regain her orientation and asks, "What is wrong with me?"

2. What is the likely diagnosis?
   Narcolepsy, a condition that involves poor control of sleep-wake cycles. Individuals with narcolepsy often experience excessive daytime sleepiness that can disrupt normal activities.

3. **What are the stages of sleep, and what happens physiologically in these stages?**
Sleep is divided into non-REM (NREM) and REM sleep. NREM sleep is divided into three stages, each being a deeper sleep. The stages are further described by fast-wave or slow-wave sleep. The earliest two stages are associated with fast-wave sleep, and stage 3 is termed slow-wave sleep based on the electroencephalogram (EEG) appearance of brain waves. REM refers to rapid conjugate eye movement. As a person falls asleep, he or she passes through stages 1 to 3 and then enters REM sleep the first time (this takes approximately 90 minutes). The first REM episode lasts typically less than 10 minutes, and then the person cycles through the stages again, with further REM episodes of about 15 to 40 minutes each.

   Physiologically, during NREM sleep, a person's pulse, respiration rate, and blood pressure are decreased and show less minute-to-minute variation. Resting muscle tone is somewhat relaxed, and there are episodic body movements. Males do not experience erection, and blood flow, including cerebral circulation, is somewhat lowered. By contrast, REM sleep is characterized by higher pulse rate, respiratory rate, and blood pressure, and EEG patterns are similar to those of one who is awake. REM sleep is also termed *paradoxical sleep* because its associated EEG findings appear similar to those found in a person who is awake. Men and women will experience penile/clitoral tumescence (engorgement). In addition, a person in REM sleep experiences near-total skeletal muscle paralysis, and movement is quite rare. Abstract and surreal dreams occur during this phase of sleep. Most REM sleep occurs in the last one-third of the night.

4. **How do nightmares differ from night terrors?**
Nightmares occur almost exclusively in REM sleep. Patients who experience nightmares are able to recall the details of these frightening events, which usually involve threats to life, security, or self-esteem. Upon awakening, the person rapidly becomes oriented. *Night terrors* occur in deep NREM sleep (stage 3). Often, the person wakes in a panicky scream. These patients are often unresponsive on awakening, have amnesia for the episode, and show signs of autonomic arousal, such as tachycardia, tachypnea, and diaphoresis. Night terrors can be treated with benzodiazepines.

5. **Using Table 24.1, cover the columns to the right, and for each stage of sleep listed in the left column, describe the EEG's appearance and associated findings.**

Table 24.1. Electroencephalographic Characteristics of Sleep Stages

STATE	EEG APPEARANCE	FREQUENCY	VOLTAGE	ASSOCIATED FINDINGS
Awake	β waves	Random fast waves	Low	
Eyes closed	α waves	8–12 cycles/s	Low	
Stage 1	θ waves	3–7 cycles/s	Low	Easy to rouse
Stage 2	Sleep spindles K complexes	12–14 cycles/s Slow, triphasic waves	Low High	
Stage 3	δ waves	2–4 cycles/s	High	Bedwetting, sleepwalking, talking, night terrors
REM sleep	β waves	Random fast waves	Low	Dreaming, muscle paralysis, penile/clitoral tumescence

EEG, Electroencephalographic; *REM,* rapid eye movement.

6. **Describe the expected EEG findings in this patient.**
The EEG in a sleep study would likely show a decreased REM latency, meaning that she rapidly progresses into REM sleep. This accounts for the restfulness these patients feel on falling asleep.
   Note: Patients with primary hypersomnia have a completely normal sleep architecture.

7. **What treatments are available for patients with narcolepsy?**
A regimen of regularly scheduled or "forced" naps during the day can be a successful treatment for some patients. In severe cases of narcolepsy, amphetamines such as methylphenidate (Ritalin) are also used. These agents cause the release of norepinephrine, dopamine, and serotonin, but all have some abuse potential. A newer agent, modafinil, has been added that has lower abuse liability. Modafinil appears to selectively decrease somnolence in patients with narcolepsy; however, the mechanism of action is unknown.

8. **This woman had been given a benzodiazepine to assist her sleep, which improved for a while, but now she reports poor sleep once more. Why have her sleep problems returned?**
She is experiencing tolerance to the effects of her medication. Benzodiazepines may be used for short-term management of insomnia, especially when there is an identifiable precipitant, but not for long-term management, because tolerance and dependence may result. Reevaluation should follow a 7- to 10-day trial of benzodiazepine use, and other agents should be considered.

9. How do benzodiazepines manifest their pharmacologic effect?

Benzodiazepines are agonists of γ-aminobutyric acid (GABA) receptors, which are bound to chloride channels. GABA is the primary inhibitory neurotransmitter in the central nervous system (CNS). This CNS inhibition leads to decreased alertness, drowsiness, and less agitation.

Note: Benzodiazepines should be avoided in the elderly because the aged population has a markedly increased (about 25%) incidence of falls when given benzodiazepines because of drowsiness and impaired balance. This effect would be especially concerning in elderly postmenopausal woman, who may have underlying osteopenia or frank osteoporosis.

10. There are now a number of drugs other than benzodiazepines that also act on the GABA benzodiazepine receptor and that reach hypnotic effects with less tolerance and less daytime sedation. What are some examples of these?

Zaleplon (Sonata), zolpidem (Ambien), and eszopiclone (Lunesta) are examples of these drugs.

Note: Sedating antidepressants such as trazodone and nefazodone (remember the z's group) may also be used.

11. When evaluating a person for sleep problems, perhaps the first and most important step is to make sure that the patient has good sleep hygiene. What does good sleep hygiene entail?

- No alcohol
- No caffeine or nicotine
- Regular exercise (but not too late in the day)
- Relaxing activity before bed (e.g., bath, reading)
- Only sleep and sex in the bedroom (no TV)
- No clockwatching
- No daytime naps
- No late meals
- Avoiding screen time before bed
- Regular bedtime

12. What changes in sleep are typical as people age?

Although this is somewhat controversial, for the purpose of boards you should assume that as people age, they experience a decrease in the amount of time in slow-wave sleep (stage 3) and REM sleep. This typically results in a reduced need for time spent sleeping. Insomnia is common in the elderly population.

SUMMARY BOX: NARCOLEPSY

- Presentation: Excessive daytime somnolence, sleep attacks, cataplexy, hypnagogic and hypnopompic hallucinations, sleep paralysis
- Diagnosis: Sleep studies will show decreased sleep latency (falls asleep faster) and earlier entry into rapid eye movement (REM) sleep.
- Complications: Can negatively affect quality of life, social isolation/withdrawal
- Treatment: Scheduled naps during the day, stimulants, and modafinil

---

CASE 24.3

An 80-year-old man with end-stage pulmonary fibrosis presents to the emergency department with multilobar pneumonia, multiorgan failure, and septic shock. He is resuscitated in the emergency department, intubated, and placed on mechanical ventilation. Later, after admission to the intensive care unit, the family arrives and the wife expresses to the admitting doctor that her husband has clearly told her many times that he would not wish to be placed on a ventilator because he knew he had end-stage lung disease. At this moment the patient's oldest son, who currently supports his parents, demands that his father be kept on mechanical ventilation indefinitely to see if he recovers.

---

1. What should the physician do?

The physician should terminate mechanical ventilation. Although the patient cannot give proper informed consent, terminating ventilation is in line with the patient's own wishes.

2. What are advance directives?

Advance directives are instructions provided by a patient in anticipation of the need for a decision to be made regarding their own medical care. They can be oral, written (e.g., living will), or in the form of a durable power of attorney. A durable power of attorney is responsibility assigned to a person by the patient to make medical decisions on their behalf in the event that they lose the capacity to do so. Statements made to others by the patient can qualify as oral advance directives. They gain more validity if they were repeated, heard by multiple persons, and recent. Although oral advance directives provide more flexibility than written directives, problems may arise from inaccurate communication of the patient's wishes or deviations in interpretation.

3. How is decision-making capacity defined?

The patient must be informed (provided with adequate insight regarding all options), able to make and communicate a stable choice, and free from the influence of others (voluntary). The decision cannot result from delusions or hallucinations. Capacity can be assessed by physicians; competence, in contrast, is a legal determination.

4. What is substituted judgment?

If a medical decision must be made on behalf of a patient lacking capacity who does not have any advance directives in place, the rule of substituted judgment can be used. The physician and the patient's surrogate decision makers (individuals who know the patient well enough to determine what he or she would have done) can make a decision for the patient based on *what they would expect the patient would have wanted*. The personal wishes of the physician or family members should not affect this decision.

STEP 1 SECRET

If substituted judgment is required, priority of surrogate decision makers is as follows: spouse, adult children, parents, adult siblings, other relatives.

5. What is the best interests standard, and when should it be used?

The *best interests standard* refers to the decision that most capable people would make in a given scenario. Unlike substituted judgment, it is used when the patient's preferences are completely unknown. Decisions made under the best interests standard should follow the principle of beneficence, which refers to a physician's responsibility to always act in the patient's best interests.

STEP 1 SECRET

Medical decisions should be made according to the following algorithm:
Autonomy (patient's own preference) → advance directives (instructions communicated by the patient to another individual) → substituted judgment (patient's anticipated desire) → best interests standard.

SUMMARY BOX: ADVANCE DIRECTIVES

- A patient is considered to have capacity if they are informed, able to make and communicate a stable decision, and free from the influence of delusions, hallucinations, or other individuals.
- Advance directives can be written, oral, or in the form of a durable power of attorney.
- Substituted judgment or the best interests standard can be used when an incompetent patient does not have any advance directives in place. Substituted judgment anticipates the decision the patient would be expected to make if they were able. The best interests standard is used when the patient's wishes are unknown.

CASE 24.4

A 15-year-old girl comes into your office asking for birth control. She admits that her parents do not know that she is sexually active, and she implores you not to tell them.

1. What should you do?

Write the prescription and agree not to tell her parents. However, you should discuss the risks and benefits of using oral contraceptives with the patient. You should also encourage the patient to communicate with her parents.

2. What are the rules regarding parental consent for minors?

Parental consent is required for minors younger than 18 years, unless the minor is emancipated (married, self-supporting, or in the military). There are, however, several situations in which parental consent is not required. These situations include emergencies, prescription of oral contraceptives, pregnancy-related medical care, and treatment of sexually transmitted infections and drug problems. Abortion generally requires parental consent, although laws vary by state.

SUMMARY BOX: CONSENT FOR MINORS

- Parental consent must be obtained unless the minor is emancipated.
- Exceptions to this rule include emergency situations, drug abuse, pregnancy-related medical care, prescription of oral contraceptives, or treatment of sexually transmitted infections.
- Laws surrounding abortion vary by state.

CASE 24.5

A patient comes into your office with depressive symptoms. You work with her over the next few months to treat her for her depression. During a follow-up visit, she expresses her gratitude for your devotion and assistance and says she would like to make it up to you by taking you out to dinner. She winks, and you understand that she intends it to be a date. Although you do not admit it to her, you find that you are indeed attracted to her as well.

1. What do you do?
   It is *never* acceptable for you to have a romantic relationship with your patients. You should politely decline her invitation and continue to see her as your patient. It is not necessary to refer her to another physician if you can continue to be professional, but it would be a good idea to invite a chaperone into the office during any future visits.

2. Is it a good idea for you to be honest and tell her that you cannot have a relationship with her while she is your patient?
   No. This would send the message that if your professional relationship were terminated, you would be willing to pursue a personal relationship with her, which goes against medical ethics.

STEP 1 SECRET

Whenever the USMLE asks you what to do in a situation similar to the one in Case 24.5, it will often try to entice you with an answer choice that suggests you refer the patient to another physician. For the purpose of boards, this will almost never be correct. The correct choice will require you to be an active participant in the solution.

SUMMARY BOX: THE PHYSICIAN–PATIENT RELATIONSHIP

- The physician–patient relationship should never extend beyond professional boundaries.
  - Under no circumstances is it acceptable to pursue a romantic relationship with a patient. This is true even if the individual is a former patient.
- In the instance that a patient breaches this boundary, your best course of action is to continue to see the patient but to clarify the professional nature of your relationship.
- It is not necessary to refer the patient to another physician, but you may want to bring a chaperone into the office during future appointments with this patient.

CASE 24.6

A patient confides to you that he has been cheating on his wife and now suspects that he may be infected with human immunodeficiency virus (HIV). You perform the appropriate tests, which turn out to be positive. You tell the patient that you will treat him for HIV, but that it is his responsibility to tell his partner. He immediately breaks down and tells you that he cannot tell his wife and all other sexual partners because his wife will leave him once she finds out that he acquired HIV while cheating on her.

1. What do you do?
   Patients who are human immunodeficiency virus (HIV) positive have a duty to protect their sexual partners from acquiring the infection. If the patient fails to do so, the physician is generally allowed (or even mandated, depending on the state of residence) to inform the partner(s).
   Note: Some states have prohibition against warning others, where the physician faces liability for any disclosures without the patient's permission.

2. Under what other conditions is it acceptable to violate patient confidentiality?
   Patient confidentiality should be maintained unless the patient is at significant risk for suicide or poses a risk to another individual. The physician can also intervene in the instance of child or elder abuse. Decisions to disclose information to family and friends should be made according to the patient's best interest if the patient is not present or is incapacitated.
   Note: The *Tarasoff* decision provides physicians with the legal ability to warn a targeted victim and notify the appropriate officials if a patient poses significant risk to another individual.

SUMMARY BOX: PATIENT CONFIDENTIALITY

- Patient confidentiality should be maintained unless a patient is at risk for suicide or harming another individual.
- The physician's role in partner notification for human immunodeficiency virus (HIV)-positive patients depends on the state.

CASE 24.7

A 70-year-old obese man with a history of congestive heart failure and newly diagnosed depression comes into your office because he can no longer sustain an erection. He seems upset because this is greatly affecting his sex life. He admits that he is too embarrassed to discuss this problem with his wife.

1. **What is the differential diagnosis for this patient's sexual dysfunction?**
   Drug effects (beta-blockers, selective serotonin reuptake inhibitors [SSRIs], ethanol), medical diseases (atherosclerosis, depression, diabetes, decreased testosterone levels), and psychological effects (e.g., performance anxiety) can lead to sexual dysfunction. Given this man's history of congestive heart failure, it is likely that he has been taking beta-blockers for some time. He was also newly diagnosed with depression and may have been given an SSRI. Side effects of both of these drugs include sexual dysfunction. This man's age and obesity put him at risk for atherosclerosis and diabetes, which can also contribute to sexual dysfunction. Performance anxiety must be included in the differential diagnosis, particularly if he can sustain erections at certain times of the day (e.g., in the absence of his partner). As the physician, you should include this question in your medical history taking.

2. **What changes occur in the elderly with regard to sexual health?**
   Men are slower to achieve erections and ejaculation and have longer refractory periods. After menopause, women may experience vaginal dryness and irritation. Unless patients are taking particular medications, libido does *not* decrease. Never assume that your elderly patients are not interested in sex or not at risk for sexually transmitted infections. If you do not include sexual health in your history and physical examination, they may be too timid to bring up their concerns on their own!

SUMMARY BOX: SEXUAL HEALTH IN THE ELDERLY

- Elderly men may be slower to achieve erections/ejaculation and may experience increased refractory time.
- Postmenopausal women may experience vaginal dryness and irritation.
- For the purpose of boards, sexual interest does not decrease in the elderly.
- Sexual dysfunction may be attributed to drug effects, diseases, or psychological effects.

CASE 24.8

A 24-year-old patient comes into your office with flulike symptoms. You suspect a viral infection and tell the patient to rest and take plenty of fluids. He becomes irritated with this advice and demands that you prescribe him antibiotics so that he can get over his sickness before his vacation the following week. You hesitate because you know that antibiotics would be of no benefit to the course of this patient's illness.

1. **What should you do?**
   Ask the patient why he feels he needs the antibiotics and politely explain why you feel that it is unnecessary to prescribe them. Although the patient may become argumentative, always keep in mind that it is your decision whether to prescribe a medication to a patient. Avoid writing unnecessary prescriptions.

SUMMARY BOX: PATIENT-REQUESTED PRESCRIPTIONS

- Avoid writing a prescription for a patient if you as the physician do not consider the medication to be an appropriate treatment.

CASE 24.9

You are working alongside a second-year resident during your inpatient medicine rotation. Over the past 2 weeks, you have noticed abrupt changes in the resident's dress and behavior. He often arrives to work late and ungroomed. You have also noticed that his breath frequently smells like alcohol. You suspect that he has been drinking heavily.

1. **What do you do?**
   It is your responsibility to protect patients from receiving inadequate or negligent care from an impaired or incompetent medical professional. You may choose to directly confront the resident in a nonthreatening manner (preferable). Alternatively, you may take a more formal approach and voice your concerns to the attending physician or the residency director.

STEP 1 SECRET

For the purpose of Step 1, you should never select an answer that suggests you do nothing.

2. What is the CAGE questionnaire?

The CAGE questionnaire is a widely used method for screening for alcohol abuse. You are expected to know this acronym for boards. If a patient responds with "yes" to more than one of the following questions, the patient should be examined further for alcohol use disorder.

- Have you ever felt like you should **C**ut down on your drinking?
- Are you ever **A**nnoyed by people criticizing you for drinking?
- Have you ever felt **G**uilty because of your drinking?
- Have you ever needed a drink first thing in the morning (**E**ye-opener) to get out of bed or start your day?

SUMMARY BOX: ALCOHOL ABUSE

- It is your responsibility to protect patients from receiving care from any medical professional who is under the influence of alcohol or drugs.
- You may choose to directly confront the colleague in question or involve others.
- The CAGE questionnaire is often used as a screening tool for alcoholism.
- You should know the components of this acronym (see text).

CASE 24.10

A mother brings her 2-year-old child to the pediatrician's office for a well-child visit. She is concerned that her child still does not speak in full sentences. She also says that despite numerous attempts, she has been unable to toilet-train her child even though her neighbor's 2-year-old child has had success.

1. Is this child developing normally?

Yes. See Table 24.2 for developmental milestones.

Table 24.2. Developmental Milestones

AGE	GROSS MOTOR	FINE MOTOR	LANGUAGE	OTHER
Infant Birth–3 months	Rolls over (3 months)	Rooting reflex	—	Orients to voice Social smile

3–6 months	Sits up (6 months)	Puts hands together
		  (3 months)
		Passes items
		  (6 months)
			Strings syllables
			  together
				Moro reflex disappears
				Stranger anxiety

6–9 months	Crawls	Pincer grasp	—	Feeds self Separation anxiety Orients to name and gestures
Toddler 12 months	Walks	Stacks 3 blocks	Speaks 1–3 words	Drinks from a cup
15 months	Runs Walks backward	—	Speaks 6 words	Babinski reflex disappears Separation anxiety
18 months	Climbs stairs Kicks ball	Stacks 4 blocks	Combines words	Brushes teeth with help

2 years	Jumps (upward)	Stacks 6 blocks
		Feeds self with
		  utensils
			Speaks >200 words
			Uses 2-word
			  sentences
				Washes hands
				Begins to engage in parallel
				  play

Continued

Table 24.2. Developmental Milestones—cont'd

AGE	GROSS MOTOR	FINE MOTOR	LANGUAGE	OTHER
Preschool				
3 years	Jumps (forward) Rides tricycle	Stacks 9 blocks Draws circles and dashes	Completely understandable	Brushes teeth Plays board games Toilet training Develops gender identity Comfortable spending a few hours away from parents
4 years	Hops on one foot	Copies stick figure	Uses prepositions and complete sentences Tells detailed stories	Dresses self Plays cooperatively and with imaginary friends
5 years	—	Draws squares and triangles Ties shoes	—	Identifies colors Counts to 5 Grooms self

2. What should you tell this concerned parent?

The mother should be told that every child develops differently, and that her child is on track for normal development. Do not automatically dismiss the mother's concerns; be sure that she feels comfortable coming to you if she notices "anything else that she considers unusual."

SUMMARY BOX: DEVELOPMENTAL MILESTONES

- You should know the information listed in Table 24.2. This is an extremely high-yield topic for boards.

CASE 24.11

A 24-year-old patient with type 1 diabetes is admitted to the hospital after an insulin overdose that resulted in hypoglycemic seizures. You go in to see the patient once she is stabilized. You ask her whether she uses her insulin regularly, and she tells you that she sometimes gives herself injections according to the doctor's instructions. When you ask her how much insulin she injects, she shrugs and tells you that it varies, depending on the food she eats. You ask her to clarify, and she tells you, "I give myself less if I skip meals and more whenever I eat junk food. I am supposed to count the carbs to determine the injection amount, but that is too much work, so I just guess."

1. How should you handle this situation?

Hypoglycemia is an inevitable situation in type 1 diabetes (it is impossible to prevent all episodes of hypoglycemia or hyperglycemia), but this patient is putting herself at increased risk for both by not following her treatment plan and dosing her insulin without being intentional about the doses for the meal she is eating. She is correct that lower-carbohydrate meals require less mealtime insulin dosing and higher carbohydrate meals require more mealtime insulin dosing, but this is typically based on calculating the amount of carbohydrates in the food (often using labels or food databases) and then calculating how much insulin to give. This is a lot of work to do correctly and patients may not adhere. The most important thing to remember when dealing with a nonadherent patient is that scolding will be ineffective in preventing future mishaps (and will never be the correct answer on boards!). Instead, you must have a discussion with the patient to figure out the reason for the nonadherence and work together to fix the problem.

Note: In severe cases, patients may be dismissed by a physician for nonadherence. For the purpose of boards, this is not likely to be the correct answer.

2. How can adherence be increased in the future?

As mentioned previously, it is crucial to determine the reason for the patient's nonadherence. Therefore, it is important to figure out whether this patient is neglecting the physician's instructions because (1) she does not understand them, (2) she does not know the importance of following them, (3) it is difficult for her to adhere to them, or (4) there are psychosocial reasons preventing her from adhering to them (e.g., lack of insurance or transportation). If you get the feeling that a patient does not understand the directions, do your best not to embarrass the patient. Instead, tell the patient that this could happen to anyone and simplify your instructions. Have the patient repeat the instructions back to you when you are done so that you know she has understood correctly (teach-back technique). Write the instructions down whenever possible. This is especially important to consider whenever the patient is not a native English speaker.

Sometimes, it is difficult for a patient to adhere to the treatment plan. Vials and pens of insulin that are not being used, for example, must be refrigerated (the current pen or vial being used can be at room temperature for up to a month). Consider a scenario in which a patient with diabetes travels a lot for work and does not always have access to a refrigerator. Similarly, patients may fear they cannot afford their medications. Reassure patients that your team will help with this and include resources such as a social worker.

It is also a good idea to make sure that the patient understands why it is important to follow a specified treatment plan. Perhaps she does not understand the reason behind regulated insulin doses. Educating the patient will more likely motivate her to follow the treatment plan correctly. Do not attempt to scare the patient into complying with a treatment plan. (For example, it is unethical to show the patient graphic pictures of gangrene and say, "This will happen to you if you don't shape up!")

SUMMARY BOX: THE NONADHERENT PATIENT

- Nonadherence is a common hurdle faced by all patients and physicians.
- Patients should not be scolded for their nonadherence. It is more important to determine the reason for the nonadherence and attempt to fix the problem.
- Never use scare tactics in an attempt to improve a patient's compliance.

CASE 24.12

A 68-year-old man is brought to your office by his wife because of abdominal pain, jaundice, and unintentional weight loss. A computed tomography scan of the abdomen reveals probable adenocarcinoma of the head of the pancreas. When you walk into the office to break the news to the patient, his wife asks to speak to you alone outside. The two of you step out of the office and she confesses that she has a feeling you are returning with bad news. "Please tell me first," she begs. "If it's really bad, I know my husband won't be able to handle it. If I know what it is, I can help break the news to him in time."

1. How should you handle this situation with the patient's wife?
   It is unlawful to disclose a patient's medical information to family or friends without the permission of the patient. Therefore you should avoid revealing any information to the patient's wife at this time. You should, however, find out why the patient's wife is so concerned about her husband's ability to handle the news. Her concerns will perhaps guide your approach to handling this patient.

2. What should you say to the patient when you walk into the room?
   You should tell the patient that you have some news to discuss with him and politely dismiss his wife for the time being. At this point, you can ask the patient whether he would like his wife to be present. If he agrees, you can invite her back into the room. Asking the patient's permission for his wife to remain in the room in her presence might pressure his decision. If the patient states when the wife is out of the room that his preference is that the wife is told for now and not him, that is permissible as the patient has the right to make this decision.

SUMMARY BOX: DISCLOSURE OF PATIENT INFORMATION

- It is unlawful to disclose any patient information to family or friends without explicit permission from the patient.
- Always ask to speak to a patient privately before discussing confidential medical information in front of others.

CASE 24.13

A 50-year-old woman presents to your clinic reporting burning pain during urination and increased urinary frequency. Already several patients behind, you quickly diagnose a urinary tract infection and prescribe a course of trimethoprim-sulfamethoxazole. The patient returns the next day with a new maculopapular rash and pruritus. On closer review of her chart, you discover she had a similar reaction in the past to trimethoprim-sulfamethoxazole. The patient asks if this reaction could have been caused by the antibiotic you prescribed.

1. What should you do?
   Physicians have an ethical obligation to inform a patient if a medical error that has caused harm has been made. Acknowledging and apologizing for medical errors improves the physician–patient relationship and can potentially decrease the likelihood of litigation. Primary motivators for patients who file lawsuits are perceived dishonesty on the part of the physician and lack of explanation for the incident.
   Note: For the purposes of the boards, you should never choose the answer choice that avoids disclosure.

CASE 24.14

A 45-year-old patient comes into your office with his wife and reports that he has been experiencing a frequent sensation of his "legs falling asleep." His discomfort causes an urge to constantly move his limbs because he feels much better when he is active. His wife states that her husband continually jerks his legs in his sleep. This activity disrupts both his and her sleep patterns, and both profess feeling tired throughout the day.

1. What is the most likely diagnosis?

   Restless legs syndrome (RLS), a disorder of unknown etiology that causes a constant urge to move in attempt to relieve unpleasant sensations in the lower limbs, is likely. It has been linked to several conditions, including Parkinson disease, rheumatoid arthritis, diabetes, kidney failure, and iron deficiency anemia. Use of certain medications may also trigger RLS. However, RLS is often idiopathic in nature.

2. What are the most common symptoms of RLS?

   Symptoms include an unpleasant sensation in the legs, urge to constantly move, relief upon movement, and worsening of symptoms when inactive. Typical leg movements associated with RLS are jiggling, pacing, tossing, rubbing, and stretching. Limb movements often occur during sleep.

3. How is RLS treated?

   The antiparkinsonian medication ropinirole, which increases synaptic dopamine availability, is first-line therapy. Although there is no direct cure for RLS, the treatment plan should involve identifying and correcting any underlying cause of the condition whenever possible. Treatment also focuses on symptom relief and includes sleep improvement, alcohol avoidance (alcohol may trigger RLS symptoms), walking, and heat/cold packs on the affected limbs.

SUMMARY BOX: RESTLESS LEGS SYNDROME

• Presentation: Unpleasant leg sensations, urge to move constantly, worsening of symptoms when inactive, limb movements during sleep
• Epidemiology: Linked to several conditions (Parkinson disease, rheumatoid arthritis, diabetes, kidney failure, iron deficiency anemia, use of certain medications) but can be idiopathic in nature
• Treatment: Dopaminergic agent ropinirole. Focus on treating the underlying cause of the disease and providing patients with symptom relief

BIOSTATISTICS

BASIC CONCEPTS

1. **What does the sensitivity of a diagnostic test measure?**

The *sensitivity* of a diagnostic test measures how effectively the test can detect disease in a patient who truly has the disease. Study and understand the layout of Table 25.1, as this 2 × 2 table will provide you the information you need to answer first-order biostatistics questions. This table can be used to organize your thoughts when attempting the basic biostatistics calculations you may be asked to perform on your USMLE Step 1 exam.

The total number of individuals who truly have the disease of interest (i.e., in whom disease is truly present) can be calculated by summing a + c. The sensitivity of a test represents the proportion of these individuals who truly have the disease (a + c) *and* who successfully tested positive for the disease (a). These individuals are called *true positives* (TP). The diseased individuals who incorrectly tested negative for the disease are categorized as *false negatives* (FN; c). In other words, sensitivity can be calculated by dividing the number of TP by the total number of truly diseased individuals: TP/(TP + FN), or a/(a + c). *Sensitivity* is also referred to as the *true-positive rate* and improves with either an increase in the percentage of a diseased population who correctly test positive or with a decrease in the number of false-negative test results. Note that sensitivity is inversely related to the false-negative rate [c/(a + c)] by the formula shown in Eq. 25.1:

$$\text{Sensitivity} = 1 - \text{False-Negative Rate} \qquad [25.1]$$

Table 25.1. Sample 2 x 2 Biostatistics Table

	PRESENCE OF DISEASE (+)	**ABSENCE OF DISEASE (−)**
(+) Test result	True positive (a)	False positive (b)
(−) Test result	False negative (c)	True negative (d)

A test with 100% sensitivity therefore, if negative, would absolutely rule out the disease because it is always positive in the presence of disease.

STEP 1 SECRET

Practice setting up tables like Table 25.1 whenever you encounter a biostatistics problem that involves sensitivity or specificity. Doing so will help you immensely on all USMLE exams, not just Step 1! It will be helpful to copy this specific table onto your whiteboard before the start of your exam, along with the basic equations for sensitivity and the other statistical values that you will learn in this chapter.

2. **What does the specificity of a diagnostic test measure?**
The *specificity* of a diagnostic test measures the ability of a test to detect absence of disease in patients who truly do not have the disease. In other words, specificity measures the percentage of truly disease-free individuals who correctly test negative for the disease. Let us again turn our attention to Table 25.1.

$$\text{Specificity} = \text{True Negatives/(True Negatives + False Positives)} = d/(d + b) \qquad [25.2]$$

Specificity is inversely related to false-positive rate as follows:

$$\text{Specificity} = 1 - \text{False-Positive Rate} \qquad [25.3]$$

Given this relationship, the specificity of a test will increase as the number of false-positive (FP) test results decreases. The utility of *specificity* when interpreting medical tests is the fact that the more *specific* the test, the more likely a positive result indicates the true presence of disease.

STEP 1 SECRET

SP(+)IN and SN(-)OUT are useful mnemonics to remember the differences between specificity and sensitivity. **SP(+) IN** reminds us that **SP**ecific tests rule **IN** disease when positive (+). The more specific a test, the more likely it is that a positive test result indicates true presence of that disease, because a highly specific test will have a small number of false-positive results. **SN(-)OUT** reminds us that Se**N**sitive tests rule **OUT** disease when negative (-). The more sensitive a test, the more likely that a negative test result correctly rules out disease, because a highly sensitive test will have a small number of false-negative results.
SP+IN: SPecific tests rule IN when positive
SN-OUT: SeNsitive tests rule OUT when negative
In serious diseases where significant differences in outcome may result from a failure of early detection, greater test *sensitivity* is often desired, even at the expense of lower specificity.

---

3. **Let us review: Cover the right column in Table 25.2, and define each of the terms in the left column.**

Table 25.2. Basic Terminology of Biostatistics Test Results

TERM	DEFINITION
True positive	A *positive* test result in someone who truly *does* have the disease
False positive	A *positive* test result in someone who truly does *not* have the disease
True negative	A *negative* test result in someone who truly does *not* have the disease
False negative	A *negative* test result in someone who truly *does* have the disease

4. **How does the sensitivity of a test relate to its specificity?**
These two statistical measures have an inverse relationship: as sensitivity increases, specificity decreases, and vice versa. Consider the example of using prostate-specific antigen (PSA) levels as a screening tool for prostate cancer. Serum PSA levels above 10 ng/dL are typically considered to be high risk, and approximately 50% of these individuals will truly have prostate cancer. On the contrary, only one in four individuals with levels between 4 to 10 ng/dL will have evidence of prostate cancer on biopsy. If the threshold for a "positive" test result was lowered from 10 ng/dL to 6 ng/dL, more individuals with prostate cancer would likely be detected, leading to *increased sensitivity*. At this lower threshold, however, the *specificity* of the test would *decrease* because there would be a greater chance that other factors unrelated to prostate cancer (e.g., benign prostatic hyperplasia) may be driving PSA levels up, therefore increasing the number of false-positive test results (Fig. 25.1). Recall that specificity is equal to 1 – false-positive rate. Because lower threshold values will increase the false-positive rate, specificity will therefore decrease.

5. **What is positive predictive value (PPV)? Negative predictive value (NPV)?**
The *positive predictive value* (PPV) is the probability that the disease in question is truly present in patients who received a positive test result. In other words, PPV = (true positives)/(true positives + false positives).
The *negative predictive value* (NPV) is the probability that the disease in question is truly absent in patients who receive a negative test result. NPV = (true negatives)/(true negatives + false negatives).
In a classic biostatistics 2 × 2 table (see Table 25.1), the PPV can be calculated by dividing the number of true positives by the total number of positive test results: PPV = a/(a + b). NPV is calculated by dividing the number of true negatives by the total number of negative test results: NPV = d/(c + d).
You should note that both PPV and NPV vary with disease prevalence. If disease prevalence increases, the numbers in the (+) disease column (TP and FN) will both increase. Because PPV = TP/(TP + FP), PPV will increase if prevalence (and therefore TP) increases, where FP = false positives. On the other hand, NPV will decrease as disease

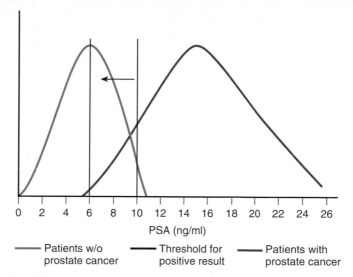

— Patients w/o   — Threshold for   — Patients with
     prostate cancer   positive result   prostate cancer

Figure 25.1. Relationship of sensitivity to specificity using the example of serum PSA levels to detect prostate cancer. Note that lowering the threshold for a positive result from 10 ng/ml to 6 ng/ml will increase sensitivity (due to fewer false negatives) and decrease specificity (due to more false positives). *PSA,* Prostate-specific antigen; *w/o,* without.

prevalence increases, because the number of FN (c) will increase. The sensitivity and specificity are characteristics of the test, but if the prevalence of disease is very low, even excellent test characteristics would have relatively low positive or negative predictive values. For instance, if you had a disease that had a prevalence of 1 in 6 billion and a test with 99% specificity, most of your positive tests would be false positives, because the true-positive rate is so low and there would be a low PPV of a positive test.

6. **What information is given by the relative risk (RR)? How is RR typically applied?**
The relative risk (RR) informs you of the ratio of the probability of a disease occurring in a group exposed to a particular risk factor versus that same disease occurring in a nonexposed group. RR is calculated by dividing the incidence of disease in the exposed group by the incidence of disease in the unexposed group. Examine Table 25.3.

Table 25.3. Sample 2 x 2 Table for Determining Relative Risk and Odds Ratio

	PRESENCE OF DISEASE (+)	ABSENCE OF DISEASE (−)
(+) Exposed	(a)	(b)
(−) Nonexposed	(c)	(d)

The percentage of exposed individuals who have developed disease can be determined by a/(a + b). Likewise, the percentage of nonexposed individuals who have developed disease can be determined by c/(c + d). Thus RR = [a/(a + b)] ÷ [c/(c + d)].

Note that this table is identical to Table 25.1 except that the "Test Result" terminology has simply been substituted for "Exposure" status.

The primary application of RR is to identify any underlying associations between a particular exposure and a particular outcome. For example, look at the sample data provided in Table 25.4. Following the calculations described previously, the incidence of lung cancer in smokers is a/(a + b) = 90/(90 + 10) = 90/100 = 0.90, and the incidence of lung cancer in nonsmokers is c/(c + d) = 10/(10 + 90) = 10/100 = 0.10. Based on this information, the RR for lung cancer in smokers is 0.90/0.10, or 9. The RR of 9 implies that smokers are nine times more likely to develop lung cancer than nonsmokers.

An RR >1 implies that the disease is *more likely* to occur in the exposed group.
An RR <1 implies that the disease is *less likely* to occur in the exposed group (i.e., that the exposure may be protective).
An RR = 1 implies that there is *no difference* in disease occurrence between exposed and non-exposed groups.

Table 25.4. Example Data Set for Lung Cancer in Smokers Versus Nonsmokers

	LUNG CANCER (+)	LUNG CANCER (−)
Smoker	90	10
Nonsmoker	10	90

7. **What information is given by the odds ratio (OR)?**

Similar to RR, the odds ratio (OR) provides a measure of association between exposure status and disease outcome. However, OR is used in case-control studies, whereas RR is used in cohort studies and randomized controlled trials. (We discuss the differences between these study types later in this chapter.) A memory trick that some students use to correctly correlate OR and RR to the appropriate study type is recognizing that the there are two "o"s in "case-control" same as in "**o**dds rati**o**." The OR is typically *retrospective*, meaning it is typically used to determine whether a past exposure was a potential risk factor for a present outcome of interest. This differs from RR, which can be used *prospectively* to determine the likelihood of future disease occurrence given a particular exposure status at the present time.

The OR is calculated by dividing the odds of exposure in the diseased group by the odds of exposure in the disease-free group. Examine Table 25.3.

$$OR = (a/c) \div (b/d) = ad/bc \qquad [25.4]$$

Let's say that you wanted to determine the odds that individuals with or without lung cancer were previously smokers. Given the information in Table 25.4, the OR would be calculated by dividing the odds of smoke exposure in individuals with lung cancer (a/c, or 90/10) by the odds of smoke exposure in those without lung cancer (b/d, or 10/90).

$$OR = \frac{90/10}{10/90} = \frac{90 \times 90}{10 \times 10} = \frac{8100}{100} = 81$$

In other words, the odds of prior smoke exposure (or smoking history) is 81 times higher in individuals with lung cancer than those without lung cancer.

An OR >1 means that the exposure occurred *more frequently* in the disease group.
An OR <1 means that the exposure occurred *less frequently* in the disease group.
An OR = 1 means that the exposure occurred with the *same frequency* in the disease and disease-free groups.

Note: For diseases that are *rare* (as well as for case-control studies where the exposure rate of the studied population is similar to that of the general population), the OR approximates the RR.

8. **What is the difference between probability and odds, and how are they measured?**

Probability and *odds* both measure the likelihood that a particular event will occur. *Probability* is expressed as a ratio from 0 to 1 and is defined by the number of results that would produce a particular outcome divided by the number of all potential outcomes. For example, the probability of rolling a six-sided die and having it land on the number 3 is 1/6 or 0.167; in this case, there are six potential outcomes (numbers 1 to 6), and only one option (the number 3) produces the desired result.

Odds are defined as the chance of a particular desired outcome occurring divided by the chance that *any* undesired outcome will occur. In the six-sided die example, the *odds* of rolling a 3 (versus not rolling a 3) are 1 to 5 or 0.2, because there is one desired option (the number 3) but five undesired options (the other five sides of the die).

The two concepts may be interconverted using the formulas shown in Eqs. 25.5 and 25.6:

$$Odds = Probability/(1 - Probability) \qquad [25.5]$$

and

$$Probability = Odds/(1 + Odds) \qquad [25.6]$$

Do the math with the six-sided die example, and see for yourself that these formulas really work!

9. **What are likelihood ratios?**

Likelihood ratios help us determine how much we should shift our degree of suspicion for a particular disease based on a given test result. Unlike PPV and NPV, likelihood ratios are *not* influenced by disease prevalence. The *positive likelihood ratio* (PLR) reflects how much a *positive* test result *increases* the probability of disease being present over the baseline prevalence. The higher the ratio, the more likely a positive test result indicates the presence of disease.

$$PLR = Sensitivity/(1 - Specificity) = (True\text{-}Positive\ Rate)/(False\text{-}Positive\ Rate) \qquad [25.7]$$

For example, if the sensitivity of a particular test is 85% and the specificity is 90%, the PLR is 0.85/(1 − 0.9) = 8.5. In this example, a positive test result means that the individual is 8.5 times more likely to have the disease in question. The more sensitive and specific the test, the higher the PLR. PLRs between 2 and 5 often indicate a small to moderate increase in the likelihood of disease given a positive test result, whereas a PLR of 10 or more generally indicates a significant increase in the likelihood of disease given a positive test result.

Negative likelihood ratio (NLR) indicates how much the probability of disease *decreases* if a test is *negative*.

$$NLR = (1 - Sensitivity/Specificity = (False\text{-}Positive\ Rate)/(True\text{-}Positive\ Rate) \qquad [25.8]$$

In the previous example, NLR = (1 − 0.85)/0.9 = 0.17, indicating that a negative test result means that the individual is 5.9 times more likely *not* to have the disease in question.

10. **What is meant by the reliability of a test?**

    Reliability (also called *precision*) is the ability to reproduce similar results with each repetition of the same test. For example, the USMLE Step 1 exam would be considered reliable if a student could take it repeatedly and get close to the same score each time. It would not be considered a reliable (or precise) exam if the same student received significantly different scores when taking the test on different dates. Precision is improved by reducing *random error*.

11. **What is meant by the validity of a test?**

    Validity (also called *accuracy*) is a measure of how closely a test's results come to the "true value," which is defined by the gold-standard test. Validity is improved by minimizing *systematic error*. *Systematic error* refers to deviations from the true value of a measurement that result from poor instrument calibration or flawed observation methods.

12. **In statistical analyses of differences between groups, a *P* value is often included to reflect how significant the difference is. What is the meaning of this *P* value?**

    P value reflects the probability that the difference observed between the experimental and control groups could occur by chance alone.

    For example, if the *P* value between an experimental and control group is .05, there is a 5% chance that the observed difference between the groups was due entirely to chance rather than the variable being tested in the experiment. In modern medical literature, the accepted convention is to consider results as "significant" if there is less than a 5% chance (e.g., $P < .05$) that the observed difference between experimental and control groups could have occurred by chance alone. Some studies will report even more stringent *P* value ranges (e.g., $P < .01$ or $P < .001$). These indicate an increasing confidence that the observed results stemmed from the experimental variable or intervention rather than mere chance.

STEP 1 SECRET

P values are very important for you to understand for both the USMLE Step 1 exam and for interpreting scientific literature during your medical career. In addition to P *values, type I and type II errors (discussed in question 13) are commonly tested board topics.*

---

13. **What are the differences between type I and type II errors? How is *statistical power* related to type II error?**

    Type I (α) error is the *false-positive error*. It is the probability of claiming that a difference exists between two groups when none truly exists. The *null hypothesis* (H_0) refers to the assertion that no meaningful difference exists between two observed groups. If a researcher claims a statistical difference between two groups when none truly exists, therefore incorrectly rejecting the null hypothesis, the researcher has committed a type I error. In contrast, a type II (β) error is the *false-negative error*. It refers to the probability of stating that no difference exists between two groups or populations when in fact there truly is a difference. Type II error is an incorrect acceptance of the null hypothesis, when in fact it should be rejected.

    Say we wish to determine the factors that influence USMLE Step 1 scores among medical students. We hypothesize that more time spent studying for the exam leads to significantly higher scores. A study is planned to test this concept by comparing scores between students who studied for 6 weeks and students who studied for 6 months. Let us suppose that we do not find that test scores differ significantly between the two groups of students despite differences in study time. If USMLE Step 1 scores are truly influenced by time spent studying among the general population of medical students, we have made a type II error by incorrectly accepting our null hypothesis.

    The term *statistical power* is the likelihood that a study can detect a difference between means (i.e., between groups) if one truly exists. Power analysis is often performed before conducting a research study to verify that the sample size is large enough to detect a significant effect of an independent variable. You certainly do not need to know how to perform a power analysis for the USMLE Step 1, but you should note that as power is increased, the likelihood of committing a type II error decreases (Eq. 25.9):

$$\text{Power} = 1 - \beta. \tag{25.9}$$

    Makes sense, right? Because β is the probability of committing a type II error (e.g., incorrectly accepting the null hypothesis by not detecting a difference that truly exists), power is inversely related to this value. This inverse relationship can be clearly observed in Table 25.5. Power increases and β decreases as sample size, precision, and expected effect size increase.

Table 25.5. Relationship Among Type I Error, Type II Error, and Power

	ACTUAL DIFFERENCE EXISTS BETWEEN GROUPS	NO ACTUAL DIFFERENCE EXISTS BETWEEN GROUPS
Significant experimental difference observed (i.e., $P < .05$)	Correct finding; study adequately powered	Type I (α error)
No significant experimental difference observed (i.e., $P > .05$)	Type II (β error)	Correct finding; increasing sample size will not alter results

14. **What are some determinants that can be used to evaluate the existence of a causal relationship between two variables?**
    - *Consistency:* Multiple studies independently support the same conclusion (e.g., six reports from different institutions provide evidence that angiotensin-converting enzyme [ACE] inhibitors reduce blood pressure).
    - *Biologic plausibility:* The proposed relationship between cause and outcome is consistent with current scientific knowledge (e.g., blocking the renin-angiotensin-aldosterone axis would be expected to decrease blood pressure).
    - *Temporality:* The cause must *precede* disease outcome (e.g., asbestos exposure precedes malignant mesothelioma of the pleura).
    - *Coherence:* Correlations between epidemiological and laboratory studies increase the likelihood of an effect (e.g., results from animal studies support the hypothesis).
    - *Dose-response relationship:* Greater exposure leads to a more severe phenotype or increased likelihood of disease (e.g., increased number of pack years in smokers directly correlates with increased risk of lung cancer).
    - *Reversibility:* Lack of exposure results in reduced likelihood of contracting disease; this is particularly powerful if a strong dose-response relationship has also been observed (e.g., reducing exposure to radiation reduces the likelihood of developing acute leukemia).
    - *Specificity:* Indicates more specific associations between an exposure and outcome with no additional explanations that enhance the probability of causation (e.g., one-to-one relationship is noted between exposure to drug X and a particular side effect).

15. **What is the difference between** *prevalence* **and** *incidence*?
    Prevalence is the percentage of the population that currently has the disease. For example, 35% of Americans are obese, so the prevalence of obesity is 35%. *Incidence* refers to how many people *develop* a disease *within a given time frame* (usually annually). For example, if 300,000 individuals are newly diagnosed with diabetes each year, the annual incidence of diabetes is 300,000.

16. **How do the incidence and duration of a disease affect its prevalence?**
    The higher the incidence and the longer the duration of the disease, the greater the prevalence of the disease.

$$\text{Prevalence} = \text{Incidence} \times \text{Duration of Disease} \qquad [25.10]$$

   Chronic diseases (e.g., arthritis, hypertension, diabetes mellitus) are unlikely to rapidly result in death, so the prevalence is typically high due to longer duration of disease. The opposite trend is true of diseases that have a short duration (e.g., meningitis), either because they rapidly result in death or because they resolve quickly, leading to a relatively high incidence but low prevalence.

MEASURES OF SPREAD

17. **The following sample distribution pattern lists the ages of 11 patients seen by a physician on a given day:**

1, 2, 3, 3, 3, 4, 5, 5, 7, 8, 80

   A. What are the mean, median, and mode for the ages of the patients seen by the physician on this day?
   The *mean* is simply the average value of the sample population, which is calculated by adding together all of the results and dividing this sum by the sample size. In this example, the mean would be 11, because (121/11 = 11). The *median* is the number in the middle of the data set when ordered sequentially. Half of the data will lie above the median and half will lie below. In this example, when the numbers are ordered sequentially (as they are given), the number 4 has equal numbers of values above and below it, making it the median. In cases in which there is an even number of results, the median is calculated by taking the average of the middle two numbers. The *mode* is the number present with the highest frequency; in this case, the mode is 3.
   B. Is the mean or the median more representative of central tendency?
   The median is less affected by outliers (e.g., 80 in this example) than the mean and is often a better representation of central tendency than the mean, particularly for small sample sizes containing multiple outliers.
   C. Is this sample "skewed" at all, and if so, in which direction?
   Yes, this sample population is positively skewed (i.e., to the right) because of the outlier value 80. In Fig. 25.2, graph A represents a positive skew and graph B a negative skew. Positive skew occurs when there are outliers that have a higher value than the numbers closer to the mean, whereas negative skew occurs when the outliers have a lower value then the numbers close to the mean.

STEP 1 SECRET

When looking at a distribution graph, an easy way to determine where the mode is located is to look at the peak of the distribution. The mode is the value that occurs at the peak because it is the outcome that appears most frequently. The mean will be located on the same side as the longer "tail" of the distribution, whereas the median is typically found in between the mean and the mode. Recall that in a normal (Gaussian) statistical distribution (i.e., the classic bell curve), mean, median, and mode will all be equal.

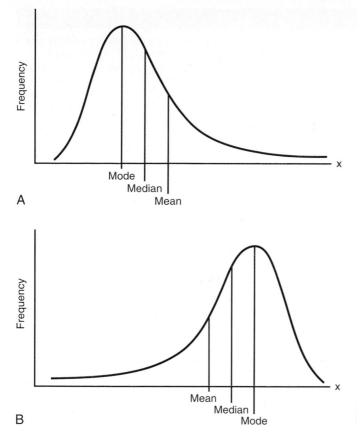

Figure 25.2. Examples of skewed data sets: (A) Positive skew, (B) negative skew.

18. What does the standard deviation of a population represent?
The *standard deviation* (σ) is a measure of how spread out the values of a test population are. If most of the values are close to the mean, the standard deviation will be small. On the other hand, if many of the values are far from the mean, the standard deviation will be larger.

In a normal distribution, all the members of a population within one standard deviation of the mean (both above and below) will constitute approximately 68% of the total population. All members within two standard deviations will constitute approximately 95% of the total population, while three standard deviations will contain approximately 99.7% of the data set. Fig. 25.3 illustrates the standard deviations along a classic Gaussian bell curve.

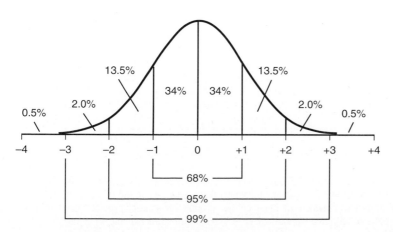

Figure 25.3. Standard deviations along a classic Gaussian bell curve.

STEP 1 SECRET

You are expected to know the percentages that fall within each standard deviation along a normal-shaped bell curve distribution for the USMLE Step 1 exam. Recall that the data are distributed evenly on both sides of the mean! Remembering the 68-95-99.7 rule for normal distributions will be extremely helpful on test day. Many students get confused by this concept on the exam, but it is a high yield topic that will net easy points when understood. For example, if you are asked to calculate how much of the data falls outside of the range of two standard deviations in a normal distribution, the answer is 5% because 95% of the data will fall within the range of two standard deviations. If you are asked to calculate how much of the data falls above two standard deviations, the answer is 2.5% because half of the 5% that is not contained within two standard deviations will fall above the curve and half will fall below. As obvious as this may sound to you now, pay close attention to the question being asked on your exam! It is easy to fall into these types of traps when you are under pressure on test day.

STUDY DESIGNS

19. What is meant by the term *bias*, and which study design best eliminates bias?

Bias is *systematic error* that affects one study group more than the other. This differs from *random error*, which typically affects both groups equally and should not adversely affect the study if there are enough participants. Randomized controlled trials (RCTs) typically control most effectively for bias, whereas case-control studies typically control bias least effectively. Other types of study designs (e.g., cohort, cross-sectional) fall somewhere between these two extremes in their ability to eliminate bias. Table 25.6 reviews concepts pertaining to study design in more detail. It is important to know which measures of association (i.e., OR or RR) are used in each study design. As discussed previously, remember that case-c**O**ntr**O**l studies use **O**dds Rati**O**, while coho**R**t and **R**andomized studies use **R**elative **R**isk.

Table 25.6. Commonly Tested Study Designs

STUDY DESIGN	SETUP	STRENGTHS	LIMITATIONS
Cohort study	A "cohort" of subjects is classified according to exposure status and then followed to determine the effect of exposure on disease outcome.	Relatively easy to set up compared with randomized studies Allows for the study of exposures that are known or suspected to be harmful Establishes a causal relationship between exposure and outcome variables	*Confounding variables*: The exposure being studied may *correlate* with the disease outcome but may not be the *cause*. There may be other "confounding" variables within the study population that make it difficult to accurately distinguish correlation from causality.
Case-control study	Subjects are classified according to the presence or absence of disease, and correlations are made between past exposures and the presence of disease.	Easiest study type to set up Allows for the study of exposures that are known or suspected to be harmful	May be affected by recall bias and interviewer bias (see Case 25.1, question 4) Does not allow for calculation of the relative risk or the percentages of those in the exposed versus unexposed groups who go on to develop disease Confounding variables are often present.
Randomized study	Participants are randomly assigned to exposure groups and followed for the development of disease.	Provides evidence for cause and not just correlation, because only one "exposure" is manipulated at a time by design.	Costly and time-consuming Cannot be used to study exposures that are known or suspected to be harmful due to ethical concerns

20. What are some of the common statistical tests used, and in what situations would you use them?

Some of the common statistical tests mentioned on USMLE Step 1 include the Student *t* test, analysis of variance (ANOVA), and the chi-square test. The *t* test is the most common statistical test mentioned on the USMLE Step 1. Its purpose is to test whether there are differences between the means of two groups. For example, you can use the *t* test to investigate mean temperatures in patients with and without influenza to see if there is a statistically significant difference in body temperature between these patient populations. The ANOVA is similar to the *t* test, but it is used in cases where there are three or more groups. Continuing with the temperature example, you can use ANOVA to see if there is a significant difference in mean temperatures between groups with malaria, influenza, and COVID-19. The chi-square test is used for categorical variables (i.e., variables that are not continuous), and it tests for differences in proportions between two or more groups. For example, you can use the chi-square test to compare the proportion of pneumonia infection between males and females. A person cannot be partially infected with pneumonia; the two categories are "infected" or "not infected."

CASE 25.1

In the mid-1800s, London was plagued by recurrent outbreaks of cholera that resulted in a high death toll. Although the cause of these outbreaks was unknown, the prevailing hypothesis was that cholera was spread by "miasma," a poisonous odor emitted from decaying organic material found in open graves, sewers, and swamps. The now-famous epidemiologist John Snow disagreed with the miasma theory and postulated instead that cholera was spread by contaminated water. He believed this in part because the initial symptoms of cholera were intestinal, and he reasoned that an inhaled poisonous odor was unlikely to manifest in this way.

To study this hypothesis, he reviewed death certificates and plotted addresses for each person for whom the death certificate implied death from cholera infection. On a map of London, he then mapped out where these people had lived before their death and compared their location to those who died of causes unrelated to cholera infection. What he found was that the incidence of cholera was much higher in London residences that obtained their water supply from a particular water pump.

1. What sort of study design was this?
   This was a *case-control* study because participants were selected on the basis of either having or not having the disease of interest (i.e., cholera).

2. How does a retrospective case-control study differ in design from a retrospective cohort study?
   These studies differ largely with respect to how subjects are classified and selected. In a case-control study, subjects are classified according to the presence or absence of *disease*. By contrast, in a retrospective cohort study, subjects are classified based on the presence or absence of *exposure*, after which disease status is determined.

3. What are the strengths of a case-control study?
   Case-control studies are relatively easy to set up because the researcher simply has to locate people who have been affected by a disease. Another strength is that case-control studies can be used to look at the effect of exposures that are known or suspected to be harmful. For example, an RCT could not determine whether having a previous history of child abuse increases the likelihood that the victim will in turn abuse their own children, because it would be unethical and illegal to randomize participants into "abused" and "not abused" groups for study. However, with a case-control study, a researcher could look at child abusers and nonabusers and compare the incidence of abuse during their childhoods.

4. What are the limitations of a case-control study?
   Although case-control studies are easy to design, they have a number of flaws. As mentioned, case-control studies simply uncover an association (i.e., correlation) between two variables but cannot establish a causal relationship. For example, if you did a case-control study and found that individuals with lung cancer have higher rates of alcoholism, you might conclude that alcoholism leads to lung cancer. However, alcoholics might be more likely than nonalcoholics to smoke cigarettes, meaning smoking could be the actual cause of their lung cancer.
   Another flaw in case-control studies is *recall bias*, which is the tendency of individuals with a disease to exaggerate or misremember their exposures and those without a disease to minimize or misremember their exposures. For example, a woman with a child who has been born with a birth defect might recall undergoing many more chest x-ray studies during her pregnancy than might a woman with healthy children, even if in reality they received the same number of chest x-rays during their respective pregnancies. *Interviewer bias* is also an issue. This occurs when an interviewer assumes a person with the disease of interest has been exposed to risk factors that the healthy person has not and thus changes the way they ask a particular question. For example, the interviewer might ask a person with lung cancer the question "How many packs per day did you smoke?" whereas they might ask a healthy person the question "You never smoked, did you?" Even though both questions ask for similar information, changes in the interviewer's wording or tone may incidentally deter the interviewee from providing accurate responses. Additional types of statistical bias are described in Table 25.7.

STEP 1 SECRET

Bias occurs when one outcome is favored over another due to systematic error. The various types of statistical bias are commonly tested on the USMLE Step 1 exam. You should know the most commonly tested types of bias, which are described in Table 25.7. Including the correct control groups is extremely important for eliminating bias.

Table 25.7. Commonly Tested Statistical Bias

BIAS TYPE	DEFINITION	EXAMPLE	METHODS TO REDUCE BIAS
Selection bias	General term for nonrandom assignment of participants to various groups within a study	Administering a survey on hospital satisfaction to the "less sick" patients	Randomize participants. Use the correct control group.
Berkson bias	A type of selection bias involving hospitalized patients, who tend to be sicker than the general population	When studying the incidence of cellulitis in diabetic patients, only hospitalized patients are examined; this rate is likely to be inflated relative to that of the general diabetic population because hospitalized patients are already more likely to have comorbidities of any kind than the general population.	Use the correct control groups (in this example, one should survey diabetics in an outpatient setting as well as nondiabetic, hospitalized patients).
Recall/responder bias	Knowledge of having a disorder distorts one's ability to recall past exposures	When surveyed for a study investigating the effect of fiber intake on colon cancer risk, patients with colon cancer provide a more detailed dietary history than patients without colon cancer.	Reduce time from exposure to follow-up. Avoid leading questions and ask specific follow-up questions (in this example, ask all subjects if they consumed specific foods in addition to asking more open-ended questions).
Confounding bias	The effect of an independent variable on a dependent variable is distorted by a third, unmeasured variable.	The association between eating more vegetables and living longer may be confounded by the fact that people who eat a lot of vegetables tend to exercise more, and regular exercise promotes longer life span.	Crossover trials (subjects receive a sequence of different exposures and act as their own controls following a washout period) Randomization Adequately control for confounding variables (in this example, one should include a group that consumes lots of fruit and vegetables but does not exercise)
Hawthorne effect	Individuals change their behavior when they know they are being studied or observed.	Participants enrolled in a dietary recall study to examine normal fiber intake within the general population may increase their fruit and vegetable intake during the study period to obtain more fiber.	Use long-term methods that make it more difficult to sustain unnatural behaviors. Be discreet with expectations to prevent subjects from altering their behaviors in order to conform to the hypothesis.
Lead-time bias	Earlier detection of a disease is incorrectly interpreted as increased survival.	Diagnosis of breast cancer with a novel technology claims to increase patient survival by 6 months, but this may be due to earlier stage diagnosis rather than any change in the course of the disease.	Normalize survival length to the severity of disease at the time of diagnosis.
Observer bias	Observer's reporting is biased because of knowledge of exposure status (not double-blinded).	Researcher reports a reduced incidence of depression in a group that he knows is currently placed on a new SSRI.	Use placebo groups and double-blinded methods.

Table 25.7. Commonly Tested Statistical Bias—cont'd

BIAS TYPE	DEFINITION	EXAMPLE	METHODS TO REDUCE BIAS
Pygmalion effect	"Self-fulfilling prophecy"; a type of observer bias in which a researcher's own expectations influence the study outcome	When investigating the effect of a new pain medication, the researcher overemphasizes the pain relief reported by subjects in the treatment group.	Use placebo groups and double-blinded methods.
Procedure bias	Subjects in different study groups are not treated equally.	In a weight loss study in which one group is placed on a diet pill + exercise routine and the second is placed on a placebo + exercise routine, the former group is trained more intensely than the latter; differences in exercise routines may account for some of the observed weight loss.	Use double-blinded methods.
Sampling bias	Selecting participants who do not represent the overall population, therefore producing results that are not generalizable	Subjects from an upper-class town are selected for participation in a study that examines factors contributing to heart attack risk. These subjects may be influenced by financial factors that do not influence the general population but may nevertheless affect heart attack risk.	Use random samples (ideal). Use population-based controls.
Late-look bias	Acquisition of data at an incorrect or inappropriate time may influence the study results.	In a study investigating the impact of stroke on quality of life, those with the most fatal form of disease (i.e., those who have passed away from stroke) will not be able to participate in the study, thus skewing the results.	Stratify groups by disease severity.
Measurement bias	Acquisition of data in a manner that distorts it	In a study that examines the effect of cold weather on weight gain, participants are weighed with clothes and shoes on; participants are more likely to be wearing bulky, heavier clothing in the winter than in the summer.	Use standardized methods of data collection. Avoid leading questions.

SSRI, Selective serotonin reuptake inhibitor.

5. **What statistical measure can be used to compare event rates in a case-control study?**

The OR can be used to compare event rates in a case-control study. Case-control studies cannot be used to calculate the RR of an exposure on the disease outcome or to define the percentage of people with a certain exposure who will go on to develop a disease. This is because the calculation of RR requires the incidence rate, which cannot be calculated from a case-control study because there is no follow-up time. As discussed previously, remember *OR is used for case-control studies, and **RR** is used for **R**CT and cohort studies.*

CASE 25.1 CONTINUED:

When John Snow charted the water supply of 100 people who died of cholera and 100 people who died of other causes, he found that 80 of the 100 people who died of cholera lived in homes supplied by a particular water pump but only 10 of the 100 people who died of other causes lived in homes supplied by this same water pump.

6. **What is the OR of developing cholera if the water supply was provided by the particular water pump in question?**

The OR is 36. The calculation is explained below:

$$OR = \frac{80/20}{10/90} = \frac{80 \times 90}{20 \times 10} = \frac{7200}{200} = 36$$

An OR greater than 1 implies that the disease is more likely to occur in the exposed group, so cholera occurred more often in those who received their water supply from this particular water pump. This does not prove that the water was the source of the infection because there may have been confounding variables that were the actual cause. For example, it may have been that individuals who lived in homes supplied by this water pump were poorer than those who had their own wells, and therefore they had jobs where they were exposed to less sanitary conditions. These unsanitary working conditions, rather than the water in their homes, may have exposed them to cholera.

SUMMARY BOX: CASE-CONTROL STUDIES

- Subjects are classified according to presence or absence of disease.
- Strengths: Easy to set up, cost efficient, can be used to study exposures that are known or suspected to be harmful
- Limitations: Risks of recall bias, interviewer bias, and confounding variables
- Cannot be used to define relative risk (RR) but can be used to calculate an odds ratio (OR)

CASE 25.2

Blood pressure is monitored regularly in a group of 500 adult men. The mean blood pressure for the group is reported as 130 ± 10 mm Hg, and the blood pressure measurements within the group follow a normal distribution.

1. **What does it mean when the blood pressure in this population is said to follow a normal distribution?**

To be *normally distributed* means that if a plot was made of the magnitude of the experimental variable (in this case, blood pressure) against the frequency of each particular magnitude, the curve takes on a "bell-shaped" form that is well described by a specific mathematical equation, which can be used to accurately calculate the standard deviation. A normal distribution (see Fig. 25.3) represents one in which the majority of participants have measurements close to the mean, *because mean, median, and mode are all equal in a normal distribution curve*. Curves are often assumed to be normal for the sake of easy calculations, but some curves differ largely from a normal curve. For example, if you asked a group of people what temperature they like their coffee, most would say either very hot or very cold. Almost no one would say that they like lukewarm coffee. This study would produce a "bimodal" distribution (Fig. 25.4) with two "humps" or modes, which would not fit the parameters of a normal distribution curve.

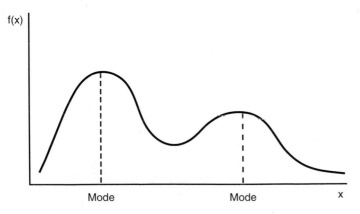

Figure 25.4. Graphical representation of a bimodal distribution.

2. **What percentage of participants had blood pressures in the range of 120 to 150 mm Hg?**

There were 81.5% of the participants with blood pressures in the range of 120 to 150 mm Hg.

Recall that in a normal distribution, 68% of the data falls within one standard deviation of the mean, 95% of the data falls within two standard deviations of the mean, and 99.7% of the data falls within three standard deviations of the mean. Therefore 68% of data will fall within the range of 130 ± 10 mm Hg (120–140 mm Hg), and 95% of the data will fall within the range of 130 ± (2 × 10) mm Hg (110–150 mm Hg). This tricky question asks what percentage of participants is in the range of 120 to 150 mm Hg. You must therefore realize that the lower value of this range (120 mm Hg) falls within *one* standard deviation of the mean, and the upper value of this range (150 mm Hg) falls within *two* standard deviations of the mean. Therefore 34% (half of 68%) of subjects will have blood pressures within the range of 120 and 130 mm Hg (i.e., the lower half of one standard deviation), while 47.5% (half of 95%) of subjects will have blood pressures within the range of 130 to 150 mm Hg (i.e., the upper half of two standard deviations). Add these two halves together, and you discover that 34% under the curve below the mean + 47.5% under the curve above the mean = 81.5% total under the curve between 120 and 150 mm Hg.

SUMMARY BOX: NORMAL DISTRIBUTION AND STANDARD DEVIATION

- Normal distributions represent bell-shaped curves in which mean, median, and mode are all equal.
- Standard deviation is used to estimate the percentage of a population that falls into a certain range, as long as the population fits a normal distribution:
  - 68% of individuals fall within one standard deviation of the mean
  - 95% of individuals fall within two standard deviations of the mean
  - 99.7% of individuals fall within three standard deviations of the mean

CASE 25.3

A 27-year-old man complains of fatigue and general malaise beginning several months earlier. Although his past medical history is unremarkable, his more recent history is significant for the use of intravenous drugs and for unprotected sex with multiple partners. With the patient's consent, you screen him for human immunodeficiency virus (HIV) infection using a test with a reported sensitivity of 95% and specificity of 75%.

1. **Why does it make sense to use a screening test with a high sensitivity, even at the cost of specificity, for this patient?**
   Screening tests in general, and particularly for life-threatening diseases such as HIV infection, should have a high sensitivity so that they maximize the possibility of detecting the disease when it is present. Because screening tests must generally be inexpensive, this high sensitivity may come at the cost of a suboptimal specificity (e.g., higher rates of false-positive results). However, because it is much more important to avoid missing a life-threatening disease (i.e., minimize false-negative results) than it is to inconvenience (or even frighten!) a patient with a false-positive result, this is considered acceptable.

   Not all screening tests have high sensitivity, however. When used as a single data point, mammograms and Papanicolaou (Pap) smears have a low sensitivity, for example. However, when performed on a regular basis (e.g., annually), these tests become much more effective screening tools because of a high *cumulative* sensitivity.

2. **If this patient tests positive, is it reasonable to tell him that you are 95% confident that he is infected with HIV?**
   No. Sensitivity and specificity values simply represent how good a test is at ruling in or ruling out a disease, and perhaps whether the test is ideal for screening large populations for a given disease. Although a positive test result will undoubtedly be concerning to the clinician and the patient, with only the information provided, there is no way of determining if this is a true-positive or a false-positive result. What is needed to calculate the PPV for this test depends on additional information (e.g., prevalence of the disease within the specific population in which the patient falls), as discussed in the next case.

3. **What if the test comes back negative? Can you tell this patient that you are 75% confident that he does not have HIV?**
   No. Again, such a statement cannot be made unless you know the NPV of the test, which was not provided.

4. **Now assume that a 90-year-old woman with no new exposures and a history of a negative HIV test in the past year and our young patient in this vignette both test positive for HIV using this test. Are they both equally likely to have the disease?**
   No. This question addresses the important concept of utilizing screening tests appropriately. The role of clinicians is to *selectively* screen only those individuals at higher risk for developing a given disease. This is because the PPV of a test depends on the prevalence of the disease in the given population being tested and on the specificity and sensitivity of the test. The prevalence of HIV in the 90-year-old female population is much lower than in young intravenous drug users. Therefore if this elderly woman tests positive for HIV, she is much more likely to have a false positive than the other patient because she had a smaller pretest probability of having HIV.

   Consider the havoc that would be created if physicians screened all women starting at the age of 20 for breast cancer by performing annual mammograms. Given that the prevalence of breast cancer in young women is low, such testing would yield numerous false positives, necessitating unnecessary referrals and expensive workups by specialists, not to mention a lot of unneeded anxiety. Using this same test to screen only women over age 40 makes a bit more sense, as the number of true positives will increase and the number of false positives will decrease due to the increased prevalence of breast cancer with aging.

SUMMARY BOX: LIKELIHOOD RATIOS, PREDICTIVE VALUES, AND PRINCIPLES OF SCREENING

- Sensitivity of screening tests should be high to avoid missing individuals with disease.
- Positive predictive value (PPV) and negative predictive value (NPV) can determine the likelihood that a person has a disease if they test positive or negative for that disease. Sensitivity and specificity cannot do this.
- PPV and NPV depend on disease prevalence and the test characteristics.

CASE 25.4

In a town of 1000 individuals, the prevalence of coronary artery disease across all age groups is 20% (as determined by angiography, the "gold standard"). You have created a wonderfully inexpensive screening test that you believe is both highly sensitive and specific for detecting coronary artery disease. Based on your test results, you create the following 2 × 2 table (Table 25.8).

Table 25.8. Example Data Set for Coronary Artery Disease

	CORONARY ARTERY DISEASE (+)	CORONARY ARTERY DISEASE (−)
(+) Test result	180 (a)	80 (b)
(−) Test result	20 (c)	720 (d)

---

1. **Given the data presented in the 2 × 2 table in Table 25.8, what is the sensitivity of this new test?**
   The sensitivity is 90%. Sensitivity can be calculated by dividing the number of true positives by the total number of persons tested who truly have the disease (i.e., true positives plus false negatives), or a/(a + c) in the 2 × 2 table. There were 180 true-positive test results and 20 false-negative test results, yielding a sensitivity of 180/200, or 90%. This means that this test detects the disease in 90% of people who truly have coronary artery disease.

2. **What is the specificity of this new test?**
   The specificity is also 90% but by a different calculation. Specificity can be calculated by dividing the number of true negatives by the total number of persons tested who truly do *not* have the disease (i.e., true negatives plus false positives), or d/(b + d) in the 2 × 2 table. There were 720 true negatives and 80 false positives, so the specificity of this test is 720/800, or 90%.

3. **What information can be obtained from calculating the PLR?**
   As described earlier in this chapter, the PLR reflects how much a positive test result increases the probability of the presence of disease (i.e., indicates posttest probability of disease). The higher the ratio, the more likely it is that the disease in question is truly present. This ratio is calculated as the sensitivity divided by 1 − specificity.

$$PLR = sensitivity/1 - specificity$$

   For this example, given that sensitivity and specificity are both 90%, the PLR can be calculated as:

$$PLR = 0.90/1 - 0.90$$
$$= 0.90/0.10$$
$$= 9$$

   A positive test result tells us that this patient's posttest probability for having the disease in question is nine times greater than his pretest probability. It is often up to the clinician to determine how to factor this new information into their management plan following the outcome of such a test.

4. **How can the PPV of this test be calculated?**
   PPV is calculated as the number of true positives divided by the total number of positive results (i.e., true positives plus false positives), or a/(a + b) in the 2 × 2 table. Without a given 2 × 2 table, this calculation requires knowledge of the sensitivity and specificity of the test and the prevalence of the disease, which gives you all the information you need to quickly generate your own 2 × 2 table and calculate the number of true positives and false positives.

$$Positive\ predictive\ value = TP/(TP + FP)$$
$$= 180/180 + 80$$
$$= 69\%$$

   Based on this PPV calculation, you would tell your patient that he is 69% likely to truly have coronary artery disease based on his positive test result.

It is very unlikely that you will be provided with a ready-made 2 × 2 table on the USMLE Step 1 exam. How can you calculate PPV if all you are given is sensitivity (90%), specificity (90%), and disease prevalence (20%)? The trick here is to create your own 2 × 2 table *by inserting sample numbers that fit the given statistics. We recommend using* very simple numbers *to do this. Let us work through an example together, using Table 25.9 to demonstrate each step of this process.*

First, presume that our sample population consists of 500 people. If disease prevalence is 20%, then 100 people in our sample population have coronary artery disease (because 20% of 500 is 100), which means that 400 people therefore do not have coronary artery disease. This is reflected in Table 25.9, part A.

Next, let us calculate the numbers for the truly diseased column (i.e., true positives and false negatives). Because the sensitivity of our test is 90%, then the number of true positives must be 90, because 90% of our 100 truly diseased individuals is 90 (a). This therefore means the number of false negatives, that is the value for (c) in our 2 × 2 table, must equal 10. This is reflected in Table 25.9, part B.

Finally, let us calculate the numbers for the disease-free column (i.e., true negatives and false positives). The specificity of our test is 90%, so the number of true negatives must be 360 because 90% of our 400 truly disease-free individuals is 360 (d). This therefore means that the number of false positives, that is the value for (b) in our 2 × 2 table, must equal 40. This is reflected in Table 25.9, part C.

Using this 2 × 2 table that we have created, we can now simply calculate the PPV based on these values, as we did for question 4:

$$PPV = TP/(TP + FP)$$
$$= 90/(90 + 40)$$
$$= 69\%$$

As you can see, we yield the same PPV result that we did in question 4!

Table 25.9. Setting Up a Sample 2 × 2 Table When Given Sensitivity, Specificity, and Disease Prevalence

	CORONARY ARTERY DISEASE (+)	CORONARY ARTERY DISEASE (−)	TOTAL
A			
(+) Test result	___ (a)	___ (b)	
(−) Test result	___ (c)	___ (d)	
Total	100	400	500
B			
(+) Test result	90 (a)	___ (b)	
(−) Test result	10 (c)	___ (d)	
Total	100	400	500
C			
(+) Test result	90 (a)	40 (b)	
(−) Test result	10 (c)	360 (d)	
Total	100	400	500

5. What is NPV for this test?

The NPV for this test is 97%. NPV is the probability that the disease is truly absent if the test result is negative. It is calculated by dividing true negatives by all negative test results (i.e., true negatives plus false negatives). The sample calculation below uses the values given in Table 25.8:

$$\text{Negative predictive value} = TN/(TN + FN)$$
$$= 720/(720 + 20)$$
$$= 0.97 \text{ or } 97\%$$

Note that the same NPV can be calculated from the values generated in our made-up 2 × 2 table (see Table 25.9), as $d/(d + c) = 360/(360 + 10) = 0.97$ or 97%.

Therefore 97% of the individuals in this sample population who had a negative test result truly do not have coronary artery disease.

SUMMARY BOX: SENSITIVITY, SPECIFICITY, LIKELIHOOD RATIOS, AND PREDICTIVE VALUES

- Sensitivity, specificity, positive predictive value (PPV), and negative predictive value (NPV) can all be calculated using a 2 × 2 table.
- It is very likely that you will have to create a 2 × 2 table for yourself if given sensitivity, specificity, and disease prevalence, so be sure you understand the example outlined in our Step 1 Secrets section for this case.
- PPV is used to express the likelihood that a positive test result indicates true presence of disease. NPV is used to express the likelihood that a negative test result indicates true absence of disease.
- Positive likelihood ratio (PLR) reflects the degree to which a positive test result increases the risk of disease. PLR = sensitivity/(1 − specificity).

CASE 25.5

In the 1940s, a study was performed on employees at a nuclear power plant to determine whether an association exists between radiation exposure and cancer rates. In this study, 500 employees with high-level radiation exposure and 500 employees with very limited exposure were followed for 10 years. The incidence rates for cancer were compared in the two groups throughout this time. The results are depicted in the 2 × 2 table shown in Table 25.10.

Table 25.10. Example Data Set of Radiation Exposure and Cancer Risk

	CANCER (+)	CANCER (−)
(+) Radiation exposure	50 (a)	450 (b)
(−) Radiation exposure	5 (c)	495 (d)

---

1. **What type of study design is this?**
   This is a (prospective) *cohort* study because individuals are classified based on *exposure*, not on the presence or absence of *disease* (as with a *case-control* study). Recall that cohort studies compare groups with or without exposure to a variable of interest to determine how that variable affects development of disease. Furthermore, this was a *prospective* study in which the complications associated with exposure were analyzed as they occurred.

2. **What is the difference between a prospective cohort study and a retrospective cohort study?**
   In a prospective cohort study, individuals with a risk factor for disease (i.e., exposure) are followed over time to see whether they do or do not develop disease. In a prospective study, disease outcome is to be determined. In a retrospective cohort study, a group of individuals who had been exposed to a variable of interest are retrospectively examined for development of disease. In other words, the study examines who already developed disease based on their past exposure status. Note that in both cases, the study population of a cohort study is grouped according to *exposure*.

3. **What is the major limitation of cohort studies?**
   The major limitation of cohort studies is the inability to distinguish correlation from causality. Although the groups may be distinct from each other according to the factor being studied, there are many other factors that may be different between the groups that could influence the outcome (i.e., *confounding* variables). For example, a cohort study found that people who eat more β-carotene have a lower incidence of lung cancer. However, this did not take into account that people who eat more β-carotene may eat substantially more fruits and vegetables in general, which itself may be protective from cancer. In fact, when a randomized trial was done, independent β-carotene supplementation actually *increased* the risk of lung cancer.

4. **Based on data presented in Table 25.10, what is the RR for cancer in the exposed group?**
   The RR for cancer in the exposed group is 10. Recall that RR is determined by comparing incidence rates in exposed individuals (I_E) to incidence rates in nonexposed individuals (I_{NE}), as shown in Eq. 25.11.

$$RR = \frac{I_E}{I_{NE}} = \frac{a/(a + b)}{c/(c + d)} = \frac{50/500}{5/500} = 10 \qquad [25.11]$$

Thus RR for the employees exposed to radiation is 10 times greater than for the nonexposed employees.

5. **What is meant by the terms attributable risk (AR), attributable risk percent (AR%), absolute risk reduction (ARR), number needed to treat (NNT), and number needed to harm (NNH)?**
AR represents the difference in disease risk between two groups based solely on exposure status. In other words, it is the risk of disease that can be *attributed* to the exposure in question. AR can be calculated as the difference in incidence rates between exposed and nonexposed groups (Fig. 25.5).
Let us calculate AR for the example data in Table 25.10:

$$AR = I_E - I_{NE}$$
$$= 50/500 - 5/500$$
$$= 45/500$$
$$= 0.09$$

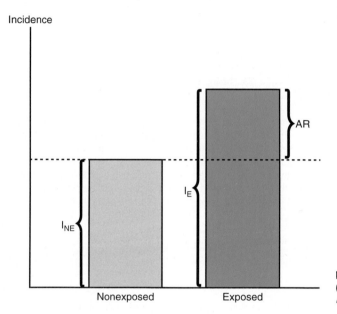

Figure 25.5. Graphical representation of attribute risk (*AR*). *I_{NE}*, Incidence of disease within a nonexposed group; *I_E*, incidence of disease within an exposed group.

This AR of 0.09 implies that 9% of people exposed to radiation developed cancer as a result of that exposure.
The AR% is a measure of the percentage of people who were exposed *and then* developed the disease. It can be calculated by dividing the AR by the incidence of disease in the exposed group:

$$AR\% = AR/I_E \times 100$$
$$= 0.09/0.10 \times 100$$
$$= 90\%$$

This AR percent of 90% implies that 90% of the workers who were exposed to radiation and later developed cancer developed their cancer as a result of the radiation.
ARR is calculated using the same variables as AR, but subtracts the incidence of exposed individuals from the incidence of nonexposed individuals to identify exposures (or interventions) that *reduce* one's chances of acquiring the disease in question.

$$ARR = I_{NE} - I_E \qquad [25.12]$$

For example, if you notice a reduction in the serum cholesterol levels of a group taking statins compared to a group not currently on statins, you would use the term *absolute risk reduction* to describe the difference in risk of developing high cholesterol between the exposed group (i.e., those taking statins) and the unexposed group (i.e., those not taking statins).
NNT refers to the average number of individuals that must be exposed to a protective factor or intervention to prevent one individual from developing the disease in question. A *smaller* NNT reflects a *more effective* treatment. It is inversely related to ARR.

$$NNT = 1/ARR \qquad [25.13]$$

NNH refers to the average number of individuals that must be exposed to a potential risk factor until one individual will develop the disease in question. A *smaller* NNH reflects a *more dangerous* exposure. It is inversely related to AR.

$$NNH = 1/AR$$

[25.14]

STEP 1 SECRET

Be sure that you know how to calculate odds ratio (OR), relative risk (RR), absolute risk reduction (ARR), attributable risk (AR), number needed to treat (NNT), and number needed to harm (NNH). These are straightforward calculations, and you are likely to be asked to calculate at least one or two of these on your USMLE Step 1 exam. These are the type of formulas you should consider adding to your whiteboard or scratch paper before your test begins, so you do not accidentally make a mistake when trying to recall each formula under the timed pressure of your exam blocks.

16. What experimental design is least susceptible to confounding factors and bias?

The experimental design that is least susceptible to confounding factors and bias is the RCT. In this study design, individuals are randomly allocated to either the treatment or control group, thereby considerably reducing the effects of any confounding factors.

The most highly regarded type of RCT is the double-blind placebo-controlled trial. *Double-blind* means that neither the investigators nor the study subjects know who is receiving the treatment. *Placebo-controlled* means that those who do not receive the intervention under investigation will receive a placebo instead, whose administration should be similar enough to the treatment such that the participants cannot tell which group they are in (e.g., the placebo for a vaccine trial is often an intramuscular injection of normal saline).

The data from an RCT may be analyzed by several different methods. Among the most common are *intention-to-treat* (ITT) and *as-treated (non–intent-to-treat)* analyses. The ITT approach includes all randomized participants in the groups to which they were initially assigned, regardless of adherence with the study criteria or withdrawal from the study. This approach reduces bias that may be introduced by patients dropping out of the study, noncompliance with treatment, or patient reassignment to another treatment arm by nonrandom means. The as-treated approach analyzes patients based on the final treatment regimen received rather than by the initial randomization. This approach is susceptible to bias from the aforementioned factors but is intended to provide a better estimate of treatment efficacy within general practice given inevitable treatment nonadherence.

SUMMARY BOX: COHORT STUDIES AND RANDOMIZED CONTROL TRIALS

- Classifies subjects based on *exposure* status
- Limitation: Presence of confounding variables
- Uses relative risk (RR) to express the magnitude of association between exposure and disease status (Only cohort studies and randomized control trials use RR; case-control studies do not use RR because incidence of disease cannot be determined.)
- Randomized double-blind placebo-controlled trial is the gold standard of experimental design

CLINICAL ANATOMY

CASE 26.1

A 68-year-old retired man presents with a 2-year history of pain and cramping of the lower extremities (LEs) with walking. This has not bothered him much, but for the past month he has noticed pain in his right foot that awakens him from sleep. He has a history of myocardial infarction (MI), type 2 diabetes mellitus, erectile dysfunction, and a 40-pack-year history of smoking.

1. What is the differential diagnosis for his foot and LE pain?

   Peripheral vascular disease (PVD), neurogenic causes (e.g., disk herniation), arthritis causing spinal stenosis, and diabetic neuropathic pain are considerations.

CASE 26.1 CONTINUED:

On further questioning, you find that the pain and cramping are absent at rest and begin after about 5 minutes of walking. Stopping for a short period relieves the pain. The right foot pain occurs only at night and is relieved by hanging the foot over the side of the bed. On physical examination, light touch, pinprick, vibration, and temperature sense are intact on the lower extremities bilaterally. He is noted to have intact femoral pulses, weak popliteal pulses, weak posterior tibial pulses, a weak left dorsalis pedis pulse, and an absent right dorsalis pedis pulse.

2. What is the most likely diagnosis?

   PVD, which is characterized by claudication symptoms (pain and cramping of the LEs with walking) that appear after a specific walking distance and resolve after a specific duration of rest. The peripheral pulse findings on physical examination also are strongly suggestive of PVD. There is also a phenomenon called pseudoclaudication from spinal stenosis that can cause pain with ambulation but is improved by leaning forward and should have a normal pulse examination.

3. Which historical features in this patient increase the likelihood of a PVD diagnosis?

   Smoking and diabetes mellitus are strong PVD risk factors. Patients with PVD often have evidence of atherosclerosis elsewhere, as demonstrated by this patient's past MI and erectile dysfunction. Other PVD risk factors include hypertension, hypercholesterolemia (most notably increased low-density lipoprotein), obesity, sedentary lifestyle, and a family history of atherosclerotic disease.

4. Why does his nocturnal right foot pain resolve when he hangs the affected foot over the bedside?

Rest pain commonly occurs in the feet at night in PVD. When a patient is supine, there is no gravitational assistance in foot blood flow. Reduced blood flow results in ischemia and pain. Hanging the foot over the side of the bed places the foot below the level of the heart; then gravity increases the flow of blood to the ischemic areas, reducing the pain.

5. Describe the path of arterial blood from the heart to the common femoral artery.

Blood leaves the heart through the aortic valve to enter the ascending thoracic aorta, arch of the aorta, and descending thoracic aorta (Fig. 26.1). The thoracic aorta passes through the aortic hiatus of the diaphragm at the level of T12 to become the abdominal aorta. The abdominal aorta bifurcates into the right and left common iliac arteries at the level of L4. Each common iliac artery bifurcates into the internal and external iliac arteries just anterior to the sacroiliac joint. The internal iliac primarily supplies pelvic structures, while the external iliac runs deep to the inguinal ligament to become the common femoral artery.

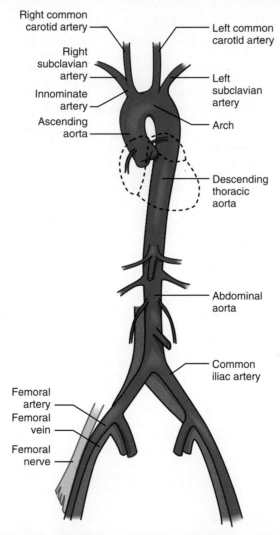

Figure 26.1. Path of arterial blood from the heart to the femoral sheath.

6. Outline the borders of the femoral triangle.

The femoral triangle is bordered by the inguinal ligament (superiorly), the sartorius (laterally), and the adductor longus (medially). From lateral to medial, it contains the femoral **N**erve, common femoral **A**rtery, femoral **V**ein, femoral canal (**E**mpty space containing lymph nodes that is the site of femoral hernias), and the deep inguinal **L**ymph nodes. The classic mnemonic is **NAVEL** (Fig. 26.2). A way to remember that NAVEL is lateral to medial is that you go from a lateral to medial direction to find your NAVEL.

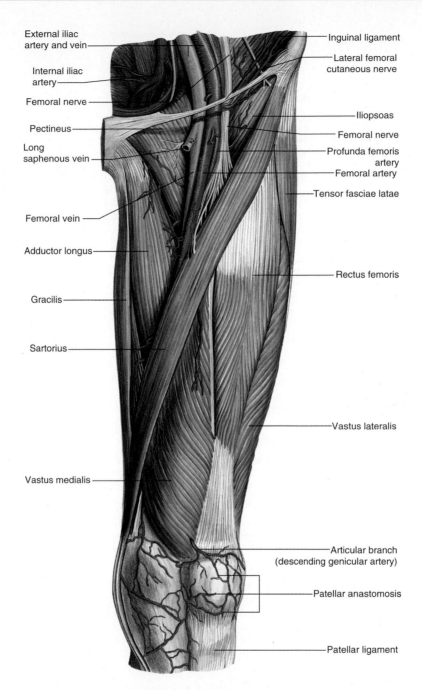

Figure 26.2. Femoral triangle. *(From Paulsen F, Waschke J. Sobotta Atlas of Human Anatomy. Vol. 1. Urban & Fischer: Elsevier; 2013.)*

7. Describe the path of arterial blood from the femoral sheath to the feet.

The common femoral artery quickly bifurcates into the profunda femoris (or deep femoral), which primarily supplies the thigh, and the superficial femoral artery, which runs through the adductor canal to the popliteal fossa (via the adductor hiatus) to become the popliteal artery. In the posterior compartment of the leg, the popliteal artery bifurcates into the tibiofibular trunk and the anterior tibial artery. The anterior tibial artery perforates the superior-most portion of the interosseous membrane and descends in the anterior compartment until it crosses the ankle joint to become the dorsalis pedis artery, which can be palpated on the dorsum of the foot lateral to the tendon of the extensor hallucis longus. The tibiofibular trunk bifurcates to become the fibular artery, which runs downward in the deep posterior compartment of the leg, and the posterior tibial artery, which can be palpated between the medial malleolus and the calcaneus before bifurcating to form the lateral and medial plantar arteries, which supply the plantar aspect of the foot (Fig. 26.3).

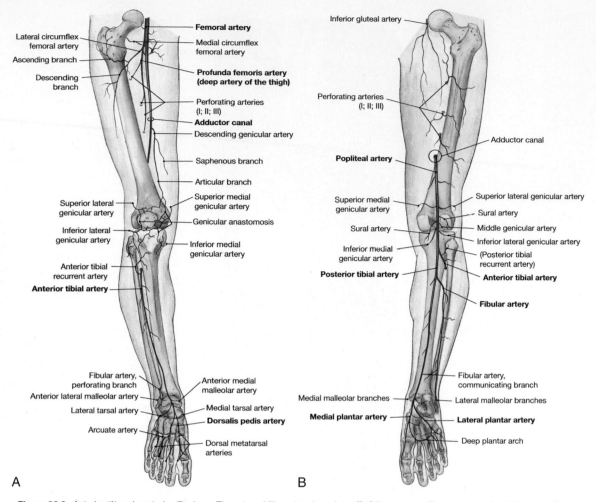

Figure 26.3. Anterior (A) and posterior (B) views. The external iliac artery branches off of the common iliac artery anterior to the sacroiliac joint and continues beneath the inguinal ligament as the femoral artery. This artery and its branches descend down the leg. *(A: From Hombach-Klonisch S, Klonisch T, Peeler J. Sobotta Clinical Atlas of Human Anatomy. Munich: Elsevier; 2019: 152-222. Fig. 4.90.)*

8. At which sites is arterial plaque formation most likely?

   The most likely sites of plaque formation are arterial branch points, such as the bifurcation of the tibiofibular trunk and anterior tibial artery, and tethered arteries, such as the superficial femoral artery in the adductor canal. Pathophysiologically, the turbulent blood flow occurring at branch points and tethering sites causes shear forces on the endothelium, increasing the likelihood of endothelial damage and potentially leading to atherosclerosis. Such changes are evident in this patient, who appears to show significant bilateral superficial femoral atherosclerotic narrowing (given intact pulses at the femoral triangle and weak pulses at the popliteal fossa) and marked right anterior tibial narrowing (supported by the absence of the dorsalis pedis pulse).

9. In Table 26.1, cover the two columns on the right and attempt to list the drug class and mechanism of action for each of the drugs commonly used in treatment of PVD.

Table 26.1. Selected Drugs Used to Treat Peripheral Vascular Disease

DRUG	CLASS	MECHANISM OF ACTION
Aspirin	Nonselective cyclooxygenase inhibitor	Irreversibly inhibits COX-1 (and COX-2), decreasing platelet production of thromboxane A_2, a vasoconstrictor and promoter of platelet aggregation
Clopidogrel	$P2Y_{12}$ antagonist	Irreversibly inhibits $P2Y_{12}$, a platelet ADP receptor necessary for activation of the glycoprotein IIb/IIIa pathway of platelet aggregation

Table 26.1. Selected Drugs Used to Treat Peripheral Vascular Disease—cont'd

DRUG	CLASS	MECHANISM OF ACTION
Statins (e.g., atorvastatin, rosuvastatin, fluvastatin, lovastatin, pravastatin, simvastatin)	HMG-CoA reductase inhibitors	Inhibit HMG-CoA reductase, the rate-limiting step in endogenous production of cholesterol, to reduce the buildup of cholesterol in atherosclerotic plaques. Results in upregulation of LDL receptor and increased clearance of circulating LDL
Cilostazol	Phosphodiesterase III inhibitor	Selectively inhibits cAMP phosphodiesterase III to reduce cAMP degradation. Increased cAMP causes vasodilation of peripheral arteries and inhibits platelet aggregation
Pentoxifylline	Phosphodiesterase inhibitor (and xanthine derivative)	Nonselective inhibitor of cAMP phosphodiesterase; increases platelet flexibility and decreases blood viscosity

ADP, Adenosine diphosphate; *cAMP,* cyclic adenosine monophosphate; *CoA,* coenzyme A; *COX-1,* cyclooxygenase-1; *HMG,* hydroxymethylglutarate; *LDL,* low-density lipoprotein.

SUMMARY BOX: PERIPHERAL VASCULAR DISEASE

- Peripheral vascular disease (PVD) is caused by atherosclerotic narrowing of peripheral arteries, usually of the lower extremities (LEs).
- Atherosclerotic lesions form preferentially at branch points and sites of tethering, because of turbulent blood flow and endothelial shear stress.
- Blood flow to the LE: aorta → common iliac → external iliac → common femoral → profunda femoris (ends in thigh) and superficial femoral → popliteal → anterior tibial (supplies anterior compartment and ends as dorsalis pedis in the dorsum of the foot) and tibiofibular trunk → fibular (supplies lateral compartment) and posterior tibial (supplies posterior compartment) → lateral and medial plantar arteries.
- From lateral to medial, the femoral triangle contains the femoral **N**erve, **A**rtery, **V**ein, canal (**E**mpty space), and the **L**ymph nodes. Remember the acronym **NAVEL**.

CASE 26.2, PART A

A 22-year-old college student presents to the emergency department (ED) after rear-ending a car while driving his new motorcycle. He claims that the major site of impact was his left shoulder, but his head and neck were wrenched to the right as well. He is clearly intoxicated and has managed to sit up, although his left upper extremity (UE) hangs by his side and is internally rotated. His forearm is extended and pronated, and his wrist is frozen in flexion. The intern on call claims to be able to diagnose his injury from across the room.

1. What structure has been injured, and how has it led to his upper extremity position?
   He has damaged nerve roots C5 and C6 (or the upper trunk) of the brachial plexus, resulting in a condition known as Erb-Duchenne palsy. His left upper extremity (UE) hangs by his side and is internally rotated because the C5 component of the axillary nerve is necessary for shoulder flexion and abduction (via the deltoid) and external rotation (via the teres minor). His forearm is extended and pronated because C5 and C6 are the main components of the musculocutaneous nerve, which supplies the two major forearm flexors (brachialis and biceps) and the major forearm supinator (biceps). His wrist is flexed because the C6 component of the radial nerve is necessary for wrist extension (via the extensor muscles of the posterior compartment of the forearm). Remember that an upper brachial plexus injury (C5–C6) gives you the "waiter's tip position" (Fig. 26.4).

2. If he had forced his UE above his head by grabbing the handlebars of the motorcycle to prevent his fall, he may have presented with a loss of sensation and impaired flexion in digits 4 and 5, impaired wrist flexion, hyperextension of the metacarpophalangeal joints, and an inability to abduct and adduct digits 2 to 5. What would be the diagnosis in this situation?
   This pattern of injury is characteristic of a tear of nerve roots C8 and T1 (or a lower trunk tear) of the brachial plexus, a condition known as *Klumpke paralysis*. The ulnar nerve is exclusively supplied by C8 and T1 and is responsible for sensory innervation to the fifth digit, the medial half of the fourth digit, and the corresponding palmar surface of the hand. It controls the majority of medial digit flexion (via the medial heads of the flexor digitorum profundus and the flexor digiti minimi muscles), as well as abduction (via the dorsal interossei) and adduction (via the palmar interossei) of digits 2 to 5. It is partially responsible for metacarpophalangeal joint flexion (via the lumbricals of digits 4 and 5) and wrist flexion (via the flexor carpi ulnaris) (Fig. 26.5).

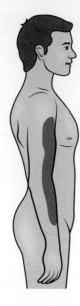

Figure 26.4. "Waiter's tip position" caused by upper brachial plexus injury.

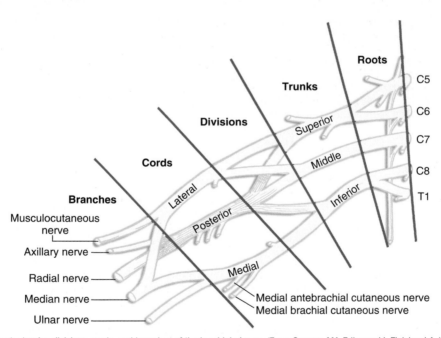

Figure 26.5. Roots, trunks, divisions, cords, and branches of the brachial plexus. *(From Gropper MA,* Eriksson LI, Fleisher LA, Wiener-Kronisch JP, Cohen NH, Leslie K. Miller's Anesthesia. *9th ed. Philadelphia: Elsevier; 2020.)*

CASE 26.2, PART B

One year later, his wild ways have continued, and he admits to twisting his ankle during an episode of extreme intoxication last weekend. He did not go to the doctor then, as he was a bit embarrassed, and his ankle feels much better. He presents today with an inability to extend his right elbow and right wrist drop since he started using crutches that a friend let him borrow.

3. What structure has he injured this time, and how has it led to his UE position?
   A compression injury to the posterior cord of the brachial plexus can occur if underarm crutches are used incorrectly. The inability to extend his wrist is due to a lack of radial nerve (a branch of the posterior cord) input to the posterior compartment of the forearm. The radial nerve also innervates the triceps brachii and anconeus muscles, which are necessary for elbow extension. Pure radial nerve palsies (which often result from injury to the nerve at the spiral groove

of the humerus) generally do not affect the triceps, because the branch of radial nerve to the triceps is very close to the origin at the posterior cord, proximal to the spiral groove.

CASE 26.2, PART C

One month later, his father, who happens to be a writer, presents to your clinic with paresthesias and pain involving his lateral palm, digits 1 to 3, and the radial half of his fourth digit. He tells you that he has been typing long hours over the past few months and now has almost finished his latest masterpiece. On physical examination, you notice mild atrophy of the thenar eminence, and tapping the middle of the wrist crease elicits paresthesias of the lateral aspect of the hand. Palmar flexion of the wrist for longer than 1 minute results in paresthesias in the radial aspect of the hand.

4. What structure has been injured and how has this happened?

Repetitive use of the hands—typing, in this case—can lead to inflammation, swelling, and subsequent compression of the structures within the carpal tunnel. This condition is known as *carpal tunnel syndrome*, and the pain, paresthesias, and muscle wasting are due to median nerve injury within the tunnel. Pain and paresthesias have arisen in the distribution of the median nerve, the lateral palm, and the radial 3½ digits. Because the median nerve also innervates the intrinsic muscles of the thumb, early thenar wasting has occurred. The classic exam findings for carpal tunnel syndrome include paresthesias of the lateral aspect of the hand when tapping on the middle of the wrist (positive Tinel sign) and paresthesias of the lateral aspect of the hand when there is palmar flexion of the wrist over 1 minute (positive Phalen test).

5. Outline the contents of the carpal tunnel.

The carpal tunnel is formed by the eight wrist (carpal) bones (also known as the deep carpal arch) and the transverse carpal ligament (superficial flexor retinaculum), which spans from the tubercles of the scaphoid and trapezium to the pisiform and the hook of the hamate. The contents include the four flexor digitorum profundus tendons, the four flexor digitorum superficialis tendons, the flexor pollicis longus tendon, and the median nerve (Fig. 26.6).

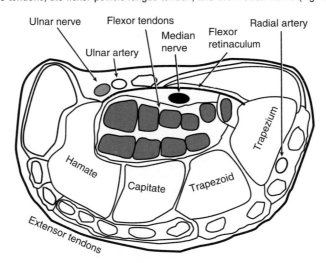

Figure 26.6. Cross-sectional anatomy of wrist. Tendons and median nerve may be compressed by inflammation or infection because they are encompassed by synovial sheath and flexor retinaculum. *(From Weiss J, Weiss L, Silver J. Easy EMG. 2nd ed. Philadelphia: Elsevier; 2016.)*

6. Describe the sensory and motor innervations of the median, ulnar, and radial nerves.

See Table 26.2 and Fig. 26.7.

Table 26.2. Sensory and Motor Innervations of the Median, Ulnar, and Radial Nerves		
NERVE	**SENSORY INNERVATION**	**MOTOR INNERVATION**
Median	Lateral palm, thumb, digits 2 and 3, and lateral half of digit 4	LOAF muscles (**L**ateral 2 lumbricals, **O**pponens pollicis, **A**bductor pollicis brevis, **F**lexor pollicis brevis)
Ulnar	Medial palm, medial dorsal hand, digit 5, and medial half of digit 4	All the intrinsic muscles of the hand except the LOAF muscles
Radial	Lateral dorsal hand, extending distally to the proximal interphalangeal (PIP) joint of digits 1 to 3 and the lateral half of digit 4	No motor innervation to the hand

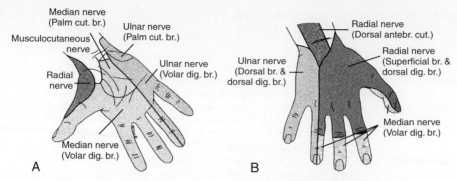

Figure 26.7. Nerves of the hand. A, Volar aspect. B, Dorsal aspect. *antebr. cut.,* Antebrachial cutaneous; *cut. br.,* cutaneous branch; *dig. br.,* digital branch. *(From Noble J.* Textbook of Primary Care Medicine. *3rd ed. St. Louis: Mosby; 2001.)*

STEP 1 SECRET

Innervation of the hand is a particularly high-yield topic. If you know nothing else about the anatomy of the hand, know the nerve innervation.

CASE 26.2, PART D

As the patient walks out of the office, he slips on icy steps and falls forward, breaking the fall with his right hand. He immediately feels severe pain in his wrist, and as his distal forearm is very obviously deformed, he carefully walks back into the clinic. You order an x-ray film, and the radiologist remarks that she sees the classic "dinner fork deformity" of a certain fracture commonly seen in patients older than 50 years, classically those with osteoporosis.

7. **What type of fracture does this patient have?**
   He has a Colles fracture, a fracture of the distal radius in which the distal fragment is displaced posteriorly/dorsally. Radiographically, the angle of the radius and the fragment in combination with the angle of the fragment and the hand resembles the curvature of a fork. This fracture is common after the age of 50 and most often occurs when one breaks a fall with an outstretched hand from the standing position.

CASE 26.2, PART E

Two months later, you are working in the emergency department (ED) again, and you come across another member of the family. He is a 20-year-old former high school starting pitcher who was getting a lesson from his brother on how to ride a motorcycle. Unfortunately, he too has taken a nasty fall. The attending at the ED says she is worried about a humerus fracture.

8. **What are the three most common sites of humerus fracture, and which nerve and artery are at risk at each of these sites?**
   See Table 26.3.

9. **On reviewing his medical history, you note that his baseball career was marred by a partially torn rotator cuff. Describe why the rotator cuff makes the glenohumeral joint different from other joints, and name its four components.**
   Most joints are stabilized primarily by a ligamentous capsule, but the glenohumeral joint is stabilized primarily by the rotator cuff, which consists of the tendons of four muscles: supraspinatus, infraspinatus, teres minor, and subscapularis (Fig. 26.8). These can be remembered by the mnemonic SITS. This design allows the glenohumeral joint to have the widest range of motion of all joints in the body, at the expense of stability and resistance to injury. The rotator cuff stabilizes the glenohumeral joint by pulling the head of the humerus toward the glenoid fossa of the scapula as other muscles flex, extend, abduct, or adduct the arm. Rapid, forceful, or repetitive movements (such as repeatedly throwing a baseball) can tear the tendons of the rotator cuff, leading to a lack of joint stability, restricted movement, and pain.

Table 26.3. Three Most Common Sites of Humerus Fracture

HUMERUS FRACTURE SITE	NERVE	ARTERY
Surgical neck	Axillary	Anterior and posterior circumflex humeral (branches of the axillary artery)
Midshaft	Radial	Profunda brachii (branch of the brachial artery)
Supracondylar	Median	Brachial

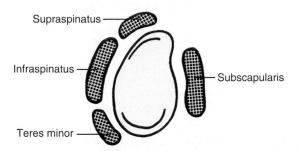

Figure 26.8. Cross-sectional view of the shoulder with humeral head stabilized in shallow scapular glenoid by rotator cuff and capsule. *(From Noble J.* Textbook of Primary Care Medicine. *3rd ed. St. Louis: Mosby; 2001.)*

STEP 1 SECRET

Upper extremity (UE) injuries, particularly those that involve the brachial plexus, are popular subjects for Step 1 anatomy questions. You should learn all of the brachial plexus components and the muscles that they innervate. Remember, board questions usually have a clinical focus! When you study the brachial plexus, spend most of your time reasoning through the various injuries that result from lesions to the different nerves, branches, trunks, divisions, and so on. You are expected to know the most common ways in which these injuries can occur, because it is likely that you will have to deduce this from the stem of the question (e.g., associate frequent computer use with median nerve damage). Lower extremity (LE) nerve injuries are also tested on boards, but not quite as commonly as UE injuries.

SUMMARY BOX: UPPER EXTREMITY INJURIES

- The musculocutaneous nerve innervates the flexors of the elbow.
- The axillary nerve innervates the deltoid and teres minor muscles, as well as the long head of the triceps brachii.
- The radial nerve innervates the extensors in the arm and forearm.
- The ulnar nerve innervates the medial heads of the flexor digitorum profundus, the flexor carpi ulnaris, medial lumbricals, interossei, and hypothenar muscles.
- The median nerve innervates the anterior forearm muscles not innervated by the ulnar nerve, the lateral lumbricals, and the thenar muscles.
- The blood supply to the upper extremity (UE) is from the brachial artery, the continuation of the axillary artery after it crosses the teres major.
- The carpal tunnel consists of the eight carpal bones and the transverse carpal ligament. It contains the median nerve and the tendons of the long flexors of the digits.
- The rotator cuff consists of the tendons of four muscles: supraspinatus, infraspinatus, teres minor, and subscapularis.

CASE 26.3, PART A

You are working in an outpatient pediatrics clinic and your next patient is a 14-day-old infant who was born 2 weeks prematurely. The mother has no concerns, and you proceed to examine the child. The infant is mildly diaphoretic, and you notice a continuous (both systolic and diastolic) "machine-like murmur" auscultated best at the second left intercostal space.

1. What is the most likely diagnosis?
   Patent ductus arteriosus (PDA) is the most likely diagnosis.

2. Describe the fetal circulation pathway.
   In fetal life, oxygenated blood from the placenta enters the fetal circulation through the umbilical vein. Roughly half of this blood enters the inferior vena cava (IVC) through the hepatic veins, while the other half bypasses the hepatic

vasculature through the ductus venosus. Because the IVC receives a mixture of oxygenated blood and deoxygenated blood (return from the fetal systemic veins), oxygen tension in the IVC is higher than that in the superior vena cava (SVC). As a result, the IVC and SVC bloodstreams follow two distinct paths on entering the right atrium. A large percentage of IVC blood entering the right atrium is shunted to the left atrium (thus bypassing the lungs) through the foramen ovale, where it mixes with poorly oxygenated blood entering the left atrium through the pulmonary veins (recall that the lungs are not ventilated in the fetus and thus simply extract oxygen from the blood). This mixed blood is directed through the left ventricle and into the ascending aorta, where it is largely distributed to the brain, upper body, and coronaries. Blood from the IVC that is not shunted to the left atrium mixes with poorly oxygenated SVC blood and passes in typical fashion to the right ventricle. This output enters the pulmonary artery and from there either enters the lungs or gets shunted through the ductus arteriosus into the descending aorta. Blood in the descending aorta supplies the lower body and eventually makes its way into the umbilical arteries, which lead back to the placenta for oxygenation (Fig. 26.9).

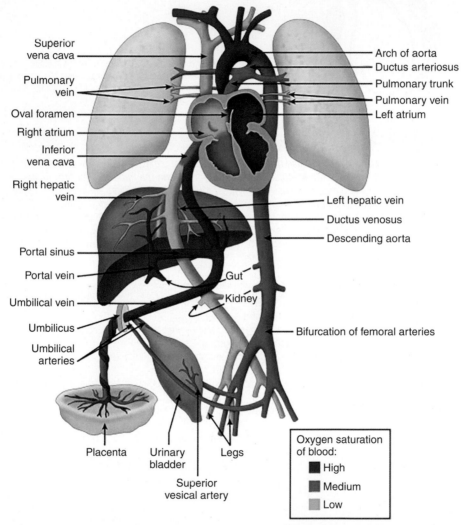

Figure 26.9. Course of fetal circulation in gestation. Note the blood flow patterns across the foramen ovale and the ductus arteriosus, and notice how blood mixes leading to a spectrum of oxygen saturations. *(From Rychik J, Tian Z.* Fetal Cardiovascular Imaging. *Philadelphia: Elsevier; 2012, Fig 1-1.)*

3. What is the utility of the ductus arteriosus?
    In utero, this connection between the aorta and the pulmonary artery acts as a right-to-left shunt. It allows most of the mixed oxygenated blood (which has entered the right side of the heart through the route of placenta → umbilical vein → ductus venosus → IVC) to bypass the developing lungs and enter the systemic circulation. Recall that bypassing the amniotic fluid-filled fetal lungs is desirable because they are incapable of gas exchange. Just after birth, the ductus arteriosus normally closes and undergoes fibrotic degeneration to become the ligamentum arteriosum.

4. **What causes the ductus arteriosus to close after birth?**

During life as a fetus, circulating prostaglandins and a low blood partial pressure of oxygen (pO_2) keeps the ductus arteriosus open. Blood pO_2 rises when breathing is initiated, signaling the newborn's ability to obtain oxygenated blood from the lungs rather than from the umbilical vein. Along with rising pO_2, decreasing levels of prostaglandins act to close the ductus arteriosus. If the ductus arteriosus remains patent after birth, it can often be closed by administering a drug that blocks the production of prostaglandin E_2, such as the cyclooxygenase (COX) inhibitor indomethacin. Alternatively, if a baby is born with a congenital defect, such as transposition of the great vessels, it is necessary to keep the ductus arteriosus open until the transposition can be surgically fixed so that oxygenated blood can still reach the systemic circulation. This can be achieved by administering alprostadil, a prostaglandin E_1 analog.

CASE 26.3, PART B

It is a slow morning on your cardiology rotation when a 32-year-old man who has a history of deep venous thrombosis (DVT) secondary to factor V Leiden thrombophilia is brought by ambulance to the emergency department (ED) with an apparent stroke. He has no history of atrial fibrillation, valvular disease, or coronary artery disease. On cardiac auscultation, you hear a mild systolic ejection murmur and wide, fixed splitting of S_2. Neurology confirms that he has had an ischemic stroke, and a transesophageal echocardiogram (TEE) indicates interatrial blood flow.

5. **What is the most likely diagnosis?**

Atrial septal defect (ASD) is most likely. A thromboembolic stroke is rare in young patients without atrial fibrillation, valvular disease, or a past MI. Although factor V Leiden produces a hypercoagulable state, it is much more likely to cause DVT than a left-sided heart or arterial thrombus. The physical examination and transesophageal echocardiogram (TEE) study findings strongly support ASD, so his stroke was most likely caused by a paradoxical embolus (in which an embolus of venous origin traveled through the ASD and then to the cerebral vasculature).

6. **Is ASD the most common congenital heart defect?**

No. Ventricular septal defect (VSD) is the most common. ASD is the second most common congenital heart defect, and PDA is the third.

7. **What are the three most common types of ASD?**

1. Ostium secundum defect

   Ostium secundum defect is the most common type of ASD. The atrial septum is formed by the septum primum and the septum secundum. In ostium secundum defect, there is usually excessive absorption of the septum primum, inadequate growth of the septum secundum, or enlargement of the foramen ovale (the opening at the inferior margin of the septum secundum). A subtype of ostium secundum defect is patent foramen ovale, in which the septum primum and septum secundum fail to fuse. This common defect may allow interatrial blood flow. Remember that this is physiologic in fetal life.

2. Ostium primum defect

   In ostium primum defect, the septum primum fails to fuse with the endocardial (atrioventricular [AV]) cushion, which leads to a communication between the atria. This is often due to an endocardial cushion defect, commonly associated with Down syndrome. Note that the endocardial cushion is the point of fusion for the atrial septum, ventricular septum, mitral valve, and tricuspid valve, and the magnitude of the defect determines the pathology. For instance, partial ostium primum defect causes an interatrial connection, but complete ostium primum defect causes an AV connection.

3. Sinus venosus defect

   Normally, the atrial septum develops completely to the left of the sinus venosus, the structure that is to become the superior and inferior venae cava and part of the right atrium. In this rare defect, the septum develops anterior to the sinus venosus, allowing interatrial flow via the sinus venosus as a result of vena cava entry straddling the septum (Fig. 26.10).

8. **How might an ASD cause right-sided heart failure?**

Left-sided heart pressures are higher than right-sided heart pressures, so an ASD allows for left-to-right shunting of blood. This increases flow volumes through the right side of the heart, leading to right ventricular (and atrial) dilation, increased work, decreased pumping ability, and eventually right-sided heart failure.

9. **What is the dreaded late complication of ASD?**

Eisenmenger syndrome refers to a situation in which pathologically increased right-sided heart flow and pressure damage the pulmonary vasculature, causing small vessel fibrosis to develop. The fibrotic vasculature exacerbates pulmonary hypertension and does not contribute to gas exchange, causing the right side of the heart to increase its output. Eventually, right-sided heart pressures become high enough to reverse the shunt of ASD to a right-to-left shunt, resulting in cyanosis and heart failure.

CASE 26.3, PART C

You are in the newborn nursery on the first day of your inpatient pediatrics rotation, and the neonatology fellow invites you in to see an infant. The infant is obviously cyanotic but seems to be having no respiratory difficulty other than mild tachypnea.

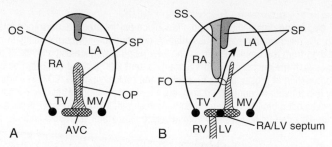

Figure 26.10. Development of atrial septum. A, The septum primum (SP) grows down from the roof of the primitive common atrium to meet the atrioventricular cushions (AVCs) and divides the primitive common atrium into right atrium (RA) and left atrium (LA). The defect below the growing free lower edge of SP is called *ostium primum* (OP) (shown here as a dotted oval). The septum primum has reached the AVCs, which have developed into tricuspid (TV) and mitral (MV) valves. The drawing shows that the upper part of the SP has (normally) degenerated to leave the large *ostium secundum* (OS) or fossa ovale defect. B, A second interatrial septum—septum secundum (SS)—grows to the *right* of the SP. The upper portions of the two septa fuse, and a portion of the upper part degenerates to form the OS. The lower edge of the SS grows downward to partially cover the OS but does not reach the AVCs. A valve-like opening—*foramen ovale* (FO)—is thereby established, permitting a shunt from RA to LA, but *not* in the reverse direction. The FO persists during fetal life (during which it transmits an essential right-to-left shunt), but after birth it usually seals off by fusion of the lower part of SP with SS. Note that the interventricular septum separates the right ventricle (RV) from the left ventricle (LV). The interventricular septum meets AVCs to the *right* of the atrial septum, so that one portion of the AVC separates RA from LV. This portion later forms the upper part of the interventricular septum, and it is through this portion that the Gerbode defect occurs. *(From Grainger RG, Allison D, Adams A. Grainger & Allison's Diagnostic Radiology: A Textbook of Medical Imaging. 4th ed. Philadelphia: Churchill Livingstone; 2001.)*

10. **What are the five cardiogenic causes of cyanosis in a newborn?**
    These five causes are known as the five Ts: **T**etralogy of Fallot, **T**ransposition of the great vessels, **T**runcus arteriosus, **T**ricuspid atresia, and **T**otal anomalous pulmonary venous return.

CASE 26.3, PART C CONTINUED:

On cardiac auscultation, you hear a 3/6 systolic crescendo-decrescendo murmur at the second left intercostal space and a loud S_2 at the fourth left intercostal space. The fellow shows you the infant's chest radiograph, which shows a "boot-shaped" heart, a classic sign of right ventricular hypertrophy.

11. **What is the most likely diagnosis?**
    The most likely diagnosis is tetralogy of Fallot, the most common congenital heart defect to cause cyanosis in infants. The murmurs of tetralogy of Fallot vary depending on the degree of pulmonary stenosis and the extent of the VSD. In this case, the pulmonary stenosis murmur overshadows any VSD murmur that might be appreciable. The loud S_2 is due to the closure of the aortic valve. Recall the four components of this disease: VSD, overriding aorta, pulmonary stenosis, and right ventricular hypertrophy.

12. **How does tetralogy of Fallot cause cyanosis?**
    Pulmonary stenosis causes a high resistance to flow through the pulmonary trunk. Coupled with concentric right ventricular hypertrophy, this leads to high right-sided heart pressures, causing right-to-left flow through the VSD (Fig. 26.11). When a critical proportion of deoxygenated blood is shunted through the VSD and mixed with oxygenated blood, cyanosis appears. It is classically seen first in the fingers and lips.

13. **What is the cause of tetralogy of Fallot?**
    The exact cause of tetralogy of Fallot is unknown, but it is believed to be multifactorial, including both environmental and genetic factors. Structurally, unequal partitioning of the primitive truncus arteriosus by the truncoconal ridges misplaces the infundibular septum, the structure that divides the two ventricular outflow tracts. The anterosuperior displacement of the infundibular septum causes pulmonary stenosis in addition to causing the aorta to override the VSD that results from failure of the truncoconal ridges to fuse with the muscular interventricular septum. Stenosis of the pulmonary trunk increases afterload, leading to concentric right ventricular hypertrophy, seen on a radiograph as a "boot-shaped" heart.

14. **What is the characteristic behavior in an infant with a later presentation of tetralogy?**
    Cyanosis that occurs with agitation, crying, or a warm bath that is corrected with squatting or "knees-to-chest" positioning. These episodes are known as *tet spells*. Crying increases pulmonary vascular resistance, and warmth decreases systemic vascular resistance, shunting blood away from the lungs and to the periphery. Squatting relieves the shunt by increasing systemic vascular resistance and forcing blood flow leaving the left ventricle to preferentially enter the lung, allowing oxygenation to resume.

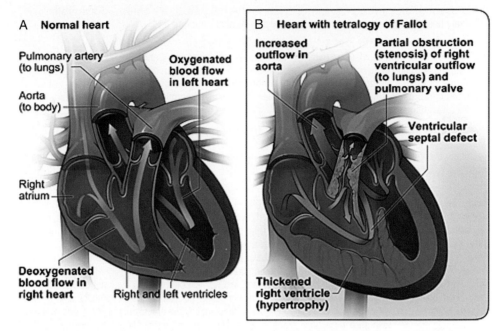

Figure 26.11. Tetralogy of Fallot. A, Normal heart. B, Heart with tetralogy of Fallot. *(From National Heart, Lung, and Blood Institute. Health Topics: Congenital Heart Defects. NHLBI website. https://nhlbi.nih.gov/health-topics/congenital-heart-defects. Accessed February 2, 2021.)*

SUMMARY BOX: CONGENITAL HEART DEFECTS

- The ductus arteriosus connects the pulmonary artery to the aorta and allows blood to bypass the developing lungs during fetal life.
- The patency of the ductus arteriosus is maintained by the presence of prostaglandin E_2 and low PO_2. It can be pharmacologically closed with indomethacin or kept open with a prostaglandin.
- During fetal life, blood also bypasses the developing lungs via the foramen ovale, which is appropriately patent at this time.
- Atrial septal defect (ASD) can be recognized on cardiac auscultation by a mild systolic ejection murmur and wide, fixed splitting of S_2.
- Ventricular septal defect (VSD) is the most common congenital heart defect, characterized by a harsh holosystolic murmur on examination.
- Eisenmenger syndrome refers to a right-to-left shunt (resulting in cyanosis) that occurred because a left-to-right shunt (VSD, ASD, or patent ductus arteriosus [PDA]) caused right-sided heart overload and pulmonary hypertension, leading to high right-sided heart pressures and shunt reversal.
- Tetralogy of Fallot is characterized by VSD, overriding aorta, pulmonary stenosis, and right ventricular hypertrophy. It is the most common cause of right-to-left cyanotic shunt in infants.

CASE 26.4, PART A

A 19-year-old college freshman presents to the emergency department (ED) with severe neck stiffness and a headache. His temperature is 38.8°C, and he has been experiencing chills. According to friends, he has become increasingly confused in the past 24 hours.

1. **What is the differential diagnosis for his symptoms?**
   Meningitis, encephalitis, mass lesion of brain (abscess or tumor), and subarachnoid hemorrhage are possible.

CASE 26.4, PART A CONTINUED:

On further questioning of his friends, it is discovered that the patient had an upper respiratory tract infection during the 3 days before his current illness. On examination, flexion of the neck while the patient is supine elicits pain and involuntary hip and knee flexion (Brudzinski sign). When the hip is flexed, attempted extension of the knee elicits pain (Kernig sign).

2. **What is the most likely diagnosis, and what is the next step to confirm this suspicion?**
He most likely has meningitis, which can be confirmed by lumbar puncture (LP).

3. **At what spinal level should an LP be performed? Why?**
In adults, the needle should be inserted between the spinous processes of L4 and L5. The space between L3 and L4 is also an acceptable choice because the conus medullaris (the terminal portion of the spinal cord) usually ends near the superior border of L2. Recall that the cauda equina continues below this level, but the free-floating nature of the nerve bundles in the cerebrospinal fluid (CSF) makes them less likely to sustain puncture damage. It should be noted that in children, an LP should be performed only between L4 and L5, because the spinal cord in children can extend to L3.

4. **Through what major structures and spaces, from superficial to deep, should the needle pass in an LP?**
Skin → subcutaneous tissue → spinal ligaments (supraspinous ligament, interspinous ligament, and ligamentum flavum) → epidural space → dura mater → arachnoid mater → subarachnoid space (from which CSF can be drawn).

5. **Describe the three layers of the meninges.**
Dura mater: This outermost layer is fused to the inside of the skull via the periosteal dural layer. The dura is double layered in the skull, allowing cranial compartmentalization and investment of the venous sinuses. In contrast, it is single layered within the vertebral canal, where it is separated from the sides by the epidural space. The dural sac extends to S2 and is attached to the coccyx via the filum terminale externum.
Arachnoid mater: This layer is fused to the inner surface of the dura and sends trabeculae to the outer surface of the pia. Between the arachnoid and the pia (the subarachnoid space) lies the CSF.
Pia mater: This is the outermost layer of the brain, spinal cord, and nerve roots because it cannot be separated from them. It invests the blood vessels of the brain and spinal cord. The pia continues after the conus medullaris as the filum terminale internum (which is not part of the cauda equina because it does not contain any axons) until the end of the dural sac at S2, where it is invested with dura to become the filum terminale externum, terminating at the coccyx (Fig. 26.12).

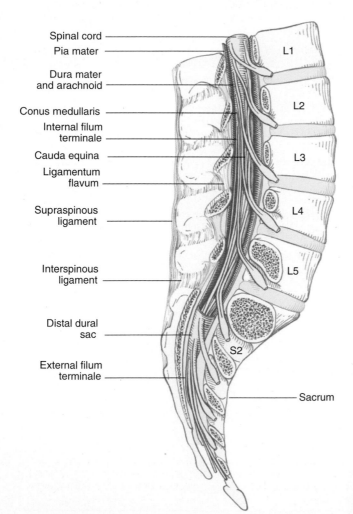

Figure 26.12. Spinal cord anatomy. Notice the termination of the spinal cord (i.e., conus medullaris) at L1–L2. *(From Miller RD, Eriksson LI, Fleisher LA, Wiener-Kronish JP, Cohen NH, Young WL. Miller's Anesthesia. 8th ed. Philadelphia: Elsevier; 2015.)*

6. **What CSF findings would you expect to find with different causes of meningitis?**
   See Table 26.4.

Table 26.4. Cerebrospinal Fluid Findings in Meningitis

PATHOGENIC CATEGORY	WHITE CELL PREDOMINANCE	PRESSURE	PROTEIN	GLUCOSE
Bacterial	PMN	↑	↑	↓
Tuberculosis	Lymphocyte	↑	↑	↓
Fungal	Lymphocyte	↑↑	↑	↓
Viral	Lymphocyte	Normal/↑	Normal/↑	Normal

PMN, Polymorphonuclear neutrophil (leukocyte).

7. **What are the most common causes of meningitis by age group?**
   See Table 26.5.

Table 26.5. Common Causes of Meningitis by Age Group

0–6 MONTHS	6 MONTHS TO 6 YEARS	6–60 YEARS	60+ YEARS
Group B streptococci *Escherichia coli* *Listeria monocytogenes*	*Neisseria meningitidis* Enteroviruses *Streptococcus pneumoniae* *Haemophilus influenzae* type b	*N. meningitidis* Enteroviruses *S. pneumoniae* Herpes simplex virus (HSV)	Gram-negative rods *S. pneumoniae* *L. monocytogenes*

STEP 1 SECRET

The information in Tables 26.4 and 26.5 is high yield for Step 1, and this knowledge will earn you easy points if you take the time to learn it well. The causes of meningitis in Table 26.5 are not listed in any particular order. The mnemonic for recalling the common causes of meningitis by age group is GEL MESH, MESH GeLS, where each word represents a separate age group (see Table 26.5).

CASE 26.4, PART B

A 1-month-old infant presents for a well-child checkup. She is developmentally normal for her age. On examination, a tuft of hair overlying a 1-cm darkly pigmented patch is found at the level of L5. The examination is otherwise entirely unrevealing.

8. **What disorder of neurologic development can be characterized by these findings?**
   Spina bifida occulta is a disorder in which the posterior neural tube fails to close, resulting in a failure of midline vertebral arch closure with intact dura. There are no associated neurologic deficits.

9. **What are the other significant disorders related to a failure of posterior neural tube closure?**
   Spina bifida cystica—meningocele: Failure of posterior midline closure of both the vertebral arch and the dura mater. The arachnoid mater herniates through the defect, creating a cyst. Neurologic deficits may or may not occur.
   Spina bifida cystica—meningomyelocele: Failure of posterior midline closure of both the vertebral arch and the dura mater, but the defect is wide enough to allow spinal cord herniation with the arachnoid. Neurologic deficits are level dependent but usually include paralysis of some degree. This disorder can be associated with Arnold–Chiari malformation type II.

CASE 26.4, PART C

A 64-year-old carpenter presents with severe lower back pain. Most of the pain is localized to a single spot in his lower back, but he has ill-defined pain and tingling that begins in the left gluteal region and courses down the lateral side of his left LE to his foot. He also has experienced left LE weakness. He reports that all these symptoms started 3 days ago, coming on suddenly while he was working in his yard. On physical examination, passive right straight leg raise causes moderate pain in the distribution (on the left) as described here.

10. **What is the most likely diagnosis?**

He has had an intervertebral disk herniation. This is supported by his severe, acute-onset lumbar back pain (upward of 90% of disk herniations involve the L4–L5 or L5–S1 disks), unilateral motor deficit, and pain and tingling that follow a spinal nerve distribution.

11. **Describe intervertebral disk anatomy and how herniation usually occurs.**

The nucleus pulposus is the central elastic cartilaginous portion of the disk. It is surrounded by the annulus fibrosus, which consists of concentric rings of fibrocartilage. With age, the nuclei pulposi become thin and lose their elasticity, and the annuli fibrosi degenerate. This makes the disk more likely to herniate, an action characterized by the nucleus pulposus breaking through a localized weakness in the annulus fibrosus. Herniations usually occur in the posterolateral direction because this is a site of relative annulus fibrosus weakness, and there is no support from the anterior or posterior longitudinal ligaments of the vertebral column. Posterolateral disk herniations occur proximal to the intervertebral foramina through which the spinal nerves pass, potentially compressing the spinal nerves and leading to radiculopathy (Fig. 26.13).

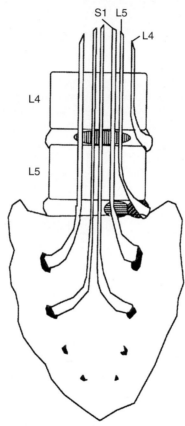

Figure 26.13. Lumbosacral disk herniation. The most common posterolateral herniation compresses the nerve root traveling downward to emerge one level below the level of the exiting root. Hence L5–S1 herniation most commonly compresses the descending S1 root *(herniation 3)*. More lateral herniation may compress the root exiting at the level of herniation *(herniation 2)*. A large central herniation may compress multiple bilateral descending roots of the cauda equina *(herniation 1)*. *(Adapted from Goetz CG.* Textbook of Clinical Neurology. *2nd ed. Philadelphia: WB Saunders; 2003.)*

12. **Describe the pattern of nerve compression seen in intervertebral disk herniations.**

Recall the scheme for numbering spinal nerves: The cervical spinal nerves C1 to C7 exit the spinal canal superior to the vertebra with the same number. The naming scheme changes at nerve C8, which exits inferior to the C7 vertebra. Thereafter, the spinal nerve roots exit below the vertebra with the same number (the L1 spinal nerve exits below the L1 vertebra). Despite the change within this numbering scheme, disk herniations tend to compress the nerve root with the same number as the vertebra below the intervertebral disk. For example, C4–C5 disk herniations result in compression of the C5 nerve root, and L4–L5 disk herniations result in compression of the L5 nerve root. This relationship is maintained because of the increasingly acute angles at which the spinal nerves come off the spinal cord as it descends (Fig. 26.14). However, this change in angle and the presence of the cauda equina allow for multiple nerve compressions to occur with a posteromedial herniation in the lower lumbar region (e.g., an L5-S1 herniation can compress both the L5 and S1 nerves).

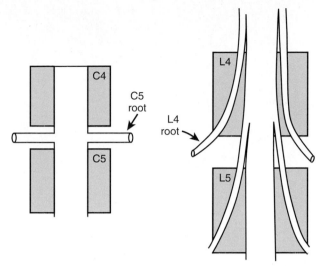

Figure 26.14. Comparison of points at which nerve roots emerge from cervical and lumbar spine. *(From Kikuchi S, Macnab I, Moreau P. Localisation of the level of symptomatic cervical disc degeneration.* J Bone Joint Surg. *1981;63B:272.)*

SUMMARY BOX: SPINAL CORD AND VERTEBRAL COLUMN

- The best site for a lumbar puncture (LP) is the L4–L5 interspace, well below the end of the spinal cord at L2.
- Spina bifida is a disorder in which the posterior neural tube fails to close.
  - Spina bifida occulta is the least severe subtype, followed by meningocele, and then by meningomyelocele.
- Intervertebral disk herniation
  - Occurs when the central nucleus pulposus herniates through the annulus fibrosus
  - Usually occurs in the posterolateral direction, where support from the anterior and posterior longitudinal ligaments is lacking
  - Usually occurs in the lower lumbar region
  - Most commonly results in compression of the nerve root named for the vertebra below the intervertebral disk

---

CASE 26.5

An 18-year-old college student presents with a 1-month history of an intermittent bulge in the right side of his scrotum. He has recently started bodybuilding and states that the bulge is more likely to appear during workouts and less likely to appear while he is lying down. There is no associated pain or scrotal erythema or edema. On physical examination, the scrotum does not transilluminate, and a soft structure can be reduced through the superficial inguinal ring.

---

1. Describe the characteristics of the most likely diagnosis.
   Indirect inguinal hernia, which is the most common type of hernia in both sexes, is characterized by a protrusion of parietal peritoneum and viscera through a part of the abdominal wall lateral to the inferior epigastric vessels. The viscera exit the abdominal cavity via the deep inguinal ring and enter the scrotum via the superficial inguinal ring, passing through the entirety of the inguinal canal. Recall that parietal peritoneum envelops the testicles during their descent out of the abdomen into the scrotum, eventually forming the tunica vaginalis. During the descent, the cavity of the tunica vaginalis is connected to the peritoneal cavity by the processus vaginalis, which is normally obliterated in the perinatal period. In some cases, a persistent processus vaginalis remains, forming a potential space within the spermatic cord through which indirect inguinal hernias can protrude. Note that this etiology means that indirect inguinal hernias are congenital (Fig. 26.15).

2. What differentiates a direct from an indirect inguinal hernia? What about a groin hernia that occurs below the inguinal ligament?
   A direct inguinal hernia is due to muscular weakness in the abdominal wall. It is characterized by protrusion of parietal peritoneum and viscera through the Hesselbach triangle, bordered laterally by the inferior epigastric artery, medially by the lateral margin of the rectus abdominis, and inferiorly by the inguinal ligament. The hernia sac is usually composed of transversalis fascia, and although it may pass through a portion of the inguinal canal, it rarely enters the scrotum and is not within the spermatic cord (Fig. 26.16). Most direct inguinal hernias are acquired. A groin hernia below the inguinal

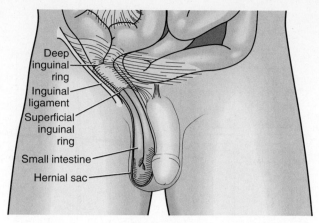

Figure 26.15. Indirect inguinal hernia. *(From Roberts JR.* Roberts and Hedges' Clinical Procedures in Emergency Medicine. *6th ed. Philadelphia: Elsevier; 2014.)*

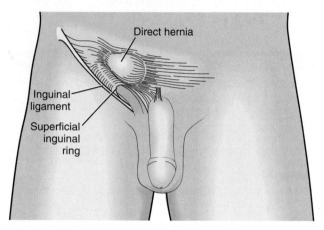

Figure 26.16. Direct inguinal hernia. *(From Roberts JR.* Roberts and Hedges' Clinical Procedures in Emergency Medicine. *6th ed. Philadelphia: Elsevier; 2014.)*

ligament is more likely a femoral hernia. These are relatively uncommon compared with inguinal hernias. They are about 10 times more common in women than men. Femoral hernias have a high incidence of incarceration and strangulation, so they usually require surgical repair.

STEP 1 SECRET

Differentiating among the various classes of hernias is commonly tested on Step 1. You should understand the relationship of the different hernia types to their respective anatomic borders. To quickly differentiate between an indirect and a direct inguinal hernia, remember that "MD's do Lie" (Medial to the epigastric vessels is associated with a Direct hernia and Lateral to the epigastric vessels is associated with an Indirect hernia). That being said, also remember that if the hernia is above the inguinal ligament and the femoral pulse is located lateral to the bulge, the patient has a direct hernia, while a femoral pulse medial to the bulge indicates an indirect hernia.

3. Describe the structure of the inguinal canal.
   The inguinal canal is an inferomedially directed passageway that connects two openings, the deep and the superficial inguinal rings. The deep inguinal ring is in the transversalis fascia, just lateral to the inferior epigastric vessels. The superficial inguinal ring is in the external oblique aponeurosis and lies just superolateral to the pubic tubercle. Two walls, a roof, and a floor delineate the canal formed between these two rings. Its major constituents are as follows: the transversalis fascia forms the posterior wall, the external oblique aponeurosis forms the anterior wall, the internal

oblique and transversus abdominis muscles form the roof, and the inguinal ligament forms the floor. It should be noted that the layers of the spermatic cord are applied via passage of the testicles through the inguinal canal. Consequently, the internal spermatic fascia is continuous with the transversalis fascia, the cremasteric fascia is continuous with the internal oblique, and the external spermatic fascia is continuous with the external oblique aponeurosis.

4. Discuss the major contents of the spermatic cord.
   - *External spermatic fascia:* Continuation of the external oblique aponeurosis.
   - *Cremasteric muscle and fascia:* Continuation of the internal oblique muscle and fascia; draws testes superiorly, often in response to cold temperatures.
   - *Internal spermatic fascia:* Continuation of the transversalis fascia.
   - *Vas deferens:* Transports sperm from the epididymis to the ejaculatory duct.
   - *Testicular artery:* Supplies testes and epididymis (testicular torsion is a medical emergency because twisting of the spermatic cord leads to occlusion of this artery).
   - *Pampiniform plexus:* A venous network that drains into the right and left testicular veins. The venous blood of the pampiniform plexus is cooler than the adjacent blood from the testicular artery. This countercurrent flow cools the blood destined for the testes, maintaining an intratesticular temperature just below the core body temperature.
   - *Genital branch of the genitofemoral nerve:* Supplies sensory innervation to the anterior aspect of the scrotum and supplies motor innervation to the cremaster muscle.
   - *Ilioinguinal nerve:* This nerve pierces the internal oblique muscle to enter the inguinal canal, thereafter traveling on the surface of the spermatic cord, rather than within it, to supply some sensory innervation to the superior aspect of the scrotum and root of the penis.
   - *Other:* Autonomic nerve fibers and lymphatic vessels that drain to the para-aortic (lumbar) and preaortic lymph nodes are also present.

5. Which lymph nodes are the most likely site of first metastasis in testicular cancer? Why is this the case?
   Testicular lymphatic fluid drains directly to the preaortic and para-aortic (lumbar) lymph nodes. Recall that during embryogenesis, each developing gonad arises from a combination of mesoderm and mesothelium called the *gonadal ridge*, which lies just medial to the mesonephros (itself, lying medial to the metanephros, which develops into the kidney). Thus, the testes (and ovaries) develop markedly superior to their position in adult life. Consequently, the blood supply and lymphatic drainage of the testes are located closer to the kidneys than to any structures of the pelvis. For example, the two testicular arteries branch directly from the aorta just inferior to the origin of the renal arteries. It should be noted that, in contrast with testicular cancer, cancer of the scrotum initially metastasizes to the superficial inguinal lymph nodes.

STEP 1 SECRET

You should expect to get a question regarding the sites of local metastasis for various types of cancer. The USMLE is especially fond of the fact that testicular and ovarian cancers metastasize to the para-aortic lymph nodes.

---

6. After a vasectomy, by what means does a male produce an ejaculate that does not include sperm? Include a summary of the path of sperm from spermatogenesis to exit from the urethra.
   Sperm makes up 5% to 10% of the semen, or ejaculate, so ejaculate after vasectomy is semen that does not contain sperm. Normally, sperm pass from their point of origin in the seminiferous tubules to the epididymis and onward into the vas deferens. The two vasa deferentia merge with the outlets of the two seminal vesicles to form the ejaculatory duct. The ejaculatory duct feeds into the prostatic urethra, where the prostate gland deposits its secretions. The prostatic urethra leads to the penile urethra, where the bulbourethral glands deposit their secretions. From the penile urethra, the ejaculate exits the body (Fig. 26.17). In a vasectomy, the vasa deferentia are ligated bilaterally, so sperm cannot pass into the ejaculatory duct, and most of them degenerate in the proximal vas deferens and epididymis. The secretions of the seminal vesicles, prostate, and bulbourethral glands enter the system distal to the ligation points at the vas deferens, and these secretions are ejaculated without sperm, which nominally contributes very little to the volume of normal ejaculate. Thus, the volume of ejaculate is not noticeably changed by vasectomy. Remember "SEVEN UP" for the pathway of the sperm: **S**eminiferous tubules → **E**pididymis → **V**as deferens → **E**jaculatory duct → **N**othing → **U**rethra → **P**enis

7. Describe the neurologic basis for erection, emission, and ejaculation.
   In the unaroused state, arteriovenous anastomoses allow most of the blood from the deep artery of the penis to bypass the helicine arteries within the corpora cavernosa. On sexual stimulation, parasympathetic input to the helicine arteries causes vasodilation and vessel straightening, greatly increasing blood flow to the corpora cavernosa, which become engorged. As the corpora cavernosa increase in volume, they compress the obliquely exiting veins against the tunica albuginea, blocking outflow of blood. Blood drainage is also restricted by contraction of the ischiocavernosus and bulbospongiosus muscles, causing a complete *erection* to occur. *Emission* occurs via sympathetic input, which causes contraction of the smooth muscle of the epididymis, vas deferens, seminal vesicles, and prostate (effectively delivering

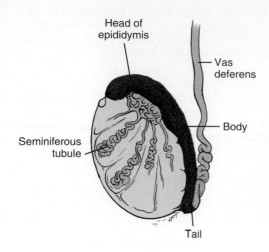

Head of epididymis

Vas deferens

Body

Seminiferous tubule

Tail

Figure 26.17. Testis and epididymis. One to three seminiferous tubules fill each compartment and drain in the rete testis in the mediastinum. Twelve to 20 efferent ductules become convoluted in the head of the epididymis and drain into a single coiled duct of the epididymis. The vas is convoluted in its first portion. *(From Parton AW, Dmochowski RR, Kavoussi LR, Peters CA. Campbell-Walsh-Wein Urology. 12th ed. Philadelphia: Elsevier; 2021.)*

sperm and secretions to the prostatic urethra). *Ejaculation* is a mixed autonomic and somatic response. As the sympathetic system closes the internal urethral sphincter to guard against backflow, the parasympathetic system causes peristalsis of the urethral muscle while the pudendal nerve causes contraction of the bulbospongiosus muscle to propel the semen forward. Remember "**P**oint and **S**hoot": **P**arasympathetic nerves are responsible for erection (**P**oint), and **S**ympathetic nerves are responsible for emission (**S**hoot)!

8. **Name the most common drugs used for treatment of erectile dysfunction and outline their mechanism of action.**
   Sildenafil (Viagra), vardenafil, and tadalafil are the drugs most commonly used to treat erectile dysfunction.
   Sexual stimulation normally results in parasympathetic-mediated endothelial cell nitric oxide (NO) release within the helicine arteries of the corpora cavernosa. NO diffuses to the adjacent vascular smooth muscle, where it causes vasodilation through a multistep pathway. NO directly activates guanylyl cyclase to produce cyclic guanosine monophosphate (cGMP). This activates protein kinase G (PKG), which then activates myosin light-chain phosphatase (MLCP), which dephosphorylates myosin light chains, leading to arterial smooth muscle relaxation and increased blood flow to the corpora cavernosa.
   Sildenafil, vardenafil, and tadalafil inhibit cGMP-specific phosphodiesterase-5 (PDE-5), which breaks down cGMP. Note that these drugs do not act in the absence of sexual stimulation, which is the initial event that causes helicine NO to be produced. Given their mechanism of action, it should be noted that these drugs should not be administered with nitrates because hypotension may result. Note that the commercial warnings of priapism represent an exceedingly rare side effect. In fact, the most common cause of drug-induced priapism is trazodone, a drug used to treat depression.

SUMMARY BOX: HERNIAS AND MALE REPRODUCTIVE FUNCTION

- Indirect inguinal hernia: Protrusion begins lateral to the epigastric vessels, runs through deep inguinal ring into inguinal canal, and often enters the scrotal sac. It is congenital.
- Direct inguinal hernia: Protrusion begins medial to the epigastric vessels, bypasses deep inguinal ring into inguinal canal, and rarely enters the scrotum. It is acquired.

CASE 26.6

A 24-year-old fishing guide presents with intermittent scrotal enlargement, which he first noticed a few months ago. He relates that the left scrotum is larger than the right, and that the swelling decreases significantly when he lies down. Occasionally, he experiences an aching scrotal pain and "heaviness." On review of systems, you discover that he and his wife have been seen in the fertility clinic because they have failed to conceive after 15 months of trying.

---

1. **What is the differential diagnosis for his symptoms?**
   Indirect inguinal hernia, varicocele, hydrocele, hematocele, testicular cancer, and infection (epididymitis or infection of the scrotal skin) are all considerations. Testicular torsion and trauma should be ruled out but are much less likely, given that the onset is not acute.

CASE 26.6 CONTINUED:

He is found to be afebrile and in no acute distress. He is not currently having testicular pain. On scrotal palpation, the left side feels like there is a ""bundle of worms" superior to the testicle. The scrotum becomes less tensely swollen when he moves from the upright to the supine position. The scrotum does not transilluminate. You are unable to appreciate a hernia sac or any focal testicular masses.

2. Which of the possibilities is now the most likely diagnosis?
   Varicocele is most likely. The infertility, aching scrotal pain and heaviness, and "bag of worms" on testicular palpation suggest this diagnosis.

3. Outline varicocele pathophysiology. Be sure to explain why varicocele is more likely to occur on the left than on the right and how this condition may lead to difficulty in having children.
   A varicocele refers to a varicosity (dilated and tortuous veins) of the pampiniform plexus. The exact cause is still debated, but there are at least three important factors. Recall that the left testicular vein drains into the left renal vein, which then crosses between the superior mesenteric artery and aorta to drain into the IVC. The angle of the testicular–renal vein junction is large enough to disturb flow, which may result in back pressure down into the pampiniform plexus. Likewise, because it runs between two arteries, the left renal vein is subject to compression (nutcracker syndrome), which results in back pressure into the distal renal vein, left testicular artery, and left pampiniform plexus (Fig. 26.18). However, although rarer, varicocele can occur on the right side as well (the right testicular vein drains directly into the IVC at an acute angle and has no major compression points), so it is likely that defective valves in the testicular veins play a role in the development of varicocele on both sides. A common board association is that right-sided varicoceles should raise suspicion of malignancy because there are no kinking or high resistance points to cause a varicocele otherwise, but only about 1 in 30 patients with a right-sided varicocele will have a malignancy. Varicoceles result in some degree of venous stasis in the pampiniform plexus, thus decreasing its ability to cool the arterial blood en route to the testes. The high intratesticular temperatures decrease sperm production and quality.

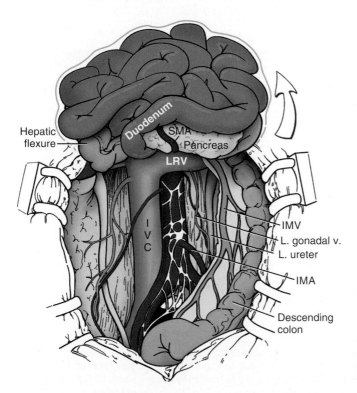

Figure 26.18. The retroperitoneal space has been exposed. The duodenum has been kocherized; its second, third, and fourth portions have been reflected superiorly, along with the pancreas and the superior mesenteric artery (SMA). The entire right colon has been mobilized and exteriorized. *IMA,* Inferior mesenteric artery; *IMV,* inferior mesenteric vein; *IVC,* inferior vena cava; *LRV,* left renal vein. (*From Wein AJ, Kavoussi LR, Novick AC, et al.* Campbell-Walsh Urology. *10th ed. Philadelphia: Saunders; 2012.*)

4. Describe the difference between hydrocele and hematocele.
   Hydrocele is a collection of excess nonsanguineous fluid within the tunica vaginalis. It can be caused by a persistent processus vaginalis that communicates between the cavity of the tunica vaginalis and peritoneal cavity, orchitis, epididymitis, and corditis, or it can be idiopathic. Scrotal transillumination is often seen on physical examination.
   Hematocele occurs when injury to the spermatic vessels leads to hemorrhage into the cavity of the tunica vaginalis.

CASE 26.6 CONTINUED:

The patient undergoes surgical correction of his varicocele. He goes on to have three children and is so pleased with how you treated him that his entire family has transferred to your care. His father, a 65-year-old bartender, first presents to your office with apparent cirrhosis and portal hypertension. He has been feeling extremely fatigued for the past 3 days. In the office, he is jaundiced and breathing rapidly (tachypnea) and has a 2/6 systolic flow murmur. You quickly send him to the emergency department (ED), where he is admitted for melena and anemia. Upper endoscopy reveals bleeding esophageal varices.

5. **What are esophageal varices?**
   Esophageal varices are dilated esophageal veins. The esophageal venous system is one of the sites of portacaval (portosystemic) anastomosis. Esophageal vein dilation occurs because of high portal pressures that force venous flow into the systemic circuit in higher volumes than normal and in the reverse direction of physiologic venous flow, to bypass the liver.

6. **How do the esophageal veins connect the portal and systemic venous systems?**
   To reach portal circulation, the esophageal veins drain into the left gastric vein. The left gastric vein feeds directly into the portal vein. To reach systemic circulation, the esophageal veins drain into the veins of the azygous system. Other portacaval anastomoses include:
   - Superior rectal veins (portal) with inferior and middle rectal veins (systemic) (dilation can lead to hemorrhoids)
   - Paraumbilical veins (portal) with superficial epigastric veins (systemic) (dilation can lead to caput medusae)
   - Various branches of the colic veins (portal) with the retroperitoneal veins of Retzius (systemic)
   - Branches of the splenic vein (portal) with the left renal vein (systemic)

7. **Describe the function of the azygos system.**
   The azygos system primarily drains the posterior walls of the thorax (via intercostal and vertebral veins) and the abdomen (via ascending lumbar and vertebral veins). It also receives the mediastinal, bronchial, and esophageal veins. The azygos system is infamous for variability, but in general, the primary vein is the azygos vein, which runs vertically along the right anterolateral aspect of the vertebral column within the thorax. It drains into the SVC.

SUMMARY BOX: ASYMMETRIES OF THE VENA CAVA

- A varicocele is characterized by varicose veins of the pampiniform plexus.
- Hydrocele and hematocele differ in that these result from fluid and blood, respectively, in the cavity of the tunica vaginalis.
- The right gonadal (testicular or ovarian) vein drains directly into the inferior vena cava (IVC), and the left gonadal vein drains into the left renal vein.
- The left renal vein runs between the superior mesenteric artery and the abdominal aorta.
- The esophageal veins are one of the five major anastomoses that connect the systemic (via the azygos system) and portal (via the left gastric vein) systems.
- The azygos system is the main venous drainage of the posterior walls of the thorax and abdomen.

CASE 26.7, PART A

You are volunteering as a team doctor for a local high school football team. You watch in horror as a player from the opposing team puts a vicious hit on your team's star running back. The primary point of impact is the lateral aspect of the right knee, which was the leg he had planted to change direction. He is unwilling to put any weight on his right leg because of the extreme pain. On examination of the knee, you note that an abnormal degree of passive tibial valgus deviation is achievable, and there is a positive McMurray test, as well as a positive anterior drawer sign.

1. **List the structures that he has injured.**
   He has the "unhappy triad" of knee injuries: he has torn his tibial (medial) collateral ligament (MCL), allowing tibial valgus deviation; lateral meniscus with a positive result on a McMurray test; and anterior cruciate ligament (ACL), associated with an anterior drawer sign. Note that the McMurray test can be used to check for both medial and lateral meniscus tears, depending on whether the medial or the lateral meniscus is stabilized by the examiner.

2. **How does the posterior cruciate ligament differ from the ACL?**
   The ACL runs from the posteromedial aspect of the lateral condyle of the femur to the anterior intercondylar area of the tibia. It is weaker than the posterior cruciate ligament (PCL), and it prevents anterior displacement of the tibia. Thus, a torn ACL yields a positive anterior drawer sign: flexing the knee to 90 degrees and pulling the tibia anteriorly under a fixed femur results in the tibia's being pulled out a short distance like a drawer. The Lachman test is where the knee is in 20 to 30 degrees of flexion and the examiner places a hand behind the tibia and another on the thigh. Subsequently,

the tibia is pulled anteriorly and tested for laxity. This is thought to be more sensitive than the anterior drawer test because on the anterior drawer test the leg is planted and the patient may be able to use their hamstrings to stabilize the knee.

The PCL runs from the medial condyle of the femur to the posterior intercondylar area of the tibia, crossing posterior to the ACL. The PCL prevents posterior displacement of the tibia. The most common way to tear the PCL is an impact to the superior tibia with a flexed knee. Consequently, a torn PCL allows the tibia to be displaced posteriorly under a fixed femur, a maneuver known as the posterior drawer sign (Fig. 26.19).

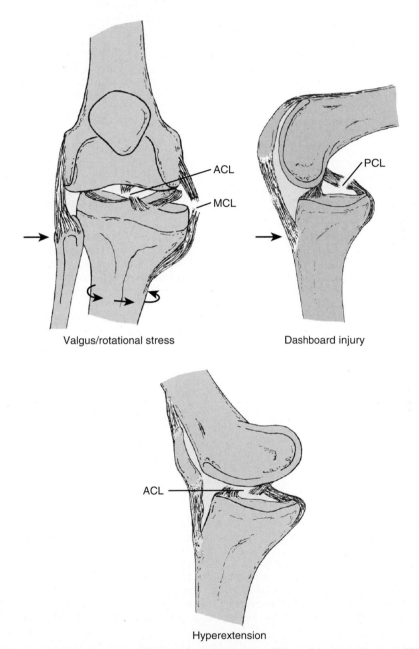

Valgus/rotational stress

Dashboard injury

Hyperextension

Figure 26.19. Common mechanisms of knee injury. *ACL,* Anterior cruciate ligament; *MCL,* medial collateral ligament; *PCL,* posterior cruciate ligament. *(From Browner BD, Jupiter JB, Levine AM, et al.* Skeletal Trauma: Basic Science, Management, and Reconstruction. *3rd ed. Philadelphia: WB Saunders; 2003.)*

3. Explain why his MCL and ACL tears led to the tear in his lateral meniscus.
   In this case, he was hit in the knee from the lateral aspect with his foot planted. The force of the hit abducted his knee joint, tearing the MCL, and propelled his tibia forward in relation to the femur, tearing his ACL. Because of the knee

abduction, the medial condyle of his femur was essentially lifted off of the medial meniscus, putting the burden of the impact onto the lateral meniscus, which tore in response to shear forces within the joint allowed by his torn ACL. It should be noted that the MCL fibers intertwine with those of the medial meniscus, making it possible for chronic damage to the MCL to extend to the medial meniscus. However, in acute injuries such as this one, medial meniscus injuries occur only in combination with lateral meniscus injuries, and lateral meniscus injuries are much more commonly included in the unhappy triad than medial meniscus injuries.

CASE 26.7, PART A CONTINUED:

He returns to you a year and a half later with issues resulting from another football injury. This past season, he had a right fibular neck fracture, and the leg was immobilized for several weeks. Since his cast was removed, he has noticed that his right foot "hangs," and that he must step higher than he did before to prevent his toes from dragging on the ground. On physical examination, testing his foot dorsiflexion reveals 5/5 strength on the left and 2/5 strength on the right. In addition, he has reduced sensation over the dorsum of his right foot.

4. This clinical picture suggests injury to what structure?
   The common fibular (or peroneal) nerve is injured. This nerve runs lateral to the fibular neck, coming from just posterior to the fibular head and coursing anterior to the fibular neck, where it divides into the deep and superficial fibular nerves. Owing to its close proximity to the fibular neck, fractures of this structure often injure the common fibular nerve.

5. How does injury to the common fibular nerve result in footdrop, as seen in this patient?
   Footdrop is characterized by difficulty with or an inability to perform dorsiflexion and eversion of the foot, leading to passive plantar flexion and inversion of the foot, especially when walking. Injury to the common fibular nerve is responsible for this dysfunction because the deep fibular nerve innervates the anterior compartment muscles. The anterior compartment muscles are tibialis anterior, extensor hallucis longus, extensor digitorum longus, and fibularis tertius, which is the distal portion of the peroneus or fibularis muscle group. The anterior compartment muscles dorsiflex the foot. The superficial fibular nerve innervates the lateral compartment muscles (fibularis longus and brevis, the proximal portion of the peroneus muscle group) that evert the foot. Note that the superficial fibular nerve has sensory branches distributed on the dorsum of the foot and the distal third of the anterior leg. Also note that the fibularis tertius acts to evert the foot, and that the actions of all of these muscles have been simplified for this discussion (Fig. 26.20).

STEP 1 SECRET

Damage to the common peroneal nerve is a favorite on boards and is commonly posed as a mononeuropathic sequela of uncontrolled diabetes. Another favorite is damage to the tibial nerve, which innervates muscles that invert and plantar flex the foot. The tibial nerve is sensory to the sole of the foot.

6. List the muscles of the posterior compartment of the leg and describe their innervation.
   The superficial muscle group consists of the gastrocnemius, soleus, and plantaris. This is separated from the deep muscle group by the fibrous transverse intermuscular septum. The deep muscle group includes the popliteus, flexor hallucis longus, flexor digitorum longus, and tibialis posterior. The primary function of the posterior compartment muscles is plantar flexion. They are all innervated by the tibial nerve, which arises just superior to the lateral femoral condyle from the divergence of the two nerve roots (L4–L5) that compose the sciatic nerve (the other being the common fibular nerve). It should be noted that the sciatic nerve is made up of five nerve roots (L4–L5 and S1–S3), but S1–S3 are involved in only sensory innervation, while L4–L5 are involved in skeletal muscle innervation.

CASE 26.7, PART A CONTINUED:

One year later, he is involved in an automobile accident and has a distal left femur fracture, which shears his popliteal artery. He undergoes emergent vascular surgery, and his popliteal artery is successfully repaired. However, 4 hours after surgery, he begins reporting severe calf pain. On examination, his leg appears pale and his calf is firm. The leg is painful with passive movement and has markedly decreased sensation and posterior tibial/dorsalis pedis pulses.

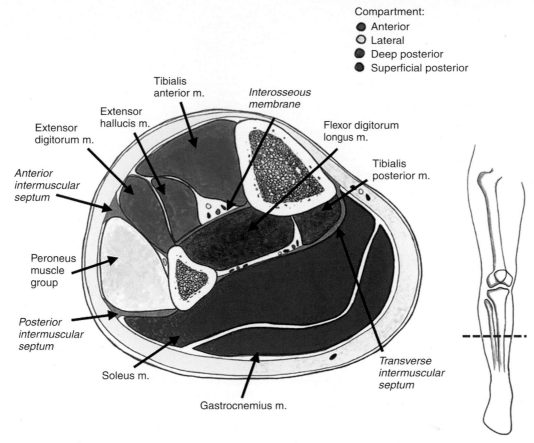

Compartment:
- ● Anterior
- ○ Lateral
- ◖ Deep posterior
- ● Superficial posterior

Tibialis anterior m.

Interosseous membrane

Extensor hallucis m.

Extensor digitorum m.

Flexor digitorum longus m.

Anterior intermuscular septum

Tibialis posterior m.

Peroneus muscle group

Posterior intermuscular septum

Transverse intermuscular septum

Soleus m.

Gastrocnemius m.

Figure 26.20. Four compartments of the leg: transverse section through middle portion of left leg. (*Illustration by Katie Carsky, MD.*)

7. What dreaded vascular surgery complication does he have?
   This patient has compartment syndrome.

8. What divides the compartments of the leg?
   The crural fascia envelops all of the muscles and bones of the leg. The four compartments (anterior, lateral, deep posterior, and superficial posterior) are separated by the anterior, posterior, and transverse intermuscular septa, as well as the interosseous membrane (which connects the tibia and fibula) (Fig. 26.21).

9. Describe the major pathophysiologic characteristics of compartment syndrome.
   The four compartments of the leg are invested with fascia that is highly resistant to stretching. Thus, relatively small volume increases, as would be seen in swelling, result in rapid increases in pressure. Because a compartment represents a closed system, an increase in intracompartmental pressure is directly transmitted to the vasculature, leading first to compression of small, thin-walled vessels. Higher pressures result in compression of progressively larger, thicker-walled vessels. If prolonged, this leads to ischemia and necrosis. In this case, his intracompartmental pressure increased because of inflammation and swelling resulting from reperfusion injury. The most common symptoms of compartment syndrome are summed up in the 6 Ps: Pain, Paresthesia, Pallor, Paralysis, Pulselessness, and Poikilothermia.

CASE 26.7, PART B

A female patient sustains a gunshot wound to the right pelvis. She undergoes emergency surgery. The surgery is successful, but the attending surgeon admits that some nerve damage was unavoidable during the procedure. Two months later, she presents to your clinic claiming that the surgery made her right leg shorter than her left leg. To prove this to you, she demonstrates that to keep the foot of her "longer leg" off the ground while walking, she must consciously lift it higher, or she must lean to the right while walking, in effect, using a waddling gait. You note that while her left foot is in the air, her left pelvis sags.

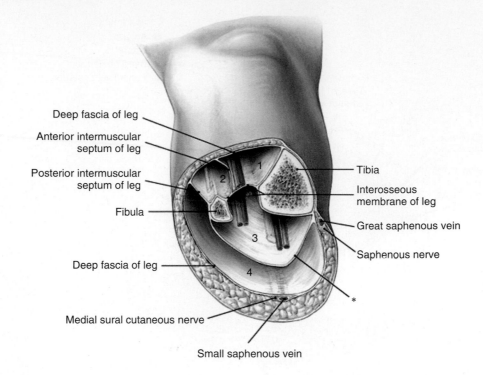

Deep fascia of leg

Anterior intermuscular septum of leg

Posterior intermuscular septum of leg

Fibula

Deep fascia of leg

Medial sural cutaneous nerve

Small saphenous vein

Tibia

Interosseous membrane of leg

Great saphenous vein

Saphenous nerve

1 Anterior compartment of leg:	**2 Lateral compartment of leg:**	**3 Posterior compartment of leg, deep part:**	**4 Posterior compartment of leg, superficial part:**
Anterior tibialis artery; vein	Superficial fibular nerve	Posterior tibial artery; vein	Triceps surae
Deep fibular nerve	Fibularis [peroneus] longus	Fibular artery; vein	Plantaris
Tibialis anterior	Fibularis [peroneus] brevis	Tibial nerve	
Extensor digitorum longus		Flexor digitorum longus	
Extensor hallucis longus		Tibialis posterior	
Fibularis [peroneus] tertius		Flexor hallucis longus	

Figure 26.21. Leg, right side; transverse section at the mid-leg level with illustration of the osteofibrous compartments; distal view. The deep fascia of leg is attached to the bones of the leg by dense connective tissue septa. *(From Paulsen F, Waschke J.* Sobotta Atlas of Human Anatomy. *Vol. 1. Urban & Fischer: Elsevier; 2013, Fig. 4.210.)*

10. What structure has been injured, and how has this led to her awkward gait?

Injury to the right superior gluteal nerve has led to paralysis of the gluteus medius and gluteus minimus muscles. These muscles abduct the thigh, and when they are not functional, the pelvis cannot be stabilized while stepping. While the patient is standing on one foot, the contralateral pelvis sags, a characteristic known as the Trendelenburg sign (Fig. 26.22). This is definitely a clinical test to know for boards.

SUMMARY BOX: LOWER EXTREMITY INJURIES

- Note the lower extremity (LE) terminology: thigh = hip joint to knee, leg = knee to ankle, foot = ankle to digits.
- The unhappy triad consists of injury to the medial collateral ligament (MCL), anterior cruciate ligament (ACL), and lateral meniscus.
- The ACL prevents anterior displacement of the tibia, while the posterior cruciate ligament (PCL) prevents posterior displacement of the tibia.
- The common fibular nerve is often injured in knee injuries or fibular neck fractures and results in footdrop.
- A functional gluteus medius and gluteus minimus (innervated by the superior gluteal nerve) are necessary for maintaining pelvic stability while walking.

CASE 26.8, PART A

A 42-year-old librarian has Graves disease and requires a thyroidectomy. She presents to your office 1 month after her surgery with a chief concern of hoarseness, which she first noticed after her surgery.

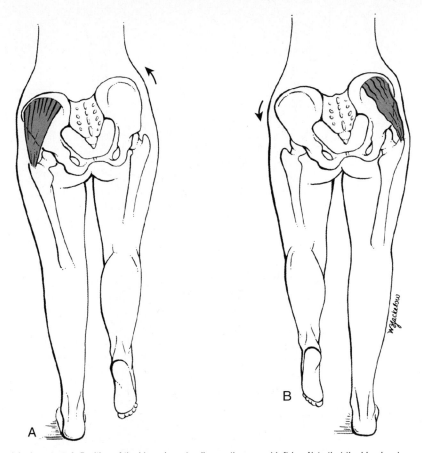

Figure 26.22. Trendelenburg test. A, Position of the hips when standing on the normal left leg. Note that the hip elevates as a result of contraction of the left hip musculature. B, Position of the hips when standing on the abnormal right leg. Note that the left hip falls as a result of lack of adequate contraction of the right hip muscles. *(From Swartz MH. Textbook of Physical Diagnosis. 8th ed. Philadelphia: Elsevier; 2021.)*

1. What is the differential diagnosis for her hoarseness?
   Vocal fold paralysis, laryngitis (infectious or as a result of gastroesophageal reflux disease [GERD]), carcinoma of the vocal folds, nodule of the vocal folds, laryngeal muscle spasm, and idiopathic origin are considerations.

2. Given the surgical history, which of these diagnoses is most likely and why?
   Vocal fold paralysis results from injury to the recurrent laryngeal nerve. The two recurrent laryngeal nerves run just posterior to the thyroid gland and are prone to injury during thyroidectomy.

3. How does injury to the recurrent laryngeal nerve result in hoarseness?
   The recurrent laryngeal nerve gives rise to the inferior laryngeal nerve, which innervates all of the intrinsic laryngeal muscles except for one, the cricothyroid muscle. An injury to either of these nerves results in nearly complete vocal cord paralysis on the side of the affected nerve, causing hoarseness. Note that dysfunction of the posterior cricoarytenoid muscle is key in the development of hoarseness because this is the only muscle that can abduct the vocal folds. Thus, bilateral injury to the recurrent laryngeal nerve can result in dyspnea and stridor, caused by an inability to abduct either vocal fold, which obstructs the airway at the larynx.

STEP 1 SECRET

Be on the lookout for damage to the recurrent laryngeal nerve that results from thyroid surgery. This is a favorite scenario on boards.

4. Describe the path of the recurrent laryngeal nerve, noting any asymmetries.
   In the developing embryo, the right and left recurrent laryngeal nerves branch off of the right and left vagus nerves and loop around the fourth aortic arches on their way back into the neck, eventually ending as the inferior laryngeal nerves.

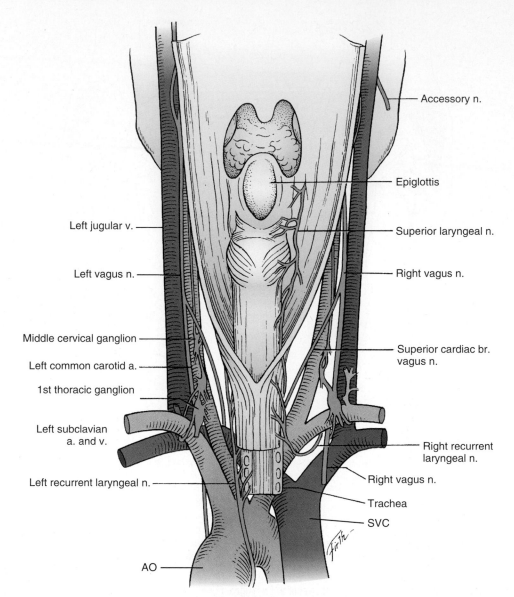

Figure 26.23. Diagram of the vagus nerve (cranial nerve X), specifically, its branch, the recurrent laryngeal nerve, and its relationship to the large vessels of the neck. The right and left nerves are not identical, and the recurrent laryngeal nerve branches at the base of the neck on the right and in the thorax on the left. *a.,* Artery; *AO,* aorta; *br.,* branches; *n.,* nerve; *SVC,* superior vena cava; *v.,* vein. *(From Goetz CG. Textbook of Clinical Neurology. 3rd ed. Philadelphia: Saunders; 2007.)*

The right fourth aortic arch becomes the right subclavian artery, so this is the artery that the right recurrent laryngeal nerve loops around when development is complete. In contrast, the left fourth aortic arch becomes the arch of the aorta, so this structure is what the left recurrent laryngeal nerve loops around when development is complete (Fig. 26.23). The recurrent laryngeal nerves most commonly run posterior to the inferior parathyroids and anterior to the superior parathyroids.

5. Describe the innervation of the lone intrinsic laryngeal muscle not innervated by the recurrent laryngeal nerve: the cricothyroid muscle.
   The cricothyroid muscle is a tensor of the vocal cords that allows high-pitched phonation. It is innervated by the external laryngeal nerve. Sometimes this nerve can be injured during thyroid surgery as well. This is one of two branches of the superior laryngeal nerve. The other branch is the internal laryngeal nerve, which supplies sensory innervation to the mucous membranes superior to the vocal folds. The superior laryngeal nerve is a direct branch from the vagus nerve.

CASE 26.8, PART B

You are at a fancy restaurant having dinner with your date. Unfortunately, the man at the table next to you begins choking on a piece of steak. You attempt the Heimlich maneuver with no success. You theorize that the piece of steak has entered the larynx and sent the intrinsic laryngeal muscles into spasm, thus tensing the vocal folds and obstructing the airway. As the man loses consciousness, you request a sharp knife from the nearest waitress.

6. To save this man's life, which structure must you incise? Why?
   The cricothyroid membrane must be cut. This fibrous membrane lies inferior to the thyroid cartilage and superior to the cricoid cartilage, connecting the two structures. Note that the thyroid gland does not overlie the thyroid cartilage, as the bulk of the gland is much more caudal, lying inferior to the cricoid cartilage. Creating an opening in the cricothyroid membrane allows the passage of lifesaving air to bypass the obstruction, because the incision site is inferior to the vocal folds, which are deep to the thyroid cartilage.

7. Describe the surface anatomy of the neck that allows one to find the cricothyroid membrane.
   The laryngeal prominence (Adams apple) is the median protrusion of the thyroid cartilage. This lies inferior to the hyoid bone at about the level of C5. By running the fingers inferior to the laryngeal prominence, down to about the level of C6, the arch of the cricoid cartilage can be palpated. The cricothyroid membrane lies just superior to the cricoid cartilage. The incision should be made here, with care not to move too far superiorly, because the thyroid cartilage lies just above. Disruption of the thyroid cartilage could damage the intrinsic laryngeal muscles (Fig. 26.24).

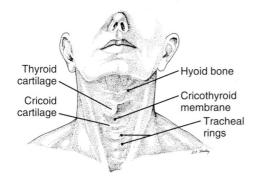

A

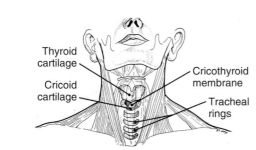

B

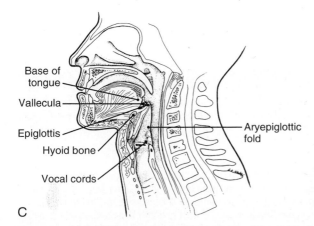

C

Figure 26.24. Anatomy of the neck. A, Surface anatomy of the neck, showing important external landmarks. B, Anterior view of the neck, showing various internal structures (overlying superficial skin and structures removed to show cricothyroid membrane). C, Lateral view of the neck, showing various structures. *(From Roberts JR. Clinical Procedures in Emergency Medicine. 4th ed. Philadelphia: WB Saunders; 2004.)*

CASE 26.8, PART C

It is Saturday night on your pediatrics rotation, and you are covering the obstetrics floor. You enter the room of the next newborn you have prepared to see and find a mother very upset about the fact that her child has two fissures running to his mouth, one from each nostril. On physical examination, you note that the fissures, just lateral to each side of the philtrum, extend into the mouth and meet at the incisive foramen, in essence creating a U-shape from the two nostrils to the incisive foramen.

8. **With what defect(s) has this child been born?**
   The child has bilateral cleft lip and cleft primary palate.

9. **Describe the embryologic basis for cleft lip.**
   Cleft lip, one of the more common developmental defects, occurs when one or both of the two maxillary processes fail to completely fuse with the corresponding medial nasal process. Note that the two medial nasal processes together make up the intermaxillary segment, the superior portion of which becomes the philtrum.

10. **Describe the embryologic basis for cleft palate.**
    Clefts of the *primary palate* occur when the palatal shelves of the maxillary processes fail to fuse with the primary palate, itself formed by the fusion of the maxillary and median nasal processes. If it is bilateral, it results in a U-shaped fissure, with the apex of the U at the incisive foramen (this lies near the three-way fusion point of the primary palate and the two palatal shelves).

    Clefts of the *secondary palate* occur when the two palatal shelves fail to fuse at the midline. The nasal septum can be visualized in the middle of the cleft secondary palate (Fig. 26.25).

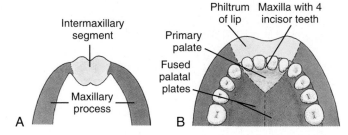

Figure 26.25. A, Schematic drawing of the intermaxillary segment and maxillary processes. B, The intermaxillary segment gives rise to the philtrum of the upper lip, the median part of the maxillary bone and its four incisor teeth, and the triangular primary palate. *(From Sadler TW. Head and neck embryology. In Sadler TW, Langman J, eds. Langman's Medical Embryology. 6th ed. Baltimore: Williams & Wilkins; 1990.)*

OTHER IMPORTANT CONCEPTS IN EMBRYOLOGY OF THE FACE AND NECK

11. **Discuss the difference between pharyngeal (branchial) pouches, arches, and clefts.**
    The six pharyngeal (branchial) arches consist of a combination of neural crest cells and mesoderm and play a role in the formation of many structures of the face and neck.
        The four pharyngeal pouches lie internally, between the pharyngeal arches, and are lined with foregut endoderm.
        The four pharyngeal clefts lie externally, between the pharyngeal arches, and are lined with ectoderm.

12. In Table 26.6, cover the right column and name the derivatives of each structure listed in the left column.

STEP 1 SECRET

Embryology in itself is a relatively low-yield subject on boards, but Table 26.6 presents extremely high-yield content. You should expect at least one question on this material. You should also remember which tissues are of neural crest origin.

---

13. **From where do the parts of the thyroid gland, other than the parafollicular C cells, originate?**
    The thyroid gland develops from a proliferation of foregut endoderm at the base of the tongue. From here, the thyroid gland descends through the thyroglossal duct to just inferior to the cricoid cartilage. It remains connected to the foramen cecum via the thyroglossal duct during development. The thyroglossal duct normally degenerates before birth, but the foramen cecum persists, marking the location of the original epithelial proliferation that formed the thyroid.

Table 26.6. Embryology of the Face and Neck

STRUCTURE	DERIVATIVE(S)
First pouch	Auditory tube and middle ear
Second pouch	Palatine tonsil
Third pouch	Inferior parathyroids and thymus
Fourth pouch	Superior parathyroids and ultimobranchial body (forms thyroid parafollicular C cells)
First arch	Malleus, incus, mandible, maxilla, zygomatic and squamous portion of the temporal bones; muscles of mastication; anterior belly of digastric, mylohyoid, tensor tympani, and tensor veli palatini muscles; innervated by cranial nerves V_2 and V_3
Second arch	Stapes, styloid, most of hyoid bone; muscles of facial expression; stapedius, stylohyoid, and posterior belly of digastric muscle; innervated by cranial nerve VII
Third arch	Greater cornu of hyoid bone, stylopharyngeus muscle; innervated by cranial nerve IX
Fourth and sixth arches	Laryngeal and upper tracheal cartilage; muscles of the soft palate, pharynx, and larynx; striated muscle of esophagus; innervated by cranial nerve X
First cleft	External acoustic meatus
Second/third/fourth cleft	Cervical sinus (eventually becomes obliterated)

SUMMARY BOX: NECK ANATOMY AND EMBRYOLOGY

- The recurrent laryngeal nerves lie just deep to the thyroid and are susceptible to injury during thyroid surgery.
  - These nerves innervate the intrinsic laryngeal muscles, except the cricothyroids.
  - The right recurrent laryngeal ascends from beneath the right subclavian artery.
  - The left recurrent laryngeal ascends from beneath the aortic arch.
- The external laryngeal nerves, direct branches off the right and left vagus nerves, innervate the cricothyroid muscles.
- The cricothyroid membrane lies inferior to the vocal cords (which are deep to the thyroid cartilage); an airway formed in this membrane can bypass a laryngeal obstruction.
- Cleft lip: Maxillary process fails to fuse with medial nasal process.
- Cleft primary palate: Palatal shelves fail to fuse with the primary palate.
- Cleft secondary palate: Palatal shelves fail to fuse at the midline.

CASE 26.9

A 20-year-old woman presents to the urgent care clinic with severe, sharp, right upper quadrant (RUQ) pain of 6 hours in duration. The pain radiates to her right shoulder, and breathing is moderately painful. She states that she had a mild RUQ ache for a few days, but it did not bother her and she saw no reason to see a doctor. A urine pregnancy test is negative.

1. What is the differential diagnosis for this patient's right upper quadrant pain?
   Cholecystitis, choledocholithiasis, cholangitis, peptic ulcer disease, hepatitis, perihepatitis, hepatic abscess or tumor, pyelonephritis, nephrolithiasis, appendicitis, right lower lobe pneumonia, ovarian cysts or tumors, and acute enteritis are possibilities.

CASE 26.9 CONTINUED:

Her medical history is unremarkable. However, her sexual history is notable for unprotected sexual intercourse with many different male partners. On physical examination, you note that on palpation, she is experiencing right lower quadrant (RLQ) pain of slightly less severity than her right upper quadrant (RUQ) pain. On pelvic examination, she has exquisite cervical motion tenderness and bilateral adnexal tenderness.

2. What is the most likely diagnosis?
   Pelvic inflammatory disease (PID) is most likely.

3. Name the two most common organisms implicated in PID.
   Chlamydia trachomatis (most common) and *Neisseria gonorrhoeae* are most commonly implicated in PID. Note that rarely PID can be caused by normal vaginal bacterial flora, as well as viruses, fungi, and parasites.

4. **How can PID lead to right upper quadrant pain?**
   PID is classically characterized by ascent of bacteria that have infected the vagina and cervix, leading to endometritis, salpingitis, and peritonitis. Peritonitis is possible because the infundibulum of the uterine tubes opens directly into the peritoneal cavity. This means that there is a direct route from the vagina to the peritoneal cavity (via the uterus and uterine tubes) by which bacteria can ascend. In rare cases, this peritonitis can lead to RUQ pain when the offending bacteria reach the liver capsule and cause perihepatitis and inflammation of the right hemidiaphragm. This condition is known as Fitz-Hugh–Curtis syndrome.

5. **Describe how the uterus and ovaries are supported.**
   The cervix is supported anteriorly by the pubocervical ligaments, laterally by the transverse cervical ligaments, and posteriorly by the uterosacral ligaments. The body of an anteverted uterus gains much of its support by resting on the bladder (note that this is not the case in patients with a retroverted uterus). The broad ligament, a double layer of peritoneum, extends laterally from the uterus and functions to support the uterus and all associated structures (note that the mesosalpinx portions of the broad ligament support the uterine tubes), as well as to carry the uterine vasculature. The round ligament, analogous to the spermatic cord, supports the uterine fundus. Each ovary is attached to the uterus via the ovarian ligament, is enveloped by the mesovarium portion of the broad ligament, and is supported laterally by the suspensory ligament of the ovary, which attaches to the lateral pelvic wall and carries the ovarian vasculature (Fig. 26.26).

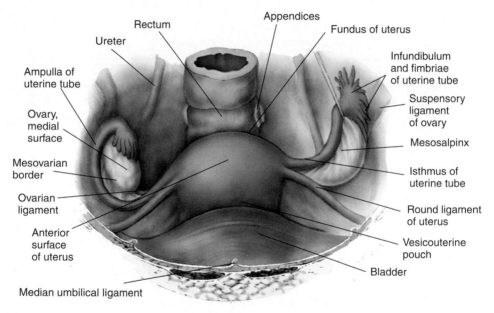

Figure 26.26. The organs of the female pelvis. The uterus is surrounded by the bladder anteriorly, the rectum posteriorly, and the folds of the broad ligaments laterally. *(Redrawn from Clemente CD. Anatomy: A Regional Atlas of the Human Body. Baltimore-Munich: Urban & Schwarzenberg; 1987.)*

6. **Can Fitz-Hugh–Curtis syndrome be seen in males?**
   Although PID and Fitz-Hugh–Curtis syndrome classically develop in females through the open connection between the vagina → uterus → fallopian tubes → peritoneal cavity, infection can occur through lymphatic, hematogenous, or direct spread from intraperitoneal infections. In males, infections can very rarely spread through these routes to the peritoneum and liver capsule, so they also can develop Fitz-Hugh–Curtis syndrome. Note that the lumina of the urethra, ejaculatory duct, vas deferens, epididymis, and seminiferous tubules are not continuous with the peritoneal cavity at any time.

7. **Outline the common drugs used in antimicrobial pharmacotherapy for PID.**
   C. trachomatis and *N. gonorrhoeae* are the most common organisms, but the normal flora of the vagina (e.g., *Gardnerella vaginalis, Streptococcus agalactiae*) or gastrointestinal (GI) tract (e.g., *Bacteroides fragilis, Peptostreptococcus, Escherichia coli*) can play a role in the infection. Infection with multiple organisms is common, so broad-spectrum antibiotics are recommended. For mild to moderately severe infections, the recommended regimen is a single intramuscular (IM) dose of a third-generation cephalosporin (such as ceftriaxone or cefoxitin) plus a 14-day course of oral doxycycline and metronidazole. An alternative and equivalent treatment is a single IM dose of ceftriaxone plus high-dose oral azithromycin weekly for 2 weeks. Severe infections (i.e., those associated with tubo-ovarian abscesses) require inpatient treatment with parenteral antibiotics. The two preferred regimens are cefotetan or cefoxitin plus oral or intravenous doxycycline and clindamycin plus gentamicin.

8. In Table 26.7, cover the column on the right and name the abdominal organs in each location.

Table 26.7. Abdominal Organs

LOCATION	ABDOMINAL ORGANS
Within the peritoneal cavity	None **Note:** The ovaries are exposed to the peritoneal cavity.
Intraperitoneal	Stomach and first part of duodenum Liver and gallbladder Spleen Tail of pancreas Jejunum and ileum Cecum and appendix Transverse and sigmoid colon
Secondarily retroperitoneal[a]	Duodenum: first, second, and third parts Ascending and descending colon Rectum Pancreas: head, neck, and body
Retroperitoneal	Kidneys (plus ureters and adrenal glands) Abdominal aorta Inferior vena cava

[a]Note that secondarily retroperitoneal organs develop intraperitoneally (covered by visceral peritoneum) but later move toward the posterior body wall and the retroperitoneal space, leaving only their anterior aspect covered by peritoneum.

SUMMARY BOX: STRUCTURE OF THE FEMALE REPRODUCTIVE SYSTEM AND THE PERITONEUM

- In most cases of pelvic inflammatory disease (PID), bacteria (usually *Chlamydia trachomatis* or *Neisseria gonorrhoeae*) from the vagina pass through the cervix into the uterus and uterine tubes, causing inflammation.
  - Peritonitis and inflammation in the liver capsule (Fitz-Hugh–Curtis syndrome) can result because the uterine tubes open directly into the peritoneal cavity.
  - In males, there is no direct connection between the lumen of the genitourinary tract and the peritoneal cavity, so Fitz-Hugh–Curtis syndrome is much rarer.
- The uterus is supported by the broad ligament (composed of peritoneum), the round ligaments, and by resting anteriorly on the bladder.
- The ovary is supported by the ovarian ligament, the mesovarium, and the suspensory ligament of the ovary.

CASE 26.10, PART A

A 64-year-old nurse had a myocardial infarction (MI) 1 month ago. He now presents to the emergency department (ED) with new-onset chest pain that is intermittent and not related to exertion. The pain is severe and is located in the left precordial and retrosternal regions, and it radiates to the neck and back.

1. What is the differential diagnosis for his chest pain?
   Unstable angina, variant (Prinzmetal) angina, MI, pulmonary embolus, aortic dissection, pericarditis, pleuritis, pneumothorax, pneumonia, costochondritis, rib fracture, anxiety/panic attack, GERD, pancreatitis, diffuse esophageal spasm, and peptic ulcer disease are possibilities.

2. An MI in what distribution would be most concerning for damage to the sinoatrial and atrioventricular nodes?
   Occlusion of the right coronary artery (RCA). The RCA supplies the atrioventricular (AV) node in nearly 100% of the population via the AV nodal branch, which originates near the origin of the posterior interventricular artery. However, it should be noted that the posterior interventricular artery, also known as the posterior descending artery, is a branch of the RCA in 80% of the population and a branch of the left circumflex artery in 5% to 10% of the population. The remaining 10% to 15% have other variations, which includes codominance (supplied by both the RCA and left circumflex artery). The sinoatrial (SA) node is supplied by the RCA in 60% of the population via the SA nodal branch, which lies near the origin of the RCA. The SA nodal branch originates from the circumflex artery in the remaining 40%.

3. Which coronary arteries supply the left ventricle?
   - *Anterior interventricular:* Shortly after originating from the ascending aorta, the left coronary artery bifurcates. One branch, the anterior interventricular artery, also known as the *left anterior descending* (LAD) *artery*, descends in the anterior interventricular groove to the apex. This artery supplies nearly the entire interventricular septum and more than half of the left ventricle.
   - *Circumflex:* The second branch of the bifurcation of the left coronary artery, this artery runs in the AV groove to the posterior side of the heart. It also supplies the left atrium.
   - *Left marginal:* This branch of the circumflex artery descends along the left heart border.
   - *Posterior interventricular:* This artery branches from the RCA, circumflex artery, or both. It descends in the posterior interventricular groove to the apex. It also supplies a small portion of the interventricular septum and part of the right ventricle (Fig. 26.27).

4. If his chest pain were caused by pleuritis (also known as pleurisy), from which pleural layer would he be sensing pain?

   He would feel pain in the parietal pleura only. In pleuritis, the inflammation involves both pleural layers. Although the visceral pleura lacks sensory innervation and cannot transmit pain sensation, the parietal pleura is exquisitely sensitive to pain because it is abundantly supplied by somatic branches of the intercostal nerves (in the areas bordering the body wall) and the phrenic nerves (in the areas bordering the mediastinum and diaphragm). Because of its differential innervation, referred pain is localized to the body wall for pleuritis in the distribution of the intercostal nerves and to the shoulder and neck for pleuritis in the distribution of the phrenic nerves.

CASE 26.10, PART A CONTINUED:

He goes on to say that this chest pain does not feel like the pain that was associated with his heart attack. He has noticed that the pain waxes and wanes with breathing, and it is position dependent: He notes that the pain is least while he sits up and leans forward. On cardiac auscultation, a friction rub is heard.

5. What is the most likely diagnosis?

   Acute pericarditis is most likely. Weeks to months after an MI, fibrinous pericarditis can occur. This phenomenon is called *Dressler syndrome* and is thought to be an autoimmune reaction to novel antigens resulting from cardiac damage, most often in the setting of MI. Preferred treatment is high-dose aspirin or ibuprofen.

6. If one were to pass a needle from outside the pericardium to the lumen of the left ventricle, through which layers would it pass, in sequence?
   1. Fibrous pericardium (unyielding, protects heart from acute volume overload; fused with the diaphragm, tunica adventitia of the great vessels, and the posterior sternal surface)
   2. Parietal layer of serous pericardium (fused to the fibrous pericardium)

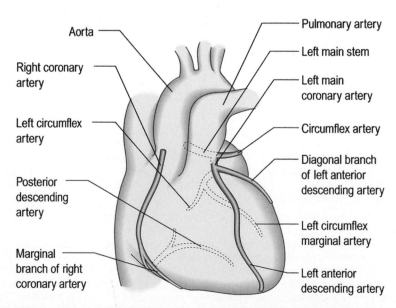

Figure 26.27. Normal coronary circulation. *(From Kumar P, Clark M. Kumar and Clark's Clinical Medicine. 9th ed. Edinburgh: Elsevier; 2017: 931-1056, Fig. 23.8.)*

3. Pericardial fluid (normally a thin lubricating film; allows the heart to move within the pericardial sac)
4. Visceral layer of serous pericardium (synonymous with the epicardium; continuous with the parietal layer at the base of the heart)
5. Myocardium (composed of cardiac muscle)
6. Endocardium (an endothelial lining; the Purkinje fibers run between this layer and the myocardium)

7. **Enlargement of which chamber of the heart is most likely to cause dysphagia?**
The left atrium, located at the base of the heart, is directly anterior to the esophagus. Marked enlargement of this chamber, as can occur with mitral stenosis, can lead to compression of the esophagus around the level of T6 through T9.

8. **What is a parasternal lift? Enlargement of which chamber of the heart is most likely to cause a parasternal lift?**
A parasternal lift is a palpable or visible pulsation of the chest wall. A parasternal lift occurs when the right ventricle, which composes the anterior-sternocostal surface of the heart, is enlarged. The elevation is usually seen or felt just to the left of the sternum (i.e., parasternally).

CASE 26.10, PART B

At the end of a long week, you leave the clinic and head to a local movie theater with friends. Soon after settling into your seat, a group of teenagers clamber into the seats directly in front of you. To entertain his buddies before the show, one of the group starts tossing his chewy fruit candies high into the air, catching them in his mouth. Before you can point out the inevitable, one of the candies lands in the boy's mouth just as he is taking a breath, and the gummy giraffe is rapidly out of sight. As the boy coughs, you recall the restaurant fiasco and prepare to start the Heimlich maneuver. However, he immediately begins to breathe, albeit with quite a bit of wheezing and dyspnea.

9. **If the candy passed into the bronchial tree, on which side would it most likely be found?**
The right main bronchus is wider and oriented more vertically as compared with the left main bronchus, so it is the more likely site of aspiration. In supine patients, aspirated contents are likely to end up in the posterior segment of the right upper lobe and/or the superior segment of the lower lobe.

10. **Describe the other major asymmetry of the bronchial tree.**
The right main bronchus divides into three lobar bronchi, one for each lobe, whereas the left main bronchus divides into only two, again one for each lobe. The right lung has superior, middle, and inferior lobes. The oblique (major) fissure separates the inferior lobe from the other two lobes, and the horizontal (minor) fissure separates the superior lobe from the middle lobe. The left lung has only superior and inferior lobes, separated by the oblique fissure. The inferior portion of the superior lobe of the left lung is called the *lingula*. It lies adjacent to the heart and is the counterpart of the right middle lobe (Fig. 26.28).

SUMMARY BOX: CARDIOTHORACIC ANATOMY

- The right coronary artery (RCA) supplies the atrioventricular (AV) node.
- The RCA supplies the sinoatrial (SA) node in 60% of the population, with the circumflex artery supplying the SA node in the other 40%.
- The anterior interventricular, circumflex, left marginal, and posterior interventricular arteries supply the left ventricle.
  - The left coronary artery bifurcates into the anterior interventricular and circumflex arteries.
  - The left marginal artery is a branch of the circumflex artery.
  - The posterior interventricular artery is a branch of the right coronary in 80% of the population and the circumflex in 15% of the population.
- In pleuritis, although both the visceral and parietal pleurae become inflamed, pain is transmitted only from the parietal pleura because the visceral pleura lacks sensory innervation.
- The outermost fibrous pericardium is fused to the parietal layer of the serous pericardium.
- The parietal and visceral layers of the pericardium are continuous near the base of the heart and contain the pericardial fluid between them.
- The left atrium is the most posterior portion of the heart, lying just anterior to the esophagus.
- The right ventricle is the anterior-most portion of the heart, and enlargement can lead to a parasternal lift.
- The right main bronchus is wider and more vertical than the left main bronchus, so an aspirated foreign body is more likely to enter it.
- The three-lobed right lung possesses a middle lobe that corresponds to the lingula of the superior lobe of the left lung, which has only two lobes.

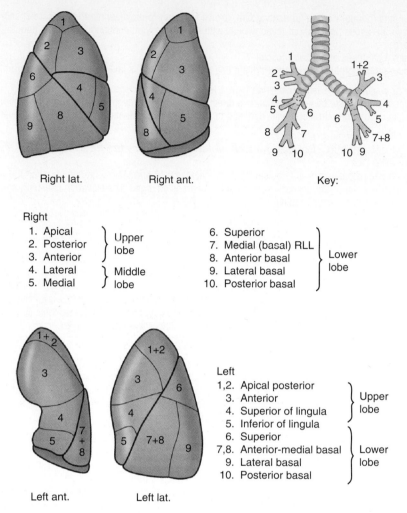

Right lat.   Right ant.   Key:

Right
1. Apical ⎫ Upper
2. Posterior ⎬ lobe
3. Anterior ⎭
4. Lateral ⎫ Middle
5. Medial ⎭ lobe

6. Superior ⎫
7. Medial (basal) RLL ⎬ Lower
8. Anterior basal ⎬ lobe
9. Lateral basal ⎬
10. Posterior basal ⎭

Left ant.   Left lat.

Left
1,2. Apical posterior ⎫
3. Anterior ⎬ Upper
4. Superior of lingula ⎬ lobe
5. Inferior of lingula ⎭
6. Superior ⎫
7,8. Anterior-medial basal ⎬ Lower
9. Lateral basal ⎬ lobe
10. Posterior basal ⎭

Figure 26.28. Segments of the pulmonary lobes. *(Modified from Jackson CL, Huber JF. Correlated applied anatomy of the bronchial tree and lungs with a system of nomenclature.* Dis Chest. *1943;9:319.)*

DERMATOLOGY

BASIC CONCEPTS

1. What are the major functions of the skin?

   The skin, which comprises the largest organ in the body, acts as a semipermeable barrier from the external environment and protects individuals from mechanical stress, fluid loss, and harmful exposures (e.g., pathogens, toxins, ultraviolet [UV] radiation). It is involved in regulating body temperature and contains a variety of nerve endings that react to heat, cold, pain, and pressure. The skin also plays an important role in the synthesis of vitamin D.

2. Describe the individual layers of the skin.

   See Table 27.1 and Fig. 27.1.

Table 27.1. Skin Layers from Superficial to Deep

	COMPOSITION	CLINICAL CORRELATIONS
Epidermis	Stratum corneum, stratum lucidum, stratum granulosum, stratum spinosum, and stratum basale, which contain: Keratinocytes: Predominant cell type of the epidermis that produces keratin, which gives strength to the skin and acts as a barrier against the outside world Merkel cells: Involved in sensory discrimination of textures and shapes Langerhans cells: Initiate processing of foreign antigens Melanocytes: Found in the stratum basale and produce melanin, which gives skin its natural pigmentation	Disruptions in the proteins involved in barrier function of the skin are responsible for diseases such as eczema. Calluses occur as a result of excess keratinocyte accumulation secondary to repeated friction. Vitiligo, a disease of skin depigmentation, occurs secondary to melanocyte destruction.
Basement membrane	Basal lamina, collagen, and connective tissue	Hemidesmosomes connecting the basement membrane to the stratum basale are the target of autoimmune destruction in bullous pemphigoid, resulting in subepidermal blisters
Dermis	Connective tissue, hair follicles, sweat glands, sebaceous glands, apocrine glands, lymphatics, blood vessels, mechanoreceptors	Site of intradermal injections (e.g., purified protein derivative [PPD] for tuberculosis screening)
Hypodermis	Primarily composed of fat; contains Pacinian and Ruffini corpuscles responsible for sensitivity to vibration/pressure and stretch/grip, respectively	Site of subcutaneous injections (e.g., insulin)

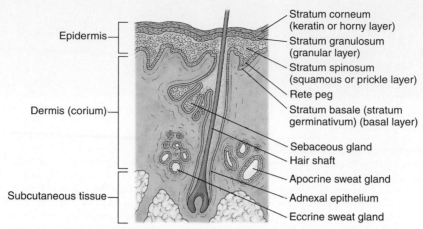

Figure 27.1. Normal layers of skin. *(From Yanoff M, Sassani JW. Ocular Pathology. 7th ed. Philadelphia: Saunders; 2015.)*

STEP 1 SECRET

*Students often use the mnemonic "**C**ome, **L**et's **G**et **S**un **B**urned!" to recall the layers of the epidermis (**C**orneum, **L**ucidum, **G**ranulosum, **S**pinosum, **B**asale).*

3. Can you describe the dermatologic terms listed in Table 27.2?
   You should have a thorough understanding of the terms mentioned in Table 27.2 because they may be used to describe lesions in a question stem.

Table 27.2. Terms Used to Describe the Appearance and Progression of Skin Lesions

Primary Morphology
Use these words to describe the appearance of the lesion.

Macule	Flat area of color change; up to 1 cm in diameter
Patch	Flat area of color change; >1 cm in diameter
Papule	Raised, round lesion above the surface of the skin; up to 1 cm in diameter
Plaque	Raised, flat-topped lesion >1 cm in diameter; often formed by coalescence of papules
Nodule	Raised or flat lesion that involves the underlying dermis and often the subcutaneous tissue; >1 cm in diameter
Cyst	A papule or nodule that contains fluid or semisolid material; gives resilient fluctuation on palpation
Vesicle	Blister containing clear fluid; <1 cm in diameter
Bulla	Blister containing clear fluid; >1 cm in diameter
Pustule	Blister filled with pus
Wheal/Hive	Evanescent (rapidly fading) papule or plaque that is typically edematous and pruritic (itchy)
Verruca	Wart

Secondary Morphology
Use these words to describe the progression of the lesion over time.

Scale	Hyperkeratosis (excess keratin or keratinocytes) within the stratum corneum
Crust	Rough exudate that dries on the lesion (can be from blood, plasma, or pus)
Excoriation	Superficial skin loss secondary to scratching or rubbing
Lichenification	Thickening caused by continuous rubbing (seen in untreated eczema)

Table 27.2. Terms Used to Describe the Appearance and Progression of Skin Lesions—cont'd

Erosion	Break in the skin that involves the epidermis only
Ulcer	Break in the skin that extends to the dermis or subcutaneous tissue
Atrophy	Thinning of skin secondary to a decrease in the underlying tissue
Hypertrophy	Excessive growth of an area of skin
Configuration *Use these words to describe the pattern or shape of lesion formation.*	
Linear	Lesion forms a line
Targetoid	Lesion has a bull's-eye appearance
Annular	Lesion forms a ring
Nummular (discoid)	Lesion is coin-shaped
Guttate	Individual, drop-like lesion
Confluent	Lesions are joined together
Generalized	Lesions are distributed diffusely over the whole body
Grouped	Lesions are clustered together
Solitary	A single lesion

CASE 27.1

A 72-year-old Caucasian man presents to the dermatologist for a lesion on his nose that his wife has been badgering him about for the past year (Fig. 27.2). He has been an avid golfer for 35 years and has never seen a dermatologist before. The dermatologist tells the patient that he is concerned about this lesion and would like to perform a biopsy of it.

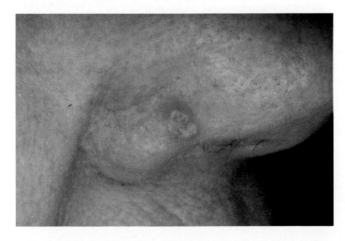

Figure 27.2. Appearance of lesion on patient in Case 27.1. *(From Lebwohl M, Heymann W, Berth-Jones J, Coulson I.* Treatment of Skin Disease: Comprehensive Therapeutic Strategies. *4th ed. Philadelphia: Saunders; 2014.)*

1. What is the most likely diagnosis?

   This is a classic presentation for a basal cell carcinoma. Basal cell carcinoma is the most common type of skin cancer. This cancer can be locally invasive but has very low metastatic potential. The lesion is most often described as a pearly, pink papule, but may also have raised borders with an area of central ulceration. Histology demonstrates groups of basal cells with peripheral palisading.

2. What are common locations for basal cell carcinomas?

   Basal cell carcinomas commonly are found on sun-exposed areas of the body, especially the face.

STEP 1 SECRET

As a rule of thumb, basal cell carcinoma will generally be found at the level of the upper lip or above because these tend to be the most sun-exposed areas of the body.

3. **How should this patient be treated?**

This patient should be treated via excisional biopsy with clear margins. This is typically sufficient because of the low metastatic potential of basal cell carcinomas.

CASE 27.1 CONTINUED:

The dermatologist also notes several small, scaly, erythematous plaques over the dorsal surface of the patient's hands, forehead, and scalp (Fig. 27.3). He states that they are precancerous lesions and recommends treating them to prevent a cancer from developing.

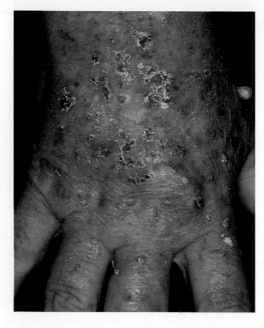

Figure 27.3. Lesions on patient in Case 27.1. *(From Habif TP. Clinical Dermatology. 6th ed. Philadelphia: Saunders; 2016.)*

4. **What is the most likely cause of these lesions?**

Excessive sun exposure caused these scaly plaques known as *actinic keratoses*. If untreated, these may progress to squamous cell carcinoma, which is the second most common type of skin cancer. Like basal cell carcinoma, squamous cell carcinoma has a predilection for the face, although it is also found below the lower lip (compared with the upper lip for basal cell carcinoma), on the ears, and on the hands. The lesions are often erythematous, ulcerative, and scaly. Like basal cell carcinoma, squamous cell carcinoma has low metastatic potential but may become severely disfiguring or metastasize to local lymph nodes and other tissue sites if left untreated. Diagnosis is typically performed using biopsy (note that this skin cancer can also be histopathologically identified by the presence of keratin pearls), and like basal cell carcinoma, treatment is primarily surgical.

CASE 27.1 CONTINUED:

Two years later, the man returns with concern about a "mole" on his left forearm that he claims has been evolving in appearance. On examination, an 8-mm, asymmetric, brown, tan, and black papule with a scalloped border is appreciated on the extensor surface of the patient's left forearm (Fig. 27.4). The dermatologist performs an excisional biopsy. The biopsy sample stains positive for S-100, a tumor marker for melanoma.

5. **What are the ABCDE characteristics suggestive of melanoma?**
   - A—Asymmetry of the lesion
   - B—Border irregularity (irregular or poorly defined)
   - C—Color variation from one area to another
   - D—Diameter greater than 6 mm
   - E—Evolution (changing in size, shape, or color over time)

6. **Who is at highest risk for melanoma?**

People with UV-damaged skin are at highest risk for melanoma. UV damage may result from excessive sun exposure or tanning bed exposure without use of sunscreen. Other risk factors include fair skin, personal or family history of melanoma, *BRAF* proto-oncogene mutation, and xeroderma pigmentosum. Although fair-skinned individuals are at greater risk than dark-skinned individuals, people with darker skin are at higher risk for acral lentiginous melanoma, which is not related to UV damage and typically appears on the palms and soles, under the nails, and in the oral mucosa.

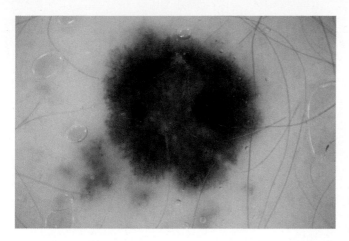

Figure 27.4. Lesion on patient in Case 27.1. *(From Bolognia J, Jorizzo J, Schaffer J.* Dermatology. *3rd ed. Philadelphia: Elsevier; 2012.)*

7. **To which locations does melanoma most commonly metastasize?**
   Melanoma most commonly metastasizes to distal skin, subcutaneous tissue, lymph nodes, brain, bone, lung, and liver. S-100 positivity of a tumor found in any of these locations is a useful way to confirm metastasis from a primary melanoma.

8. **What is the most important factor in determining this patient's prognosis?**
   Likelihood of metastasis, which is dependent on tumor depth (Breslow thickness), is important in determining prognosis. The deeper a melanoma extends into the dermis, the more likely it is to have metastasized.

9. **How should this patient be managed?**
   Primary treatment includes surgical excision with clean, wide margins. Lymph node biopsy should also be performed for medium- to high-risk lesions, and imaging may be necessary for the purposes of staging. Unfortunately, metastatic melanoma is devastating and often deadly. Although chemotherapy and radiation are traditionally used for metastatic melanoma, they have not been incredibly successful. In recent years, several biologic therapies have been developed for melanoma, including ipilimumab, an anti-CTLA-4 antibody, and vemurafenib, a BRAF kinase inhibitor that may be used in patients positive for the BRAFV600E mutation. Note that although melanoma only accounts for about 1% of all skin cancer cases, it is responsible for the most skin cancer deaths.

SUMMARY BOX: BASAL CELL CARCINOMA

- Epidemiology: Most common type of skin cancer
- Presentation: Typically found on the sun-exposed portions of the body, especially above the upper lip
- Diagnosis: Skin biopsy
- Treatment: Surgical (e.g., excisional biopsy)
- Prognosis: Excellent, as this tumor rarely metastasizes

SUMMARY BOX: SQUAMOUS CELL CARCINOMA

- Epidemiology: Second most common type of skin cancer
- Presentation: Typically found on the sun-exposed portions of the body, especially the face, lower lip, ears, and hands. Actinic keratosis is a precursor lesion.
- Diagnosis: Skin biopsy. Note that this tumor can be distinguished from other skin cancers by the presence of keratin pearls.
- Treatment: Surgical (e.g., excisional biopsy)
- Prognosis: Very good if detected at earlier stages because of low metastatic potential, although does have the capacity to become disfiguring and metastasize if left untreated

SUMMARY BOX: MELANOMA

- Epidemiology: Most common cause of skin cancer death but accounts for only 1% of skin cancers; often seen in patients with excessive ultraviolet (UV) damage or fair-skinned individuals
- Presentation: Positive for ABCDE characteristics
- Diagnosis: Skin biopsy
- Treatment: Surgical excision, chemoradiation, and biologics
- Prognosis: Varied, although does result in a significant number of fatalities; tumor depth is correlated with likelihood of metastasis

CASE 27.2

A 73-year-old man with a history of Parkinson disease presents with several large blisters on his extremities and trunk (Fig. 27.5). He describes severely itchy skin, which started 2 weeks before the onset of his blistering. On physical examination, several tense bullae are appreciated. Thorough examination of the oral cavity is negative for any lesions.

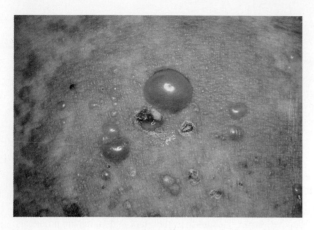

Figure 27.5. Appearance of vesicles and bullae in patient in Case 27.2. *(From Goldman L, Schafer A. Goldman-Cecil Medicine. 25th ed. Philadelphia: Elsevier; 2016.)*

1. **What is the most likely diagnosis in this patient?**

   The most likely diagnosis is bullous pemphigoid, an autoimmune disorder caused by the development of immunoglobulin G (IgG) antibodies against hemidesmosomes, which anchor basal epithelial cells to the basement membrane. As a result, this condition leads to the development of tense, subepithelial blisters as opposed to the flaccid blisters seen in patients with pemphigus vulgaris. This condition most commonly develops in patients older than 70 years and has been associated with several neurologic disorders, including Parkinson disease, stroke, and dementia. A prodromal phase marked by development of a skin rash and/or pruritus may precede the development of bullae.

2. **How is bullous pemphigoid differentiated from pemphigus vulgaris?**

   Pemphigus vulgaris is an autoimmune skin disorder marked by the formation of IgG antibodies against desmoglein, a component of desmosomes, which attach adjacent epidermal cells to one another. As a result of autoantibodies attacking desmoglein, cells become separated from one another, leading to significant acantholysis (loss of intracellular connections between keratinocytes) and subsequent formation of intraepithelial, flaccid blisters. The epidermal surface is easily separated in response to gentle mechanical pressure (Nikolsky sign). Unlike bullous pemphigoid, pemphigus vulgaris typically involves both mucosal and cutaneous sites and may make eating uncomfortable. Although the incidence of pemphigus vulgaris is very low (approximately 0.5 per 100,000 people annually), Ashkenazi Jews and people of Indian, southeast European, and Middle Eastern descent are at greater risk for this condition.

   For more information to help differentiate blistering disorders, see Table 27.3, which reviews presentations of the most common blistering skin disorders.

Table 27.3. Blistering Skin Disorders				
BLISTERING DISORDER	**GROSS PRESENTATION**	**HISTOLOGY**	**PATHOPHYSIOLOGY**	**DIRECT IMMUNOFLUORESCENCE**
Bullous pemphigoid	Tense blisters, usually spares mucous membranes	Subepidermal separation	IgG autoantibodies against hemidesmosomes	Linear pattern
Pemphigus vulgaris	Flaccid blisters, mucous membranes often involved, positive Nikolsky sign	Intradermal separation	IgG autoantibodies against desmoglein	Reticular pattern
Dermatitis herpetiformis	Small vesicles often on extensor surface	Subepidermal separation	IgA autoantibodies deposit in papillary dermis; typically associated with celiac disease	Granular pattern

Table 27.3. Blistering Skin Disorders—cont'd

BLISTERING DISORDER	GROSS PRESENTATION	HISTOLOGY	PATHOPHYSIOLOGY	DIRECT IMMUNOFLUORESCENCE
Erythema multiforme	Multiple types of lesion, including macules, papules, vesicles, targetoid lesions	Varies based on lesion type	Delayed type IV hypersensitivity reaction to infections (typically HSV, *Mycoplasma*) or drugs (typically sulfa drugs and β-lactam antibiotics)	Nonspecific
Stevens-Johnson syndrome	Prodrome followed by macules that become flaccid bullae that slough off, mucous membranes affected, positive Nikolsky sign	Necrotic epithelium	Delayed type IV hypersensitivity reaction usually to drugs (typically sulfa drugs, antibiotics, and antiepileptics)	Nonspecific

HSV, Herpes simplex virus; *IgA,* immunoglobulin A; *IgG,* immunoglobulin G.

CASE 27.2 CONTINUED:

The dermatologist performs a skin biopsy from the perilesional area of an intact bulla, and direct immunofluorescence is performed. A linear staining pattern at the dermoepidermal junction is seen (Fig. 27.6).

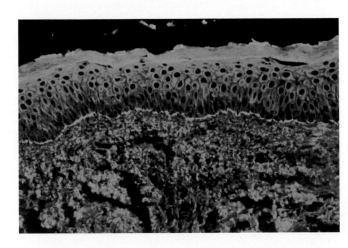

Figure 27.6. Direct immunofluorescence showing linear immunoglobulin G (IgG) along the dermoepidermal junction. *(From Brinster NK, Liu V, Diwan AH, McKee PH. Dermatopathology: High-Yield Pathology. Philadelphia: Elsevier; 2011.)*

3. How do these results affect your diagnosis?
   They confirm the diagnosis of bullous pemphigoid, which is associated with a linear band of IgG autoantibodies that deposit at the dermoepidermal junction. Similar to bullous pemphigoid, the definitive diagnosis of pemphigus vulgaris is also made by direct immunofluorescence of a skin biopsy sample. However, because pemphigus vulgaris involves deposits of IgG antibodies along the connections *between* cells, the immunofluorescence pattern throughout the epidermis is said to be reticular or resemble "chicken wire" (Fig. 27.7).

4. How should this patient be treated?
   Treatment of bullous pemphigoid involves either topical or oral corticosteroids, the latter of which is typically reserved for more difficult to manage cases. Immunomodulatory drugs, including rituximab (anti-CD20 antibody), have also been used for refractory cases. Although this condition is chronic and may wax and wane over the course of several months or years, it is usually self-limited in nature.

Clinical Pearl
If not treated, pemphigus vulgaris carries a high risk for secondary infection. Patients are typically administered high-dose oral steroids or immunomodulatory agents.

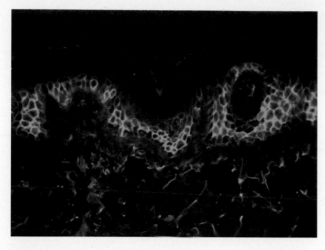

Figure 27.7. Direct immunofluorescence of pemphigus vulgaris. *(From High WA.* Dermatopathology. *2nd ed. Philadelphia: Elsevier; 2014.)*

SUMMARY BOX: BULLOUS PEMPHIGOID

- Epidemiology: More commonly seen in elderly individuals and in patients with certain neurologic disorders
- Presentation: Tense, subepithelial blisters; typically spares mucosal sites
- Pathophysiology: Immunoglobulin G (IgG) autoantibodies against hemidesmosomes, resulting in separation of the dermoepidermal junction
- Diagnosis: Direct immunofluorescence demonstrating a linear pattern
- Treatment: Topical or oral steroids, immunomodulatory drugs

SUMMARY BOX: PEMPHIGUS VULGARIS

- Epidemiology: Very rare; increased incidence in Ashkenazi Jews and individuals of Indian, southeast European, and Middle Eastern descent
- Presentation: Flaccid blisters involving mucosal and cutaneous sites, positive Nikolsky sign
- Pathophysiology: Immunoglobulin G (IgG) autoantibodies against desmoglein (a component of desmosomes), leading to acantholysis
- Diagnosis: Direct immunofluorescence demonstrating a reticular pattern
- Treatment: Oral steroids, immunomodulatory drugs

STEP 1 SECRET HIGH-YIELD DERMATOLOGY

The rashes discussed in subsequent cases are known to appear very frequently on Step 1. Learn their appearance, patterns, and epidemiologic presentations well!

5. A 34-year-old man presents with itchy, silvery plaques on his elbows, knees, and buttock region. He states that his mother had a similar condition.
   Psoriasis is a multifactorial autoimmune disorder involving excessive growth and accumulation of keratinocytes. Patients commonly report pruritus. On examination, look for the erythematous, silvery-scaled appearance of these plaques that may wax and wane over time. Pinpoint bleeding occurs after removal of the scales (Auspitz sign). Note that these plaques are classically found on the extensor surfaces of the skin (e.g., elbows, knees) as shown in Fig. 27.8. The disorder is also associated with nail pitting and psoriatic arthritis.

6. A 6-year-old asthmatic child presents with an itchy, irritated rash on his arms, inner surface of his elbows, and stomach (Fig. 27.9). His mother asks you why his rash is so much worse in the winter.
   Atopic dermatitis (eczema) is a condition marked by poor skin barrier function that results in transepidermal water loss. Eczema is often found in conjunction with other allergic disorders (e.g., asthma, allergic rhinitis) and tends to be worse during times of the year when humidity is low. Eczema is classically found on the flexural regions of the skin but commonly presents on the cheeks in infants. Treat with moisturizing lotions and topical steroids.

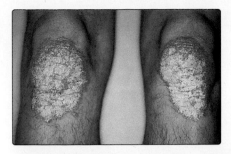

Figure 27.8. Psoriasis on the knees. *(From Gawkrodger, DJ, Ardern-Jones MR.* Dermatology: An Illustrated Colour Text. *5th ed. Philadelphia: Churchill Livingstone; 2012.)*

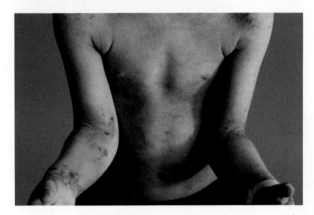

Figure 27.9. Appearance of rash on patient in question 6. *(From Lyons JJ, Milner JD, Stone KD. Atopic dermatitis in children: clinical features, pathophysiology, and treatment.* Immunol Allergy Clin North Am. *2015;35(1):161-183.)*

7. A 42-year-old gardener presents with a 2-day history of an itchy rash marked by erythema and blisters on his arms (Fig. 27.10). He states that this has happened to him twice before.

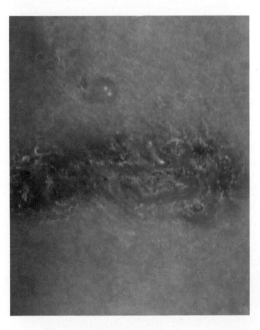

Figure 27.10. Note the acute eczematous rash with vesicle formation. *(Courtesy of the Honickman Collection of Medical Images in memory of Elaine Garfinkel and the Jefferson Clinical Images Collection [through the generosity of JMB, AKR, LKB, and DA].)*

The patient has a poison ivy rash, an example of contact dermatitis. As the name implies, contact dermatitis results from direct skin contact with an irritating substance, leading to a type IV hypersensitivity response that occurs 24 to 72 hours after exposure. Poison ivy and similar plants such as poison oak and poison sumac precipitate acute contact dermatitis reactions, which (as opposed to chronic dermatitis) are commonly associated with erythematous vesicles and extreme pruritus. Precipitating factors for chronic contact dermatitis include metals (e.g., jewelry, especially nickel), soaps, detergents, and cosmetics.

STEP 1 SECRET

Contact dermatitis may also be presented in the context of a patient with a rash that perfectly underlies the button on their jeans. This button often contains nickel, a classic skin irritant.

8. A 7-year-old child presents to the emergency department (ED) with a whole-body rash (Fig. 27.11) that developed 15 minutes after consuming shellfish for the first time. His parents deny any known allergies to foods or medications.

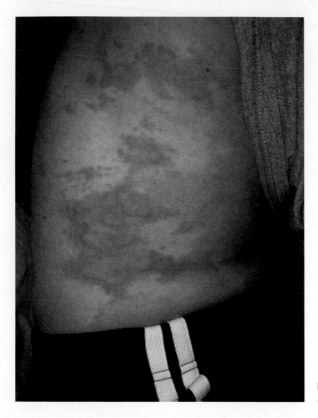

Figure 27.11. Rash of child in question 8. *(From Amar SM, Dreskin SC. Urticaria. Prim Care. 2008;35(1):141-57.)*

Urticaria (hives) is most frequently triggered by a systemic allergic reaction to environmental or food substances that results in histamine release from mast cells. However, there are many nonallergic causes for urticaria that you should be aware of, including viral infections, drugs, cold temperature, and autoimmune conditions. Pay attention to time intervals, as chronic urticaria is not likely to be allergic in nature. Although this patient did not present with other symptoms of anaphylaxis, he should be given a prescription for an epinephrine autoinjector for any future emergency situations.

9. A 3-year-old girl presents with 2 days of rash that has spread from her head down to her trunk (Fig. 27.12A). Before the development of this rash, the girl had spiked a 104°F fever and developed a cough, runny nose, and red, watery eyes. Her mom also noticed some tiny white spots inside her daughter's mouth that were not there a week ago (Fig. 27.12B).
This presentation is very suspicious for measles, a highly contagious virus that presents with a prodromal phase consisting of high fever and the 4 Cs (**c**ough, **c**oryza, **c**onjunctivitis, and **K**oplik spots). This is followed by the development of a characteristic maculopapular rash that spreads from head to toe. Koplik spots (see Fig. 27.12A) are white lesions that appear on the buccal mucosa before the development of the rash; they are pathognomonic for measles infection but are not required to make the diagnosis.

10. A 4-year-old boy presents with 7 days of high fever and refusal to walk. On examination, you note that the child's extremities are swollen and covered by an erythematous, maculopapular rash that is also present on his trunk. His tongue and oral mucosa are bright red (Fig. 27.13), and his lips are cracked. You note the presence of large lymph nodes on the right side of his neck and bilateral conjunctivitis.
Kawasaki disease is a medium vessel vasculitis that commonly affects children younger than 5 years. To make this diagnosis, the patient must have a fever for a minimum of 5 days along with the presence of at least four of the

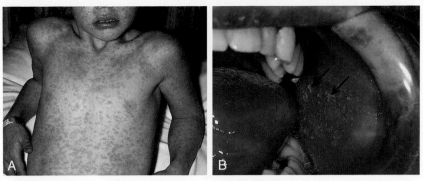

Figure 27.12. Rash of patient in question 9. *(From Dockrell DH, Sundar S, Angus, BJ, Hobson RP.* Davidson's Principles and Practice of Medicine. *22nd ed. Philadelphia: Elsevier; 2014.)*

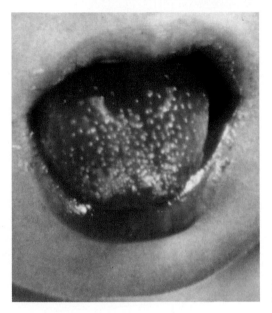

Figure 27.13. Tongue of patient in question 10. *(From Crawford M, Di-Marco J, Paulus W.* Cardiology. *3rd ed. Philadelphia: Mosby; 2010.)*

following five **CRASH** symptoms: **C**onjunctivitis, **R**ash, unilateral cervical **A**denopathy, **S**trawberry tongue, and **H**and and/or foot erythema or swelling. This is one of the rare occasions where children should be treated with high-dose aspirin to prevent thrombosis, as well as intravenous immunoglobulin G (IVIG). Recall that the most severe consequence of this disease is coronary artery aneurysm, for which these patients must be monitored extensively during the course of their illness. There is also incomplete Kawasaki disease where only two to three clinical criteria are met (instead of four or more). In this case, labs are obtained (erythrocyte sedimentation rate [ESR] and C-reactive protein [CRP]), and if elevated, additional laboratory workup is needed to confirm the diagnosis.

STEP 1 SECRET

A popular mnemonic for recalling the criteria for Kawasaki disease is CRASH and Burn, *the latter of which will remind you of the need for at least 5 days of fever to make this diagnosis.*

11. A 2-year-old boy presents with a crusty-looking golden rash on his face for 2 days (Fig. 27.14). Impetigo is a superficial skin infection of early childhood that is most commonly caused by *Staphylococcus aureus* and *Streptococcus pyogenes*. As a result, this rash is often seen below the nares (secondary to colonization from rubbing) and around the mouth but can be found anywhere on the body. You can recognize this rash by its yellow, crusted appearance. Impetigo is typically treated with topical antibiotics, such as mupirocin, but may require systemic antibiotics if invasive complications (e.g., abscess formation from methicillin-resistant *S. aureus*) occur. Be on the lookout for poststreptococcal glomerulonephritis, which is a potential complication that can occur after development of this rash.

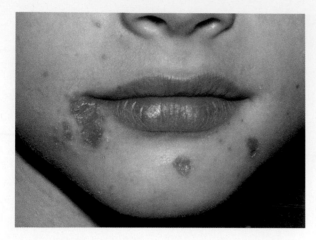

Figure 27.14. Rash of patient in question 11. *(From Bolognia J, Schaffer J, Duncan K, Ko C. Dermatology Essentials. Philadelphia: Saunders; 2014.)*

12. A 2-year-old boy is brought in for a rash by his concerned babysitter (Fig. 27.15). You note that he has a low-grade fever and clear discharge from his nose and are reassured that this rash is not secondary to abuse, despite appearing as though the child has been hit across the cheeks.

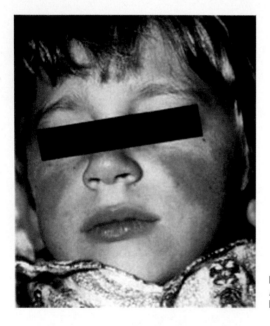

Figure 27.15. Rash of patient in question 12. *(From Cherry J, Demmler-Harrison G, Kaplan SL, et al. Feigin and Cherry's Textbook of Pediatric Infectious Diseases. 7th ed. Philadelphia: Saunders; 2014.)*

This patient is infected with parvovirus B19, resulting in erythema infectiosum, or fifth disease, a common viral exanthem of childhood. The bright red rash that appears after the onset of fever and upper respiratory infection (URI) symptoms often occurs on the cheeks, giving the child a slapped-cheek appearance. The rash is also commonly seen on the torso, arms, and legs but is generally more reticular in appearance in these locations.

13. A 6-month-old infant is found to have a 5-day rash on her genitals, upper thighs, and buttocks (Fig. 27.16).
Diaper dermatitis (diaper rash) is an extremely common condition that is found on the skin surfaces in direct contact with a child's diaper (note that the skinfolds, which do not typically come in contact with the diaper, are often spared). Excessive moisture in the diaper area secondary to the constricting effects of the diaper itself, along with the presence of fecal and urinary contents, disturbs the upper layers of the skin, making it increasingly susceptible to frictional damage. This damage then permits the secondary growth of bacterial and fungal organisms, such as *Candida albicans*, which may then spread to the skinfolds. Treatment involves keeping the skin dry and use of topical steroids and barrier creams, as well as topical antifungals in more severe cases.

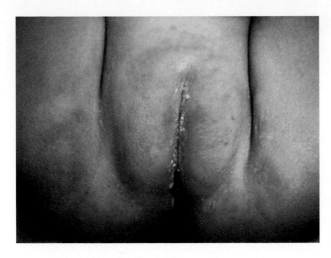

Figure 27.16. Rash of patient in question 13. *(From Lebwohl M, Heymann W, Berth-Jones J, Coulson I.* Treatment of Skin Disease: Comprehensive Therapeutic Strategies. *4th ed. Philadelphia: Saunders; 2014.)*

14. A 65-year-old woman with a history of diabetes (HbA1c 12%) presents to the ED with fever and severe pain over her right foot, which is extremely tender to palpation. Range of motion is limited secondary to swelling. Several hours later, she develops deep reddish-purple discoloration of the skin overlying her foot as her pain continues to increase (Fig. 27.17). She denies any known trauma or injuries but admits that her sensation in her feet is not well preserved.

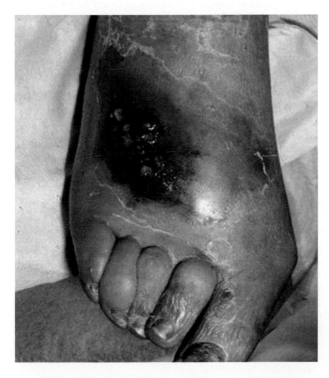

Figure 27.17. Foot of patient in question 14. *(From Torok ME. Skin and soft tissue infections. Conlon CP.* Medicine. *2009;37(11):603-609.)*

Necrotizing fasciitis is a severe soft tissue infection that results in destruction of underlying subcutaneous fat and fascial layers. Incidence is higher in diabetic individuals than the general population and is usually the result of a mixed aerobic and anaerobic infection. Because inflammation is typically deep within the tissue, patients often present with pain and fever before the onset of skin changes. Crepitus is present in approximately half of all patients with necrotizing fasciitis and is secondary to bacterial gas formation. Necrotizing fasciitis is an emergency that must be treated with broad-spectrum antibiotics and aggressive surgical debridement.

15. An 8-year-old child presents to your office for a well-child check. You note the presence of several shiny, dome-shaped papules on his trunk that his mother states have been present for 5 weeks (Fig. 27.18). Your patient affirms that the rash is not bothersome to him. You find out that the patient's younger brother has a similar rash on his abdomen that began 3 months ago.

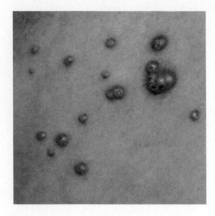

Figure 27.18. Rash of patient in question 15. *(From Habif TP. Clinical Dermatology. 6th ed. Philadelphia: Saunders; 2016.)*

Molluscum contagiosum is a highly contagious skin rash that results from infection by poxvirus. Although this rash is most common in young children, it can be transmitted sexually in adolescents and adults. This condition is typically diagnosed by its classic appearance of flesh-colored, waxy, dome-shaped papules that may persist for months before resolving. Be on the lookout for the central indentation/umbilication of these papules, which can be key to identifying molluscum.

16. An 8-year-old boy presents with a 2-day history of diffuse, erythematous rash. His mother tells you that the rash first appeared in his armpits and then spread down his trunk and to his extremities. On physical examination, you note a blanching rash with numerous small papules that gives the skin a rough textural appearance (Fig. 27.19). The patient had a fever, chills, and sore throat 3 days before the onset of the rash.
Scarlet fever is a classic sequela of streptococcal A pharyngitis that typically occurs in children from 5 to 15 years old. As a result, patients classically report fever and sore throat before the onset of the rash a few days later. Scarlet fever can be identified by its fine, erythematous, maculopapular appearance. Because these papules are so small and clustered together, the skin tends to adopt a rough "sandpaper-like" texture characteristic of this rash. Four to seven days after its onset, the rash will begin to desquamate. Patients should be treated with antibiotics (e.g., amoxicillin) as soon as possible.

17. A 75-year-old man presents with a 3-day history of burning sensation over his left shoulder. On physical examination, you note a vesicular rash arranged in a band-like pattern over the left shoulder blade that does not extend past his neck (Fig. 27.20).
Shingles/herpes zoster is a condition that results from reactivation of latent varicella-zoster (VZV) virus within the sensory ganglia, leading to the onset of a painful vesicular rash that follows a dermatomal distribution. *This rash is easily recognizable by the fact that it does not cross the midline.* It typically begins to crust 1 to 2 weeks after its onset. Treatment for herpes zoster consists of oral acyclovir, valacyclovir, or famciclovir. The most common complication of this condition is postherpetic neuralgia, which leads to chronic and often debilitating pain, as well as altered sensation over the involved areas. If the rash crosses midline or presents bilaterally, this is evidence of disseminated disease and should raise suspicion for immunocompromise (e.g., HIV/AIDS).

18. A 34-year-old woman with a history of systemic lupus erythematosus (SLE) is prescribed trimethoprim/sulfamethoxazole (TMP-SMX) for a urinary tract infection. Two days later, she develops a fever of 103°F, malaise, joint pain, sore throat, itchy eyes, and targetoid lesions on her chest and face (Fig. 27.21). The following day, she develops painful vesicles and bullae on her chest and neck, and her lips become cracked and ulcerated. Her mouth hurts so badly that she cannot eat or drink. You notice that the surrounding mucosa and distinct areas of her skin have begun to slough off. You advise her to discontinue the medication immediately.

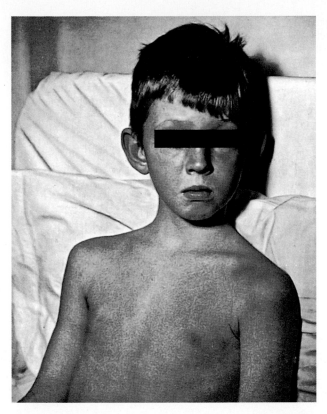

Figure 27.19. Rash for patient in question 16. *(Courtesy Dr. Franklin H. Top, Professor and Head of the Department of Hygiene and Preventive Medicine, State University of Iowa, College of Medicine, Iowa City, IA; and Parke, Davis & Company's Therapeutic Notes. From Gershon AA, Hotez PJ, Katz SL.* Krugman's Infectious Diseases of Children. *11th ed. Philadelphia: Mosby; 2004.)*

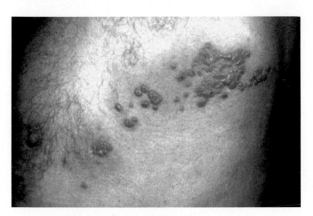

Figure 27.20. Shoulder of patient in question 17. *(From High WA.* General Dermatology. *Philadelphia: Saunders; 2009.)*

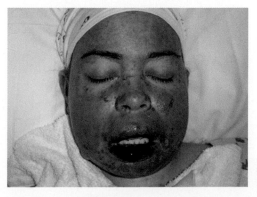

Figure 27.21. Appearance of patient in question 18. *(From Ferri F, Studdiford J, Tully A.* Ferri's Fast Facts in Dermatology: A Practical Guide to Skin Disease and Disorders. *Philadelphia: Saunders; 2010.)*

Stevens-Johnson syndrome (SJS) is a life-threatening rash that is thought to result from a hypersensitivity reaction that causes apoptosis of keratinocytes and separation of the epidermis from the dermis. Although SJS resembles toxic epidermal necrosis (TEN) in disease pathogenesis, the latter is considered to be a more severe form of the illness, involving greater than 30% of body surface area. SJS involves less than 10% of body surface area, and 10% to 30% involvement suggests a combination of SJS and TEN. Mucous membrane involvement and targetoid lesions are hallmarks of the disease. The most common causes of SJS include infections, medications (particularly sulfa drugs, penicillin, analgesics, and anticonvulsant agents), and malignancy. Patients with SLE are at increased risk for this condition.

Clinical Pearl

Erythema multiforme (EM) is a self-limited condition that occurs as a hypersensitivity reaction to drugs and infections. Although it typically presents with localized papules and targetoid lesions, unlike Stevens-Johnson syndrome (SJS), the mucosa is seldom involved. However, even EM can present with a wide spectrum of severity.

---

19. A 54-year-old woman presents for her annual preventative care visit. Your preceptor tells you to examine her before he comes into the room. You note a morbidly obese but otherwise well-appearing woman with thick, dark brown plaques around her neck (Fig. 27.22) and in her axillary folds.

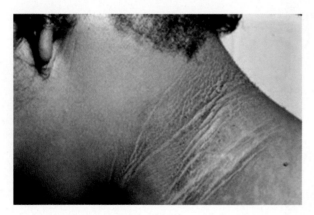

Figure 27.22. Neck of patient in question 19. *(From Murphy-Chutorian B, Han G, Cohen SR. Dermatologic manifestations of diabetes mellitus: a review.* Endocrinol Metab Clin North Am. *2013;42(4):869-898.)*

Acanthosis nigricans is a common condition marked by hyperpigmentation of intertriginous areas of the skin (e.g., neck, axillae, groin, skinfolds of the breasts). It is linked to conditions that result in insulin resistance, including obesity, type 2 diabetes mellitus, and polycystic ovarian syndrome. This rash can easily be recognized by its velvety, hyperpigmented appearance in patients with comorbid conditions.

20. A 65-year-old man presents for his annual preventative care visit. His wife is concerned about the red spots on his back (Fig. 27.23), though he states that they have been present for years and have not changed in appearance or caused him any pain.

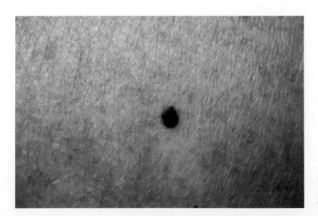

Figure 27.23. Appearance of skin lesion for patient in question 20. *(From Brinster NK, Liu V, Diwan AH, McKee PH.* Dermatopathology: High-Yield Pathology. *Philadelphia: Elsevier; 2011.)*

Campbell de Morgan spots are benign skin growths that result from abnormal proliferation of endothelial cells within capillary beds and increase in frequency with age. As they are easily recognizable by their bright red papular appearance, they are more commonly referred to as *cherry hemangiomas*. Although they may bleed if scratched or ruptured, they are generally not concerning so long as they remain stable in appearance.

21. A 70-year-old Caucasian man presents to your office for a rash on his back. He recently went to the beach with his brother, who noticed the lesions on his back and told him that he may have skin cancer. On physical examination, you note several well-demarcated, scaly, and hyperpigmented lesions with a "stuck-on" appearance (Fig. 27.24).

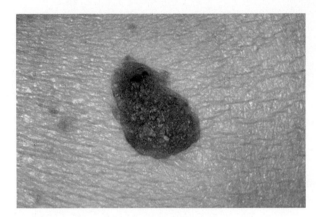

Figure 27.24. Appearance of skin lesion for patient in question 21. *(From Brinster NK, Liu V, Diwan AH, McKee PH.* Dermatopathology: High-Yield Pathology. *Philadelphia: Elsevier; 2011.)*

Seborrheic keratoses are common growths of middle-aged and elderly individuals that result from benign proliferation of immature keratinocytes. This condition is typically marked by the presence of several well-demarcated, round or oval hyperpigmented lesions on the back, trunk, arms, or face, although singular lesions may also be present. Because these are slow-growing, noncancerous lesions, treatment is not generally indicated unless they cause pain or cosmetic issues. However, biopsy should be performed if the diagnosis is uncertain or if there is suspicion of malignancy. Abrupt onset of multiple seborrheic keratoses, also known as the Leser-Trélat sign, raises suspicion for an underlying gastrointestinal malignancy.

22. A 20-year-old woman presents with an intensely itchy rash on her knees, ankles, and feet (Fig. 27.25). When you ask her about associated symptoms, she states that over the past 6 months, she has been experiencing significant abdominal pain, bloating, and diarrhea with meals.

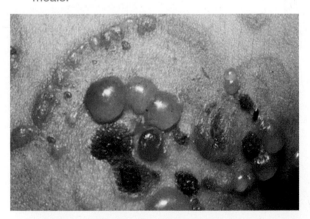

Figure 27.25. Appearance of rash for patient in question 22. *(From Bolognia J, Jorizzo J, Schaffer J.* Dermatology. *3rd ed. Philadelphia: Elsevier; 2012.)*

Dermatitis herpetiformis is a highly pruritic, symmetrically distributed blistering condition of the skin that results from deposition of IgA autoantibodies in the subepidermal layers of the skin. Most patients with this condition have an associated history or symptoms of celiac disease. This condition responds extremely well to a gluten-free diet.

23. A 55-year-old man presents with facial flushing and an intense skin eruption on his face, especially around the tip of the nose (Fig. 27.26). He reports a history of severe acne during his teenage years, which eventually resolved during high school. The facial flushing is exacerbated when consuming spicy foods.

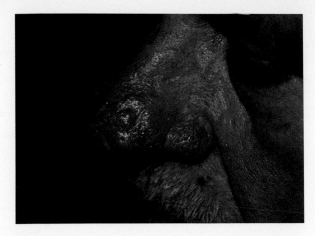

Figure 27.26. Appearance of skin eruption for patient in question 23. *(From Webster GF. Rosacea.* Med Clin North Am. *2009;93(6):1183-1194, Fig. 3.)*

Rosacea is a facial skin eruption characterized by scattered red papules and pustules on the face, similar to acne, but without comedones; it typically affects adults aged 30 years and older. Involvement of the nose can cause rhinophyma (large, bulbous nose). Facial flushing is common with triggers, including spicy foods, hot foods or drinks, heat, sun exposure, and alcohol consumption.

24. A 40-year-old woman with a history of hepatitis C and intravenous (IV) drug use presents with an itchy skin rash over her jawline and wrists (Fig. 27.27). On examination, there are web-like-appearing white lines over the buccal mucosa.

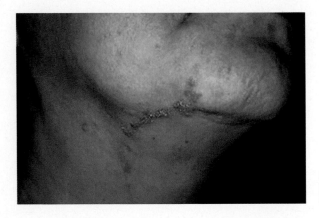

Figure 27.27. Appearance of skin rash for patient in question 24. *(From Bolognia J, Schaffer J, Duncan K, Ko C.* Dermatology Essentials. *Philadelphia: Saunders; 2014.)*

Lichen planus is characterized by the six Ps (pruritic, planar, polygonal, purple papules, and plaques). It is associated with Wickham striae, or reticular white lines along the oral mucosa. Histology shows a "saw tooth" appearance of the dermal–epidermal junction. You should recognize its association with chronic hepatitis C infection. Management is typically with antihistamines and topical corticosteroids.

PATHOLOGY

CASE 28.1

A 17-year-old Caucasian woman is seen by her gynecologist for her yearly exam. She reports regular but heavy menstrual periods that last 7 to 8 days. She also reports feeling "tired a lot." When discussing her diet, she states that she eats "a normal amount" but does not like meat. She takes no medications or supplements. Physical examination is unremarkable. The following image was obtained from a smear of her peripheral blood (Fig. 28.1).

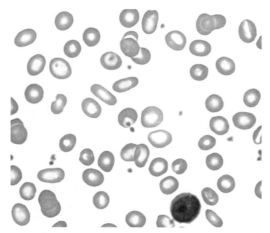

Figure 28.1. Peripheral blood smear of patient in question 1. *(From Aster J, Pozdnyakova O, Kutok J.* Hematopathology: A Volume in the High Yield Pathology Series. *Philadelphia: Saunders; 2013: 19.)*

What laboratory tests would confirm the likely diagnosis in this patient?
Low hemoglobin (female normal: 12–16 g/dL), low ferritin (female normal: 12–150 ng/mL), low mean corpuscular volume (MCV; 80–100 μm^3), and normal to high total iron-binding capacity (TIBC; normal: 250–350 $\mu g/dL$) would likely confirm the diagnosis of iron-deficiency anemia (IDA). The peripheral blood smear in Fig. 28.1 shows the classic picture of IDA consisting of red blood cells (RBCs) that are hypochromic (increased central pallor) and microcytic (small). Inadequate intake of dietary iron or increased blood loss can lead to IDA. Young females with heavy menses are at particularly increased risk because of ongoing losses, as well as lower overall stores compared with men. This patient also reports a diet that includes little to no meat, and although vegetables do contain free ferric iron, it is inefficiently absorbed compared with the heme-bound iron found in meat products. Often, patients with IDA have vague symptoms such as fatigue and weakness, or they can be completely asymptomatic. An iron supplement may be of benefit to this patient.

CASE 28.2

A 23-year-old African-American man is brought to the emergency department with intense chest pain. He reports the chest pain is constant, 10/10 in severity, and has only been partially relieved by opioid analgesics given in the emergency department. He states that the pain began this morning and has progressively gotten worse throughout the day. Recently, he was treated for an upper respiratory tract infection. On presentation, his only other symptoms include a cough and a low-grade fever. He states that he has been to the hospital before with similar symptoms. His chest x-ray film is remarkable for bilateral pulmonary infiltrates. During his workup, the peripheral blood smear shown in Fig. 28.2 was obtained.

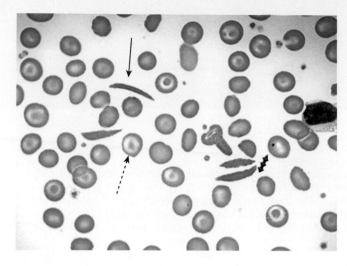

Figure 28.2. Peripheral blood smear of patient in question 2. *(From Barth D. Approach to peripheral blood film assessment for pathologists.* Semin Diagn Pathol. *2012; 29:31-48.)*

What complication is this patient most likely experiencing?

This patient is most likely experiencing acute chest syndrome, a vaso-occlusive crisis of the lungs typically seen in the setting of respiratory infections in patients with sickle cell anemia. The peripheral smear shows classic sickle-shaped RBCs (see Fig. 28.2, solid arrow), frank anemia, occasional target cells (also known as codocyte; dashed arrow), and Howell-Jolly bodies (nuclear RBCs remnants caused by hyposplenism; thick three-point arrow). Tissue hypoxia is the main cause of sickle cell formation in patients with the HbS variant of hemoglobin beta chain. Precipitators of sickle cell pain crises are often difficult to ascertain; however, in this case, the patient is recently getting over an upper respiratory tract infection, which can promote sickling through hypoxemia. The mainstay of treatment is pain management; hydration to achieve euvolemia; broad-spectrum antibiotics; and, depending on severity, simple transfusion or exchange transfusion.

CASE 28.3

A 45-year-old Caucasian woman is seen by her primary care physician for concerns of general fatigue and weakness. She also is concerned that her tongue "looks different." Her medical history includes a sleeve gastrectomy 15 years ago for morbid obesity. With this procedure, as well as a strict postoperative dietary regimen, she was able to significantly decrease her body mass index. Since that time, she has had intermittent follow-up because of problems keeping insurance. On physical examination, she is noted to have a slightly enlarged, "beefy," magenta-colored tongue. Fig. 28.3 shows a peripheral blood smear from this patient.

What is the most likely etiology of her fatigue?

Vitamin B_{12} deficiency is the most likely cause of her fatigue. The cellular abnormality in question is a hypersegmented neutrophil (polymorphonuclear leukocyte; see Fig. 28.3, arrow), which is commonly seen in megaloblastic anemias.

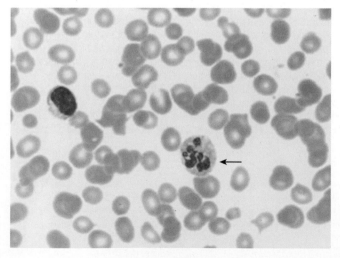

Figure 28.3. Peripheral blood smear of patient in question 3. *(From Shah DR, Daver N, Borthakur G, et al. Pernicious anemia with spuriously normal vitamin B12 level might be misdiagnosed as myelodysplastic syndrome.* Clin Lymphoma Myeloma Leuk. *2014;14:e141-e143.)*

Megaloblastic changes are seen in situations that interfere with DNA synthesis, and thus a dyssynchrony between cytoplasmic and nuclear development exists. Common causes of megaloblastic anemias include vitamin B_{12} and folate deficiencies and treatment with medications that interrupt folate synthesis, such as methotrexate. In this case, the patient underwent sleeve gastrectomy, which has reduced her overall levels of intrinsic factor production, a glycoprotein necessary for vitamin B_{12} absorption. The patient's glossitis is also a hallmark of vitamin B_{12} deficiency, although the exact mechanism of its development is incompletely understood.

CASE 28.4

A 75-year-old Caucasian woman is evaluated for increasing fatigue, unintentional weight loss, night sweats, and a sense of fullness in her left upper abdomen. Her examination is benign except for some dullness to percussion in the left upper quadrant. During her workup, a peripheral blood smear shows teardrop-shaped RBCs (dacrocytes) and many immature granulocytes and RBCs (leukoerythroblastosis). Subsequently, the patient was sent for a bone marrow biopsy, which resulted in the image shown in Fig. 28.4B when stained for reticulin.

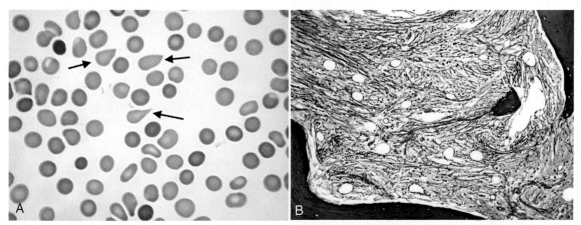

Figure 28.4. A, Peripheral blood smear from patient in question 4. B, Bone marrow biopsy stained for reticulin. *(A: Adapted from Bain BJ.* Goldman-Cecil Medicine, *26th ed. Philadelphia: Elsevier; 2020; B: From Hudnall S.* Hematology: A Pathophysiologic Approach. *Philadelphia: Mosby; 2012: 209, Fig. 12-30.)*

What is the likely diagnosis in this patient?

A marrow-infiltrating disorder such as myelofibrosis is the likely diagnosis. The marked increase in reticulin-stained marrow (Fig. 28.4B) is consistent with the diagnosis of myelofibrosis. The peripheral smear will often show dacrocytes (arrows in Fig. 28.4A, caused by RBC damage in the marrow) and the premature release of immature forms (leukoerythroblastosis). Myelofibrosis is classified as a myeloproliferative disease (MPD), which includes conditions such as chronic myelogenous leukemia (CML), essential thrombocytosis, and polycythemia vera. The disease is most likely caused by the inappropriate release of fibrogenic factors (transforming growth factor β [TGF-β]/platelet-derived growth factor [PDGF]) from megakaryocytes, which are often seen as large and dysplastic cells within the marrow. Like other MPDs, activating *JAK2* mutations have been implicated as a causative derangement and provide a unique therapeutic target for ongoing clinical trials. The presentation of classic "B symptoms" (fever, night sweats, weight loss) is likely due to the vast amount of extramedullary hematopoiesis that occurs in the spleen as a result of an obliterated bone marrow. This process is ultimately disordered for unknown reasons, eventually lagging behind and resulting in pancytopenia as the disease progresses.

CASE 28.5

An 86-year-old woman with Alzheimer dementia lives in a long-term nursing facility. She also has a history of urinary retention, and she has a urine catheter in place. Today, she is rushed to the emergency department with a temperature of 102.5°F and rigors. In the emergency department, she has a white blood cell count of 20,000/mm³, her blood pressure is 80/60 mm Hg, her heart rate is 122 beats/min, and she has an elevated serum D-dimer. Fig. 28.5 shows the image of the peripheral smear taken during her workup.

What process is occurring in this patient?

Disseminated intravascular coagulation (DIC), exemplified by schistocytes on the peripheral smear (arrows) and elevated D-dimer in the context of evolving urosepsis, is the most likely diagnosis in this patient. DIC can be initiated by many factors, but the most common mechanisms involve widespread endothelial cell injury leading to microangiopathic hemolytic anemia or systemic release of tissue factor and/or thromboplastic substrates (e.g., in placental products, retained dead fetus, acute promyelocytic leukemia, and some adenocarcinomas).

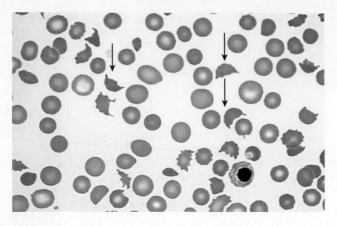

Figure 28.5. Peripheral blood smear of patient in question 5. *(From Carey WD. Cleveland Clinic: Current Clinical Medicine. 2nd ed. Philadelphia: Saunders; 2011: 579, Fig. 1.)*

CASE 28.6

A 66-year-old Black man is evaluated for increased weakness, lethargy, constipation, body aches, and polyuria. His physical examination is completely unremarkable. Laboratory workup reveals an elevated serum calcium, elevated blood urea nitrogen and creatinine, and mild anemia. A urinalysis is unremarkable except for 3+ proteinuria, and a skeletal survey is done (Fig. 28.6). A bone marrow biopsy and serum protein electrophoresis (SPEP) are ordered to confirm the diagnosis. A peripheral blood smear from the patient is shown in Fig. 28.7.

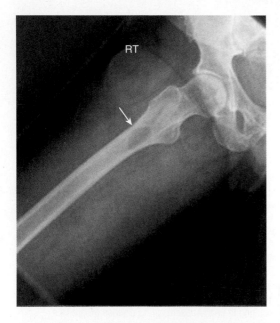

Figure 28.6. X-ray of right femur of patient in question 6. *(From Punja M, McWey RP, Heller M. Lytic lesion. J Emerg Med. 2013;44:179-180.)*

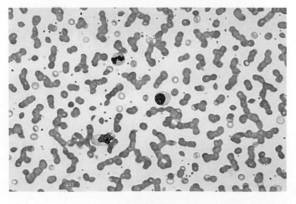

Figure 28.7. Peripheral blood smear of patient in question 6. *(From Jaffe ES. Hematopathology. 2nd ed. Philadelphia: Elsevier, Fig. 26-3.)*

What is the likely diagnosis for this patient?

Multiple myeloma (MM) is the likely diagnosis. MM is a plasma cell neoplasm that causes clinical features as a result of occupying lesions in bone marrow, excessive production of immunoglobulin, and interference with normal humoral immunity. The important clinical sequelae are compiled in the CRAB criteria: elevated serum **C**alcium, **R**enal disease (secondary to glomerular damage from excessive light chain aggregates sometimes referred to as Bence-Jones proteins), **A**nemia, and lytic **B**one lesions. The "punched-out" bone lesions shown in Fig. 28.6 are a result of upregulation of receptor activator of nuclear transcription factor-κB ligand (RANKL) by myeloma-derived *CCL3*, which in turn activates osteoclasts and leads to bone resorption and hypercalcemia. The rouleaux formation, or large stacks of RBCs, shown in Fig. 28.7 are caused by the large M protein in MM.

CASE 28.7

A 32-year-old Caucasian man is seen in the emergency department for right upper quadrant pain, which he describes as constant and sharp. He reports a recent history of similar pain that was transient and was especially noticeable after eating at fast food restaurants. His only other pertinent medical history is long-standing anemia. His physical examination is remarkable for tenderness to palpation in the right upper quadrant, splenomegaly, and yellow discoloration under his tongue. A right upper quadrant ultrasound demonstrates gallstones, one of which is in the common bile duct. His complete blood count shows a low hemoglobin and hematocrit and a high mean corpuscular hemoglobin concentration (MCHC).

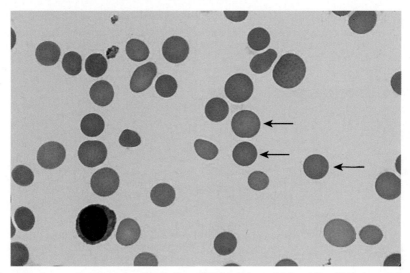

Figure 28.8. Peripheral blood smear of patient in question 7. *(From Klatt E.* Robbins and Cotran Atlas of Pathology. *3rd ed. Philadelphia: Saunders; 2015, Fig. 4-7.)*

An image from his peripheral smear is shown in Fig. 28.8. How can his current condition be explained?

This patient has hereditary spherocytosis (HS). HS is due to an inherited defect in proteins important for RBC skeleton structure—namely, spectrin and ankyrin. Seventy-five percent of cases are autosomal dominant, with the remaining 25% being compound heterozygotes with much more severe disease. The loss or dysfunction of these proteins lowers the deformability of the RBCs, causing these cells to adopt the shape with the smallest diameter for any given volume: a sphere. These spherocytes (Fig. 28.8, arrows) are hyperchromic and have a high mean corpuscular hemoglobin concentration (MCHC). In HS, the normal lifespan of the RBC is decreased from 120 days to 10 to 30 days because these cells are more susceptible to both rupture and destruction in the spleen, resulting in anemia. Three important clinical sequelae are aplastic crisis in patients with *Parvovirus* infections (which halts normal erythropoiesis by infecting RBC progenitors), hemolytic crisis with any inciting event that increases hemolysis of RBCs, and biliary colic or choledocholithiasis from indirect hyperbilirubinemia and subsequent formation of bilirubin pigment stones (as is seen in this patient). Patients may benefit from therapeutic splenectomy.

CASE 28.8

A 21-year-old woman presents to her primary care physician for a lump on her neck. She has had a low-grade fever for several weeks, night sweats, and unintentional weight loss. The patient has large, painless cervical lymphadenopathy. Her medical history includes infectious mononucleosis but is otherwise unremarkable. A biopsy of her lymph node is taken and the slide appears as shown in Fig. 28.9. A minority of cells appear to be large and bilobed and are shown by immunohistochemical analysis to be CD15+.

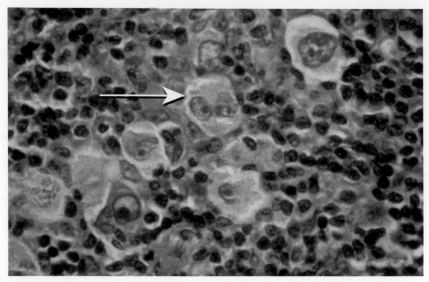

Figure 28.9. Biopsy of lymph node of patient in question 8. This high-power photomicrograph shows the characteristic Reed-Sternberg cell (*arrow*) of Hodgkin lymphoma, identified by its "owl-eye" nucleus. *(From Neville BW, Damm DD, Allen C, et al. Oral and Maxillofacial Pathology, 4th ed. St Louis: Elsevier; 2016, Fig. 13-25.)*

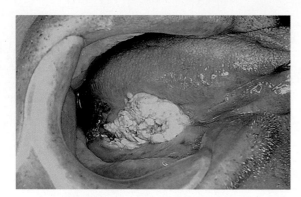

Figure 28.10. Tongue lesions of patient in question 9. *(From Shah JP, Patel S, Singh B, et al. Jatin's Head and Neck Surgery and Oncology, 5th ed. Elsevier; 2020, Fig. 8.9.)*

What is the most likely diagnosis in this patient?

Hodgkin lymphoma is the most likely diagnosis. Hodgkin lymphoma has a bimodal distribution, presenting in young adults or the elderly, and progresses in a predictable fashion. B symptoms, such as night sweats, weight loss, and low-grade fevers are the first to appear, and as the disease continues, lymph nodes, spleen, liver, bone marrow, and other organs become involved. Because of the predictable progression, staging is useful because it will inform decisions about treatment plans. Hodgkin lymphoma is associated with Epstein-Barr virus (EBV) infections because EBV-infected tumor cells express a protein from the EBV genome that allows for upregulation of NF-κB and other genes that prompt lymphocyte proliferation. In addition, Reed-Sternberg (RS) cells (Fig. 28.9, arrow) release factors that lead to an accumulation of reactive lymphocytes, macrophages, and granulocytes, which account for most of the mass in Hodgkin tumors. RS cells are positive for the marker CD15 and can be seen on histology as bilobed or binucleated cells. Although they are critical for diagnosis, they alone are not pathognomonic for Hodgkin lymphoma, because they can be seen in infectious mononucleosis, other cancers, and large-cell non-Hodgkin lymphoma. Several subtypes of Hodgkin lymphoma exist, including nodular sclerosis type (most common), mixed cellularity type, lymphocyte-rich type, and lymphocyte-deplete type. Another related disease moiety, referred to as *lymphocyte-predominant Hodgkin*, also exists, but it acts very differently from classic Hodgkin and has a different immunophenotype. Each of these different types has characteristic features that are beyond the scope of USMLE Step 1.

CASE 28.9

A 58-year-old man is seeing his primary care physician for a nonhealing lesion on the lateral surface of his tongue (Fig. 28.10) and some unusual oral bleeding. He is otherwise asymptomatic. The patient has no significant medical or family history of malignancy, but he consumes three to four beers daily and has smoked two packs of cigarettes per day for the past 25 years. The patient is referred to a dermatologist, who performs a biopsy, which yields the image shown in Fig. 28.11.

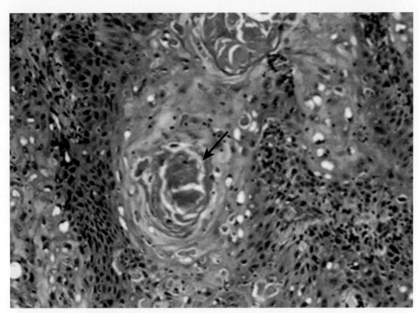

Figure 28.11. Biopsy sample of the patient in question 9. *(From Ojha J, Kossak E, Mangat S, et al. Recurrent pain and swelling associated with impacted maxillary third molar. J Am Dent Assoc. 2015;146:840-844.)*

What is the likely diagnosis?

Oral squamous cell carcinoma (SCC) is the likely diagnosis. SCC is a cancer of stratified squamous epithelium and is usually a disease found in older people that is also more commonly seen in men. Although SCC is often found on *sun-exposed* areas such as the face and outer lip, the most significant contributors to the risk for development of *oral* SCC are excessive smoking and alcohol consumption. Persistent red or white patches, ulcers, overlying swelling, and hyperkeratosis, as shown in Fig. 28.10, are classic patterns for oral SCC. Oral SCC is often asymptomatic or associated with oral bleeding at the time of presentation but may progress to cause pain with movement of the tongue, tooth pain, dysarthria, and dysphagia. On biopsy, circular eosinophilic keratin pearls (see Fig. 28.11, arrow) and intercellular bridging (unable to be appreciated at low magnification) are two histologic features that may be helpful for diagnosis. If localized (i.e., no lymph node involvement), 5-year survival rates typically exceed 75%.

CASE 28.10

A 54-year-old man with a history of chronic obstructive pulmonary disease is evaluated for several weeks of cough, dyspnea, unintentional weight loss, occasional hemoptysis, and significant muscle weakness. Examination is significant for decreased breath sounds in the right lung field and muscle weakness that seems to improve with serial measurement. Specialized testing reveals high levels of an antibody to presynaptic calcium channels. Imaging shows a central lung mass obstructing the right main bronchus. A biopsy of the mass is performed and stains positive for synaptophysin and chromogranin. The biopsy is shown in Fig. 28.12.

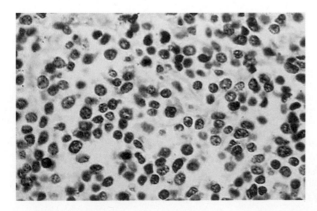

Figure 28.12. Biopsy sample of the patient in question 10. *(Adapted from Skarin A. Atlas of Diagnostic Oncology. 4th ed. Philadelphia: Mosby; 2010, Fig 5.21.)*

What is the likely diagnosis?

Small cell carcinoma is the likely diagnosis. Small cell carcinoma of the lungs (also referred to as *oat cell carcinoma*) is primarily seen in males with a history of smoking. It is found centrally within the lungs (e.g., in the main bronchus, as in this case). On biopsy, round to oval cells with little cytoplasm can be visualized. Cells are arranged in clusters without glandular or squamous organization, and necrosis is common and substantial. Small cell carcinoma originates from neuroendocrine progenitor cells lining the bronchial epithelium, and some have the ability to produce neurosecretory granules containing adrenocorticotropic hormone (ACTH) or antidiuretic hormone (ADH), causing paraneoplastic syndromes of Cushing syndrome and syndrome of inappropriate secretion of antidiuretic hormone (SIADH). Tumors are often positive for chromogranin and synaptophysin as a result of their neuroendocrine origins. Recall that patients with small cell carcinoma of the lungs may also present with Lambert-Eaton syndrome as in this case because of the production of antibodies against presynaptic calcium channels. This leads to symptoms of muscle weakness that improve with use.

CASE 28.11

A 32-year-old woman is evaluated for a lump on her throat. Medical history is remarkable only for undergoing successful treatment for head and neck cancer as a child. She feels well otherwise and has no other concerns. On examination, there is a small nodule protruding from the thyroid that moves freely during swallowing. Scintigraphy reveals poor uptake of radioactive iodine by the nodule. A fine needle aspirate and biopsy are taken. The aspirate shows empty-appearing nuclei, and the biopsy is shown in Fig. 28.13.

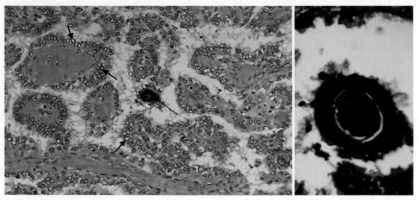

Figure 28.13. Biopsy sample of the patient in question 11. *(From Klatt E. Robbins and Cotran Atlas of Pathology, 3rd ed. Philadelphia: Elsevier; 2015, Fig. 15-29.)*

What environmental exposures may have contributed to her current condition?

Previous exposure to radiation may have contributed to this patient's presenting with papillary thyroid carcinoma. Papillary carcinomas are the most common type of thyroid cancer found in the United States, and they are often associated with a mutation in the *RET* proto-oncogene or ionizing radiation (this patient was presumably treated with ionizing radiation for her head and neck cancer as a child). On histology, the hallmarks of this disease are psammoma bodies (Fig. 28.13, left panel, thin arrow, and right panel) and orphan Annie eye nuclei (thick arrows). Psammoma bodies are circular calcifications and are rarely found in other thyroid cancers, so they are a good indication for papillary carcinoma. Orphan Annie eyes (Fig. 28.13, thick arrows) are empty-appearing nuclei that are created by dispersed chromatin. They may also be evident as intranuclear grooves, which are thin, hypochromatic lines traversing the nucleus. Papillary thyroid cancer has an excellent prognosis in most patients.

CASE 28.12

A 28-year-old woman presents to her gynecologist for infertility. The patient has had spotting that began a few years after menarche, and she has been trying to conceive for nearly 2 years with no success. On examination, the physician palpates a pelvic mass. Ultrasound reveals several round masses in the uterus (see Fig. 9.9 in Chapter 9 [Male and Female Reproductive Systems] for reference), and the patient is sent for surgery. The surgeon discovers multiple round, well-circumscribed masses of various sizes within the myometrium and excises them. Biopsies of the masses are performed, and a representative image is shown in Fig. 28.14.

What is the most likely diagnosis in this patient?

Leiomyoma is the most likely diagnosis. Leiomyomas, or fibroids, are a very common neoplasm in women, consisting of a benign growth of well-differentiated smooth muscle cells and a capsule. It is not uncommon to find multiple leiomyomata within the myometrium of a patient's uterus. The masses have a characteristic whorled pattern that can be seen both grossly on bisection and microscopically. Cells have long nuclei and cytoplasmic processes with a low

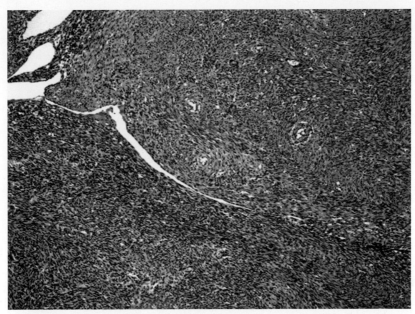

Figure 28.14. Biopsy sample of the patient in question 12. *(From Oliva E, Baker PM. Endometrial/ioid stromal tumors and related neoplasms of the female genital tract.* Surgical Pathol Clin. *2009;2:679-705.)*

mitotic index, making them nearly indistinguishable from normal smooth muscle. Leiomyomata are often asymptomatic; however, they can present with abnormal vaginal bleeding and impaired fertility because implantation is less likely to occur at a site containing a fibroid mass. Growth can change over time because these tumors are sensitive to estrogen, causing them to shrink after menopause. Fibroids are generally not considered precancerous and rarely convert to a malignant neoplasm (leiomyosarcoma).

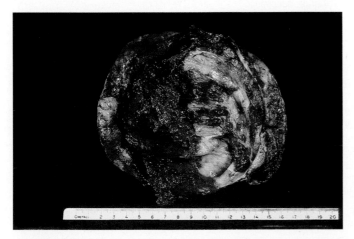

Figure 28.15. Gross pathology of ovary for patient in question 13. *(From Goldblum RG, Lamps LW, McKenney J, et al.* Rosai & Ackerman's Surgical Pathology. *11th ed. Philadelphia: Elsevier; 2018, Fig. 35.16.)*

CASE 28.13

A 32-year-old woman presents to her gynecologist for infertility. She has pain with intercourse (dyspareunia), as well as dysmenorrhea. On examination, her cervix and uterus are within normal limits; however, her ovaries are somewhat enlarged on palpation. Ultrasound shows cystic dilations in both ovaries. Surgery is performed; a depiction of one of her ovaries if additional dissection and examination were to be performed is as shown in Fig. 28.15.

What is the likely etiology of this patient's infertility?
Endometriosis is the likely cause of the infertility. When endometrial tissue is found outside of the uterus, it is referred to as *endometriosis*. The ovary and fallopian tube are commonly affected sites. There are several hypotheses for the development of endometriosis, including retrograde menstruation through the fallopian tubes, lymphatic or vascular

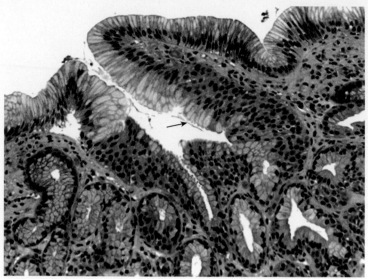

Figure 28.16. A biopsy from the lower esophageal segment of patient in question 14. *(From Lisovsky M, Srivastava A. Barrett esophagus: evolving concepts in diagnosis and neoplastic progression. Surg Pathol Clin. 2013;6:475-496.)*

spread of endometrial tissue, and development of multiprogenitor cells into endometrial cells that seed in abnormal locations. The tissue responds to estrogen the same way that endometrium in the uterus does by entering a proliferative state. During menstruation, foci of endometriosis also bleed and cause painful menstrual cycles by inducing a strong inflammatory response. Chocolate cysts, or endometriomas, of the ovaries represent sites of previous hemorrhage. Scarring may also occur in these locations, leading to infertility. Because the ectopic tissue responds to estrogen, foci enlarge during pregnancy and decrease in size after menopause.

CASE 28.14

A 42-year-old man with a history of gastroesophageal reflux disease is evaluated for persistent heartburn. Upper endoscopy reveals red patches extending from the gastroesophageal junction. A biopsy from the lower esophageal segment is shown in Fig. 28.16.

For what condition is this patient at increased risk?
This patient is at increased risk for esophageal adenocarcinoma secondary to Barrett esophagus. Long-term acid stress from chronic gastroesophageal reflux disease (GERD) leads to intestinal metaplasia, in which the nonkeratinized stratified squamous epithelium in the lower esophagus becomes nonciliated columnar with interspersed goblet cells. Intestinal metaplasia in the esophagus is called *Barrett esophagus*. The risk for dysplasia and adenocarcinoma is increased in patients with Barrett esophagus, and periodic endoscopy with biopsy is recommended for this population. This patient's biopsy (see Fig. 28.16) reveals multilayered epithelium (arrow) with mixed squamous and columnar features.

CASE 28.15

A 3-year-old boy, accompanied by his mother, is seen by his pediatrician for an abdominal lump. The mother explains that as she was holding her son, she noticed a hard lump on the right side of his abdomen. She also reports that she has noticed dark urine over the past week. On examination, the patient has elevated blood pressure and a large, smooth, right-sided mass that extends across the midline. Urinalysis reveals hematuria. The boy is sent for imaging, and a photo of the radiologic findings is presented in Fig. 28.17.

What is the most likely diagnosis in this patient?
Wilms tumor is the most likely diagnosis. The most common primary renal tumor found in childhood is Wilms tumor. Most cases occur before the age of 10 years. Symptoms include hematuria, hypertension, and a large, palpable abdominal mass caused by a well-circumscribed tumor that can become so large that it crosses the midline. These

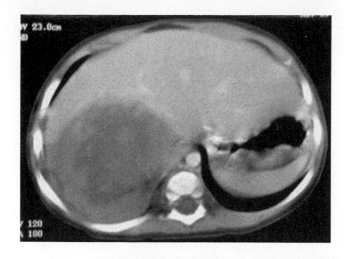

Figure 28.17. Abdominal computed tomography scan of the patient in question 15. *(From Ehrlich PF. Wilms tumor: progress and considerations for the surgeon. Surg Oncol. 2007;16:157-171.)*

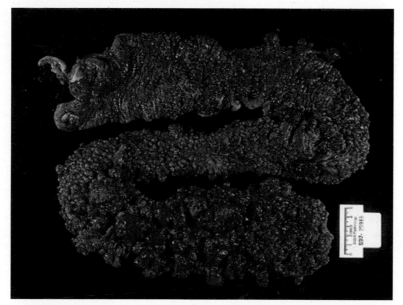

Figure 28.18. Adenomatous polyposis coli. *(From Skarin AT. Atlas of Diagnostic Oncology. 4th ed. St. Louis: Mosby; 2010.)*

masses are often accompanied by deletions or mutations in the *WT1* gene, which is important for both kidney and genital formation. *WT1* insults may also result in *WAGR* complex, which causes Wilms tumor, aniridia, genital malformations, and mental retardation.

CASE 28.16

A 16-year-old girl is evaluated for bloody stool. The patient has had several episodes of hematochezia, abdominal pain, and diarrhea in the past few weeks. Her father has a history of colorectal carcinoma, and her grandfather had a history of colonic polyps. On imaging, there are multiple nodular hypodensities in her colon. Endoscopy confirms the diagnosis, and resection of the colon is performed. The gross appearance of the resected colon appears in Fig. 28.18.

What gene mutation is most likely responsible for this patient's condition?
The *APC* gene, which leads to this patient's condition of familial adenomatous polyposis (FAP), is most likely responsible for this patient's condition. FAP is an autosomal dominant condition leading to the generation of hundreds to thousands of colonic polyps or adenomas. The risk for colorectal carcinoma is 100% in untreated patients and warrants resection of the colon. Common presenting symptoms are hematochezia, abdominal pain, and diarrhea. Symptoms appear early

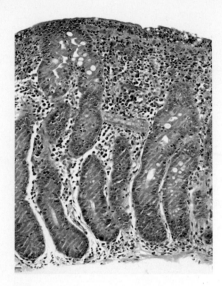

Figure 28.19. Gastrointestinal tract. *(From Rosai J.* Rosai & Ackerman's Surgical Pathology. *11th ed. Philadelphia: Elsevier; 2018, Fig. 15.12B.)*

in life, usually in the teens, and colorectal carcinoma develops before the age of 40. Intestinal polyps can also be seen in Gardner syndrome, along with osteomas of the mandible or skull. Turcot syndrome is similar, presenting with intestinal polyps and central nervous system (CNS) tumors.

CASE 28.17

A 43-year-old woman is evaluated for several weeks of fatigue, unintentional weight loss, and diarrhea. She is also concerned about an itchy rash on her elbows. On examination, there are grouped vesicles on the extensor surfaces of her arms. Laboratory tests indicate anemia, and serum is positive for anti-gliadin antibodies. The patient is sent for a duodenal biopsy, the results of which are shown below (Fig. 28.19).

What is the most likely diagnosis in this patient?

Celiac disease is the most likely diagnosis. The biopsy shows *villous atrophy* and intraepithelial lymphocytes along with crypt hyperplasia, indicating a diagnosis of celiac disease. Gluten, a component of wheat, barley, and rye, is the inciting factor in celiac disease. Gluten is digested into gliadin and subsequently to component peptides that are recognized by CD4$^+$ T cells, resulting in their activation in susceptible individuals. Gliadin can also cause T cell–mediated enterocyte damage and produce the characteristic flattened appearance of villi. The damaged villi are unable to properly absorb nutrients in the proximal small intestine, leading to weight loss, fatigue, and deficiencies in iron and fat-soluble vitamins. Laboratory findings will often show the presence of immunoglobulin A (IgA) antibodies against gliadin, tissue transglutaminase, or endomysium. IgA is also deposited at the tips of dermal papillae, causing a pruritic rash on extensor surfaces called *dermatitis herpetiformis* (see Fig. 27.25).

CASE 28.18

A 38-year-old man with a history of type 2 diabetes mellitus is evaluated for several weeks of fatigue, abdominal pain, and joint pain. His examination is significant for nontender hepatomegaly, testicular atrophy, and skin bronzing. On cardiac examination, the patient has a new, irregular heart rhythm. Laboratory test results show high iron, high ferritin, and low TIBC. A liver biopsy is performed and stained with Prussian blue as shown in Fig. 28.20.

What is the most likely diagnosis in this patient?

Hemochromatosis is the most likely diagnosis. The patient presents with a triad of hepatomegaly, skin pigmentation, and diabetes mellitus, which are consistent with hemochromatosis, also known as *bronze diabetes*. Prussian blue stains iron, which accumulates in the liver, as illustrated in the biopsy image (see Fig. 28.20). Hemochromatosis can be caused by repeated blood transfusions or a genetic defect, most commonly in the *HFE* gene. Because there is no physiologic mechanism for iron to leave the body, iron uptake must be well controlled. Hepcidin is the main regulator of iron homeostasis and works by causing ferroportin to be internalized and cleaved, preventing iron release into serum. In hereditary hemochromatosis, hepcidin is deficient and ferroportin is free to release iron into the serum. Iron accumulates in tissues and organs, leading to free radical damage, particularly in the liver. The heart is also susceptible to iron deposition, leading to arrhythmias, restrictive cardiomyopathy, and congestive heart failure (CHF). Patients are also at an increased risk for hepatocellular carcinoma. Hemochromatosis is diagnosed more frequently in men because menstruation is protective against iron overload in women.

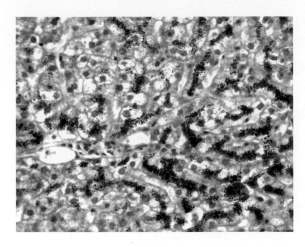

Figure 28.20. Liver biopsy of the patient in question 18. *(From Kumar V, Abbas AK, Aster JC. Robbins and Cotran Pathologic Basis of Disease. 9th ed. Philadelphia: Elsevier; 2015, Fig. 18-25.)*

CASE 28.19

An obese 35-year-old woman with a history of diabetes is seen for a routine physical. She has no concerns. On examination, there is mild hepatomegaly, and laboratory workup indicates elevated serum bilirubin and alkaline phosphatase. A liver biopsy is taken and is shown in Fig. 28.21.

What process is likely taking place in this patient?

Hepatic steatosis is likely occurring. The patient's biopsy demonstrates microvesicular droplets and macrovesicular lipid globules within hepatocytes, indicating hepatic steatosis. The disease mechanism is incompletely understood, but it is believed that oxidative stress on the hepatocytes leads to lipid peroxidation and reactive oxygen species that over time can lead to cirrhosis. Hepatic steatosis can be seen in alcoholic steatohepatitis, nonalcoholic fatty liver disease (NAFLD), or nonalcoholic steatohepatitis (NASH). NAFLD is associated with obesity, insulin resistance, and diabetes, as seen in this case. However, patients are often asymptomatic. The histology in NASH is similar but also includes lobular inflammation.

CASE 28.20

A 45-year-old man presents in the emergency department after a minor motor vehicle accident. The patient admits to drinking five alcoholic drinks that evening, and he has up to three cans of beer each night after work. When an intravenous (IV) line is started, the IV site bleeds profusely. His examination is significant for jaundice, scleral icterus, gynecomastia, and ascites. Laboratory workup reveals elevated alanine transaminase, aspartate transaminase, bilirubin, prothrombin time (PT), and anemia. An ultrasound reveals nodular hepatic architecture. A liver biopsy is ordered, and the trichrome stain is presented in Fig. 28.22.

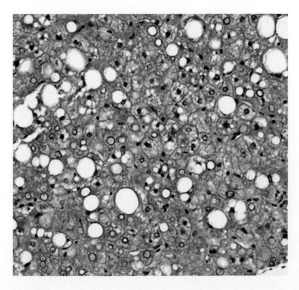

Figure 28.21. Liver. *(From Rosai J. Rosai & Ackerman's Surgical Pathology. 11th ed. Philadelphia: Elsevier; 2018: 726-802, Fig. 19.35.)*

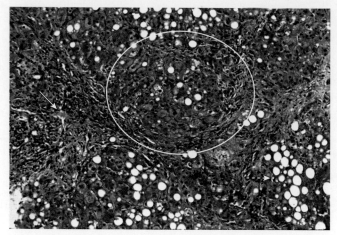

Figure 28.22. Alcoholic liver disease. *(From Carey WD. Cleveland Clinic: Current Clinical Medicine. 2nd ed. Philadelphia: Saunders; 2011: 508, Fig. 3.)*

What is the most likely diagnosis in this patient?

Cirrhosis is the most likely diagnosis. The patient's history of alcohol use and presenting symptoms are consistent with hepatic cirrhosis. Alcohol metabolism creates excess NADH, the reduced form of nicotinamide adenine dinucleotide (NAD), increasing the NADH/NAD$^+$ ratio, which is a positive regulator for lipid synthesis. In addition, creation and secretion of lipoproteins are impaired, trapping lipids inside hepatocytes (see Fig. 28.22, dashed arrow). Lipid peroxidation leads to production of reactive oxygen species, promoting hepatocyte damage and eventually fibrosis (see Fig. 28.22, solid arrow). Parenchymal hepatocytes entrapped in the fibrosis create regenerative nodules, which may be visible on imaging. On trichrome stain, biopsy demonstrates these nodules with surrounding blue collagen bands (see Fig. 28.22, circle), which is the hallmark of chronic liver insult. The patient's symptoms can all be explained by hepatocyte damage. Loss of albumin and other proteins leads to loss of oncotic pressure, which is demonstrated by his ascites. Jaundice and scleral icterus are products of elevated serum bilirubin, which cannot be taken out of circulation by the liver. Gynecomastia is a result of increased estrogen, which would normally be metabolized by hepatocytes. Clotting factors are also in short supply, which accounts for the elevated PT.

CASE 28.21

A 51-year-old man presents to his primary care physician with a skin rash. The patient explains that he has had several blisters on the inside of his mouth, and that recently his chest and head have developed scabbing and blisters as well. The physician notes vesicles distributed on the patient's trunk, scalp, and oral mucosa. The vesicles rupture when gentle pressure is applied. A skin biopsy is taken and is shown in Fig. 28.23.

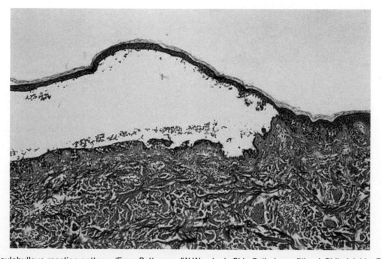

Figure 28.23. The vesiculobullous reaction pattern. *(From Patterson JW. Weedon's Skin Pathology. 5th ed. Philadelphia: Elsevier; 2021, Fig. 7.7.)*

What laboratory test will confirm his suspected diagnosis?

Elevated anti-desmoglein levels would confirm that this patient likely has pemphigus vulgaris. Flaccid vesicles that rupture easily and are found on the oral mucosa indicate pemphigus vulgaris. Crusting erosions may also be observed on examination. In pemphigus vulgaris, IgG autoantibodies against desmogleins cause damage to desmosomes, forcing the epithelial cells to separate from each other and the basal cell layer, which leads to intraepidermal blistering. This is called *acantholysis*. The row of basal cells left behind are described as having a "tombstone" appearance. In addition to the hematoxylin and eosin (H&E) stain, direct immunofluorescence will demonstrate a reticular or fish-net pattern where the IgG has deposited on the surface of epithelial cells (see Fig. 27.7).

CASE 28.22

A 64-year-old woman, accompanied by her son, is being seen by her primary care physician. The son explains that a year ago she began repeatedly forgetting where she placed her jewelry and keys. Beginning a few months ago, she would get lost on her way home and is having difficulty paying for groceries and bills. Physical examination is unremarkable. On mental status examination, the patient is oriented to person but not place or time and cannot recall three unrelated words after a 5-minute interval. If a postmortem biopsy were taken, it would appear as shown in Fig. 28.24.

What is the most likely diagnosis in this patient?

Alzheimer disease (AD) is the most likely diagnosis. AD is the most common cause of dementia in elderly patients and is usually a diagnosis of exclusion. Although imaging can aid in determining the cause of dementia, a definitive diagnosis can only be made using a biopsy showing neurofibrillary tangles (see Fig. 28.24, asterisks) and neuritic plaques (NP). Neurofibrillary tangles are formed when tau protein, normally involved in microtubule assembly, becomes abnormally hyperphosphorylated, resulting in an insoluble protein that is resistant to clearance in the extracellular space. The tangles display a characteristic flame shape around pyramidal neurons (see Fig. 28.24). Even after neuron death, the protein can leave a "ghost" image visible on microscopy. Neuritic plaques are derived from amyloid precursor protein (APP) that is broken down into various components, including Aβ amyloid. Aβ amyloid accumulates extracellularly and forms characteristic rounded structures (see NPs in Fig. 28.24).

CASE 28.23

A 27-year-old woman is evaluated for impaired vision in her left eye. Several months ago she experienced a sudden visual deficit in her right eye along with an episode of lower extremity weakness, both of which resolved on their own. On examination, the patient has a left-sided visual field deficit, but vision in her right eye remains intact. A radiograph of the brain is taken and is shown in Fig. 28.25.

What is the most likely diagnosis in this patient?

Multiple sclerosis (MS) is the most likely diagnosis. MS usually presents in women between the ages of 20 and 40 years. In the most common disease course, lesions are separated by time and space, meaning symptoms recur and resolve on their own, and the lesions are not found in a single location in the CNS. Common symptoms include visual disturbances caused by optic neuritis and motor or sensory deficits in the limbs. Symptoms occur as a result of T cells reacting to antigens found in myelin. Plaques can be viewed on imaging where white matter has been demyelinated. Histologically, these regions will display low oligodendrocyte numbers and reactive astrocytosis. The radiograph shows periventricular plaques, which is a classic location for demyelination in multiple sclerosis. Cerebrospinal fluid (CSF) analysis will typically demonstrate elevated IgG levels.

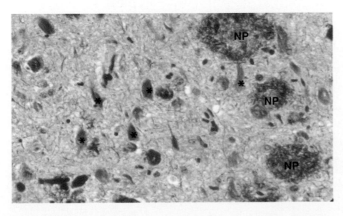

Figure 28.24. Biopsy sample of patient in question 22. NP, neuritic plaque. *(From Stern T, Fava M, Wilens T, Rosenbaum J.* Massachusetts General Hospital Psychopharmacology and Neurotherapeutics. *London: Elsevier; 2016, Fig. 14-1.)*

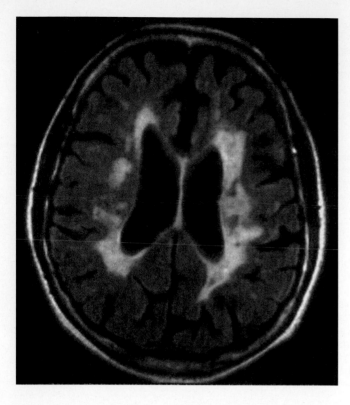

Figure 28.25. Brain imaging of patient in question 23. *(From Perkin G, Miller D, Lane R, Patel M, Hochberg F. Atlas of Clinical Neurology. 3rd ed. Philadelphia: Saunders; 2011: 343-359, Fig. 13-30.)*

CASE 28.24

A 56-year-old woman is evaluated for several months of fatigue, weakness, unintentional weight gain, and constipation. Examination reveals brady-cardia, dry skin, diminished (1+) patellar reflexes, and an enlarged thyroid. The patient is sent for a thyroid biopsy, the results of which are shown in Fig. 28.26. Laboratory workup is performed prior to biopsy.

Thyroid testing is most likely to reveal what findings?

Testing would reveal a high thyroid-stimulating hormone (TSH), low T_3, and low T_4 secondary to hypothyroidism as a result of Hashimoto thyroiditis. Weight gain, bradycardia, cold intolerance, and hyporeflexia are indicative of hypothyroidism. In parts of the world where iodine levels are adequate, Hashimoto thyroiditis is the most common cause of hypothyroidism.

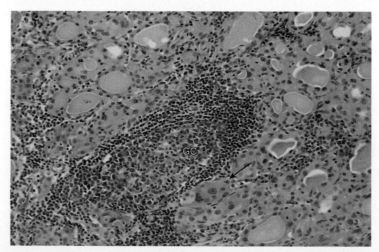

Figure 28.26. Thyroid gland. GC, germinal center. *(From Gray W, Kocjan G. Diagnostic Cytopathology. 3rd ed. Edinburgh: Churchill Livingstone; 2010, Fig. 17-14.)*

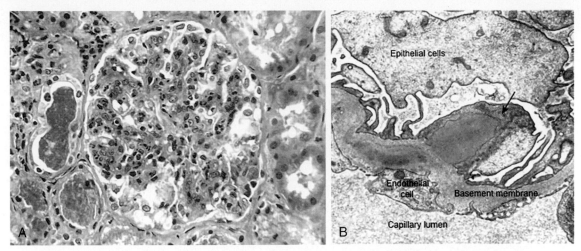

Figure 28.27. A, Glomerular hypercellularity on hematoxylin and eosin stain. B, Kidney biopsy sample showing an electron microscopy image of patient in question 25. *(Adapted from Vinay K. Robins Basic Pathology. 10th ed. Philadelphia: Elsevier; 2018: 549-581, Fig. 14.9.)*

Hashimoto thyroiditis is an autoimmune condition that destroys the thyroid gland and is associated with circulating antibodies against thyroid antigens, thyroglobulin, and thyroid peroxidase. Continuous injury to the cuboidal epithelium causes metaplasia, producing Hürthle cells, which are characterized by profuse eosinophilic cytoplasm (see Fig. 28.26, arrow). Biopsies will also demonstrate well-developed germinal centers (GCs).

CASE 28.25

A 2-year-old boy accompanied by his father is evaluated for fever and dark, cloudy urine. The father notes that his son had a sore throat about 2 weeks ago, but otherwise his history is unremarkable. On examination, the child has a temperature of 101°F and periorbital edema. His urinalysis shows proteinuria, hematuria, and red cell casts. A kidney biopsy is taken, and an electron microscopy image is presented in Fig. 28.27.

What is the likely etiology of this patient's condition?

Poststreptococcal glomerulonephritis (PSGN) is the likely etiology. The patient's laboratory values and presentation 1 to 2 weeks after a sore throat are consistent with PSGN. During a streptococcal infection, antibodies form immune complexes with bacterial antigens that are deposited beneath the basement membrane—that is, subepithelially. The depositions appear as dense "humps" or "meatballs" on electron microscopy (Fig. 28.27B, arrow). On immunofluorescence, the immune complex accumulations appear granular, and on H&E, the glomerulus will appear larger and hypercellular because of leukocyte infiltration (Fig. 28.27A). Alterations in the filtering ability of the kidney cause protein to leak into the urine, accounting for the patient's proteinuria and periorbital edema. Because this is a nephritic process, hematuria and RBC casts will also be seen.

CASE 28.26

A 61-year-old man is evaluated for a 1-month history of fatigue, fever, and unintentional weight loss and a new painful "rash" on his fingers and toes. The patient's history includes rheumatic fever as a child. Three weeks ago, he underwent an uncomplicated dental procedure. On examination, the patient has red streaks on his nail bed (Fig. 28.28) and tender, raised, erythematous lesions on the pads of his fingers and toes (Fig. 28.29). The physician notes circular, hemorrhaged spots on the retina and a new cardiac murmur. Blood cultures demonstrate gram-positive cocci. If the patient's heart were to be dissected on autopsy, it would appear as the photo provided in Fig. 28.30.

What is the most likely diagnosis in this patient?

Bacterial endocarditis is the most likely diagnosis. Most cases of bacterial endocarditis present with fever, fatigue, weight loss, and a new murmur. Additional symptoms include red streaks on the nail bed called *splinter hemorrhages* (Fig. 28.28, arrow); tender, raised red lesions on the finger and toe pads (Osler nodes); erythematous nontender lesions on the palms and soles (Janeway lesions; see Fig. 28.29); and white spots on the retina surrounded by erythema (Roth spots), all of which are the result of bacterial emboli. The patient's dental procedure caused viridans group Streptococci to enter the blood and infect a cardiac valve, leading to deposition of fibrin and additional bacteria. The depositions are evident as the friable vegetations shown in Fig. 28.30 and are the reason for the murmur. The insidious development of symptoms indicates that the infection is subacute. Subacute bacterial endocarditis causes infections on previously damaged or abnormal valves, such as in rheumatic fever, by low-virulence organisms. Acute bacterial endocarditis

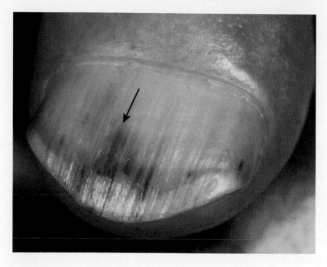

Figure 28.28. Red streaks on nail bed of patient in question 26. *(From Swartz M.* Textbook of Physical Diagnosis. *8th ed. Philadelphia: Elsevier; 2021, Fig. 8.10.)*

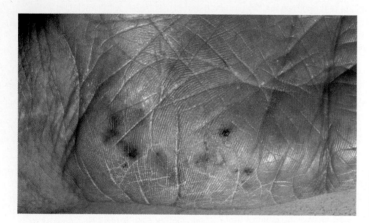

Figure 28.29. Janeway lesions of patient in question 26. *(From James WD, Elston D, Treat JR, et al.* Andrews' Diseases of the Skin. *13th ed. Philadelphia: Elsevier; 2020, Fig. 14.1.)*

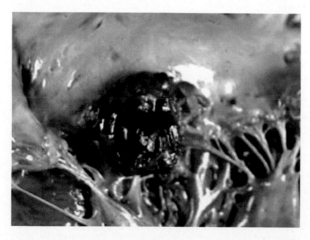

Figure 28.30. Patient's dissected heart on autopsy showing friable vegetation of patient in question 26. *(From Sanaiha Y, Lyons R, Benharash P. Infective endocarditis in intravenous drug users.* Trends Cardiovasc Med. *2020;30:491-497.)*

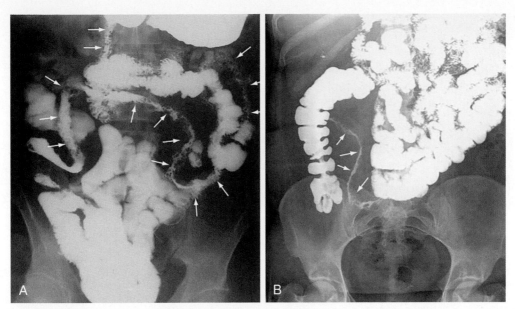

Figure 28.31. Barium swallow procedure for patient in question 27. *(From Sands BE, Siegel CA. Sleisenger and Fordtran's Gastrointestinal and Liver Disease, 10th ed. Philadelphia: Elsevier Saunders; 2016: 1990-2022, Fig. 115-4.)*

occurs more rapidly, damages previously healthy cardiac valves, and is caused by high-virulence organisms, such as *Staphylococcus aureus*. Given its normal placement on skin, patients who abuse IV drugs are more susceptible to acute bacterial endocarditis.

CASE 28.27

A 23-year-old woman with a body mass index of 19 is evaluated for fatigue, periodic fever, abdominal pain, and bloody diarrhea, which she has had for nearly 1 year. She has also recently developed tingling in her feet. Her examination is positive for right lower quadrant tenderness, conjunctival pallor, and 1+ ankle reflexes. Barium swallow (Fig. 28.31) and small bowel biopsy are performed; results are shown in Fig. 28.32.

What is the most likely diagnosis in this patient?
Crohn disease is the likely diagnosis. Crohn disease can occur anywhere in the gastrointestinal (GI) tract but is commonly found in the terminal ileum, ileocecal valve, and cecum. Transmural inflammation is a distinguishing feature that helps differentiate this disease from ulcerative colitis (UC), which involves only the mucosa and submucosa. Fistulas and strictures are common complications that occur in patients with Crohn disease as a result of full-thickness wall involvement. In addition to leukocyte infiltration, another histologic feature of Crohn disease is the presence of noncaseating granulomas (see Fig. 28.32, arrow) in the involved areas of the intestine. The inflammation in the

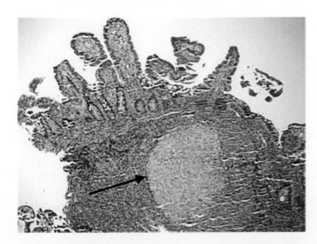

Figure 28.32. Small bowel biopsy sample of patient in question 27. *(Adapted from Feuerstein JD, Cheifetz AS. Crohn disease: epidemiology, diagnosis, and management. Mayo Clin Proc. 2017;92(7):1088-1103.)*

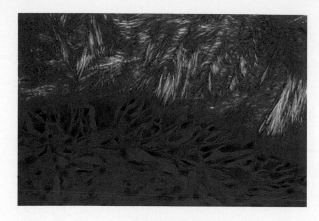

Figure 28.33. Synovial fluid under polarized light in the patient in question 28. *(From O'Dowd G, Bell S, Wright S.* Wheater's Pathology: A Text, Atlas and Review of Histopathology. *6th ed. Philadelphia: Elsevier; 2020: 303-319, Fig. 22.10B.)*

intestinal wall damages villi and leads to symptoms of malabsorption, weight loss, and vitamin B_{12} deficiency in cases that involve the terminal ileum (as suggested by this patient's neurologic symptoms). Anemia is also a concern in patients with Crohn disease as a result of blood loss in stool and/or chronic inflammation (as suggested by this patient's fatigue and conjunctival pallor). On gross examination of the GI tract, skip lesions may be present, which are characterized by multiple sharply demarcated lesions with normal areas in between, leading to a "cobblestoned" appearance that classically spares the rectum. This can be contrasted with UC, in which lesions always involve the colon/rectum and are continuous in the caudal-to-cranial direction. Note that the bowel wall may be thickened in Crohn disease, which narrows the intestinal lumen (Fig. 28.31A, arrows), leading to a string sign on barium swallow (Fig. 28.31B, arrows).

CASE 28.28

A 46-year-old man with a history of hypertension is evaluated for a painful, inflamed toe. The patient's symptoms began the previous night after he consumed a large meal and several alcoholic drinks at a dinner celebration with his family. On examination, the patient's right great toe is erythematous, swollen, and tender around the first metatarsophalangeal joint. Blood is drawn, and laboratory analysis shows hyperuricemia. Joint aspiration is performed at the affected joint, and a sample of the synovial fluid is shown in Fig. 28.33 under polarized light.

How would you explain these findings?

This patient has gout, as is demonstrated by needle-shaped monosodium urate (MSU) crystals, which are negatively birefringent under polarized light (thus causing the crystals to appear yellow). The crystals are formed under conditions that lead to hyperuricemia, such as overproduction of uric acid (e.g., cancer or tumor lysis syndrome), or when excretion is reduced. MSU has low solubility at low temperatures and in synovial fluid, which allows supersaturation to occur more readily in joints that are accustomed to colder temperatures, including toes, ankles, knees, and wrists. The crystals develop in the synovium and cartilage around the joint, and a precipitating event releases them into the synovial fluid. The MSU crystals initiate an inflammatory response via activation of the NLRP3 inflammasome, causing pain and swelling at the affected joint. Acute attacks are often precipitated by large meals, purine-rich foods (e.g., shellfish), and/or alcohol consumption.

CASE 28.29

A 37-year-old man is evaluated for several months of weakness, unintentional weight loss, and tongue swelling. On examination, there is hepatomegaly, several bruises on the arms and legs, and the sides of the tongue have indentations. Laboratory findings include proteinuria and elevated serum immunoglobulin light chains. A biopsy sample is stained with Congo red and examined under polarized light (Fig. 28.34).

What is the most likely diagnosis in this patient?

Amyloidosis (AL) is the most likely diagnosis. Congo red staining and the apple green birefringence of extracellular hyaline material indicate AL. AL occurs when there are excessive, abnormally folded proteins that form beta-pleated sheets that deposit extracellularly. Accumulation of the abnormal proteins causes crowding and pressure atrophy of nearby cells, leading to damage in a variety of organs, including the kidneys, GI tract, and heart, which accounts for the multisystem symptoms seen in this disease. The most common form of AL is due to the depositions of free immunoglobulin light chains from monoclonal plasma cells; however, less common forms of the disease can also be seen that involve other proteins, such as serum amyloid A and transthyretin.

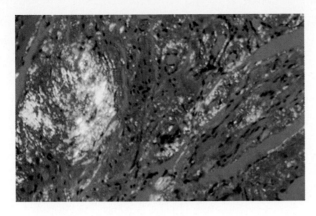

Figure 28.34. Biopsy sample of the patient in question 29. *(From Neville BW, Damm DD, Allen C, Chi AC. Oral and Maxillofacial Pathology. 4th ed. St. Louis: Elsevier; 2016: 761-800, Fig. 17-10.)*

CASE 28.30

A 15-year-old man is evaluated for dyspnea, hemoptysis, and dark urine. On chest imaging, the patient has several focal consolidations. Urinalysis reveals hematuria, and a kidney biopsy stained with H&E shows crescentic lesions (Fig. 28.35, dotted line). Immunofluorescence of the biopsy is also performed and is shown in Fig. 28.36.

What is the most likely diagnosis in this patient?

Goodpasture syndrome is the most likely diagnosis. Goodpasture syndrome is caused by accumulations of antibodies against type IV collagen in alveolar and glomerular basement membranes (GBMs), leading to hematuria, edema, hemoptysis, dyspnea, and/or dry cough. Recall that deposition of antibodies along the GBM leads to the linear pattern seen on immunofluorescence. Goodpasture syndrome is a rapidly progressive glomerulonephritis that creates crescent-shaped lesions around the glomeruli on H&E staining (see Fig. 28.35, dotted line and Fig. 28.36, arrows).

CASE 28.31

A 59-year-old woman with a history of smoking is evaluated for several weeks of worsening dyspnea. On a previous visit, her body mass index was 24; however, today her body mass index is 20. She is barrel-chested and she is breathing through nearly closed lips. Total lung capacity and reserve volume are both increased. Forced expiratory volume/forced vital capacity ratio and diffusing capacity of the lung for carbon monoxide (D_{LCO}) are markedly decreased. A chest radiograph (Fig. 28.37) and lung biopsy (Fig. 28.38) are shown.

What is the most likely diagnosis?

Emphysema is the most likely diagnosis. Smoking increases the number of neutrophils in the alveolar spaces and stimulates release of protease-containing granules. α1-Antitrypsin is the protein responsible for inhibiting

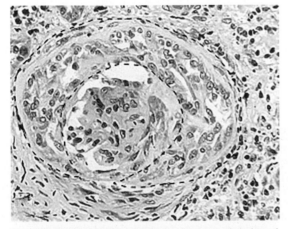

Figure 28.35. Kidney biopsy sample showing crescentic lesions of the patient in question 30. *(Adapted from Phelps RG, Turner AN. Comprehensive Clinical Nephrology. 6th ed. Philadelphia: Elsevier; 2019: 281-289, Fig. 24.5.)*

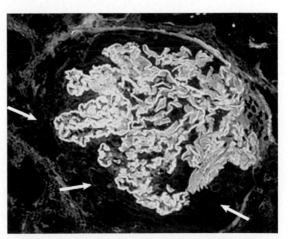

Figure 28.36. Immunofluorescence of the biopsy sample of the patient in question 30. *(From Phelps RG, Turner AN. Comprehensive Clinical Nephrology. 6th ed. Philadelphia: Elsevier; 2019: 281-289, Fig. 24.5.)*

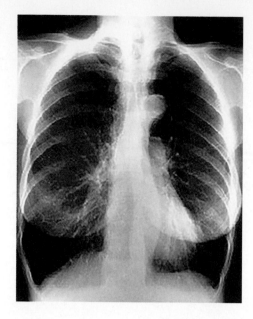

Figure 28.37. Chest radiograph of patient in question 31. *(From Kemp SV, Polkey MI, Pallav LS. The epidemiology, etiology, clinical features, and natural history of emphysema.* Thor Surg Clin. *2009;19(2):149-158.)*

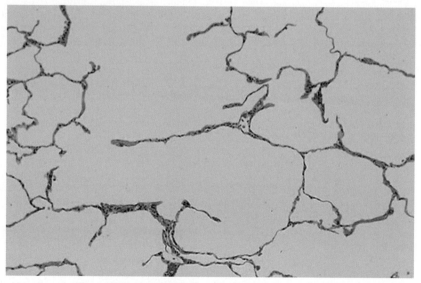

Figure 28.38. Lung biopsy sample of the patient in question 31. *(From Klatt E.* Robbins and Cotran Atlas of Pathology. *3rd ed. Philadelphia: Saunders; 2015, Fig. 5-24.)*

proteases, and when the ratio of α1-antitrypsin to protease is low, elastin begins to degrade and alveolar spaces become enlarged, leading to emphysema. Smokers typically demonstrate a centrilobular pattern of destruction, predominantly in the upper lobes, because alveoli in these areas are most frequently contacted by particles from cigarette smoke (note the enlargement of alveoli secondary to destruction of alveolar walls in Fig. 28.38). In cases of α1-antitrypsin deficiency, destruction is more evenly distributed in a panacinar pattern (uniformly enlarged) more commonly in the lower lobes. However, these cases present at a younger age than the patient in this vignette. As damage to elastin accumulates and elastic recoil diminishes, the patient loses the ability to fully exhale, leading to air trapping. This increases the patient's reserve volume and total lung capacity. The patient's vital capacity has also decreased, causing her to take quick, short breaths that increase the work of breathing and lead to weight loss. Air trapping can be visualized as an expanded barrel chest (see Fig. 28.37) and diaphragm flattening, as shown in the radiograph.

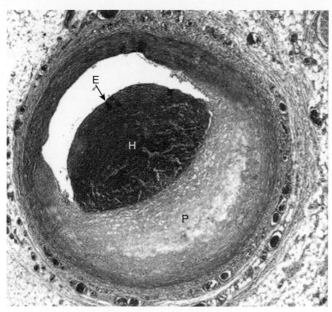

Figure 28.39. Artery biopsy sample of patient in question 32. E, endothelial; H, hemorrhage; P, stable plaque. *(From O'Dowd G, Bell S, Wright S. Wheater's Pathology: A Text, Atlas and Review of Histopathology. 6th ed. Philadelphia: Elsevier; 2020: 92-100.e7, Fig. 8.6.)*

CASE 28.32

A 54-year-old man with a history of diabetes is evaluated for leg pain. The patient explains that he takes his dog for a walk every morning, but the past few weeks he has experienced leg pain while walking that is relieved with rest. His father had two myocardial infarctions (MIs) before the age of 55. On examination, the patient has a body mass index of 27, and his blood pressure is 135/70 mm Hg. The sample lipid profile reveals elevated low-density lipoprotein and low high-density lipoprotein. If an artery biopsy were to be taken, it may appear as the slide shown in Fig. 28.39.

What process is occurring in this patient?

Atherosclerosis is likely occurring in this patient. This patient's history of diabetes, hypertension, and dyslipidemia, along with his first-degree family history of premature heart disease, points to the development of atherosclerosis. The inciting event in atherosclerosis is endothelial (Fig. 28.39, E) injury, which allows inflammatory cells into the vessel lumen and lipoprotein accumulations on the wall. Macrophages accumulate with these lipoproteins and become foam cells. Platelet adhesion occurs on the lesion and, along with the foam cells, releases factors that allow for smooth muscle proliferation and extracellular matrix production in the lumen, creating a cap over the lipid accumulations. This structure is called a *stable plaque* (Fig. 28.39, P). When a hemorrhage (Fig. 28.39, H) occurs within the plaque, blood can track beneath the endothelium, which causes it to bulge farther into the artery. This narrowing of the lumen on top of the preexisting plaque can lead to a decreased oxygen supply to the tissues that receive blood flow through this artery. This patient's leg claudication could have been caused by the hemorrhage decreasing blood supply or by progression of his atherosclerotic disease. When atherosclerotic plaques occur in the popliteal artery, they can cause leg pain on exertion, also known as *claudication*. Note that myocardial perfusion abnormalities caused by stable plaques can cause stable angina, whereas perfusion abnormalities associated with unstable plaques can cause unstable angina.

CASE 28.33

A 58-year-old man is evaluated in the emergency department for a 2-hour history of dyspnea associated with severe left-sided chest pain radiating to the left arm. He has a history of hypertension and diabetes. On examination, the patient is obese, diaphoretic, and has a pulse of 120. Electrocardiogram shows ST-segment elevation in the anterior leads. Blood work reveals elevated CK-MB and troponin I. An image from cardiac catheterization is shown in Fig. 28.40, along with an image of how the patient's heart would appear on autopsy (Fig. 28.41) if he were to die a few days later.

What is the most likely diagnosis in this patient?

Acute ST-elevation myocardial infarction (STEMI) is the most likely diagnosis. Hypertension, diabetes, and obesity are associated with coronary artery disease, which can lead to an MI. The patient's current presentation (radiating chest pain, diaphoresis, and rapid heart rate) is consistent with an MI. MIs occur when a coronary artery becomes 100% occluded by an embolus or thrombus. Unstable atherosclerotic plaques can rupture, causing platelet adhesion and degranulation. Production of microthrombi allows the plaque to completely block the flow of blood, causing the

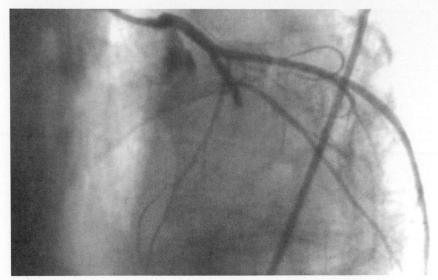

Figure 28.40. Cardiac catheterization image of the patient in question 33. *(From Zheng Y, Mao JY. Typical coronary artery aneurysm exactly within drug-eluting stent implantation region in a patient with rheumatoid arthritis. J Cardiovasc Dis Res. 2012;3(4):329-331.)*

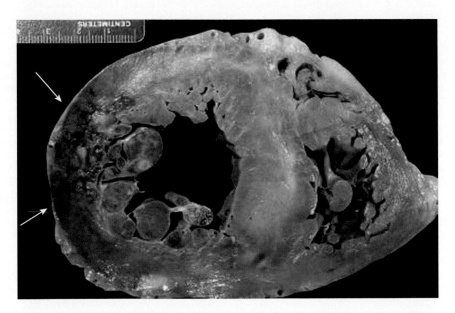

Figure 28.41. Image of patient's heart during autopsy discussed in question 33. *(From Burke AP. Pathology of Acute Myocardial Infarction, Medscape. http://emedicine.medscape.com/article/1960472-overview.)*

underlying myocytes to become ischemic. An area of ischemia appears in the gross image as a region of dark and damaged tissue (see Fig. 28.41, arrows), and the catheterization image depicts an occluded coronary artery. In this case, ST elevations in the anterior leads, plus the location of the ischemic area and the blockage of flow in the catheterization, point to total occlusion of the left anterior descending (LAD) artery (see Fig. 28.40). Damage to the myocytes allows for release of cytoplasmic proteins, allowing proteins such as CK-MB and troponins to be released into the blood. Troponin I is the most sensitive and specific biomarker for MI because it is specifically found in cardiac cells. When cardiac myocyte damage extends through the entire thickness of the heart wall, ST elevations appear on electrocardiogram (ECG), causing STEMI. If damage occurs (elevated troponin) *without* transmural ischemia, diagnostic ST elevations will not be present, and the patient has a *non-STEMI* (NSTEMI). Common ECG findings in NSTEMI include T-wave inversions and ST depressions.

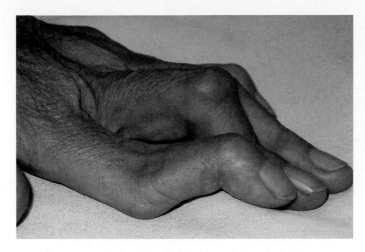

Figure 28.42. Patient's affected finger joint discussed in question 34. *(From Cifu D.* Braddom's Physical Medicine and Rehabilitation. *5th ed. Philadelphia: Elsevier; 2016, Fig. 31-1B.)*

CASE 28.34

A 48-year-old woman is evaluated for 2 to 3 months of fatigue and joint pain. She has joint stiffness in the morning, which improves as the day progresses. On examination, the joints in her hands, feet, and wrists are swollen, warm, and tender, with limited range of motion. There is radial deviation of the wrists and ulnar deviation of the fingers. On plain films, there is narrowing of the joint space. Laboratory tests show elevated anti-cyclic citrullinated protein (anti-CCP) antibodies. A photo of the affected finger joints is shown in Fig. 28.42.

What do these findings indicate?

Rheumatoid arthritis (RA) is indicated. RA is an autoimmune disorder in which T lymphocytes react against an unknown antigen in the joint synovium. The T cells release cytokines that cause inflammation and macrophage activation, leading to destruction of collagen and bone in the joint space. In addition, certain subsets of T lymphocytes can be directly cytotoxic to components of the joints. The diagnosis of RA can be supported by laboratory tests through the presence of anti-CCP and rheumatoid factor (IgM to the Fc portion of IgG). Although the sensitivities of these two tests are nearly identical, the specificity of anti-CCP antibodies (90%–98% sensitivity) exceeds that of rheumatoid factor, making it a better diagnostic test for RA. Radiographic tests may show joint effusions, erosions, and narrow joint spaces in patients with RA. Unlike osteoarthritis (OA), in which symptoms improve with rest, RA presents with joint stiffness after rest that improves with use as the inflammatory infiltrate in the joints is mechanically cleared. Other symptoms of RA include ulnar deviation of fingers and symptoms of synovitis (joint tenderness, swelling, and hard lumps). Note the finger adduction and "swan-neck" deformation (in which the proximal finger joints are extended and the distal finger joints are flexed) in Fig. 28.42.

CASE 28.35

A 56-year-old man with a history of hypertension presents to the emergency department with intense chest pain. The pain occurred without warning and radiates to his back, between the scapulae. On examination, he is noticeably tall and slender, with very long extremities and digits. His femoral pulses are diminished bilaterally. The ECG is unremarkable. Chest x-ray film shows mediastinal widening. A histologic image of the aortic wall in a patient with this condition is as shown in Fig. 28.43.

What is the most likely diagnosis?

Aortic dissection is the most likely diagnosis. Aortic dissections in older patients with high blood pressure occur when there is hypertrophy of the vasa vasorum and loss of blood flow to the myocytes in the tunica media, leading to atrophy. The atrophic smooth muscle layer is prone to tearing and can progress distally or proximally toward the heart, leading to cardiac tamponade. Often the damage extends through the adventitia, causing massive hemorrhage. In young patients, aortic dissections can often be attributed to diseases that affect normal collagen homeostasis and produce abnormal vasculature, such as Marfan syndrome or Ehlers-Danlos syndrome. This is the case in the patient described, as illustrated by the histologic image of the aortic wall (see Fig. 28.43). The elastic pink fibers typically run in parallel, but they are disrupted by a mucinous ground substance (stained blue) as a result of cystic medial necrosis. This is how Marfan syndrome weakens the tissues that contain elastin.

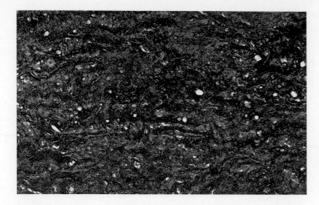

Figure 28.43. Mucin stain of a portion of the wall of the aorta of the patient in question 35, demonstrating pools of mucoid material. *(From Klatt E. Robbins and Cotran Atlas of Pathology. 3rd ed. Philadelphia: Saunders; 2015: 1-26.e3, Fig. 1-29.)*

CASE 28.36

A 28-year-old female ballet dancer accidentally falls and hits her head on the stage floor when her dance partner fails to catch her. Outside of a headache, she states that she feels fine but decides to leave early for the day. That afternoon, her husband returns home from work to find her sleeping on the couch and very difficult to rouse. He quickly calls emergency response, and she is rushed to the hospital, where she is put on mechanical ventilation and other life-supportive measures. The patient dies several hours later. If a computed tomography scan had been performed near the time of her injury, the image shown in Fig. 28.44 would have been obtained, led to the diagnosis, and could have saved her life.

What is the most likely cause of this patient's death?
An epidural hematoma caused this patient's death. This unfortunate patient has the classic presentation of an epidural hematoma. This includes a lucid interval where the patient experiences little to no symptoms for several hours after the initial injury. If the pathology goes unrecognized, it can quickly lead to altered mental status, coma, and death secondary to herniation of the brainstem. Epidural hematomas are a result of injury to meningeal arteries, which will bleed into the space between the dura mater and the skull (the epidural space), causing the dura mater to separate off of the calvarium and impinge on brain parenchyma (see Fig. 28.44, arrows). The middle meningeal artery is the most likely to

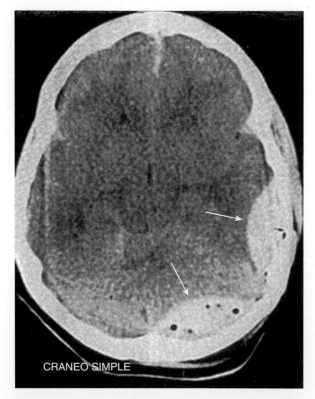

CRANEO SIMPLE

Figure 28.44. Computed tomography (CT) scan of the patient in question 36. *(From Ferri F. Ferri's Clinical Advisor 2020. Philadelphia: Elsevier; 2020, 517-518.e1.)*

be injured because the overlying pterion region is relatively weak and susceptible to traumatic damage. Note that epidural hematomas appear as bright, almond-shaped regions on computed tomography (CT) as they create a space between the outside of the dura and the inside of the skull, and therefore are limited by the suture lines at which the dura inserts to the skull. In contrast, subdural hematomas form crescent-shaped lesions.

CASE 28.37

A 66-year-old man is brought to the emergency department after a fall at home. His wife reports that he slipped on the kitchen floor and fell and hit the side of his head. She reports he experienced a brief loss of consciousness, and on waking he reported complained of a headache but was following commands. In the emergency department, he has somewhat altered mental status and right-sided upper extremity weakness. His wife reports no other medical problems except for atrial fibrillation for which he receives warfarin and a daily "baby aspirin" for heart health. She also states that his dose of warfarin was recently increased because his last international normalized ratio value was subtherapeutic. His CT scan is shown in Fig. 28.45.

What is the most likely diagnosis?

Subdural hematoma is the most likely diagnosis. The patient's presentation of loss of consciousness, headache, altered mental status, and focal neurologic symptoms in the context of anticoagulation is strongly suggestive of an intracranial hemorrhage. The CT scan shows a left-sided, crescent-shaped hemorrhage that crosses suture lines (see Fig. 28.45, arrow), which classifies this as a subdural hematoma. These lesions are a result of shear force on bridging veins after head trauma or rapid accelerating/decelerating force. Because the bleed is venous rather than arterial, the signs and symptoms tend to come on more slowly than an epidural hematoma. Subdural hemorrhages do not typically have an associated lucid interval.

CASE 28.38

A 71-year-old man with a history significant for atrial fibrillation, hypertension, and hyperlipidemia is rushed to the emergency department after his wife noticed a facial droop. Once there, the patient is awake, alert, and oriented to person, place, and time; however, he has a noticeable right-sided facial droop with forehead sparing, loss of sharp and dull sensation in both his upper and lower extremities on the right, as well as substantial loss of motor strength (2/5). An emergent CT scan is negative for an acute bleed but shows a loss of gray-white differentiation on the right cortex, and because his last seen normal time was determined to be less than 3 hours ago, he receives tissue plasminogen activator. A magnetic resonance image taken the following day demonstrates the lesion shown in Fig. 28.46.

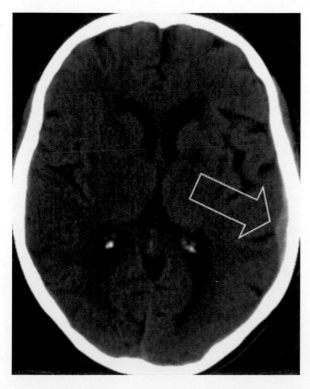

Figure 28.45. Computed tomography (CT) scan of patient in question 37. *(From Dharsono F, Constantine CP. Arterial origin subdural hematoma and associated pial pseudoaneurysm following minor head trauma. Clin Imag. 2013;37:750-752.)*

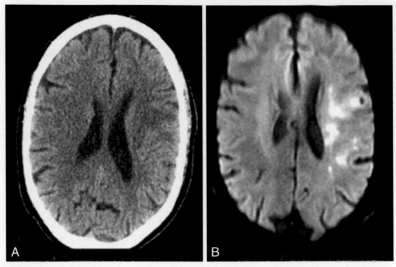

Figure 28.46. Computed tomography (CT) (A) and magnetic resonance imaging (MRI) (B) of patient in question 38 after intra-arterial throm-bolysis for a left middle cerebral artery (MCA) stroke. *(From Lövblad KO, Altrichter S, Mendes Pereira V, et al. Imaging of acute stroke: CT and or MRI. J Neuroradiol. 2015;42:55-64.)*

What is the most likely diagnosis?

Middle cerebral artery (MCA) ischemic stroke is the likely diagnosis. This patient is exhibiting focal neurologic signs consistent with a stroke of MCA distribution of the left cortical hemisphere. In the emergent setting, a CT is always ordered to rule out the possibility of intracranial hemorrhage and to look for early signs of ischemic stroke. The patient's acute CT (Fig. 28.46A) demonstrates slight hypodensity in the left hemisphere as a result of ischemia. The diffusion-weighted magnetic resonance imaging (MRI) (Fig. 28.46B) taken after the CT reveals a large lesion in the left hemisphere. Ischemic strokes are much more common than hemorrhagic strokes and can be either thrombotic or embolic. Although this patient's stroke is ischemic in nature (negative for acute bleed on CT), the precise etiology is unclear because he has risk factors for both subtypes: hypertension and dyslipidemia (thrombotic secondary to atherosclerotic disease) and atrial fibrillation (embolic). It is important to differentiate the etiology before treatment to avoid further morbidity. Thrombolysis with tissue plasminogen activator (tPA) is the appropriate treatment for ischemic stroke, but it has a time-sensitive window of use. In a subset of patients outside of the thrombolytic window, thrombectomy can be performed within 24 hours as long as there is a large vessel occlusion (e.g., can be accessed with a mechanical thrombectomy device) and most of the brain is ischemic penumbra (e.g., salvageable if reperfused) rather than infarct.

CASE 28.39

A 48-year-old man, a former marine, is seen by his primary care physician for joint pain. He states that the pain is located in both knees without radiation, started several years ago, and has progressively worsened with the most excruciating pain occurring in the evenings. He now finds himself using 8 to 10 200-mg tablets of ibuprofen per day, which helps with the pain. He denies any fever, chills, recent infection, or other symptoms. He has an unremarkable medical history. On examination, his knees are slightly swollen but otherwise appear grossly normal. An x-ray of the patient's knee is shown in Fig. 28.47.

What is the most likely diagnosis?

OA is the most likely diagnosis. The patient's plain film x-ray shows classic hallmarks of OA—namely, marked joint space narrowing caused by loss of fibrocartilage. Bony outgrowths called *osteophytes* may also be present. OA is a very common condition that results from chronic wear and tear on a joint leading to bone-on-bone contact, inflammation, and associated pain. Pain is worsened by exertion/use and is often most pronounced later in the day. Patients usually can be managed conservatively with anti-inflammatory agents. In advanced cases, total joint replacement may be required.

CASE 28.40

A 67-year-old man with a medical history significant for CHF is seen in the emergency department for a 1-day history of increasing dyspnea on exertion, pleuritic chest pain, leg swelling, orthopnea, and paroxysmal nocturnal dyspnea. On examination, he has dullness to percussion and decreased breath sounds over the lung bases bilaterally. A chest x-ray (Fig. 28.48A) and chest CT scan (Fig. 28.48B) are performed to confirm the diagnosis. The patients' at-home dose of furosemide is increased, and he is admitted to the hospital to monitor his respiratory status.

What is the most likely diagnosis?

Congestive heart failure causing a transudative plural effusion. The recumbent chest x-ray (CXR; see Fig. 28.48A) shows blunting of the right costophrenic angle with diffuse haziness of the right lung field (black arrow). The normal cardiac outline is obscured (silhouette sign). The upright CXR (see Fig. 28.48B) reveals that the pleural fluid is gravity dependent (white arrow). It is important to be aware of how position affects imaging of pleural effusions so that the impression is not mistakenly lessened or worsened. Effusions can be either transudative or exudative depending on the etiology. Situations that increase intracapillary pressure or decrease plasma oncotic pressure will lead to a transudative process (e.g., CHF, cirrhosis). Exudative effusions will be seen in states of increased vascular permeability (e.g., infection, malignancy, collagen vascular diseases). Evaluation of the pleural fluid by thoracentesis can determine whether the process is transudative or exudative using the Light criteria (pleural fluid/serum protein ratio > 0.5, lactate dehydrogenase [LDH] ratio > 0.6, or LDH greater than two-thirds the upper limit of normal favoring the latter diagnosis of an exudative process), although this concept is most likely beyond the scope of the USMLE Step 1.

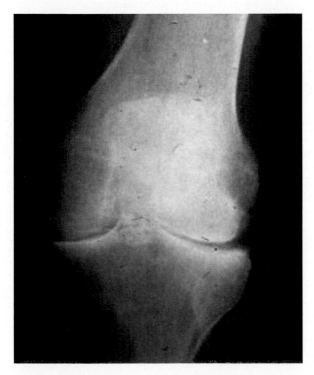

Figure 28.47. X-ray film of the patient's knee discussed in question 39. *(From Ralston SH, Penman I, Strachan M, Hobson R. Davidson's Principles and Practice of Medicine. 23nd ed. Philadelphia: Elsevier; 2018: 981-1060, Fig. 24-19.)*

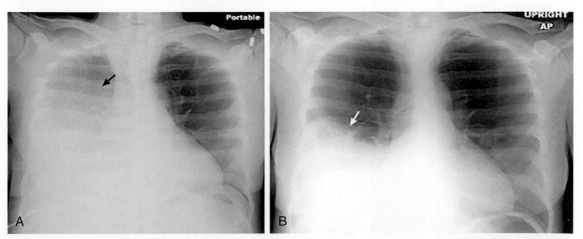

Figure 28.48. Chest X-ray film of the patient in question 40. *(From Herring W. Learning Radiology: Recognizing the Basics. 4th ed. Philadelphia: Saunders; 2020: 60-69, Fig. 8.8.)*

CASE 28.41

A 70-year-old man is being seen for an annual Medicare wellness visit. He has a known history of hypertension and hyperlipidemia and is a past smoker (45 pack-years). He also has a notable family history, with multiple family members having MI and stroke at relatively young ages. Examination is significant for a small pulsatile nontender mass near the umbilicus. His examination is otherwise normal, and he has no symptoms to report. The patient is sent for an abdominal CT scan with angiography, which is shown in Fig. 28.49.

What is the most likely diagnosis?

Abdominal aortic aneurysm (AAA) is the most likely diagnosis. AAAs are usually asymptomatic unless ruptured and often present as a pulsatile nontender abdominal mass or abdominal "fullness" on routine examination. Risk factors for AAA development are similar for that of atherosclerosis with the addition of hereditary conditions that affect the integrity of vessel walls (e.g., vasculitis, diseases of collagen). Smoking is among the strongest risk factors, so the U.S. Preventive Services Task Force (USPSTF) recommends that all men between 65 and 75 years of age who have a history of smoking receive a one-time screening for AAA. If rupture occurs, the patient can destabilize quickly secondary to massive hemorrhage and can present with severe low back pain, hypotension, syncope, or cardiovascular collapse. Important diagnostic signs that may indicate aortic rupture include Grey Turner sign (ecchymosis on the flank) or Cullen sign (ecchymosis near the umbilicus). Diagnosis in the acute setting is made with ultrasound, which is quick and has a nearly 100% sensitivity for identifying AAAs. Otherwise, the preoperative planning imaging of choice involves abdominal CT with or without angiography. AAAs larger than 5.5 cm in diameter are repaired either openly or endovascularly with graft placement. Smaller AAAs can wait with surveillance unless they are high rupture risk with low operative risk.

CASE 28.42

A 44-year-old man is brought to the emergency department by his wife for an acute onset of severe lower back pain, nausea, and vomiting. He reports that the pain is located on his left side and has been intermittent for the past several days. He states that when it comes on "I can't get comfortable." Today, the pain became sharp, constant, and severe and is radiating into his groin. His exam is benign, except for some tenderness at the left costovertebral angle. He is started on IV fluids and analgesia for his pain. A CT scan is ordered and is shown in Fig. 28.50.

What process is most likely to have occurred in this patient?

Nephrolithiasis is likely. This patient presents with classic renal colic secondary to a kidney stone (sudden, severe, writhing pain) that progressed from his flank to his groin. Patients may also experience nausea and vomiting, urinary tract infection (UTI), or frank hematuria. Kidney stones occur most commonly at the ureterovesicular junction, renal calyx, and ureteropelvic junction. Calcium (oxalate/phosphate) stones make up about 80% to 85% of cases and are radiopaque (obstruct the passage of radiation, thereby appearing white/opaque on plain film). Other less common stones include uric acid stones, struvite stones, and cystine stones. Risk factors for stone development include dehydration, family history, medications, male gender, UTI, and a low-calcium/high-oxalate diet. If sufficiently large, the stone can cause urinary obstruction leading to hydronephrosis.

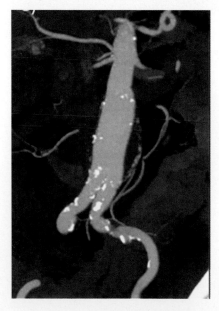

Figure 28.49. Abdominal computed tomography (CT) scan of the patient in question 41. *(From Villard C, Hultgren R. Abdominal aortic aneurysm: Sex differences. Maturitas. 2017;109:63-69.)*

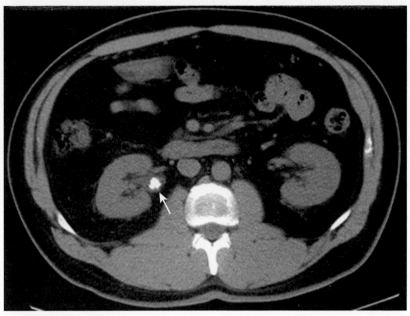

Figure 28.50. Computed tomography (CT) scan of abdomen for the patient in question 42. *(From Curhan GC. Clinical crossroads: a 44-year-old woman with kidney stones. JAMA. 2005;293:1107-1114.)*

CASE 28.43

A 50-year-old woman is evaluated for several weeks of headache. Review of systems is positive for slight bilateral nipple discharge and several months of irregular menses. She also notes being in three car accidents in recent months but denies head trauma. Medical history is unremarkable. Her examination is significant for bilateral outer visual field deficits and the ability to express a white discharge from her nipples. A magnetic resonance image of the brain is ordered and is shown in Fig. 28.51.

What is the most likely diagnosis?

Pituitary adenoma (prolactinoma) is the likely diagnosis. The MRI scan demonstrates a mass expanding from within the sella turcica and compression of the underlying optic chiasm, most consistent with a pituitary tumor (see Fig. 28.51, arrow). Pituitary adenomas account for 10% of intracranial neoplasms, most of which are benign. Symptomatology is driven by excessive hormone secretion (which varies depending on the cell type of origin), hypopituitarism (if the infundibular stalk is compressed), and compression of the optic chiasm that lies just above the pituitary fossa, which

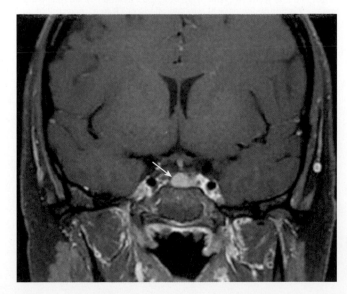

Figure 28.51. Magnetic resonance image (MRI) of the brain of the patient in question 43. *(From Oh MC, Kunwar S, Blevins L, Aghi MK. Medical versus surgical management of prolactinomas. Neurosurg Clin N Am. 2012;23(4): 669-678.)*

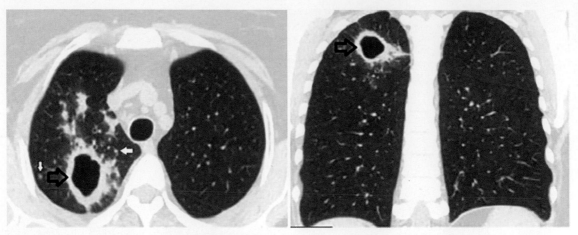

Figure 28.52. Computed tomography (CT) slices with cavitary lesions in lung apex. *(From Kumru G, Akturk S, Erdogmus S, et al. Cavitary lung disease in renal transplant recipients: A single center experience.* Transplantation Reports. *2017;2(4):19-21.)*

leads to bitemporal hemianopsia. In this vignette, the patient presents with signs and symptoms of a prolactinoma (galactorrhea, amenorrhea), the most common type of hypersecreting pituitary adenoma. Other manifestations of hypersecreting pituitary adenomas include acromegaly (excess growth hormone [GH]), Cushing disease (excess ACTH), and hyperthyroidism (excess TSH). MRI and hormone levels are included in the standard diagnostic workup of pituitary tumors. Transsphenoidal excision is the surgical option for pituitary adenomas, although prolactinomas can often be treated medically with dopamine agonists (e.g., bromocriptine).

CASE 28.44

A 20-year-old woman from Bosnia presents to the emergency department after a motor vehicle accident. The patient undergoes an urgent CXR and CT scan of the head and neck. The incidental findings, noted in the apices of the lung, are shown in the CT scan (Fig. 28.52). The emergency physician immediately puts the patient on airborne precautions and orders a sputum sample as seen in Fig. 28.53.

Why was this done?

The patient's immigrant status and incidental radiographic findings are suspicious for active *Mycobacterium tuberculosis* (tuberculosis [TB]) infection. This diagnosis is confirmed by the presence of bacteria on the acid-fast stain, which resist decolorization by acid as a result of the high mycolic acid content of their cell walls. Primary TB infection is acquired through inhalation of droplets containing the active bacilli, which then deposit in the lungs and are ingested by alveolar macrophages. The surviving bacteria, which as obligate aerobes prefer the oxygen-rich areas of the lung, are sequestered and kept dormant by the formation of granulomas within the lung. However, the bacteria can be reactivated by any circumstance that weakens the immune system, leading to the clinical manifestations of TB (e.g., fever, night sweats, weight loss, hemoptysis) and potential for hematogenous or lymphatic dissemination. Risk factors for TB include an immunocompromised state, recent immigrant status, and employment within the health care system. Note that although the tuberculin skin test (PPD) is used to screen for TB exposure, CXR (or CT) is required to distinguish active

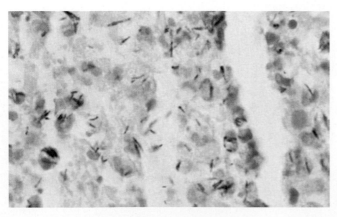

Figure 28.53. Acid-fast stain of sputum for the patient in question 44. *(From Walter N, Daley CL.* Clinical Respiratory Medicine. *4th ed. Philadelphia: Elsevier; 2012, Fig. 31-9.)*

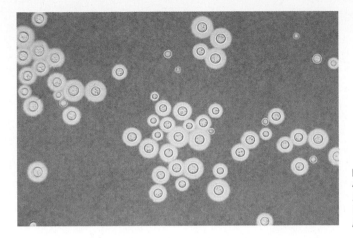

Figure 28.54. Cerebrospinal fluid of the patient in question 45. *(From Haley L; CDC. Centers for Disease Control and Prevention's Public Health Image Library (PHIL), with identification number #3771: Nov 24, 2016. Available at: http://phil.cdc.gov/phil/home.asp. Accessed May 18, 2020.)*

TB from latent infection and will classically demonstrate upper lobe infiltrates with cavitations if the former is present (see Fig. 28.52, black arrows). CT may also show centriacinar nodules (see Fig. 28.52, white arrow). It is important to realize that cavitary pulmonary lesions do not confirm the diagnosis of pulmonary TB because these lesions can be seen in association with other species of *Mycobacterium*; however, the presence of cavitary lesions in a patient with likely exposure should elicit isolation precautions until the patient has undergone appropriate screening for *Mycobacterium tuberculosis*, and the results are sufficiently negative.

CASE 28.45

An 8-year-old boy whose status is 4 months post-bone marrow transplant for acute myeloid leukemia presents to the emergency department with 3 hours of altered mental status and a fever of 103.4°F. A workup for a fever of unknown origin is initiated, which includes a spinal tap. The cerebrospinal fluid is stained with India ink, and the histologic findings are shown in Fig. 28.54.

What is the most likely diagnosis?

Cryptococcus neoformans is the likely diagnosis. This dimorphic fungus can cause an asymptomatic pulmonary infection, which is later followed by the development of meningitis, as is seen in this case. *Cryptococcus* is an opportunistic infection that preferentially infects individuals who are immunocompromised, such as those with AIDS, leukemia, or lymphoma and transplant recipients treated with immunosuppressive agents to prevent tissue rejection. *Cryptococcus* is best visualized by India ink stain, which outlines the cell wall of the yeast and allows for visualization of its polysaccharide capsular halo as shown in Fig. 28.54. A CSF cryptococcal antigen test is more sensitive than India ink staining.

CASE 28.46

A 22-year-old woman presents to the OB/GYN with symptoms of increased vaginal discharge and a vaginal odor that is predominant after intercourse. The physician performs a vaginal swab and prepares a wet mount to perform a "bedside" examination (Fig. 28.55).

What is the most likely diagnosis?

Bacterial vaginosis is the most likely diagnosis. This infection is most commonly associated with *Gardnerella vaginalis* but represents multimicrobial overgrowth in the vaginal environment. The diagnosis is made by the presence of thin white-gray discharge, pH > 4.5, positive whiff test (amine odor with the addition of potassium hydroxide [KOH]), and "clue cells" on the vaginal swab (see Fig. 28.55), which represent vaginal squamous epithelial cells that are covered by coccobacilli. These are a pathognomonic feature of bacterial vaginosis and warrant treatment with metronidazole in symptomatic women. If this is detected incidentally on a Papanicolaou test, and the woman is asymptomatic, the decision to treat is not as clear and should not simply be reflexive.

CASE 28.47

A 66-year-old patient presents to the emergency department with a "cut" on his penis (Fig. 28.56). He asks whether this may have resulted from the fact that he sometimes catches his zipper on his foreskin without noticing because his sensation has been blunted by his long-standing history of poorly controlled diabetes.

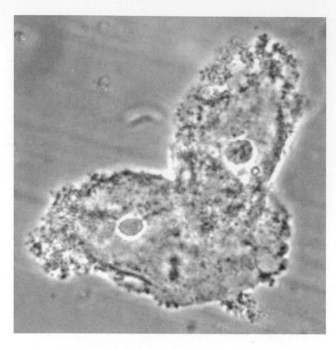

Figure 28.55. Vaginal swab sample of the patient in question 46. *(From Rein M; CDC. Centers for Disease Control and Prevention's Public Health Image Library (PHIL), with identification number #3720: Nov 24, 2016. Available at: http://phil.cdc.gov/phil/home.asp. Accessed May 20, 2020.)*

What is the appropriate next step in diagnosis?

Laboratory testing for syphilis is the appropriate next step because this lesion is not likely to have resulted from a zipper laceration. The penile chancre demonstrated in Fig. 28.56 is associated with primary syphilis and is a painless, hard, and indurated (punched-out base) lesion that results from infection with the *Treponema pallidum* spirochete. Symptoms in the secondary stage include a maculopapular rash on the palms and soles and condyloma lata (painless, wart-like lesions) on the genitals. The tertiary stage is defined by the formation of soft growths with necrotic centers on other areas of the body, aortic aneurysms, and Argyll-Robertson pupils, which accommodate but do not react to light. Traditional algorithms suggest two-step testing for definitive diagnosis of syphilis and include rapid plasma reagin (RPR) followed by fluorescent treponemal antibody absorption (FTA-Abs) for confirmation of results. However, you should note that syphilis polymerase chain reaction (PCR) is the preferred testing method in most clinical practices. Penicillin G is the treatment of choice for all stages of syphilis.

CASE 28.48

A 45-year-old man comes to the emergency department after returning from central Africa 2 weeks ago to volunteer at a nonprofit medical clinic. He admits that he did not take "those pills they prescribed me before I left" because he was told they may cause lucid dreams. He has been having paroxysmal fevers up to 104°F but is otherwise asymptomatic. Laboratory testing reveals anemia; blood smear is shown in Fig. 28.57.

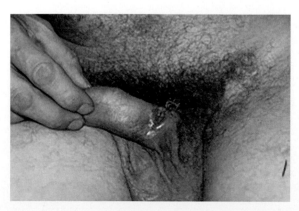

Figure 28.56. Patient's penis showing a cut as discussed in question 47. *(From Dombrowski JC, Celum C, Baeten J. The Travel and Tropical Medicine Manual. 5th ed. Philadelphia: Elsevier; 2017: 535-544, Fig. 43.1.)*

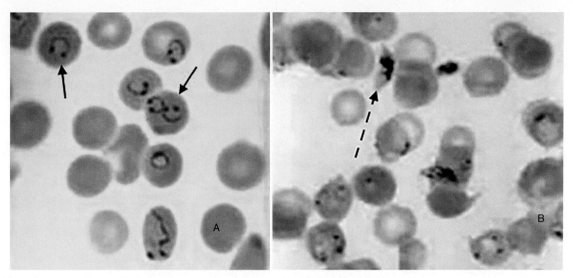

Figure 28.57. Blood smear of the patient in question 48. *(Adapted from Khan S, Zia A, Gupta ND, Bey A. Acute gingival bleeding as a complication of falciparum malaria: a case report.* Oral Surg Oral Med Oral Pathol Oral Radiol. *2012;113(5):e19-e22.)*

What is the most likely diagnosis?

Plasmodium falciparum is the most likely diagnosis. The incubation period for malaria can be between 2 and 5 weeks, which explains this patient's delayed presentation. A blood smear with a Giemsa stain is the gold standard for laboratory diagnosis of malaria. As shown in Fig. 28.57, trophozoite "rings" can be visualized within RBCs (Fig. 28.57A, solid arrows). The trophozoites age into multinucleated schizonts that eventually release individual merozoites, causing red cell lysis as they are released into the vasculature, accounting for this patient's anemia. The gametocyte stage (Fig. 28.57B, dashed arrow) is the cell that is responsible for transmission between the human and mosquito host. Rapid antigen testing is often combined with smear results for a final clinical interpretation. Treatment for malaria is with artemisinin-combination therapy (ACT) using artemisinins and other antimalarial agents such as quinine derivatives.

STEP 1 SECRET

A good rule of thumb to remember for your exam: If an infection is not caused by bacteria (i.e., it is viral or parasitic in etiology), confirmatory testing is usually done via PCR or antigen detection assays.

CASE 28.49

A 26-year-old man from Connecticut is evaluated for several days of fever, chills, and arthralgias. He normally enjoys hiking and rock climbing but has not felt well enough in recent days to perform these activities. An image of the patient's peripheral smear is shown in Fig. 28.58.

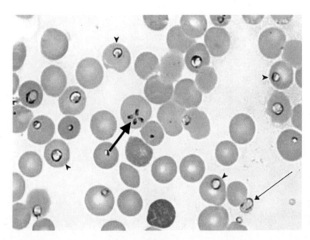

Figure 28.58. Peripheral smear of the patient in question 49. *(Adapted from Long SS, Prober CG, Fischer M.* Principles and Practice of Pediatric Infectious Diseases. *5th ed. Philadelphia: Elsevier; 2018: 1298-1303.e2, Fig. 258.2.)*

What is the most likely diagnosis?

Babesiosis, which is a malaria-like parasitic disease caused by infection with the protozoan *Babesia*, is the most likely diagnosis. The new-onset anemia and a history of outdoor activity in an endemic area should lead you to suspect babesiosis in this patient. In a *Babesia* infection, ringed-shaped parasites can be seen both intracellularly within erythrocytes (see Fig. 28.58, arrowheads) as well as extracellularly (thin arrow), and they vary in size. Maltese crosses (thick arrow), which are pathognomonic for babesiosis, are formed by multiple *Babesia* within a single erythrocyte. Although it is rare to visualize Maltese crosses on smears, it is often possible to see multiple parasites within a single cell, which is uncommon for malaria infection.

CASE 28.50

A 9-year-old boy accompanied by his mother presents to his pediatrician for a routine physical examination. On questioning, the mother recalls seeing a rash on his face about 1 month ago (Fig. 28.59), but otherwise there is no new information to report. Examination at this time is entirely unrevealing.

The infectious agent that causes the rash pictured in the figure is also responsible for which bone marrow abnormality?

Aplastic anemia (crisis) is caused by infection with parvovirus B19 (also known as *fifth disease* or *erythema infectiosum*). Aplastic crisis can occur in patients with a preexisting hemolytic anemia (sickle cell disease, thalassemia) because the virus preferentially destroys erythroid progenitor cells in bone marrow. Healthy, immunocompetent people with the infection are asymptomatic. Adults may experience arthralgias while children can display the "slapped cheek" rash shown in the figure. An intrauterine infection during pregnancy may result in spontaneous abortion, stillbirth, or hydrops fetalis because of red cell destruction in the fetus.

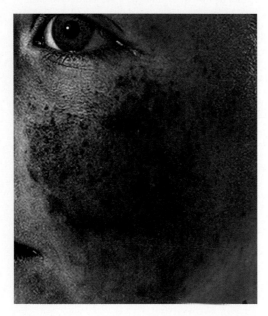

Figure 28.59. Facial rash of the patient in question 50. *(From Ralston SH, Penman I, Strachan M, Hobson R. Davidson's Principles and Practice of Medicine, 23rd ed. Philadelphia: Elsevier; 2018:215-304, Fig. 11.9.)*